Movie Star Choice

by Barry Bendel

Eloquent Books

An imprint of AEG Publishing Group

845 Third Avenue, 6th Floor – # 6016

New York, NY 10022

www.eloquentbooks.com

ISBN: 978-1-60860-329-9

Printed in the United States of America

Foreword

A warm welcome to the First Edition of "Movie Star Choice" – a comprehensive biographical history of international film stars – major and minor – who acted on the silver screen during the past eighty years of Talking Pictures.

My experience doesn't stretch back quite that far, but ever since I first visited a London movie theater in 1944 to see Walt Disney's *Bambi,* I have been fanatical about film.

In those early days I was dependent on the generosity of a visiting aunt who was serving in the British Army. Because she was stationed some distance from where I lived, those magical escapes were rare then. With Dad away on duty with the secret service my mother was much too busy raising my young sister and baby brother to take me. Nonetheless, the seed had been sown and by 1947 I started generating my own income with a morning paper-round. Most of the money I earned was spent on tickets to the movies.

Double-bills, in those days, were the norm and there were often two feature films. During World War II the distribution from Hollywood was severely disrupted, so the backlog was immense. In the late 1940s there was no real TV in Britain. The "cinema" as we called it, ruled. Despite the age-restrictions, I saw about two hundred films each year. That habit intensified during the early 1950s and it went up several notches when, in 1956, I emigrated with my family to California.

Long before movie guides were even thought of, I kept a record of, and rated, every movie I ever saw and continued to do so throughout my working life. It was purely a hobby, and the idea of writing a book on the subject barely flickered across my mind during the next forty years or so. Now retired, I have been able to devote the past two and a half years or so to a project which I consider a labor of love.

It is almost exclusively about the 'sound' period. The silent era is mentioned in some of the early biographies and I only refer to television and stage work where it is relevant to the career. The list of titles below each biography is my personal selection of what I consider to be their best work.

The individuals who fill these pages virtually selected themselves, but since starting this project with the aim of including my personal favorites, I've added stars of some film genres whom I wasn't too familiar with. I've included the vital statistic of height, along with the other details, because it always fascinated me. In the old days, whether or not it was due to vanity on the part of an actor (usually males) the studios would add inches where they felt it was necessary – even if people could see their built-up shoes.

It was the same with birth dates, but usually in reverse. Today, things are much more transparent, with actors frequently keeping their birth-names, however awkward-sounding.

Where the child stars are concerned, in the cases where they didn't progress to significant adult roles I have given their height at the peak of their juvenile careers. Margaret O'Brien, Freddie Bartholomew and Bobby Driscoll are three examples.

In order to control the time taken to research and write the biographies, I have had to limit the number of stars covered in this book by imposing a rule for inclusion: other than rare exceptions, such as James Dean, all fifteen hundred and sixty five stars have appeared in a minimum of six worthwhile films.

Which raises the question – how do I actually judge what is a "worthwhile" movie? My definition is it's one you can watch and enjoy – more than once.

By making those selections, I am not attempting to compete with the many excellent movie guides on the market. To begin with, I would find it extremely difficult to work within their four-star system of ratings. Since I first started rating films back in 1956, I've given marks out of a maximum of ten for every one of almost 30,000 titles I have seen.

To give readers a further insight regarding my taste in movies, I've listed my choice two hundred favorites on a following page. Their score is between 8.5-10 – meaning excellent, unmissable, or a classic. In my opinion, none of the titles listed in "Movie Star Choice" are worth less than 5 out of 10 – meaning worthwhile.

As far as movie guides go, I appreciate that the ratings given are to a large extent a reflection of the author's personal tastes. This book is no exception. The difference is that I am not publishing star ratings – only my choice of what is worth watching from the output of each actor and actress. Everyone disagrees with the critics or experts at times and I've no doubt that it will be the same with some of my recommendations. During my many years of being a fan, I have rarely come across a group of people who all reacted in the same way after seeing a film.

The one thing I am sure of is this; whether you are a regular moviegoer, watch films on DVDs, videos, on your computer, or catch the oldies at Turner Classic Movies, you will find "Movie Star Choice" entertaining, interesting, informative and useful.

Barry Bendel
Portsmouth
England
– 2009

Acknowledgments

Firstly to my wife, Doris, who has not only been supremely patient and supportive during the past two years, she has been a priceless source of information regarding the history and the stars of the German and Italian Cinema – both past and present. She has also spent many hours reading through proofs. I shouldn't forget my son, Marc, whose tough opinions and constructive criticisms I have valued greatly. I would also like to express my appreciation to the publishers, Eloquent Books, who showed remarkable patience as I neared the end of this mammoth task. The people who helped me to complete this project by reading the text, commenting on my written work, and most importantly, spotted mistakes include:- Chris Carrell, an Arts Director, who cast his eagle eye over my grammar; David Eliades, a playwright and author, who took the time to read my first draft; Michael Cox, who helped me improve it; Gian and Binder Gil, an Indian couple, who lent me DVDs of Bollywood movies from their extensive collection and read my finished text; Dominique Ivanyi, who checked French spelling and accents; Mercé Perera, who helped with Spanish stars; Ingrid Reed, who scrutinized the Swedish selections; Robert Smith, owner of a bookshop, who is both an avid reader and film buff, checked dates and titles; Jeff Wallder, an advertising copywriter, who edited the manuscript; Graham Thomas, from Design Agency Evoke, and Jackie Plummer from i-i-design.com, whose suggestions and technical advice were invaluable; and last, but not least, eleven-year-old Alexis Watkins, who recommended a number of new names on the scene and drew my attention to many of the recent movies for younger audiences.

My Choice Movies

ACE IN THE HOLE (1951)
ADVENTURES OF ROBIN HOOD The (1938)
AFRICAN QUEEN The (1951)
ALL THE PRESIDENT'S MEN (1976)
AMERICAN BEAUTY (1999)
AMERICAN HISTORY X (1998)
AN AMERICAN IN PARIS (1951)
ANATOMY OF A MURDER (1959)
ASHES AND DIAMONDS (1958)
ASPHALT JUNGLE The (1950)
BABETTE'S FEAST (1987)
BAD DAY AT BLACK ROCK (1955)
BALL OF FIRE (1941)
BAND WAGON The (1953)
BELLE ET LA BÊTE La (1946)
BEST YEARS OF OUR LIVES The (1946)
BÊTE HUMAIN La (1938)
BICYCLE THIEVES (1948)
BIG SLEEP The (1946)
BILLY LIAR (1963)
BLACK BOOK (2006)
BLACK SWAN The (1942)
BODY AND SOUL (1947)
BOURNE ULTIMATUM (2007)
BRIDGE ON THE RIVER KWAI (1957)
CALL ME MADAM (1953)
CASABLANCA (1942)
CHARIOTS OF FIRE (1981)
CINEMA PARADISO (1988)
CITIZEN KANE (1941)
CRASH (2004)
CRIMES AND MISDEMEANORS (1989)
CROSSFIRE (1947)
DARLING (1965)
DAY FOR NIGHT (1973)
DAY THE EARTH STOOD STILL The (1951)
DEER HUNTER The (1978)
DELIVERANCE (1972)
DIE HARD (1988)
DIRTY HARRY (1972)
DR. STRANGELOVE (1963)
DOUBLE INDEMNITY (1944)
DUEL (1971)
ENGLISH PATIENT The (1996)
ERIN BROKOVICH (2000)
EXORCIST The (1973)
EYES WITHOUT A FACE (1959)
FALLING DOWN (1992)
FAREWELL MY CONCUBINE (1993)
FISHER KING The (1991)
FLIRTING (1989)
FRENCH CANCAN (1955)
FRENCH CONNECTION The (1971)
FROM HERE TO ETERNITY (1953)
GANDHI (1982)
GENEVIEVE (1953)
GILDA (1946)
GLADIATOR (2000)
GODFATHER The (1972)
GONE WITH THE WIND (1939)
GOODFELLAS (1990)
GOOD WILL HUNTING (1997)
GRAPES OF WRATH (1940)
GUNFIGHT AT THE OK CORRAL (1957)
GUNFIGHTER The (1950)
HAIL THE CONQUERING HERO (1944)
HARVEY (1950)
HEAVEN CAN WAIT (1943)

HILARY AND JACKIE (1998)
HIROSHIMA MON AMOUR (1959)
HISTORY OF VIOLENCE (2005)
HOLIDAY (1938)
HOLLYWOOD OR BUST (1956)
HOW TO MARRY A MILLIONAIRE (1953)
HUD (1963)
HUSTLER The (1961)
I AM A FUGITIVE FROM A CHAIN GANG (1932)
IN BRUGES (2008)
IN THE HEAT OF THE NIGHT (1967)
INSIDER The (1999)
INVASION OF THE BODYSNATCHERS (1956)
IT HAPPENED ONE NIGHT (1934)
IT'S A GIFT (1934)
IT'S A WONDERFUL LIFE (1946)
JAWS (1975)
JEAN DE FLORETTE (1986)
JERRY MAGUIRE (1996)
JULES ET JIM (1961)
JULIUS CAESAR (1953)
KRAMER VS KRAMER (1979)
KIND HEARTS AND CORONETS (1949)
KING KONG (1933)
KILLERS The (1946)
KISS ME DEADLY (1955)
LADY FROM SHANGHAI The (1948)
LADYKILLERS The (1955)
LAURA (1944)
LAWRENCE OF ARABIA (1962)
LOLA MONTÈS (1955)
LOLITA (1961)
L.A. CONFIDENTIAL (1997)
LOVERS The (1958)
MAGNIFICENT SEVEN (1960)
MAGNOLIA (1999)
MALTESE FALCON The (1941)
MAN WHO WOULD BE KING The (1975)
MANCHURIAN CANDIDATE The (1962)
MAN FROM LARAMIE (1955)
MANHATTAN (1979)
MATRIX The (1999)
MATTER OF LIFE AND DEATH A (1946)
MEET ME IN ST LOUIS (1944)
MEMOIRS OF A GEISHA (2005)
MIDNIGHT (1939)
MILDRED PIERCE (1945)
MIRACLE ON 34TH STREET (1947)
MR SMITH GOES TO WASHINGTON (1939)
MONSIEUR HULOT'S HOLIDAY (1953)
MY DARLING CLEMENTINE (1946)
NETWORK (1976)
NIGHT AT THE OPERA A (1935)
NIGHT OF THE HUNTER (1955)
NIGHTMARE ALLEY (1947)
NINOTCHKA (1939)
NO COUNTRY FOR OLD MEN (2007)
NORTH BY NORTH WEST (1959)
NOTORIOUS (1946)
ODD MAN OUT (1946)
OKLAHOMA! (1955)
OLIVER TWIST (1948)
OLIVADOS Los (1950)
OMEN The (1976)
ONCE UPON A TIME IN AMERICA (1984)
ONLY ANGELS HAVE WINGS (1939)
ON THE TOWN (1949)
ON THE WATERFRONT (1954)

OUTLAW JOSEY WALES The (1976)
OUT OF THE PAST (1947)
PACK UP YOUR TROUBLES (1932)
PANDORA AND THE FLYING DUTCHMAN (1951)
PAN'S LABYRINTH (2006)
PATHS OF GLORY (1957)
PAWNBROKER The (1965)
PLACE IN THE SUN A (1951)
POSTMAN ALWAYS RINGS TWICE The (1946)
PRISONER OF ZENDA The (1937)
PSYCHO (1960)
RAGING BULL (1980)
RAIDERS OF THE LOST ARK (1981)
RAILWAY CHILDREN The (1971)
RAISE THE RED LANTERN (1991)
READER The (2008)
REBECCA (1940)
REBEL WITHOUT A CAUSE (1955)
RED RIVER (1948)
RED SHOES The (1948)
RED SORGHUM (1987)
ROMAN HOLIDAY (1953)
ROSEMARY'S BABY (1968)
SCARFACE (1932)
SE7EN (1995)
SEVEN SAMURAI The (1954)
SHANGHAI GESTURE The (1941)
SHAWSHANK REDEMPTION (1994)
SILENCE OF THE LAMBS The (1991)
SINGIN' IN THE RAIN (1953)
SLUMDOG MILLIONAIRE (2008)
SMILES OF A SUMMER NIGHT (1955)
SOME LIKE IT HOT (1959)
STAR WARS (1977)
STRANGERS ON A TRAIN (1951)
SULLIVAN'S TRAVELS (1941)
SUPERMAN (1978)
SWEET SMELL OF SUCCESS (1957)
SWING TIME (1936)
TAXI DRIVER (1976)
THAT OBSCURE OBJECT OF DESIRE (1977)
THELMA & LOUISE (1991)
THIEF The (1997)
THIRD MAN The (1949)
TOP HAT (1935)
TRISTINA (1970)
TRUE ROMANCE (1993)
TRUMAN SHOW The (1998)
12 ANGRY MEN (1957)
TWELVE O'CLOCK HIGH (1950)
TWENTIETH CENTURY (1934)
UGETSU MONOGATARI (1953)
UNTOUCHABLES The (1987)
VERA CRUZ (1954)
VIVA ZAPATA (1952)
WAGES OF FEAR The (1953)
WAY OUT WEST (1937)
WEST SIDE STORY (1961)
WHITE HEAT (1949)
WILD BUNCH The (1969)
WILD STRAWBERRIES (1957)
WINCHESTER '73 (1950)
WIZARD OF OZ The (1939)
WOMAN IN THE DUNES (1963)
YEARLING The (1946)
YELLOW SKY (1948)
YOU ONLY LIVE TWICE (1967)

Movie Star Choice

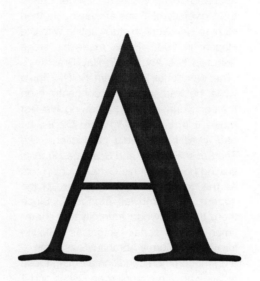

Bud **Abbott**
5ft 8in
(WILLIAM ALEXANDER ABBOTT)

Born: **October 2, 1895**
Asbury Park, New Jersey, USA
Died: **April 24, 1974**

Bud's parents were both circus people – his mother was a bareback rider with Ringling Brothers. As a boy, Bud worked at Coney Island Amusement Park. After leaving school at fourteen he was employed in carnivals. By the 1920s he was supporting his wife Betty, in Minsky's Burlesque Shows. Bud subsequently worked as a substitute "straight man" for various vaudeville stars – which is how, in around 1933, he met Lou Costello. The pair clicked immediately and the new duo established itself in burlesque and minstrel shows. Following a guest spot on a national radio show hosted by Kate Smith, they were given a contract by Universal. In 1940, they made their screen debut in a film called *One Night in the Tropics*. They were intended to be comic support for the stars Allan Jones, Nancy Kelly and Robert Cummings, but they completely stole the show with their slick routines. From 1942-51, they were rarely out of the top ten box office attractions. Early hits were *Hold That Ghost* and *Ride 'em Cowboy*. When their popularity began to wane in the 1950s, they did radio and TV shows until an acrimonious split in 1957 – fighting over money – caused by Lou's habit of taking the lion's share. Although Bud was an alcoholic and an epileptic, he outlived Lou, who died in 1959. In the early 1960s, Bud's attempt to start a new double act with the vocalist Candy Candido, failed. After his death from cancer, Bud's ashes were scattered, as he had wished – into the Pacific Ocean.

Buck Privates (1941)
In the Navy (1941)
Hold That Ghost (1941)
Ride 'em Cowboy (1942)
Who Done It? (1942)
It Ain't Hay (1943)
Here Come the Co-Eds (1945)
Abbott and Costello
Meet Frankenstein (1948)
Abbott and Costello
Meet the Invisible Man (1951)

F. Murray **Abraham**
5ft 11in
(FAHRID MURRAY ABRAHAM)

Born: **October 24, 1939**
Pittsburgh, Pennsylvania, USA

Frank was the son of an Assyrian, Fahrid Abraham and his wife, Maryan. His father worked as an auto mechanic. Frank was brought up in El Paso, near the Mexican border – where in his youth, he became a member of a teenage gang. As he grew older, his attitude changed and he focused his attention on education. He attended Texas Western College, before the University of Texas at Austin. He then went to New York to study acting with Uta Hagen. In 1966, Frank made his stage debut in Los Angeles in Ray Bradbury's "The Wonderful Ice Cream Suit". For a while, he was content to concentrate on theater work. In 1971, following his first movie role, in *They Might Be Giants,* he had small parts in big productions, like *The Sunshine Boys* and *Scarface*. Frank's shining hour is still his Oscar winning role as the composer, Antonio Salieri, in the superb 1984 movie, *Amadeus*. Since then, the Hollywood fraternity will sometimes refer to certain actors as suffering from the "F. Murray Abraham Syndrome" – a not uncommon condition afflicting those artists who, after winning an Oscar, find it almost impossible to repeat that level of film performance – or ever get the chance to. It's not something that bothers the man himself. Frank's private life is a very happy one. He has been married to the same woman, Kate Hannan, since 1962. They have two grown children.

The Prisoner of Second Avenue (1975)
The Sunshine Boys (1975)
The Big Fix (1978)
Scarface (1983)
Amadeus (1984)
The Name of the Rose (1986)
Last Action Hero (1993)
Nostradamus (1994)
Mighty Aphrodite (1995)
Children of the Revolution (1996)
Star Trek: Insurrection (1998)
Finding Forrester (2000)
Joshua (2002) Ticker (2002)
Quiet Flows the Don (2006)
Carnera: The Walking Mountain (2006)

Joss **Ackland**
6ft 1in
(SIDNEY EDMOND JOCELYN ACKLAND)

Born: **February 29, 1928**
North Kensington, London, England

Joss was the son of Sydney and Ruth Ackland. He attended the London School of Speech and Drama before making his stage debut at the age of seventeen, in "The Hasty Heart". His first film appearance was an uncredited one, in the 1950 thriller, *Seven Days to Noon*. He spent the next four years acting with British regional theaters. In 1955, he went to Kenya to run a tea plantation outside Nairobi, and then moved down to Cape Town, in South Africa, where he worked on local radio and also wrote plays. Two years later, he returned to England to join the Old Vic, where he acted with Paul Scofield and Tom Courtenay. In the early 1960s, in London, Joss appeared on the West End stage and was an associate director of the Mermaid Theater. He worked a lot on TV, then in 1966, had his first featured movie role in the Hammer Horror film, *Rasputin: The Mad Monk*. Until the 1970s, he was unknown to movie audiences. After that, he made a good career as a character actor and is still active in his eighty-first year. Joss had seven children with the actress Rosemary Kirkcaldy. In 1963, she saved five of them and only just escaped alive during a fire at their home. The injuries sustained ended her acting career. She died in 2006.

Mr. Forbush and the Penguins (1971)
The House That Dripped
Blood (1971) Villain (1971)
England Made Me (1973)
The Three Musketeers (1973)
Royal Flash (1975)
Operation Daybreak (1975)
Saint Jack (1979)
Lady Jane (1986)
White Mischief (1987)
The Hunt for Red October (1990)
Giorgino (1994)
Surviving Picasso (1996)
Firelight (1997)
Asylum (2005)
These Foolish Things (2006)
Flawless (2007)
How About You? (2007)

Amy **Adams**
5ft 5in
(AMY LOU ADAMS)

Born: **August 20, 1974**
Vicenza, Vicenza, Italy

Born to American parents on a U.S. Army base in Italy, where her father had been stationed, Amy then grew up in Castle Rock, Colorado. She was one of a large family of seven children who were raised as Mormons. She was eleven when her parents divorced, and following that, the family's church-going ceased. After she graduated from Douglas County High school in Castle Rock, where she sang in the choir, she trained seriously for a career as a ballerina but appeared in shows at a Denver dinner theater. She next moved to Chanhassen, in Minnesota, where she danced and sang in a similar set-up and starred in musicals such as "Brigadoon", "A Chorus Line" and "Good News". She was spotted by a movie producer and in 1999, made her film debut, in *Drop Dead Gorgeous,* which was actually filmed on her home turf, in Minnesota. Amy then went to live in Los Angeles, where she soon had a leading role in the Fox TV-series, 'Manchester Prep'. In 2000, she was seen in episodes of such shows as 'Buffy the Vampire Slayer', 'Providence' and 'Charmed'. Far from neglecting the big screen, she also appeared in some independent films before making an impact in the A-List movie, *Catch Me If You Can.* She was first nominated for a Best Supporting Actress Oscar for *Junebug.* For her recent movie, *Doubt,* she was Oscar-nominated in the same category. She's currently dating the actor, Darren Le Gallo.

Catch Me if You Can (2002)
Junebug (2005) The Wedding
Date (2005) Standing Still (2005)
Moonlight Serenade (2006)
Talladega Nights: The
Ballad of Ricky Bobby (2006)
Tenacious D in
The Pick of Destiny (2006)
Enchanted (2007)
Charlie Wilson's War (2007)
Sunshine Cleaning (2008)
Miss Pettigrew Lives for a Day (2008)
Doubt (2008)

Brooke **Adams**
5ft 5in
(BROOKE ALLISON ADAMS)

Born: **February 8, 1949**
New York City, New York, USA

Brooke was the daughter of Robert K. Adams, who was a producer and actor, and a descendant of two American Presidents – John Adams and John Quincy Adams. Her mother was actress Rosalind Gould. As an aspiring young actress, Brooke went to the High School for Performing Arts and the School of American Ballet – both in New York. She started her stage career by playing juvenile leads on the New York theater scene. That led to TV plays and low-budget films. Brooke moved into another league when two performances – in *Days of Heaven* and *Invasion of the Bodysnatchers* (which were released in 1978), got her positive reviews. But by 1995, due partly to a dearth of good roles, and a need to spend more time with her two young daughters, Brooke retired. When she came back six years later, she had lost her little girl looks but began to appear in some interesting adult roles. One of the first of that type was when she was sensitively directed by her husband Tony Shalhoub, in the film *Made-Up,* a moving story of a woman dealing with the problems of growing old. The screenplay was written by her sister, Lynne Adams. On Broadway in recent years, Brooke has starred in "The Heidi Chronicles" and Anton Chekhov's "The Cherry Orchard". She has recently been seen on television in the comedy drama 'Monk' – which stars her husband. Brooke is also currently working with Tony on an untitled comedy drama which is about to be shot in Indiana.

Shock Waves (1977)
Invasion of the Body
Snatchers (1978)
Days of Heaven (1978)
Cuba (1979)
Tell Me a Riddle (1980)
The Dead Zone (1983)
Gas, Food, Lodging (1992)
Made-Up (2002)
At Last (2005)
The Legend of
Lucy Keyes (2006)

Julie **Adams**
5ft 6in
(BETTY MAY ADAMS)

Born: **October 17, 1926**
Waterloo, Iowa, USA

Julie grew up in Arkansas, where as a child, she acted in a school play "Hansel and Gretel". When she was in her late teens she decided to seek her fame and fortune in Hollywood – working as a secretary for a time to pay for her acting and speech lessons. Her first part was in 1949, playing a young starlet in the Betty Hutton and Victor Mature vehicle for Paramount, *Red, Hot and Blue.* Julie then starred in seven B-movie westerns which included the excellent, Don 'Red' Barry film, *The Dalton Gang.* Not long after that, Julie found herself signing a contract for Universal Pictures and starring with Tom Ewell – in the 1951 comedy, *Finders Keepers.* In 1954 – the same year she encountered *The Creature from the Black Lagoon* – she changed her name for the third time in her life when she became Mrs. Ray Danton. She and Danton acted together in *The Looters* for Universal, and before they divorced in 1981, Ray directed Julie in his own horror-movie – *Psychic Killer.* Even though officially retired since 2000, the acting bug was still in her. Five years later, she made a welcome come-back – and is currently keeping busy on TV. Only a couple of years ago, it was great to see Julie again – in a chilling short, titled *Lost,* and also in a supporting role in a big movie – *World Trade Center.* In 2008, she appeared (for the second time) in an episode of an Emmy-nominated television series 'Lost: Missing Pieces'.

Bright Victory (1951)
Bend of the River (1952)
The Treasure of the Lost
Canyon (1952)
The Lawless Breed (1953)
The Mississippi Gambler (1953)
The Creature from the
Black Lagoon (1954)
Six Bridges to Cross (1954)
The Private War of
Major Benson (1955)
Away All Boats (1956)
Slaughter on 10th Avenue (1957)
World Trade Center (2006)

Nick **Adams**
5ft 9in
(NICHOLAS ALOYSIUS ADAMSCHOCK)

Born: **July 10, 1931**
Nanticoke, Pennsylvania, USA
Died: **February 7, 1968**

Nick was born into a poor family. His father, Peter Adamschock, who was from the Ukraine, was an anthracite coal miner. His mother's name was Catherine. From an early age, Nick was totally obsessed with the idea of making it in the competitive world of show business. Before he set out to take that world by storm he served with the United States Coastguards. Then, when he auditioned for a part in the New York stage production of *Mister Roberts*, its star, Henry Fonda, advised him to get some training as an actor – advice he totally ignored. A year later, Nick acted in the film version – with Fonda. Once described as a Hollywood hustler – he certainly worked the pool halls when he first arrived in California and established close friendships with James Dean and Natalie Wood, with whom he acted in the teen classic, *Rebel Without a Cause*. Later, he hung out with Elvis Presley and his Memphis Mafia. But Nick rarely got more than supporting parts – albeit in some top movies. He was probably most famous for his role as Johnny Yuma in the 1959 TV series 'The Rebel'. Around that time, Nick was on the CBS Quiz program *What's My Line,* but just like his film career, it wasn't a winner. He became more and more disappointed with his lack of real success. He spent his own money promoting his Oscar nomination for *Twilight of Honor,* but lost. By 1964 his career was on the skids and he was reduced to acting in Japanese B-movies. Four years later, in what was suspected as suicide, he died of a drug overdose at his home.

Mister Roberts (1955)
Rebel Without a Cause (1955)
Picnic (1955)
The Last Wagon (1956)
No Time For Sergeants (1958)
Pillow Talk (1959)
The FBI Story (1959)
Hell is for Heroes (1962)
The Interns (1962)
Twilight of Honor (1963)

Dawn **Addams**
5ft 5½in
(VICTORIA DAWN ADDAMS)

Born: **September 21, 1930**
Felixstowe, Suffolk, England
Died: **May 7, 1985**

Dawn was the daughter of Captain James Addams and his wife, Ethel. After starting school in England, she went with her father to India following her mother's early death. They lived near Calcutta, where she went to school until, during the partition of India in 1947, things became dangerous for British citizens. She and her father then took the long boat journey home. Her great beauty – a cross between Elizabeth Taylor and Jean Simmons, soon caught the eye of a movie talent scout, but when Dawn told her very old-fashioned father that she wanted to become an actress, he took her with him to Rio de Janeiro. But it didn't change her mind – Dawn was a very determined young woman. From 1949, she was studying at the Royal Academy of Dramatic Art in London and living with another girl in a rented apartment, a short walk from the West End's theaterland. In 1951, she acted in her first Hollywood movie, *Night Into Morning* – filmed in and around the University of California, at Berkeley. Bit parts in films followed but in 1954, Dawn returned to Europe, married an Italian Prince – Don Vittorio Emanuele Massimo and had a son named Prince Stefano. Dawn reached the peak of her popularity around the time of Chaplin's *A King in New York*. In the 1960s she starred in several mostly forgettable European productions and eventually, in B-horror movies. In 1974, she remarried briefly. Dawn was only fifty-four when she died of cancer, at her home in London.

Night Into Morning (1951)
The Unknown Man (1951)
A King in New York (1957)
The Silent Enemy (1958)
Temptation (1959)
The Black Chapel (1959)
**The Thousand Eyes of
Dr. Mabuse** (1960)
L'Education sentimentale (1962)
La Tulipe noire (1964)
The Vampire Lovers (1970)
Vault of Horror (1973)

Isabelle **Adjani**
5ft 4½in
(ISABELLE YASMINE ADJANI)

Born: **June 27, 1955**
Paris, France

The daughter of an Algerian father, Mohand Crif Adjani and a German mother, named Augusta, Isabelle grew up with German as her first language. And, along with French and English, was soon fluent in three. Isabelle began acting in amateur theater productions when she was twelve, and by the age of fourteen she had appeared in her first movie – *Le Petit Bougnat*. She joined the famous Comédie Française in Paris, from where she was able to project herself into the world of French cinema via television productions such as 'Ondine', in 1974. That same year, her film career took off following her role in the film *La Gifle* (The Slap). Not long after that, she was hired by François Truffaut to star in his magnificent film *The Story of Adèle H* – a biographical story about Victor Hugo's daughter. Isabelle's fine performance transformed her into an international star and earned her a Best Actress Oscar nomination. She received a second nomination for *Camille Claudel*. After good plastic surgery to improve her features, she became one of the most beautiful of French actresses. Her life off screen has been as passionate as on it. She was engaged to composer Jean Michel Jarre, but they separated in 2004 and she now spends much of her time raising her two sons – one of whom is from a relationship with the English actor, Daniel Day-Lewis. In 2008, she was seen on French TV in 'Figaro' by 18th century French playwright, Beaumarchais.

La Gifle (1974)
The Story of Adèle H (1975)
The Driver (1978)
Possession (1981)
Quartet (1981)
L'été meurtrier (1983)
Subway (1985)
Camille Claudel (1988)
La Reine Margot (1994)
Adolphe (2002)
Bon Voyage (2003)
**Monsieur Ibrahim et les
fleurs du Coran** (2003)

Mario **Adorf**
5ft 10in
(MARIO ADORF)

Born: **September 8, 1930**
Zurich, Switzerland

Mario's father was an Italian surgeon named Matteo Menniti, who was resident in a Zurich hospital. Although Matteo was a married man, he had an affair with a German nurse, then left her holding the baby – Mario. When he was still a small boy she took him to her home in Mayen/Eifel, Germany, where he grew up during the rise of Adolf Hitler. Luckily for him, he was too young to become a young Nazi. When World War II ended, Mario was still at secondary school. After that, he attended Mainz University, where he studied several subjects including Literature, and was a member of the boxing team. Mario was also keenly involved in their theatrical productions – appearing in a variety of plays – which made up his mind to become an actor. This led him to Munich, in 1953, to study Drama at the Otto-Falckenberg-Schule. He appeared on stage and was spotted by a German film studio scout. After a few bit parts Mario's career took off with a featured role in *The Devil Strikes at Night*. He became popular in German, French, Italian and English-language films. His most famous roles were Matzerath, in *The Tin Drum*, and Schukert, in the hit Rainer Werner Fassbinder movie, *Lola*. Much of his recent work has been on TV. Mario has lived with his second wife, Monique, since 1968. They tied the knot in 1985.

The Devil Strikes at Night (1958)
Lulu (1962)
Major Dundee (1965)
Paralyzed (1971)
Execution Squad (1972)
La Faille (1975) **The Lost Honor of Katharina Blum** (1975)
Bomber & Paganini (1976)
The Tin Drum (1979)
Lola (1981)
State buoni...se potete (1984)
Momo (1986)
I Ragazzi di Via Panisperna (1989)
La luna negra (1989)
Amigomío (1994) **Rossini** (1997)
Epstein's Night (2002)

Ben **Affleck**
6ft 2½in
(BENJAMIN GEZA AFFLECK-BOLDT)

Born: **August 15, 1972**
Berkeley, California, USA

Ben's father, Timothy Affleck was a former actor who worked as a social worker and drug counselor. His mother, Christine, was a schoolteacher. At the age of eight he moved with his parents to Cambridge, Massachusetts. He met and befriended Matt Damon, with whom he attended the local high school – Cambridge Rindge and Latin. Ben worked in children's TV shows before appearing together with Damon in a movie called *School Ties*, in which he played a very unpleasant, anti-semitic character. Both actors, who are Boston Red Sox Baseball fanatics, were extras in Kevin Costner's movie, *Field of Dreams*. Along with Damon, Ben received a Best Screenplay Oscar in 1997 – for *Good Will Hunting*. They then founded their own production company "Live Planet". After a couple of critically panned movies, Ben lay low for the whole of 2005, partly because, in June, he married the beautiful actress Jennifer Garner. He made what could be termed a comeback in 2006, when he was named Best Actor at the Venice Film Festival for his role as the tragic 1950's TV Superman, George Reeves, in the movie *Hollywoodland*. It also earned him a Golden Globe nomination for Best Supporting Actor. Ben completed his third project as a film director – *Gone Baby Gone*. His next acting role, in the comedy, *He's Just Not That Into You*, wasn't in the same league as the superior, *State of Play*.

Chasing Amy (1997)
Good Will Hunting (1997)
Armageddon (1998)
Shakespeare in Love (1998)
Dogma (1999)
Boiler Room (2000)
Bounce (2000)
Pearl Harbor (2001)
Changing Lanes (2002)
The Sum of all Fears (2002)
Paycheck (2003)
Jersey Girl (2004)
Man About Town (2006)
Hollywoodland (2006)
State of Play (2009)

Casey **Affleck**
5ft 9in
(CALEB CASEY AFFLECK)

Born: **August 12, 1975**
Falmouth, Massachusetts, USA

Ben's younger brother kept a lot of pets when he was a small boy. At certain times when the house was filled with his cats, snakes, guinea pigs and turtles, he used to drive his mother mad. He was always a talented and expressive kid who, when he was twelve, played Kevin Bacon's brother in a television film, 'Lemon Sky'. After high school, he moved to California, where he got a part in the movie *To Die For,* and he became good friends with one of its cast, Joaquin Phoenix. Casey then went to New York, where he majored in Physics, Astronomy and Western Philosophy at Columbia University. During that period he lived with his grandmother in Manhattan. Casey appeared with his brother in the hit film *Good Will Hunting,* and by 2000, he was not only established as an actor, he had also fallen in love with Joaquin's sister, Summer. They were married in 2006 and now have two children. Casey still has a great love of nature – he is deeply involved with animal rights movements and campaigns for PETA and Farm Sanctuary. Recently, he featured in a couple of good A-list movies – *Ocean's Thirteen* and *The Assassination of Jesse James by the Coward Robert Ford* – for which he was nominated for a Best Supporting Actor Oscar. Another worthwhile addition to his acting credits is *Gone Baby Gone,* a well-received drama, which was directed by brother, Ben. Casey's fans look forward to his upcoming movie – *The Killer Inside Me.*

To Die For (1995)
Chasing Amy (1997)
Good Will Hunting (1997)
Drowning Mona (2000)
Hamlet (2000)
Ocean's Eleven (2001)
Gerry (2002)
Lonesome Jim (2005)
The Last Kiss (2006)
Ocean's Thirteen (2007)
The Assassination of Jesse James by the Coward Robert Ford (2007)
Gone Baby Gone (2007)

John **Agar**
6ft 1in
(JOHN G. AGAR)

Born: **January 31, 1921**
Chicago, Illinois, USA
Died: **April 7, 2002**

John was the eldest of four children born to a meat packer, John Agar Sr., and his wife, Lillian. He was a keen sportsman during his schooldays at Harvard School for Boys' and Lake Forest Academy – in Chicago. Following his father's death in 1942, his family moved to Los Angeles. The following year John joined the Army Air Corps, where he achieved the rank of sergeant. Towards the end of World War II, as a tall and very handsome PT instructor, John was on official escort duty for "America's Sweetheart" the sixteen-year-old Shirley Temple, who was visiting the base. They fell in love and their Hollywood wedding in 1945 was front-page news around the globe. All this media attention turned John into a celebrity. He was signed by David O. Selznick, who quickly organized acting lessons, and in 1948, John made his film debut, in John Ford's classic western *Fort Apache* – which co-starred Shirley. That year, a daughter was born to the couple. John's heavy drinking put an end to the marriage, and a drink-driving conviction in 1951, almost ended his career. But he bounced back, with the help of a new wife, the model Loretta Combs. They had two sons and were together until her death in 2000. He had kept working as a movie actor – becoming a leading man in a series of low-budget sci-fi and horror films. John remained on friendly terms with his hero, John Wayne, who got him supporting parts in three of his later films – *The Undefeated, Big Jake* and *Chisum*. John died of emphysema, two years after his wife.

Fort Apache (1948)
She Wore a Yellow Ribbon (1949)
Sands of Iwo Jima (1949)
Breakthrough (1950) Revenge of the
Creature (1955) Tarantula (1955)
Star in the Dust (1956)
The St. Valentine's Day Massacre (1967)
Chisum (1970) Big Jake (1971)
Divided We Fall (1982)
Miracle Mile (1988)

Jenny **Agutter**
5ft 8in
(JENNIFER ANN AGUTTER)

Born: **December 20, 1952**
Taunton, Somerset, England

Jenny's mother Catherine, was known to everyone as "Kit". Her father Derek, was a British Army officer. Because of her dad's overseas postings, she spent much of her early life in Kuala Lumpur, Malaysia, and Cyprus. While at Elmhurst Ballet School in Camberley, near London, Jenny was seen there by a casting agent and she made her film debut at the age of twelve in *East of Sudan* – a rather modest effort starring Anthony Quayle and Sylvia Syms. During 1966 she appeared in the television series called 'Ballerina'. It was soon followed by a BBC television production of 'The Railway Children'. She also starred in the movie version four years later *and* the 2000 re-work. In 1971 Jenny had her first adult role – appearing nude for the first time, in *Walkabout,* a tense drama about stranded children, directed by Nicolas Roeg and filmed on location in the Australian outback. Jenny went to Hollywood in 1973, where she had a good ten-year spell – most notably in *Logan's Run* and *An American Werewolf in London.* A talented photographer, "Snap", a book of her best work, was published in 1983. Jenny has kept busy in films, on stage – including several Shakespeare plays, and on TV. She's been married to Swedish hotelier, Johan Tham since 1990. They have a son together and the family divides its time between their home in Camberwell, in South East London, and the greater peace and quiet of Cornwall. It doesn't mean retirement: Jenny's recently been enjoying acting in films again.

The Railway Children (1970)
Walkabout (1971) Logan's Run (1976)
The Eagle Has Landed (1976)
Equus (1977)
The Riddle of the Sands (1979)
An American Werewolf
in London (1981)
King of the Wind (1990)
At Dawning (2001)
Heroes and Villains (2006)
Irina Palm (2007)
Act of God (2008)

Brian **Aherne**
6ft 2in
(WILLIAM BRIAN DE LACY AHERNE)

Born: **May 2, 1902**
Cambridge, England
Died: **February 10, 1986**

Brian was the son of William de Lacy Aherne and his wife Louise. Having made his stage debut aged nine in Birmingham, Brian showed such great promise that he was sent to the 'Italia Conti Academy' in London. Its founder, whose name *was* Italia Conti, was an established actress who believed in giving students a broader education, which included opportunities for youngsters to act in plays. At eighteen, after leaving Malvern College – which was close to his home, he began studying to be an architect, but soon realized that the theater was the life he wanted. He made his senior stage debut in London, in 1923, in "Paddy The Next Best Thing" at the Savoy Theater. Seven British silent films led to his first starring talkie film, in 1931's *Madame Guillotine*. He went to America in 1933 and after his debut in *Song of Songs* – with Marlene Dietrich, he appeared in over thirty Hollywood movies and was nominated for a Best Supporting Actor Oscar in *Juarez*. He was married for six years to Joan Fontaine. After retiring in 1967, Brian took up writing. He called his autobiography "A Proper Job". Ten years later he published a biography of his pal, George Sanders, who, fortunately for him, was dead. He had given it the less than flattering title of "A Dreadful Man". Brian lived for another ten years – in Venice, Florida, before dying of heart failure.

What Every Woman Knows (1934)
Sylvia Scarlett (1935)
Beloved Enemy (1936)
The Great Garrick (1937)
Juarez (1939) Captain Fury (1939)
Vigil in the Night (1940)
The Lady in Question (1940)
Hired Wife (1940) Skylark (1941)
A Night to Remember (1943)
Forever and a Day (1943)
Smart Woman (1948)
I Confess (1953) The Swan (1956)
The Best of Everything (1959)
Susan Slade (1961) Lancelot and
Guinevere (1963) Rosie (1967)

Danny **Aiello**
6ft 3in
(DANIEL LOUIS AIELLO JR.)

Born: **June 20, 1933**
New York City, New York, USA

Danny was born to a poor Italian American couple during the Great Depression. His father Daniel Aiello Sr., was a laborer. His mother, Frances, worked as a seamstress. When times got tough his father abandoned the family and Danny shone shoes in Grand Central Station to help supplement the family income. He dropped out of James Monroe High School in the Bronx, and at sixteen, lied about his age when he joined the Army. He then worked for the Greyhound Bus Company, and after ten years, he became their Union representative. He married his sweetheart, Sandy, in 1955 and they had four children. In 1972, he was a bouncer in a night club when the regular emcee at a comedy night didn't show up. Danny took over as entertainer with such success, friends persuaded him to give acting a go. His stage debut in "Lamp Post Reunion" won a Theatrical World Award. In 1973, he made his film debut in *Bang the Drum Slowly* and began to build a new career as a tough character actor, with small parts in Woody Allen films and *The Godfather: Part II.* He was then Oscar nominated for his supporting role as the owner of a pizzeria in *Do the Right Thing* and by the early 1990s, he had featured in several top films including *Moonstruck, Jacob's Ladder* and *Léon.* Danny is both the director and the star of *Anyone's Son,* which will be released in 2009.

Fingers (1978) Defiance (1980)
Fort Apache the Bronx (1981)
Once Upon a Time in America (1984)
The Purple Rose of Cairo (1985)
Moonstruck (1987)
January Man (1989)
Do the Right Thing (1989)
Jacob's Ladder (1990)
Once Around (1991) Ruby (1992)
Léon (1994) Lieberman in
Love (1995) City Hall (1996)
2 Days in the Valley (1996)
Dinner Rush (2000)
Brooklyn Lobster (2005)
The Last Request (2006)

Anouk **Aimée**
5ft 8in
(FRANÇOISE SORYA DREYFUS)

Born: **April 27, 1932**
Paris, France

Anouk was the daughter of Henri Dreyfus and the much admired Jewish actress, Geneviève Sorya. Although showing early promise when training as a dancer and actress at the Bauer-Therond Dramatic School in Paris, she became one of the most reluctant of movie stars. Anouk had several golden opportunities to become a really big name, but for some reason, she didn't choose to follow up. When she was fourteen, she made her first screen appearance in *La Fleur de L'âge.* At sixteen Anouk was a charming Juliet, in *Les Amants de Vérone.* In 1951, she had a daughter with her second husband. After a British film with Trevor Howard – *The Golden Salamander,* she established herself as a star in France and the Continent throughout the 1950s. She looked to be spreading her wings with appearances in two of the Italian master, Federico Fellini's film classics – *La Dolce Vita* and *8½.* Then in 1966, after acting in *Un homme et une femme* and being nominated for a Best Actress Oscar, Anouk seemed close to international stardom at last. A couple of years later however, she was almost forgotten. A disappointing sequel made twenty years later with the same stars, did little to revive interest in her. Her recent films – in which she has strong supporting roles, have helped bring her back into focus. She was married four times; the last being from 1970 until 1978, to the English acting legend, Albert Finney.

The Man Who Watched
Trains Go By (1952)
La Rideau Cramoisi (1953)
Les Amants de Montparnasse (1958)
La Tête contre les murs (1959)
La Dolce Vita (1960)
Lola (1961) 8½ (1963)
Un homme et une femme (1966)
Un soir, un train (1968)
Mon premier amour (1978)
Festival In Cannes (2001)
The Birch-Tree Meadow (2003)
And They Lived Happily
Ever After (2004)

Jessica **Alba**
5ft 6½in
(JESSICA MARIE ALBA)

Born: **April 28, 1981**
Pomona, California, USA

Jessica is the daughter of Mark Alba – who is Mexican American – and his wife Catherine – who is of Danish descent. Her father was in the United States Air Force, which meant living in Biloxi, Mississippi and Del Rio, Texas, when she was small. It's hard to believe it now, but Jessica was a sickly child – suffering from collapsed lungs, a ruptured appendix and pneumonia. A move back to California when she was nine saw a big improvement in her health and enough confidence to look for work as a model. She was signed by an agent when she was thirteen. In 1994, Jessica made her film debut with a small role in a family movie entitled *Camp Nowhere.* Her next assignments were TV commercials for Nintendo and J.C. Penney. There was one more movie part during the next five years and several in television shows – most notably, ten episodes of 'Flipper', where she was able to use her ability as a scuba diver. Jessica took acting classes at the Atlantic Theater Company in New York City. She then had a featured role in a really sparkling teen comedy, *Idle Hands.* That film, and *The Sleeping Dictionary,* for which she won a Golden Globe, were good, as was "Dark Angel' – a TV drama for which she was also nominated. It was two years later, in the big budget, *Sin City,* that she really made her mark – it won her the MTV Award for the "Sexiest Performance". Her subsequent films show plenty of evidence that she is a beautiful, emerging star. Her younger brother, Joshua, is an actor. Jessica and her husband, Cash Warren (son of Michael) welcomed their first baby, a girl, in the summer of 2008. A rare error of judgement saw Jessica in the mediocre movie, *The Love Guru,* but she has three promising titles ready for release.

Idle Hands (1999)
The Sleeping Dictionary (2003)
Sin City (2005)
Fantastic Four (2005) 4: Rise of the
Silver Surfer (2007) Bill (2007)
Awake (2007) The Eye (2008)

Eddie **Albert**
5ft 10in
(EDWARD ALBERT HEIMBERGER)

Born: **April 22, 1906**
Rock Island, Illinois, USA
Died: **May 26, 2005**

Eddie's parents were unmarried when he was born. Due to the social stigma at that time, his birth date was given as 1908 – the year they married. When he was two, the family moved to Minneapolis, where they had a very tough time. During World War I, his life was made miserable when classmates victimized him because of his German surname. In 1929 he graduated from the University of Minnesota with a business degree – which wasn't of much use when the stock market crashed. Eddie did any job he could get – including working as a trapeze artist in a circus. He was given a Warners' contract, but soon after his film debut in *Brother Rat,* World War II intervened. He served in the US Navy, and was awarded the *Bronze Star* for rescuing seventy wounded marines while under fire. His post-war screen persona was darker, as demonstrated in the film *Smash-Up,* but in 1945, his private life was bright. He married Mexican actress, Margo. They had two children and were happy together until her death forty years later. For six decades, until his ninetieth birthday, he worked as a character actor in movies, TV, and on stage. Eddie was nominated for Best Supporting Actor Oscars for *Roman Holiday* and *The Heartbreak Kid.* He died of pneumonia eleven months short of his 100th birthday at his home in Pacific Palisades, California.

Brother Rat (1938)
The Wagons Roll at Night (1941)
Out of the Fog (1941)
Strange Voyage (1946)
Rendezvous with Annie (1946)
Smash-Up (1947)
Meet Me after the Show (1951)
Carrie (1952)
Roman Holiday (1953)
Oklahoma! (1955)
I'll Cry Tomorrow (1955)
Attack! (1956)
The Sun Also Rises (1957)
The Heartbreak Kid (1972)
Dreamscape (1984)

Lola **Albright**
5ft 5in
(LOLA ALBRIGHT)

Born: **July 20, 1925**
Akron, Ohio, USA

Her parents were both valued members of the choir at the local Evangelical church. They passed their vocal talent on to Lola, who would entertain visitors to their home with cute renditions of popular songs. After World War II ended, Lola took a job as a part-time model for a department store. She then worked on the switchboard at an Akron radio station where her sexy voice was noted by a Hollywood talent scout who happened to be tuning in. When he saw Lola in the flesh he was completely bowled over and began sending her photo to the studios. His efforts led to small parts in big MGM musicals like *Easter Parade,* and *The Pirate.* In 1950, Lola had a featured role in the great boxing movie *Champion,* but during the 1950s her twenty films were mostly 'B' westerns. Lola was married to actor, Jack Carson, from 1952-58, but it didn't really help her career. After her divorce, things improved: her key role as nightclub singer Edie Hart, in the TV series *Peter Gunn* (produced by Blake Edwards and directed by Robert Altman) was nominated for an Emmy. She used her own voice for the Edie character – resulting in a couple of smoochy record albums including the sublime "Dreamsville"conducted by Henry Mancini. That proved to be a productive period for her – she not only replaced Dorothy Malone (albeit temporarily) in the popular television soap opera, 'Peyton Place', but in 1966 she won the "Best Actress" Silver Bear, at the Berlin Film Festival for her performance in the drama *Lord Love A Duck.* Her few later films were disappointing but she was a regular on TV during the 1970s. Lola retired from acting in 1984 and now lives quietly in California.

Champion (1949)
The Good Humor Man (1950)
The Tender Trap (1955)
A Cold Wind in August (1961)
Kid Galahad (1962)
Lord Love a Duck (1966)
The Way West (1967) **Where Were You When the Lights Went Out** (1968)

Alan **Alda**
6ft 2in
(ALFONSO JOSEPH D'ABRUZZO)

Born: **January 28, 1936**
New York City, New York, USA

Alan is the son of another movie actor, Robert Alda, and a former "Miss New York" beauty contest winner, Joan Brown. His early life was far from easy. At seven years of age he contracted polio during an epidemic and he was bedridden for over two years. He fully recovered – did really well at the Archbishop Stepinac High School, in White Plains – and eventually received a bachelor's degree from Fordham University. He started acting when he was in Europe during his junior year, but any thespian ambitions he may have had were put on hold when, on leaving University, he received his draft papers. Significantly, Alan served in Korea (after the war had ended) as a gunnery officer in the US Army Reserve. The experience influenced his portrayal of Hawkeye Pierce in the TV-series 'M*A*S*H'. After he left the Army he joined the 'Compass Players' comedy revue – mainly active in Chicago and St. Louis. He made his movie debut in the 1963 comedy *Gone Are the Days,* and his Broadway starring debut in 1966, in "The Apple Tree". He wrote the screenplay and starred in *The Seduction of Joe Tynan,* and played cameo roles in several Woody Allen films. Alan's still acting, writing and directing as he moves into his 70s. He has been nominated for an Emmy thirty-one times, and won a Best Supporting Actor Oscar for *The Aviator.* A devout Catholic, he has been married for more than forty years to author and photographer, Arlene Weiss. The couple live in Leonia, New Jersey.

California Suite (1978)
The Seduction of Joe Tynan (1979)
The Four Seasons (1981)
Crimes and Misdemeanors (1989)
Manhattan Murder Mystery (1993)
Everyone Says I Love You (1996)
Mad City (1997)
What Women Want (2000)
The Aviator (2004)
Resurrecting the Champ (2007)
Flash of Genius (2008)
Nothing But the Truth (2008)

Robert **Alda**
5ft 11in
(ALPHONSO GIUSEPPE G. R. S'ABRUZZO)

Born: February 26, 1914
New York City, New York, USA
Died: **May 3, 1986**

The son of Anthony and Frances D'Abruzzo, Robert showed early promise as an entertainer when he was a student at Stuyvesant High School. After graduating in 1930, he won a talent contest and began his career as a singer and dancer in vaudeville and then moved to a successful period in burlesque. In 1932, he married a former 'Miss New York', Joan Brown – four years later, their son Alan was born. Times were tough, and in the summer months, Robert kept his young family going by working in stock on the Catskills circuit in New York State. By the late 1930s, Robert was working on the radio and in 1937, he was one of the first performers to appear on TV. He was just starting a serious stage career when World War II spoilt his plans. When peace returned he'd established himself sufficiently to be chosen by Warner brothers to star as George Gershwin in *Rhapsody in Blue*. Why it didn't result in fully-fledged stardom is a mystery, because he went on to play leading roles in successful films like *Cloak and Dagger,* and *The Beast with Five Fingers.* In 1950, Robert, along with Stubby Kaye and Vivian Blaine, was in the original Broadway cast of "Guys and Dolls" and won the 1951 Tony as Best Actor. Although a Roman Catholic, he divorced Joan and married Flora Martino. Until his death from the effects of a stroke, in Los Angeles, Robert's later film work was mainly in Italy. He acted in American television productions until 1983.

Rhapsody in Blue (1945)
Cloak and Dagger (1946)
The Beast with Five Fingers (1946)
The Man I Love (1947)
Nora Prentiss (1947)
April Showers (1948)
Mr. Universe (1951)
Beautiful But Dangerous (1956)
Imitation of Life (1959)
Totò e Peppino divisi a
Berlino (1962)
The Serpent (1973)

Jane **Alexander**
5ft 6½in
(JANE QUIGLEY)

Born: October 28, 1939
Boston, Massachusetts, USA

Jane was born into a medical family. Her father Thomas Quigley was an orthopedic surgeon and her mother Ruth was a nurse. Jane discovered her love of acting during her time at Beaver Country Day School for Girls. She then attended the Sarah Lawrence college in New York where she concentrated on theater and mathematics – the latter with a computer career in mind. Jane then spent her junior year at Edinburgh University in Scotland where she was a member of the Dramatic Society. After splitting up from her first husband, Robert Alexander (whose name she kept) Jane concentrated on theater work – in 1967 she was in the original cast of "The Great White Hope" in Washington, D.C. She then met the producer/director Edwin Sherin, in Washington, and when they were both free in 1975, they married. Highly regarded in New York theater circles before making her first film at the age of thirty, Jane knocked on Oscar's door four times during her early years in Hollywood – she was nominated for *The Great White Hope, All The President's Men, Kramer vs Kramer* and *Testament.* For her brilliant stage and television work, Jane won a Tony *and* two Emmys – the first in 1981, for 'Playing for Time' and the second for the 2005 miniseries, 'Warm Springs'. Since the turn of the century, Jane has had several good supporting roles in movies. In their leisure time she and her husband are active in arts, wildlife and world peace organizations.

The Great White Hope (1970)
All The President's Men (1976)
Kramer vs Kramer (1979)
Brubaker (1980) Testament (1983)
Square Dance (1987)
The Cider House Rules (1999)
Sunshine State (2002)
The Ring (2002)
Fur: An Imaginary
Portrait of Diane Arbus (2006)
Feast of Love (2007)
Gigantic (2008)
The Unborn (2009)

Joan **Allen**
5ft 10in
(JOAN ALLEN)

Born: August 20, 1956
Rochelle, Illinois, USA

The youngest of four children, Joan's first early step towards her future profession was to take ballet lessons. She didn't do any acting until she starred in plays at Rochelle Township High School and was voted 'most likely to succeed'. She began the process of doing so during her time at Northern Illinois University where she got to know John Malkovich and helped him form the Steppenwolf Theater Company. Malkovich became a close friend and introduced her to the works of Harold Pinter, Edward Albee and Jean Ionesco. In 1983, he co-starred with her in the TV drama 'Say Goodnight, Gracie'. Joan's first movie (in a strong supporting role) was in *Compromising Positions,* a 1985 comedy/drama. On her Broadway debut in 1988, she won a Tony for her performance in "Burn This". She also starred in the Pulitzer Prize winning play "The Heidi Chronicles". Joan had been in a dozen movies before she received her first Oscar nomination, for playing Pat Nixon opposite Anthony Hopkins in the biopic *Nixon.* The other two were for *The Crucible* and *The Contender.* More recently, Joan has featured in the action-packed *Bourne* series. A model of consistency, she's highly-rated among her peers. She has a daughter, from a ten-year marriage to the actor Peter Friedman – which ended in 2002.

Manhunter (1986)
Peggy Sue Got Married (1986)
Ethan Frome (1993)
Searching for Bobby Fischer (1993)
Nixon (1995)
The Crucible (1996)
The Ice Storm (1997) Face/Off (1997)
Pleasantville (1998)
When the Sky Falls (2000)
The Contender (2000)
Off the Map (2003)
The Notebook (2004)
The Bourne Supremacy (2004)
Yes (2004) The Upside
of Anger (2005) Bonneville (2006)
The Bourne Ultimatum (2007)
Death Race (2008)

Karen **Allen**
5ft 7in
(KAREN JANE ALLEN)

Born: **October 5, 1951**
Carrolton, Illinois, USA

Because of her husband's work as an FBI agent, Karen's mother had to ferry her three daughters all around the United States. They settled in Washington D.C. when she was eleven and Karen went over the border, to DuVal High School in Glenn Dale, Maryland. After graduating in 1969, she enrolled at the Fashion Institute of Technology in New York, to study Art and Design. Following that, she wrote short stories, travelled all around South America and ran a boutique. In 1973, after a successful audition for a role in "Saint" she toured the UK. On her return, she joined the Washington Theater Laboratory before studying at the Lee Strasberg Institute. Karen's first film was the award-winning short *Whidjitmaker*, in 1976. Two years later she made her feature debut in *Animal House* and had a small part in Woody Allen's *Manhattan*. She achieved stardom and won a Saturn Award for Best Actress, in *Raiders of the Lost Ark*. The following year, Karen made her Broadway debut in "The Monday after the Miracle" and continued acting in films and on TV. In 1987, she married Kale Browne – who, three years later, acted with her in the TV drama 'Challenger'. They had a son, but divorced in 1997. Apart from acting, she created her own knitware brand and taught at Karen Allen Fibre Arts. In 2008, she made a return to the scene of one of her early films, in *Indiana Jones and the Kingdom of the Crystal Skull*.

Raiders of the Lost Ark (1981)
Shoot the Moon (1982)
Starman (1984)
The Glass Menagerie (1987)
Scrooged (1988)
Malcolm X (1992)
The Sandlot (1993)
King of the Hill (1993)
Wind River (1998)
The Perfect Storm (2000)
In the Bedroom (2001)
Poster Boy (2004) **Indiana Jones and the Kingdom of the Crystal Skull** (2008)

Woody **Allen**
5ft 5in
(ALLEN STEWART KONIGSBERG)

Born: **December 1, 1935**
Brooklyn, New York City, New York, USA

Woody went to a Hebrew school for eight years. By the age of nine he was already mesmerizing his classmates with magic tricks. At fifteen, at his high school in Brooklyn, he produced one-liners to spice up the work of local newspaper gossip columnists; at sixteen he was writing gags for Sid Caesar and three years later, was working on scripts for the *Ed Sullivan Show*. He studied communication and film at New York University, and developed his great admiration for the work of Ingmar Bergman. After that he began earning a living as a stand-up comedian in New York night clubs. In 1965, he was hired to write the screenplay and made his acting debut in *What's New Pussycat?* Four years later he made his directorial debut with *Take the Money and Run*. In 1969 his face was on the cover of *Life Magazine*. Apart from his screen credits, Woody is an excellent traditional jazz clarinetist who has toured Europe with his own band and often sits in at jam sessions in New York. Woody has won Oscars – for Best Screenplay and Best Director for *Annie Hall* and *Hannah and Her Sisters* and has been nominated for them on eighteen other occasions - in various categories – including Best Actor for *Annie Hall*. His genius is still burning brightly, as demonstrated by *Cassandra's Dream* and *Vicky Cristina Barcelona* – both of which he wrote and directed.

Take the Money and Run (1969)
Bananas (1971)
Play it Again Sam (1972)
Sleeper (1973)
Love and Death (1975)
The Front (1976) **Annie Hall** (1977)
Manhattan (1979) **Zelig** (1983)
The Purple Rose of Cairo (1985)
Hannah and her Sisters (1986)
Crimes and Misdemeanors (1989)
Husbands and Wives (1992)
Sweet and Lowdown (1999)
The Curse of the Jade Scorpion (2001)
Hollywood Ending (2002)
Anything Else (2003)
Scoop (2006)

June **Allyson**
5ft 1in
(ELEANOR GEISMAN)

Born: **October 17, 1917**
Lucerne, New York, USA
Died: **July 8, 2006**

June's alcoholic father, Robert Geisman, abandoned her and her mother, Clara, when she was only six year old. For the next couple of years, they lived close to poverty. Following a very serious accident when June was eight, doctors said she might be crippled for life – she spent four years confined within a steel brace. Luckily they were wrong. Swimming therapy got her fit and she developed a big passion for the nimble footwork of dancers Fred Astaire and Ginger Rogers. Immediately on leaving high school she took up dancing and got a chorus job in a Broadway show by Rogers and Hart, called "Sing Out the News". June's talent was recognized by Hollywood and she was used by Warners to perform speciality dance numbers in Vitaphone shorts, starting in 1937, with *Swing For Sale*. Her first full length movie *Best Foot Forward* – in 1943, impressed MGM enough to give her a speciality dance number in *Girl Crazy* – a vehicle for Mickey Rooney and Judy Garland – made that same year. She had to wait until 1947 before getting really *Good News*, after which, for ten years or so, she was a moviegoers' favorite – playing the sweet girl next door, or the sweet wife of successful men – in biopics such as *The Stratton Story* and *The Glenn Miller Story*. Her real-life successful man was the first of her four husbands – the singer/actor/director, Dick Powell. After he died in 1963, she struggled with alcoholism, but appeared on TV until retiring in 2001. June died at her home in Ojai, California, of respiratory failure and acute bronchitis.

Good News (1947)
The Three Musketeers (1948)
Words and Music (1948)
The Stratton Story (1949)
Too Young to Kiss (1951)
The Glenn Miller Story (1953)
Executive Suite (1954)
Woman's World (1954)
The Shrike (1955)
The McConnell Story (1955)

Mathieu **Amalric**
5ft 6in
(MATHIEU AMALRIC)

Born: **October 25, 1965**
Neuilly-sur-Seine, France

Mathieu's father, Jacques Amalric, was a journalist and editorialist who worked for the French newspapers "Le Monde" and "Libération". His mother, Nicole, who was born in Poland, was "Le Monde's" literary critic. After completing his school studies, Mathieu got a job as a trainee assistant director with a film production company. It gave him opportunities to direct his own short films, and although he prefers that to acting, he hasn't done too badly. He made his screen debut in 1984, with a small role in the successful movie, *Les Favoris de la lune,* and whilst he valued the experience, it didn't give him a burning desire to become a film star. In fact, he spent more than ten years behind the camera before he was offered an interesting role in *Le Journal du séducteur.* Mathieu was good enough to be nominated as Best Actor at the Acteurs à l'Écran festival. For the next few years, he had roles in films which were mainly seen in Art House theaters. He made his feature debut as a director, in 2001, with *Wimbledon Stage.* For acting, he's won three Césars – the last being for the highly acclaimed film, *Le Scaphandre et le papillon.* Mathieu has two children, but is separated from his wife.

Le Journal du séducteur (1996)
Genealogies of a Crime (1997)
Trois ponts sur la rivière (1999)
False Servant (2000)
L'Affaire Marcorelle (2000)
Roland's Pass (2000)
Boyhood Loves (2001)
A Real Man (2003)
Kings and Queen (2004)
The Moustache (2005)
Munich (2005)
Un lever de rideau (2006)
Michou d'Auber (2007)
Un secret (2007)
Le Scaphandre et le papillon (2007)
57,000 km entre nous (2008)
Un conte de Noël (2008)
La Guerre (2008)
Quantum of Solace (2008)

Don **Ameche**
5ft 11in
(DOMINIC FELIX AMICI)

Born: **May 31, 1908**
Kenosha, Wisconsin, USA
Died: **December 6, 1993**

Don was one of five children born to Felix Amici, an Italian immigrant, and his wife Barbara, who was of Irish/German origin. He left school at fifteen and had a spell in vaudeville early on. It was a disaster and he was sacked by his employer for being "too stiff." He was much more successful when he joined a Chicago radio station. After five years, he was well-known enough to transfer to Los Angeles, where as the master of ceremonies, he presented guest stars like Nelson Eddy, Dorothy Lamour and ventriloquist Edgar Bergen – with Charlie McCarthy. Hollywood studios beckoned, and following his debut (in a dual role) in 1936's *The Sins of Man* he was cast as a romantic lead in a dozen or so films. After playing Alexander Graham Bell, his name was used for some time, in a U.S. slang expression – an "Ameche" – meaning a telephone. By that time, he'd firmly established himself as a charming, amusing leading man. Films like *Heaven Can Wait* ensured his popularity throughout the war years but from the 1950s onwards, he was seen mostly on TV. In the 1980s he made a welcome film comeback and picked up a deserved Oscar for his work in the comedy hit *Cocoon.* For more than fifty years, Don was married to a nice supportive lady, Honore Prendergast. They had six children together. He worked up until the year he died – in Scottsdale, Arizona, of prostate cancer.

One in a Million (1936)
In Old Chicago (1938)
Happy Landing (1938)
Alexander's Ragtime Band (1938)
Midnight (1939)
The Story of Alexander Graham Bell (1939) **Swanee River** (1939)
Down Argentine Way (1940)
Moon Over Miami (1941)
Heaven Can Wait (1943)
Wing and a Prayer (1944)
Slightly French (1949)
Trading Places (1983)
Cocoon (1985)

Leon **Ames**
5ft 8in
(LEON WAYCOFF)

Born: **January 20, 1902**
Portland, Indiana, USA
Died: **October 12, 1993**

Leon's parents were Russian immigrants. He decided to become an actor after watching theatrical performances when he was at high school. He learned to act by going on tour with a troupe of players and eventually joined a theater company in Cincinnati, Ohio. He then went to New York, where he worked in a shoe store while gaining experience with stock companies. In 1931, he made his film debut – playing a small role of a hood in the crime drama, *Quick Millions.* His Broadway debut, was in 1933, in "It Pays to Sin". He was third-billed below Sidney Fox and Bela Lugosi, in *Murders in the Rue Morgue* – which began a busy film career for him. He kept his birth name, Waycoff all through around thirty mostly forgettable pictures. He became Leon Ames in 1936 when firmly established as a character actor. He could afford to get married, and in 1938 he did, to Christine Gossett, with whom he had two children. The quality of his films remained very mixed, until he got the plum role of Alonzo Smith, in Judy Garland's classic *Meet Me in St. Louis.* It started a run of movies for MGM which was Leon's best period. From 1957-1958, he was President of the SAG. He died at Laguna Beach following a stroke.

Charlie Chan on Broadway (1937)
Suez (1938) **Mysterious Mr. Moto** (1938)
Mr. Moto in Danger Island (1939)
Crime Doctor (1943)
Thirty Seconds Over Tokyo (1944)
Meet Me in St. Louis (1944)
The Thin Man Goes Home (1944)
Son of Lassie (1945)
Anchors Aweigh (1945)
Weekend at the Waldorf (1945)
They Were Expendable (1945) **The Postman Always Rings Twice** (1946)
Lady in the Lake (1947) **A Date with Judy** (1948) **Little Women** (1949)
On Moonlight Bay (1951)
Angel Face (1952) **By the Light of the Silvery Moon** (1953)
Peyton Place (1957)

Gillian **Anderson**
5ft 3in
(GILLIAN LEIGH ANDERSON)

Born: August 9, 1968
Chicago, Illinois, USA

Soon after she was born, Gillian's mother, Rosemary, a computer analyst, moved her young family to Puerto Rico. By the time Gillian was nearly two, her father Edward Anderson, had taken the decision to go to England so he could attend the London Film School. Gillian was sent to Fortismere School in Crouch End and later attended a school in Harringay. Ten years later her dad set up his own film post-production company in the United States. Gillian was eleven when the Andersons moved to Grand Rapids, Michigan. She attended the local Fountain Elementary School and then the City High-Middle School, which ran a program with an emphasis on the humanities. As a teenager, she was a little way out. To deflect attention away from the London accent which embarrassed her, she had her nose pierced and would frequently change the color of her hair. At school she was voted "Most Likely to be Arrested". This awkwardness was better channeled when she acted in a school production of "Arsenic and Old Lace". She was soon appearing in plays at the Grand Rapids Community Theater – another step closer to an acting career. In 1990, she received a Bachelor of Fine Arts from the Goodman School of Drama in Chicago. Gillian made her pro stage debut that year in "Absent Friends" at the Manhattan Theater Club. In 1992, she made her film debut in *The Turning*. After moving to Los Angeles she acted reluctantly in television dramas, but they led to the role of Dana Scully in 'The X-Files', and a Golden Globe in 1997. Since then, the twice-married Gillian has appeared in high-profile movies including *The Last King of Scotland*.

The X Files (1998)
Playing by Heart (1998)
The House of Mirth (2000)
The Mighty Celt (2005)
A Cock and Bull Story (2005)
The Last King of Scotland (2006)
Straightheads (2007)
How to lose Friends &
Alienate People (2008)

Dame Judith **Anderson**
5ft 6in
(FRANCES MARGARET ANDERSON)

Born: February 10, 1897
Adelaide, South Australia, Australia
Died: January 3, 1992

The daughter of James and Jessie Anderson, Judith was educated at Norwood High School in Adelaide. She made her stage debut at seventeen (as Francee Anderson), in the play "A Royal Divorce" in Sidney. American actors in the cast saw her potential, and persuaded her to try her luck in the USA. She had no success in California – her Australian accent was still strong, so she went to New York. In 1922, after three tough years of attending casting sessions and touring with stock companies, she appeared on Broadway. The following year with her name changed to Judith, she co-starred with Louis Calhern in the hit play "Cobra". By the early 1930s she'd established herself as a great classical actress, and was regularly in plays starring notables like Lilian Gish, John Barrymore – and even Humphrey Bogart. Judith's looks were hardly those of a movie star, so the few parts she got were character roles. Following her debut in 1933's *Blood Money*, she had to wait eight years for her next opportunity - which she grabbed with both hands. The sinister Mrs Danvers, in *Rebecca* – for which she was nominated for a Best Supporting Actress Oscar – is one of the most memorable characters in movie history. Judith was made a British Dame in 1959. Her relatively few film roles were usually special – as a viewing of any of those listed here will prove. Her last role was in an episode of TV's 'Santa Barbara' in 1987. She died of pneumonia.

Rebecca (1940)
Free and Easy (1941)
King's Row (1942)
Edge of Darkness (1943)
Laura (1944)
And Then There Were None (1945)
The Diary of a Chamber Maid (1946)
Specter of the Rose (1946)
Pursued (1947)
The Red House (1947)
The Ten Commandments (1956)
Cat on a Hot Tin Roof (1958)

Bibi **Andersson**
5ft 5¼in
(BERIT ELISABETH ANDERSSON)

Born: November 11, 1935
Kungsholmen, Stockholm, Sweden

Bibi looked up to her older sister, Gerda, who became a ballet dancer at the Royal Opera and appeared in Ingmar Bergman's *Summer Interlude* and *Waiting Women*. It inspired her to study hard at Stockholm's Royal Dramatic Theater School, and she became a member of the Royal Dramatic Theater. In 1951, she acted in a detergent commercial shot by Ingmar Bergman and would go on to appear in thirteen of his works. At eighteen years old, after three uncredited film roles, she made her first official appearance in a dull Nils Poppe comedy called *Dum-Bom*. She had an affair with Bergman and joined him at the Malmö theater, where she acted in a Strindberg play he was directing. This led to a very small part in his film, *Smiles of a Summer Night*. By 1957, Bibi had not only become a star in Sweden, she was well known as one of Bergman's regular players. She had opportunities abroad – her most successful efforts being the western film *Duel at Diablo;* the critically acclaimed Danish production *Babette's Feast;* and the American drama *I Never Promised You a Rose Garden*. In 1996 she published her autobiography, "A Blink of the Eye". Apart from regular TV and stage work during the past twenty years, she's made appearances in good films like *As if I Didn't Exist*. Since May 2004, Bibi's been married to her third husband, Gabriel Mora Baeza.

The Seventh Seal (1957)
Wild Strawberries (1957)
So Close to Life (1958)
The Face (1958)
The Devil's Eye (1960)
Now About These Women (1964)
Duel at Diablo (1966) **Persona** (1966)
The Girls (1968)
A Passion (1969)
The Kremlin Letter (1970)
Scenes from a Marriage (1973)
I Never Promised
You a Rose Garden (1977)
Babette's Feast (1987)
As if I Didn't Exist (2002)
When Darkness Falls (2006)

Harriet **Andersson**
5ft 4½in
(HARRIET ANDERSSON)

Born: **January 14, 1932**
Stockholm, Sweden

Having watched her parents struggle to make ends meet during the worldwide Great Depression, by the time she was fourteen, Harriet had a burning desire to succeed in the competitive, but highly-paid world of show business. She first trained as a dancer, and when she left school, she sought to use those skills to make a living in the entertainment industry, beginning with the Stockholm music hall. To make contacts she worked as an elevator attendant in the Malmö Stadsteater. One fine day, who should walk in but Ingmar Bergman! They had a short and sweet affair and through his influence she managed to land a series of bit parts in films. In 1952, Harriet took a giant career step forward with a sensational role in *Summer with Monika* – written for her by Bergman. It was the first of eight she made for him. Like Bibi Andersson (who is no relation) Harriet has had a rather brief international career and her best movie work is essentially Swedish. In the 1960s, she was living with Finnish director Jörn Donner. It was Harriet's starring role in his film *To Love,* which won her the Best Actress award (the Volpi Cup) at the 1964 Venice Film Festival. In 1975, Harriet won the Best Actress Award for *The White Wall.* As with many stars, the roles started to dry up, but her fifty-five year career must be applauded by lovers of Swedish movies. Harriet was still acting in 2007.

Summer With Monika (1952)
Sawdust and Tinsel (1953)
A Lesson in Love (1954)
Journey into Autumn (1955)
Smiles of a Summer's Night (1955)
Through A Glass Darkly (1961)
To Love (1964)
Loving Couples (1964)
Now About These Women (1964)
The Deadly Affair (1966)
Cries and Whispers (1972)
The White Wall (1975)
Fanny and Alexander (1982)
Beyond the Sky (1993)
Dogville (2003)

Ursula **Andress**
5ft 5in
(URSULA ANDRESS)

Born: **March 19, 1936**
Berne, Switzerland

Ursula's father was a German diplomat who married a Swiss woman. He fathered five daughters and a son, before going missing without trace during World War II. Fluent in four languages, Ursula was able to enjoy life all around Europe in her teens after running away with a young Italian actor. When working as a model in a Rome art college she was spotted by scouts from Cinecittà Studios, outside the city, and made her first film, *Sins of Casanova,* in 1954. Three years later, she met and married American actor, John Derek, and for a while, settled down to domestic life with him. Ursula had become one of the most famous movie icons of all time with her memorable appearance as Honey Ryder in the very first James Bond movie, *Dr. No.* A subsequent role in the 1967 Bond spoof, *Casino Royale,* wasn't successful. She co-starred with Elvis Presley in *Fun in Acapulco,* but after that, she had few opportunities to break away from the stereotype. In her private life, things weren't working. John Derek took pictures of her for Playboy in 1965, but they divorced in 1966, following her well-publicized affair with French heart-throb, Jean-Paul Belmondo. Her last big role was in the 1981 film *Clash of the Titans,* when she not only had an opportunity to work with Sir Laurence Olivier, but she had her only child (a son) with her co-star in the movie, Harry Hamlin. Since then, she's worked on European TV and in the occasional film. She remained good friends with John Derek until his death in 1998.

Dr. No (1962)
Fun in Acapulco (1963)
4 for Texas (1963) **Nightmare in the Sun** (1965) **She** (1965)
What's New Pussycat (1965)
Up to His Ears (1965)
The 10th Victim (1965)
The Blue Max (1966)
Perfect Friday (1970)
Clash of the Titans (1981)
Cremaster 5 (1997)
The Bird Preachers (2005)

Dana **Andrews**
5ft 10in
(CARVER DANA ANDREWS)

Born: **January 1, 1909**
Collins, Mississippi, USA
Died: **December 17, 1992**

The third of thirteen children – the last of whom became actor, Steve Forrest, Dana was born on a farm on the outskirts of Collins, where his father, the Rev. Charles Andrews, preached as a Baptist minister. After World War I, the family moved to Huntsville, Texas. He later studied business administration in Houston. Dana was an accountant for Gulf & Western until he became unemployed during the Great Depression. In the hope of making a career out of his good singing voice, he hitch-hiked to California in 1931. To pay for his singing lessons and drama studies at the Pasadena Community Playhouse, Dana dug ditches, picked oranges, and pumped gas . He was eventually offered a contract by Sam Goldwyn and made his debut in *The Westerner* in 1940. Declared unfit for war service, he suffered at the box-office. Then, because so many actors were away, he got the chance to star in some great movies – *The Ox-Bow Incident, Laura* and *A Walk in the Sun* are prime examples. They were matched by *The Best Years of Our Lives,* but during the mid-1950s his career stalled and he turned to drink. After *Night of the Demon,* things got worse. He was nearly killed on the highway and had to quit. In 1972, he made a TV film for Alcoholics Anonymous. He appeared in supporting roles until retiring in 1985 to live with his wife Mary. In his final years Dana suffered from Alzheimer's Disease. He died at his home in Los Alimitos, California, of pneumonia.

The Ox-Bow Incident (1943)
The North Star (1943) **Up In Arms** (1944)
The Purple Heart (1944)
A Wing and a Prayer (1944)
Laura (1944) **Fallen Angel** (1945)
A Walk in the Sun (1945)
Canyon Passage (1946)
The Best Years of Our Lives (1946)
Daisy Kenyon (1947)
Boomerang (1947)
Night of the Demon (1957)
In Harm's Way (1965)

Edward **Andrews**
5ft 10in
(EDWARD ANDREWS)

Born: **October 9, 1914**
Griffin, Georgia, USA
Died: **March 8, 1985**

Ed was the son of a busy Episcopalian minister, whose various postings took his family to Pittsburgh, Cleveland and finally, Wheeling, in West Virginia. In Pittsburgh, young Ed witnessed first-hand the magic of acting, when he attended plays at the Nixon Theater. At the age of twelve, he had his first taste of the stage with a walk-on part in a stock company production, starring James Gleason. After high school, he spent three years at the University of Virginia in Charlottesville. Ed graduated, then joined a stock company. For a while he was exclusively a stage actor – making his first Broadway appearance in 1935, in "How Beautiful With Shoes". Three years later, he acted in the Pulitzer Prize-winning play, "The Time of Your Life". After making his film debut in 1936, in *Rushin' Art* – as Ed Andrews, he didn't try the medium again for nearly twenty years. Following a few TV appearances, he was cast in the film-noir drama, *The Phenix City Story*. In his early forties, he became famous – as Edward Andrews – acting in films with Bogart, Cagney and Esther Williams and appearing in TV shows such as 'Sergeant Bilko', 'Studio One' and 'The US Steel Hour'. Ed completed his last film, *Gremlins* – before dying of a heart attack, at his home in Santa Monica, California.

The Phenix City Story (1955)
The Harder They Fall (1956)
These Wilder Years (1956)
Tea and Sympathy (1956)
Tension at Table Rock (1956)
The Unguarded Moment (1956)
Three Brave Men (1956)
Hot Summer Night (1957)
The Tattered Dress (1957)
Trooper Hook (1957) Elmer Gantry (1960)
The Absent Minded Professor (1961)
The Young Savages (1961)
Advise & Consent (1962)
The Thrill of It All (1963)
Send Me No Flowers (1964)
Tora! Tora! Tora (1970) Avanti! (1972)
Sixteen Candles (1984) Gremlins (1984)

Harry **Andrews**
5ft 10in
(HARRY FLEETWOOD ANDREWS)

Born: **November 10, 1911**
Tonbridge, Kent, England
Died: **March 6, 1989**

The youngest of five children and son of a doctor, Harry was educated at Wrekin College, in Shropshire. He had intended to work for the police, but after a friend had introduced him to the Liverpool Repertory Company, he began a stage career as a Shakespearean actor in 1933. It was interrupted by the outbreak of World War II, during which he served as a 2nd Lieutenant with the London Scottish Regiment. Although he returned to the stage in 1946, his army experience provided him with the ideas for many of his future film roles. On his film debut, in *The Red Beret,* in 1953, he plays a regimental sergeant major! In the 1960s, he did it again – as R.S.M. Wilson in *The Hill.* For over a quarter of a century, Harry was a very popular featured character actor in a host of big movies – 1978 was his last big year - he appeared in both *Death on the Nile* and *Superman.* He was bi-sexual and had a long-term relationship with the actor Basil Hoskins. Harry died at his home in Salehurst, Sussex, from a viral infection complicated by asthma.

Moby Dick (1956)
A Hill in Korea (1956)
I Accuse! (1958)
Ice-Cold in Alex (1958)
The Devil's Disciple (1959)
A Touch of Larceny (1959)
A Circle of Deception (1960)
Reach for Glory (1962)
The Best of Enemies (1962)
Nine Hours to Rama (1963)
55 Days at Peking (1963)
The Informers (1963)
The Truth About Spring (1964)
Nothing But the Best (1964)
The Hill (1965)
Sands of the Kalahari (1965)
I'll Never Forget What'isname (1967)
The Seagull (1968)
The Charge of the Light Brigade (1968)
The Ruling Class (1972)
Death on the Nile (1978)
Superman (1978)

Dame Julie **Andrews**
5ft 8in
(JULIA ELIZABETH WELLS)

Born: **October 1, 1935**
Walton-on-Thames, Surrey, England

Julie's father, Edward Wells, was a teacher, and her mother, Barbara was a pianist who loved show business. She divorced the first 'Ted' while Julie was still very young and in 1939, she married Ted Andrews, with whom she had started working in a show called "The Dazzle Company". Before that she sent Julie to dancing classes and watched her perform at the age of three in "Winken, Blinken and Nod". Julie's step-father was aware of the little girl's talent and paid for her to take voice lessons at the Cone-Ripman School and privately with Madame Stiles-Allen. Julie made her professional debut at ten years of age in the musical "Starlight Roof" at the London Hippodrome. A year later, she became the youngest artist to appear in a Royal Command Performance at the London Palladium. For the next seven years, she worked on radio shows and in West End musicals. Julie made her Broadway debut in 1954, in the London hit, "The Boy Friend". Two years later, she became a star name in "My Fair Lady". In 1957, she co-starred with Vic Damone in Richard Rogers and Oscar Hammerstein's television musical, 'Cinderella'. Ignoring Julie's fine Eliza Doolittle (and her great voice) for the film *My Fair Lady* – in 1964, Jack Warner opted for the guaranteed box-office appeal of Audrey Hepburn. Julie won a Best Actress Oscar for *Mary Poppins,* and was nominated for *The Sound of Music* and *Victor/Victoria*. In 1969, she married Blake Edwards. After botched throat surgery in 1998, she is unlikely to sing again, but she has starred in *The Princess Diaries* and is due to star in a comic/fantasy called *Tooth Fairy.*

Mary Poppins (1964)
The Americanization of Emily (1964)
The Sound of Music (1965)
Thoroughly Modern Millie (1967)
10 (1979) S.O.B. (1981)
Victor/Victoria (1982)
Duet for One (1986)
Relative Values (2000)
The Princess Diaries (2001)

Heather **Angel**

5ft 2in

(HEATHER GRACE ANGEL)

Born: **Febuary 9, 1909**
Oxford, Oxfordshire, England
Died: **December 13, 1986**

Daughter of an Oxford don, Heather grew up on the family farm before going to boarding school. She began her stage career at the Old Vic in London – acting in a number of Shakespeare plays before turning her attention to the movies. At that point in time with the advent of the talkies, actors with trained voices were much in demand. Heather's film debut was in *City of Song* in 1931, but it was the Hollywood film *Berkeley Square,* with Leslie Howard, which made her a star. It was followed by *Mystery of Edwin Drood,* and a key role opposite the film's Oscar winner, Victor McLaglen, in *The Informer.* She was in five of the *Bulldog Drummond* series, from 1937 to 1939, but by then she was beginning to be pushed into B-pictures. Her confidence was still sufficient for her to be screen-tested for the part of Melanie, in *Gone with the Wind,* which she lost to Olivia de Havilland. From the late thirties she played supporting roles in some good movies including *Pride and Prejudice.* She was rarely seen on the screen after 1950, but provided voices for two Walt Disney animated classics – *Alice in Wonderland* and *Peter Pan.* Heather did a fair amount of television work which included the soap opera 'Peyton Place'. Her last movie was *Gone with the West,* in 1975. She made her final appearance on the small screen – as Harry Truman's mother-in-law, in the 1979 TV mini-series, 'Backstairs at the White House'. That year, Heather retired to Santa Barbara, and died there of cancer.

Berkeley Square (1933)
Mystery of Edwin Drood (1935)
The Informer (1935)
The Perfect Gentleman (1935)
The Three Musketeers (1935)
The Last of the Mohicans (1936)
Pride and Prejudice (1940)
That Hamilton Woman (1941)
Suspicion (1941)
Cry Havoc (1943)
Lifeboat (1944)
Premature Burial (1962)

Pier **Angeli**

5ft 1in

(ANNA MARIA PIERANGELI)

Born: **June 19, 1932**
Cagliari, Sardinia, Italy
Died: **September 10, 1971**

Pier's family moved up to Rome when she was in her early teens. After completing secondary school, she went to art college. Her delicate beauty was something to inspire any would-be painter, but it was appreciated by somebody involved in another art form. She was 'discovered' by the Russian-born film director, Léonide Moguy, who was a friend of her family. Although she had no previous acting experience, Moguy cast her as Mirella in his beautiful film, *Domani é Troppo Tardi* (Tomorrow Is Too Late), which starred Vittorio de Sica. Pier was impressive and her name was duly noted by MGM in Hollywood. When she was just nineteen, she went there to be directed by Fred Zinnemann in *Teresa,* a film about a World War II veteran bringing his young Italian bride to live in the United States. From then on, she was tried in historical and modern settings, but her screen persona never developed the range to make her a big star. Her best work was in the boxing drama, *Somebody Up There Likes Me* as the loving wife of Paul Newman. She had once been engaged to Kirk Douglas, but after a doomed love for James Dean she married the Italian-American singer, Vic Damone, following strong urging from her mother. The couple had a son and Damone recorded a lovely album called "Angela Mia", dedicated to Pier. But she never forgot her big love and was divorced in 1959. The following year, she came to Britain to make her last good film – *The Angry Silence.* In 1962, she began a seven-year marriage to the Italian composer, Armando Trovajoli, with whom she had a son. Nearing forty, and depressed, she committed suicide – she said she was unable to face the idea of growing old.

Tomorrow is Too Late (1950)
Teresa (1951) **The Light Touch** (1951)
The Story of Three Loves (1953)
Mam'zelle Nitouche (1953)
Somebody Up There Likes Me (1956)
The Angry Silence (1960)

Jennifer **Aniston**

5ft 4in

(JENNIFER ANISTON)

Born: **February 11, 1969**
Sherman Oaks, California, USA

The daughter of a Greek-American actor, John Aniston, and actress, Nancy Dow, Jennifer spent a year of her childhood in Greece. Her godfather was her dad's best friend, Telly Savalas. The family relocated to New York where her dad appeared in television soaps – as well as 'Kojak'. Her parents sent her to the Rudolf Steiner School, where she began to develop her creative thinking and love of the arts. After Jennifer graduated from the High School of Performing Arts, in New York, she appeared in off-Broadway shows such as "For Dear Life" and "Dancing on Checker's Grave". Between shows, she supported herself in tele-sales and was for a short time, a bike messenger. She moved to Los Angeles in 1989 and in 1990, got her first television role, in a comedy, 'Camp Cucamonga'. She followed it with nine episodes of 'Ferris Bueller'. After that, progress was painfully slow and she was seriously disillusioned when, three years later, after some unsuccessful television shows, she made her film debut in the rather poor horror movie, *Leprechaun.* Luckily, she didn't give up. From 1994, buoyed by the role of Rachel in the long-running 'Friends', she was in a stronger position to choose movie roles. Jennifer's good run began with the comedy, *Dream for an Insomniac* and progressed to the even better, *The Good Girl.* From 2000-2005, Jennifer was Mrs. Brad Pitt. She overcame that sad ending with films like *The Break-Up,* and we are now beginning to see the best of her as a movie actress.

Dream for an Insomniac (1996)
She's the One (1996)
The Object of My Affection (1998)
Office Space (1999) **Rock Star** (2001)
The Good Girl (2002)
Bruce Almighty (2003) **Derailed** (2005)
Rumor Has It... (2005)
Friends With Money (2006)
The Break-Up (2006)
Management (2008)
Marley & Me (2008)
He's Just Not That Into You (2008)

Annabella
5ft 3in
(SUZANNE GEORGETTE CHARPENTIER)

Born: **July 14, 1909**
La Varenne St. Hilaire, Val-de-Marne, France
Died: **September 18, 1996**

Annabella was married before she was twenty. She had a baby daughter named Anne, who would later become the wife of the actor, Oscar Werner. Her ambition for a film career resulted in her divorce and then a second marriage to the actor Jean Murat, who was more than twenty years her senior. She had made her film debut in 1927, in the silent classic *Napoléon.* By the mid-thirties she was a popular and well-established star in France. She won the Best Actress Award at the Venice Film Festival in 1935, for *Veille d'armes,* and was a favorite of the director, René Clair. Murat's career was on the wane at that time, and they began to drift apart. In 1937 her performance in the British film *Wings of the Morning,* was admired by the Hollywood actor, Tyrone Power, who insisted on her for the film *Suez,* in which he was set to star. Following her divorce from Murat, Power married her a year later in the garden of Charles Boyer's home. Don Ameche was Best Man. Studio boss Darryl F. Zanuck did not approve of the marriage and even though Annabella had a contract with 20th Century Fox, he starved her of movie roles. Power did absolutely nothing to influence the situation – their years as a married couple did her surprisingly few favors in Hollywood. This put a strain on the marriage and after they divorced in 1949, Annabella returned to France. She acted on the stage and made her final film, *Bonaparte et la révolution.* After that, she lived in retirement at Neuilly-sur-Seine, outside Paris – where she died of a heart attack.

Le Million (1931)
Paris Méditerranée (1932)
Gardez le sourire (1933)
Variétés (1934) La Bandera (1934)
Veille d'armes (1935)
Hôtel du nord (1937)
Wings of the Morning (1937)
Suez (1938)
13 Rue Madeleine (1946)
Bonarparte et la révolution (1971)

Francesca **Annis**
5ft 4in
(FRANCESCA ANNIS)

Born: **May 14, 1944**
London, England

The daughter of an English actor, father and a Brazilian/French actress, mother, Mariquita Annis, Francesca spent her first seven years in Brazil, where her parents ran a nightclub on Copacabana beach. On her return to London, speaking fluent Portuguese, Francesca soon settled down in the English way of life. She received her education at a Roman Catholic convent school and even contemplated becoming a nun! Although she enjoyed ballet, she studied drama at the Corona Academy Stage School at Turnham Green, in West London. In 1958 she made her screen debut in a children's film titled *The Cat Gang.* When she was eighteen, Francesca was cast as one of Elizabeth Taylor's handmaidens in *Cleopatra.* She was most certainly a swinging 'sixties girl, but her stardom didn't happen overnight. In 1970 she had a strong supporting role in the critically acclaimed *The Walking Stick.* She was sensational a year later, in Roman Polanski's *Macbeth* – beautifully acted and fondly remembered for her nude sleep-walking during the soliloquy. A year earlier, Polanski's wife, Sharon Tate had been murdered by Charles Manson, but he impressed Francesca with his strength and calm demeanor. Her co-star in the film, Jon Finch, was her lover and regular companion until she began a relationship with the photographer, Patrick Wiseman and had his three children. That ended when, in 1994 she acted in "Hamlet" with Ralph Fiennes and lived with him for eleven years. Francesca celebrated half-a-century in films during 2008 – when she had a good role in the thriller, *Shifty.*

Cleopatra (1963)
Murder Most Foul (1964)
The Walking Stick (1970)
The Tragedy of Macbeth (1971)
Dune (1984)
El Río de oro (1986)
The Debt Collector (1999)
Milk (1999) Onegin (1999)
The Libertine (2004)
Revolver (2005) Shifty (2008)

Ann-Margret
5ft 5in
(ANN-MARGRET OLSSON)

Born: **April 28, 1941**
Valsjöbyn, Jämtlands län, Sweden

How do you move from a tiny village in Sweden called Valsjöbyn, to become a big star in Hollywood? Ann-Margret knows the answer. She was taken to Valsjöbyn from Stockholm as a six-month-old baby. Shortly after that, her father left to work in the United States. When World War II was over, she and her mother joined him in Fox Lake, Illinois. Ann-Margret learned English and when she was eight she took dancing lessons. She was a cheerleader at fourteen and in 1957, won talent contests. In 1960, after being discovered by George Burns when she was in a campus musical at Northwestern University, she was given a job in his show at the Dunes Lounge, in Las Vegas. She made a few recordings for RCA – an LP called *Beauty and the Beard* with trumpeter Al Hirt, did rather well. After appearing on the Jack Benny Show, she met Frank Capra, who provided her with her first movie role. After starring with Elvis Presley in *Viva Las Vegas,* she had an affair with him and remained his friend until his death. There is little doubt that in an earlier era, Ann-Margret would have been a big star in musicals. Not only was she drop-dead gorgeous, but when she was given the opportunity, she proved she could act as well – she was twice Oscar-nominated – for *Carnal Knowledge* and *Tommy.* Since 1967, she's been married to the actor, Roger Smith, and is still acting on a regular basis.

Pocketful of Miracles (1961)
Bye Bye Birdie (1963)
Viva Las Vegas (1964)
The Cincinnati Kid (1965)
Carnal Knowledge (1971)
The Train Robbers (1973)
Tommy (1975) Magic (1978)
Twice in a Lifetime (1985)
52 Pick-Up (1986)
Grumpy Old Men (1993)
Any Given Sunday (1999)
Interstate 60 (2002)
Memory (2006)
The Loss of a
Teardrop Diamond (2008)

Susan **Anspach**
5ft 4in
(SUSAN ANSPACH)

Born: **November 23, 1942**
New York City, New York, USA

Susan was raised in the Queen's district of New York, where a neighbor of hers was the singer/songwriter, Paul Simon. Susan graduated from William Cullen Bryant High School, in Long Island City, then studied at the Actors' Studio, where she appeared on the same stage as Al Pacino. Susan began her career in Broadway and off-Broadway shows, including a spell as the female lead in the rock-musical "Hair". In 1965, she had a featured role with Robert Duvall, Jon Voight and Dustin Hoffman in "A View From the Bridge". That same year, she made her first television appearances starting in an episode of 'The Defenders'. In 1970, Susan made her film debut in *The Landlord,* which marked Hal Ashby's directorial debut. It was quickly followed by the important supporting role of Catherine, in one of Jack Nicholson's early classics, *Five Easy Pieces.* She and Jack became an item and they had a son called Caleb. After his one and only attempt at marriage had failed, Jack said goodbye and she married the actor Mark Goddard. The future looked bright for her – she was even described by Vincent Canby, in the 'New York Times' as "one of the most charming and talented actresses in America". Despite this highly promising start to Susan's career, by the end of the 1970s she was finding it difficult to get good film roles. Frustratingly for her fans, her performance in *Montenegro* was truly outstanding, but there was little in the way of follow-up. In 1996, Susan was giving acting lessons to the animation artists at Dreamworks, to prepare for the studio's feature, *The Prince of Egypt.* She will be seen again on film as the star of the 2008 drama, *American Primitive.*

The Landlord (1970)
Five Easy Pieces (1970)
Play It Again Sam (1972)
Blume in Love (1973)
The Big Fix (1978) **Running** (1979)
Montenegro (1981)
Misunderstood (1984)
Alien X Factor (1997)

Anne **Archer**
5ft 7in
(ANNE ARCHER)

Born: **August 24, 1947**
Los Angeles, California, USA

Anne was born into a well-known show business family – her parents were John Archer (who appeared in over sixty films from the late 1930s until the 1970s) and Marjorie Lord, who did lots of stage and television work in the same period. After leaving college, Anne herself worked on television and in the theater. She made her debut on the small screen in 1970 – in an episode of 'Storefront Lawyers'. Her first film appearance was in *The Honkers,* in 1972 – she was fourth-billed below James Coburn. There was a supporting role in a weak Bob Hope comedy, *Cancel My Reservation* – which did nothing to enhance her film career. Apart from *Lifeguard,* not much happened for her on the movie front for ten years. After reaching the short-list for the Lois Lane part in *Superman* (and losing out to Margot Kidder) she had to wait a while for her breakthrough, which came in 1987, with *Fatal Attraction.* Anne's performance was nominated for a Best Supporting Actress Oscar, a BAFTA, and a Golden Globe. In 1991 she caused controversy when she came out with the story of her abortion. Since *Mojave Moon,* her best roles have been in the exciting action film, *Rules of Engagement,* and a fine comedy/drama, *Uncle Nino.* In 2001, Anne got good reviews when she played Mrs. Robinson in "The Graduate" on the London West End stage. She keeps busy acting on television and her many fans are looking forward to her new film, *Felon.* In 2009, Anne will be celebrating her 30th wedding anniversary with her husband, Terry Jastrow.

Lifeguard (1976)
Fatal Attraction (1987)
Narrow Margin (1990)
Patriot Games (1992)
Short Cuts (1993)
Clear and Present Danger (1994)
Mojave Moon (1996)
Rules of Engagement (2000)
Uncle Nino (2003)
November (2004)
Felon (2008)

Fanny **Ardant**
5ft 8½in
(FANNY MARGUERITE JUDITH ARDANT)

Born: **March 22, 1949**
Saumur, Maine-et-Loire, France

Fanny's father was a cavalry officer in the French army. When she was little, he moved his family to Monaco where he was adviser to Prince Rainier's personal guard. They got to know the family including the former film star Princess Grace (Kelly). She moved to Aix-en-Provence when she was seventeen and studied political science. Her interest turned to acting, so she took drama lessons from Jean Périmony. She made her stage debut in 1974 in a play entitled "Corneille's Polyeucte". Her first film was *Marie-poupée* in 1976. Her work in a popular television series, 'Les dames de la côte' brought her wider recognition and was admired by François Truffaut who following her supporting role in Claude Lelouch's *Les Uns et les autres,* gave her the lead in the appropriately named *La Femme de côté* – co-starring Gérard Depardieu. Fanny's performance not only resulted in her first César nomination but international acclaim as well. She then became Truffaut's partner and in 1982, they became the proud parents of a baby daughter. Their relationship brought out the best in her – resulting in a Best Actress Silver Ribbon for *La Famiglia,* a César for *Pédale douce* and a shared Silver Bear for *8 femmes* – with 7 other women. Fluent in Italian and Spanish, Fanny is one of Europe's most admired actresses.

Les Uns et les autres (1981)
La Femme de côté (1981)
Vivement dimanche (1983)
L'été prochain (1985) **Mélo** (1986)
La Famiglia (1987)
Afraid of the Dark (1991)
Le Colonel Chabert (1994)
**Les Cent et une nuits de
Simon Cinéma** (1995)
Pédale douce (1996)
Ridicule (1996) **Elizabeth** (1998)
La Débandade (1999) **Le Libertin** (2000)
8 femmes (2002) **Callas Forever** (2002)
Nathalie (2003) **Crossed Tracks** (2007)
The Secrets (2007)
L'Ora di punta (2007)
Hello Goodbye (2008)

Eve **Arden**
5ft 7¹/₂in
(EUNICE QUEDENS)

Born: **April 30, 1908**
Mill Valley, California, USA
Died: **November 12, 1990**

Eve quit school at sixteen and under her real name, made her stage debut with a stock company in San Francisco. She got a part in an early sound film – a musical called *Song of Love,* but she waited four years before her next role – uncredited in Joan Crawford's *Dancing Lady.* She then became Eve Arden and things started to move for her. A hit revue at the Pasadena Playhouse led to a golden opportunity one year later in "Ziegfeld Follies" of 1934. In the 1936 edition of that Broadway show, she deservedly won a part in a Hollywood movie on the strength of her hilarious comedy sketch. The film, *Oh Doctor!* was only so-so, but she began getting work from various studios as a wise-cracking supporting player – her Eve, in *Stage Door* being an early example. She had talent and sparkle, typified in *Mildred Pierce* – for which she was nominated for a Best Supporting Actress Oscar. But probably because she had a complex about her mother being much prettier than she was, she rarely attempted to get leading roles. In fact, although she built her reputation as a supporting player, Eve was regarded throughout her film career in Hollywood, as being a 'scene stealer.' Her many television appearances during the 1970s and 80s, proved she continued to be exactly that – right up to her final show in 1987. Eve died of cardiac arrest, in Los Angeles three years later.

Stage Door (1937)
Eternally Yours (1939)
At the Circus (1939) **Ziegfeld Girl** (1941)
Whistling in the Dark (1941)
Manpower (1941)
Bedtime Story (1941)
Cover Girl (1944) **Doughgirls** (1944)
Mildred Pierce (1945)
The Voice of the Turtle (1947)
We're Not Married! (1952)
Our Miss Brooks (1956)
Anatomy of a Murder (1959)
**The Dark at the Top of
the Stairs** (1960) **Grease** (1978)

Asia **Argento**
5ft 6in
(ARIA MARIA VITTORIA ROSSA ARGENTO)

Born: **September 20, 1975**
Rome, Italy

Asia is the daughter of Dario Argento, an Italian director, producer and screenwriter, who specializes in the "giallo" genre. Her mother, the actress Daria Nicolodi, starred in several of his films. Because of her parents' busy schedule, Asia was a lonely child, who found it hard to make friends and spent most of her time reading books and writing poems. When she was nine years old, she featured in an episode of a TV series, 'Sogni e bisogni'. Her film debut was in 1986, in the horror movie, *Demoni 2...L'Incubo ritorna,* and she was given her first starring role in 1989, in *Zoo.* She did alright as a child actress, but she needed experience. She was first directed by her father in his 1993 film *Trauma,* but it took Carlo Verdone to make her a star, in his *Perdiamoci di vista!* – for which she was awarded the David di Donatello as Best Actress. Her fluent French got her the role of Charlotte de Sauve, in *La Reine Margot* and in 1994, she began directing, with two short films – *Prospettive* and *A Ritroso.* Asia shared a Best New Director Award at Williamsburg Brooklyn Film Festival, for her feature, *Scarlet Diva.* Internationally, she made *The Heart Is Deceitful Above All Things,* filmed in Tennessee. She directed, acted and wrote the screenplay. Asia is the mother of Anna Lou, from her relationship with musician Marco Castoldi, who acted in two of her movies.

Palombella (1989)
Perdiamoci di vista! (1994)
Stendhal's Syndrome (1996)
Scarlet Diva (2000)
Love Bites (2001)
La Sirène rouge (2002)
Triple X (2002)
**The Heart Is Deceitful Above
All Things** (2004) **Last Days** (2005)
Marie Antoinette (2006)
Transylvania (2006)
Boarding Gate (2007)
Go Go Tales (2007)
The Last Mistress (2007)
La Terza madre (2007)
De la guerre (2008)

Alan **Arkin**
6ft 2in
(ALAN WOLF ARKIN)

Born: **March 26, 1934**
New York City, New York, USA

Alan grew up in a typically Jewish family home in Brooklyn. He was movie crazy from an early age. His father, David, was a teacher, and a talented writer and painter. His mother, Beatrice, whose parents were immigrants from the Ukraine, was a schoolteacher. Before and during World War II Alan admired the great movie character actors, such as Charles Laughton and Spencer Tracy. The family moved to Los Angeles in 1946, when his father was offered a job as a set designer. From the age of ten, Alan attended drama schools. While at Franklin High School in L.A. he studied with a former pupil of Stanislavsky. At around that time both his parents were accused of being communists, and his dad was barred from taking a job he'd been offered as a set designer. After Los Angeles City College Alan went to Bennington, a Liberal Arts college in Vermont. It might have been too liberal – in 1955 he dropped out to join a folk-trio called "The Tarriers", as both singer and composer. Over the next twelve years, Alan performed and recorded (on a recorder) and made four albums of children's folk songs with "The Baby Sitters". After a spell on Broadway, he became a movie actor in the 1960s. After a short called *That's Me,* in 1963, he burst onto the screen in *The Russians Are Coming the Russians Are Coming* and was Oscar-nominated. A second nomination as Best Actor came his way for *The Heart is a Lonely Hunter.* He would have been well pleased when, thirty-eight years later, he was named Best Supporting Actor for *Little Miss Sunshine.* Alan has three sons from his three marriages.

**The Russians Are Coming,
the Russians Are Coming** (1966)
Wait Until Dark (1967)
The Heart is a Lonely Hunter (1968)
Four Days In September (1997)
Little Miss Sunshine (2006)
The Novice (2006) **Rendition** (2007)
Sunshine Cleaning (2008)
Get Smart (2008)

Richard **Arlen**
5ft 11in
(CORNELIUS RICHARD VAN MATTIMORE)

Born: **September 1, 1898**
Charlottesville, Virginia, USA
Died: **March 28, 1976**

Richard was educated at St. Paul High School in Minnesota, St. Thomas College, and the University of Pennsylvania. He started his working life in a variety of jobs – including sports editor at a local newspaper. After serving as a pilot in the Royal Canadian flying corps, during World War I, he drifted into silent films in 1920 - initially as a busy extra. He was given his first featured role in the spring of 1923, in a South Seas adventure titled *Vengeance of the Deep.* His flying experience resulted in a role which brought him stardom in the 1927 Academy Award winner, *Wings.* It also brought him into contact with his future wife, the actress, Jobyna Ralston. When sound became the norm, Richard had just the right kind of voice. Jobyna wasn't so lucky. She retired from films after her first two 'talkies' revealed her pronounced lisp. Richard kept busy in leading roles in action movies throughout the early 1930s. He freelanced from the end of the decade and then joined Paramount. During World War II, he made a dozen movies – mostly with a war theme. In 1948, he began to lose his hearing, which affected his career. An operation sorted it out, and he was close to his 150th film when he made his final appearance in *A Whale of a Tale,* in 1976, just before he died of emphysema.

The Virginian (1929)
Caught (1931) Touchdown (1931)
Guilty as Hell (1932)
Island of Lost Souls (1932)
Come on Marines (1934)
Let 'em Have It (1935)
Artists & Models (1937)
Minesweeper (1943)
Timber Queen (1944)
Storm Over Lisbon (1944)
When My Baby
Smiles at Me (1948)
Kansas Raiders (1950)
The Mountain (1956)
Warlock (1959)
The Best Man (1964)

Arletty
5ft 3½in
(LÉONIE MARIE JULIE BATHIAT)

Born: **May 15, 1898**
Courbevoie, Seine, France
Died: **July 23, 1992**

Arletty's first connection with the world of show business was in the early part of the twentieth century, when she hung around outside the local music hall to hear a chanteuse entertaining the poor people of her town. Her own family were poor and like many girls from her background, she started work at fourteen. She had begun studying at secretarial school when her father was killed in a mining accident in 1914. To help support her family, she worked in a munitions factory during World War I. When it was over she went to live in Paris, where she worked as a mannequin, posed nude for the great painter, Henri Matisse, and acted in the theater. She then caught the eye of a film producer, and in 1931, appeared in her first film *Un Chien qui Rapporte.* By 1936, now called Arletty, she was the toast of Paris and a star of the city's stage, with celebrated roles in the plays "Les Joirs du Capitole" and "Fric-Frac". On screen, her reputation soared after her appearance in Marcel Carné's *Hôtel du Nord.* Seven years later, he starred her in his masterpiece – *Les Enfants du Paradis.* Despite a scandalous affair with a German officer during World War II – for which she had to serve four months in prison, Arletty was still worshiped in France. For another ten years she made films and worked on the Paris stage. In 1960, an unlucky accident with some eye-drops left her nearly blind. After that she appeared only in roles which required little or no physical movement. For the final twenty years of her life she was a sad and lonely woman and that's the way she died – alone and in her sleep.

Hôtel du Nord (1938)
Le Jour se lève (1939)
Circonstances atténuantes (1939)
Tempête (1940)
Les Enfants du Paradis (1945)
Portrait d'un assassin (1949)
L'Air de Paris (1954)
Huis-Clos (1955)
Maxime (1958)

Pedro **Armendáriz**
5ft 9in
(PEDRO GREGORIO ARMENDARIZ HASTINGS)

Born: **May 9, 1912**
Mexico City, Distrito Federal, Mexico
Died: **June 18, 1963**

Born to a Mexican father and an American mother during the Mexican revolution, Pedro was raised in the Mexico City suburb of Churubusco. To protect him from the violence, his mother facilitated a move to relatives in Laredo, Texas, where he stayed until both parents died in 1921. Pedro went to live with an uncle who encouraged him to study engineering at the California Polytechnic State University. After graduating in 1931, he returned to Mexico City, where he did various jobs until he was discovered by the director Miguel Zacarías, who starred him in his 1935 film, *Rosario.* Pedro worked for all the Mexican directors in films which were aimed at the huge local market. When he acted opposite the returning Hollywood star, Dolores Del Rio, in *María Candelaria,* he became known abroad. John Ford gave him his first American film role in *The Fugitive,* and Pedro began commuting between Mexico and the United States on a regular basis. He remained a big star in Mexico throughout the 1950s and once in a while, made French and American films. He developed cancer after exposure to radiation while filming *The Conqueror.* He suffered terrible pain in his hips during the following seven years. In 1963, shortly after finishing work on *From Russia with Love,* he used a shotgun to kill himself.

María Candelaria (1944)
Bugambilia (1945)
Enamorada (1946)
The Fugitive (1947)
Fort Apache (1948)
3 Godfathers (1948)
We Were Strangers (1949)
La Malguerida (1949)
Rosario Castro (1950)
La noche avanza (1952)
El Robozo de Soledad (1952)
El Bruto (1953) La Rebelión
de los colgados (1954)
La Escondida (1956)
Flor de Mayo (1959)
From Russia with Love (1963)

Robert **Armstrong**

5ft 10in

(ROBERT ARMSTRONG)

Born: **November 20, 1890**
Saginaw, Michigan, USA
Died: **April 20, 1973**

When Bob was a boy, his father was lured by the prospect of gold in Alaska. He took the family West and made his base in Seattle. After a short spell in the US Army during World War I, Bob studied law at the University of Washington, but dropped out when he was made aware of a new and exciting money-making prospect. Pointing to the rapidly developing movie industry, an uncle persuaded him to consider an acting career. He did so, and joined James Gleason's stock company. Bob's acting improved as they toured the country with various productions. In New York, in 1925, he was given his first starring role in a play Gleason had written, called "Is Zat So". He made his film debut two years later, in the silent, *The Main Event*. His rasping voice and pugnacious appearance were ideal for the Talkies. At the time of his most famous role – as Carl Denham, in *King Kong,* Bob was a movie veteran. Later supporting roles in films like *'G' Men* and *The Fugitive* ensured regular employment. From the early 1950s onwards, Bob made his living mainly on television. During his career he acted in over a hundred films – the last one being *For Those Who Think Young,* in 1964. From 1939, Bob was married to his third wife, Louise de Bois, who was with him when he died of cancer at his home in Santa Monica, California.

The Lost Squadron (1932)
The Most Dangerous Game (1932)
Billion Dollar Scandal (1933)
King Kong (1933)
'G' Men (1935)
The Ex-Mrs. Bradford (1936)
The Girl Said No (1937)
Man of Conquest (1939)
Dive Bomber (1941)
Gang Busters (1942)
Blood on the Sun (1945)
The Sea of Grass (1947)
The Fugitive (1947)
The Paleface (1948)
Mighty Joe Young (1949)
The Peacemaker (1956)

Edward **Arnold**

6ft 1in

(GUNTHER EDWARD ARNOLD SCHNEIDER)

Born: **February 18, 1890**
New York City, New York, USA
Died: **April 26, 1956**

The son of German immigrants, Ed was interested in acting from the age of twelve when he played Lorenzo in "The Merchant of Venice". He was seventeen when he made his professional stage debut – opposite Ethel Barrymore, in "Dream of a Summer Night". In 1916, he made his film debut (first of thirty-five appearances for Essanay studios) in a comedy/drama, *The Misleading Lady*. By 1920, he stopped making films in order to concentrate on stage work. With the advantage of sound, which suited his superb baritone, Ed made his screen come-back in 1932, in a Warner Bros. short subject, *Murder in the Pullman*. That same year he was rubbing shoulders (on the screen at least) with Bette Davis, Bogart and all three of the Barrymores. One of his most memorable roles was Diamond Jim Brady, in *Diamond Jim*. The stars he supported in his films would serve as a Hollywood 'Who's Who. From 1940-42, Ed served as President of the Screen Actors Guild. In the 1950s, he was happy to work on TV and continued to lend his considerable presence as a supporting actor in movies. Married three times, he had two daughters and a son, who had a brief acting career. Ed died of a cerebral hemorrhage in Encino, California, a few months after completing his final film, *Miami Exposé*.

Whistling in the Dark (1933)
The Barbarian (1933)
Roman Scandals (1933)
The Glass Key (1935)
Diamond Jim (1935)
Crime and Punishment (1935)
You Can't Take It with You (1935)
Mr. Smith Goes to Washington (1939)
Johnny Apollo (1940)
Meet John Doe (1941)
The Devil and Daniel Webster (1941)
Johnny Eager (1942)
Take Me Out to the Ball Game (1949)
Annie Get Your Gun (1950)
City That Never Sleeps (1953)
Living It Up (1954)

Françoise **Arnoul**

5ft 2in

(FRANÇOISE GAUTSCH)

Born: **June 3, 1931**
Constantine, Algeria

Françoise spent her early life in Algeria and Morocco with her parents and her two brothers. Her father was a career soldier and her mother had given up an acting career to marry him – which might explain why Françoise couldn't wait to become an actress. When she was seven, her mother sent her to dancing lessons in Rabat. During World War II she appeared in shows organized to aid the Red Cross. Her father was then posted to Casablanca where she and her brothers went to school. In 1945, he remained in Morocco while the rest of his family went to settle in Paris. Young Françoise went to a local school where she was friendly with Michele Morgan's sister. She kept up with the latest movies by reading "Cinémonde" and eventually, after drama school, made her film debut in 1949 in the well received *L'épave*. In the mid-1950s, she was, in my teenage fantasy, the sexiest creature to appear on cinema screens – in films like *Le Mouton a cinque pattes* (The Sheep Has Five Legs), *French Cancan* and *La Chatte*. Her secret weapons were her burning dark eyes ! In the 1960s, her film career faded in terms of quality, but she kept plugging away – occasionally turning up in worthwhile movies such as *Violette & François*. French movie queens don't worry much about growing old. Françoise continues playing character roles in films and on television, at the age of seventy-seven, in 'Le Voyageur de la Toussaint'.

Forbidden Fruit (1952)
La Rage au corps (1954)
Secrets d'alcôve (1954)
Le Mouton a cinq pattes (1954)
French Cancan (1954)
Les Amants du Tage (1955)
No Sun in Venice (1957)
La Chatte (1958)
Le Testament d'Orphee (1960)
Le Diable et les dix
commandements (1962)
Violette & François (1977)
Les Années campagne (1992)
Merci pour le geste (2000)

Patricia **Arquette**
5ft 1in
(PATRICIA T. ARQUETTE)

Born: **April 8, 1968**
Chicago, Illinois, USA

Her father, Lewis Arquette, was an actor and her grandfather was the well-known comedian, Cliff Arquette. Her mother, who died in 1997, was the daughter of a Jewish Holocaust refugee from Poland. Patricia's father converted to Islam and shortly after she was born, the family joined a Hippy commune in Virginia. When she was fifteen, Patricia ran away from home to live with her sister, Rosanna, in Los Angeles. She attended the Mid-City Alternative School and the Los Angeles Center for Enriched Studies before making her movie debut, in A *Nightmare on Elm Street 3*. Her progress continued via TV work and supporting roles in films, which climbed to another level when Sean Penn gave her a featured role in his drama, *The Indian Runner*. By the end of the decade, she was a respected actress – having starred in several critically acclaimed films – the pick of which were *True Romance, Ed Wood,* and *Beyond Rangoon*. In 1995 she made the big mistake of marrying Nicolas Cage. They separated after nine months, acted as a couple in public, and finally divorced in 2001! After a four-year long engagement, she married the actor Thomas Jane, in 2006, in Venice, Italy. Although there has been a shortage of good movie roles recently, Patricia is currently starring in NBC TV's popular series "Medium", for which she was nominated for a Golden Globe – three years running.

A Nightmare on
Elm Street 3 (1987)
The Indian Runner (1991)
Trouble Bound (1993)
Ethan Frome (1993)
True Romance (1993)
Ed Wood (1994)
Beyond Rangoon (1995)
Flirting With Disaster (1996)
Lost Highway (1997)
Bringing Out the Dead (1999)
Stigmata (1999)
The Badge (2000)
Holes (2003)
Fast Food Nation (2006)

Rosanna **Arquette**
5ft 3in
(ROSANNA LAUREN ARQUETTE)

Born: **August 10, 1959**
New York City, New York, USA

Like her sister, Patricia, Rosanna is a descendant of the American explorer, Meriwether Lewis, who led the Corps of Discovery at the beginning of the nineteenth century. That adventurous spirit was soon apparent to her. In 1963, her family moved to Chicago where her father managed The Second City Theater. He took them to live in a commune when Rosanna was eleven – which was really bad for the youngster's schooling. She was fifteen when she left home and hitch-hiked with a group of teenagers to San Francisco. After three years of working in odd jobs she made her professional stage debut in 1977 in a Story Theater musical, "The Metamorphoses", in Los Angeles. She got some TV parts during that year, and in 1979 had a small role in the sequel movie *More American Graffiti*. She played troubled teenagers in several films until she got her first starring role four years later, in *Baby It's You*. It was followed by *Desperately Seeking Susan* – opposite Madonna. In the 1990s, Rosanna's career peaked in films like *Pulp Fiction, Crash,* and *Buffalo '66*. She has been married three times and has a daughter, Zoe Blue Sidel. Once expected to become a great screen comedienne, that promise has not yet been fulfilled. A taste of what she may still achieve is demonstrated in *I-See-You.Com*. A lot of Rosanna's talent is on show in the selections listed below.

Desperately Seeking
Susan (1985) Silverado (1985)
After Hours (1985)
Nobody's Fool (1986)
The Big Blue (1988)
Black Rainbow (1989)
Pulp Fiction (1994)
Crash (1996)
Buffalo '66 (1998)
Sugar Town (1999)
The Good Advice (2001)
Dead Cool (2004)
Iowa (2005)
I-See-You.Com (2006)
Ball Don't Lie (2008)

Jean **Arthur**
5ft 3in
(GLADYS GEORGIANNA GREENE)

Born: **October 17, 1900**
Plattsburgh, New York, USA
Died: **June 19, 1991**

Being a professional photographer, Jean's father was able to use his daughter to model for beauty product ads. In 1922, her picture was seen by a Fox talent scout and she was given her first film role – a small part in an early John Ford film called *Cameo Kirby*. She lacked confidence in her acting ability, but the studio had faith in her. For her part, she went back to New York and worked in the theatre. They changed her name to Jean Arthur and she made slow but steady progress from a rather timid-looking girl with dark hair to a striking blonde. With the advent of sound, she was recognized as one of the few great individualists. Despite a rather nasal sounding voice, she made an effortless transition from silent films. In 1935, it was her comedic ability in another John Ford movie *The Whole Town's Talking* that put her on the map. Jean Arthur was a big star for ten years - she was said to be Frank Capra's favorite actress. Under George Stevens' strong direction, she earned a Best Actress Oscar nomination in 1943, for *The More the Merrier*. Like the true star she was, Jean left the screen on a high note, at the age of fifty-two, in the classic western, *Shane*. She made a brief return in 1965 – appearing in one episode of the TV western, 'Gunsmoke' and then eleven episodes of 'The Jean Arthur Show'. Jean was twice married and divorced. She lived in quite retirement in Carmel, California, before dying of heart failure.

Whirlpool (1934)
If You Could Only Cook (1935)
Mr Deeds Goes to Town (1936)
The ex-Mrs Bradford (1936)
The Plainsman (1936)
History Is Made at Night (1937)
You Can't Take It With You (1938)
Only Angels Have Wings (1939)
Mr Smith Goes to Washington (1939)
The Devil and Miss Jones (1941)
The More the Merrier (1943)
A Foreign Affair (1948)
Shane (1953)

Armand **Assante**
5ft 10in
(ARMAND ANTHONY ASSANTE)

Born: **October 4, 1949**
New York City, New York, USA

Armand came from a creative, arts-related family background. His father, Armand Assante Sr., was a painter from an Italian background. His mother, Katherine, who was from Irish stock, was a poet and a music teacher. Armand was raised in a devoutly Roman Catholic environment. After graduating from Cornwall Central High School, he enrolled at the American Academy of Dramatic Arts. He finally made his off-Broadway debut in 1971, in "Lake of the Woods". In 1974, he had a small role in an early Sylvester Stallone movie, *The Lords of Flatbush*. When he made his directorial debut, in 1978, Sly gave Armand a good featured role as his crippled, war veteran brother in *Paradise Alley*. Armand's movie breakthrough was two years later when he had fun playing Goldie Hawn's French admirer, in *Private Benjamin*. After returning to Broadway in the choice role of Emperor Napoléon I, in "Kingdoms" he was a very very macho Mike Hammer, in *I, the Jury,* and gave his support to Dudley Moore and Nastassja Kinski, in *Unfaithfully Yours*. For the five years, until 1989, he was mainly seen on TV including a Golden Globe nominated role in 'Jack the Ripper.' Apart from *Q & A,* for which he was nominated for a Golden Globe, there wasn't a big film role worthy of his talent until *The Mambo Kings* – in 1992. Things got better for him, but he then experienced seven lean years. The new millennium, starting with the excellent *Looking for an Echo,* has seen a lot more consistency and some quality roles.

The Mambo Kings (1992)
1492: Conquest of Paradise (1992)
Hoffa (1992)
Looking for an Echo (2000)
Tough Luck (2003)
Two for the Money (2005)
Funny Money (2006)
Mexican Sunrise (2007)
California Dreamin' (Nesfarsit) (2007)
When Nietzsche Wept (2007)
American Gangster (2007)
La Linea (2008)

Fred **Astaire**
5ft 9in
(FREDERIC AUSTERLITZ JR)

Born: **May 10, 1899**
Omaha, Nebraska, USA
Died: **June 22, 1987**

Fred's father, who was from an Austrian background, was in the brewing industry, but the boy had no desire to follow in his footsteps. With his mother's tireless encouragement, beginning with dancing lessons, Fred was in show business from the age of five. His first dancing partner was his younger sister Adele. They toured together in vaudeville and in 1916, were offered a chance to appear in a Broadway show "Over The Top". They achieved great fame on both sides of the Atlantic but when Adele retired to marry into British aristocracy, Fred traveled to Hollywood, where in 1933, he was teamed for the first time with Ginger Rogers, in the film *Flying Down to Rio*. Their partnership proved to be extra special and they were together in ten films – all box-office winners – *Top Hat* and *Swing Time* being the *crème de la crème*. Despite the handicap of not being born tall, dark and certainly not handsome, he overcame it with an abundance of sheer style and true class in a glamour-obsessed Hollywood. Fred was married to Phyllis Livingston Potter, from 1933 until her death in 1954. Fred was nominated for a Supporting Oscar, for *The Towering Inferno*. His interest in racing introduced him to his second wife, the jockette, Robyn Smith. She was with him when he died of pneumonia, in Los Angeles.

Flying Down to Rio (1933)
The Gay Divorcee (1934)
Top Hat (1935)
Swing Time (1936)
Follow the Fleet (1936)
Shall We Dance? (1937)
Broadway Melody of 1940 (1940)
Holiday Inn (1942)
Easter Parade (1948)
The Belle of New York (1952)
The Band Wagon (1953)
Daddy Long Legs (1955)
Funny Face (1957)
Silk Stockings (1957)
On the Beach (1959)
The Towering Inferno (1974)

Nils **Asther**
6ft 0½in
(NILS ANTON ALFHILD ASTHER)

Born: **January 17, 1897**
Hellerup, Copenhagen, Denmark
Died: **October 13, 1981**

Nils was born in Denmark to wealthy Swedish parents, who raised him in the Swedish seaport of Malmö. After finishing his secondary schooling, Nils then attended the Royal Dramatic Theater School, in Stockholm. He started his stage career in Sweden and also in Copenhagen. He was nineteen when he made his film debut – in *Vingarne,* directed by Mauritz Stiller, and shot in Lidingö, near Stockholm. During the 1920s, Nils made movies in Sweden, Denmark and Germany. But he had his eye on the big film industry of Hollywood. In 1927, he made his debut there with a supporting role in *Topsy and Eva*. Nils had the good looks and the height to become a big star, and things looked promising until the advent of sound. At first he was okay – especially when playing foreigners, as in *The Bitter Tea of General Yen,* but by 1934, his unattractive accent finished his career as a star. In 1930, he had married the American actress, Vivian Duncan with whom he had a daughter. The marriage was over in less than two years. He kept his name in the cast list of Hollywood films but they were usually small roles. In 1958, he went back to Scandinavia and settled in Sweden. Nils died there, in Stockholm, twenty-three years later.

The Sea Bat (1930)
– But the Flesh Is Weak (1932)
The Washington Masquerade (1932)
The Bitter Tea of General Yen (1933)
Storm at Daybreak (1933)
The Right to Romance (1933)
If I Were Free (1933)
By Candlelight (1933)
Dr. Kildare's Wedding (1941)
Night of January 16th (1941)
Sweater Girl (1942)
Night Monster (1942)
Submarine Alert (1943)
Mystery Broadcast (1943)
Bluebeard (1944)
The Man in Half Moon Street (1945)
Son of Lassie (1945)
Jealousy (1945)

Mary **Astor**
5ft 6in
(LUCILE VASONCELLOS LANGHANKE)

Born: **May 3, 1906**
Quincy, Illinois, USA
Died: **September 25, 1987**

Mary's parents, who were teachers, were fanatical film fans. Her dad would fantasize about little Lucile becoming a movie star one day. After the family had moved to New York he became friendly with a photographer who knew Lillian Gish. Lucile was pushed into entering beauty contests and her dad's determination resulted in a short-lived Hollywood contract at the age of fourteen. After several bit parts and with her name changed to Mary Astor, she got her first big chance in 1924, (opposite John Barrymore, with whom she had an affair) in *Beau Brummel*. She signed a contract with First National and by the time the Talkies started she was already a veteran of nearly forty films. She initially failed the test for sound so she made use of being out of favor by acting in a Los Angeles theater. The play brought rave reviews and she was soon back in front of the cameras. Mary became an actress of the highest order, offering first class support in *Dodsworth* and *The Prisoner of Zenda*, and winning a Best Supporting Actress Oscar for *The Great Lie*. During a career which spanned over forty-five years, she appeared in around 100 films including *The Maltese Falcon* and *Meet Me In St. Louis.* From 1950, she was mainly seen in TV dramas. She did make one last film, *Hush...Hush, Sweet Charlotte,* and in 1965 retired to write her memoirs (which became a best-seller) and a couple of novels. Mary died of a heart attack at Woodland Hills, California.

Red Dust (1932)
Easy to Love (1934)
Page Miss Glory (1935)
Dodsworth (1936)
The Prisoner of Zenda (1937)
Midnight (1939) **The Great Lie** (1941)
The Maltese Falcon (1941)
The Palm Beach Story (1942)
Meet Me in St Louis (1944)
Cass Timberlane (1947)
Act of Violence (1948)
Little Women (1949)

William **Atherton**
6ft 1in
(WILLIAM ATHERTON KNIGHT)

Born: **July 30, 1947**
Orange, Connecticut, USA

Bill first started acting when he was at high school – appearing in the original off-Broadway production of John Guare's "The House of Blue Leaves". After he had become the youngest person to be accepted into the Long Wharf Theater Repertory, in New Haven, Connecticut, Bill went on to study at the Pasadena Playhouse and Carnegie Institute of Technology, in Pittsburgh. This led to stage work starting with his debut in "The Boy Friend" at the Clinton Playhouse, in 1964. In 1972, he made his film debut in *The New Centurions.* Bill's big break came two years later, in Steven Spielberg's *The Sugarland Express.* In 1980, he married Bobbi Goldin, who's been his companion for nearly forty years. During that decade, he specialized in sleazy film characters, but still kept his options open with good work on TV series such as 'The Twilight Zone' and 'The Equalizer'. Bill also shone in other on and off-Broadway productions - including his one-man show – "William Atherton: Acting, Ethics, Person" – and Arthur Miller's "The American Clock". Bill hit the movie big-time in the hit comedy *Ghostbusters,* but he was injured on the set when 200 pounds of shaving cream was accidentally dropped on him from a crane. He recovered and later scored high marks in the *Die Hard* films, *The Pelican Brief* and *The Last Samurai.* His recent work includes the exciting crime dramas – *Hacia la oscuridad,* (which was shot in Panama City) and *The Girl Next Door.*

The Sugarland Express (1974)
The Day of the Locust (1975)
Looking for Mr. Goodbar (1977)
Ghost Busters (1984)
Real Genius (1985)
Die Hard (1988)
Die Hard 2 (1990)
Oscar (1991)
The Pelican Brief (1993)
Hoodlum (1997) **Mad City** (1997)
The Last Samurai (2003)
Hacia la oscuridad (2007)
The Girl Next Door (2007)

Rowan **Atkinson**
6ft 1in
(ROWAN SEBASTIAN ATKINSON)

Born: **January 6, 1955**
Consett, County Durham, England

The son of a successful Durham farmer, Eric Atkinson, and his wife, Ella, Rowan had two elder brothers. He was educated at St. Bees School, in Cumbria, and at Newcastle University, where he studied Electrical Engineering before getting an MSc degree from Queen's College, Oxford. Rowan soon became a part of the University's Dramatic Society and he appeared at the Edinburgh Fringe Festival in 1976. He then formed a double act with Angus Deayton as his straight man – the inspired result was filmed for television and its success led to Rowan being offered his own show on ITV, in 1978. He chose instead to work on 'Not the Nine O'Clock News'. Within three years, he was known around the world as Edmund 'Blackadder'. He made his movie debut in 1983, in the short comedy, *Dead on Time.* That same year, he had a small but visible supporting role in Sean Connery's Bond 'comeback' – *Never Say Never Again.* As encouraging as that was, he continued the 'Blackadder' series until making the Oscar-winning short, *The Appointments of Dennis Jennings,* in 1988. His first important feature was Mel Smith's *The Tall Guy,* in which he co-starred with Jeff Goldblum and Emma Thompson. He played supporting roles in international hits like *Four Weddings and a Funeral* and has had success with his *Mr. Bean* movies – strongly influenced by Chaplin and Tati. His best film by far is *Keeping Mum,* which benefits from the presence of Maggie Smith. Since 1990, Rowan's been married to Sunetra Sastry. They have two children.

Never Say Never Again (1983)
The Tall Guy (1989)
The Witches (1990)
Hot Shots! Part Deux (1993)
Four Weddings and a Funeral (1994)
Bean (1997)
Rat Race (2001)
Johnny English (2003)
Love Actually (2003)
Keeping Mum (2005)
Mr. Bean's Vacation (2007)

Sir Richard **Attenborough**
5ft 7in
(RICHARD SAMUEL ATTENBOROUGH)

Born: **August 29, 1923**
Cambridge, England

Richard went to school in Leicester, where his father was head of University College. He later won a scholarship to RADA and impressed one of London's biggest theatrical agents, who took him on. He made his professional stage debut in the play "Ah Wilderness!". He was nineteen when he appeared in his first movie *In Which We Serve,* which starred Noel Coward and was directed by David Lean. Richard served in the RAF during World War II. When it was over he continued in small movie roles, usually playing small-time crooks or cowards, until his breakthrough role in 1947 (playing a small-time crook) in *Brighton Rock.* Richard was a youthful-looking star of British films throughout the late 1940s and most of the 1950s. In 1952 he and his wife, actress, Sheila Sim were in the original cast of "The Mouse Trap" in London's West End. So as to concentrate on directing, Richard took fewer acting roles after 1970. A supporter of the British Film Industry, he was very successful behind the camera. In 1983 he won the Best Director Oscar for his epic movie *Ghandi.* Richard appeared to have given up acting in 2002, and was only seen at award ceremonies. But the passion was still burning. He will be seen on the screen in 2009, in Jonathan English's *Ironclad.*

The Man Within (1947)
Brighton Rock (1947)
London Belongs to Me (1948)
The Guinea Pig (1948)
Morning Departure (1950)
Gift Horse (1952)
The Ship That Died of Shame (1955)
Private's Progress (1956)
I'm All Right Jack (1959)
The Angry Silence (1960)
The League of Gentlemen (1960)
The Great Escape (1963)
Guns at Batasi (1964)
Seance on a Wet Afternoon (1964)
Only When I Laugh (1968)
10 Rillington Place (1971)
Jurassic Park (1993)
Elizabeth (1998)

Lionel **Atwill**
5ft 10in
(LIONEL ALFRED WILLIAM ATWILL)

Born: **March 1, 1885**
Croydon, Surrey, England
Died: **April 22, 1946**

Lionel was born into a wealthy family and attended Mercers School, in London, before studying to be an architect. Lionel (who was nicknamed "Pinky") then went on the stage. His debut, in 1905, was at the Garrick Theater in "The Walls of Jericho". By the age of thirty his reputation had crossed the Atlantic and so had he and his first wife, Phyllis. He went to New York in 1915 and acted with Lily Langtry in several Broadway productions. From 1918, when he made his screen debut in *Eve's Daughter,* he was occasionally tempted to act in silent movies. But his marvellous voice was ideal for the Talkies and in 1927, he made two experimental sound pictures for Fox. In 1932, with a starring role in *Doctor X,* a twelve-year run of success began, including worthy titles such as *Captain Blood, The Great Garrick* and *The Hound of the Baskervilles.* It all stopped in 1943, when a sex scandal which had taken place at his home three years earlier, resurfaced. He had perjured himself to protect the identities of his guests and got five years on probation. His third wife divorced him and he was no longer in demand. Lionel was reduced to acting in Poverty Row films – which was, for a man of his acting pedigree – 'The End'. He died of pneumonia at his home in Pacific Palisades, California.

Mystery of the Wax Museum (1933)
Captain Blood (1935)
The Devil is a Woman (1935)
The Great Garrick (1937)
Three Comrades (1938)
The Great Waltz (1938)
Son of Frankenstein (1939)
The Three Musketeers (1939)
The Hound of the
Baskervilles (1939)
The Great Profile (1940)
Boom Town (1940)
Sherlock Holmes and the
Secret Weapon (1943)
House of Frankenstein (1944)
Crime, Inc. (1945)

Stéphane **Audran**
5ft 6in
(COLETTE SUZANNE DACHEVILLE)

Born: **November 2, 1932**
Versailles, Seine-et-Oise, France

Not much is known about Stéphane's early life other than the fact that she grew up in the town southwest of Paris, which is renowned for its splendid baroque palace. After leaving school at eighteen, she embarked on a course of drama lessons and began working in stage productions during the early 1950s. After getting romantically involved with the actor Jean-Louis Trintignant, (a top star in France at the time) she made her movie debut in 1957, in Daniel Costelle's *Le Jeu de la Nuit.* She then had a small uncredited role in Jacques Becker's *Montparnasse 19,* which was noticed by new wave director, Claude Chabrol. He gave her a good part in *Les Cousins* and she was suddenly on the scene. Stéphane was one of a cool and different breed of French actresses epitomized by Catherine Deneuve. In 1964, after she'd split with Trintignant, she married Claude Chabrol and appeared in most of his films up to and beyond their divorce, in 1980. Her essential titles from that time must include *Les Biches, La Femme Infidèle* and *Le Boucher.* Their son is the young actor, Thomas Chabrol. Stéphane, who is a great French film star, is bi-lingual. In 1974, she won a Best Actress BAFTA for two films – *Juste avant la nuit* and *The Discreet Charm of the Bourgeoisie.* She's appeared in more than fifty movies over the past forty years and is excellent in *La Fille de Monaco.*

Les Bonnes Femmes (1960)
Les Biches (1968)
La Femme Infidèle (1969)
Le Boucher (1970)
La Rupture (1970)
Juste avant la nuit (1971)
The Discreet Charm of
the Bourgeoisie (1972)
Violette Noziére (1978)
The Big Red One (1980)
Coup de torchon (1981)
Poulet au vinaigre (1985)
Babette's Feast (1987)
Au petit Marguery (1995)
La Fille de Monaco (2008)

Jean-Pierre **Aumont**
6ft
(JEAN-PIERRE PHILLIPE SALOMONS)

Born: January 5, 1911
Paris, France
Died: January 30, 2001

Jean-Pierre was the son of Alexandre and Suzanne Salomons, who owned a Paris department store called La Maison du Blanc. His father, a Dutchman who had settled in France, was Jewish. When he was sixteen Jean-Pierre began studying drama at the Paris Conservatoire. He made his stage debut in 1930. A year later, his screen career started when he appeared in the film Jean de la Lune. He continued in both mediums throughout the 1930s, and became a star of the Paris stage in 1934, when he appeared in Jean Cocteau's play – "La Machine Infernale". Two of Marcel Carné's classics, Drôle de drame and Hôtel du Nord, ensured his place in screen history. He was forced to flee France in 1942 when the German occupation began and then went to Hollywood. After shooting had finished on The Cross of Lorraine, he joined the Free French in North Africa where he participated in 'Operation Torch' and later joined the Allied Army in Italy. He was wounded and awarded the Legion d'Honneur and the Croix de Guerre for bravery. He went back to acting and for many years was a regular face on TV and cinema screens and in Broadway productions. In 1952, his wife, the Dominican actress (three-times his co-star) Maria Montez – whom he loved very much – died from a heart attack in the swimming pool of their home in France. Four years later Jean-Pierre married the Italian actress Marisa Pavan, who was the twin-sister of Pier Angeli. They had two sons and were together until he died of a heart attack, at Gassin, in France.

Maria Chapdelaine (1934)
Drôle de drame (1937)
Hôtel du Nord (1938)
The Cross of Lorraine (1943)
Song of Scheherazade (1947)
Lili (1953) **The Seven**
Deadly Sins (1962)
La nuit américaine (1973)
Giorgino (1994)
The Proprietor (1996)

Daniel **Auteuil**
5ft 7in
(DANIEL AUTEUIL)

Born: January 24, 1950
Algiers, Algeria

Although Daniel's parents, Henri and Yvonne Auteuil, were professional opera singers in France, it soon became clear (despite his attempt at operetta) that his voice was better suited to the stage and screen. This he confirmed himself when, during his teenage years, he accompanied them to the concert halls of Europe and vowed that one day he would be a great actor. He enrolled in classes with François Florent, at the drama school, Cours Florent, in Paris. Daniel began his career in musical productions including "Godspell". Following a very small role in the film L'Agression in 1974, he was a featured player two years later, in the charming comedy Monsieur Papa. He kept working hard in the theater and in films - getting bigger and better parts every time. By the mid-1980s, following roles in Jean de Florette and Manon des Source, he was without question, a French super-star – tackling any kind of role with equal panache. His movie career has progressed smoothly, while his private life has been less so. Daniel has two daughters from his former wives (both actresses) Anne Jousset, and Emmanuelle Béart. The latter co-starred with him in three of his early movies. In 2006, he married the sculptress, Aude Ambroggi.

L'Arbalète (1984)
Jean de Florette (1986)
Manon des sources (1986)
Un coeur en hiver (1992)
Ma saison préférée (1993)
La Séparation (1994)
Une femme française (1995)
La Fille sur le pont (1999)
Le Placard (2001)
L'Adversaire (2002)
Après vous (2003) Sotto falso
nome (2004) 36 Quai des
Orfèvres (2004) Caché (2005)
Peine ou faire l'amour (2005)
My Best Friend (2006)
The Second Wind (2007)
Me Two (2008)
MR 73 (2008)

Dan **Aykroyd**
6ft 1in
(DANIEL EDWARD AYKROYD)

Born: July 1, 1952
Ottawa, Ontario, Canada

Dan's father, Samuel, was a civil engineer who worked as a policy adviser to former Canadian Prime Minister Pierre Trudeau. Dan's mother Lorraine, was a French Canadian. Dan was brought up as a Roman Catholic and until he was seventeen, intended to become a priest. In a complete change of direction, he studied criminology and sociology at Carleton University before deciding to drop out and concentrate on becoming an entertainer. To begin with, he worked in the post office before getting a start as a comedian in night clubs. It was there that he perfected his talent for impersonating celebrities. He then gained experience in the "Second City" comedy troupe and during that same period, moonlighted as an announcer on a Toronto television station. For its first four seasons (1975-79) Dan was both writer and cast member on the American television show – 'Saturday Night Live'. The show's massive popularity made him famous and led to television and movie opportunities. In 1977, Dan made his first movie appearance (as star) in Love at First Sight. This was followed by 1941 – which was directed by Steven Spielberg, and The Blues Brothers. That film, along with Trading Places, and Driving Miss Daisy – for which Dan was Oscar-nominated as Best Supporting Actor, mark the high points of his career. Recent film work has been of a more supporting nature. Since 1983, he's been married to the actress Donna Dixon. They have three children.

Love at First Sight (1977)
The Blues Brothers (1980)
Trading Places (1983)
Indiana Jones and
the Temple of Doom (1984)
Ghost Busters (1984)
Into the Night (1985)
The Great Outdoors (1988)
Driving Miss Daisy (1989)
Pearl Harbor (2001)
Bright Young Things (2003)
I Now Pronounce You Chuck &
Larry (2003) War Inc. (2008)

Lew **Ayres**
5ft 9in
(LEWIS FREDERICK AYRE III)

Born: **December 28, 1908**
Minneapolis, Minnesota, USA
Died: **December 30, 1996**

Perhaps in anticipation of his future employment – as Doctor Kildare, young Lew studied medicine at the University of Arizona. But he soon dropped out - much preferring to sit in at jazz gigs, where he could perform equally well on the piano, guitar, or banjo. He got a job with Henry Halstead's band at the Coconut Grove in Los Angeles, and was playing banjo one night when Pathé executive Paul Bern, (who eventually went to MGM) asked to meet him. Bern got him a small part in an uninspiring film *The Sophomore* and then a better one, in the Greta Garbo silent movie *The Kiss.* It was Bern who in 1929, recommended Lew for the key role of a young German soldier, Paul Bäumer, in one of the greatest anti-war movies off all time, *All Quiet on the Western Front.* It guaranteed Lew a place in cinema history. Ten years later it was revealed that Lew had been so deeply affected by the story, he elected to be a conscientious objector when World War II started. For some time, the American movie-going public and exhibitors registered their disapproval of his pacifist stance by boycotting his films. Lew was later nominated for a Best Actor Oscar in *Johnny Belinda.* His co-star, Jane Wyman, fell in love with him and left her husband – the actor and future U.S. President, Ronald Reagan! From 1950, Lew acted in TV shows. His last was a 1994 episode of 'Hart to Hart'. Two years later, he died in his sleep in Los Angeles after being in a coma for several days.

**All Quiet on the
Western Front** (1930)
Common Clay (1930)
Holiday (1938)
Young Doctor Kildare (1938)
Doctor Kildare Goes Home (1940)
The Dark Mirror (1946)
The Unfaithful (1947)
Johnny Belinda (1948)
The Capture (1950)
Advise & Consent (1962)
The Carpetbaggers (1964)

Charles **Aznavour**
5ft 3in
(CHAHNOUR VARINAG AZNAVOURIAN)

Born: **May 22, 1924**
Paris, France

Charles was the youngest of two children born to Armenian immigrants. His father had a fine baritone voice with which he used to entertain customers in restaurants in Paris. His mother was a former actress who earned money during the depression by working as a seamstress. Charles and his sister contributed by waiting on tables and selling newspapers. He was only nine years old when he made his stage debut in the play, "Emil and the Detectives". He took singing and dancing lessons and after making his film debut as an extra, in *La Guerre des gosses,* in 1937, he quit school to join a theatrical troupe which toured France and Belgium. When World War II began, he was singing at the "Club de la Chanson", in Paris, and met the songwriter, Pierre Roche – later his partner in the concert duo known as "Roche and Aznamour". Charles befriended Edith Piaf and lived with her on a platonic basis. After the war, he established a career as a solo singer and began to get regular work in films – many of them musical offerings such as *Paris Music Hall.* His talent as a dramatic actor emerged in *Les Dragueurs* and *Un taxi pour Tobrouk,* but importantly, it had been noticed by the great François Truffaut, who cast Charles as the leading man in his classic, *Shoot the Pianist.* Film roles like that one are hard to come by, but he was an even better singer/songwriter and was loved all over the world. Charles has six children from his three marriages – three with his current wife, Ulla.

Les Dragueurs (1959)
Un taxi pour Tobrouk (1960)
Le Passage du Rhin (1960)
Shoot the Pianist (1960)
**The Devil and the Ten
Commandments** (1962)
Les Vierges (1963)
Rat Trap (1963) **High Fidelity** (1964)
Cloportes (1965)
Un Beau monstre (1971)
The Tin Drum (1979)
Viva la viel (1984)
Mon colonel (2006)

B

Lauren **Bacall**
5ft 8¹/₂in

(BETTY JOAN PERSKE)

Born: **September 16, 1924**
New York City, New York, USA

Lauren was the only child of a Jewish immigrant couple. Her father was related to former Israeli Prime Minister, Shimon Peres. Her parents divorced when she was six years old and Lauren never saw her father again. She established a close relationship with her mother, who encouraged her to study dancing at the American Academy of Dramatic Art. She worked as a fashion model in her late teens, and made her acting debut on Broadway, as Betty Bacall, in "Johnny Two By Four". "Slim", the wife of Howard Hawks, spotted her picture on the cover of Harper's Bazaar. She told her husband, who arranged a screen test. He liked her, changed her name to Lauren, and cast her in Hemingway's *To Have and Have Not*. She and Bogart fell in love and after his divorce in 1945, they married. They remained soul-mates until his death in 1957. Lauren's filmography is relatively short – she had a reputation for turning down parts she didn't fancy. During the 1960s she appeared on Broadway, and won Tony awards for "Applause" and "Woman of the Year". Lauren was once romanced by Sinatra and for eight years was married to Jason Robards. Lauren is a genuine living (and working) legend from the Golden Age of Movies.

To Have and Have Not (1944)
Confidential Agent (1945)
The Big Sleep (1946)
Dark Passage (1947) Key Largo (1948)
Young Man with a Horn (1950)
Bright Leaf (1950)
How to Marry a Millionaire (1953)
Woman's World (1954)
The Cobweb (1955)
Written on the Wind (1956)
Designing Woman (1957)
The Gift of Love (1958)
North West Frontier (1959)
Shock Treatment (1964)
Murder on the Orient Express (1974)
Dogville (2003) Manderlay (2005)
These Foolish Things (2006)
The Walker (2007)

Amitabh **Bachchan**
6ft 0¹/₂in

(AMITABH HARIVANSH)

Born: **October 11, 1942**
Allahabad, British India

Amitabh was the son of Harivansh Rai Bachchan, a well-known Hindi poet, and his wife, Teji – a Sikh from Karachi. She was an actress who had film offers before allowing her maternal instincts to dictate her future. Amitabh was educated at Jhana Prabodhini and Boys' High school in Allahabad and Sherwood College in Nainital. He left the University of Delhi with a BA in science and worked as a freight broker for a shipping firm. After deciding on an acting career, he made his film debut in *Saat Hindustani* and won a 1969 National Film Award as Best Newcomer. He married the actress Jaya Bhadari in 1973 and the couple appeared in films together as well as raising two children. Amitabh became the action-man hero of Bollywood during the 1970s. He went on to receive six Filmfare Best Actor Awards and was nominated for more than twenty other roles. During the shooting of *Coolie,* he narrowly escaped death when he badly injured his intestines during a fight scene. He took a break from movies, got involved with politics and hosted 'Who Wants to Be a Millionaire?' on Indian TV. It helped his comeback in 2003, and he's still a star.

Deewar (1975)
Parvarish (1977)
Jurmana (1979)
Kaala Patthar (1979)
Dostana (1980) Shaan (1980)
Kaalia (1981) Yaarana (1981)
Naseeb (1981) Laawaris (1981)
Silsila (1981) Satte Pe Satta (1982)
Bemisal (1982) Shakti (1982)
Pukar (1983) Mahaan (1983)
Coolie (1983) Sharaabi (1984)
The Last Option (1986)
Main Azaad Hoon (1989)
The Path of Fire (1990)
Hum (1991) Khuda Gawah (1992)
Baghban (2003) Khakee (2004)
Dev (2004) Lakshya (2004)
Deewaar (2004) Black (2005)
Bunty Aur Babli (2005)
Sakar (2005) Eklavya (2007)
The Last Lear (2007)

Alicja **Bachleda**
5ft 7in

(ALICJA BACHLEDA-CURUS)

Born: **May 12, 1983**
Tampico, Tamaulipas, Mexico

The daughter of a Polish mother and a Mexican father, Alicja was taken back to Poland to live in Cracow soon after she was born. She went to the local junior school and even at the age of six, she was displaying a remarkable early talent as a performer – with a special emphasis on singing and reading poetry. She was a hit at children's music festivals and by the age of eleven, she started winning prizes in Cracow, Czestochowa and Tuchola. She began representing her country at music festivals all over Europe – releasing half-a-dozen singles. Alicja also took acting classes and in 1995, made her debut with the female lead in 'Zwierzocziekouplór' – a television movie. Despite all this activity, Alicja didn't neglect her studies - graduating from the General V School in Cracow and also attending advanced classes in Spanish and English. In 1999, Alicja was cast by the legendary film director Andrzej Wajda, in *Pan Tadeusz*. She continued her progress in Polish films and in a popular television series – 'Na dobre i na zie'. In 2004, she made her first foray into foreign films with a trip to Germany to act in *Heart Over Head,* and three years after that, returned there to work for the famous gay director, Marco Kreuzpaintner in his slick comedy drama *Summer Storm*. The film won a number of awards at European festivals. Marco used Alicja's talents again in his highly-praised thriller, *Trade,* which starred Kevin Kline. In one of the final scenes, she did her own stunt – a very high jump. After a German drama, *The Beheaded Rooster,* Alicja traveled to Ireland to star opposite Colin Farrell in Neil Jordan's new film, *Ondine*.

Pan Tadeusz (1999)
The Gateway of Europe (1999)
Syzyfowe prace (2000)
Heart Over Head (2001)
Summer Storm (2004)
Comme des voleurs (2006)
Trade (2007)
The Beheaded Rooster (2007)
Ondine (2008)

Jim **Backus**

5ft 11in

(JAMES GILMORE BACKUS)

Born: **February 25, 1913**
Cleveland, Ohio, USA
Died: **July 3, 1989**

Jim was privately educated. When he was in grade school, his teacher was Margaret Hamilton – later the 'Wicked Witch of the West' in the movie, *The Wizard of Oz.* She didn't have much influence on the boy, whose first step towards a career was to attend the Kentucky Military Institute, in Lyndon. Somebody who did influence him was fellow cadet, Victor Mature. By the time Jim went to the famous University School in Cleveland, he began appearing on the stage. He then studied at the American Academy of Dramatic Arts before using his distinctive voice to get work on the radio. In 1943, he married the actress, Henrietta Kaye. His first movie work was as narrator for a short animated film about the nuclear threat, called *Where Will You Hide?* A year later, in 1949, he made his first screen appearance in the comedy *One Last Fling* and that same year – the first of many, he was Mr. Magoo's voice in *Ragtime Bear.* When he played James Dean's father in *Rebel Without A Cause,* his face was little known. After nearly seventy appearances, the short-sighted Magoo was more famous than Jim, who'd done most of his work as the voice. He died of pneumonia in Los Angeles shortly after finishing work on a 'Bugs Bunny' television show.

Father was a Fullback (1949)
Bright Victory (1951)
His Kind of Woman (1951)
The Man with a Cloak (1951)
I'll See You in My Dreams (1951)
I Want You (1951)
Don't Bother to Knock (1952)
Angel Face (1952)
I Love Melvin (1953)
Rebel Without a Cause (1955)
You Can't Run Away from It (1956)
Ask Any Girl (1959)
Boy's Night Out (1962)
It's a Mad Mad
Mad Mad World (1963)
Crazy Mama (1975)
Peter's Dragon (1977)

Kevin **Bacon**

5ft 11in

(KEVIN NORWOOD BACON)

Born: **July 8, 1958**
Philadelphia, Pennsylvania, USA

Kevin was the youngest of six children. His mother was a teacher, and his father a city planner. All six were taught to be independent, but Kevin soon proved he was thinking even further. He was one of the youngest students ever admitted to Broadway's Circle in the Square Theater School, but even then, it was a hard fight to get where he wanted to be. He waited on tables and took small parts in stage productions. Kevin's film debut in *Animal House,* hardly set the studios clamoring for his signature. He felt uneasy about Hollywood, and for a time, resisted it. In 1982, following his movie role in the hit comedy, *Diner,* things began to look up. Two years later, Kevin starred in the smash-hit, *Footloose,* but he was beginning to be type-cast. In 1988 he married the actress Kyra Sedgwick, who provided him with a couple of lovely children and an unlimited amount of encouragement. Kevin then re-invented himself as a character actor. Starting with *JFK,* in 1991, he has continued to steal the rave reviews from the stars. In 1994 Kevin inspired a trivia game 'Six Degrees of Kevin Bacon' which was played on American college campuses. After some TV work behind the camera, Kevin directed his first movie, *Loverboy* – which starred his wife.

Friday the 13th (1980)
Diner (1982) Footloose (1984)
The Big Picture (1989)
Tremors (1989) JFK (1991)
A Few Good Men (1992)
The River Wild (1994)
Murder in the First (1995)
Apollo 13 (1995)
Telling Lies in America (1997)
Trapped (2002)
Mystic River (2003)
Loverboy (2005)
Where the Truth Lies (2005)
The Air I Breathe (2007)
Death Sentence (2007)
Rails and Ties (2007)
New York, I Love You (2008)
Frost/Nixon (2008)

Fay **Bainter**

5ft 5in

(FAY OKELL BAINTER)

Born: **December 7, 1893**
Los Angeles, California, USA
Died: **April 16, 1968**

Encouraged by her parents, Fay began her acting career at the age of six, when she appeared with stock companies in the Los Angeles area. At eighteen, her effort to take Broadway by storm failed and she returned to California. In 1922, Fay married a career soldier, Reginald Venable, with whom she had a son and would remain with until his death. Experience in summer stock eventually led to a triumphant debut in New York, and by the mid-twenties she was a big Broadway favorite. Fay bided her time before entering the movies – she was forty-three when making her movie debut opposite another stage legend, Lionel Barrymore, in *This Side of Heaven.* In 1938, she won a Best Supporting Actress Oscar for *Jezebel,* and she was narrowly beaten by its star, Bette Davis for the Best Actress Award – Fay's nomination being for *White Banners.* For a decade, she'd featured in some big movies including *Woman of the Year* and *The Secret Life of Walter Mitty,* but by 1950, her screen career slackened off. In a rare later film appearance, Fay was Oscar-nominated for *The Children's Hour,* and she went on working – mainly on TV, until 1965, when she retired. She died of pneumonia, at her home in Los Angeles.

This Side of Heaven (1934)
Quality Street (1937)
Make Way for Tomorrow (1937)
White Banners (1938)
Jezebel (1938)
The Shining Hour (1938)
Young Tom Edison (1940)
Our Town (1940)
Babes on Broadway (1941)
Woman of the Year (1942)
Journey for Margaret (1942)
The Human Comedy (1943)
Presenting Lily Mars (1943)
Dark Waters (1944) State Fair (1945)
Deep Valley (1947)
The Secret Life
of Walter Mitty (1947)
The Children's Hour (1961)

Carroll **Baker**
5ft 5in
(CARROLL BAKER)

Born: May 28, 1931
Johnstown, Pennsylvania, USA

The daughter of William Watson Baker, a traditional travelling salesman, and his wife, Virginia, Carroll worked as a dancer when she left school and then as a very decorative assistant to a magician. Her beauty deserved a little more exposure and in 1949, she was crowned "Miss Florida Fruits and Vegetables". Following an unsuccessful marriage, she set her sights on an acting career. In 1953, she began working in TV commercials, and was studying at New York's Actors Studio. She was given a small role in the Esther Williams musical, *Easy to Love,* which encouraged her to believe that a future lay ahead. Carroll then had a role in the Broadway show "All Summer Long". In the theater audience one night, was the movie director Elia Kazan. He was so impressed, he cast Carroll in the title role of the Tennessee Williams-scripted movie, *Baby Doll,* for which she was nominated for a Best Actress Oscar. That same year, she appeared in James Dean's final film, *Giant.* During a peak period in the 1960s, she starred on Broadway, in Garson Kanin's "Come on Strong". In 1969 she went to live in Europe, where she made several Italian giallo thrillers. In 1978 she starred in Andy Warhol's film *Bad.* Married to an Englishman, Donald Burton, Carroll has published her autobiography which is aptly titled "Baby Doll". Burton passed away in December 2007. Since the film *Nowhere to Go,* in 1998, Carroll has been seen in a few episodes of TV dramas.

Baby Doll (1956)
Giant (1956)
The Big Country (1958)
Station Six-Sahara (1962)
How the West Was Won (1962)
The Carpetbaggers (1964)
Cheyenne Autumn (1964)
Sylvia (1965)
The Greatest
Story Ever Told (1965)
Ironweed (1987)
Kindergarten Cop (1990)
The Game (1997)

Diane **Baker**
5ft 8in
(DIANE CAROL BAKER)

Born: February 25, 1938
Hollywood, California, USA

Having started life right on the doorstep of Filmdom's capital city, Diane began preparing herself for an acting career when she was eighteen. She moved to New York, where she studied drama with Charles Conrad, and ballet with Nina Fonaroff. When she returned to Los Angeles in 1958, she continued her acting education at Estelle Harman's Workshop. Through that exposure, she was offered a contract by 20th Century Fox. One year later, Diane made her film debut in *The Diary of Anne Frank*. In the 1960s she moved to Universal. She was nominated for a Best Supporting Actress Golden Globe for *The Prize,* and she soon had an opportunity to work with Alfred Hitchcock in *Marnie*. At the end of the 1970s, Diane formed Artemis Productions – setting herself up as a producer of independent films – including TV and the movie, *Never Never Land,* which was filmed in Britain in 1980. As an actress, Diane has continued to appear in carefully selected television roles. In 2000 she was highly praised for her portrayal of Rose Kennedy in the CBS mini-series – 'Jackie Bouvier Kennedy Onassis'. In 2005, she appeared in five episodes of the HBO series, 'Unscripted,' which was directed by George Clooney. For three years, Diane has been Director of Acting at the School of Motion Pictures and Television – at the Academy of Art University, in San Francisco. Diane last acted in a movie four years ago, but was seen on TV in 2008, in 'House M.D.'

The Diary of Anne Frank (1959)
Journey to the Center
of the Earth (1959)
The Prize (1963)
Marnie (1964)
Mirage (1965)
Baker's Hawk (1976)
The Silence of the Lambs (1991)
The Cable Guy (1996)
Harrison's Flowers (2000)
A Mighty Wind (2003)
The Keeper: The Legend of
Omar Khayyam (2005)

Joe Don **Baker**
6ft 2½in
(JOE DON BAKER)

Born: February 12, 1936
Groesbeck, Texas, USA

The son of Doyle Charles Baker and his wife, Edna, Joe was studying business administration at North Texas State when he was persuaded to act in a play. After serving two years in the U.S. Army, he studied at the Actors' Studio in New York. He enjoyed an early taste of success when in 1963, he appeared on Broadway in an Actors' Studio production of "Marathon 33". His first professional acting job was in an episode of the TV-series 'Honey West' in 1965. Bit parts in television westerns and an uncredited appearance in the film *Cool Hand Luke* kept Joe employed until his full movie debut in 1969, in *Guns of the Magnificent Seven.* On Christmas day of that year, Joe married Maria Dolores Rivero-Torrens, whom he has since divorced. He was in another western, *Wild Rovers,* but much more importantly, he played Steve McQueen's brother, in *Junior Bonner,* which secured his position as a supporting player – he was then a private detective in Martin Scorsese's *Cape Fear.* His two James Bond films – *GoldenEye* and *Tomorrow Never Dies* are of unusual interest because Joe was actually tested for the starring role (which went to Roger Moore) in *Live and Let Die.*

Wild Rovers (1971)
Junior Bonner (1972)
Walking Tall (1973)
Charley Varrick (1973)
The Outfit (1973)
Framed (1975) **The Pack** (1977)
The Natural (1984)
Fletch (1985)
The Living Daylights (1987)
Cape Fear (1991)
The Distinguished Gentleman (1992)
Reality Bites (1994)
Underneath (1995)
The Grass Harp (1995)
GoldenEye (1995)
Mars Attacks! (1996)
Tomorrow Never Dies (1997)
The Commission (2003)
Strange Wilderness (2008)

Sir Stanley **Baker**
6ft
(WILLIAM STANLEY BAKER)

Born: **February 28, 1928**
Ferndale, Rhondda Valley, UK
Died: **June 28, 1976**

Growing up in a tough Welsh mining area may have contributed to Stanley's on-screen persona. At school Stanley was encouraged to take up acting by the same teacher who had influenced Richard Burton, two years earlier. The two became close friends and drinking companions. When Stanley was sixteen – having just finished secondary school in London, he got a small part in a rather poor Ealing Studios war drama, *Undercover,* which was shot on location near his birthplace. Nevertheless, Stanley developed the acting bug from that experience. After the war ended, he did bits of theater work, and in 1949, got a small uncredited part in an excellent Robert Newton movie, *Obsession.* The film was directed by the black-listed American, Edward Dmytryk, and young Stanley learned a hell of a lot from just being on the set with two such masters of their crafts. His first big break came in 1951, when he had a featured role in the Gregory Peck movie, *Captain Horatio Hornblower R.N.,* and two years later, he firmly established his snarling, unpleasant character, in *The Cruel Sea.* At his best in tough, aggressive roles – especially when playing opposite heroic leading men, he could project a powerful air of menace with a single glance. His later career yielded top performances in *Zulu* and *Accident.* His final film was *Zorro,* in 1975. He died at his home in Màlaga, Spain, of lung cancer and pneumonia.

The Cruel Sea (1953)
Richard III (1955) Hell Drivers (1957)
Yesterday's Enemy (1959)
Hell Is a City (1959)
The Criminal (1960)
The Guns of Navarone (1961)
Eva (1962) A Prize of Arms (1962)
In the French Style (1963)
Zulu (1964) Dingaka (1965)
Sands of the Kalahari (1965)
Accident (1967) Robbery (1967)
Perfect Friday (1970)
Zorro (1970)

Adam **Baldwin**
6ft 4in
(ADAM BALDWIN)

Born: **February 27, 1962**
Chicago, Illinois, USA

Adam, who is no relation to the Baldwin brothers acting dynasty, spent his early years in Chicago. He attended New Trier Township High School in Winnetka, Illinois, which produced several top movie actors – including Ann-Margret, Ralph Bellamy, Bruce Dern, Charlton Heston, Rock Hudson and Virginia Madsen. Adam soon followed the starry alumni into the movie world and was a hit on his debut, in *My Bodyguard* – a small budget production, shot in Chicago by director Tony Bill, who is credited with discovering him. Adam's work in the movie received a lot of praise, but after his next role, a small part in the same year's *Ordinary People,* he had to wait four years for his next opportunity, in the critically panned, *D.C. Cab.* In 1986, after some modest success, he moved to Los Angeles, where he worked as a truck driver while awaiting his big break. It came in the form of a dream role – as "Animal Mother" in Stanley Kubrick's powerful war movie, *Full Metal Jacket.* It establish Adam in Hollywood and led to roles in the high-profile films, *Radio Flyer, Wyatt Earp, Independence Day* and *The Patriot* – among others. He also appeared in some good television series including 'The Cape' and most recently, 'Chuck'. Adam is married to the actress, Ami Julius. They have three children.

My Bodyguard (1980)
Hadley's Rebellion (1984)
Full Metal Jacket (1987)
The Chocolate War (1988)
Cohen and Tate (1989)
Predator 2 (1990)
Radio Flyer (1992)
Where the Day Takes You (1992)
Wyatt Earp (1994)
Independence Day (1996)
The Patriot (2000)
Jackpot (2001)
Double Bang (2001)
The Keyman (2002)
Serenity (2005)
Gospel Hill (2008)
Drillbit Taylor (2008)

Alec **Baldwin**
6ft 1in
(ALEXANDER RAE BALDWIN III)

Born: **April 3, 1958**
Massapequa, Long Island, USA

One of six children from a Catholic family, Alec is best known of the four Baldwin brothers – who are all actors. They all went to Alfred G. Berner High School, where Alec and the youngest, Daniel, were coached at football by Hall of Famer, Bob Reifsnyder. In 1979, Alec attended New York University. Then, after a break to study acting at the Lee Strasberg Theater Institute, he graduated in 1994. For two years, until 1982, he was a regular in the daytime soap 'The Doctors' and two years after that, he achieved national prominence through his role in 'Knots Landing'. He made his movie debut in 1987, in *Forever Lulu,* and followed up with several good roles in successful films such as *Beetle Juice* and *Married to the Mob.* In 1991 he met Kim Basinger when they co-starred in *The Marrying Man.* He married her, and it lasted until 2000, when they divorced after a protracted legal battle. In 2004, he was nominated for a Best Supporting Actor Oscar for *The Cooler.* Alec is said to fancy a career in politics when he quits acting. His criticism of the Bush administration provided newspapers with many column inches. If his present good run – including *The Departed, The Good Shepherd* and *Lymelife* continues, it'll be a while before he does so.

Beetle Juice (1988)
Married to the Mob (1988)
The Hunt for Red October (1990)
Glengarry Glen Ross (1992)
Malice (1993) The Shadow (1994)
Ghosts of Mississippi (1996)
Pearl Harbor (2001)
The Cooler (2003)
Along Came Polly (2004)
Elizabethtown (2005)
Mini's First Time (2006)
The Departed (2006)
Running with Scissors (2006)
The Good Shepherd (2006)
Suburban Girl (2007)
Brooklyn Rules (2007) Lymelife (2008)
My Best Friend's Girl (2008)
My Sister's Keeper (2009)

Christian **Bale**
6ft 1¼in
(CHRISTIAN CHARLES PHILIP BALE)

Born: **January 30, 1974**
Haverfordwest, Pembroke, Wales

Christian's mother worked as a circus clown. The youngest of four children, he left Wales with his family when he was two. Because of their father's job as a commercial pilot, they lived in several countries before settling for a time in Bournemouth, where at school he took an active interest in junior rugby. When he was eight, Christian acted in a television commercial, and in 1984, made his West End stage debut in "The Nerd" which starred Rowan Atkinson. Christian's father became his manager and in 1986, he appeared in a film made for television, 'Anastasia: The Mystery of Anna'. His co-star, Amy Irving was married to Steven Spielberg, and she helped the thirteen-year-old get his movie career under way with an important role in *Empire of the Sun*. Initially, he was overcome by the attention he received and considered giving up. Two years later, director Kenneth Branagh changed his mind by offering him a part in *Henry V.* Disney work followed, and by the time Wynona Ryder insisted that he starred in *Little Women* he was a veteran. As an adult his acting skills, good looks and personality have won him many fans. In 2008, Christian shared the Robert Altman Award with nine others for *I'm Not There.* Since 2000, he's been married to the actress, Sibi Blazic. The couple have a daughter named Emmaline.

Empire of the Sun (1987)
Newsies (1992) **Swing Kids** (1993)
Prince of Jutland (1994)
Little Women (1994)
The Portrait of a Lady (1996)
Metroland (1997) **Velvet Goldmine** (1998)
American Psycho (2000) **Laurel**
Canyon (2002) **Equilibrium** (2002)
El Maquinista (2004)
Harsh Times (2005) **Batman**
Begins (2005) **The New**
World (2005) **Rescue Dawn** (2006)
The Prestige (2006) **3:10 to Yuma** (2007)
I'm Not There (2007)
The Dark Knight (2008)
Public Enemies (2009)

Lucille **Ball**
5ft 6in
(LUCILLE DÉSIRÉE BALL)

Born: **August 6, 1911**
Jamestown, New York, USA
Died: **April 26, 1989**

Lucy's father was Henry Ball, a telephone lineman. Her mother, Desiree was known as "DeDe". Lucy appeared in amateur theater productions when she was a little girl. Her grandfather took her to vaudeville shows and encouraged her to take part in school plays. At fifteen, Lucy attended a drama school, but she didn't like it, so she took to the road. By the time she was twenty, she'd become a Hattie Carnegie model. In 1933, with some of the other girls, she went to Hollywood to appear in the Samuel Goldwyn movie *Roman Scandals*. Goldwyn gave her a contract, then sacked her. She wasn't much luckier at Columbia, and for three years, the parts were all but invisible. A recommendation from Ginger Rogers, whose mother was Lucille's drama coach, turned the tide. It resulted in a decent role in *Stage Door,* which led to a series of better and bigger parts. When she was filming *Too Many Girls* in 1940, she met the Cuban band-leader Desi Arnaz and they married that same year. Lucy could act seriously, as proved in the film noir, *The Dark Corner,* but it wasn't really in her nature. She was soon the funniest woman to be seen on the screen (including – starting in 1951 with a hit television show – 'I Love Lucy'). Although Lucy was really quite pretty, she got lots of laughs (especially on television) through her unique facial contortions and her vocal reactions. Lucy died in Beverly Hills, from acute aorta aneurism.

Stage Door (1937)
Room Service (1938)
The Joy of Living (1938)
The Big Street (1942)
Dubarry was a Lady (1943)
Ziegfeld Follies (1946)
The Dark Corner (1946)
Lured (1947)
Fancy Pants (1950)
The Fuller Brush Girl (1950)
The Long Long Trailer (1953)
The Facts of Life (1960)
Mame (1974)

Martin **Balsam**
5ft 7in
(MARTIN HENRY BALSAM)

Born: **November 4, 1919**
The Bronx, New York City, New York, USA
Died: **Febuary 13, 1996**

Marty was the eldest of three children born to Jewish parents, Albert and Lillian Balsam. He was in the drama club at DeWitt High School and studied at New York's New School until he was twenty. World War II interrupted his acting career and he served in the Army Air Corps. From 1947, he was selected by Elia Kazan to train at the famous Actors' Studio, and in 1949, appeared in a series of dramas produced by the studio for television. Marty really started to get regular work when Lee Strasberg took over in 1952. Through Elia Kazan and method actors he befriended such as Marlon Brando and Rod Steiger, Marty, appeared in significant films, beginning with his debut in the Kazan-directed classic *On the Waterfront.* For the next forty years, he proved a totally reliable man to have on the set. In 1959, he married the actress, Joyce Van Patten, but they divorced four years later. Their daughter, Talia, is an actress. Marty won a Best Supporting Actor Oscar for *A Thousand Clowns.* Two years later, he won a Tony Award for 'You Know I Can't Hear You When the Water's Running'. Marty married Irene Miller in 1963, and they were happy together until his sudden death from a heart attack, in Rome, Italy.

On the Waterfront (1954)
12 Angry Men (1957)
Time Limit (1957)
Al Capone (1959)
Psycho (1960)
Breakfast at Tiffany's (1961)
Cape Fear (1962)
Seven Days in May (1964)
The Carpetbaggers (1964)
The Bedford Incident (1965)
A Thousand Clowns (1965)
Hombre (1967)
The Anderson Tapes (1971)
The Taking of Pelham
One Two Three (1974)
All the President's Men (1976)
The Delta Force (1986)
Cape Fear (1991)

Eric **Bana**
6ft 3in
(ERIC BANADINOVICH)

Born: August 9, 1968
Melbourne, Victoria, Australia

The youngest of two brothers, Eric's father, Ivan, was a Croatian who worked as a logistics manager for Caterpillar Inc. His mother Eleanor, a hairdresser, was born in Germany. By the age of seven, Eric showed precocious talent as a mimic. To start off he impersonated family members and later he had his classmates in an uproar when he mimicked his teachers. He decided to become an actor after he saw the movie *Mad Max,* but did nothing about it until he was twenty-three, when he became a stand-up comic in bars and pubs. After two years of hard work, he was invited on to Steve Vizard's 'Tonight Live' and stayed for four years. By 1996 he was hosting his own comedy sketch series, 'The Eric Bana Show'. It failed and was withdrawn after eight episodes, but Eric turned his attention to films, making his debut in the Australian hit comedy, *The Castle.* That year, he married Rebecca Gleeson, the daughter of an Australian High Court Chief Justice. They have since had two children. Following more television exposure, Eric was approached to play a serious role – as the legendary psychopathic criminal Mark "Chopper" Read in *Chopper.* It won him an Australian Film Institute Award and a 'Best Actor' at the Stockholm Film Festival. Its success was a breakthrough for Eric – landing him a top role in Ridley Scott's *Black Hawk Down,* an action drama filmed in Morocco. He has recently won a second AFI Award as Best Lead Actor in *Romulus, My Father.* In the early part of the new millennium Eric was a regular in the Australian TV series, 'Something in the Air'.

The Castle (1997)
Chopper (2000)
Black Hawk Down (2001)
The Nugget (2002)
Hulk (2003) Troy (2004)
Munich (2005) Lucky You (2007)
Romulus, My Father (2007)
The Other Boleyn Girl (2008)
Star Trek (2009)
The Time Traveler's Wife (2009)

Ann **Bancroft**
5ft 8in
(ANNA MARIA ITALIANO)

Born: September 17, 1931
The Bronx, New York City, New York, USA
Died: **June 6, 2005**

It wasn't until she was persuaded to appear in a high school play, that Anne even considered an acting career. One of her teachers was so impressed, he arranged an audition for a part in the television dramatization of 'Torrents of Spring' by Turgenev. She got the part and did well enough to be given a role in the TV soap opera 'The Goldbergs', where she used the name Anne Marno. She accepted an offer of a contract from 20th Century Fox and in 1952, made her movie debut as a cabaret singer in *Don't Bother to Knock.* A dozen films later, with no stardom in sight (despite some favorable reviews) she turned her back on Hollywood. Working in the theater gave her new confidence. She was thought to be perfect as a Jewish girl in 'Two for the See-Saw'. And the reviews (and a second Tony) for her part as Helen Keller's mother in 'The Miracle Worker', made her essential for the movie version – for which she won a Best Actress Oscar. She proved an equally good actress in comedy and drama and will be remembered for her seductive Mrs. Robinson in *The Graduate.* She was Oscar-nominated for that role, as well as for *The Pumpkin Eater* and *The Turning Point.* Anne married Mel Brooks (whom she met on a TV chat show in 1964) and converted to Judaism. They had one son, Max, who was born in 1971. Ann died from uterine cancer, at her home in New York.

The Miracle Worker (1962)
The Pumpkin Eater (1964)
The Graduate (1967)
The Prisoner of
Second Avenue (1975)
The Turning Point (1977)
To Be or Not to Be (1983)
Agnes of God (1985)
'Night Mother (1986)
84 Charing Cross Road (1987)
Malice (1993)
Home for the Holidays (1995)
Critical Care (1997)
Heartbreakers (2001)

Antonio **Banderas**
5ft 9in
(JOSÉ ANTONIO DOMINGUES BANDERAS)

Born: August 10, 1960
Málaga, Andalusia, Spain

He was brought up in a typical Spanish Catholic family – his father José was a policeman in the Guardia Civil, and his mother, Ana was a schoolteacher. As a boy, Antonio was soccer mad and is still remembered as a young player of great promise. In fact he only gave up his dream of a professional career when he broke his leg at the age of fourteen. When he was eighteen, he moved to Madrid, to try his luck in the Spanish film industry. He got his first movie role in 1982, and that same year, began a fruitful collaboration with the director, Pedro Almodóvar. For . seven years, his reputation grew until a major world-wide hit called *Tie Me Up! Tie Me Down!* enabled him to make the move to Hollywood. In 1996 Antonio divorced his Spanish wife, and married the American actress Melanie Griffith, with whom he has a daughter. He was nominated for Golden Globes for *Evita* and *The Mask of Zorro.* In 2003 Antonio made a critically successful Broadway appearance in the hit musical, "Nine" – which was based on Fellini's $8^{1}/_{2}$ – and he was nominated for a Tony. His effort at directing, a 1999 film starring his wife, called *Crazy in Alabama,* failed. But Antonio's a positive guy and in 2006, he tried again, with *El Camino de los ingleses* – which was better. On the acting front, maybe the batch of movies in production, including the crime drama – *Thick as Thieves* and his portrayal of the Spanish painter, *Dali,* will produce the hit he needs.

Pestanos postizas (1982)
Women on the Verge of a
Nervous Breakdown (1988)
The Mambo Kings (1992)
Philadelphia (1993)
Desperado (1995) Evita (1996)
The Mask of Zorro (1998)
Frida (2002) Once Upon a
Time in Mexico (2003)
Imagining Argentina (2003)
The Legend of Zorro (2005)
Take the Lead (2006)
Bordertown (2006)
The Other Man (2008)

Tallulah **Bankhead**
5ft 3in
(TALLULAH BROCKMAN BANKHEAD)

Born: **January 31, 1902**
Huntsville, Alabama, USA
Died: **December 12, 1968**

Tallulah was the daughter of Democratic politician, William Bankhead, and his wife Adelaide – who died of blood poisoning three weeks after giving birth to her. A decision to send her to the Convent of the Sacred Heart, in New York, was a bit strange considering that her mother had been Episcopalian and her father was a Methodist. Four schools later, she finished her education anyway. At fifteen, Tallulah won a beauty contest run by Picture Play film magazine and persuaded her dad to let her go and live in New York. She made her stage debut at the Bijou Theater, with a bit part in "The Squab Farm". Tallulah's theatrical career took off after she moved to England in 1923. After making her West End debut at Wyndham's Theater, in "The Dancers", she acquired a reputation for both her acting skills and her countless lovers. After eight years in London, she returned to New York City and in tandem with a brief new film career, starting with *Tarnished Lady,* she conquered Broadway. She quickly became bored with movies and its people. After 1932, her life was one big series of parties and affairs – there were suggestions that she swung both ways. She still worked in the theater, was rejected by David O. Selznick after a poor screen test for *Gone with the Wind* and made two more films after a twelve-year absence from the screen – one of which, Alfred Hitchcock's *Lifeboat,* won her the New York Film Critics Circle Award. In the 1950s she returned to the stage. Her last appearances were in two 1967 episodes of the television series 'Batman'. Tallulah, a heavy drinker and smoker all her adult life, died in New York of pneumonia and influenza, complicated by emphysema.

Tarnished Lady (1931)
My Sin (1931) **The Cheat** (1931)
Devil and the Deep (1932)
Faithless (1932)
Lifeboat (1944)
A Royal Scandal (1945)
Fanatic (1965)

Ian **Bannen**
6ft 2in
(IAN BANNEN)

Born: **June 29, 1928**
Airdrie, Lanarkshire, Scotland
Died: **November 3, 1999**

Ian's father was a successful lawyer who was hoping his son would follow him into the profession. Until he was eighteen, he attended Ratcliffe College boarding school in Leicestershire. He did eighteen months National Service in the Army before he began his stage career in Dublin in 1947. From there he went to London, where he made a name for himself. Ian's film debut was in 1950, when he had a small role in *Pool of London,* and it was six years before he had his first featured role – in the comedy *Private's Progress.* In 1960, he became a member of Peter Hall's Royal Shakespeare Company. He worked in British films up until 1964, and in 1965, he was nominated for a Best Supporting Actor Oscar for *The Flight of the Phoenix.* In 1971, he was cast to replace Alan Bates in *Sunday Bloody Sunday,* but couldn't cope with the homosexual nature of the role. His replacement in that film, Peter Finch, was nominated for an Oscar. Ian's career continued with supporting roles in some big films, and he worked steadily on stage and TV. In 1995, he was given a BAFTA Lifetime Achievement Award. Ian had just finished work on his final two movies, in 1999, when he was killed in a car accident near Loch Ness.

A Tale of Two Cities (1958)
The Hill (1965)
The Fight of the Phoenix (1965)
Too Late the Hero (1970)
The Offence (1972)
Bite the Bullet (1975)
Sweeney (1977)
Gorky Park (1983)
Defence of the Realm (1985)
Circles in the Forest (1990)
Speaking of the Devil (1991)
Damage (1992)
Braveheart (1995)
Something to Believe in (1998)
Waking Ned (1998)
To Walk with Lions (1999)
The Testimony of
Taliesin Jones (2000)

Javier **Bardem**
6ft
(JAVIER ÁNGEL ENCINAS BARDEM)

Born: **March 1, 1969**
Las Palmas de Gran Canaria, Spain

The son of Carlos Encinas and the actress Pilar Bardem, Javier came from a long line of actors and filmmakers who were active since the early days of Spanish cinema. His older brother and sister continued the tradition with Javier not far behind. When he was six years old, he made his film debut in *El Pícaro* and was regularly seen in TV-series as he grew older. His interest turned to sport in his teens when he was good enough for the Spanish junior rugby fifteen. He was twenty when he made his first movie as an adult – *Las Edades de Lulú* and together with Penélope Cruz, was in the international success, *Jamón, jamón* – two years later. He became a star worldwide after his appearance as the Cuban poet, Reinaldo Arenas, in Julian Schnabel's *Before Night Falls.* It was his first English language role and he received an Oscar nomination – as Best Actor. In 2004, Javier was voted Best Actor at the Venice Film Festival for *The Sea Inside.* A cameo in Tom Cruise's *Collateral,* that same year was followed by a quieter spell – leading to his towering performance as the ruthless killer, in *No Country for Old Men.* He was unanimously judged to be the year's Best Supporting Actor with a Golden Globe, a BAFTA, a Critics' Choice Award and an Oscar. Since appearing with Penélope Cruz in *Vicky Cristina Barcelona,* the two have become close.

Las Edades de Lulú (1990)
Tacones lejanos (1991)
Amo tu cama rica (1992) **Jamón,
jamón** (1992) El Amante bilingüe (1993)
Golden Balls (1993) **The Detective
and Death** (1994) **Numbered Days** (1994)
La Madre (1995) **Ecstasy** (1996)
Live Flesh (1997) Entre las piernas (1999)
Second Skin (1999) **Before Night
Falls** (2000) **The Dancer Upstairs** (2002)
Los Lunes al sol (2002)
Collateral (2004)
The Sea Inside (2004)
Goya's Ghosts (2006)
No Country for Old Men (2007)
Vicky Cristina Barcelona (2008)

Brigitte **Bardot**
5ft 7in
(BRIGITTE BARDOT)

Born: **September 28, 1934**
Paris, France

Born in a luxurious apartment close to the River Seine, Brigitte enjoyed all the privileges provided by her wealthy Roman Catholic family. Her mother had at one time dreamed of a theatrical career, and perhaps as an outlet for her own disappointment, she encouraged Brigitte to take ballet lessons. A sister was born just as the war was starting and the family lived through five years of German occupation. Brigitte was not pretty or popular as a little girl. She was skinny, wore spectacles and a brace on her teeth. In her teens, her outlet was dancing. In 1947, Brigitte was accepted at the National Conservatory of Music and Dance. Her mother then opened a fashion boutique, which was around the time that Brigitte blossomed into a chic beauty. At fifteen, she featured in a fashion show, and a year later, appeared in the magazines Elle and Jardin des Modes. Her photo was seen by the director Marc Allegret, and she was given a screen test (which she failed) in the presence of young Roger Vadim, who she fell for. Brigitte married him in 1952 and he sent her to acting classes before she made her film debut in that year's *Le Trou Normand*. With Roger's help, her career took off – along with most of her clothes – in films like *And God Created Woman* and *The Night Heaven Fell*. Brigitte was always a rather limited actress, but her popularity outlasted her career. She lives with her fourth husband, Bernard d'Ormale and various pets, near the resort of St. Tropez, in the south of France.

Les Grande manoeuvres (1955)
Cette sacré gamine (1955)
Mi figlio Nerone (1956)
Et Dieu créa la femme (1956)
La Parisienne (1957)
The Night Heaven Fell (1958)
En cas de malheur (1958)
Babette Goes to War (1959)
Come Dance With Me! (1959)
La Vérité (1960)
Le Mépris (1963)
Viva Maria! (1965)

Lynn **Bari**
5ft 7in
(MARGARET SCHUYLER FISHER)

Born: **December 18, 1917**
Roanoke, Virginia, USA
Died: **November 20, 1989**

Known for much of her early life as Peggy, she was the second child born to John and Marjorie Fisher – her brother John having arrived three years earlier. When their father, who had worked in the automotive industry, died in 1925, the two young children were taken by their widowed mother to live in Boston. Two years later, she remarried, and in 1928, Peggy's new stepfather took the family to Los Angeles where she went to the Horace Mann Grade School and then Beverly Vista High. When she was fifteen, and looking for a summer job, she saw an ad seeking tall showgirls to appear in a Joan Crawford musical for MGM, known as *Dancing Lady*. Peggy got a part in the chorus and changed her name to Lynn Bari. Two bit parts later, she was signed by Fox. She completed her education at the studio school while playing small roles in movies. She got her first featured part in 1938 in *Mr. Moto's Gamble,* and that year, played the 'other woman' in a film with Barbara Stanwyck. She featured in strong supporting roles in big films such as *Blood and Sand, Sun Valley Serenade* and *Orchestra Wives,* but true stardom proved elusive. She married Walter Kane, an aide to Howard Hughes, but it didn't change Lynn's status. Her second husband, Sid Luft, ended up as a Mr. Judy Garland. During World War II, she was just behind Betty Grable as the Armed Forces favorite pin-up. Lynn was on TV for fifteen years – ending her career in 1968, in the movie, *The Young Runaways*. She died of a heart attack, at her home in Santa Barbara.

The Great Ziegfeld (1936)
Blood and Sand (1941)
Sun Valley Serenade (1941)
The Magnificent Dope (1942)
Orchestra Wives (1942)
Home, Sweet Homicide (1946)
Margie (1946)
Has Anybody Seen My Gal? (1952)
I Dream of Jeanie (1952)
Damn Citizen (1958)

Ellen **Barkin**
5ft 7in
(ELLEN RONA BARKIN)

Born: **April 16, 1954**
The Bronx, New York City, New York, USA

Ellen grew up in a middle-class Jewish home and had a happy childhood. Her student years were spent at the High School of the Performing Arts, Hunter's College, where she received degrees in history and drama, and the Actor's Studio. She studied acting for seven years before stage work in mostly off-Broadway plays, and a good part in a 1981 television soap opera, 'Search for Tomorrow' helped get her movie debut, in *Diner*. She had some great notices for her role as a neglected wife, and it led to more of the same. She often played the kind of woman who ended up with the wrong kind of man. Sadly for her, in real life, this also appears to be the case. Her two marriages ended in divorce. The first to the Irish actor Gabriel Byrne, whom she met when filming *Siesta* in 1987 – the year she made one of her best movies – *Sea of Love*. Byrne left her with two children to raise, but she battled on. In 1992, Ellen was nominated for a Best Actress Golden Globe award for the top comedy/musical, 'Switch'. A six-year marriage to Ronald Perelman, a wealthy businessman, ended in 2006. For a few years, things had gone very quiet for Ellen, but recently she's been getting a few nice juicy supporting roles in A-List movies such as *Ocean's Thirteen*.

Diner (1982)
Harry & Son (1984)
Desert Bloom (1986)
Down by Law (1986)
The Big Easy (1987)
Siesta (1987)
Johnny Handsome (1989)
Sea of Love (1989)
Switch (1991)
Mac (1992)
This Boy's Life (1993)
Wild Bill (1995)
The Fan (1996)
Drop Dead Gorgeous (1999)
Mercy (2000)
Palindromes (2004)
Trust the Man (2005)
Ocean's Thirteen (2007)

Binnie **Barnes**
5ft 5in
(GITTEL ENOYCE BARNES)

Born: May 25, 1903
Islington, London, England
Died: July 27, 1998

Leaving school at fifteen, Binnie worked for a local dairy and even helped to deliver the milk. She then trained as a nurse, but gave it up in order to concentrate on an acting career. Binnie was spotted by comedian, Stanley Lupino (Ida's father), who employed her in a series of short films. In 1929, she made her stage debut with Charles Laughton and, after her film debut in *A Night in Montmartre* was one of his wives, Katherine Howard – in *The Private Life of Henry VIII*. Binnie began to get bigger roles and (in his final film) she acted with Doug Fairbanks Senior in *The Private Life of Don Juan*. Binnie went to Hollywood and played Lillian Russell in *Diamond Jim* the following year, before supporting big stars including Jeanette MacDonald, Nelson Eddy, Cary Grant and Katherine Hepburn. In 1940 she married producer, Mitchell Frankovich. One of their sons became a screenwriter. At the end of World War II, they moved to Italy where her voice was dubbed in films, including the popular *Pirates of Capri*. Binnie retired from movies in 1954, but reappeared in a few of her husband's productions. Finally in 1973 – in *40 Carats* – with Gene Kelly in the line-up. Binnie worked for charities until her death from natural causes, at her home in Beverly Hills.

The Private Life of Henry VIII (1933)
Diamond Jim (1935)
Small Town Girl (1936)
The Last of the Mohicans (1936)
Magnificent Brute (1936)
Three Smart Girls (1936)
Broadway Melody of 1938 (1937)
Holiday (1938) **Always Goodbye** (1938)
The Three Musketeers (1939)
Man About Town (1939)
Frontier Marshal (1939)
Day-Time Wife (1939)
'Til We Meet Again (1940)
This Thing Called Love (1940)
Three Girls About Town (1941)
Skylark (1941)
The Spanish Main (1945)

Drew **Barrymore**
5ft 4in
(DREW BLYTH BARRYMORE)

Born: February 22, 1975
Culver City, California, USA

The daughter of John Drew Barrymore, she has a pedigree background, with Lionel, John, and Ethel as relatives. Her career began before her first birthday, when she appeared in a dog commercial and was bitten by its star. She had her first movie role in *Altered States,* when she was four. A year later, Drew shot to fame as Gertie, in *E.T. the Extra-Terrestrial.* In 1984 she was nominated for a Golden Globe as Best Supporting Actress in *Irreconcilable Differences.* As a nine-year-old kid, the fame went to her head. She started drinking, smoking marijuana and snorting cocaine, which brought a virtual halt to her career. In 1990, she published her autobiography "Little Girl Lost". She had her first adult role in 1992, in *Poison Ivy.* Later, in the January 1995 issue of Playboy, Drew appeared nude – and was undressed in five movies around that time. In 1996, she made a serious comeback in the popular horror film, *Scream.* Since then, things have continued on an upward path for her. Drew has had success with several action thrillers, horror films, and romantic comedies. She now runs her own production company, Flower Films. In 2002, she featured in *Confessions of a Dangerous Mind* – which marked George Clooney's directorial debut. A recent film, *Music and Lyrics* is a good example of Drew's adult charm and her confidence with romantic comedy.

E.T. the Extra-Terrestrial (1982)
Firestarter (1984)
Boys on the Side (1995)
Scream (1996)
Charlie's Angels (2000)
Donny Darko (2001)
Confessions of a Dangerous Mind (2002)
Duplex (2003)
50 First Dates (2004)
Fever Pitch (2005)
Music and Lyrics (2007)
Lucky You (2007)
He's Just Not That Into You (2009)

Ethel **Barrymore**
5ft 7in
(ETHEL MAE BLYTH)

Born: August 15, 1879
Philadelphia, Pennsylvania, USA
Died: June 18, 1959

Ethel was the second of three children destined for a life in the theater. Her father, Maurice Blyth, was an immigrant from England who married Georgina Drew of Philadelphia. Both were actors, who together joined Augustin Daly's New York company and performed with most of the great names of the English and American Victorian theater. Despite this influence, Ethel originally planned a career as a concert pianist. She changed her mind and made her stage debut in 1894 and became a big star on both sides of the Atlantic. She married in 1909 and had three children, but it hardly interrupted her stage work. In 1914, Ethel made her first movie *The Nightingale* – but it was the theater she truly loved. She also worked for the Actors Equity Union. By 1930 her film roles reflected the fact that she was fifty, but influenced by the success of her brothers in the medium, she really came into her own when she was of pensionable age. In 1944 she won the Best Supporting Actress Oscar for her role as Cary Grant's mother in *None But the Lonely Heart.* Some of her later efforts – especially *The Spiral Staircase, Pinky,* and *Young at Heart,* are superior. In 1955, she published her charming autobiography "Memories". She retired in 1957, after starring in a modest film called *Johnny Trouble.* Ethel lived quietly until eighteen months later, when she died of a heart condition, at her home in Beverly Hills.

Rasputin and the Empress (1932)
None But the Lonely Heart (1944)
The Spiral Staircase (1946)
The Farmer's Daughter (1947)
The Paradine Case (1947)
Moonrise (1948)
Portrait of Jennie (1948)
The Great Sinner (1949)
Pinky (1949)
The Secret of Convict Lake (1951)
The Story of Three Loves (1953)
Young at Heart (1954)

John **Barrymore**
5ft 9in
(JOHN SIDNEY BLYTH BARRYMORE)

Born: **February 15, 1882**
Philadelphia, Pennsylvania, USA
Died: **May 29, 1942**

The youngest of the three Barrymore children, John achieved greater fame (and infamy) than his two competitive siblings. When he was a young man, he went with his sister to study at the *Beaux Arts* in Paris – they both thought of becoming painters or journalists. John was the first to tread the boards – establishing himself as a leading actor of his generation in 1909 in "The Fortune Hunter". After John made his movie debut in 1913, in *An American Citizen,* he signed for Famous Players. Continuing to work in the theater, including a famous stage "Hamlet" and films, his fame grew, but so did his heavy drinking. He moved to Hollywood in 1925, where even the fact that he was in his early forties did not distract from his star rating, his huge salary and his opulent lifestyle. By 1927 he had come top of the first U.S. box-office survey, and his salary from United Artists was $150,000 per film. He made his first talkie, *General Crack,* for Warner Bros., but moved to MGM, where Lionel was already a star. By the late 1930s, he looked old and overweight, like the broken-down drunks he played on screen. His long period of popularity and huge earnings made it very hard to understand why the 'Great Profile' was virtually penniless when he died of cirrhosis of the liver. Perhaps it was the alimony paid to his quartet of wives – his fourth divorce was eighteen months before his death.

Svengali (1931)
The Mad Genius (1931)
Grand Hotel (1932)
A Bill of Divorcement (1932)
Rasputin and the Empress (1932)
Topaze (1933)
Dinner at Eight (1933)
Counsellor-at-Law (1933)
Twentieth Century (1934)
Romeo and Juliet (1936)
Maytime (1937)
The Great Man Votes (1939)
Midnight (1939)
The Invisible Woman (1940)

Lionel **Barrymore**
5ft 11in
(LIONEL HERBERT BLYTH BARRYMORE)

Born: **April 28, 1878**
Philadelphia, Pennsylvania, USA
Died: **November 15, 1954**

Lionel began his stage career in 1903. After several years living in Paris, where he studied painting, he made his film debut in 1911, for Biograph, in *Fighting Blood*. He went to Broadway in 1917, and carved out a big career on the stage with highly-rated performances in many of the classic plays. By the time the talkies started, Lionel had already acted in around 130 films – many of them shorts. A part talkie *The Lion and the Mouse* was the first time audiences had heard his voice. In 1931, he won a Best Actor Oscar for his role as alcoholic Defense Attorney Stephen Ashe, in *A Free Soul.* The previous year he had also been nominated, as Best Director, for *Madame X.* He appeared only once with *both* Ethel and John, in the film *Rasputin and the Empress,* and with John in four other movies. Lionel never re-married after his second wife's death in 1936. He acted from a wheelchair after breaking his hip following a bad fall in 1937 – including his role as Dr. Gillespie in ten movies. From 1946 he wrote classical-style pieces of music, including a one-act opera. He also wrote a novel – "Mr. Cantomwine". In 1944, he and Ethel became the first Oscar winning brother and sister. He made his final film *Lone Star,* in 1952. His retirement was a short one – he died of a heart attack less than two years later.

A Free Soul (1931)
Broken Lullaby (1932)
Grand Hotel (1932)
Dinner at Eight (1933)
Treasure Island (1934)
David Copperfield (1935)
The Little Colonel (1935)
Ah Wilderness! (1935) The Road to
Glory (1936) Camille (1936)
Captains Courageous (1937)
A Yank at Oxford (1938)
You Can't Take It With You (1938)
A Guy Named Joe (1943)
It's a Wonderful Life (1946)
Duel in the Sun (1946)
Key Largo (1948)

Freddie **Bartholomew**
5ft
(FREDERICK LLEWELLYN MARCH)

Born: **March 28, 1924**
Dublin, Ireland
Died: **January 23, 1992**

Freddie's Irish parents were so poor, they abandoned him when he was two years old. His mother took him to London to live with her sister, Millicent Bartholomew. Millicent gave him her surname and encouraged him to appear in school plays. She paid for his acting classes at the Italia Conti School, where he showed sufficient promise to get bit parts in English films. A message was sent to David O. Selznick who, after refusing MGM's selection of American actors, was in Britain casting the young lead for his planned film of Charles Dickens' *David Copperfield.* Eventually, after difficulties due to British government restrictions on child actors, Freddie was taken to Hollywood by his aunt and was a highly-paid star following the success of that film. He was given a seven year contract, but after playing Garbo's son in *Anna Karenina,* he was loaned out to other studios. His success resulted in his parents attempting to gain custody of him. Movies like *Captains Courageous* earned big money, but the legal battle raged for three years – and much of his fortune was wasted on lawyer's fees. As he reached his teens, he lost his appeal at the box-office. In 1944, he served in the United States Air Force. There was little interest in him after that, and by 1950, he decided against an adult career and was working in advertising. Freddie lived in peaceful retirement in Sarasota, Florida, until dying of emphysema.

David Copperfield (1935)
Anna Karenina (1935)
Professional Soldier (1935)
Little Lord Fauntleroy (1936)
The Devil is a Sissy (1936)
Lloyd's of London (1936)
Captains Courageous (1937)
Kidnapped (1938)
Lord Jeff (1938)
Listen, Darling (1938)
Swiss Family Robinson (1940)
Tom Brown's Schooldays (1940)
A Yank at Eton (1942)

Mischa **Barton**
5ft 8½in
(MISCHA ANNE MARSDEN BARTON)

Born: **January 24, 1986**
Hammersmith, London, England

Mischa's father, Paul Barton, was a foreign exchange broker in London. Her mother, Nuala, who was Irish, worked as a photographer. Along with her two sisters, Mischa was taken to live in New York City when she was four years old. She began acting when she was eight – in an off-Broadway production of Tony Kushner's "Slavs". Mischa appeared in other stage plays before attending the Professional Children's School in Manhattan – from where she graduated in 2004. She was by then a seasoned veteran of plays and films. She made her movie debut in the award winning, *Lawn Dogs* and then appeared in small roles in hits such as *Notting Hill, The Sixth Sense,* and *Lost and Delirious.* She worked as a model during that period – in ads for Calvin Klein and Neutrogena skincare products among several others. In 2003, Mischa reached a huge audience in the Fox TV drama series, 'The O.C'. It lifted her to potential star status and she helped make that happen by attending classes at The Royal Academy of Dramatic Art, in the summer of 2006. While she was there, Mischa appeared on British television as a guest host on 'The Friday Night Project'. After returning to America she played the role of Marissa Cooper in the TV comedy drama, 'The O.C.' In 2006 she won the Teen Choice Award for her acting in the show. She was soon back on the movie track in *The Oh in Ohio, Closing the Ring* and more recently, a starring role in the highly-rated comedy, *Assassination of a High School President.*

Lawn Dogs (1997)
Notting Hill (1999) **The Sixth Sense** (1999) **Skipped Parts** (2000)
Lost and Delirious (2001)
Julie Johnson (2001)
The Oh in Ohio (2006)
Closing the Ring (2007)
St.Trinian's (2007)
Assassination of a High School President (2008)
You and I (2008)
Walled In (2009)

Richard **Basehart**
5ft 9in
(JOHN RICHARD BASEHART)

Born: **August 31, 1914**
Zanesville, Ohio, USA
Died: **September 17, 1984**

Before leaving high school, Richard set out to be a newspaper reporter like his father, who was editor of the Zanesville Ohio Times. By the early 1930s, America was experiencing a bad recession which made it difficult to get a job. Richard had begun acting when he was only thirteen – appearing with the local Wright Players Stock Company – so, being a realistic man, he turned his attention to the stage – transferring to Philadelphia, where he joined the Hedgerow Theater Company. After six years, he went to New York, where he quickly made an impact in the play, "Counterattack". In 1945, his convincing portrayal of a young Scotsman in "The Hasty Heart", earned him the New York Critics' Award as the year's most promising newcomer. Throughout the 1940s he was often seen in Broadway plays. He made his movie debut in 1946 in *Cry Wolf.* When he was filming *Fourteen Hours,* his wife, Stephanie, was taken to hospital with a brain tumor which killed her. Richard went to Italy where he met his second wife, Valentina Cortese. Three years later he appeared in two Fellini films including the classic, *La Strada.* In 1984 Richard hosted the Los Angeles Olympic Games. Shortly after they were over, he died from a series of strokes.

Repeat Performance (1947)
He Walked by Night (1948)
Tension (1949)
Fourteen Hours (1951)
The House on Telegraph Hill (1951)
Fixed Bayonets (1951)
Decision Before Dawn (1951)
The Stranger's Hand (1953)
La Strada (1954)
The Swindle (1955)
Moby Dick (1956)
Time Limit (1957)
The Brothers Karamazov (1958)
5 Branded Women (1960)
Portrait in Black (1960)
The Satan Bug (1965) **Rage** (1972)
Being There (1979)

Kim **Basinger**
5ft 7½in
(KIMILA ANN BASINGER)

Born: **December 8, 1953**
Athens, Georgia, USA

Kim was the third of five children. Her father, Don, was a musician in a big-band during the 1940s and 50s, and landed in Normandy on D-Day, during World War II. Her mother Ann had been a model and appeared in Esther Williams musicals – performing in water ballet. Considering those achievements, it isn't surprising to learn that Kim was painfully shy as a little girl. To overcome this, Ann encouraged her to study classical ballet. She grew in confidence as she became more beautiful, and when she was sixteen, she won the 'Junior Miss Georgia' title. She was offered a contract by the Ford Modeling Agency in New York. By the time she was twenty, she was a top photographic model – appearing in ads and magazines. In the early 1970s, Kim took acting classes at the Neighborhood Playhouse and performed and sang in Greenwich Village clubs. It took a year or so before she felt ready to tackle Hollywood, so she moved to Los Angeles. She started in television, including work in the hit series 'Charlie's Angels' and got married. In 1981, Kim made her movie debut in *Hard Country.* She followed it as a Bond girl, and by the end of the decade, became a star in the blockbuster, *Batman.* Her marriage to Alec Baldwin didn't last. She took time off to take care of their daughter, and made a Best Supporting Actress Oscar-winning comeback in *LA Confidential.* Kim's work since then has been consistently good.

Never Say Never Again (1983)
The Natural (1984)
Fool for Love (1985)
No Mercy (1986) **Batman** (1989)
LA Confidential (1997)
8 Mile (2002)
People I Know (2002)
The Door in the Floor (2004)
Elvis Has Left the Building (2004)
Cellular (2004)
Even Money (2006)
The Sentinel (2006)
The Burning Plain (2008)
The Informers (2008)

Angela **Bassett**
5ft 4in
(ANGELA EVELYN BASSETT)

Born: August 16, 1958
New York City, New York, USA

When Angela was a little girl, her mother Betty, a social worker, relocated to St. Petersburg, Florida, where she and her sister, D'nette grew up. The two girls loved putting on shows to entertain their friends and family, but Angela was academic too. Through encouragement from a teacher, at Boca Ciega High School, she was able to get a scholarship to Yale University from where she received a BA in African-American studies in 1980. She went on to earn a Master of Fine Arts Degree from the Yale School of Drama. At Yale, she met her future husband, Courtney B. Vance. After Yale, Angela worked as receptionist in a beauty salon before acting work came along in 1984, in the form of "Ma Rainey's Black Bottom" and in 1985 (along with TV work) "Black Girl", at the off-Broadway, Second Stage Theater. In 1986, she made her film debut with a small role as a TV reporter in the thriller, *F/X*. For the next six years, most of her roles were in television series. Angela became better known to movie audiences after John Singleton's *Boyz n the Hood*. A series of impressive film roles led to her co-starring with Denzel Washington in *Malcolm X,* and a Best Actress Oscar nomination for her uncanny portrayal of Tina Turner, in *What's Love Got to Do with It* lifted her to new heights. *Strange Days* confirmed her star status and she has continued to progress.

Boyz n the Hood (1991)
City of Hope (1991)
Passion and Fish (1992)
Innocent Blood (1992)
Malcolm X (1992)
What's Love Got to Do
with It (1993)
Panther (1995)
Strange Days (1995)
Contact (1997)
Music of the Heart (1999)
The Score (2001)
Sunshine State (2002)
Akeelah and the Bee (2006)
Gospel Hill (2008)
Nothing But the Truth (2008)

Sir Alan **Bates**
5ft 11in
(ALAN ARTHUR BATES)

Born: February 17, 1934
Allestree, Derbyshire, England
Died: **December 27, 2003**

Alan grew up very happily in a lovely old village in the middle of a picturesque farming area. Both his parents were amateur musicians who taught him to appreciate music. When he was a boy, his visits to the local cinema made him dream of becoming an actor. His parents supported his ambition and he was awarded a scholarship to the Royal Academy of Dramatic Art, in London. But when that was over, his career was interrupted by National Service in the Royal Air Force. In 1956 he made his professional stage debut in John Osborne's "Look Back in Anger" at the Royal Court Theater. His role as Jimmy Porter made him a star of the stage and propelled him towards his first film *The Entertainer,* in 1960. Alan was nominated for a Best Actor Oscar and a Golden Globe for *The Fixer* and he became a truly international star in *Women in Love, The Go-Between* and *An Unmarried Woman.* His wife, actress Victoria Ward, suffered a fatal heart attack in 1992. Only two years earlier, their son Tristan, died of an asthma attack. The tragedies affected Alan deeply, but he kept on working and he was the winner of two Tony Awards. Joanna Pettet was Alan's companion until he died in London, of pancreatic cancer.

The Entertainer (1960)
Whistle Down the Wind (1961)
A Kind of Loving (1962)
The Caretaker (1963)
Nothing But the Best (1963)
Zorba the Greek (1964)
Georgy Girl (1966)
Far from the Madding Crowd (1967)
The Fixer (1968)
Women in Love (1969)
The Go-Between (1970) Butley (1974)
An Unmarried Woman (1978)
The Return of the Soldier (1982)
Force majeure (1989)
Hamlet (1990)
Gosford Park (2000)
The Sum of All Fears (2002)
Hollywood North (2003)

Kathy **Bates**
5ft 3in
(KATHLEEN DOYLE BATES)

Born: **June 28, 1948**
Memphis, Tennessee, USA

Kathy, her two older sisters, and their stay-at-home mother, lived a reasonably comfortable life provided by their father, a mechanical engineer. After graduating from high school, Kathy attended the Southern Methodist University in Dallas, Texas, where she majored in theater and in 1969, graduated with a Bachelor of Fine Arts degree. She then went to New York, where for several years, she appeared in off-Broadway productions, which included "Vanities". She was nominated for a Tony for her role in "Night Mother" for which she received the Outer Circle Award. In 1990, nineteen years after her film debut, in *Taking Off,* Kathy increased her audience considerably with her starring role in *Misery,* and won both a Best Actress Oscar and a Golden Globe. She married Tony Campasi, with whom she had lived for twelve happy years – the marriage only lasted six! Broadening her repertoire, in 1995, she won an American Comedy award, a Screen Actors Guild award and another Golden Globe for the HBO TV movie 'The Late Shift'. She was nominated for a Best Supporting Actress Oscar for *About Schmidt.* She is now a governor for the Academy Awards. After gaining plenty of experience on television, Kathy directed and acted in the 2006 feature movie, *Have Mercy* and was seen recently in the very good film, *Revolutionary Road.*

Misery (1990)
Fried Green Tomatoes (1991)
Dolores Clairborne (1995)
Titanic (1997)
Primary Colors (1998)
The Waterboy (1998)
Baby Steps (1999)
About Schmidt (2002)
Unconditional Love (2002)
The Ingrate (2004)
3 & 3 (2005) Solace (2006)
Relative Strangers (2006)
Bonneville (2006)
P.S. I Love You (2007)
The Day the Earth Stood Still (2008)
Revolutionary Road (2008)

Anne **Baxter**
5ft 4in
(ANNE BAXTER)

Born: **May 7, 1923**
Michigan City, Indiana, USA
Died: **December 12, 1985**

Anne's father was an executive with the Seagrams Distillery. Her mother had the distinction of being the daughter of the famous architect, Frank Lloyd Wright. When she was ten, the family moved to New York City. Shortly after that, she was taken to a Broadway play, starring the great actress Helen Hayes. It was an exciting time – the talkies had been around for half a dozen years, and Anne developed the acting bug through going to movies and starring in plays at her school. When she was fifteen, she was lucky enough to be sent to the School of Dramatic Art, where she was taught her craft by the legendary Russian stage actress, Maria Ouspenkaya. Through the school she began getting small parts in Broadway plays. By the late thirties, her reputation was growing, but a trip to Hollywood to audition for the role of Mrs. de Winter in Hitchcock's *Rebecca,* received a 'too young' verdict – she was sixteen! 20th Century Fox signed her, although her movie debut in 1940, was on loan to MGM, in *Twenty Mule Train.* Anne worked hard in all her roles, and by the time she married the actor John Hodiak (the first of three husbands) in 1946, she was a Best Supporting Actress Oscar winner for *The Razor's Edge.* Other good parts followed – *Yellow Sky* and *All About Eve* were among them, but her later work was mostly on TV. Anne's final bow was a television film, 'The Masks of Death'. A year later she passed away in New York, after a stroke.

The Magnificent Ambersons (1942)
Five Graves to Cairo (1943)
The North Star (1943)
The Razor's Edge (1946)
Yellow Sky (1949)
A Ticket to Tomahawk (1950)
All About Eve (1950)
I Confess (1953)
The Blue Gardenia (1953)
The Ten Commandments (1956)
Walk on the Wild Side (1962)
The Busy Body (1967)

Warner **Baxter**
5ft 11in
(WARNER LEROY BAXTER)

Born: **March 29, 1889**
Columbus, Ohio, USA
Died: **May 7, 1951**

Warner's mother was widowed when he was only nine. When they moved to San Francisco in 1906, their building was destroyed by the earthquake. So for two weeks, with fires raging around them, they lived in a tent. Having experienced drama for real, the seventeen-year-old had no alternative but to be an actor. Four years later, he was appearing in vaudeville and from there, graduated to the stage and Broadway. Looking just like a perfect American model from a mail-order catalogue got him work as a Hollywood extra. After his first starring role in *Sheltered Daughters* in 1921, he became a popular star of silent films – top-billed in no less than 48 features in that decade. His first talkie, *In Old Arizona,* where he played the Cisco Kid, won him a Best Actor Oscar. He was signed by Fox, and for ten years was one of Hollywood's highest-paid stars. By the time the US entered World War II, his career as a top movie star was on the slide. Most of his later films were poor features or mediocre Bs. But he had made over one hundred – some of them – especially the gripping *Prisoner of Shark Island* and *Kidnapped,* were excellent. Warner Baxter made his last film, *State Penitentiary,* in 1950. He spent his final few months in Malibu, suffering from chronic arthritis, and died of pneumonia.

The Squaw Man (1931)
42nd Street (1933)
Penthouse (1933)
Grand Canary (1934)
Broadway Bill (1934)
King of Burlesque (1936)
The Prisoner of Shark Island (1936)
The Road to Glory (1936)
To Mary with Love (1936)
Slave Ship (1937)
Kidnapped (1938)
Wife, Husband and Friend (1939)
Barricade (1939)
Adam Had Four Sons (1941)
Lady in the Dark (1944)
The Crime Doctor's Diary (1949)

Nathalie **Baye**
5ft 6in
(NATHALIE BAYE)

Born: **July 6, 1948**
Mainneville, Eure, France

Nathalie's parents were both painters who instilled in their daughter a love of art and music. By the time she was fourteen, she had developed a passion for dancing. She took lessons in Monaco, but the serious stuff began three years later, when she went to New York to train as a ballerina. During that time, Nathalie perfected her English and also became interested in an acting career. After returning to France, she studied drama at the National Conservatory of Dramatic Art, in Paris. She made her film debut in 1971, with a small part in the comedy *Faustine,* which starred Isabelle Adjani. She had an important supporting role in Francois Truffaut's *Day for Night,* and in 1974, was one of the stars in the highly regarded, *La Guele Ouverte.* Films for Truffaut and Jean-Luc Goddard increased both her skill and her popularity. Recognition of her acting talent has included nine César nominations – four of which she won – most notably for *Sauve qui peut (la vie)* and *La Balance.* A relationship with French singer Johnny Hallyday produced a daughter, the actress Laura Smet. Her career stalled briefly but 1999 marked a comeback. Nathalie was superb in *Venus Beauty Institute* – when she played a forty-year-old beautician, in a Paris salon. Her star has continued to shine ever since. Nathalie won another Best Actress César, for *Le Petit lieutenant.*

Sauve qui peut (la vie) (1980)
Beau-pére (1981)
La retour de Martin Guerre (1982)
La Balance (1982)
La Baule-des Pins (1990)
Venus Beauty Institute (1999)
Catch Me If You Can (2003)
La Fleur du mal (2003)
Le Petit Lieutenant (2005)
Mon fils à moi (2006)
Tell No One (2006)
Michou d'Auber (2007)
Prix à payer (2007)
Passe-passe (2008)
Les Bureaux de Dieu (2008)
Cliente (2008)

Jennifer Beals
5ft 8¹/₂in
(JENNIFER BEALS)

Born: **December 19, 1963**
Chicago, Illinois, USA

The impressively beautiful Jennifer is from a mixed race family. Her father, Alfred Beals, was an African American who died when she was ten. Her mother Jeanne, was Irish. Jennifer and her two brothers were raised by her and their stepfather, Edward Cohen. It was always clear that Jennifer was a very bright child. After graduating from the Francis W. Parker High School, she worked as a fashion model and when she was seventeen, made her first film appearance, in *My Bodyguard.* But she was soon studying again – at Yale University, where she received a BA – in American Literature. While still there she starred as Alex Owens in the hit movie *Flashdance* and won a Golden Globe. After graduation, she took a while to get her career moving. In 1986 she married the independent filmmaker Alexandre Rockwell and acted in several of his films during their ten-year marriage. In one of them, *Four Rooms,* Jennifer appeared with her good friend, Quentin Tarantino. The 1990s gave her a couple of very good years, but there was little consistency. Since 2004, Jennifer has starred as the lesbian, Bette Porter, in the popular television series 'The L Word'. Besides being stepmother to his two children, she has a daughter – born in 2005 – with her second husband, Ken Dixon.

Flashdance (1983)
The Bride (1985)
La Partita (1988) **Sons** (1989)
Vampire's Kiss (1989)
Blood and Concrete (1991)
In the Soup (1992)
Mrs. Parker and the
Vicious Circle (1994)
Four Rooms (1995)
Devil in a Blue Dress (1995)
Let It Be Me (1995)
The Last Days of Disco (1998)
13 Moons (2002)
Roger Dodger (2002)
Runaway Jury (2003)
Break a Leg (2005)
Joueuse (2009)

Sean Bean
5ft 10in
(SHAWN MARK BEAN)

Born: **April 17, 1959**
Sheffield, South Yorkshire, England

Sean grew up with an obsession with soccer – especially his beloved Sheffield United. He played for his school, Brook Comprehensive, but didn't quite have the skill or ambition to make it a career. He led a gang called 'The Union' and was often involved in fighting. It led to him joining a boxing club at fifteen – and giving up drinking and smoking for two years. After leaving school, he took a welding course at Rotherham College, where he switched to drama. Sean shone immediately and won a scholarship to RADA. In 1983 he made his professional stage debut (as Shaun Behan) in "Romeo and Juliet". The next year included a TV-commercial and his film debut in *Winter Flight.* After some impressive performances at the Young Vic, he joined the world famous Royal Shakespeare Company. Sean's first really important movie was Derek Jarman's *Caravaggio.* In 1996, he was in familiar territory in a movie about Sheffield football supporters called *When Saturday Comes.* From then on, he's kept up a very high standard – the pick of which are *Patriot Games, GoldenEye* and *National Treasure.* Sean considers himself "rough" but he's a real softy when it comes to his three daughters, from two of his four marriages.

Caravaggio (1986)
Stormy Monday (1988)
How to Get Ahead in
Advertising (1989)
The Field (1990)
Prince (1991)
Patriot Games (1992)
Black Beauty (1994)
GoldenEye (1995) **Ronin** (1998)
Bravo Two Zero (1999)
The Fellowship of the Ring (2001)
Tom & Thomas (2002)
Equilibrium (2002)
National Treasure (2004)
The Island (2005)
Silent Hill (2006)
The Hitcher (2007)
Outlaw (2007)
Far North (2007)

Emmanuelle Béart
5ft 4¹/₄in
(EMMANUELLE BÉART)

Born: **August 14, 1963**
St. Tropez, Var, France

Her father, the French singer and poet, Guy Béart, firmly believed in keeping little Emmanuelle and her brothers away from the influences of city life. They grew up on a farm near St.Tropez, and with the sea not far away, they were a happy family. Her mother, Geneviève, had been an actress, and in 1976, she took her daughter to see a movie called *Mado,* which starred Romy Schneider. It left such an impression on her, she decided that she too would be an actress when she grew up. When she was eighteen, her parents sent her to work as an au pair in Montreal, where they thought she could learn English. On her return to France, Emmanuelle took drama classes in Paris and got a role in the film *Premiers désirs,* which was directed by the famous beauty photographer, David Hamilton. She then worked in television dramas before meeting her first husband, Daniel Auteuil, who helped her film career take off. She won a Best Supporting Actress César in 1987 for her role in *Manon des Sources.* Her biggest successes have been *Un coeur en hiver* and *La Belle noiseuse.* Never afraid to support a cause – be it popular or extremely controversial – Emmanuelle is now an ambassador for UNICEF, and politically active on behalf of illegal immigrants in France. During 2006 she was a lingerie model for H&M.

L'Amour en douce (1985)
Manon des sources (1986)
Date with an Angel (1987)
La Belle noiseuse (1991)
Un coeur en hiver (1992)
Une femme française (1995)
Mission Impossible (1996)
Le Temps retrouvé (1999)
La Répétition (2001)
8 femmes (2002)
Les Égarés (2003)
The Story of Marie and
Julien (2005)
L'Enfer (2005)
Les Témoins (2007)
Vinyan (2008)
Mes Stars et mois (2008)

Ned **Beatty**
5ft 7in
(NED THOMAS BEATTY)

Born: **July 6, 1937**
Louisville, Kentucky, USA

When he was ten, Ned began singing in gospel choirs and barbershop quartets. He also sang at his local church. When he was at high school he was interested in acting, but his first appearance on a stage was in 1956, when he was in the cast of "Wilderness Road" but it wasn't a quick and easy road to success. The first ten years of his career were spent at the Barter Theater in Abington, Virginia. In the late 1960s, he appeared in Shakespeare plays and "The Great White Hope" on Broadway. His movie debut was in the harrowing role of Bobby Trippe, in *Deliverance*. After that, he was in demand as a character actor both in movies and on television. He was Oscar nominated for *Network* in 1976, and his acting is always first class. His description by 'Daily Variety' as the "busiest actor in Hollywood" is no exaggeration. In 2001, Ned returned to the stage as the star of the London West End revival of "Cat on a Hot Tin Roof" and transferred with it to Broadway in 2003. Ned has eight children from his four marriages. He relaxes between acting roles by playing golf, and the bass guitar.

Deliverance (1972)
Nashville (1975)
All the President's Men (1976)
Network (1976)
Silver Streak (1976)
Gray Lady Down (1978)
Superman (1978)
Wise Blood (1979)
Superman II (1980)
The Big Easy (1987)
The Fourth Protocol (1987)
After the Rain (1988)
Chattahoochee (1989)
Hear My Song (1991)
Rudy (1993) **Just Cause** (1995)
He Got Game (1998)
Cookie's Fortune (1999)
Spring Forward (1999)
Where the Red Fern Grows (2003)
The Walker (2007) **Shooter** (2007)
Charlie Wilson's War (2007)
In the Electric Mist (2008)

Warren **Beatty**
6ft 2in
(HENRY WARREN BEATY)

Born: **March 30, 1937**
Richmond, Virginia, USA

The son of a professor of psychology, Ira Owens Beaty, and his wife Kathlyn – a drama teacher – Warren grew up in the Bellevue district of Richmond with his older sister, Shirley. The family moved to Arlington, where he became a star footballer at Washington-Lee High School. He considered taking it up professionally. In 1956, his sister, by then known as Shirley Maclaine, was making a name for herself in Hollywood. She had enough influence on her handsome brother to persuade him to consider an acting career. He took a job as a stagehand in Washington D.C. during the summer, and after graduating, turned down several football scholarships and opted for drama school. TV and radio work followed until 1960, when he made his film debut, in Elia Kazan's *Splendor in the Grass.* For about six years he did not become the box-office success that many people anticipated. Then, in 1967, it all changed. He produced and starred in the mammoth artistic and commercial hit, *Bonnie and Clyde.* Although Warren won the Best Director Oscar for *Reds* and was nominated for Best Actor Oscars for *Bonnie and Clyde, Heaven Can Wait* and *Reds,* his love life appeared to be more prolific than his films. In 1992 that all changed when he married Annette Bening. The couple, who now have four children, co-starred in *Love Affair.* Warren retired from acting and directing films after starring in the very disappointing *Town & Country,* in 2001.

All Fall Down (1962)
Lilith (1964)
Bonnie and Clyde (1967)
McCabe and Mrs Miller (1971)
The Parallax View (1974)
Shampoo (1975)
The Fortune (1975)
Heaven Can Wait (1978)
Reds (1981)
Dick Tracy (1990)
Bugsy (1991)
Love Affair (1994)
Bulworth (1998)

Kate **Beckinsale**
5ft 8in
(KATHRYN BAILEY BECKINSALE)

Born: **July 26, 1973**
London, England

Kate's father, actor Richard Beckinsale, died in 1978. Her mother is the actress Judy Loe. When she was eleven, Kate was sent to the exclusive Godolphin and Latymer School, in Hammersmith, on the outskirts of London. She hated Physical Education, but did so well at English, that in her teens, she was twice winner of the W.H.Smith 'Young Writers Competition' for short stories and poems. After making her television debut in the 1991 drama 'One Against the Wind', Kate went to New College, at Oxford University, where she majored in French and Russian literature. She had already decided on an acting career, and in 1993, she appeared in Kenneth Branagh's film version of *Much Ado About Nothing.* Because it was filmed in Italy, Kate dropped out of her studies and concentrated on her career. The TV production of 'Cold Comfort Farm' and the title role, in 'Emma' got things off to a good start. She won a Spanish award for *Shooting Fish,* and after she'd played the female lead in *Pearl Harbor,* she was named 'England's Number One Beauty' by "Hello!" Magazine. She earned praise for her portrayal of Ava Gardner, in *The Aviator.* Kate had a daughter with the actor Michael Sheen, but wasn't married. In 2003, after she worked with the director Len Wiseman on *Underworld,* Kate made up her mind that she'd found the ideal husband. They've since made a sequel together – called *Underworld Evolution.*

Haunted (1995)
Shooting Fish (1997)
The Golden Bowl (2000)
Pearl Harbor (2001)
Serendipity (2001)
Laurel Canyon (2002)
Underworld (2003)
Van Helsing (2004)
The Aviator (2004)
Underworld Evolution (2006)
Click (2006) **Snow Angels** (2007)
Vacancy (2007)
Winged Creatures (2008)
Nothing But the Truth (2008)

Bonnie **Bedelia**
5ft 4in
(BONNIE BEDELIA CULKIN)

Born: **March 25, 1948**
New York City, New York, USA

Bonnie comes from a family bristling with talent – her brother Kit, became the father of Macaulay Culkin. From an early age, Bonnie loved performing in front of an audience. She went to ballet lessons when she was four, and three years later, she studied with the famous George Balanchine. She was only nine when she made her off-Broadway debut in "Tom Sawyer" and from 1959, spent four years as a professional with the New York Ballet. While she was still at High School, she appeared in the television soap-opera, 'Love of Life'. She then enrolled at Uta Hagen's Quintano School of Acting – appearing in four Broadway productions during her time there. Bonnie joined Martin Sheen and Louis Gossett Jr. in forming a classical acting group in Los Angeles. She finally made her film debut – in John Frankenheimer's *Gypsy Moths,* in 1969, but after three films – one of which was *They Shoot Horses Don't They?* Bonnie spent most of the next ten years working on television. She got good notices and a Golden Globe nomination for *Heart Like a Wheel,* and her movie career was back on track. Five years later, she starred with Bruce Willis in one of the best action films of all time – *Die Hard* and its sequel, two year's later, wasn't far behind. Bonnie has been married to her third husband, Michael McRae, since 1995.

The Gypsy Moths (1969)
They Shoot Horses,
Don't They? (1969)
The Big Fix (1978)
Heart Like a Wheel (1983)
Violets Are Blue (1986)
The Boy Who Could Fly (1986)
Die Hard (1988)
Fat Man and Little Boy (1989)
Die Hard 2 (1990)
Presumed Innocent (1990)
Bad Manners (1997)
Anywhere But Here (1999)
Sordid Lives (2000)
Manhood (2003)
Berkeley (2005)

Wallace **Beery**
6ft 1in
(WALLACE FITZGERALD BEERY)

Born: **April 1, 1885**
Kansas City, Missouri, USA
Died: **April 15, 1949**

The son of an Irish policeman and half-brother to actor, Noah Beery, Wallace ran away from home at fifteen to join the Ringling Brothers Circus, where became assistant to the elephant trainer. By 1903 he was a chorus boy in New York shows. Wallace continued singing and appearing in summer stock until his 1913 film debut in *His Athletic Wife.* Despite a rugged build and a craggy face, he became known for his role in a series of films, as a dumb Swedish housemaid. At the age of thirty, he moved to Hollywood, where among other things, he directed for Universal, and was married for a short time to Gloria Swanson. Before the advent of the talkies, Wallace had appeared in over a hundred films, including shorts and serials, and even directed a movie in Japan. Initially, he wasn't thought to have a big future in sound films. Paramount dropped him, but luckily, MGM signed him and gave him a good part in *The Big House,* which earned him a Best Actor Oscar nomination. He won one for *The Champ.* He was forty-five, but a new career as an even bigger star was just beginning. It lasted ten years before he ended up in second features for his loyal employer, MGM. Wallace's last movie *Big Jack,* was a good western, but he died of a heart attack in Beverly Hills, a few months later.

The Big House (1930) Min and
Bill (1930) The Secret Six (1931)
The Champ (1931) Hell Divers (1931)
Grand Hotel (1932) Flesh (1932)
Tugboat Annie (1933) Dinner at
Eight (1933) Viva Villa! (1934)
Treasure Island (1934) China
Seas (1935) Ah Wilderness! (1935)
A Message to Garcia (1936)
Slave Ship (1937)
The Bad Man of Brimstone (1937)
Stablemates (1938)
Stand Up and Fight (1939)
Barnacle Bill (1941)
A Date With Judy (1948)
Big Jack (1949)

Ed **Begley**
5ft 11in
(EDWARD JAMES BEGLEY)

Born: **March 25, 1901**
Hartford, Connecticut, USA
Died: **April 28, 1970**

The son of Irish immigrants, Ed was born into extreme poverty. His life was so miserable, he ran away from home several times before making the break permanent when he was thirteen. In 1931, after years of hardship, which included a spell in the Navy, he landed a job as an announcer with a Hartford radio station. He developed his voice skills to such an extent, he was able to move to New York in the late 1930s, where he became a radio actor. Ed played the title role in the 'Charlie Chan' series which ran from 1944 to 1948. He made his Broadway debut at the age of forty-three, in the short-lived "Land of Fame" – which brought him none. In 1947 Arthur Miller's "All My Sons" did. Ed made his film debut in the excellent *Boomerang* for 20th Century Fox. He had roles in an average of two or three TV or theater films a year right up to the year of his death. They included the classic, *12 Angry Men,* and an Oscar winning performance as Best Supporting Actor, in *Sweet Bird of Youth.* He was so proud of his Oscar, he carried it with him wherever he went. He had three wives and three children. His son, Ed Jr. is star of the TV show 'Living With Ed'. He died while enjoying himself at a party given by his Hollywood agent.

Boomerang! (1947)
Sorry, Wrong Number (1948)
Sitting Pretty (1948)
It Happens Every Spring (1949)
The Great Gatsby (1949)
Backfire (1950)
Dark City (1950)
The Turning Point (1952)
Patterns (1956)
12 Angry Men (1957)
Odds Against Tomorrow (1959)
Sweet Bird of Youth (1962)
The Unsinkable Molly Brown (1964)
The Oscar (1966)
Warning Shot (1967)
Billion Dollar Brain (1967)
Hang 'Em High (1968)
Road to Salina (1970)

Barbara **Bel Geddes**
5ft 3½in
(BARBARA BEL GEDDES)

Born: **October 31, 1922**
New York City, New York, USA
Died: **August 8, 2005**

Born into a theatrical family, Barbara was the daughter of stage and industrial designer, Norman Bel Geddes, and his wife, Helen Belle Sneider. Her parents were wealthy and she was educated at private schools where she first acted in plays. When she was eighteen, Barbara made her stage debut in a summer-stock production of "The School for Scandal". In 1941, she made her Broadway debut in "Out of the Frying Pan". She continued on the stage for six years – winning the first Clarence Derwent Award for outstanding young performer. In 1944, she married her first husband, Carl Schreuer. The following year, Barbara won the New York Drama Critics Award for "Deep Are the Roots". She made her film debut in *The Long Night* – the first of five films (including her Best Supporting Oscar-nominated role in *I Remember Mama*) before starting a long, successful TV career, in an episode of 'Robert Montgomery Presents'. Whether it was a case of good judgement on her part, or good luck, Barbara's relatively few movie appearances were nearly always in winners – notably *Panic in the Streets, Fourteen Hours* and *Vertigo,* which would stand up very well on anyone's list of film credits. In 1978, Barbara accepted the biggest role of her career – as Eleanor Southworth – 'Miss Ellie' Ewing, in the record-breaking soap opera, 'Dallas' – for which she won an Emmy. Barbara retired in 1990 and lived her last fifteen years at her home in Northeast Harbor, Maine. She died there of lung cancer.

The Long Night (1947)
I Remember Mama (1948)
Blood on the Moon (1948)
Caught (1949)
Panic in the Streets (1949)
Fourteen Hours (1951)
Vertigo (1958)
The Five Pennies (1958)
5 Branded Women (1960)
By Love Possessed (1961)
Summertree (1971)

Harry **Belafonte**
6ft
(HAROLD GEORGE BELAFONETE JR.)

Born: **March 1, 1927**
New York City, New York, USA

Harry was born in Harlem. He was the son of Harold Belafonete Sr., a chef in the British Royal Navy, who came from Martinique. His mother, Melvine, took him to live in her country Jamaica when he was eight. Four years later, Harry returned to New York, where he attended George Washington High School. In 1944, he served in the United States Navy and when the war was over, joined young actors, Curtis, Brando and Poitier, at the New York Dramatic Workshop. To pay for his classes, Harry worked as a singer in New York clubs, often backed by the Charlie Parker Quintet. He also performed with the American Negro Theater and eventually appeared on Broadway. In 1952, he signed a record contract with RCA Victor and began to get roles in movies, starting with *Bright Road.* Harry's albums were very popular. "Calypso", cut in 1956, earned him the epithet "King of Calypso" and sold over one million copies. Harry's early recordings are still sought after. In 1959 he became the first African American to win an Emmy – for his television special, 'Tonight with Belafonte'. In 1961, Harry performed at President Kennedy's inaugural Gala. Like many of his people he had been a victim of racial prejudice and refused to perform in the southern states. An early supporter of Civil Rights, in 1963 he helped organize the historic march on Washington. He has appeared only infrequently in films and was last seen on screen in *Bobby.* Since 1957, Harry's been married to the former dancer, Julie Robinson. Three of his four children are in show business.

Bright Road (1953)
Carmen Jones (1954)
Island in the Sun (1957)
The World, the Flesh and the Devil (1959)
Odds Against Tomorrow (1959)
Buck and the Preacher (1972)
Uptown Saturday Night (1974)
Kansas City (1998)
Bobby (2006)

Ralph **Bellamy**
6ft 1½in
(RALPH REXFORD BELLAMY)

Born: **June 17, 1904**
Chicago, Illinois, USA
Died: **November 29, 1991**

As soon as he left high school in 1922 Ralph started his acting career on stage in Chicago. By 1927 he even owned his own theater. In 1931 he made his film debut, in a Wallace Beery gangster movie, *The Secret Six*. He soon established himself as a reliable supporting actor, and he didn't play a leading role until *Straight from the Shoulder,* five years later. Ralph acted in a couple of "Screwball Comedies" which starred Cary Grant. For one of them, *The Awful Truth,* he was nominated for a Best Supporting Actor Oscar. Ralph played the detective, Ellery Queen in four films during the war years, and in 1945 he married the Hammond organist, Ethel Smith, whose recording of *Tico Tico* had reached Number 14 in the U.S. charts and was featured in the 1944 film, *Bathing Beauty*. But Ethel and Ralph were not in harmony – they divorced less than two years later. For a while, he returned to the stage, and served four terms as President of the Actors' Equity. Ralph continued to act in plays on both stage and TV. His long career in the movies was recognized in 1987, when he was presented with an honorary Academy Award. He made his final screen appearance in *Pretty Woman*. The following year, Ralph died of a lung ailment in Santa Monica, California.

Airmail (1932)
Picture Snatcher (1933)
Once to Every Woman (1934)
The Wedding Night (1935)
Hands Across the Table (1935)
The Awful Truth (1937)
Carefree (1938) **His Girl Friday** (1940)
Brother Orchid (1940)
Dive Bomber (1941)
The Wolf Man (1941)
Lady on a Train (1945)
The Court Martial of Billy Mitchell (1955)
Rosemary's Baby (1968)
Trading Places (1983)
The Good Mother (1988)
Pretty Woman (1990)

Maria **Bello**
5ft 5in
(MARIA ELAINA BELLO)

Born: **April 18, 1967**
Norristown, Pennsylvania, USA

Maria was the daughter of Joe Bello, an Italian American, who worked as a contractor. Her mother, Kathy, who was of Polish ancestry, taught in a school. Maria was raised as a Roman Catholic. After junior church schools, she was educated at Archbishop Carroll High School, in Radnor, Pennsylvania. After graduation, Maria majored in political science at Villanova University, in the same town. Although it was her intention to become a lawyer, she took acting classes during her senior year. She went to New York City, to look for a job, but was soon getting parts in off-Broadway plays – such as "The Killer Inside Me" and "Small Town Gals With Big Problems". In 1992, she made her film debut in an independent production titled *Maintenance,* but for most of the decade, she was acting in TV-series, including 'Mr. & Mrs. Smith' and 'ER'. Her film career really began in *Permanent Midnight,* and among several strong roles she received two nominations for Best Actress Golden Globes – for *The Cooler* and *A History of Violence.* Maria has a son, Jackson, from a relationship with Dreamworks Executive, Dan McDermott. Her new film, *The Private Lives of Pippa Lee,* should be good.

Permanent Midnight (1998)
Payback (1999)
Coyote Ugly (2000)
Duets (2000)
Auto Focus (2002)
100 Mile Rule (2002)
The Cooler (2003)
Secret Window (2004)
Silver City (2004)
Assault on Precinct 13 (2005)
The Sisters (2005)
The Dark (2005)
A History of Violence (2005)
Thank You for Smoking (2005)
World Trade Center (2006)
Flicka (2006)
Butterfly on a Wheel (2007)
Nothing Is Private (2007)
The Jane Austin Book Club (2007)
Yellow Handkerchief (2008)

Monica **Bellucci**
5ft 10in
(MONICA BELLUCCI)

Born: **September 30, 1964**
Città di Castello, Umbria, Italy

Monica is the daughter of Luigi Bellucci, who ran a trucking company, and his wife, Maria, who was a painter. Coming from a small Italian village was no obstacle to the ambitious Monica. She paid her way for law studies at the University of Perugia, by modeling for art schools. Halfway through the course she changed her mind about what she wanted to do. She went to Milan, where she joined the Elite Model Agency. She was signed by Dolce & Gabbana – featuring in the French fashion magazine, *Elle.* This exposure resulted in a small part in the 1990 Italian television drama 'Vita coi figli', and that same year, a starring role in the Italian hit movie, *Briganti.* Within three years, she'd added American experience to her credits as one of an all-star cast in Francis Ford Coppola's *Dracula.* Monica is not only a welcome modern edition to the list of great Italian screen beauties, she has acted in four languages – Italian, French, English and Persian. In 1999, she managed to disappoint a large number of the world's men, by marrying the French actor Vincent Cassel. They have a daughter named Deva. Monica has been able to combine motherhood with a film career – she's been kept busy and was in the recent hit, *Shoot 'Em Up.*

Briganti (1990) Dracula (1992)
L'Appartement (1996)
Come mi vuoi (1997)
L'Ultimo capodanno (1998)
A los que aman (1998)
Under Suspicion (2000)
Malèna (2000)
Le Pacte des loups (2001)
Irréversible (2002)
Ricordati di me (2003)
Tears of the Sun (2003)
Matrix Reloaded (2003)
The Passion of the Christ (2004)
The Brothers Grimm (2005)
Shoot 'Em Up (2007)
Wild Blood (2008)
The Man Who Loves (2008)
The Private Lives of Pippa Lee (2009)

Jean-Paul **Belmondo**
5ft 10½in
(JEAN-PAUL BELMONDO)

Born: **April 9, 1933**
Neuilly-sur-Seine, France

The son of the famous French sculptor Paul Belmondo, J-P was blessed with a face which looked like it was hewn out of stone – ideal for his tough-guy roles in movies. Bébel, as he was nicknamed, was a poor pupil at school, but he excelled at soccer and boxing. The latter gave him a broken nose, which added to his appeal as an actor. By the early 1950s, J-P was studying dramatic art at the Conservatoire in Paris, from where he narrowly missed being selected for the Comédie Française. He toured with actor friends and, following a few small stage roles, he was given a part in a film. Unfortunately, his scenes were cut from the release print. For the next three years, his films were forgettable until *A bout de souffle* – 'Breathless'. The film was a breakthrough for Belmondo, his American co-star, Jean Seberg, and it's young French New Wave director, Jean-Luc Goddard. J-P enjoyed a good long run at the top in the French Cinema, but reverted to theater work as he grew older. He won a César in 1988, for *Itinéraire d'un enfant gâté,* but refused it because the sculptor whose name it bares had once criticized his father's work. He did accept the Legion d'Honneur he was awarded in 2007. J-P lives with his second wife, Natty, but he has not been seen on stage or screen since suffering a stroke while in Corsica – in 2001.

A bout de souffle (1959)
Classe Tous Risques (1960)
La Viaccia (1961) Leon Morin,
Priest (1961) Le Doulos (1962)
L'homme de Rio (1964)
Pierrot le fou (1965)
Is Paris Burning? (1966)
Love Is a Funny Thing (1969)
Borsalino (1970) La Casse (1971)
La Scoumoune (1972)
Le Magnifique (1973)
Fear Over the City (1975)
Flic ou Voyou (1979)
Le Marginal (1983)
Hold Up (1985)
L'Itiniraire d'un enfant gâté (1988)

William **Bendix**
5ft 10½in
(WILLIAM BENDIX)

Born: **January 14, 1906**
New York City, New York, USA
Died: **December 14, 1964**

William (never called Bill) first acted in a silent film at the Vitagraph movie studio in Brooklyn, when he was five years old. He took a job as a bat boy with the New York Giants – running errands for his big hero, Babe Ruth and then proving good enough to play minor league baseball. He flirted with show business until getting married in 1928. The small grocery store he was managing then went bust during the Depression, so he moved into cabaret, where he would sing for his supper. By 1939, he had appeared in several stage productions including a good performance on Broadway, in "The Time of Your Life". Producer Hal Roach got a close-up of William's ugly mug from the front stalls, and offered him a contract. He made his film debut in 1942 – appearing in several scenes with Spencer Tracy, in *Woman of the Year.* Throughout a ten year period in movies, his supporting roles were never less than memorable. He was nominated for a Best Supporting Actor Oscar for *Wake Island.* Towards the end of the war, he starred in the radio series 'The Life of Riley'. When TV began to compete with the movies, he transferred successfully to the small screen, where it ran until 1958. He still appeared in movies – the best of which were *A Connecticut Yankee* (when he sang with Bing Crosby), *The Big Steal, The Dark Corner,* and *Detective Story.* He died in Los Angeles of lobar pneumonia.

Woman of the Year (1942)
The Glass Key (1942) **Wake Island** (1942)
Guadalcanal Diary (1943)
Lifeboat (1944) The Hairy Ape (1944)
A Bell for Adano (1945)
The Blue Dahlia (1946) **A Connecticut Yankee in King Arthur's Court** (1949)
The Life of Riley (1949)
The Streets of Laredo (1949)
The Big Steal (1949)
The Dark Corner (1950)
The Web (1950) Gambling House (1950)
Detective Story (1951)
Macao (1952)

Roberto **Benigni**
5ft 6in
(ROBERTO BENIGNI)

Born: **October 27, 1952**
Misericordia, Arezzo, Tuscany, Italy

Roberto's father, Luigi, was a prisoner in a concentration camp until 1945. After his release, he and his wife had three daughters before Roberto arrived. The boy was destined for the priesthood – attending a seminary in Florence, but leaving after a flood seriously damaged the school. He then went to Prato, in Tuscany, to study accountancy. Roberto became interested in acting – making his stage debut in Prato in 1972. Later that year, he transferred to Rome, where he appeared in plays and began directing. In 1975, he enjoyed big success with Giuseppe Bertolucci's play, "Cioni Mario di Gaspare fu Giulia". During the 1970s, he became infamous in Italy for the TV series 'Televacca' which was suspended due to censorship. Roberto made his film debut in 1977, in another Bertolucci creation, *Berlinguer ti voglio bene.* He upset some and was cheered by others for criticizing the Pope on a TV show. He concentrated on Italian films before starring in three by the American director, Jim Jarmusch – including *Coffee and Cigarettes.* In 1997, he won the Best Actor Oscar for *La vita è bella,* – also voted 'Best Foreign Film'. Since 1991, Roberto's been married to the actress Nicoletta Braschi. His readiness to get involved with political statements hasn't changed. In 2005, he led thousands of people in a TV protest against Berlusconi's plan to cut state arts funding. It appears to have been his last performance.

I Love You (1977) La Luna (1979)
Clair de femme (1979)
Il Pap'occhio (1980)
Il Minestrone (1981)
You Disturb Me (1983)
Down by Law (1986)
Coffee and Cigarettes (1986)
The Little Devil (1988)
Night on Earth (1991)
Johnny Stecchino (1991)
Il Mostro (1994)
La Vita é bella (1997)
Coffee and Cigarettes (2003)
La Tigre e la neve (2005)

Annette **Bening**
5ft 8½in
(ANNETTE CAROL BENING)

Born: **May 29, 1958**
Topeka, Kansas, USA

Annette was the youngest of four children. When she was a year old, her father, who worked in the insurance business, took up a job in Wichita, Kansas. Six years later, the family moved again, when he was transferred to San Diego, California. Rather shy as a youngster, Annette didn't take much interest in drama, other than watching movies, until at junior high school, she played the lead in "The Sound of Music". She then studied drama at Patrick Henry High School. After a year working as a cook on a charter boat, she finished college in San Diego, and three years later, graduated from San Francisco State University. Annette began her stage career at the American Conservatory Theater, but eventually moved to New York where, for a time, she concentrated on the stage. In 1987 she was nominated for a Tony for the Broadway play, "Coastal Disturbances". Her movie debut came the following year in the rather dull, *The Great Outdoors,* but a trio of films including *The Grifters,* for which she was Oscar nominated, led to a role in *Bugsy,* and future husband, Warren Beatty. Annette then became world-famous as the lady who landed that perennial Hollywood bachelor. Annette's second Oscar nomination came seven years later, for *American Beauty.* After a quiet couple of years, she was recently one of *The Women* – a remake of George Cukor's classic 1939 film. It also marked the directing debut for the writer/producer, Diane English.

Valmont (1989)
Postcards from the Edge (1990)
The Grifters (1990)
Bugsy (1991)
Guilty by Suspicion (1991)
Love Affair (1994)
Richard III (1995)
The American President (1995)
The Siege (1998)
American Beauty (1999)
Open Range (2003)
Being Julia (2004)
Running With Scissors (2006)

Richard **Benjamin**
6ft 2in
(RICHARD BENJAMIN)

Born: **May 22, 1938**
New York City, New York, USA

Raised in the Jewish religion, Richard attended the New York High School of Performing Arts, and during those years, he made his first stage appearances. He then studied for a BA in Drama, at Northwestern University, near Chicago. It was there that he met the love of his life Paula Prentiss, and married her in 1961. They had a son and a daughter in the 1970s. Although they were exactly the same age, Richard's career took longer to develop – especially on the movie front, where Paula was in demand. Richard's work was mainly in television series like 'Dr. Kildare', but in 1965, he had a golden opportunity – as director of the London production of "Barefoot in the Park". A year later, he made his Broadway debut (as an actor) in Neil Simon's "The Star Spangled Girl". He and his wife then starred together in the 1967 TV sitcom, 'He and She'. It was said to be too "New Yorkish" for national success, but it got him noticed. He was given the lead in the movie *Goodbye Columbus* in 1969, and for most of the next decade, his was a familiar face in movies. Richard has made his mark in Hollywood, both as an actor and as a director. Both he and his wife Paula continue to act in television dramas and Richard also directs TV plays. He made a welcome return to movies in the highly amusing comedy, *Keeping Up with the Steins,* and continues to work.

Goodbye Columbus **(**1969)
Catch-22 (1970)
Diary of a Mad
Housewife (1970)
The Marriage of a Young
Stockbroker (1971)
Portnoy's Complaint (1972)
The Last of Sheila (1973)
Westworld (1973)
The Sunshine Boys (1975)
House Calls (1978)
Scavenger Hunt (1979)
Deconstructing Harry (1997)
Keeping Up with the Steins (2006)
Henry Poole Is Here (2008)

Bruce **Bennett**
6ft 3in
(HAROLD HERMAN BRIX)

Born: **May 19, 1906**
Tacoma, Washington, USA
Died: **February 24, 2007**

A bright, clever child, Bruce was also a natural athlete. He played football for the University of Washington, where he majored in Economics. In 1926, he was in the team beaten 20–19 by Alabama at the Rose Bowl. The cause of the upset was a young man called Johnny Mack Brown (later a movie star) who scored two of his side's three touchdowns. Two years after that, as Herman Brix, Bruce won a silver medal in the Shot-Putt at the Olympic Games in Amsterdam. He was forced to pull out of the 1932 Games because of an injury sustained while making his film debut, in *Touchdown*. It also delayed his role as a screen Tarzan – having to wait until 1935, when he was the choice of the author, Edgar Rice Burroughs, for *The New Adventures of Tarzan*. Right up to the war, Bruce worked mainly in serials and 'B'-pictures. After serving in the U.S. Army, he changed his name and enjoyed a period of success – working with big stars like Joan Crawford – in *Mildred Pierce,* and Humphrey Bogart, with whom he was outstanding as the prospector Cody, in *The Treasure of the Sierra Madre*. He gave up acting in 1973, but enjoyed a success-ful career in business. At ninety-six years of age, Bruce skydived from 10,000 feet over Lake Tahoe. It was no big surprise when he died in Santa Monica, of compli-cations from a broken hip!

The Heckler (1940)
The More the Merrier (1943)
Sahara (1943)
Mildred Pierce (1945)
A Stolen Life (1946)
The Man I Love (1947)
Nora Prentiss (1947)
Dark Passage (1947)
The Treasure of
the Sierra Madre (1948)
Undertow (1949) Sudden Fear (1952)
Strategic Air Command (1955)
Three Violent People (1956)
Love Me Tender (1956)
The Outsider (1961)

Constance **Bennett**
5ft 4in
(CONSTANCE CAMPBELL BENNETT)

Born: **October 22, 1904**
New York City, New York, USA
Died: **July 24, 1965**

Connie and her younger sisters, Barbara and Joan, grew up in a theatrical family. Their father, Richard, was a well-known stage actor who occasionally did film work – in 1931, he appeared with her when she starred in *Bought*. By her early teens, she had acted in some New York-produced silent films, starting with *Valley of Decision* in 1916. She put her career on hold when she got married in 1925 and then lived overseas for a couple of years. After her divorce in 1929, she started again, along with the talkies and a hit film called *This Thing Called Love*. Connie's nice voice and sophisticated acting style suited the new medium, especially comedy, at which she was most adept. As early as 1931, she was only behind Greta Garbo in a U.S. exhibitors poll. She moved from Warner Bros. to RKO, where she had a huge hit with the George Cukor-directed *What Price Hollywood?* which contains her best performance – at the peak of her career. Connie remained popular, and she was co-starring opposite such leading lights as Frederic March and Clark Gable. She ended a dozen years at the top with her utterly charming supporting role in Garbo's swan-song, *Two-Faced Woman*. Connie completed what proved to be her last film, *Madame X*, in 1965. She died at Fort Dix, New Jersey a short time later of a cerebral hemorrhage. Her fifth husband, Theron Coulter, was by her side.

This Thing Called Love (1929)
Son of the Gods (1930)
Common Clay (1930)
Lady with a Past (1932)
What Price Hollywood? (1932)
Bed of Roses (1933)
The Affairs of Cellini (1934)
After Office Hours (1935)
Topper (1937)
Merrily We Live (1938)
Two-Faced Woman (1941)
Centennial Summer (1946)
The Unsuspected (1947)
As Young as You Feel (1951)

Joan **Bennett**
5ft 4in
(JOAN GERALDINE BENNETT)

Born: **February 27, 1910**
Palisades Park, New Jersey, USA
Died: **December 7, 1990**

As a child, Joan had small roles in a few silent films. She was sent to a French finishing school in Versailles, near Paris, but on her return home, a career as an actress seemed unlikely when, at barely sixteen years of age, she ran away with a young millionaire and got married. After two unhappy years, and a baby (which later provided Joan with the title 'Hollywood's youngest, most beautiful grandmother') she divorced him and resumed her movie career. Joan secured a contract with Goldwyn and acted in the popular Ronald Colman film, *Bulldog Drummond.* After that, she was dropped by the studio, but had plenty of offers. The fact that she was Constance Bennett's sister helped her at that early stage when she appeared, like Connie, in leading roles as a blonde (her natural color) ingenue. Eventually, the comparison between the two did her no favors. It was after she became a brunette in 1939, that she established herself. She was tested unsuccessfully for the role of Scarlett O'Hara, in *Gone With the Wind,* but top films such as *The Man I Married, Manhunt,* and *The Woman in the Window,* gave her ten years of popularity. After a scandal in 1951, when husband, Walter Wanger, took a pot-shot at her agent, her film career petered out. After that she made a living from TV. Joan died from a heart attack in Scarsdale, New York.

Bulldog Drummond (1929)
Little Women (1931)
The Pursuit of Happiness (1934)
Private Worlds (1935)
She Couldn't Take It (1935)
Trade Winds (1939)
The House Across the Bay (1940)
The Man I Married (1940)
Manhunt (1941)
The Woman in the Window (1944)
Scarlet Street (1946)
The Reckless Moment (1949)
Father of the Bride (1950)
For Heaven's Sake (1950)
We're No Angels (1955)

Jack **Benny**
5ft 8in
(BENJAMIN KUBELSKY)

Born: **February 14, 1894**
Chicago, Illinois, USA
Died: **December 26, 1974**

The son of a Jewish haberdasher, Jack was encouraged by his mother to study the violin. By fourteen, he was playing in the high school orchestra, and earning extra money in local dance bands. He became so proficient, he entered vaudeville immediately after finishing high school. It was a good decision. He was learning from the best: in the same theater was a young team of comedians called the Marx Brothers. In 1912, he was part of a double-act, but within a year he'd gone solo, and was billed as 'Ben Benny, the Fiddlin' Kid'. Towards the end of World War I, he served in the United States Navy, where he would sometimes entertain. His violin playing was booed one evening and he began to tell jokes instead. He didn't give up the fiddle, but included jokes in his act from there on. In 1922 Jack went with Zeppo Marx to a Passover seder. There he met a girl called Sadye, who after they married, adopted the stage name Mary Livingstone. Jack's career took off with the 'Jack Benny Program', running from 1932 until 1948. His bad violin playing became his trademark, and the show featured Mary, Dennis Day, Phil Harris and Eddie 'Rochester' Anderson. His humor never quite transferred to the big screen but the films listed – especially *Buck Benny Rides Again* and his best, *To Be or Not To Be* are well worth a look. A guest appearance in *A Guide for the Married Man* in 1967 was his last film. He died of stomach cancer, in Holmby Hills, California.

The Big Broadcast of 1937 (1936)
College Holiday (1936)
Artists and Models (1937)
Artists and Models Abroad (1938)
Man About Town (1939)
Buck Benny Rides Again (1940)
Love Thy Neighbor (1940)
Charley's Aunt (1941)
To Be or Not to Be (1942)
George Washington
Slept Here (1942)
The Horn Blows at Midnight (1945)

Tom **Berenger**
5ft 11in
(THOMAS MICHAEL MOORE)

Born: **May 31, 1949**
Chicago, Illinois, USA

Tom, whose father was a travelling salesman, grew up in an Irish Catholic family. In 1972, after he had graduated from the University of Missouri – where he majored in journalism, he decided to pursue an acting career, working in regional theaters to gain experience. In the mid-1970s, Tom moved to New York where, while taking acting classes at the Herbert Berghof Studios, he got a starring role in the television soap, 'One Life to Live'. His first film opportunity was as the star of a little-known independent production, *Rush It,* in 1976. A year later, he had a supporting role in Michael Winner's star-packed, but disappointing, *The Sentinel.* Tom played heroes or villains with equal facility for about five years without a major breakthrough. That came in 1983, when he starred opposite Glenn Close, in *The Big Chill.* He built a reputation as a fine actor and in 1986, won a Golden Globe and was nominated for a Best Supporting Actor Oscar for his memorable portrayal of Sergeant Barnes, in *Platoon.* Through Tom Cruise, whom he met when acting in *Born on the Fourth of July,* he got involved with the Church of Scientology. After divorcing his second wife, (who was active in the movement) he denounced it and has had no more connection with the Church. Tom is the father of six children from three marriages. He's been married to Patricia Alvaran, since 1998.

Looking for Mr Goodbar (1977)
The Big Chill (1983) Platoon (1986)
Someone to Watch Over Me (1987)
Betrayed (1988)
Born on the Fourth of July (1989)
The Field (1990) Shattered (1991)
Sniper (1993) Gettysburg (1993)
The Substitute (1996)
The Gingerbread Man (1998)
One Man's Hero (1999)
Takedown (2000)
Training Day (2001)
The Christmas Miracle of
Jonathan Toomey (2007)
Stiletto (2008)

Marisa **Berenson**
5ft 8in
(MARISA BERENSON)

Born: **February 15, 1947**
New York City, New York, USA

The daughter of an American diplomat and a European countess, Marisa was also the granddaughter of the famous Italian-born Parisian fashion designer, Elsa Schiaparelli. With such a glamorous background and the looks to go with it, she became one of the world's highest paid fashion models during the 1960s. Marisa made her film debut in Luchino Visconti's beautiful film, *Death in Venice*. She gained further movie experience in Bob Fosse's *Cabaret* and formed a long-standing friendship with Liza Minelli. Because of her beauty, Marisa wasn't taken seriously as an actress and her social circle, which included high profile Andy Warhol and Diane von Furstenberg, tended to get more media attention than her films. Even so, she really wanted to act. She then appeared on stage in Williamstown and Los Angeles, in Philip Barry's "Holiday", in 1980, and was frequently seen in TV dramas. She made films and TV programs in Italy, Germany and France with varying success. Since the 1990s, Marisa has based herself in Paris, acting in French films with an occasional trip to America, including a featured role in the six-parter, 'The Hollywood Detective'. Her sister Berry, who was a noted photographer and the former wife of Anthony Perkins, was killed aboard the hijacked plane which crashed into the World Trade Center on 9/11. Currently single, Marisa has been twice married and divorced.

Death in Venice (1971)
Cabaret (1972)
Barry Lyndon (1975)
S.O.B. (1981)
White Hunter Black Heart (1990)
**Le Grand blanc
de Lambaréné** (1995)
Tonka (1997) **Elles** (1997)
Retour à la vie (2000)
Lisa (2001)
Lonesome (2001)
**Color Me Kubrick:
A True...ish Story** (2005)
24 mesures (2007)

Candice **Bergen**
5ft 7½in
(CANDICE PATRICIA BERGEN)

Born: **May 9, 1946**
Beverly Hills, California, USA

Candy's father was the ventriloquist Edgar Bergen. When she was a child she was often referred to as Charlie McCarthy's little sister. Charlie was the dummy. She got her looks from her mother – former Powers Model, Frances Westcott. Candy first appeared before an audience when she was eleven, on the Groucho Marx quiz show, 'You Bet Your Life'. As she grew up, she studied photography, becoming a photo-journalist, then a professional model. She started at the University of Pennsylvania, but was expelled due to her casual attitude towards education. She turned to acting and made her film debut at the age of twenty, in *The Group*. She reached the peak of her fame as a movie star in the early 1970s, but kept herself in the public eye with television work. In 1975, she was the first female host of 'Saturday Night Live'. She was nominated for a Best Supporting Actress Oscar, for *Starting Over*. Fluent in French, she married the famous film director Louis Malle in 1981 and they had a daughter named Chloe. After his death in 1995, she married Marshall Rose, a New York real estate magnate. She continues to act: in 2005 Candy was nominated for an Emmy as Supporting Actress for her television work in 'Boston Legal', in which she has been seen in eighty episodes. On the film front, Candy recently appeared in the critically panned "Chick-Flick", *Sex and the City*, and has been no luckier with *The Women* and *Bride Wars*.

The Sand Pebbles (1966)
Vivre pour vivre (1967)
Soldier Blue (1970)
Carnal Knowledge (1971)
The Hunting Party (1971)
11 Harrowhouse (1974)
The Wind and the Lion (1975)
Bite the Bullet (1975)
Starting Over (1979)
Rich and Famous (1981)
Gandhi (1982)
Miss Congeniality (2000)
Sweet Home Alabama (2002)

Patrick **Bergin**
6ft 3in
(PATRICK CONNOLLY BERGIN)

Born: **February 4, 1951**
Dublin, Ireland

Patrick was the son of a senator in the Irish parliament, but he took little interest in politics – preferring to appear in theatrical productions when still at high school. When he was seventeen, he moved to London, where he studied for a bachelor's degree in education at North London Polytechnic. He funded it by working as a laborer and postman before starting his working life teaching juvenile delinquents and children with learning difficulties. He still kept his interest in the theater alive, and in 1980, decided to concentrate on full-time acting. The following year, he met his future wife, Paula Frazier. He got small roles with repertory theater companies and in 1984, made his debut on British TV – as a Tottenham Hotspurs player, in the soccer drama, 'Those Glory Days'. Patrick's first big screen appearance was in 1988, when he had a supporting role in the Irish-made independent film, *Taffin* which starred Pierce Brosnan. His first Hollywood film was in Bob Rafelson's *Mountains of the Moon*. By 1991, Patrick was co-starring with Julia Roberts in one of her less successful films, *Sleeping with the Enemy* – his performance was fine – he was nominated for a Saturn Award – but the storyline sucked. It didn't impede his progress, and he soon had *Patriot Games* and *Map of the Human Heart* to add to his resumé. In 1992, he married Paula. The couple have one child. Patrick's upcoming movie – *Gallowwalk*, sounds like it could be a winner.

Mountains of the Moon (1989)
Highway to Hell (1992)
Patriot Games (1992)
Map of the Human Heart (1993)
The Proposition (1996)
The Island on Bird Street (1997)
One Man's Hero (1999)
When the Sky Falls (2000)
The Boys from County Clare (2003)
Ella Enchanted (2004)
Johnny Was (2006)
The Black Pimpernel (2007)
Strength and Honor (2007)

Ingrid **Bergman**
5ft 9in
(INGRID BERGMAN)

Born: August 29, 1915
Stockholm, Sweden
Died: **August 29, 1982**

Ingrid's mother died when she was two, and her father, before she was twelve. This experience made her a fiercely independent young woman. After she left school at sixteen, she studied at the Royal Dramatic Theater, in Stockholm. She worked as an extra in a film called *Landskamp,* in 1932, and the national Svensk Filmindustri gave her a contract. She then played a hotel maid, in *Munkbrogreven* and, by around 1935, she was a star in Sweden. Two films, both solid tear-jerkers, and both to be remade in Hollywood, put her on the international movie map. *Intermezzo* and *A Woman's Face* found their way to the USA, and she was given a one-film contract to appear in the American version of the former. It was a terrific success and Ingrid was crowned Queen of Hollywood. Then it all changed. In 1950, she had a baby son, out of wedlock, with the Italian film director Roberto Rossellini. American movie audiences were horrified and they ostracized her. It took them six years to forgive her, but they did. Despite her three Oscars – for *Gaslight, Anastasia* and *Murder on the Orient Express,* some folk believe she was not as good an actress as Greta Garbo (who never won), but she was certainly much better loved. She had three daughters from her three marriages – actress Isabella Rossellini being most famous. She died in London of lymphoma complications following breast cancer. Ingrid's last acting role was on TV as 'A Woman called Golda' (Meir).

Intermezzo (1939)
Adam Had Four Sons (1941)
Dr. Jekyll and Mr. Hyde (1941)
Casablanca (1942)
Gaslight (1944) **Spellbound** (1945)
The Bells of St. Mary's (1945)
Notorious (1946) **Anastasia** (1956)
Indiscreet (1958)
**The Inn of the Sixth
Happiness** (1958) **The Visit** (1964)
Murder on the Orient Express (1974)
Autumn Sonata (1978)

Halle **Berry**
5ft 7in
(HALLE MARIA BERRY)

Born: August 14, 1966
Cleveland, Ohio, USA

Halle's parents selected her christian name from the popular Halle's Department Store in Cleveland. Her mother, Judith Hawkins, a lovely lady from Liverpool, who was a psychiatric nurse, got divorced from Jerome J. Berry when Halle was four. She was educated at Bedford High School and Cuyahoga Community College. Halle decided to become an actress after she'd entered some beauty contests and been crowned "Miss Ohio USA" and "Miss Teen All-American". She was runner-up in the 1986 "Miss USA" contest and sixth in the "Miss World" competition that same year. It was great exposure for her – opening the door to a modeling career in Chicago, and a first professional acting role, in a local cable television series called "Chicago Force". This led to a weekly television series in 1989, "Living Dolls". In 1991, Halle moved up a gear when she appeared in Spike Lee's *Jungle Fever.* Bigger parts followed including a Best Breakthrough performance, the following year, in the Eddie Murphy comedy, *Boomerang.* She was highly praised for her role opposite Warren Beatty, in *Bulworth* and a year after that, won a Golden Globe for Best Actress in a TV Movie, "Introducing Dorothy Dandridge". In 2001, Halle was awarded a Best Actress Oscar for *Monster's Ball.* Since then she shone as a Bond Girl and starred in the hit movie, *X-Men: The Last Stand.* Halle's two marriages ended in divorce.

The Last Boy Scout (1991)
Boomerang (1992)
The Flintstones (1994)
Executive Decision (1996)
Bulworth (1998)
Why Do Fools Fall in Love (1998)
X-Men (2000)
Swordfish (2001)
Monster's Ball (2001)
Die Another Day (2002)
X2 (2003)
X-Men: The Last Stand (2006)
Perfect Stranger (2007)
Things We Lost in the Fire (2007)

Richard **Beymer**
6ft 2in
(GEORGE RICHARD BEYMER)

Born: February 20, 1938
Avoca, Iowa, USA

After moving to Los Angeles in the late 1940s, Dick began his acting career while still a student at North Hollywood High School. Through acting in school plays he progressed to small parts on television – starting with the series 'Sandy Dreams'. Following a walk on part in the Richard Basehart movie, *Fourteen Hours,* Dick made his official movie debut in 1953 (as Dick Beymer) supporting Jennifer Jones and Montgomery Clift, in Vittorio de Sica's *Indiscretion of an American Wife.* Even though he got regular TV work and the occasional film role, it took seven years to achieve stardom. In 1961, he acted with Natalie Wood, George Chakiris and Rita Moreno, in his biggest success, *West Side Story.* He had a brief relationship with Sharon Tate, when she worked with him on Hemingway's *Adventures of a Young Man.* In 1962 Dick shared a Golden Globe for 'Most Promising Newcomer' along with Bobby Darin and Warren Beatty. Mindful of some of the criticism levelled at him for the way he'd played Tony in *West Side Story,* Dick took classes at the Actor's Studio in New York. It was interrupted by his decision to travel south to take part in the civil rights struggle and make a documentary of that experience. He was mostly seen on TV during the past three decades and was in thirty episodes of 'Twin Peaks'. After appearing in a strange movie called *Home the Horror Story* and an episode of TV's 'Family Law', Dick retired from acting in 2001. He lives in Fairfield, Iowa, where he paints, takes photographs, and in 2007, completed his first book, "Imposter: Or Whatever Happened to Richard Beymer?" He acted in a short, *Sadie's Waltz* in 2008.

So Big (1953)
Johnny Tremain (1957)
The Diary of Anne Frank (1959)
West Side Story (1961)
Bachelor Flat (1962)
**Hemingway's Adventures of a
Young Man** (1962)
The Longest Day (1962)
The Stripper (1963)

Charles **Bickford**
6ft 1in
(CHARLES AMBROSE BICKFORD)

Born: **January 1, 1891**
Cambridge, Massachusetts, USA
Died: **November 9, 1967**

Born in the very first minute of 1891, Charles was the fifth of seven children. When he was only nine, he was tried and acquitted for attempting to murder a man who had run over his dog. His first job was as a lumberjack in Canada when he was sixteen. In San Francisco three years later, he was pursuing a burlesque actress who offered him a job as a performer in her touring show. He appeared on Broadway in "Outside Looking In" and Cecil B. DeMille liked him enough to star him in his first talkie, the 1929 film, *Dynamite*. It was good enough to earn Charles an MGM contract, but his battles with studio boss, Louis B. Mayer, made life difficult for him. In 1935, he was offered a contract by 20th Century Fox, but it was withdrawn after he was mauled by a lion during the filming of *East of Java*. The studio did not want a leading man who had bad scarring on his neck. Nevertheless, he was top-billed in several other movies. He was up for a Best Supporting Actor Oscar three times – for *The Song of Bernadette*, *The Farmer's Daughter* and *Johnny Belinda*. The Best Actress Oscar went to the star of his film on all three occasions! Charles appeared in *A Star Is Born*, and *The Big Country*, during the 1950s, and was active up until his death from a blood infection.

Anna Christie (1930)
The Squaw Man (1931)
Little Miss Marker (1934)
East of Java (1935)
The Plainsman (1936)
High, Wide, and Handsome (1937)
Of Mice and Men (1939) The Song of
Bernadette (1943) Wing and a
Prayer (1944) Duel in the Sun (1946)
The Farmer's Daughter (1947)
Brute Force (1947)
Johnny Belinda (1948)
A Star is Born (1954)
The Court-Martial of Billy Mitchell (1955)
The Big Country (1958)
The Unforgiven (1960)
Days of Wine and Roses (1962)

Jessica **Biel**
5ft 9in
(JESSICA CLAIRE BIEL)

Born: **March 3, 1982**
Ely, Minnesota, USA

Jesse is the daughter of Jon Biel, who is described as an entrepreneur. Her mother, Kimberly, created a warm home for Jesse and her younger brother, Justin. That was easier said than done because of the Biel's frequent moves. They did eventually settle down – in Boulder, Colorado. Jesse won a scholarship to the Young Actors Space in Los Angeles at the age of eleven. She attended the International Modeling and Talent Association Conference in Los Angeles a year later and was signed by a talent agent. Jesse was soon working in TV commercials for DeLuxe Paints and Pringles. Around that time she appeared in an unreleased musical short film titled *It's a Digital World*. She made her feature film debut in *Ulee's Gold,* as Peter Fonda's granddaughter – which won her a Young Artist Award. At fourteen, Jesse was cast as Mary Camden, in the long-running TV series '7th Heaven' and remained with the show for several years. She had her first grown-up film role in a so-so romantic comedy called *Summer Catch,* before scoring high marks in *Rules of Attraction* and a very good remake of *The Texas Chainsaw Massacre* – for which she was nominated for a Best Actress Saturn. Most of Jesse's later films have confirmed that promise. Her performance in *Easy Virtue* is nothing short of magical. Jesse has a very good singing voice and Justin Timberlake is a recent boyfriend.

Ulee's Gold (1997)
I'll Be Home for Christmas (1998)
The Rules of Attraction (2002)
The Texas Chainsaw
Massacre (2003)
Cellular (2004)
Blade: Trinity (2004)
Stealth (2005) London (2005)
Elizabethtown (2005)
The Illusionist (2006)
Home of the Brave (2006)
Next (2007)
I Now Pronounce You
Chuck & Larry (2007)
Easy Virtue (2008)

Juliette **Binoche**
5ft 6in
(JULIETTE BINOCHE)

Born: **March 9, 1964**
Paris France

At four years of age, Juliette experienced the trauma of her parents' divorce. Even so, they passed on their artistic talent. Her father was a sculptor and her mother, an actress. Juliette showed great ability as a painter long before becoming an actress. Both she and her sister Marion were sent to a boarding school where there were opportunities to act in student productions of well-known plays such as Ionesco's "Le roi se meurt". After leaving school, Juliette studied acting at the Paris Conservatoire. During summer vacation she toured with a theater company in France, Belgium and Switzerland, using the pseudonym Juliette Adrienne. After her graduation, she continued on the stage but also took small parts in feature films and television dramas. Her first big screen appearance was in 1983, in a film about student opposition to the French Algerian war – *Liberty Belle.* In the space of just two years, she had acted in a Jean-Luc Godard movie and was nominated for a César. Her Oscar as Best Supporting Actress, in *The English Patient,* confirmed her growing stature as an international star and she has gone on impressing her many fans. Juliette never married, but has had relationships with the actors Olivier Martinez, Benoît Magimel (with whom she had a daughter, Hannah), Mathieu Amalric, and currently, the writer, Santiago Amigorena.

Rendez-vous (1985)
Mauvais sang (1986)
The Unbearable
Lightness of Being (1988)
Les Amants du Pont-Neuf (1991)
Les Trois coleurs bleu (1993)
Damage (1993) Le Hussard sur
les toit (1995) The English
Patient (1996) Chocolat (2001)
Décalage horaire (2002)
Caché (2005)
Breaking and Entering (2006)
Désengagement (2007)
Dan in Real Life (2007)
Paris (2008)
L'Heure d'été (2008)

Jane **Birkin**
5ft 8½in
(JANE MALLORY BIRKIN)

Born: **December 14, 1946**
London, England

Jane's father, David, was an espionage hero during World War II, when he served in the Royal Navy as a Lieutenant-Commander. Her mother, Judy Campbell, had been an actress and singer in Noel Coward's musical comedies. Jane grew up in a fairly conventional way until the 'sixties began to swing. She left school at sixteen, and with some guidance from her mother, she began her acting career on the stage. Composer John Barry saw and liked her and cast her in his 1965 musical, "Passion Flower Hotel". They fell in love and their daughter, Kate was born in 1967. Before that happened, Jane made her film debut with an uncredited part in the comedy, *The Knack...and How to Get It,* but more sensationally, for a British film she'd featured (nude) in, Michelangelo Antonioni's landmark film, *Blow-Up.* The movie was loved by the French and in 1968, she went to Paris to audition for *Slogan,* starring Serge Gainsbourg. Jane got the part, Serge got Jane, and John Barry became consigned to history. The couple made a record – "Je t'aime...moi non plus" and appeared together in some very poor movies. From a filmgoer's point of view, the best thing to come out of the relationship was their daughter, Charlotte Gainsbourg. As she matured, Jane has become a very good actress. She was nominated for Césars, for *La Pirate, La Femme de ma vie* and *La Belle noiseuse.* Jane has recently been directing films.

L'Animal (1977) Death on the
Nile (1978) Melancholy Baby (1979)
Evil Under the Sun (1982)
La Pirate (1984)
La Femme de ma vie (1984)
Daddy Nostalgie (1990)
La Belle Noiseuse (1991)
Black for Remembrance (1995)
The Same Old Song (1997)
A Soldier's Daughter Never Dies (1998)
The Last September (1999)
Hell of a Day (2001)
Merci Docteur Rey (2002)
La Tête de maman (2007)

Jacqueline **Bisset**
5ft 6½in
(WINIFRED JACQUELINE FRASER-BISSET)

Born: **September 13, 1944**
Weybridge, Surrey, England

Her mother was French, so Jacqueline was bi-lingual long before she started school, at the Lycée Français Charles de Gaulle, in London. She was encouraged to go to ballet lessons. When she was in her teens, her father left the family and she worked as a fashion model to help her mother and brother, Max. Jacqueline kept her eyes open for work opportunities and in 1966 made her film debut, in Roman Polanski's *Cul-de-sac.* The following year she had a good role in the Audrey Hepburn movie, *Two for the Road.* The parts then came thick and fast – some of them, like *Bullitt,* and *Airport,* were very high profile. In 1973, she used her French in François Truffaut's *Day for Night,* and with heart throb Jean-Paul Belmondo, in *Le Magnifique.* In 1977, she set a fashion for wet T-shirts when she went swimming in *The Deep.* Jacqueline was nominated for Golden Globes – for three of her films, *The Sweet Ride, Who Is Killing the Great Chefs of Europe?* and *Under the Volcano,* but has yet to win. She's still a beautiful lady, but she doesn't always get the roles she would like. All the fans who hoped that her new film, *Death in Love* would be a special treat, were rewarded.

Two for the Road (1967)
The Detective (1968)
The Mephisto Waltz (1971)
The Life and Times of
Judge Roy Bean (1972)
Bullitt (1973)
La Nuit Américaine (1973)
Le Magnifique (1973)
Murder on the
Orient Express (1974)
Der Richter und sein
Henker (1975)
Who Is Killing the
Great Chefs of Europe? (1978)
Rich and Famous (1981)
La Cérémonie (1995)
Dangerous Beauty (1998)
Latter Days (2003)
Swing (2003)
Death in Love (2008)

Gunnar **Björnstrand**
6ft 3in
(KNUT GUNNAR JOHANSON)

Born: **November 13, 1909**
Stockholm, Sweden
Died: **May 26, 1986**

As the son of the Swedish stage actor, Oscar Johanson, Gunnar was attracted to a theatrical career, but somehow, he became an apprentice baker. He was drafted into military service for eighteen months and it made him consider his future. He took acting lessons from his dad and made his stage debut at the Hippodrom Theater in Malmö. He had a small part in a play featuring the distin-guished actor, Gösta Ekman. From then on, he was determined to become a star. Gunnar enrolled at Stockholm's Royal Dramatic School at the same time as Signe Hasso and Ingrid Bergman. It was there that he met and fell in love with his lifelong partner, Lillie. After they finished studying they found work for two years at the Swedish Theater in Vasa, Finland. There were periods of hardship after that, but things improved to the point where Gunnar made his first film, *Natt i hamn* in 1943. Very soon, he established himself by acting on stage in August Strindberg's "Spöksonaten" – directed by Ingmar Bergman. Gunnar was first introduced to movie audiences by Bergman in 1953, in *Gycklarnas Afton.* Although he was never as well known as others in the Swedish master's incredible repertory company, Gunnar appeared in more of his films than any other actor. He died of natural causes.

Gycklarnas Afton (1953)
A Lesson in Love (1954)
Smiles of a Summer Night (1955)
The Seventh Seal (1956)
Wild Strawberries (1957)
The Face (1958)
The Devil's Eye (1960)
Through a Glass Darkly (1961)
Winter Light (1962)
Loving Couples (1964)
My Sister, My Love (1966)
Persona (1966)
Violenza al sole (1968)
The Girls (1968) Shame (1968)
Autumn Sonata (1978)
Fanny and Alexander (1982)

Jack **Black**
5ft 7in
(THOMAS JACK BLACK)

Born: **August 28, 1969**
Santa Monica, California, USA

Jack was the son of a couple of satellite engineers – Thomas Black Sr., and his wife Judith – who worked on the Hubble Space Telescope. Jack's mother was Jewish and his father converted to Judaism, but they divorced when Jack was ten years old. Around that time, he did a bit of work as a child model – appearing in a commercial for Artari "Pitfall!". After being bullied at his school, Jack transferred to Poseidon, in Santa Monica. Later, he attended Crossroads High School for Arts and Sciences, where he was tops at Drama. He dropped out of UCLA during his sophomore year to concentrate on his career. He began to get small roles in TV shows – the first of which was in 1991 – as an Ice-Hockey player in 'Our Shining Moment'. The following year, Jack made his film debut, in *Bob Roberts*. He kept plugging away as a Supporting Actor, and eventually *High Fidelity* launched him into leading roles – in such hits as *School of Rock, King Kong* and *Holiday*. All this time, he didn't neglect the music scene, where he was lead singer in the comedy rock band, "Tenacious D", which released two albums of songs. On March 24, 2006 he married Tanya Hayden, the cello-playing daughter of the great jazz bassist, Charlie Hayden. The couple now have two sons.

Dead Man Walking (1995)
The Cable Guy (1996)
Mars Attack! (1996) The Jackal (1997)
Enemy of the State (1998)
Cradle Will Rock (1999)
Jesus' Son (1999)
High Fidelity (2000)
Frank's Book (2001)
Shallow Hal (2001)
Orange County (2002)
The School of Rock (2003)
King Kong (2005) Nacho Libre (2006)
Tenacious D in
The Pick of Destiny (2006)
The Holiday (2006)
Margot at the Wedding (2007)
Be Kind Rewind (2008)

Karen **Black**
5ft 7in
(KAREN BLANCHE ZIEGLER)

Born: **July 1, 1939**
Park Ridge, Illinois, USA

Karen and her sister, (later actress Gail Brown), were the daughters of Norman A. Ziegler and his wife, Elsie, who was the prize-winning author of children's books. Her paternal grandfather Arthur Ziegler, a noted classical musician, was first violinist with the Chicago Symphony Orchestra. Unsurprisingly, young Karen was a brilliant child prodigy, who entered Northwestern University, in Evanston, near Chicago, at the age of fifteen. She dropped out after two years and in 1958, went to New York to study acting with Lee Strasberg. She had her first taste of movie acting two years later, in an independent film, *The Prime Time,* in which little acting skill was required of her. In 1965, she received high praise for her Broadway debut, in "The Playroom" – for which she was nominated for a Drama Circle Critics Award. A year later, she had a leading role in the film, *You're a Big Boy Now* – directed by young Francis Ford Coppola. Karen's big break came in 1969, when she appeared in *Easy Rider.* She reached her peak when she was nominated for an Oscar for *Five Easy Pieces* – which won her a Golden Globe, and she was nominated again, four years later, for *The Great Gatsby.* She and her fourth husband, Stephen, are active in the Church of Scientology. Karen has been seen in over a hundred movies and has recently turned her hand to scriptwriting.

Easy Rider (1969) Five Easy
Pieces (1970) The Outfit (1973)
The Great Gatsby (1974)
Nashville (1975) The Day of
the Locust (1975) Family Plot (1976)
Capricorn One (1978)
Come Back to the Five and Dime,
Jimmy Dean, Jimmy Dean (1982)
Can She Bake a Cherry
Pie? (1983) The Children (1990)
Rubin and Ed (1991)
Cries of Silence (1993)
America Brown (2004)
Firecracker (2004)
Read You Like a Book (2006)
Suffering Man's Charity (2007)

Honor **Blackman**
5ft 6in
(HONOR BLACKMAN)

Born: **December 12, 1927**
West Ham, London, England

The daughter of a statistician and his wife, Honor was still a schoolgirl when the war started. She left at sixteen to work as a Home Office dispatch rider – often with bombs exploding nearby. She persuaded her dad to pay for her acting lessons as a birthday gift before beginning her studies at the Guildhall School of Music and Drama, in London. She made her stage debut in "The Gleam" in 1946, and was recruited as a Rank starlet shortly after that. Her first credited film role was in *Daughter of Darkness,* in 1948. Honor then appeared in Somerset Maugham's *Quartet.* Her roles got bigger as the British public warmed to her good looks. By 1954, she'd starred in half a dozen films and been featured with the likes of Elizabeth and Robert Taylor, as well as a young Richard Burton. As the decade wore on however, she suffered a nervous breakdown following a painful divorce. After recovering, she was mostly seen in B-movies and on TV. Honor had a strong role in a good film about the Titanic – *A Night to Remember.* It didn't turn her into an international star – it took the TV series 'The Avengers' to do that. After that, she got the part of Pussy Galore, in the James Bond movie, *Goldfinger,* and for a few years, she in demand. Honor was married and divorced twice. She still appears on TV and in movies as a supporting actress.

Quartet (1948)
A Boy, a Girl and a Bike (1949)
So Long at the Fair (1950)
A Night to Remember (1958)
A Matter of WHO (1961)
Serena (1962)
Jason and the Argonauts (1963)
Goldfinger (1964)
Life at the Top (1965)
Moment to Moment (1965)
The Last Roman (1968)
The Virgin and the Gypsy (1970)
Age of Innocence (1977)
To Walk with Lions (1999)
Bridget Jones's Diary (2001) Colour Me
Kubrick: A True...ish Story (2005)

Rubén **Blades**
5ft 10in
(RUBÉN BLADES BELLIDO DE LUNA)

Born: **July 16, 1948**
Panama City, Panama

He was named after his grandfather from St. Lucia, who came to Panama to work on the canal. Rubén's father was a percussionist and his mother was a singer. When he was a student at the Universidad Nacional, he began writing songs and performing as a singer with Latin bands. After he had graduated with degrees in political science and law he followed his parents to the United States. He eventually settled in New York where he got a job in the mailroom at Fania Records. It led to work on the salsa music scene and the recording of several albums with Willy Colón's band. Rubén's first hit was "Pablo Pueblo" in 1977. He later used it as his campaign anthem when he ran (unsuccessfully) for the Presidency of Panama. The 1978 album "Siembra" by Colón and Blades became the biggest-selling salsa record in history. In 1982, Rubén made his film debut in a boxing movie called *The Last Fight,* for which he wrote the title song. In 1985 he gained much wider recognition when he wrote the screenplay and acted in the superb independent film, *Crossover Dreams.* His film roles became more frequent after that, but it will take time before his movie credits outnumber his fifty or so record albums. In 2004, Rubén became Minister of Tourism for Panama, which kept him quiet on the movie front for three years. He also had a new wife, Luba Mason, whom he married in 2006. After a three-year gap, Rubén will be back on the movie screen in the role of a doctor in the Panamanian production *Granpa.*

Crossover Dreams (1985)
The Milagro Beanfield War (1988)
Disorganized Crime (1989)
Predator 2 (1990)
Chinese Box (1997)
Cradle Will Rock (1999)
All the Pretty Horses (2000)
**Once Upon a Time
in Mexico** (2003)
Imagining Argentina (2003)
Spin (2003)
Secuestro Express (2005)

Robert **Blake**
5ft 4in
(MICHAEL JAMES VINCENZO GUBITOSI)

Born: **September 18, 1933**
Nutley, New Jersey, USA

Robert's father, Giacomo Gubitosi, came to America from Italy in 1907. He married Elizabeth Cafone, who was an American born Italian, and formed a song and dance act featuring their children as "The Three Little Hillbillies". In 1938, they took the family to Los Angeles, where they were able to get the children work as film extras. Robert's career really began at the age of five, when, as Mickey Gubitosi, he appeared in MGM's *Our Gang* series of shorts. His first feature film appearance was in 1939's *Bridal Suite.* In 1942, he adopted the stage name, Bobby Blake – appearing in Red Ryder westerns and Laurel and Hardy's *The Big Noise.* In 1948, he was the Mexican boy who sells the down-and-out Humphrey Bogart a winning lottery ticket in *Treasure of the Sierra Madre.* Robert's home life was so miserable he ran away at sixteen. He served in the United States Army in 1950 before studying acting with Jeff Corey. In 1956, he was first billed as Robert Blake. In 1962, he married actress, Sondra Kerr, and the couple had two children, including the actor Noah Blake. Robert's portrayal of the murderer Perry Smith in, *In Cold Blood* and the cop, in *Electra Glide in Blue* are career highlights. In 2002 there was real-life drama when he was charged with the murder of his second wife, the ten-times married, Bonnie Lee Bakley. Robert was acquitted, but he went bankrupt and is currently working as a ranch hand.

The Black Rose (1950)
Three Violent People (1956)
Pork Chop Hill (1959)
Town Without Pity (1961)
PT 109 (1963)
**The Greatest Story
Ever Told** (1965)
In Cold Blood (1967)
Tell Them Willie Boy Is Here (1969)
Electra Glide in Blue (1973)
**Second-Hand
Hearts** (1981)
Money Train (1995)
Lost Highway (1997)

Cate **Blanchett**
5ft 8½in
(CATHERINE ELISE BLANCHETT)

Born: **May 14, 1969**
Melbourne, Victoria, Australia

Cate's father, who was an American from Texas, died from a heart attack when she was ten. She has an older brother who works in the computer industry, and a younger sister who is a theatrical designer. After secondary education at a Methodist Ladies' College, she studied economics and fine art at the University of Melbourne. On a visit to Egypt, she was invited to be an extra in a local film, but walked off the set when she found that she was the only person cheering an American boxer who was being beaten by an Egyptian. Back in Australia, she attended the National Institute of Dramatic Art – from where she graduated in 1992. There were TV roles, before Cate made her film debut in 1997, in *Paradise Road.* She was nominated for an Oscar a year later, portraying Elizabeth I of England. It won her a BAFTA and a Golden Globe. In 2005, she won the Best Supporting Actress Oscar for her role as legend, Katherine Hepburn, in the Martin Scorsese biopic, *The Aviator.* She has a real prospect of becoming a great screen actress, but it isn't only films she's involved with. From 2008 onwards, Cate and her playwright husband, Andrew Upton, will be artistic co-directors of the Sydney Theater Company. Cate is never far away when it comes to awards. She won an Italian Volpi Cup, a Golden Globe, and an Independent Spirit, for *I'm Not There.*

Elizabeth (1998)
The Talented Mr Ripley (1998)
The Shipping News (2000)
Charlotte Gray (2000) **The Gift** (2000)
The Fellowship of the Ring (2001)
Bandits (2001)
The Two Towers (2001)
The Return of the King (2002)
Veronica Guerin (2003)
The Aviator (2004) **Babel** (2005)
Notes on a Scandal (2006)
Elizabeth: The Golden Age (2006)
I'm Not There (2007)
**Indiana Jones and the Kingdom of
the Crystal Skull** (2008) **The Curious
Case of Benjamin Button** (2008)

Brian **Blessed**
5ft 9in
(BRIAN BLESSED)

Born: **October 9, 1937**
Mexborough, Yorkshire, England

The son of a miner, William Blessed, and his wife, Hilda, Brian started life in a small coalmining community, but was raised in the nearby town of Goldthorpe, South Yorkshire. His family was poor, so Brian finished his education early, at Bolton-on-Dearne Secondary Modern School, in 1952. He spent several frustrating years working for a firm of undertakers and later, as a plasterer for a builder. After National Service in the RAF, he suffered a nervous breakdown. When he recovered, he went to the Bristol Old Vic Theater School to train as an actor. He got television work in shows like 'The Avengers' and 'Z Cars' and in 1966 was effectively cast – as a policeman in his first film, *The Christmas Tree.* In the four years that followed, he must have wondered when his break would come. The Michael Caine, Omar Sharif vehicle – *The Last Valley,* provided it. Brian was frequently employed in historical films, but didn't seem to mind. He was even cast as Richard IV in the first 'Black Adder' series. For a change of pace he decided, aged fifty-six, to climb up Mount Everest. He held his age-group record for nearly ten years! In 1999 he acted in and directed, *King Lear,* but for some people, three hours proved a little too long. Apart from climbing mountains and acting, Brian is something of an expert on soccer. He lives in Surrey with his wife, the actress Hildegarde Neil Zimmermann. They have a daughter and several dogs.

Henry VIII and His Six Wives (1972)
Man of La Mancha (1972)
King Arthur, the Great
Warlord (1975)
Flash Gordon (1980)
Henry V (1989) **Robin Hood:**
Prince of Thieves (1991)
Much Ado About Nothing (1993)
Hamlet (1996)
Star Wars Episode I:
The Phantom Menace (1996)
Days of Wrath (2006)
As You Like It (2006)
The Conclave (2006)

Bernard **Blier**
5ft 8in
(BERNARD BLIER)

Born: **January 11, 1916**
Buenos Aires, Argentina
Died: **March 29, 1989**

Bernard grew up in Buenos Aires with his French-born parents. His father was a researcher at L'Institut Pasteur. When Bernard was thirteen, the family returned to Paris where he spent an unhappy three years at the Lycée Condorcet. In 1931 he began to study acting, and three years later he made his debut at Ciotat, in a half empty theater. He wasn't discouraged. From 1934, he studied with Louis Jouvet at the Paris Conservatoire, becoming life-long friends with François Périer and Gerard Oury. Before graduating in 1937 he made his film debut in *Trois, six, neuf.* After a couple of stage appearances, Bernard acted in the 1938 Marcel Carné classic, *Hotel du Nord.* He married his sweetheart, Gisele that year and in 1939, their son Bertrand (the future film director) was born. During the making of *Le Jour se lève,* he struck up a friendship with the film's star, Jean Gabin. Bernard joined the infantry at the outbreak of war, but after the French surrender, he was in Paris, acting in films and plays. After the war, he provided regular support in top French films such as *Quai des Orfèvres, Crime et chatiment, Les Misérables* and *Buffet froid* – directed by Bertrand. After a forty year film career, Bernard died of cancer, at Saint-Cloud, Hauts-de-Seine, France.

Hotel du Nord (1938)
Le Jour se léve (1939)
La Nuit fantastique (1942)
Quai des Orfèvres (1947)
Dédée d'Anvers (1948)
L'École buissonnière (1949)
Manèges (1950)
Avant le déluge (1954)
Crime et chatiment (1956)
Les Misérables (1958)
Le Président (1961)
Crimen (1961)
Les Tontons flingeurs (1963)
Lo Straniero (1967)
My Uncle Benjamin (1969)
Le Distrait (1970)
Buffet froid (1979)

Joan **Blondell**
5ft 3in
(ROSE JOAN BLONDELL)

Born: **August 30, 1906**
New York City, New York, USA
Died: **December 25, 1979**

Joan's father was the vaudeville comedian Eddie Blondell. Her mother, Katie Cain provided support for Eddie. Joan had a younger sister, Gloria, with whom she joined her parents' vaudeville act when they were children. They were billed as the "Katzenjammer Kids". She went with them on a world tour, but in Australia, she made the decision to go it alone. When she got back home, she joined a stock company in Dallas. She was crowned "Miss Dallas" of 1926 and placed fourth in the "Miss America" contest that year. At the age of twenty, she rejoined her family act in New York. The movies were already killing vaudeville, so Joan decided 'if you can't beat 'em, join 'em'. But first, she made her Broadway debut in the "Ziegfeld Follies". In 1927 she got her first film part in *The Trial of Mary Dugan.* Two years later, she was in two plays with James Cagney. "Penny Arcade", was bought (along with it's two stars) by Warners for filming. It was renamed *Sinner's Holiday* and it earned Joan a five year contract. The epitome of the big-hearted American 'dame', Joan began a long spell of popularity. From 1936-1944, she was married to co-star, Dick Powell. Her second husband was Mike Todd. She was Oscar-nominated, as Best Supporting Actress for *The Blue Veil.* When she went to the big movie house in the sky, after dying of leukemia, in Santa Monica, California, Joan had completed fifty years in the movie business.

Sinner's Holiday (1930)
Public Enemy (1931)
The Greeks Had
a Word for Them (1932)
Gold Diggers of 1933 (1933)
Footlight Parade (1933)
Stage Struck (1936)
The Perfect Specimen (1937)
Cry Havoc (1943)
Nightmare Alley (1947)
The Blue Veil (1951)
The Desk Set (1957)
The Cincinnati Kid (1965)

Claire **Bloom**
5ft 5in
(PATRICIA CLAIRE BLUME)

Born: **February 15, 1931**
Finchley, London, England

Claire was born in North London, to Edward and Elizabeth Blume, who were descended from Jewish immigrants. She received her secondary education at the independent Badminton School, in Bristol. After studying for the stage at London's Guildhall School of Music and Drama, and the Central School, she changed her name to Claire Bloom. Her dulcet tones were heard on BBC radio before, in 1946, she made her stage debut with the Oxford repertory in a play entitled "It Depends What You Mean." Three years later, she appeared in London's West End, in "The Lady's Not For Burning" – with Richard Burton. It impressed enough to get the Rank Organization excited, and they signed her up for their charm school at £25 per week. In 1952, Charles Chaplin chose her to star as a young ballerina, in his sentimental drama, *Limelight.* After that world-wide exposure, she concentrated on the theater – joining the Old Vic for two seasons. In 1955, Laurence Olivier cast her as Lady Anne in his *Richard III.* She then had movie opportunities on more modern themes including *Look Back in Anger,* and *The Spy Who Came in from the Cold* – re-uniting her with Richard Burton. She had three husbands, one of whom was the late Rod Steiger. Claire can still be seen on the stage and in television dramas. In 2006, she co-starred with Billy Zane on the London stage in "Six Dance Lessons in Six Weeks".

Limelight (1952)
The Man Between (1953)
Richard III (1955)
Look Back in Anger (1958)
The Brothers Karamazov (1958)
The Buccaneer (1958)
The Wonderful World of
the Brothers Grimm (1962)
The Haunting (1963)
The Spy Who Came in
from the Cold (1965) Charly (1968)
Crimes and Misdemeanors (1989)
Imagining Argentina (2003)
Kalamazoo? (2006)

Orlando **Bloom**
5ft 11in
(ORLANDO JONATHAN BLANCHARD BLOOM)

Born: **January 13, 1977**
Canterbury, Kent, England

He was four when the man he believed to be his father (the South African civil rights activist, Harry Bloom) died. Orlando was then raised by his real dad, Colin Stone, and his mother Sonia. At St. Edmund's School in Canterbury, Orlando suffered from slight dyslexia, but revealed an aptitude for the Arts. He acted in school plays and also got involved with the local theater. He and his sister gave poetry readings at the Kent Festival and Orlando was ready to embark on his career. He spent two years at the National Youth Theater before winning a scholarship to the British American Drama Academy in London. He landed a television role, in 'Midsomer Murders' and in 1997, made his film debut in *Wilde.* The following year, after he had transferred to the Guildhall School of Music and Drama, he fell three storeys from a rooftop terrace and broke his back. Not only did he completely recover, he got a part in the film, *Black Hawk Down,* because of that experience – his character also breaks his back! One evening in a theater, he was contacted by the movie director, Peter Jackson. Peter invited him to work on his *Lord of the Rings* trilogy. By the time Orlando finished eighteen months of filming in New Zealand, he was a star. Since then, that position has been fortified by his appearances in the *Pirates of the Caribbean* trilogy.

The Fellowship of the Ring (2001)
Black Hawk Down (2001)
The Two Towers (2002)
Ned Kelly (2003)
Pirates of the Caribbean:
The Curse of
the Black Pearl (2003)
The Return of the King (2003)
Kingdom of Heaven (2005)
Elizabethtown (2005)
Pirates of the Caribbean:
Dead Man's Chest (2006)
Love and Other Disasters (2006)
Pirates of the Caribbean:
At World's End (2007)
New York, I Love You (2008)

Eric **Blore**
5ft 8in
(ERIC BLORE)

Born: **December 23, 1887**
London, England
Died: **March 2, 1959**

After leaving school at fourteen, Eric worked as a junior at a London insurance firm. When he was twenty, he decided to seek his fortune in Australia. Over there he cultivated an interest in theater and acted in local amateur productions. He returned to Europe at the end of World War I and began to pursue a career as an entertainer. He developed a Music Hall personality of the 'silly-ass' variety and appeared in his first film, in 1920, *A Night Out and a Day In.* Eric went to New York three years later, where he acted in musical comedies. In 1926, he played Lord Digby in the silent version of *The Great Gatsby.* His first Astaire and Rogers movie, *Flying Down to Rio,* established him as a great character and his role in "The Gay Divorcee", on Broadway, made him a must for the film version. His accent, pregnant pauses, facial expressions and outbursts of wit, made him an essential ingredient of a number of musical comedy films. In 1959, Eric's premature obituary appeared in The New Yorker. It caused the poor man such distress that his lawyer forced the magazine to print a retraction and an apology. By the time it appeared, The New Yorker was the only publication to get it wrong - Eric had actually passed away – at his home in Hollywood!

The Gay Divorcee (1934)
Folies Bergère de Paris (1935)
Top Hat (1935)
The Ex-Mrs. Bradford (1936)
Piccadilly Jim (1936)
Swing Time (1936)
Quality Street (1937)
Shall We Dance (1937)
It's Love I'm After (1937)
Swiss Miss (1938)
Island of Lost Men (1939)
The Lady Eve (1941)
Sullivan's Travels (1941)
Holy Matrimony (1943)
Kitty (1945)
Romance on the High Seas (1948)
Fancy Pants (1950)

Emily **Blunt**
5ft 7½in
(EMILY OLIVIA LEAH BLUNT)

Born: **February 23, 1983**
London, England

Emily was one of four children born to a barrister and his wife, who was a teacher. She was raised in the middle-class leafy suburb of Roehampton, in South West London – attending a local private school, Ibstock Place. She suffered from a stammer until she was twelve – curing it when her teacher asked her to play a character in a play – using a different accent. When she was sixteen, Emily attended boarding school at Hurtwood House – where she played cello, sang, and excelled at sport. She also benefited from two years of drama studies on the school's theater course. In August 2000, she was chosen to appear at the Edinburgh Festival in "Bliss", which was commissioned by the National Theater. The following year, she made her London West End debut at the Haymarket Theater, in "The Royal Family" with Judi Dench and won the Evening Standard's Best Newcomer Award. Emily made her film debut in 2003, as Isolda, in *Warrior Queen*. She was praised for her portrayal of Catherine Howard in the TV play 'Henry VIII' later that year. Her first important film role was as Tamsin, in *My Summer of Love*. In 2005, she started a three-year relationship with singer Michael Bublé and lived for much of the time with him in Vancouver. She provided a backing vocal on his recording of "Me and Mrs. Jones", but the couple split up due to busy work schedules. Emily's biggest hit film to date was *The Devil Wears Prada,* but she also features strongly in *The Jane Austen Book Club, Charlie Wilson's War* and *Sunshine Cleaning*. She will soon be seen as *The Young Victoria*.

Boudica (2003)
My Summer of Love (2004)
Irresistible (2006)
The Devil Wears Prada (2006)
Wind Chill (2007)
The Jane Austen Book Club (2007)
Dan in Real Life (2007)
Charlie Wilson's War (2007)
Sunshine Cleaning (2008)
The Great Buck Howard (2008)

Ann **Blyth**
5ft 2in
(ANN MARIE BLYTH)

Born: **August 16, 1928**
Mount Kisco, New York, USA

Ann was the daughter of Harry and Nan Blyth. Following her parents' divorce just after she was born, her mother turned to religion and brought her daughter up as a devout Catholic. Ann went to school in New York, and at the age of nine joined the New York Children's Opera. She began her acting career on Broadway in 1941. Performing at the Biltmore Theater in Los Angeles in 1943, she was spotted by film director Henry Koster, who got her a contract with Universal. She dropped the 'e' from her first name and made her film debut in 1944, in *Chip off the Old Block*. On loan to Warners, to play Joan Crawford's cruel, ungrateful daughter Veda in *Mildred Pierce* she was nominated for a Best Supporting Actress Oscar. After that film she went on a winter sports vacation to Lake Arrowhead in California and broke her back when she was thrown from a speeding toboggan. Her recovery took more than a year, so she was unable to capitalize on her success. She used her sweet singing voice in films for the next ten years – the best of which was *The Great Caruso*. In 1953, Ann married Dr. James McNulty, the brother of the singer-comedian, Dennis Day – who introduced them. In 1957, she retired from films to raise their five children and from 1960, she concentrated on television work. She later did musical theater and last appeared in a TV version of 'Murder She Wrote', in 1985. After fifty-four years of happy marriage, Ann became a widow in 2007. She lives near San Diego, California.

Mildred Pierce (1945)
Brute Force (1947)
Another Part of the Forest (1948)
Mr. Peabody and the Mermaid (1948)
Our Very Own (1950)
The Great Caruso (1951)
The World in his Arms (1952)
The Student Prince (1954)
The King's Thief (1955)
Kismet (1955)
Slander (1956)
The Helen Morgan Story (1957)

Sir Dirk **Bogarde**
5ft 8½in
(DEREK VAN DEN BOGAERDE)

Born: **March 28, 1921**
Hampstead, London, England
Died: **May 8, 1999**

Starting life as Derek, he spent his early years with his brother and sister – at the family home in Sussex. Their father, a Dutchman, was the arts correspondent for "The Times" newspaper in London. When he was eleven, Derek was sent to a boarding school in Glasgow. He became a student at the Chelsea Polytechnic – in preparation for a career in commercial art, but he was more interested in the theater. He went to drama lessons before making his London West End debut in 1939. At the start of World War II, Dirk joined the Queen's Royal Regiment. During his five years service, he achieved the rank of major and was awarded seven medals. The paintings he produced now hang in the Imperial War Museum. He was quite traumatized by what he saw in Belsen – describing it as "Looking into Dante's Inferno". In 1947, he was re-christened Dirk Bogarde and signed by Rank. They gave him his first leading role in *Esther Waters* in 1948, but it was *The Blue Lamp* which made him a household name. The 1950s was his heart-throb period, but from then on, he was simply a fine actor with great credit due for his performances in *Victim, The Servant, Darling* and *Death in Venice*. His several autobiographical books are entertaining, if not very revealing about a very complex man. Dirk died of a heart attack at his home in London.

So Long at the Fair (1950)
Hunted (1952)
Appointment in London (1953)
Desperate Moment (1953) Simba (1955)
Libel (1959) Victim (1961)
I Could go on Singing (1963)
The Servant (1963) King and
Country (1964) Darling (1965)
Accident (1967) The Fixer (1968)
The Damned (1969)
Death in Venice (1971)
The Night Porter (1974)
A Bridge Too Far (1977)
Despair (1979)
Daddy Nostalgie (1990)

Humphrey **Bogart**
5ft 8½in
(HUMPHREY DEFOREST BOGART)

Born: **December 25, 1899**
New York City, New York, USA
Died: **January 14, 1957**

Unlike his often rough film personality, 'Bogie' grew up with all the trappings of wealth and privilege. His father was a surgeon who always hoped that his son would study medicine at Yale. He was very disappointed. 'Bogie' served in the US Navy at the end of World War I, and while there, he had an accident which gave him his trademark snarl. He was friendly with the brother of actress Alice Brady, who got him small parts in a couple of her films. In 1930 he was signed by Fox, who put him in his first feature, *A Devil With Women*. That, and two films for Warners were a bit lightweight so he went home disillusioned. He played Duke Mantee on stage in "The Petrified Forest" and in the film version. It earned him a Warners contract, but he struggled to overcome studio indifference. The turning point came with *High Sierra*. He married Lauren Bacall in 1945 and they had twelve happy years together. *The Maltese Falcon, Casablanca, The Big Sleep,* and *The Treasure of the Sierra Madre* were only a few of his career highlights. An Oscar for *The African Queen* was less than he deserved. To many, 'Bogie' was the biggest star in Hollywood – admired by other actors as well as his millions of fans. A heavy smoker for most of his life, Bogie died of throat cancer.

The Petrified Forest (1936)
Kid Galahad (1937)
Angels With Dirty Faces (1938)
They Drive by Night (1940)
High Sierra (1941)
The Maltese Falcon (1941)
Casablanca (1942) Sahara (1943)
To Have and Have Not (1944)
The Big Sleep (1946)
Dead Reckoning (1947)
The Treasure of the Sierra Madre (1948)
In a Lonely Place (1950)
The African Queen (1951)
The Caine Mutiny (1954)
The Barefoot Contessa (1954)
The Desperate Hours (1955)
The Harder They Fall (1956)

Ray **Bolger**
5ft 10½in
(RAYMOND WALLACE BULAO)

Born: **January 10, 1904**
Dorchester, Massachusetts, USA
Died: **January 15, 1987**

Ray's father, James Bulcao, was a painter and decorator who was born in Portugal. His mother, Anne, was Irish, and it was she who chose to live in the mainly Irish neighborhood of Dorchester, where young Ray grew up. Naturally, he was raised as a Roman Catholic. When he was a small boy, his parents took him to vaudeville shows – which he absolutely loved. When he got home, he'd entertain his family with impressions of what he'd seen and heard. By the time Ray left school at sixteen, he had decided he wanted a career in show business. He began in vaudeville as one half of the Sanford and Bolger Duo. In 1922, he made his stage debut in Boston with the Bob Ott Musical Comedy Repertory Company. Two years later, he made his film debut in the silent, *Carrie of the Chorus.* It was a while later, before he was spotted by the promoter, Gus Edwards and given a starring role in the Broadway musical, "A Merry Word". The lead in Rogers and Hart's 1936 show, "On Your Toes" made him a star and won him an MGM contract and his first sound film appearance in *The Great Ziegfeld.* With Nelson Eddy and Jeanette MacDonald he did *Sweethearts,* but it was with his role as the Scarecrow, in the wonderful *Wizard of Oz* – that Ray achieved everlasting fame. He toured with the USO during World War II but didn't make many movies after that. Best are the *Harvey Girls* and *Where's Charley?* – also a Broadway success. Ray was married to Gwendolyn Rickard from 1929 until his death from cancer in Los Angeles. There were no children.

Rosalie (1937)
Sweethearts (1938)
The Wizard of Oz (1939)
The Harvey Girls (1946)
Look for the Silver Lining (1949)
Where's Charley? (1952)
April in Paris (1952)
Babes in Toyland (1961)
The Daydreamer (1966)
Just You and Me, Kid (1979)

Ward **Bond**
6ft 1in
(WARDELL E. BOND)

Born: **April 9, 1903**
Benkelman, Nebraska, USA
Died: **November 5, 1960**

When Ward was sixteen, his family moved to Denver. Two years later, Ward graduated from East Denver High School before attending the University of Southern California. He played in the University football team alongside a guy called Marion Morrison – later known as the Hollywood star, John Wayne. The entire Southern Cal team were hired to appear in John Ford's *Salute* in 1929 – the beginning of a long association for the three men. Ward acted in Wayne's first film as a leading man, *The Big Trail* – the very first movie to be shot in 70mm wide screen, and they became great friends and drinking buddies. He also did some good work for Frank Capra, beginning with *It Happened One Night.* According to the American Film Institute, he was in more of their list of the "100 Greatest American Movies" than any other actor. When he made his first TV appearance, he had 233 movies behind him. In the 1950s, Ward starred in the popular 'Wagon Train' series. He was in Dallas to watch a football game when he suffered a massive heart attack. At Ward's funeral John Wayne read the eulogy.

The Man Who Lived Twice (1936)
Conflict (1936) Dead End (1937)
Bringing Up Baby (1938)
Drums Along the Mowhawk (1939)
Gone With the Wind (1939)
The Grapes of Wrath (1940)
Tobacco Road (1941)
Sergeant York (1941)
The Maltese Falcon (1941)
Gentleman Jim (1942)
A Guy Named Joe (1943)
The Sullivans (1944)
My Darling Clementine (1946)
It's a Wonderful Life (1946)
The Fugitive (1947) Fort
Apache (1948) 3 Godfathers (1948)
Wagonmaster (1950)
The Quiet Man (1952)
Johnny Guitar (1954)
Mister Roberts (1955)
The Searchers (1956) Rio Bravo (1959)

Beulah **Bondi**

5ft 6in

(BEULAH BONDY)

Born: **May 3, 1888**
Chicago, Illinois, USA
Died: **January 1, 1981**

She was the daughter of Adolphe Bondy, who was of Hungarian stock, and his wife, Eva. Beulah began her stage career when she was seven – in the title role of "Little Lord Fauntleroy" at the Memorial Opera House, in Valparaiso. From 1916 to 1918, she attended University there – graduating with both a Bachelor's and a Master's degree in Oratory. Beulah worked on the stage for twelve years before she made her film debut in *Street Scene* – reprising her earlier stage role. She became a big favorite of directors – never giving less than her best in dozens of character roles. She was nominated as Best Supporting actress for *The Gorgeous Hussy* and *Of Human Hearts.* She was James Stewart's mother in four movies, including *It's a Wonderful Life,* but she never married or had children. She portrayed Martha Walton in the TV series and won an Emmy for her final episode of the show in 1976. Four years later, Beulah died of pulmonary complications after breaking her ribs when she tripped over her beloved cat.

Street Scene (1931) **Rain** (1932)
The Stranger's Return (1933) **The Good
Fairy** (1935) **The Invisible Ray** (1936)
The Trail of the Lonesome Pine (1936)
The Case Against Mrs. Ames (1936)
Hearts Divided (1936) **The Gorgeous
Hussy** (1936) **The Buccaneer** (1938)
Of Human Hearts (1938)
The Sisters (1938) **Mr. Smith Goes to
Washington** (1939) **Our Town** (1940)
The Captain Is a Lady (1940)
Penny Serenade (1941)
Watch on the Rhine (1943)
Our Hearts Were Young and Gay (1944)
The Very Thought of You (1944)
And Now Tomorrow (1944)
The Southerner (1945)
Sister Kenny (1946)
It's a Wonderful Life (1946)
The Snake Pit (1948)
So Dear to My Heart (1948)
Reign of Terror (1949)
Track of the Cat (1954)

Helena **Bonham-Carter**

5ft 3½in

(HELENA BONHAM-CARTER)

Born: **May 26, 1966**
Golders Green, London, England

Helena's family tree is full of celebrated and interesting people. Her paternal great-grandfather was Herbert Henry Asquith, the Liberal Prime Minister of Britain from 1908 until 1916. Her maternal grandfather was a Spanish diplomat, who was based in Washington, D.C. Helena is also related to Anthony Asquith, the film director. She was educated at a top private school, Westminster. She won a national writing contest when she was fourteen, and used the cash prize to pay for her entry in "Spotlight," the actors' directory. It yielded a part in a television commercial when she was sixteen and in 1983, a role in a TV film called 'A Pattern of Roses'. Helena's first starring role was in 1984, in *Lady Jane*, but it was released after her breakthrough film, *A Room with a View*. That and some of her early work for Merchant-Ivory, earned her a reputation as a Victorian-style English rose. She broke away from that to some extent in the Edwardian-era, *Wings of a Dove,* which contained a nude scene and earned an Oscar nomination. Later work has been more varied, but she has yet to strike gold. Meanwhile she has diversified by launching her own fashion line "The Pantaloonies". Helena has a son, Billy-Ray and a daughter, Nell, with the film director Tim Burton. They met in 2001.

A Room With a View (1986)
Lady Jane (1986)
Francesco (1989)
Getting It Right (1989) **Hamlet** (1990)
Where Angels Fear to Tread (1991)
Howard's End (1991)
Frankenstein (1994)
Mighty Aphrodite (1995)
Twelfth Night (1996)
Wings of the Dove (1997)
Fight Club (1999) **Charlie and
the Chocolate Factory** (2003)
**Conversations with Other
Women** (2005) **Sixty Six** (2006)
The Order of the Phoenix (2007)
Sweeney Todd (2007)
**Harry Potter and the Half-Blood
Prince** (2009)

Richard **Boone**

6ft 2in

(RICHARD ALLEN BOONE)

Born: **June 18, 1917**
Los Angeles, California, USA
Died: **January 10, 1981**

Dick was one of three children of a corporate lawyer – who was a direct descendant of famous frontiersman, Daniel Boone. After high school, Dick went to Stanford University, but he dropped out before graduating. He joined the U.S. Navy in 1941, to serve as an aviation ordnance man and he saw action in the South Pacific. When the war was over, he used the G.I.Bill to pay for lessons at the Actor's Studio in New York. In 1947 he made his Broadway debut in "Medea" and in 1950, he landed his first film role in *Halls of Montezuma*. Dick was a regular on television during the 1950s – starring in 'Medic' for which he was Emmy nominated, and the even more successful, 'Have Gun Will Travel'. His own 'Richard Boone Show' ran for two years from 1964 and won a Golden Globe. Even though Dick rarely starred, movies were still a big part of his life. He appeared in three John Wayne films and in 1968, at Brando's insistence, he directed the final scenes of the disastrous *Night of the Following Day*. By the mid-1970s, he was teaching at the Neighborhood Playhouse. In 1981, Dick made his final film, *The Bushido Blade*. Following Dick's death from throat cancer his ashes were scattered in the ocean off the coast of Hawaii.

Halls of Montezuma (1951)
The Desert Fox (1951)
Man on a Tightrope (1953)
The Robe (1953) **Dragnet** (1954)
The Raid (1954)
Man Without a Star (1955)
Battle Stations (1956)
Star in the Dust (1956)
Away All Boats (1956)
The Garment Jungle (1957)
The Alamo (1960)
Rio Conchos (1964)
The War Lord (1965)
Hombre (1967)
The Arrangement (1969)
The Kremlin Letter (1970)
The Shootist (1976)

Shirley **Booth**
5ft 3in
(THELMA MARJORIE FORD)

Born: **August 30, 1898**
New York City, New York, USA
Died: **October 16, 1992**

When she was fifteen she was thrilled by the arrival of a baby sister, Valentine – who was born on February 14th. By that time, Shirley was already active in school plays and at seventeen, she joined a stock company. For about ten years she toured the country – gaining valuable experience in all manner of theatrical productions. It was early January 1925, when Shirley made her Broadway debut, opposite Humphrey Bogart, in "Hell's Bells". Never a glamour girl and not really interested in stardom she kept on working within the limited scope of the theater, where she was much admired. In 1929, she married the actor/writer, Ed Gardner. In 1935, her stage fame started to spread when she appeared in the long-running comedy hit, "Three Men on a Horse". Even after acting with Katherine Hepburn on stage in "The Philadelphia Story" she wasn't expecting a screen career. In fact, her next project was playing Miss Duffy, in the popular radio show, 'Duffy's Tavern' – which ran until 1943, the year she had a stage hit with Ralph Bellamy in "Tomorrow the World". In 1949 she received her first Tony Award for "Goodbye My Fancy". The likelihood of Shirley making a film seemed remote until she was asked to repeat her Broadway stage triumph in Come Back, Little Sheba. She was fifty-four and we can only admire her incredible command of the medium in the four movies she made. From 1961-66 she won new fans – as Hazel in the TV series, 'Hazel'. Shirley retired in 1974 after recording the voice of Mrs. Santa, in an animated TV film, 'The Year Without a Santa Claus'. Eighteen years later she died of natural causes at her home in North Chatham, Massachusetts. Shirley was married twice – the second time to William H. Baker, who died in 1951. There were no children.

Come Back, Little Sheba (1952)
About Mrs. Leslie (1954)
Hot Spell (1958)
The Matchmaker (1958)

Powers **Boothe**
6ft 1¹⁄₂in
(POWERS ALLEN BOOTHE)

Born: **June 1, 1948**
Snyder, Texas, USA

The son of Merril Vestal Boothe, and his wife, Emily Reeves, Powers received his early schooling in Scurry County and was later educated at Southwest Texas State College, in San Marcos. He was twenty-one when he married his sweetheart, Pam Cole. They had two children and are still happily married. Their daughter, Parisse, is a young actress. In 1972, he received his Master of Fine Arts Degree, from the Southern Methodist University, in Dallas. He then joined the repertory company connected to the Oregon Shakespeare Festival and appeared in the title role of "Henry IV, Part 2", "Troilus and Cressida" and several other highbrow offerings. He made his New York stage debut in 1974, in the Lincoln Center production of William Shakespeare's "Richard III". It was in a role as a member of the cast of that very play that he made his movie debut – in Neil Simon's The Goodbye Girl. Five years later, Powers made his Broadway debut in the one-act play, "Lone Star". He came to national attention in 1980, with his Emmy Award winning portrayal of Jim Jones in the CBS-TV film, 'Guyana Tragedy: The Story of Jim Jones'. It lead to more movie work, starting with the exciting drama, Southern Comfort, in which he co-starred with Keith Carradine. His classical training made him ideal for serious, authority figure roles, and led to him being cast in two excellent films shot in the old Soviet Union – Stalingrad, and Angely smerti.

Southern Comfort (1981)
Red Dawn (1984)
The Emerald Forest (1985)
Extreme Prejudice (1987)
Stalingrad (1989)
Rapid Fire (1992)
Angely smerti (1993)
Tombstone (1993)
Blue Sky (1994)
Nixon (1995)
U Turn (1997)
Men of Honor (2000)
Frailty (2001) **Sin City** (2005)
The Final Season (2007)

Ernest **Borgnine**
5ft 9in
(ERMES EFFRON BORGINO)

Born: **January 24, 1917**
Hamden, Connecticut, USA

The only child of Italian immigrants, Ernest was more interested in playing games and watching sports (especially boxing) than academic endeavors. Following high school, Ernest spent ten years in the US Navy. After the war, he worked in factories and was getting nowhere fast until his mother suggested that his personality might be suited to an acting career. He enrolled at the Randall School of Drama in Hartford, and after that, had four years' invaluable experience with the famous Barter Theater, in Abingdon, Virginia. In 1949, he made his Broadway debut, as the male nurse, in "Harvey". Two years later, he moved to Los Angeles and got his first film role in The Whistle at Eaton Falls. Ernest's career took off when, at the age of thirty-eight, he was given the plum role of Sergeant "Fatso" Judson, in the award-winning, From Here to Eternity. His own award – a Best Actor Oscar, came his way in 1955, for his sensitive performance in Marty. He has been awarded doctorates from colleges all around the USA. In 1996 he toured the country by bus in order to meet his fans. Ernest is still very active – he recently completed more than sixty years as a professional actor.

From Here to Eternity (1953)
Johnny Guitar (1954)
Vera Cruz (1954)
Bad Day at Black Rock (1955)
Marty (1955) **Jubal** (1956)
The Catered Affair (1956)
The Best Things in Life Are Free (1956)
The Vikings (1958) **Barabba** (1961)
McHale's Navy (1964)
The Flight of the Phoenix (1965)
The Dirty Dozen (1967)
The Wild Bunch (1969)
Hannie Caulder (1971)
The Poseidon Adventure (1972)
Emperor of the North (1973)
Hustle (1975)
Escape From New York (1981)
High Risk (1981)
BASEketball (1998)
La Cura del Gorilla (2006)

Kate **Bosworth**
5ft 5in
(CATHERINE ANN BOSWORTH)

Born: **January 2, 1983**
Los Angeles, California, USA

Kate had a difficult childhood – growing up in different parts of the country due to her father's job as an executive with the retail company, Talbots. She always felt like the 'new girl' at school and she remembers being extremely shy and not very popular. Later at Cohasset High School, in Massachusetts, she learned Spanish and played both representative soccer and lacrosse. She became more confident, showing exceptional skill in becoming a fine horsewoman. It got her a supporting role in the 1998 film, *The Horse Whisperer*. In 2000, Kate was accepted at Princeton University, but because of her desire to establish herself as an actress she deferred her attendance. She moved to Los Angeles and soon got her first leading role in the surfing move, *Blue Crush*. Kate took the role seriously and in order to add fifteen pounds of muscle to her slim frame, she trained six hours a day for several months. The result was a more curvy Kate and a popular movie. After that big film's success, parts in such hits as *The Rules of Attraction* and *Wonderland* came her way with growing frequency. She played Sandra Dee in Kevin Spacey's biopic of his idol, Bobby Darin, *Beyond the Sea,* and worked with the actor again in *21*. In 2006 Kate landed the plum role of Lois Lane in the blockbuster *Superman Returns*. Kate's on-off relationship with the actor Orlando Bloom is now in its fifth year. She also has two cats – Louise and Dusty and a dog named Lila.

The Horse Whisperer (1998)
Remember the Titans (2000)
Blue Crush (2002)
The Rules of Attraction (2002)
Wonderland (2003)
Advantage Hart (2003)
Win a Date with
Tad Hamilton (2004)
Beyond The Sea (2004)
Bee Season (2005)
Superman Returns (2006)
The Girl in the Park (2007) 21 (2008)
The Laundry Warrior (2009)

Timothy **Bottoms**
5ft 11in
(TIMOTHY JAMES BOTTOMS)

Born: **August 30, 1951**
Santa Barbara, California, USA

Tim is one of four brothers – all of whom became actors. His father was an art teacher who had a passion for music, which he passed on to his family. When he was seventeen, Tim, who had a fine voice, toured Europe with the Santa Monica Madrigal Society. At high school he performed in stage productions and was the first in his family to pursue an acting career. He was in "Romeo and Juliet" when he was selected by writer/director, Dalton Trumble, for the 1971 film version of *Johnny Got His Gun*. Shortly after that, Tim starred as the teenager, Sonny Crawford in Peter Bogdanovich's masterpiece, *The Last Picture Show,* which also featured his brother Samuel. Towards the end of the 1970s, Tim's film career stalled, but he had strong television roles such as in the 1981 miniseries version of 'East of Eden'. In 1987, he co-starred with his brothers Samuel and Joseph, in the TV pilot, 'Favorite Son'. In 1990, he starred in a belated sequel to *The Last Picture Show – Texasville*. Tim's Broadway debut came in 1991, in "The 5th of July". With an uncanny resemblance to the man, Tim has played President Bush three times in television dramas, including the series, 'That's My Bush!' in 2001. In the past six years he has had an enviable strike rate – with six very good films to his credit.

Johnny Got His Gun (1971)
The Last Picture Show (1971)
Love and Pain and the
Whole Damn Thing (1973)
The Paper Chase (1973)
The White Dawn (1974)
Operation: Daybreak (1975)
Horses and Champions (1994)
The Haven (2000)
The Hiding Place (2000)
Elephant (2003)
The Girl Next Door (2004)
Paradise, Texas (2005)
Shanghai Kiss (2007)
Along the Way (2007)
Chinaman's Chance (2008)
Parasomnia (2008)

Carole **Bouquet**
5ft 8in
(CAROLE BOUQUET)

Born: **August 18, 1957**
Neuilly-sur-Seine, France

Carole started life on the outskirts of Paris, in the comfortable middle-class district of Neuilly. Her father, who was an aeronautical engineer was literally 'left holding the babies' when his wife left to return to her village near Toulon. Carole and her older sister were raised by their dad, who was not the world's greatest communicator. It was particularly difficult as she only saw her mother during visits, and Carole had a bad time at school – being expelled from several including a boarding school run by Dominican nuns. Carole was a stunning looking teenager, but her reaction to being stared at was to give the impression of being aloof. After she had passed her baccalauréat she briefly began reading philosophy at the Sorbonne, but switched to the Conservatoire d'Art Dramatique. She spent her spare time at museums and in cinemas, which is where she first became aware of the films of Luis Buñuel. By sheer coincidence, she was spotted in the street and offered the leading role of Conchita in *That Obscure Object of Desire*. Carole had a small role in *Buffet Froid* and, following a trip to New York, where she acted in a piece of rubbish – *Blank Generation,* she became a Bond girl in *For Your Eyes Only*. Her big love, Jean-Pierre Rassam, died in 1985. In 1996, she began an eight-year relationship with Gérard Depardieu. She starred on stage in "Bérénice" in 2007.

That Obscure Object of Desire (1977)
Buffet froid (1979) For Your Eyes
Only (1981) Day of the Idiots (1981)
Mystère (1983) Rive droite, rive
gauche (1984) Double messieurs (1986)
Jenatsch (1987) Bunker Palace
Hôtel (1989) Tango (1993)
Lucie Aubrac (1997) En plein
coeur (1998) The Bridge (1999)
Wasabi (2001) Summer Things (2002)
Red Lights (2004)
Bad Spelling (2004)
Nordeste (2005) L'Enfer (2005)
Perfect Match (2007)
Les Hauts murs (2008)

Stephen **Boyd**
6ft 1in
(WILLIAM MILLAR)

Born: **July 4, 1931**
Glengormley, Northern Ireland
Died: **June 2, 1977**

Stephen was one of nine children who were supported by a truck driver father. After leaving secondary school, he studied bookkeeping at a commercial college in Belfast. He was employed by an insurance firm and then a travel agency. After work, he rehearsed with a semi-professional theater company. He moved to the Ulster Theater Group and changed his name to Stephen Boyd. During a three year stay with the group, he also refined his voice by doing radio work. London proved less friendly and he fell ill when reduced to washing-up jobs and busking in the streets. When Stephen was working as a doorman at the Odeon Theater, Michael Redgrave saw him one night and was impressed enough by his looks and personality to introduce him to the Windsor Repertory Company. BBC TV roles, radio work, and a couple of small parts in movies showcased his talent and in 1956 he signed a seven-year contract with 20th Century-Fox. His debut for them was in *The Man Who Never Was* – playing a member of the IRA. Big parts in big movies like *Ben Hur* and *The Fall of the Roman Empire* gave Stephen a dozen years at the top. By the late 1960s, he was earning a living in European B-movies. In 1977, when appearing to be making a comeback, Stephen suffered a massive heart-attack while playing a round of golf in California. Both his two marriages survived less than a year.

The Man Who Never Was (1956)
Seven Waves Away (1957)
Island in the Sun (1957)
The Night Heaven Fell (1958)
The Bravados (1958) **Woman Obsessed** (1959) **The Best of Everything** (1959) **Ben-Hur** (1959)
Lisa (1962) **The Third Secret** (1964)
The Fall of the Roman Empire (1964)
Genghis Khan (1965)
The Bible: In the Beginning (1966)
Fantastic Voyage (1966)
The Squeeze (1977)

Charles **Boyer**
5ft 9in
(CHARLES BOYER)

Born: **August 28, 1899**
Figeac, Midi-Pyrénées, France
Died: **August 26, 1978**

From early childhood, Charles Boyer dreamed that, one day, he would be an actor. After leaving the Sorbonne in Paris, where he read philosophy, he studied drama at the Conservatoire. He made his stage debut in 1919, and the following year, made his first movie appearance in *L'Homme du large*. For seven years, he enjoyed huge success on the Paris stage and in French films, but it was the long-running hit play "Mélo" which first brought him to the attention of Hollywood. Initially, he did French versions of American films, but the audiences were missing out on his beautiful voice. MGM only gave him small supporting parts, so he got released from his contract and returned to Paris. In 1935, US audiences liked him in *Private Worlds* – co-starring Claudette Colbert. Walter Wanger gave him a contract, and from then on he kept French fans happy and secured new admirers. He was twice Oscar-nominated – for *Algiers* and for *Gaslight*. In 1942, Charles took out US citizenship. Although he appeared like a Casanova, he was happily married to British actress Pat Paterson, for over forty-five years. Two days after she died, he committed suicide.

Mayerling (1936)
History is Made at Night (1937)
Conquest (1937)
Algiers (1938) **Love Affair** (1939)
When Tomorrow Comes (1939)
All This And Heaven Too (1940)
Back Street (1941)
Hold Back the Dawn (1941)
Appointment For Love (1941)
Tales of Manhattan (1942)
The Constant Nymph (1943)
Gaslight (1944) **Cluny Brown** (1946)
The Cobweb (1955)
Une Parisienne (1957) **Fanny** (1961)
A Very Special Favor (1965)
How to Steal a Million (1966)
Paris brûle-t-il? (1966)
Barefoot in the Park (1967)
The April Fools (1969)

Peter **Boyle**
6ft 2in
(PETER BOYLE)

Born: **October 18, 1935**
Norristown, Pennsylvania, USA
Died: **December 12, 2006**

His father, Peter Boyle Sr. was well-known in Philadelphia as a host on children's TV shows. Both he and his wife, Alice, were of Irish descent, and strict Catholics. They educated Peter with a view to the priesthood – at St. Francis de Sales School and for three years, as a novice at the Institute of the Brothers. While he was living there, he attended La Salle University – graduating with a BA in 1957. By sheer coincidence, it was also the year he quit the order – believing finally that he wasn't cut out for religious life. He then worked as a cameraman on a TV cooking show, before being commissioned as an ensign in the U.S. Navy. Peter suffered a nervous breakdown which ended that career and he went to New York and worked as a postal clerk to pay for acting classes with Uta Hagen. He toured in "The Odd Couple" and made his film debut with an uncredited role in *The Group* in 1966. He put himself on the map in the excellent *Medium Cool* and enjoyed a successful career. When Peter married Loraine Alterman, in 1977, John Lennon was best man. Peter died in New York City of multiple myeloma (bone-marrow cancer) and heart disease.

Medium Cool (1969) **Joe** (1970)
T.R. Baskin (1971) **The Candidate** (1972)
Steelyard Blues (1973) **Slither** (1973)
The Friends of Eddie Coyle (1973)
Kid Blue (1973) **Crazy Joe** (1974)
Young Frankenstein (1974)
Taxi Driver (1976) **Swashbuckler** (1976)
F.I.S.T (1978) **The Brink's Job** (1978)
Hardcore (1979)
Where the Buffalo Roam (1980)
Outland (1981)
Hammett (1982) **Yellowbeard** (1983)
Johnny Dangerously (1984)
Walker (1987) **Red Heat** (1988)
The Dream Team (1989)
Honeymoon in Vegas (1992)
Nervous Ticks (1993)
The Shadow (1994) **Killer** (1994)
While You Were Sleeping (1995)
Monster's Ball (2001)

Lorraine **Bracco**
5ft 8in
(LORRAINE BRACCO)

Born: October 2, 1954
Brooklyn, New York City, New York, USA

The daughter of an Italian American father, Sal Bracco – who was a fishmonger, and an English mother, called Sheila, Lorraine grew up in the town of Hicksville in New York State. She has an older brother, Sal Jr., and a younger sister, Elizabeth, who also became an actress. When she was at a Long Island grade school, around the age of twelve, Lorraine was voted the "Ugliest girl in the 6th grade". Happily, that all changed as she grew older and by the time she was attending high school, she had begun a successful modeling career with the Wilhelmina Agency. At nineteen, she was working in Paris, France, for Jean-Paul Gaultier. While there, she acted in several extremely poor French movies – starting in 1979, with *Duos sur canapé*. She had a short-lived first marriage to Daniel Guerard, with whom she had a daughter and added the French language to her armory. She returned to the United States to study with Stella Adler and at the Actors Studio in New York City. Lorraine married actor, Harvey Keitel in 1982. Their daughter, Stella, was born four years later. Lorraine's studies were rewarded when the American thriller, *Someone to Watch Over Me,* got her movie career under way. She acted in the classic, *Goodfellas,* for which she was nominated for a Best Supporting Actress Oscar. Her divorce from Keitel led to a custody battle and bankruptcy, in 1999. She was rescued by the popular TV series, 'The Sopranos'. Another marriage and divorce caused her clinical depression, but she'll be back.

Someone to Watch Over Me (1987)
Sing (1989)
The Dream Team (1989)
In una notte di chiaro di luna (1989)
Goodfellas (1990)
Talent for the Game (1991)
Medicine Man (1992)
Radio Flyer (1992)
The Basketball Diaries (1995)
Hackers (1995)
Les Menteurs (1996)
Riding in Cars with Boys (2001)

Eddie **Bracken**
5ft 7in
(EDWARD VINCENT BRACKEN)

Born: February 7, 1915
Astoria, New York, USA
Died: November 14, 2002

Eddie started early in show business – he was already singing and dancing on stage at the age of nine. The Knights of Columbus in New York considered him professional enough to perform at their functions. His parents enrolled him at New York's Professional Children's School for Actors and he began to pick up some work. He appeared in four of Hal Roach's *Our Gang* two-reelers and performed on Broadway and in traveling shows – which is where he met a young girl called Connie Nickerson. They got married and were together for sixty-three years. It was tough at first: in 1933 he made his stage debut in "The Lady Refuses". Audiences refused to see it and it closed after seven performances. Three years later, he did slightly better; he starred on Broadway in "So Proudly We Hail". It lasted twice as long! Eddie didn't give up. In 1939, his success in "Too Many Girls" won him the role in the movie version, a year later. For a time he established himself in parts where his character was only envied by guys who looked as goofy as he did. But as, in the end, he usually got the girl, he was envied by other guys too. His Preston Sturges movies, *The Miracle of Morgan's Creek* and *Hail the Conquering Hero* are rightly regarded as comedy classics. Eddie's last Broadway appearance was in 1992, in "Dreamtime" when he was seventy-seven. His wife Connie, whom he'd been married to since 1939, passed away in August 2002 – three months before Eddie himself died after complications from surgery in Montclair, New Jersey.

Too Many Girls (1940)
Caught in the Draught (1941)
The Fleet's In (1942)
Sweater Girl (1942)
Star Spangled Rhythm (1942)
The Miracle of Morgan's Creek (1944)
Hail the Conquering Hero (1944)
Out of this World (1945)
Summer Stock (1950)
Two Tickets to Broadway (1951)

Scott **Brady**
6ft 2in
(GERARD KENNETH TIERNEY)

Born: September 13, 1924
Brooklyn, New York City, New York, USA
Died: April 16, 1985

Scott was referred to as 'Jerry' by his parents when he was a kid. His father Lawrence, who was chief of New York's aqueduct police force, had had show business ambitions as a young man. Scott's two brothers, Lawrence and Ed went on to become actors. Despite their dad's background, all three would be in serious trouble with the law at one time or another. Scott was a superb athlete at high school – excelling at basketball, football, track and boxing. When the USA entered World War II, he enlisted and served overseas as a naval aviation mechanic. In 1945, Scott headed for Hollywood, where his brother Lawrence was already making a name for himself. Scott was offered a screen test by Hal Wallis, which he failed. He then used the G.I.Bill to study acting and smooth out his Brooklyn accent. He signed with the poverty-row studio Eagle Lion and made his debut, as a boxer, in the 1947 movie *Born to Kill,* starring his brother. His fourth film, *He Walked By Night,* was his breakthrough. He graduated to Fox and then Universal – making a living from a lot of 'B' pictures and once in a while, a good feature, before becoming a character actor on television. In 1984, Scott made his last film appearance, in *Gremlins*. He died of emphysema a year later – in Los Angeles.

He Walked By Night (1948)
Port of New York (1949)
Undercover Girl (1950)
Kansas Raiders (1950)
The Model and the
Marriage Broker (1951)
Bronco Buster (1952)
Bloodhounds of Broadway (1952)
Johnny Guitar (1954)
The Vanishing American (1955)
The Storm Rider (1957)
Marooned (1969)
The Heist (1971)
The Night Strangler (1973)
The China Syndrome (1979)
Gremlins (1984)

Zach **Braff**
6ft
(ZACHARY ISRAEL BRAFF)

Born: **April 6, 1975**
South Orange, New Jersey, USA

Zach is the youngest of four children born to Jewish parents. His father, Hal Braff, was a trial attorney, who had dabbled in amateur theatricals. His mother, Anne, worked as a clinical psychiatrist. They divorced and then remarried during his childhood. Zach believes that it may have triggered an obsessive-compulsive disorder, which was first diagnosed when he was ten. Quite early on, he had a desire to work in films. With this end in mind he attended Stagedoor Manor Performing Arts Training Center in upstate New York. He graduated from Columbia High School in Maplewood, New Jersey and later, he earned a Bachelor of Arts Degree in Film, from Northwestern University, in Illinois. He began his career at New York's Public Theater – acting in Shakespeare's "Twelfth Night" and "Macbeth". In 1993, Zach appeared in an episode of TV's 'The Baby-Sitters Club', and made his film debut in Woody Allen's *Manhattan Murder Mystery*. Apart from a short – *Lionel on a Sunday,* which Zach wrote and directed in 1997, six years went by before his next film – a starring role in the comedy, *Getting to Know You*. His real career-making break was as Andrew Largeman in *Garden State* – which he wrote and directed, and was voted Best New Director by the Chicago Film Critics. Since 2001, Zach has played Dr. John 'J.D.' Dorian in over one hundred and fifty episodes (directing six of them), of a hugely popular, hospital-set, TV comedy drama series, 'Scrubs'. In 2005 Zach was the voice of animated film star, *Chicken Little.* He collaborated with writer brother, Adam on a recent television drama called 'Night Life'. Still single, he has yet to find the right girl to settle down with.

Manhattan Murder Mystery (1993)
Getting to Know You (1999)
Blue Moon (2000)
The Broken Hearts Club:
A Romantic Comedy (2000)
Garden State (2004)
The Last Kiss (2006)
Fast Track (2006)

Kenneth **Branagh**
5ft 9½in
(KENNETH CHARLES BRANAGH)

Born: **December 10, 1960**
Belfast, Northern Ireland

The son of a carpenter, Ken was raised by his Protestant parents in one of Belfast's toughest areas. His early schooldays were miserable because of the sectarian violence. Luckily for him, his dad moved the family to Reading, in England. Although not a great scholar, Ken loved to read. He was also good enough to captain his school's rugby and soccer teams. When Ken was fifteen, he went to see Derek Jacobi play "Hamlet" on stage – and he knew he wanted to become an actor. He graduated from RADA in 1981, with the prized 'Bancroft Gold Medal.' His own 'Hamlet' during his final year was highly praised. In 1984 Ken joined the famous Royal Shakespeare Company. He formed his own company called 'Renaissance' and brought the Bard's work to the masses. He was the original choice for the movie *Amadeus* until it was decided to go 'all-American'. He was D.H. Lawrence in 1985's *Coming Through*. His *Henry V* brought him a pair of Oscar nominations – Best Director and Best Actor. It co-starred his wife Emma Thompson, and his hero, Jacobi. In 2001, he starred in a fine TV movie, 'Conspiracy'. Ken's current wife, Lindsay Brunnock, was introduced to him by his friend, Helena Bonham Carter.

Coming Through (1985)
A Month in the Country (1987)
Henry V (1989)
Dead Again (1991)
Peter's Friends (1992)
Much Ado About Nothing (1993)
Frankenstein (1994)
Othello (1995) Hamlet (1996)
The Gingerbread Man (1998)
The Proposition (1998)
Celebrity (1998)
The Theory of Flight (1998)
Love's Labour's Lost (2000)
How to Kill Your Neighbor's Dog (2000)
Rabbit-Proof Fence (2002)
Harry Potter and the
Chamber of Secrets (2002)
5 Children and It (2004)
Valkyrie (2008)

Neville **Brand**
5ft 8in
(NEVILLE BRAND)

Born: **August 13, 1920**
Griswold, Iowa, USA
Died: **April 16, 1992**

One of seven children, Neville moved with his family to Kewanee, Iowa, when he was still a kid. He graduated from the local high school in 1939, and then joined the Illinois National Guard. Eighteen months later, Corporal Neville Brand, as he'd become, began infantry training in preparation for being sent to Europe. Neville fought in Belgium and Germany, and in 1944, he was awarded the Silver Star medal – for gallantry in combat when single-handedly, he destroyed a German command post. He was promoted to Sergeant and just before the Nazis surrendered, he was shot and almost killed. Neville's other decorations included the Purple Heart. With the help of the G.I. Bill, he studied acting, but no role he played would ever be like his real-life experiences. He made his film debut in *D.O.A.* and worked steadily in movies – mainly in supporting roles – in top titles such as *Halls of Montezuma, Stalag 17, The Tin Star,* and *Birdman of Alcatraz.* When film work dried up, he appeared on TV until his retirement in 1985 – having just acted in the dreadful *Evil of the Night* – which surely must have clinched his decision. His only wife, Mae, with whom he had two children, was at his bedside when he died of emphysema in Sacramento, California.

D.O.A. (1950)
Halls of Montezuma (1950)
Only the Valiant (1951)
The Mob (1951)
Red Mountain (1951)
The Turning Point (1952) Kansas City
Confidential (1952) Stalag 17 (1953)
The Charge at Feather River (1953)
The Man from the Alamo (1953)
Riot in Cell Block 11 (1954)
Love Me Tender (1956)
The Tin Star (1957) Cry Terror! (1958)
The Last Sunset (1961)
Birdman of Alcatraz (1962)
That Darn Cat! (1965)
Tora! Tora! Tora! (1970)
The Ninth Configuration (1980)

Klaus Maria **Brandauer**
5ft 9in
(KLAUS GEORG STENG)

Born: **June 22, 1943**
Bad Aussee, Austria

When he became an actor, Klaus took his mother's maiden name, Maria Brandauer, as his stage name. He was nineteen when he decided on a stage career and went to Germany to study acting at the Stuttgart Academy of Music and Performing Arts. In 1963, he made his debut in "Measure for Measure" at the State Theater, Tübingen and married his first love, Karin, who died in 1992. Klaus acted on the stage for five years before working on Austrian and German television – firstly in the historical drama, 'Das Käthchen von Heilbronn', in 1968. He made his film debut four years later, in *The Salzburg Connection,* which was shot on his home territory, but didn't start a stampede for his services among the world's casting agents. Klaus very wisely continued his TV career before a role in a German-Hungarian production – *A Sunday in October,* gave him a taste for filmmaking once more. The vehicle for a new start was *Mephisto* – directed by István Szabó. It won him a David di Donatello Award as Best Foreign Actor and a Best Foreign Language Film Oscar. Suddenly casting agents were beating a path to his door. He worked on a Bond movie and *Out of Africa* – for which he was nominated for a Best Supporting Actor Oscar, and he was in demand. In 1987, he was Head of Jury at the Berlin Film Festival. In 2006, he directed "The Threepenny Opera" in Berlin. In 2007, he married his second wife, Natalie Krenn. Klaus has two big films in post-production including Coppola's *Tetro.*

Mephisto (1981) **Kindergarten** (1983)
Never Say Never Again (1983)
Colonel Redl (1985) **Out of Africa** (1985)
The Lightship (1986) **Streets of Gold** (1986) **Hanussen** (1988) **Burning Secret** (1988) **Spider's Web** (1989)
Georg Elser (1989) **The French Revolution** (1989) **The Russia House** (1990) **White Fang** (1991)
Rembrandt (1999)
Belief, Hope and Blood (2000)
Between Strangers (2002)

Marlon **Brando**
5ft 10in
(MARLON BRANDO JR.)

Born: **April 3, 1924**
Omaha, Nebraska, USA
Died: **July 1, 2004**

His father, Marlon Sr., was a pesticide and chemical feed manufacturer. His mother, Julia, was an actress. Marlon's parents had a stormy relationship. By the time he was thirteen, they'd been separated for three years and come back together. At that point, he and his brother and sister went to live in Libertyville, near Chicago. Their mother suffered from alcoholism, but she was a kind and talented woman who had helped Henry Fonda start his acting career. Marlon was expelled from high school and then sent to Shattuck Military Academy, where he soon showed a talent for drama. By the time he returned home in 1943, he had decided, because sister Jocelyn was already appearing on Broadway, to try to follow in Hank Fonda's footsteps. In New York, he studied the Stanislavski System with Stella Adler and joined the Actors' Studio. He got his chance on Broadway in "I Remember Mama" and became a star in 1947, as Stanley Kowalski, in the stage version of Tennessee Williams' "A Streetcar Named Desire". He used 'the method' in *The Men,* a sensational film debut, in 1950, and became an all-time great screen-actor, in *Viva Zapata, Julius Caesar,* and Oscar winning performances – in *On the Waterfront* and *The Godfather,* which will influence future generations. Two of his three wives acted in different versions of *Mutiny on the Bounty* – 27 years apart. He died in Los Angeles of pulmonary fibrosis.

The Men (1950) **A Streetcar Named Desire** (1951) **Viva Zapata** (1952)
Julius Caesar (1953) **On the Waterfront** (1953) **Guys and Dolls** (1955)
The Young Lions (1958) **The Fugitive Kind** (1959) **One-Eyed Jacks** (1961)
Mutiny on the Bounty (1962) **The Chase** (1966) **The Godfather** (1972)
Last Tango in Paris (1973)
The Missouri Breaks (1976)
Superman (1978)
A Dry White Season (1989)
The Brave (1997)

Benjamin **Bratt**
6ft 2in
(BENJAMIN G. BRATT)

Born: **December 16, 1963**
San Francisco, California, USA

Ben was one of five children. His father, who was of German/English descent, was a sheet metal worker. His mother, Eldy, is a Quechua Indian from Peru. On his dad's side, there was a theatrical connection in the person of Ben's grandfather, the Broadway actor, George Cleveland Bratt. Ben was educated at Lowell High School, where he first took a keen interest in drama and oratory – as a member of the Lowell Forensic Society – the oldest high school speech and debating society in the entire nation. During his time there he was nicknamed "Scarecrow" by classmates because of his somewhat undernourished appearance. Ben filled out and went on to earn a Bachelor of Fine Arts from the University of California at Santa Barbara. He began a program at the American Conservatory, but left to make his television debut in 'Juarez', which was never aired. He made his film debut in 1988, in *Lovers, Partners & Spies.* In 1999, Ben was nominated for an Emmy for his work on the TV show, 'Law & Order'. After he'd dated Julia Roberts for three years, Ben married the actress, Talisa Soto, with whom he worked when he won an ALMA as Outstanding Actor, in *Piñero.* The couple have a daughter and a son. His latest film project, *La Mission,* is written and directed by Ben's brother, Peter.

One Good Cop (1991)
Bound by Honor (1993)
Demolition Man (1993)
Clear and Present Danger (1994)
The River Wild (1994)
Follow Me Home (1996)
Red Planet (2000)
Miss Congeniality (2000)
Traffic (2000)
Piñero (2001)
The Woodsman (2004)
Thumbsucker (2005)
The Great Raid (2005)
Love in the Time of Cholera (2007)
Trucker (2008)
La Mission (2009)

Rossano **Brazzi**
6ft
(ROSSANO BRAZZI)

Born: **September 18, 1916**
Bologna, Italy
Died: **December 24, 1994**

When Rossano was four, the Brazzi family moved to Florence. The boy had a fine voice which was much admired by the church choir he sang in. After leaving school at the beginning of the world recession, Rossano worked as a street singer to earn a few extra Lire. He began studying law at San Marco University, but abandoned it when both his parents were murdered by fascists. He then turned his attention to acting and in 1939, made his movie debut, in *Processo e morte di Socrate*. During World War II, he was still acting, but at night he was working for the Resistance. His singing ability proved useful when, in 1943, he appeared with the Swedish soprano, Zarah Leander, in *Damals*, filmed in Nazi Germany. Rosanno acted in Italian films until 1948, when he was offered a part in the Hollywood film, *Little Women*. His looks and charm were just what audiences were yearning for. He became an international star in *Three Coins in the Fountain, The Barefoot Contessa* and *South Pacific*. He went out of fashion as he reached his fifties, but worked up until 1993, when he made his last film. Rossano claimed to have been in over 200 movies, but many were of poor quality. After his first wife Lydia died, he married Ilse Fischer, who was with him until his death in Rome from a neural virus.

The King's Jester (1941)
We the Living (1942)
Damals (1943)
Il Passatore (1947)
Little Women (1948) **Volcano** (1950)
La corona negra (1951)
Milady and the Musketeers (1952)
Carne de horca (1953)
Three Coins in the Fountain (1954)
The Barefoot Contessa (1954)
Summertime (1955)
The Story of Esther Costello (1957)
South Pacific (1958)
A Certain Smile (1958)
Light in the Piazza (1962)
The Italian Job (1969)

Walter **Brennan**
5ft 11in
(WALTER ANDREW BRENNAN)

Born: **July 25, 1894**
Swampscott, Massachusetts, USA
Died: **September 21, 1974**

Walter's parents were Irish immigrants. Apart from being an engineer, his father had a passion for inventing gadgets which never saw the light of day. When Walter was a boy, he acted in school plays and was considered by his fellow pupils to be naturally amusing, with a gift for mimicry. Walter performed in vaudeville until World War I and served with the American volunteers in Belgium, where he was said to have suffered damage to his vocal chords in a mustard gas attack. The result was premature ageing and a squeaky voice which wasn't helped by the early loss of most of his teeth. During the 1920s, Walter made and lost a fortune in real estate. He was so broke, he began taking bit-parts in silent films and having liked the steady income, became a character actor in the talkies. He was likeable in all his films except when playing 'Old Man Clanton' in *My Darling Clementine*. Walter won his three Best Supporting Actor Oscars – for *Come and Get It, Kentucky* and *The Westerner* and was also nominated for *Sergeant York* – in a purple patch lasting five years. He was especially good in westerns. In a career spanning about fifty years, he appeared in over 230 films and television productions. Walter died in Oxnard, California, of emphysema. He was married to Ruth Wells from 1920 until his death. They had three children.

Come and Get It (1936)
Kentucky (1938) **The Westerner** (1940)
Sergeant York (1941)
To Have and Have Not (1944)
A Stolen Life (1946)
Nobody Lives Forever (1946)
My Darling Clementine (1946)
Red River (1948)
Blood on the Moon (1948)
A Ticket to Tomahawk (1950)
Bad Day at Black Rock (1955)
Rio Bravo (1959)
How the West was Won (1962)
Who's Minding the Mint? (1967)
Support Your Local Sheriff! (1969)

George **Brent**
6ft 1in
(GEORGE BRENDAN NOLAN)

Born: **March 15, 1899**
Shannonbridge, Offaly, Ireland
Died: **May 26, 1979**

George started acting when he was a child, playing small roles at Dublin's Abbey Theater. Although his family had a history of service with the British Army, George joined the IRA in 1920, and fled the country with a price on his head. He ended up in Canada, where he spent two years with a stock company. He moved to New York and, by the late 1920s was appearing in Broadway plays. He was thirty when he made his film debut in *The Sacred Flame*, and he played opposite Greta Garbo, in *The Painted Veil*. But it was his easy charm and mature personality that made him appealing to film makers, and to Bette Davis, with whom he did twelve films and had a long lasting affair. George certainly proved to be a ladies' man of the highest order – his six wives included actresses Ruth Chatterton and Ann Sheridan. He was also a licensed pilot – doing all his own flying scenes in *The Great Lie*. By the start of the 1950s, his star had faded and he made "B" pictures and did television work. A year before he died of emphysema, at Solana Beach, California, George came out of retirement to play the part of a judge in the movie, *Born Again*.

42nd Street (1933)
Female (1933)
The Painted Veil (1934)
Front Page Woman (1935)
Special Agent (1935)
The Case Against Mrs. Ames (1936)
Mountain Justice (1937)
Jezebel (1938)
Dark Victory (1939)
The Old Maid (1939)
'Til We Meet Again (1940)
The Great Lie (1941)
In This Our Life (1942)
The Affairs of Susan (1945)
The Spiral Staircase (1945)
My Reputation (1946)
Out of the Blue (1947)
The Corpse Came C.O.D. (1947)
FBI Girl (1951)

Abigail **Breslin**
5ft 1in
(ABIGAIL KATHLEEN BRESLIN)

Born: **April 14, 1996**
New York City, New York, USA

Abbie is the youngest person in this book, but she's no less deserving of inclusion. She is the daughter of Michael Breslin, a telecommunications expert and his wife, Kim, who manages her career. Abbie has two older brothers – Ryan and Spencer, who is twelve years older than her, and also a movie actor. The family live in New York, where she continues her schooling in tandem with her career. She started working in front of cameras when she was three years old – appearing in television commercials – most memorably for Toys 'R' Us. Abbie's film debut was a small but impressive role in *Signs* – with stars Mel Gibson and Joaquin Phoenix for company. Two years later, she starred with her brother in *Raising Helen*. The first sign that she had a big future in movies came when she was nominated for a Best Supporting Actress Oscar for her role as Olive Hoover, in *Little Miss Sunshine*. Three or four of her subsequent films have confirmed that great promise. In October 2007, Abbie made her stage debut, at New York City's Guggenheim Museum, in "Right You Are (If You Think You Are)" in a starry ensemble cast which included Cate Blanchett, Natalie Portman, Diane Wiest and Peter Sarsgaard. Abbie loves animals and wants to be a vet when she grows up – that is, if she isn't too busy making films. Most of her movies so far have been worthwhile – the only really dud during her six-year-long career was *The Santa Clause 3: The Escape Clause.*

Signs (2004)
Raising Helen (2004)
Keane (2004)
**Chestnut: Hero
of Central Park** (2004)
Little Miss Sunshine (2006)
Imaginary Friend (2006)
The Ultimate Gift (2006)
No Reservations (2008)
Definitely Maybe (2008)
Nim's Island (2008)
Kit Kittredge: An American Girl (2008)
My Sister's Keeper (2009)

Jean-Claude **Brialy**
5ft 11in
(JEAN-CLAUDE BRIALY)

Born: **March 30, 1933**
Aumale, Algeria
Died: **May 30, 2007**

The son of a colonel in the French Army, Jean-Claude lived in Algeria until the age of nine. During the war his family moved around all over France before settling in Strasbourg. He took his baccalaureate there before entering the city's Centre of Dramatic Art. He appeared on stage in the classics as well as performing modern works by Jean-Paul Sartre and Jean Cocteau. Because his parents did not share his enthusiasm for the stage, he went to Paris in 1954. He made some friends in the cinema world before doing his military service. In 1956, he made his film debut in a short called *Le Coup du Berger,* and after several small roles, he impressed in 1958, in Claude Chabrol's *Le Beau Serge* and in 1959, in *Les Cousins.* He was in his element with the French new wave and became an international star of the genre in Jean-Luc Goddard's *Une Femme est une Femme.* Unlike some of his contemporaries, he never ventured into the world of Hollywood. One of the few French actors to be openly gay, he was a national icon in films, television and the theater, right up until his death from cancer in Monthyon, France.

Le Beau Serge (1958)
Les Cousins (1959)
Une femme est une femme (1961)
**Le Diable et les dix
commandements** (1962)
The Bride wore Black (1968)
Claire's Knee (1970)
Le Juge et l'assassin (1976)
Robert et Robert (1978)
Le Maître-nageur (1979)
La Banquière (1980)
La Nuit de Varennes (1982)
Inspecteur Lavardin (1986)
S'en fout la mort (1990)
La Reine Margot (1994)
Il Mostro (1994)
Portraits chinois (1996)
Kennedy et moi (1999)
Unfair Competition (2001)
Special Delivery (2002)

Beau **Bridges**
5ft 10in
(LLOYD VERNET BRIDGES III)

Born: **December 9, 1941**
Los Angeles, California, USA

Born within a couple of days after the attack on Pearl Harbor, and delivered by candlelight because of a blackout, his parents called him 'Beau' after Ashley Wilkes' son in *Gone with the Wind.* In 1949, he had a juvenile role in the movie, *The Red Pony.* In 1951, he was in baby brother Jeff's first movie, *The Company She Keeps.* Surprisingly for his height, Beau was an excellent basketball player who represented UCLA during his freshman year. He transferred to the University of Hawaii, but dropped out to embark on a career as an actor. In thirty years of making movies, Beau has been in enough 'bomb' movies to wipe out Iraq, but he has shone in some really good TV dramas – winning Golden Globes for 'Without Warning: The James Brady Story', and 'The Positively True Adventures of the Alleged Texas Cheerleader-Murdering Mom'. In fairness, he has made a few first-class films – most notably *Norma Rae, Heart Like a Wheel,* and *The Fabulous Baker Boys.* He takes an active interest in environmental causes, loves swimming and surfing, and is an advocate of handgun control. Beau plays guitar to a high standard and pursues his hobby of collecting Native American percussion instruments. He and his second wife Wendy have been married since 1984. They have three children. In 2006, Beau was one of the voices in the live-action, computer-animated *Charlotte's Web.*

The Incident (1967)
The Landlord (1970)
The Other Side of the Mountain (1975)
Norma Rae (1979) **Love Child** (1982)
Heart Like a Wheel (1983)
The Iron Triangle (1988)
The Fabulous Baker Boys (1989)
The Wizard (1989)
Rocket Man (1997)
Sordid Lies (2000)
The Ballad of Jack and Rose (2005)
I-See-You.Com (2006)
The Good German (2006)
Max Payne (2008)

Jeff **Bridges**
6ft 1in
(JEFFREY LEON BRIDGES)

Born: **December 4, 1949**
Los Angeles, California, USA

Born into a family where both parents were actors made Jeff's future career path very clear. Like his older brother, Beau, Jeff had an early taste of movie making when he was still a baby. In 1958, he was in a couple of episodes of his dad's television series, 'Sea Hunt'. His first movie role as an adult was in *Halls of Anger,* when he was twenty-one. The following year, he starred in Peter Bogdanovich's classic, *The Last Picture Show,* for which he was Oscar-nominated – the first of four – the others were for *Thunderbolt and Lightfoot, Starman,* and *The Contender.* Unlike Beau, Jeff's film career has been liberally sprinkled with hit movies. The only big disappointment of his early days was a poor remake of *King Kong,* in 1976. He is able to take starring roles and cameos in his stride, and always offers value for money. Jeff is a gifted cartoonist, whose work has been used in films. He's also a keen photographer and a good guitarist and songwriter, who has released his own album, 'Be Here Soon'. Since 1977, Jeff's been happily married to Susan Geston, and has three grown-up daughters. On the acting front, his recent work – as Obadiah Stane in *Iron Man* – is something special.

The Last Picture Show (1971)
Fat City (1972)
Bad Company (1972)
Thunderbolt and Lightfoot (1974)
Rancho de Luxe (1975)
Heaven's Gate (1980)
Cutter's Way (1981)
The Fisher King (1983)
Starman (1984)
Jagged Edge (1985)
The Fabulous Baker Boys (1989)
American Heart (1992)
Fearless (1993)
The Big Lebowski (1998)
The Contender (2000) **K-Pax** (2001)
Seabiscuit (2003) **Tideland** (2005)
Stick It (2006) **A Dog Year** (2008)
Iron Man (2008)
How to Lose Friends &
Alienate People (2008)

Lloyd **Bridges**
6ft
(LLOYD VERNET BRIDGES JR.)

Born: **January 15, 1913**
San Leandro, California, USA
Died: **March 10, 1998**

Lloyd's father, Lloyd Bridges Sr., was involved in the hotel business, and he once owned a movie theater. He wanted his son to become a lawyer, but when he was studying political science at UCLA, Lloyd became interested in acting. He appeared with a classmate, Dorothy Dean Simpson in a play called "March Hares". In 1936, he made his film debut – a small part in a "B" musical called *Freshman Love.* By the late-1930s, he was appearing on Broadway and eventually founded his own off-Broadway theatre as well as becoming a member of the Actors Lab. During that time, he took a scholarly interest in Communism. It was to affect his career for a while during the 1950s, when he was blacklisted. He married Dorothy in 1939, and they remained together for more than fifty years. In 1941, the year Lloyd signed a contract with Columbia, the first of their actor-sons, Lloyd Vernet Bridges III – now known as Beau, was born. Lloyd worked hard for the studio and appeared in everything they threw at him, including Three Stooges comedies as well as frequently uncredited bit parts in films like *Here Comes Mr. Jordan.* Lloyd freelanced from 1945 and appeared in three excellent movies – *A Walk in the Sun, Home of the Brave* and *High Noon* – before becoming famous for his deep-sea diver role – in the popular TV series – 'Sea Hunt'. The year before he died in Los Angeles Lloyd made his final film – *Jane Austen's Mafia.*

Sahara (1943)
A Walk in the Sun (1945)
Abilene Town (1946)
Canyon Passage (1946)
Home of the Brave (1949)
High Noon (1952)
The Rainmaker (1956)
The Goddess (1958)
The Happy Ending (1969)
Airplane! (1980) **Cousins** (1989)
Hot Shots! (1991)
Blown Away (1994)

Jim **Broadbent**
5ft 7in
(JAMES BROADBENT)

Born: **May 24, 1949**
Lincoln, Lincolnshire, England

Jim was the son of Roy Broadbent – an artist, sculptor, interior designer and furniture maker. His mother, Doreen, was also a sculptress. Both were amateur actors. Jim's dad took over a former church and converted it into a theater. During World War II, the couple, who were conscientious objectors, worked the land to provide food for Britain. Jim was educated at the Quaker School, in Leighton Park, in Reading. For a short time, he went to art college before transferring to the London Academy of Music and Dramatic Art. He began his acting career at the National Theater of Brent, and in 1978 appeared at the Edinburgh Fringe. Jim made his film debut with a very small role in Jerzy Skolimowski's *The Shout.* He worked on television and low-profile movies until his breakthrough in Mike Leigh's *Life Is Sweet.* He established himself as a character actor in such varied fare as *The Crying Game, Bullets Over Broadway,* and *Little Voice.* Later came box-office hits like *Bridget Jones's Diary* – for which he won a BAFTA. Jim's portrayal of John Bayley, in *Iris,* won him a Best Supporting Actor Oscar and a Golden Globe. His uncanny resemblance to Lord Longford in the television film, 'Longford' earned him another BAFTA and second Golden Globe. Jim is married to the painter and former theater designer, Anastasia Lewis.

The Crying Game (1992)
Enchanted April (1992)
Bullets Over Broadway (1995)
Richard III (1996) **The Borrowers** (1997)
Topsy-Turvy (1999)
Bridget Jones's Diary (2001)
Moulin Rouge (2001) **Iris** (2001)
Gangs of New York (2002)
Nicholas Nickleby (2002)
Bright Young Things (2003)
Art School Confidential (2006)
Hot Fuzz (2007) **When Did You Last**
See Your Father? (2007)
Indiana Jones and the Kingdom of
the Crystal Skull (2008)
The Half-Blood Prince (2009)

Matthew **Broderick**
5ft 8in
(MATTHEW BRODERICK)

Born: **March 21, 1962**
New York City, New York, USA

Matthew is the son of a professional actor – the late James Broderick, and a talented painter mother, Patricia. At Walden School in New York, Matthew took up acting by accident – literally! A serious knee injury put an end to his endeavors as a soccer player and athlete, so he focussed his attention on the somewhat less physical art of drama. Through his father's theater connections, Matthew made his stage debut at the age of seventeen. It was a workshop production of "On Valentine's Day." His boyish charm was loved by all who saw it. By the age of twenty-one, Matthew had been in two Neil Simon projects: the stage play "Brighton Beach Memoirs" and what became his feature film debut, *Max Dugan Returns*. He proved to be a very good comic actor and his services were soon in demand. In 1994, he was the voice of the adult Simba in Disney's *The Lion King*. A year later, he was involved in a car crash while driving through Ireland. The accident killed a woman and her daughter. Matthew only broke his leg but he suffered mentally for some time. In 1995, he gave a Tony Award winning performance on television in 'How to Succeed in Business Without Even Trying'. Matthew is married to the 'Sex in the City' actress, Sarah Jessica Parker. He provides the voice in the animated feature, *The Tale of Despereaux*.

War Games (1983)
Ladyhawke (1985)
Ferris Bueller's Day Off (1986)
Project X (1987)
Biloxi Blues (1988) **Glory** (1989)
The Freshman (1990)
The Cable Guy (1996)
Addicted to Love (1997)
Election (1999)
You Can Count on Me (2000)
The Stepford Wives (2004)
The Last Shot (2004)
The Producers (2005)
Then She Found Me (2007)
Diminished Capacity (2008)
Finding Amanda (2008)

Steve **Brodie**
6ft 0½in
(JOHN STEVENS)

Born: **November 21, 1919**
El Dorado, Kansas, USA
Died: **January 9, 1992**

After leaving school, Steve became a property boy in a Kansas City theater. He took every opportunity to learn from the professional actors who appeared there. He made his stage debut when he was twenty, but just as he was beginning his career, World War II came along and he served in the U.S. armed forces until he was invalided out. In 1944, he auditioned for Universal Pictures, in Hollywood. He adopted the stage name, Steve Brodie after reading about a bookie of that name, who jumped off Brooklyn Bridge, in 1886. The new Steve made his movie debut with an uncredited role in *Ladies Courageous* and followed up as an Australian pilot, in *Follow the Boys* – which starred George Raft – who had played a character called Brodie in *The Bowery*. Steve had a good role in the classic war movie, *A Walk in the Sun* and for a few years, seemed to attract quality. The future looked bright and he married actress Lois Andrews, with whom he had a son, and would remain with until her death in 1968. Steve began working on TV in 1951, and although he still got roles in movies such as *The Caine Mutiny*, TV provided most of his income. He died of cancer in West Hills, California.

A Walk in the Sun (1945) **Badman's Territory** (1946) **Desperate** (1947)
Crossfire (1947) **Out of the Past** (1947)
The Arizona Ranger (1948)
Return of the Bad Men (1948)
Station West (1948) Bodyguard (1948)
Home of the Brave (1949)
Tough Assignment (1949)
Armored Car Robbery (1950)
Winchester '73 (1950)
Kiss Tomorrow Goodbye (1950)
The Admiral Was a Lady (1950)
The Steel Helmet (1951)
Only the Valiant (1951) M (1951)
Two Dollar Bettor (1951)
The Story of Will Rogers (1952)
White Lightning (1953)
The Beast from 20,000 Fathoms (1953)
The Caine Mutiny (1954)

Adrien **Brody**
5ft 10¾in
(ADRIEN BRODY)

Born: **April 14, 1973**
New York City, New York, USA

Adrien was the only child of Elliott Brody – a history teacher who had lost several family members in the Holocaust, and Sylvia Plachy – a lady photo-journalist, who had fled Hungary during the 1956 uprising. Adrien grew up in Queens and using the title "The Amazing Adrien" he would perform magic tricks at children's parties. He often accompanied his mother on assignments for the 'Village Voice' which taught him to be comfortable in front of cameras. To get him away from rough neighborhood kids, his folks encouraged him to pursue an acting career and sent him to acting classes. From the age of eighteen, Adrien attended the American School of Dramatic Arts and LaGuardia High School for the Performing Arts. He made his film debut in 1989, in *New York Stories*. In 1992, his daredevil antics resulted in a motorcycle accident which sidelined him for several months. He'd had ten years of small parts in movies when he appeared in *The Thin Red Line*. Richard Shepard's *Oxygen,* and *Dummy* – in which he was able to draw on his childhood box of magic tricks – helped put Adrien's name on the radar. In 2002, he was world famous after winning the Best Actor Oscar for Roman Polanski's *The Pianist*. Since then, apart from a short, *The Tehuacan Project,* about deaf children in Mexico, he's worked on lighter themes, like the blockbuster *King Kong* and the amusing movies – *The Darjeeling Limited* and *The Brothers Bloom*.

The Thin Red Line (1998)
Oxygen (1999)
Summer of Sam (1999)
Liberty Heights (1999) Bread and Roses (2000) Harrison's Flowers (2000) Love the Hard Way (2001) Dummy (2002)
The Pianist (2002) The Village (2004)
The Jacket (2005) King Kong (2005)
Hollywoodland (2006) Manolete (2007)
The Darjeeling Limited (2007)
The Brothers Bloom (2008)
Cadillac Records (2008)

James **Brolin**
6ft 4in

(CRAIG KENNETH BRUDERLIN)

Born: **July 18, 1940**
Los Angeles, California, USA

Jim was the eldest of four children born to Henry Bruderlin, a building contractor, and his wife, Helen Sue. They settled in Westwood, California, where Jim's hobby was model airplanes. He first became interested in acting after seeing James Dean's movies and when he became friendly with Ryan O'Neal, the pair enrolled at University High School in Los Angeles, where they took acting classes. Following graduation in 1958, Jim's parents urged him to follow his new friend into show business. He began his career with a role in the TV series 'Bus Stop' and changed his name to James Brolin. He was given a contract by 20th Century Fox, and had small roles in films, starting with *Take Her, She's Mine,* in 1963. By the end of the decade, Jim was combining films with TV work – after three nominations, he won an Emmy for 'Marcus Welby M.D.' In terms of movies, he didn't get the kind of break which would take him into the top division until *Skyjacked* – with Charlton Heston and *Westworld* – with Yul Brynner. In 1983, he tested for the Bond film *Octopussy,* when Roger Moore was talking about quitting, but changed his mind. Jim's television work has been the more successful – he was twice nominated for Golden Globes for his work in the popular soap, 'Hotel'. Since 1998, Jim has been married to the singer and movie actress, Barbra Streisand.

Von Ryan's Express (1965)
Fantastic Voyage (1966)
The Boston Strangler (1968)
Skyjacked (1972)
Westworld (1973) The Car (1977)
Capricorn One (1978)
The Amityville Horror (1979)
Night of the Juggler (1980)
High Risk (1981)
Gas, Food Lodging (1992)
Relative Fear (1994)
Traffic (2000)
Catch Me If You Can (2002)
The Hunting Party (2007)
Last Chance Harvey (2008)

Josh **Brolin**
5ft 11½in

(JOSH J. BROLIN)

Born: **February 12, 1968**
Los Angeles, California, USA

Josh is the son of James Brolin and Jane Cameron Agee, who was described as an aspiring actress. Despite his pedigree Josh wasn't attracted to acting – he was happy among the horses on his parents' ranch. He had his mind changed for him after being praised for his acting in a high school production of "A Streetcar Named Desire". When his parents were on the brink of divorce, he went to live with his dad in Los Angeles. He took acting lessons from Stella Adler and at seventeen, made his film debut in the very popular, *The Goonies.* For ten years, most of his work was on television – he starred in the western series, 'The Young Riders'. In 1989, he married Alice Adair and started a family. He then co-founded the Reflection Festival with Anthony Zerbe and enjoyed the chance to both act *and* direct. Movie stardom didn't come easy and in 1995, he had to contend with the death of his mother, who died when her car crashed into a tree. He was low-profile as a movie actor, but in 1996, debuted on Broadway, in Sam Shephard's "True West". Twenty-two years after his dad's success in the event, Josh won the Toyota Pro/Celebrity Race at Long Beach. In 2004, he married actress Diane Lane. In 2005 – he got good notices for the TV mini-series 'Into the West'. He hit a purple patch, beginning with *Grindhouse* and shared a Screen Actors Guild Award with the cast of *No Country for Old Men.* He was nominated for a Supporting Actor Oscar for *Milk.*

The Goonies (1985)
Bed of Roses (1996)
Nightwatch (1997) Mimic (1997)
Best Laid Plans (1999)
Hollow Man (2000) Coastlines (2002)
Milwaukee, Minnesota (2003)
Melinda and Melinda (2004)
The Dead Girl (2006) Grindhouse (2007)
No Country for Old Men (2007)
Planet Terror (2007)
In the Valley of Elah (2007)
American Gangster (2007)
W. (2008) Milk (2008)

Charles **Bronson**
5ft 10in

(CHARLES DENNIS BUCHINSKY)

Born: **November 3, 1921**
Ehrenfeld, Pennsylvania, USA
Died: **August 30, 2003**

The son of poor Lithuanian immigrants, Charles was one of a family of fifteen children. He grew up in a tough coal-mining area near Pittsburgh. When he was ten and his father died, he was sent, like his older brothers, to work in the mines. In 1943, he joined the United States Army Air Force and served as a tail-gunner aboard B-29 bombers in the Pacific theater. After the war, he took advantage of the G.I. Bill to study art. Then, when he and his room-mate, Jack Klugman read what actors were being paid, they decided to give it a go. Charles enrolled at the Pasadena Playhouse in California. His enthusiastic efforts impressed a teacher, who recommended him to the film director, Henry Hathaway. The result was his film debut in 1951, in *You're in the Navy Now.* He used his own name to begin with, but when the McCarthy hearings began, he changed it to Bronson. His weatherbeaten, slightly Mexican looks, gave him plenty of work as red-indians and tough guys. He was hugely popular during the 1960s and 70s due to his work in *The Magnificent Seven, The Dirty Dozen, Once Upon a Time in the West* and *Death Wish.* He was married three times – two of his wives, Kim Weeks and Jill Ireland – were actresses. Charles kept on working until 1999, when ill health and Alzheimer's disease slowed him down and resulted in his death in Los Angeles, from pneumonia.

House of Wax (1953)
Apache (1954) Vera Cruz (1954)
Jubal (1956) Run of the Arrow (1957)
Machine-Gun Kelly (1958)
The Magnificent Seven (1960)
The Great Escape (1963)
The Dirty Dozen (1967) Once Upon a Time in the West (1968) The Valachi Papers (1972) Chato's Land (1972)
The Mechanic (1972) Mr.Majestyk (1974)
Death Wish (1974) Hard Times (1975)
Breakheart Pass (1975)
St. Ives (1976) Telefon (1977)
The Indian Runner (1991)

Geraldine **Brooks**
5ft 2in
(GERALDINE STROOCK)

Born: **October 29, 1925**
New York City, New York, USA
Died: **June 19, 1977**

Geraldine's Dutch American parents had theatrical connections. Her father, James Stroock, ran a busy costume company. Her mother, Bianca, was a set stylist and costume designer. One of her aunts had been a Ziegfeld Girl and another was a member of the Metropolitan Opera Company. Her older sister, Gloria, became an actress. Geraldine began dancing lessons at the age of two and received every kind of encouragement from her extended show business family. In her early teens, she attended the Hunter Modeling School in New York and, at Julia Richman High School – from where she graduated in 1942 – she was president of the drama club. After high school, Geraldine studied at the American Academy of Dramatic Art and the Neighborhood Playhouse. She then gained experience in summer stock plays before, in 1944, she appeared on Broadway, in "Follow the Girls". After her success as Perdita, in Shakespeare's "A Winter's Tale" at the Theater Guild, she was offered a contract by Warner Bros and made her debut – with Errol Flynn and Barbara Stanwyck, in Cry Wolf. Following three meaty supporting roles, she lost her appeal somewhat and acted in European films, one of which, Vulcano, starred the great Anna Magnani. From 1952 until 1976, she was mostly seen on TV in shows like 'Gunsmoke', 'The Fugitive' and 'Ironside'. Her second husband was the screenwriter, Bud Schulberg. Geraldine died of cancer in Riverhead, New York.

Cry Wolf (1947)
Possessed (1947)
Embraceable You (1948)
An Act of Murder (1948)
Streets of Sorrow (1949)
The Younger Brothers (1949)
The Reckless Moment (1949)
Challenge to Lassie (1949)
Vulcano (1950)
The Green Glove (1952)
Street of Sinners (1957)
Johnny Tiger (1966)

Pierce **Brosnan**
6ft 1in
(PIERCE BRENDAN BROSNAN)

Born: **May 16, 1953**
Navan, County Meath, Ireland

Pierce was an only child. He grew up in Navan, which is close to his birthplace, but in County Meath. When his father left just after his first birthday, Pierce stayed in Ireland with his grandparents . His mother went to live in London and when he was eleven, he joined her there. She'd married a man called William Charmichael who soon became a father-figure and mentor – taking the boy to his first Bond film, Goldfinger. Pierce attended a school in Putney and at sixteen, began training as a commercial artist. A year later, he was a student at the Drama Center, in London, where he completed a three-year acting course. After that, like any young actor, he struggled to find work and mainly got small parts on the stage. In 1979, he starred in an Irish TV drama, 'Murphy's Stroke'. That led, in 1980, to a small role in a highly rated British film, The Long Good Friday, which was admired in America. His good looks brought him a television role in 'Mansions of America', and popularity, in 'Remington Steele'. Visiting his wife Cassandra Harris, on the set of For Your Eyes Only, Pierce was seen by "Cubby" Broccoli, who picked him as his new James Bond. NBC would not release him, and he waited fourteen years for international stardom – which arrived with Golden Eye and has continued.

The Lawnmower Man (1992)
Mrs. Doubtfire (1993)
Golden Eye (1995)
Mars Attacks! (1996)
Dante's Peak (1997)
Tomorrow Never Dies (1997)
The Nephew (1998)
The Thomas Crown Affair (1999)
The World is Not Enough (1999)
Evelyn (2002) Die Another
Day (2002) Laws of Attraction (2004)
After the Sunset (2004)
The Matador (2005)
Seraphim Falls (2006)
Butterfly on a Wheel (2007)
Married Life (2007)
Mamma Mia! (2008)

Joe E. **Brown**
5ft 7½in
(JOSEPH EVANS BROWN)

Born: **July 28, 1892**
Holgate, Ohio, USA
Died: **July 6, 1973**

Joe dispensed with education at the age of ten to join a group of tumblers known as the 'Five Marvelous Astons'. They performed at circuses and vaudeville shows where he added comedy to his repertoire. He made his Broadway debut in the early 1920s, in the musical comedy "Jim Jam Jems". In 1928, Joe appeared for the first time in a movie, in Crooks Can't Win, and shot to stardom a year later, in the first color and talkie musical, On with the Show. By 1931, he was important enough for Warners to put his name above the movie title. For three years – 1933-36, he was among the top ten box-office earners in the United States. In 1935, he was 'Flute' in Max Reinhardt's magical screen version of A Midsummer Night's Dream. More than thirty starring roles in seven years didn't stop movie audiences from abandoning him. After his contract with Warners ended in 1937, he was relegated to 'B'-pictures and guest spots. During World War II, he toured extensively to entertain the servicemen overseas and at the famous Hollywood Canteen. His son Don, was killed when his military plane crashed in 1941. He made a handful of films during the 1950s – playing Cap'n Andy in Showboat – and topping everything he'd ever done, as Osgood Fielding III, in Billy Wilder's Some Like It Hot. Joe was a keen sports fan, and his son Joe L. Brown, was the General Manager of the Pittsburgh Pirates for twenty years. Joe died of a stroke, in Brentwood, California.

Top Speed (1930) Sit Tight (1931)
Fireman Save My Child (1932)
You Said a Mouthful (1932)
Elmer the Great (1933)
Alibi Ike (1935) Bright Lights (1935)
A Midsummer Night's Dream (1935)
Fit for a King (1937)
The Gladiator (1938)
The Daring Young Man (1942)
Pin Up Girl (1944)
Show Boat (1951)
Some Like It Hot (1959)

Nigel **Bruce**
6ft
(WILLIAM NIGEL ERNEST BRUCE)

Born: **February 4, 1895**
Ensenada, Baja California, Mexico
Died: **October 8, 1953**

Nigel was the son of Sir William Waller Bruce who was a descendant of Robert the Bruce. He was born while his parents were on holiday in Mexico, but he was raised as an Englishman and educated at the famous Abingdon School near Oxford. He was not academic and when he joined the army at the beginning of World War I, it was as a humble private. He saw action in France, but after he sustained a serious leg injury in 1915, he sat out the rest of the war in a wheelchair. When he was fully recovered, he took a keen interest in the theater. Although he would never be anything more than a character actor, he was encouraged by friends to make his stage debut in the London production of "Why Marry" in 1920. Nigel then married a lady called Violet. After that, his speciality, the silly bumbling fool, was much in demand in London's West End theaters. Eventually he built up enough of a reputation to go to Hollywood in 1934. Nigel never tried to play anything other than himself, but he appeared in a string of hit movies among which were *Rebecca, The Charge of the Light Brigade* and *Suspicion,* and he was the definitive Dr. Watson. He died of a heart attack in Santa Monica, California, shortly after completing his final movie, *World for Ransom.*

Treasure Island (1934) **The Scarlet Pimpernel** (1935) **Becky Sharp** (1935) **The Charge of the Light Brigade** (1936) **Under Two Flags** (1936) **The Last of Mrs. Cheyney** (1937) **Thunder in the City** (1937) Kidnapped (1938) **The Adventures of Sherlock Holmes** (1939) **The Hound of the Baskervilles** (1939) Rebecca (1940) **Suspicion** (1941) **Sherlock Holmes Faces Death** (1943) **Lassie Come Home** (1943) **The Scarlet Claw** (1944) **The Pearl of Death** (1944) **The Corn Is Green** (1945) **Terror by Night** (1946) **The Two Mrs. Carrolls** (1947) **The Exile** (1947) Julia Misbehaves (1948) **Limelight** (1952)

Virginia **Bruce**
5ft 6in
(HELEN VIRGINIA BRIGGS)

Born: **September 29, 1910**
Minneapolis, Minnesota, USA
Died: **February 24, 1982**

Virginia grew up in Fargo, North Dakota, where her dad was an insurance broker. Her mom was a women's' golf champion, who encouraged her daughter to take dancing, singing and piano lessons during her early years. In 1928, Virginia left high school and traveled to Los Angeles, where she enrolled at UCLA. While waiting for the semester to start, she joined a group of students who were getting work as extras at Hollywood studios. She appeared in walk on roles in *Fugitives* and four other films released in 1929. On the strength of the rushes, she was called to the studio to test for a part in *Woman Trap*. She never did go to UCLA. In 1930, she made her Broadway debut in "Smiles" and that was followed by another hit show, "America's Sweetheart". By the time she married the fading star, John Gilbert – after they acted together in *Downstair* – Virginia's own star was in the ascendancy. She wasn't outshone by Oscar-winning Luise Rainer, in *The Great Ziegfeld,* and played opposite Spencer Tracy in *The Murder Man,* and Frederic March in *There Goes My Heart.* After Gilbert, she married three more times and made her final film, *Madame Wang's,* in 1981. One year later, Virginia died of cancer at Woodland Hills, California.

The Miracle Man (1932)
Winner Take All (1932)
Downstairs (1932) **Kongo** (1932)
The Mighty Barnum (1934) **Society Doctor** (1935) **Shadow of Doubt** (1935) **Let 'em Have It** (1935) **The Murder Man** (1935) **The Garden Murder Case** (1936) **The Great Ziegfeld** (1936) **Born to Dance** (1936) **Between Two Women** (1937) **Wife, Doctor and Nurse** (1937) **The Bad Man of Brimstone** (1937) **Yellow Jack** (1938) **There Goes My Heart** (1938) **Let Freedom Ring** (1939) **Hired Wife** (1940) **Brazil** (1944) **Night Has a Thousand Eyes** (1948) **Strangers When We Meet** (1960)

Yul **Brynner**
5ft 8in
(YULI BORISOVICH BRYNER)

Born: **July 11, 1920**
Vladivostok, Primorsky province, Russia
Died: **October 10, 1985**

He was the son of an inventor called Boris Brynner, who abandoned the family when Yuli and his sister were very young. Their mother took them to live in a small town in Manchuria until early in 1934, when they settled in Paris. They were not poor – they lived in a smart apartment in a good district of the city. Yuli enrolled at the Lycée Moncelle, but with a limited knowledge of French he was not a good student. He could play the guitar, so he dropped out to play with Russian musicians in nightclubs. He got to know the poet Jean Cocteau – who persuaded him to become an apprentice at the Theatre des Mathurins. In 1941, he went to the United States to study with the Russian actor, Michhail Chekhov – a nephew of the playwright. Yuli made his New York stage debut in "Twelfth Night". In 1944, he married the actress Virginia Gilmore, who starred with him in the first TV talk show, 'Mr. and Mrs.' He made his film debut (as Yul Brynner) in *Port of New York* in 1949, but two years later, after Mary Martin got him the role of the Siamese King, in Rogers and Hammerstein's "The King and I," he shaved his head, transferred the role to the screen, won an Oscar, and achieved world stardom in films such as *The Ten Commandments, Anastasia, The Brothers Karamazov,* and *The Magnificent Seven.* Yul was married four times and had four children. He died of lung cancer caused by heavy smoking. His ashes were buried in the grounds of an Abbey in France.

The King and I (1956)
The Ten Commandments (1956)
Anastasia (1956)
The Brothers Karamazov (1958)
The Buccaneer (1958)
The Journey (1959)
Once More with Feeling (1960)
The Magnificent Seven (1960)
Taras Bulba (1962)
Invitation to a Gunfighter (1964)
The Serpent (1973) **Westworld** (1973)
Futureworld (1976)

Geneviève **Bujold**
5ft 4in
(GENEVIÈVE BUJOLD)

Born: **July 1, 1942**
Montréal, Québec, Canada

Having been confined for twelve very unhappy school years in the Hochelaga Convent, in Montreal, Geneviève was expelled for reading a forbidden novel. Any form of self-expression was frowned upon, so it was not surprising that she sought to express herself by seeking an acting career. Geneviève enrolled in the Conservatoire d'Art Dramatique, where she was trained in classical French drama, and in 1963, did a TV series and a Canadian movie, *Amanita Pestilens*. With a local theater company called Rideau Vert, she went on a tour to Paris in 1965. While there, she was offered a role opposite Yves Montand, in *La Guerre est finie* and in a matter of months had appeared in two more French movies – the second directed by the great Louis Malle. She worked on Canadian TV, married a producer and because her English was very good, began to get opportunities in top international films. For her Hollywood debut role, in *Anne of the Thousand Days* there were both Oscar and Emmy nominations. In 1971, she was praised for her performance in the very dull, Greek-filmed drama, *The Trojan Women*. Her best films are *Coma, Trouble in Mind* and *Dead Ringers*. Geneviève keeps busy acting in Canadian films and TV. Her son, Matt Almond, from her first marriage, is an actor/director. She has a son with her longtime companion, Dennis Hastings.

La Guerre est finie (1966)
Le Roi de Coeur (1966) **Le Voleur** (1967)
Anne of the Thousand Days (1969)
Kamouraska (1973) **Earthquake** (1974)
Swashbuckler (1976)
Obsession (1976) **Coma** (1977)
Murder by Decree (1979)
Tightrope (1984) **Choose Me** (1984)
Trouble in Mind (1985)
Dead Ringers (1988)
Mon amie Max (1994)
The House of Yes (1997)
Last Night (1998)
Mon petit doigt m'a dit (2005)
Déliverez-moi (2006)

Sandra **Bullock**
5ft 7½in
(SANDRA ANNETTE BULLOCK)

Born: **July 26, 1964**
Arlington, Virginia, USA

Sandy's father was a Pentagon contractor and her mother, Helga Meyer, was a German opera singer. When she lived in Nuremberg during her early childhood, Sandy sang in a children's' chorus and took parts in her mother's productions. The family returned to the Washington area when she was a teenager, and she attended high school there. In 1982, she enrolled at East Carolina University, in Greenville, NC, where in her senior year, she took time out to pursue an acting career. Sandy eventually completed her course and got a bachelor's degree. By 1986 in New York, she was studying acting at the Neighborhood Playhouse. She was in an off-Broadway play called "No Time Flat". She made her film debut in 1987 in *Hangmen* and moved to Los Angeles, where she did a lot of television work. In 1993, her mother's voice coaching proved invaluable when Sandy got a singing role in *The Thing Called Love.* Her first important movie was later that year, when she had the leading female role in *Demolition Man* – opposite Sylvester Stallone and Wesley Snipes. It took *Speed,* for which she won a Saturn Award, *Miss Congeniality* – in which she played comedy – and *Crash* – to secure star status. She's now one of Hollywood's most popular actresses. Sandy is married to the producer Jesse James, who is most famous for manufacturing the hand-made motorcycles, "West Coast Choppers".

Demolition Man (1993)
Wrestling Ernest Hemingway (1993)
Speed (1994)
While You Were Sleeping (1995)
A Time to Kill (1996)
In Love and War (1996)
Miss Congeniality (2000)
**Divine Secrets of the Ya-Ya
Sisterhood** (2002)
Two Weeks Notice (2002)
Crash (2004)
The Lake House (2006)
Infamous (2006)
Premonition (2007)

George **Burns**
5ft 7in
(NATHAN BIRNBAUM)

Born: **January 20, 1896**
New York City, New York, USA
Died: **March 9, 1996**

George was the ninth of twelve children of Louis Birnbaum, a substitute cantor, and his wife, Dorothy, who tolerated his lack of ambition. Her son was a different kettle of fish. When he was just six years old, he formed a close harmony group, The Peewee Quartet. He left school early to concentrate on a show business career and adopted the stage name, George Burns – which may have referred to the marks he left on sofas with his cigars, but was better than "Peartree" (Birnbaum). In 1923, he met an Irish Catholic girl named Gracie Allen, who became his stage partner and his wife. The duo began to appear in short films and made their feature debut in *The Big Broadcast.* The Burns and Allen radio show was first aired that year – featuring Artie Shaw and Tony Martin. George and Gracie provided comedy in several films including Fred Astaire's *A Damsel in Distress.* Their 'Burns and Allen Show' ran on TV from 1950-58, when Gracie began suffering from heart problems. When she died, George kept as busy as possible – touring in a nightclub act with Carol Channing, Dorothy Provine, and Jane Russell at different times. He reappeared in movies and won a Best Supporting actor Oscar for *The Sunshine Boys.* His last role, as a 100-year-old comedian in *The Radioland Murders* was two years before he died in Beverly Hills, of cardiac arrest – aged 100 years and 49 days. He's buried with his beloved Gracie.

The Big Broadcast (1932)
International House (1933)
College Humor (1933)
We're Not Dressing (1934)
Love in Bloom (1935)
Here Comes Cookie (1935)
A Damsel in Distress (1937)
College Swing (1938)
Honolulu (1939)
The Sunshine Boys (1975)
Oh, God! (1977) **Just You and Me,
Kid** (1979) **Going in Style** (1979)
Radioland Murders (1994)

Raymond **Burr**
6ft 1½in
(RAYMOND WILLIAM STACY BURR)

Born: **May 21, 1917**
New Westminster, British Columbia, Canada
Died: **September 12, 1993**

Ray spent much of his early life traveling. At one stage his family went to China, where his father worked as a trader. After their return to Canada, his parents divorced and his mother took him to live in Vallejo, California. As he grew up, Ray helped his family by taking odd jobs, working as a ranch hand and even as a nightclub singer. He was serving in the Navy in Okinawa during the war, when he was shot in the stomach and sent home. He made his film debut in 1946, in the prison drama, *San Quentin*. In 1947, he was married, but it was later revealed as a studio cover-up to hide the fact that he was gay. He made around fifty films, including *A Place in the Sun,* and *Rear Window* before becoming Perry Mason in the television series of that name. It ran from 1957-1966 and was resurrected in 1985. After that, he was the invalided ex-police chief 'Ironside.' He won an Emmy for Perry Mason and he was nominated several times for both series. He worked with top stars and directors such as Alfred Hitchcock, but he will probably be best remembered for his image as the man in the wheelchair. Ray's last acting role was in 'Perry Mason' on television, in 1993. He died of liver cancer later that year, in Sonoma, California.

Desperate (1947)
Ruthless (1948)
Station West (1948)
Black Magic (1949)
Abandoned (1949)
Red Light (1949)
Key to the City (1950) M (1951)
A Place in the Sun (1951)
His Kind of Woman (1951)
The Blue Gardenia (1953)
Rear Window (1954)
You're Never Too Young (1955)
Count Three and Pray (1955)
Great Day in the Morning (1956)
A Cry in the Night (1956)
Ride the High Iron (1956)
Crime of Passion (1957)

Ellen **Burstyn**
5ft 7in
(EDNA RAE GILLOOLY)

Born: **December 7, 1932**
Detroit, Michigan, USA

Ellen was the daughter of John Gillooly, a building contractor, and his wife, Correine. Although she was raised as a Catholic, her parents divorced when she was small. She started earning her own money when she was fourteen. After graduating from Cass Technical High School, in Detroit, Ellen went to Texas, where she worked as a photo model. In 1952, she became a dancer on 'The Jackie Gleason Show' on television. She made her Broadway debut in "Fair Game " in 1957 and began getting regular TV work starting with the 'Hallmark Hall of Fame'. In 1964, after six years on the small screen, she became serious about an acting career and studied with Lee Strasberg at the Actors Studio. She was thirty-seven, when she made her film debut in *Pit Stop* and could hardly have dreamed of the incredible career ahead. She was nominated for Best Actress Oscars, for *The Last Picture Show, The Exorcist, Same Time Next Year, Resurrection,* and *Requiem for a Dream.* She won it for *Alice Doesn't Live Here Anymore.* Married and divorced three times – Ellen's acting successes should be ample compensation for those failures.

The Last Picture Show (1971)
The King of Marvin Gardens (1972)
The Exorcist (1973) Harry and
Tonto (1974) Alice Doesn't Live Here
Anymore (1974) Same Time Next
Year (1978) Resurrection (1980)
Silence of the North (1981)
The Cemetery Club (1993) When a
Man Loves a Woman (1994)
Roommates (1995) The Spitfire
Grill (1996) Deceiver (1997)
Playing by Heart (1998)
Walking Across Egypt (1999)
The Yards (2000)
Requiem for a Dream (2000)
Divine Secrets of the
Ya-Ya Sisterhood (2003)
The Elephant King (2006)
The Fountain (2006)
The Stone Angel (2007)
Lovely, Still (2008) W. (2008)

Richard **Burton**
5ft 9in
(RICHARD WALTER JENKINS)

Born: **November 10, 1925**
Pontrhydyfen, South Wales
Died: **August 5, 1984**

The son of a miner, Richard was the twelfth of thirteen children – the strain of which shortened his poor mother's life. When she died, he was brought up by an older sister. At twelve, Richard was given encouragement to read Shakespeare by a teacher at his secondary school. That teacher, who recognized his talent, had never managed to escape the depressing environment himself. In 1941, Richard answered an ad placed in the local paper by the actor Emlyn Williams, for a Welsh boy to appear in his London production of "The Druid's Rest". He got the part, then went to Oxford University on a scholarship. In 1947, following his National Service, Richard soon established himself as a stage actor with the potential to be another Olivier. His early movie roles didn't interfere with his theater work, and they were mostly unmemorable. Despite a superb voice, his potential remained unfulfilled. Even so, he was nominated for six Best Actor Oscars – for *The Robe, Becket, The Spy Who Came in from the Cold, Who's Afraid of Virginia Woolf?, Anne of the Thousand Days* and *Equus.* As he got more desperate to win an Oscar, the more physically dissipated he became, but it could have been worse – imagine how Peter O'Toole must feel. Heavy drinking and his life with Liz Taylor provided a lot more drama than most of his later movies but it led to his early death – aged fifty-nine – in Geneva, from a cerebral hemorrhage.

My Cousin Rachel (1952)
The Robe (1953)
Look Back in Anger (1958)
Becket (1964)
The Night of the Iguana (1964)
The Spy Who Came in from
the Cold (1965)
Who's Afraid of Virginia Woolf (1966)
The Taming of the Shrew (1967)
Where Eagles Dare (1969)
Anne of the Thousand Days (1969)
Equus (1977) The Wild Geese (1978)

Steve **Buscemi**
5ft 9in
(STEVEN VINCENT BUSCEMI)

Born: December 13, 1957
Brooklyn, New York City, New York, USA

Steve is of Italian Irish ancestry through his parents, John Buscemi – a veteran of the Korean war, and Dorothy, who worked for the Howard Johnson restaurant chain. As you might expect, Steve and his three brothers were raised in the Catholic faith. In 1975, he graduated from Valley Stream Central High School, in New York. During those years, he represented the school at wrestling and during his final year, became interested in acting. After attending the Nassau Community College he made his mind up to pursue an acting career and went to live in Manhattan, where he began to study at the Lee Strasberg Institute. To pay for his fees, he served as a firefighter in New York's Little Italy, for four years. Steve began writing and performing original works for the stage together with his fellow actor/writer, Mark Boone Jr. In 1986, he made his feature film debut in *Parting Glances*. After that, he has worked for most of Hollywood's top film-makers, including Quentin Tarantino – *Reservoir Dogs* and *Pulp Fiction,* and Joel Coen – *Fargo* and *The Big Lebowski* – appearing in more Coen Brothers movies than any other actor. Since 1987, Steve's been married to film-maker, Jo Andres. They have a teenaged son named Lucien.

King of New York (1990)
Miller's Crossing (1990)
Barton Fink (1991)
Reservoir Dogs (1992)
Pulp Fiction (1994) Desperado (1995)
Things to Do in Denver
When You're Dead (1995)
Fargo (1996) Trees Lounge (1996)
Con Air (1997)
The Big Lebowski (1998)
Ghost World (2001)
The Grey Zone (2001)
Coffee and Cigarettes (2003)
Big Fish (2003) The Island (2005)
Romance & Cigarettes (2005)
Delirious (2006) Interview (2007)
I Think I Love My Wife (2007)
I Now Pronounce You
Chuck & Larry (2007)

Gary **Busey**
6ft
(WILLIAM GARETH JACOB BUSEY SR.)

Born: June 29, 1944
Goose Creek, Texas, USA

Gary was the son of Delmer Lloyd Busey, a construction design manager, of Native American ancestry. His mother, Virginia, was Irish. He grew up in Oklahoma, where he attended Nathan Hale High School, in Tulsa. He graduated from Pittsburg State University, in Kansas, where he became interested in acting and went to Oklahoma State, but quit before graduating. Gary had a career as a professional drummer in a number of Country-Western bands led by Willie Nelson, Leon Russell and Kris Kristofferson. Gary played with various bands and also appeared on a local Tulsa television comedy show. In 1968, he made his first film appearance, as an extra in *Wild in the Streets,* and also got married to his first wife, Judy. Three years later, their son Jake was born and Gary's movie career took off. He appeared with his pal, Kristofferson in *A Star Is Born* and acted with Dustin Hoffman in *Straight Time.* Gary reached the heights in *The Buddy Holly Story* – for which he was nominated for a Best Actor Oscar and won a BAFTA. Since 2000, good roles have proved hard to come by. But every once in a while...

The Last American Hero (1973)
Thunderbolt and Lightfoot (1974)
The Gumball Rally (1976) A Star Is
Born (1976) Straight Time (1978)
The Buddy Holly Story (1978)
Big Wednesday (1978) Carny (1980)
Barbarosa (1982) The Bear (1984)
Insignificance (1985) Silver Bullet (1985)
Lethal Weapon (1987)
Hider in the House (1989)
Predator 2 (1990)
My Heroes Have Always Been
Cowboys (1991) Point Break (1991)
Under Siege (1992) The Firm (1993)
Surviving the Game (1994)
Sticks & Stones (1996)
Carried Away (1996)
Lost Highway (1997) Fear and
Loathing in Las Vegas (1998)
The Hard Easy (2005) A Sight for Sore
Eyes (2005) Blizhiniy Boy (2007)
Nite Tales: The Movie (2007)

Gerard **Butler**
6ft 2in
(GERARD JAMES BUTLER)

Born: November 13, 1969
Glasgow, Scotland

The son of Scottish-born parents, Edward and Margaret Butler – Gerard's great-grandparents hailed from Ireland and he was raised as a Catholic. He was taken to Canada to live in Montreal when he was small, but after his parents divorced, he accompanied his mother to her home-town of Paisley. Gerard was exceptionally good at school and eventually graduated from Glasgow University Law School. But his love of drama was strong. After some acting lessons, he made his debut in "Coriolanus" and also acted in the stage version of "Trainspotting". He made his film debut as Archie Brown in *Mrs. Brown* and had a small role in the Bond movie, *Tomorrow Never Dies.* For two years, he appeared in the TV series, 'Lucy Sullivan Is Getting Married' and in a trio of independent movies – *The Cherry Orchard, One More Kiss,* and *Harrison's Flowers.* With his reputation growing, he starred in the American TV miniseries, 'Attila' and played the title role in Wes Craven's *Dracula.* He was praised for his work in 'The Jury' on British TV and was 'The Phantom' in the film of Andrew Lloyd Webber's musical. Gerard showed he had a flair for romantic comedy, in *P.S. I Love You*, then featured in the box-office hit, *300.* In *Nim's Island,* Gerard uses Scottish and American accents in a dual role. His personal life is a well-guarded secret, but he has been linked with both actress, Cameron Diaz, and the dancer, Cheryl Burke.

Mrs. Brown (1997)
Tomorrow Never Dies (1997)
One More Kiss (1999)
The Cherry Orchard (1999)
Harrison's Flowers (2000)
Shooters (2002)
Reign of Fire (2002)
Timeline (2003) Dear Frankie (2004)
The Phantom of the Opera (2004)
The Game of their Lives (2005)
Beowulf & Grendel (2005) 300 (2006)
Butterfly on a Wheel (2007)
P.S. I Love You (2007)
Nim's Island (2008)

Red **Buttons**
5ft 6in
(AARON CHWATT)

Born: **February 5, 1919**
New York City, New York, USA
Died: **July 13, 2006**

The son of poor Jewish immigrants, Red began working at twelve – entering every amateur talent contest he could in order to compete for the $5 first prize. He acquired his stage name at the age of sixteen when he worked as a bell hop at Ryan's Tavern, in the Bronx. Band leader, Charles "Dinty" Moore named him because of his red hair and shiny buttoned uniform. That summer, Red worked at the Beerkill Lodge in the Catskills for $1.50 a week plus room and board. His straight man was Robert Alda, whose wife was about to give birth to Alan. In 1939, Red was the youngest comic in the business when appearing at Minsky's. In 1941, José Ferrer chose him to star in a farce, but as it was set in Pearl Harbor, it was abandoned following the Japanese attack. Red did make his Broadway debut with Ferrer a year later, in "Vickie". He joined the Army Air Corps in 1943 – entertaining the troops in Europe with Mickey Rooney. After the war he appeared with Big Bands and did Broadway shows. Ten years after his first (uncredited) film role in 1947, he appeared in *Sayonara* – winning a Best Supporting Actor Oscar and a Golden Globe. His movie career yielded two Golden Globe nominations – for *Harlow,* and *They Shoot Horses, Don't They?* He acted until his eightieth year. His last role was as Jules 'Ruby' Rubadoux in a 2005 episode of the television series, 'ER'. He died of vascular disease, in Century City, California.

Sayonara (1957)
Hatari! (1962)
The Longest Day (1962)
Your Cheatin' Heart (1964)
Harlow (1965)
They Shoot Horses,
Don't They? (1969)
The Poseidon Adventure (1972)
Pete's Dragon (1977)
Movie Movie (1978)
The Ambulance (1990)
It Could Happen to You (1994)
The Story of Us (1999)

Spring **Byington**
5ft 3in
(SPRING DELL BYINGTON)

Born: **October 17, 1886**
Colorado Springs, Colorado, USA
Died: **September 7, 1971**

The eldest of two daughters born to Professor Edwin Byington, and his wife, Helene, Spring was brought up by her grandparents in Port Hope, Ontario after her father died. She rejoined her mother, who had graduated from the Boston University School of Medicine and set up a practice in Denver. She herself graduated from North High School in 1904 where she had begun to take a serious interest in acting – touring mining camps in the Colorado Springs area with a troupe of other young hopefuls. In South America, she married touring company director, Roy Chandler. Four years later they were divorced. She returned home with their two children. In 1924 she appeared on Broadway, in "A Beggar on Horseback". After several years on the stage, she was signed by RKO to play Marmee, in *Little Women.* She was cast as motherly types, without a bad bone in her body, but that *was* Spring. She was nominated for a Best Supporting Actress Oscar for *You Can't Take It with You* and went on to enchant audiences in virtually every film she made. A bi-sexual, she was a long-time companion of actress, Marjorie Main. Spring died of cancer, in Hollywood.

Little Women (1933)
Ah, Wilderness! (1935)
Dodsworth (1936)
The Charge of the Light Brigade (1936)
Green Light (1937)
It's Love I'm After (1937)
Jezebel (1938)
You Can't Take It with You (1938)
The Devil and Miss Jones (1941)
Meet John Doe (1941)
Roxie Hart (1942)
Heaven Can Wait (1943)
The Enchanted Cottage (1945)
Dragonwyck (1946)
In the Good Old
Summertime (1949)
Angels in the Outfield (1951)
Because You're Mine (1952)
Please Don't Eat the Daisies (1960)

Gabriel **Byrne**
5ft 10in
(GABRIEL JAMES BYRNE)

Born: **May 12, 1950**
Dublin, Ireland

Gabriel was the first child of a devoutly Roman Catholic couple. He was educated at the strict Christian Brothers school in Dublin and, as is usual for the eldest son, was expected to prepare for the priesthood. But it wasn't what he wanted to do, so he studied archaeology and the Irish language, at University College, Dublin. He tried his hand as an archaeologist then worked as a cook, and because of his love of language, went to Spain to teach. Gabriel then embarked on a much more dangerous pursuit – bullfighting. He was twenty-nine when he began his acting career, on stage with the Abbey Theater, in Dublin. From 1989 he appeared at the Royal Court and National Theaters in London and achieved further prominence on a very popular Irish television show – 'The Riordans'. He made his film debut in the Arthurian epic, *Excalibur.* After co-starring with her in the previous year's *Siesta,* he married Ellen Barkin, in 1988. They had two children, but separated in 1993 – and finally got divorced six years later. He was seen recently in the excellent Australian drama, *Jindabyne.* Gabriel also produces films and has written an autobiography called 'Pictures in My Head'.

Excalibur (1981)
Defence of the Realm (1985)
Lionheart (1987)
Shipwrecked (1990)
Miller's Crossing (1990)
Into the West (1992)
The Usual Suspects (1995)
Dead Man (1995)
Polish Wedding (1998)
Enemy of the State (1998)
Stigmata (1999) Canone
inverso - making love (2000)
Virginia's Run (2002) Spider (2002)
Emmett's Mark (2002)
Shade (2003) P.S. (2004)
Assault on Precinct 13 (2005)
Wah-Wah (2005)
Jindabyne (2007)
Emotional Arithmetic (2007)
Leningrad (2007)

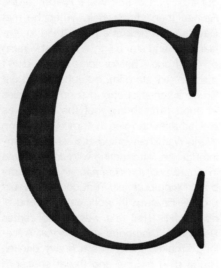

James **Caan**
5ft 11in
(JAMES EDMUND CAAN)

Born: March 26, 1940
The Bronx, New York City, New York, USA

The son of German Jewish immigrants, Jim spent most of his early life playing sports. He was a good swimmer – earning extra money during vacation time as a lifeguard. While studying economics at Michigan State University, he was good enough to consider a professional career as a footballer, but opted for acting instead. He enrolled in New York's Neighborhood Playhouse, where he was coached by teachers such as Sanford Meisner. By the early 1960s, Jim was appearing in popular television shows like 'The Untouchables' and 'Alfred Hitchcock Presents'. He made his movie debut in *Irma La Douce*. A short-lived marriage (the first of four) was followed by film roles which were unsatisfactory too. In 1969, he starred in a commercial failure, *The Rain People* and in 1971, a good television film 'Brian's Song'. A dream role in *The Godfather* and a nomination for a Best Supporting Actor Oscar, and Jim was close to stardom, but good movies were cancelled out by too many flops. After the death of his sister, he became very depressed, and wasn't seen in films for five years. He later underwent treatment for a cocaine problem. He came back in *Misery,* and has kept on going. For the past five years, Jim's been starring in the hit TV series, "Las Vegas".

The Rain People (1969)
T.R.Baskin (1971)
The Godfather (1972)
Cinderella Liberty (1973)
The Gambler (1974) Another Man,
Another Chance (1977) Thief (1981)
Alien Nation (1988)
Misery (1990) Honeymoon in
Vegas (1992) Flesh and Bone (1993)
Bottle Rocket (1996) Eraser (1996)
This Is My Father (1998)
The Yards (2000)
The Way of the Gun (2000)
Viva Las Nowhere (2001)
City of Ghosts (2002) Jericho
Mansions (2003) Dogville (2003)
Get Smart (2008)

Bruce **Cabot**
6ft 1½in
(ETIENNE PELISSIER JACQUES DE BUJAC)

Born: April 20, 1904
Carlsbad, New Mexico, USA
Died: May 3, 1972

The son of a French Colonel, the future actor's American mother died shortly after giving birth to him. Bruce was raised in Tennessee and attended University in Sewanee. In his early twenties, he was a sailor on a merchant ship and became an insurance salesman before trying his luck in Hollywood at the beginning of 1931. He got a bit part in that year's *Heroes of the Flames* then struck lucky when he met David O. Selznick at a party. It led to regular work and star billing in the first version of *King Kong*. That for some reason didn't result in real stardom, but it helped to get Bruce a series of strong supporting roles in good films throughout the 1930s, as well as starring roles in B-movies. During World War II he worked overseas for Army Intelligence. After acting with John Wayne in *Angel and the Badman,* they became big drinking buddies. That contact would provide Bruce with work until the end of his life. His final role was in the James Bond film, *Diamonds Are Forever.* A lifelong smoker as well as a heavy drinker, Bruce died of lung and throat cancer in Woodland Hills, at the age of sixty-eight.

King Kong (1933)
Disgraced (1933) Ann Vickers (1933)
Holiday (1938)
Murder on the Blackboard (1934)
Let 'em Have It (1935) Fury (1936)
The Last of the Mohicans (1936)
Smashing the Rackets (1938)
Dodge City (1939)
Susan and God (1940)
The Flame of New Orleans (1941)
Fallen Angel (1945)
Angel and the Badman (1947)
Sorrowful Jones (1949)
Best of the Badmen (1951)
The Comancheros (1961)
Hatari! (1962) McLintock! (1963)
Cat Ballou (1965)
The Chase (1966)
The War Wagon (1967)
Chisum (1970) Big Jake (1971)
Diamonds Are Forever (1971)

Nicolas **Cage**
6ft
(NICHOLAS KIM COPPOLA)

Born: January 7, 1964
Long Beach, California, USA

The son of Professor August Coppola, and Joy – a dancer/choreographer, Nick's uncle is Francis Ford Coppola. His two brothers have ended up in show business. Nick attended Beverly Hills High School, where his first taste of the theater was in a school production of "Golden Boy". He changed his name to avoid any suggestion of nepotism and made his film debut in 1982, in *Fast Times at Ridgemount High,* but the part was so small, he was hardly noticed. He was certainly noticed two years later – when he co-starred with Matthew Modine in a good movie – *Birdy.* After that, he was in the fast lane. By early in the new Millennium, Nick had starred in several top movies. He'd won an Oscar for *Leaving Las Vegas* and found time to marry and divorce Patricia Arquette – as well as his hero Elvis Presley's daughter – Lisa Marie. Now in his early forties, he seems better able to handle the pressures of being a star and directing and running his own production company. Since 2004, Nick has been married to Alice Kim, who was working as a waitress in a sushi bar when he met her. She appeared in his film *Next.* They have a son named Kal-el.

Birdy (1984)
Peggy Sue Got Married (1986)
Raising Arizona (1987)
Moonstruck (1987)
Wild at Heart (1990)
It Could Happen to You (1994)
Leaving Las Vegas (1995)
The Rock (1996) Con Air (1997)
Face Off (1997)
City of Angels (1998)
8mm (1999)
Bringing Out the Dead (1999)
Captain Corelli's Mandolin (2001)
Adaptation (2002)
Matchstick Men (2003)
The Weather Man (2005)
World Trade Center (2006)
Grindhouse (2007) Next (2007)
National Treasure:
Book of Secrets (2007)
Knowing (2009)

James **Cagney**
5ft 6½in
(JAMES FRANCIS CAGNEY)

Born: **July 17, 1899**
New York City, New York, USA
Died: **March 30, 1986**

Raised on New York's lower East Side, Jimmy left school early to start earning a living. During World War I, he worked in vaudeville – and in a show called "Every Sailor" – in which he was one of the chorus girls! He created speciality dances and toured extensively with his wife, Frances (with whom he remained married for sixty-two years). In 1930, after starring with Joan Blondell in "Penny Arcade", he went to Hollywood to make the movie version, called *Sinner's Holiday*. He was then employed in several pictures as a gangster, because he wasn't considered an actor, like Muni or Tracy. He was in fact, always James Cagney, and movie audiences loved him being tough with women and even tougher with men. For a change, he played Bottom, in *A Midsummer Night's Dream* and won an Oscar for the all-singing, all-dancing, *Yankee Doodle Dandy*. In 1949, aged fifty, he was his old self in the dynamic *White Heat,* but it was to be the last of its kind. During the 1950s, Jimmy made a few good films including a couple of comedies and a musical. After a twenty year gap,he made his final movie bow in *Ragtime*. He lived in retirement with Frances until dying of a heart attack in Stanfordville, New York, after an illness caused by diabetes.

The Public Enemy (1931) Blonde
Crazy (1931) Taxi! (1932)
Footlight Parade (1933) Lady
Killer (1933) "G" Men (1935)
A Midsummer Night's Dream (1935)
Angels with Dirty Faces (1938)
Each Dawn I Die (1939) The Roaring
Twenties (1939) City for Conquest (1940)
The Strawberry Blonde (1941) Yankee
Doodle Dandy (1942) Blood on
the Sun (1945) White Heat (1949)
Kiss Tomorrow Goodbye (1950)
Run for Cover (1955) Love Me or Leave
Me (1955) Mister Roberts (1955)
Shake Hands with the Devil (1959)
The Gallant Hours (1960)
One, Two, Three (1961) Ragtime (1981)

Sir Michael **Caine**
6ft 2in
(MAURICE JOSEPH MICKLEWHITE)

Born: **March 14, 1933**
Rotherhithe, London, England

The son of a fish-market porter, Mike grew up street-wise, in a tough area of South East London. After serving in the Korean war he started his acting career. The stage name he'd adopted, Michael Scott, was already being used, so he changed it after watching *The Caine Mutiny*. He acted in amateur theater and joined a Horsham repertory company. This early experience resulted in television roles and work with Sam Wanamaker. In 1956, he got a small role in *A Hill in Korea* – the first of thirty such parts – until Stanley Baker, who had seen him in the West End play "Next Time I'll Sing To You", asked him to test for his upcoming movie, *Zulu*. Mike played the part of an upper-class English army officer to good reviews. He made his name in Len Deighton's thriller, *The Ipcress File*. Success in that led to *Alfie,* and since then, the world has been his oyster. Mike's likeable personality and natural style has kept him at the top much longer than many people predicted. He's won two Best Supporting Actor Oscars from six nominations – for *Hannah and Her Sisters* and *The Cider House Rules* – and he still has plenty of gas left in the tank. Since 1973, Mike's been married to Shakira Baksh. They have a daughter.

Zulu (1964) The Ipcress File (1965)
Alfie (1966) The Italian Job (1969)
Get Carter (1971) Sleuth (1972)
The Man Who Would Be King (1975)
The Eagle Has Landed (1976)
Educating Rita (1983) Hannah and Her
Sisters (1984) Mona Lisa (1986)
Without a Clue (1988) Dirty Rotten
Scoundrels (1988) Noises Off... (1992)
Little Voice (1998) The Cider House
Rules (1999) Last Orders (2001)
Secondhand Lions (2003)
Around the Bend (2004)
The Weather Man (2005)
Children of Men (2006)
The Prestige (2006)
Flawless (2007) Sleuth (2007)
The Dark Knight (2008)
Is There Anybody There? (2008)

Louis **Calhern**
6ft 4in
(CARL HENRY VOGT)

Born: **February 19, 1895**
Brooklyn, New York City, New York, USA
Died: **May 12, 1956**

Lou was brought up in St. Louis, Missouri. While at high school, he was hired by a theatrical company to do menial work and appeared on stage as an extra. The whole atmosphere was magic and he caught the acting bug. He changed his name using two sources – the first from his adopted city and the second, an anagram of the first seven letters of his christian names. Initially he worked in burlesque and with touring companies, but it was interrupted by three years in the US Army during World War I. In 1919 he first established himself on Broadway. His performance in a hit play "The Cobra" aroused interest in the film world and in 1921, Lou made his film debut in *What's Worth While?* He then concentrated on stage work and the first two of four actress wives. His voice was too good to be lost to the talkies, so from 1930 onwards he supported stars like Cagney, Tracy, and the Marx Brothers. Reaching fifty, he stepped up a gear. He was Oscar nominated for his portrayal of Oliver Wendell Holmes, in *The Magnificent Yankee* and had the title role in a superb version of *Julius Caesar*. Three years later, Lou died suddenly – of a heart attack in Tokyo, Japan – while filming *Teahouse of the August Moon.*

Duck Soup (1933)
The Man with Two Faces (1934)
The Count of Monte Cristo (1934)
Woman Wanted (1935)
The Life of Emile Zola (1937)
Fast Company (1938)
Juarez (1939) Heaven Can Wait (1943)
Up in Arms (1944) Notorious (1946)
The Red Pony (1949)
The Magnificent Yankee (1950)
Annie Get Your Gun (1950)
The Asphalt Jungle (1950)
Two Weeks with Love (1950)
The Prisoner of Zenda (1952)
Julius Caesar (1953)
Executive Suite (1954)
Blackboard Jungle (1955)
High Society (1956)

Rory **Calhoun**
6ft 3in
(FRANCIS TIMOTHY MCCOWN DURGIN)

Born: **August 8, 1922**
Los Angeles, California, USA
Died: **April 28, 1999**

After a difficult childhood when he was often in trouble with the law, Rory worked as a lumberjack in Santa Cruz, California. He was discovered by Alan Ladd, who told him to give Hollywood a try. He was nineteen when he got a small role in the western *Sundown,* and signed a contract with 20th Century Fox. It didn't last long and he was soon freelancing. His agent arranged a movie premier date with the beautiful starlet, Lana Turner. She wore a white fur and the contrasting couple gave photographers plenty of material. Rory played 'Gentleman Jim' Corbett in *The Great John L,* but it was the thriller, *The Red House,* that started female fan-mail pouring in. Rory starred in his next film – a B-picture called *Adventure Island* and was then third-billed below Ronald Reagan and Shirley Temple in *That Hagen Girl.* In 1950, Fox were impressed enough to offer him another contract. He made some good movies for the studio, but after two helpings of Marilyn Monroe, they let him go. Rory smiled and galloped off into the sunset – frequently acting in westerns – including TV's 'Bonanza', 'Gunsmoke', 'Rawhide', and 'Wagon Train'. After his health declined around 1994, Rory lived in retirement with his second wife, Sue Rhodes, in Burbank, California, until he died of emphysema and diabetes.

The Great John L. (1944)
The Red House (1947)
Sand (1949)
A Ticket to Tomahawk (1950)
I'd Climb the Highest Mountain (1951)
Meet Me After the Show (1951)
With a Song in My Heart (1952)
Way of a Gaucho (1952)
The Silver Whip (1953)
How to Marry a Millionaire (1953)
River of No Return (1954)
Dawn at Socorro (1954)
The Spoilers (1955)
The Big Caper (1957) Dayton's
Devils (1968) Motel Hell (1980)
Pure Country (1992)

Simon **Callow**
5ft 7in
(SIMON PHILIP HUGH CALLOW)

Born: **June 13, 1949**
Streatham, London, England

Simon's French mother raised him as a Roman Catholic. He studied at Queen's University in Belfast, but switched to an acting course at the Drama Centre, in London. He did stage work and some TV – the first, a 'Carry On Laughing' episode called "Orgy and Bess". There were then several episodes of the sitcom 'Chance in a Million' – as Tom Chance. Simon played Mozart in the original stage production of "Amadeus", but in the film version in 1984, he had a minor role. He is successful as a writer – with biographies of Charles Laughton and Orson Welles. A critique "Being An Actor" caused controversy. He then had a good role, as the Reverend Beebe, in the Merchant Ivory film, *A Room With a View.* He was BAFTA-nominated for that and *Four Weddings and a Funeral.* His attempt to direct a stage version of the classic French movie, *Les Enfants du Paradis,* was a huge failure. Since then he has directed operas which were successful. He played the villainous Count Fosco in "The Woman in White" and he reprised the role eight years later for Andrew Lloyd Webber. In 1999, he was awarded the CBE. In December 2004, Simon hosted the well-attended, 'Gay Men's Christmas Show', at London's Barbican concert hall. No one's been able to follow that!

Amadeus (1984)
A Room with a View (1985)
The Good Father (1986)
Postcards from the Edge (1990)
Four Weddings and a Funeral (1994)
Jefferson in Paris (1995)
The Scarlet Tunic (1997)
Shakespeare in Love (1998)
No Man's Land (2001)
Merci Docteur Rey (2002)
Bright Young Things (2003)
George and the Dragon (2004)
The Phantom of the Opera (2004)
Bob the Butler (2005)
The Civilization of Maxwell Bright (2005)
The Best Man (2005)
The Knight Templar (2007)
Chemical Wedding (2008)

Phyllis **Calvert**
5ft 5in
(PHYLLIS HANNAH BICKLE)

Born: **February 18, 1915**
London, England
Died: **October 8, 2002**

When Phyllis was a little girl in Chelsea, she showed remarkable talent as a dancer. When she was seven, she was enrolled at the Margaret Morris School, near her home. Sadly for Phyllis and her parents, an ankle injury finished her career four years later. She switched to acting classes, and in 1927, after a few minor stage appearances, had an uncredited bit part in the comedy movie, *The Arcadians.* Throughout the 1930s she concentrated on stage work and in 1939 she met her husband, the actor Peter Murray-Hill. Phyllis co-starred with George Formby in the 1940 Ealing comedy film *Let George Do It!* and in 1941, she had a decent role in *Kipps,* starring Michael Redgrave. Having established herself as a star of some Gainsborough Studios costume dramas, she made the mistake in 1947, of signing a four year deal with Paramount, in Hollywood. She made three US movies – only one was okay. She was too English and returned home to earn a BAFTA nomination for *Mandy.* After her husband died while she was filming *Indiscreet,* she raised their two children on her own and never remarried. Phyllis made her final appearance – on TV, in an episode of 'Midsomer Murders', in 2000. She died of natural causes in London, two years later.

Kipps (1941)
The Young Mr. Pitt (1942)
The Man in Grey (1943)
Fanny by Gaslight (1944)
Madonna of the Seven Moons (1945)
They Were Sisters (1945)
The Magic Bow (1946)
Root of All Evil (1947)
Broken Journey (1948)
The Golden Madonna (1949)
Appointment with Danger (1951)
Mr. Denning Drives North (1951)
Mandy (1952) The Net (1953)
Indiscreet (1958)
Oscar Wilde (1960)
Oh! What a Lovely War (1969)
The Walking Stick (1970)

Neve **Campbell**
5ft 7in
(NEVE ADRIANNE CAMPBELL)

Born: October 3, 1973
Guelph, Ontario, Canada

Neve's dad, Gerry – a Scot from Glasgow – taught high school drama classes. Her mother Marnie, is a yoga instructor and psychologist, from Amsterdam, whose parents ran a theater company in the Netherlands. Neve's parents divorced when she was two and she and brother, Christian, lived mainly with Gerry. When she was nine, she moved into residence at the National Ballet School of Canada, in Toronto. After a catalog of bad injuries sustained during the rigorous training schedule she switched to acting while attending Earl Haig Secondary School. She was eighteen when she first had small roles in a trio of TV shows. In 1994, Neve made her film debut, in the independent Canadian production, *The Dark,* which won her no acting plaudits. For praise she had to wait until she crossed the border and starred in Wes Craven's *Scream,* for which she won a Saturn Best Actress Award. She hosted 'Saturday Night Live' before the equally good sequel. Neve was hot at that point and even scored unseen in 1998, when she did the speaking voice of the adult Kiara in the animated feature, *The Lion King II.* It was also the year that she got divorced from her first husband, the actor John Colt. From that time on, her movie career has continued along nicely, with rare forays into the theater. In 2006, she appeared at London's Old Vic, in Arthur Miller's "Resurrection Blues". In 2007, in Malibu, she married her second husband – the English actor, John Light.

Scream (1996)
Scream 2 (1997)
Wild Things (1998) 54 (1998)
Drowning Mona (2000)
Panic (2000) Scream 3 (2000)
Lost Junction (2003)
The Company (2003)
Blind Horizon (2003)
Reefer Madness: The Movie
Musical (2005)
Partition (2007)
I Really Hate My Job (2007)
Closing the Ring (2007)

John **Candy**
6ft 2¹/₂in
(JOHN FRANKLIN CANDY)

Born: October 31, 1950
Toronto, Ontario, Canada
Died: March 4, 1994

John's family background was Scottish. His father's early death should have warned him to be careful with his diet. At Neil McNeil Catholic High School, he was reasonably athletic and a good footballer, but with a big appetite. After working on local television, he had his first film role in 1973, in the disappointing drama, *Class of '44.* Three years later, he had a supporting role in the late-night television talkshow 'Ninety Minutes Live'. It was short-lived, but he got lucky almost immediately with the popular comedy-show, 'Second City Television'. His impressions of celebrities from all walks of life were high spots. In 1976, he was in a film worthy of his talents – *The Silent Partner* – which featured a great soundtrack by Oscar Peterson. In 1979 he married Rosemary Hobor (with whom he had two children) and his career took off. He worked for Stephen Spielberg's *1941,* before he appeared in the mammoth hit, *The Blues Brothers,* and hosted 'Saturday Night Live' on US TV. Films like *Planes, Trains and Automobiles* and *Home Alone,* varied his portrayals – from hilarious comedy to drama. John's last film – aptly-titled, *Canadian Bacon* – was released the year he died. Despite frequent warnings from doctors, he would refuse to diet or give up smoking. He died in his sleep after suffering a massive heart attack when he was preparing to film in Durango, Mexico.

The Blues Brothers (1980)
Stripes (1981)
National Lampoon's
Vacation (1983)
Splash (1984)
Follow That Bird (1985)
Little Shop of Horrors (1986)
Planes, Trains and
Automobiles (1987)
Uncle Buck (1989)
Home Alone (1990)
JFK (1991) Only the Lonely (1991)
Cool Runnings (1993)
Canadian Bacon (1995)

Dyan **Cannon**
5ft 5in
(SAMILLE DIANE FREISEN)

Born: January 4, 1937
Tacoma, Washington, USA

Dyan's father was a Baptist, who met her Jewish mother when she first arrived from Russia during the mid-1930s. After high school, Dyan made her film debut in 1959, in the racially themed, *This Rebel Breed.* Billed as Diane Cannon at that time, she made one more film before disappearing for about nine years. She went to live with Cary Grant, who didn't like his women to work. They married in 1965 and had a daughter. A 33-year age difference meant a troubled relationship and, in 1968, a divorce and a protracted custody battle followed. When Dyan as she was then known, was free, she set about rebuilding her movie career. The groundbreaking *Bob & Carol & Ted & Alice,* was a dream start – she was nominated for an Oscar for Best Supporting Actress. Unfortunately, it opened the way for a series of roles as a buxom blonde. Tiring of the situation, she took a break. In 1976 she wrote, directed and produced *Number One,* which was nominated for an Oscar as Best Short Film in the 'Live Action' category. There was also an Oscar nomination for her supporting role in *Heaven Can Wait.* A directing effort in 1990 was probably her last. Dyan still acts in films – she was most recently seen in *The Boynton Beach Bereavement Club.* She is a Born-Again Christian.

The Rise and Fall of Legs
Diamond (1960) This Rebel
Breed (1969)
Bob & Carol & Ted
& Alice (1969)
The Anderson Tapes (1971)
Le Casse (1971)
Such Good Friends (1971)
Shamus (1973) The Last
of Sheila (1973)
Heaven Can Wait (1978)
Revenge of the Pink
Panther (1978)
Honeysuckle Rose (1980)
Deathtrap (1982)
Author! Author! (1982)
The Boynton Beach
Bereavement Club (2005)

Eddie **Cantor**
5ft 7½in
(EDWARD ISRAEL ISKOWITZ)

Born: **January 31, 1892**
New York City, New York, USA
Died: **October 10, 1964**

Eddie grew up in a poor Jewish ghetto, in New York. He was the son of Russian immigrants, Mechel and Meta Iskowitz. His mother died of lung cancer when he was two. As a boy, Eddie attended the Jewish-run, Surprise Lake Camp, in New York State. In 1906, he left school to start a job as an office boy. Most evenings he'd head for theaters in different parts of the city, where they held amateur shows. It gave him the chance to perform in front of audiences and he was soon offered a job in a burlesque show. He formed a double act with his pal Sammy Kessler, but after touring together they quarreled and broke up. In 1914, Eddie married Ida Tobias, who was his wife and mother of his 5 kids until her death. Three years later, he joined the Ziegfeld Follies for three seasons. After going it alone, he returned to star in the Ziegfeld production of "Kid Boots". Its success led to Eddie's movie debut in 1926, in the film of the same name. Another hit Ziegfeld show, "Whoopee!" was turned into a two-tone Technicolor movie, and with Eddie's radio programs going well, he became very hot property. Goldwyn loved him – starring him in several big budget productions. By 1933, he was the most popular American star overseas – ahead of Garbo. In 1943, he moved to 20th Century Fox, where he had one hit before his career plummeted. His final movie, in 1948, failed, as did his biopic, *The Eddie Cantor Story* – seven years later. He was awarded a special Oscar in 1956 – the year he retired – after a role in TV's 'Matinee Theater'. Eddie died of a heart attack in Beverly Hills.

Whoopee! (1930) **Palmy Days** (1931)
The Kid from Spain (1932)
Roman Scandals (1933)
Kid Millions (1934)
Strike Me Pink (1936)
Ali Baba Goes to Town (1937)
Thank Your Lucky Stars (1943)
Show Business (1944)
If You Knew Susie (1948)

Capucine
5ft 7in
(GERMAINE LEFEBVRE)

Born: **January 6, 1931**
Saint-Raphaël, Var, France
Died: **March 17, 1990**

The daughter of a wealthy industrialist, she went to private schools in the south of France before receiving a BA degree in foreign languages from the University of Samur. She went to Paris, where she was discovered by a fashion photographer as she was walking along a boulevard. She changed her name to Capucine – French for 'nasturtium' – and she became a top model around the same time as Audrey Hepburn. The two became great friends when they worked for the big fashion houses, such as Givenchy and Christian Dior. In 1949, Capucine made her movie debut, with an uncredited role in a good jazz-themed comedy drama, *Rendez-vous de juillet.* Fourth-billed was actor, Pierre Trabaud, who became her husband for exactly six months. She continued modeling until 1957 when, working in New York, she was seen by producer, Charles K. Feldman, who took her to study acting with Gregory Ratoff. It led to her co-starring with Dirk Bogarde in *Song Without End.* In 1962, after they worked together on *The Lion,* she started a two-year affair with William Holden. As both a bi-sexual and a manic depressive, she was a most unhappy girl. Professionally, her last fifteen years were a disaster – highlighted by her ill-judged part in *Curse of the Pink Panther,* in 1983. After a number of botched suicide attempts, Capucine finally succeeded by throwing herself from the balcony of her eighth-floor apartment in Lausanne. Her only known survivors were her three cats.

North to Alaska (1960)
Walk on the Wild Side (1962)
The Lion (1962)
The Pink Panther (1963)
What's New Pussycat? (1965)
The Honey Pot (1967)
Fräulein Doktor (1969)
Fellini Satyricon (1969)
Soleil Rouge (1971)
L'Incorrigible (1975)
Nest of Vipers (1977)
Arabian Adventure (1979)

Claudia **Cardinale**
5ft 6in
(CLAUDE JOSÉPHINE ROSE CARDINALE)

Born: **April 15, 1938**
Tunis, Tunisia

This daughter of a Sicilian father and a Tunisian-born mother, whose own parents were Sicilian, Claudia grew up in Tunisia. She was judged to be 'The Most Beautiful Italian Girl in Tunisia', in 1957. The prize was a trip to Venice, but having been raised in French, she spoke no Italian. She then spent two months learning to act and was given a seven year contract with Vides Films. She made her debut a year later, in *Goha*. Producer Franco Cristaldi became her mentor, and from 1966 – for nine years – her husband. In 1960, Claudia worked for the first time with Visconti, and three years later, she was starring in his movie *The Leopard,* with Burt Lancaster. She also appeared in the Fellini masterpiece *8½.* It was the first time her own voice had been heard by Italian audiences but her voice was dubbed again in *The Pink Panther.* During the 1960s, Claudia made a few films outside Italy, the best of which – *The Professionals* – re-united her with Burt Lancaster. In 1968, she became internationally famous in the Sergio Leone movie *Once Upon a Time in the West.* It is in Italian films that she has done best and won awards. At sixty-nine, Claudia looks great, is still making movies, but in recent years, little of value. Like Capucine, she made the mistake of appearing in one of the later *Pink Panthers.* But on a personal level, they have nothing in common. She's written a couple of books and is also an ambassador for Women's Rights. She has two children – Patrizio and Claudia – from different relationships, and lives in Paris.

Upstairs and Downstairs (1959)
Rocco and His Brothers (1960)
The Leopard (1963)
The Pink Panther (1963)
Vaghe stelle dell'Orsa (1965)
The Professionals (1966)
Once Upon a Time in the West (1968)
Il Prefetto di ferro (1977) **Claretta** (1984)
La Révolution Française (1989)
**And Now...Ladies
and Gentlemen** (2002)

Harry **Carey**
6ft
(HENRY DEWITT CAREY II)

Born: **January 16, 1878**
The Bronx, New York City, New York, USA
Died: **September 21, 1947**

Harry's father was a New York judge, and his mother was the president of a sewing machine company. He attended Hamilton Military Academy, and studied law at New York University. Harry caught pneumonia after a boating accident. While recovering, he wrote a play titled "Montana" and he toured with it for three years. He joined Biograph Studios and went to Hollywood with D.W. Griffith – making his first film appearance in 1908 – in *Bill Sharkey's Last Game.* Harry became one of the greatest cowboy stars of the silent screen – making the first of twenty-six films with John Ford – *Straight Shooting,* in 1917. With the coming of sound, Harry was fifty. For a while he tried vaudeville with his third wife Olive, but hated touring. In 1929, he made a come-back when Irving Thalberg gave him the title role in MGM's hit, *Trader Horn.* With his film earnings, Harry bought a ranch in Saugus, California. He was nominated for a Best Supporting Actor Oscar for *Mr. Smith Goes to Washington.* His actor son, Harry Carey Jr., appeared with him in *Red River.* Harry had just completed work on *So Dear to My Heart,* when he died at his home in Brentwood, California, from a combination of coronary thrombosis, lung cancer and emphysema.

Trader Horn (1931)
Law and Order (1932)
Barbary Coast (1935)
The Prisoner of Shark Island (1936)
Ghost Town (1936)
The Last Outlaw (1936)
Valiant Is the Word for Carrie (1936)
Aces Wild (1936)
Kid Galahad (1937)
Souls at Sea (1937)
The Law West of Tombstone (1938)
Mr. Smith Goes to Washington (1939)
The Shepherd of the Hills (1941)
The Spoilers (1942)
Duel in the Sun (1946)
Angel and the Badman (1947)
Red River (1948)
So Dear to My Heart (1948)

MacDonald **Carey**
6ft
(EDWARD MACDONALD CAREY)

Born: **March 15, 1913**
Sioux City, Iowa, USA
Died: **March 21, 1994**

Mac's father, Charles Carey, was an Irish Catholic who worked as an investment counselor. Elizabeth MacDonald Carey – his mother – inspired his stage name. At high school, he had a melodic baritone voice and was the driving force behind the choir. He studied at the University of Iowa, from where he graduated in 1936. His first intention had been to become a drama teacher, but he was so passionate about acting, he changed his mind. To start with, he worked on radio in New York, where he met Elizabeth Heckacher, a socialite from Philadelphia, who was at drama school. They married in 1941 – going on to have six children – three boys and three girls. Before that he joined a stage company – acting in short versions of Shakespeare. After his Broadway debut in "Lady in the Dark", Paramount bought the screen rights and signed Mac to act in it, after his debut in a 1942 comedy, *Take a Letter, Darling.* By the time they filmed it, he was serving with the U.S. Marines in World War II. He did complete a featured role in Hitchcock's *Shadow of a Doubt* before that happened, but when he re-emerged, in 1947, his big chance had gone. For the next forty years, he made his living mainly from television work. Two years after making his last appearance, in a television drama called 'A Message from Holly', Mac died of lung cancer, in Beverly Hills.

Take a Letter Darling (1942)
Wake Island (1942)
Shadow of a Doubt (1943)
Suddenly It's Spring (1947)
Streets of Laredo (1949)
The Great Gatsby (1949)
Comanche Territory (1950)
The Lawless (1950)
The Great Missouri Raid (1951)
Excuse My Dust (1951)
Let's Make It Legal (1951)
John Paul Jones (1959)
The Damned (1963)
Tammy and the Doctor (1963)
American Gigolo (1980)

Richard **Carlson**
5ft 11in
(RICHARD CARLSON)

Born: **April 29, 1912**
Albert Lea, Minnesota, USA
Died: **November 21, 1977**

Richard's father, a lawyer, was Danish, and his mother was born in France. He was the last of four children. When he was nine, they all moved to Minneapolis. He was always keen on writing, and by the time he left high school, Richard's mind was set on becoming a playwright. At the University of Minnesota he wrote and directed plays. He graduated with honors and accepted a post there as an English teacher, but it didn't take long for him to feel frustrated so he quit. He invested his savings in a repertory company, but after incurring big losses, he headed for Los Angeles, in 1936. After some small roles at the Pasadena Playhouse, Richard went East. He soon landed parts in Broadway shows – most notably in "The Ghost of Yankee Doodle Dandy" – with the great Ethel Barrymore. He made his screen debut in *The Young in Heart.* Four years in the Navy interrupted his career and caused him hardship on his return to civilian life, but Richard kept plugging away – acting, directing and writing for films and television. His last film appearance was in 1969, in the Elvis Presley crime drama, *Change of Habit.* He retired in 1975, but he had only two more years to live before he died in Encino, California, of a cerebral hemorrhage. Richard was survived by his wife, Mona and their two sons.

The Young in Heart (1938)
Too Many Girls (1940)
The Ghost Breakers (1940)
The Little Foxes (1941)
Back Street (1941)
The Magnificent Ambersons (1942)
A Stranger in Town (1943)
So Well Remembered (1947)
King Solomon's Mines (1950)
The Blue Veil (1951)
The Magnetic Monster (1953)
It Came from Outer Space (1953)
Creature from the
Black Lagoon (1954)
The Helen Morgan Story (1957)
The Power (1968)

Robert **Carlyle**
5ft 8in
(ROBERT CARLYLE)

Born: April 14, 1961
Glasgow, Scotland

After his mother left when he was four, Bobby was raised by his father Joe, who worked as a painter and decorator in Glasgow. While he was still at school, Bobby attended acting classes at the Glasgow Arts Centre, and went on to graduate from the Royal Scottish Academy of Music and Drama – also in the city. Together with four of his friends, Bobby founded the Raindog Theater Company – named after one of his favorite Tom Waits' albums – "Rain Dog". The first time Bobby was seen on screen was on television, in a March 1991 episode of 'The Bill', although he had already starred in Ken Loach's film, *Riff-Raff* – which was made in 1990 – but not released until three years later. He first made an impact as a vicious killer in an episode of TV's 'Cracker' in 1994, but was even nastier playing the psychopath Francis Begbie, in *Trainspotting*. Bobby's ability to change appearance and persona to suit the roles he plays, has won him many admirers. In total contrast to Begbie, was his gentle 'Gaz' in the hit comedy, *The Full Monty*. In real life he's really as nice as that. Since 1997, Bobby's been married to the make-up artist, Anastasia Shirley, whom he met when he worked on 'Cracker'. They have three children.

Go Now (1995)
Trainspotting (1996)
Carla's Song (1996)
The Full Monty (1997)
Face (1997)
The World Is Not Enough (1999)
Angela's Ashes (1999)
The Beach (2000)
There's Only One Jimmy Grimble (2000)
To End All Wars (2001)
The 51st State (2001)
Black and White (2002)
Marilyn Hotchkiss Ballroom Dancing & Charm School (2005)
The Mighty Celt (2005)
28 Weeks Later (2007)
Stone of Destiny (2008)
Summer (2008)

Art **Carney**
5ft 11in
(ARTHUR WILLIAM MATTHEW CARNEY)

Born: November 4, 1918
Mount Vernon, New York, USA
Died: **November 9, 2003**

Art was the son of a newspaperman, Edward Carney, and his wife, Helen. He was the youngest of six sons and grew up in an Irish American Catholic family. Art was educated locally at the A.B.Davis High School, where he first developed his natural talent for mimicry and appeared in school drama productions. Without any formal training he began his career in show business at the age of nineteen, with the Horace Hiedt Orchestra. In 1939, it was featured in the first big-money give-away radio show, 'Pot of Gold'. With Art as its host, the program was so popular that in 1941, the band appeared in the film version – providing him with his movie debut. For two years he was a regular in radio shows such as 'Land of the Lost' and 'Joe and Ethel Turp' – and became famous for his impersonations of Franklyn D. Roosevelt and Dwight D. Eisenhower. In 1944 he was drafted into the U.S. Army, and during the Battle of Normandy, he was hit in the leg and limped for evermore. He returned to radio with Henry Morgan and was 'seen' for the first time, on 'The Morey Amsterdam Show' – on TV, in 1948. He remained a television performer until making his feature film debut, aged forty-five, in the comedy *The Yellow Rolls Royce*. He won a Best Actor Oscar for *Harry and Tonto*. The last words he spoke on screen were "I'm outta here..." in *Last Action Hero*. He died later that year with his third wife, Jean, at his bedside.

The Yellow Rolls-Royce (1964)
Harry and Tonto (1974)
Scott Joplin (1977)
The Late Show (1977)
House Calls (1978)
Movie Movie (1978)
Steel (1979) **Going in Style** (1979)
Defiance (1980)
St. Helens (1981) **Firestarter** (1984)
The Naked Face (1984)
The Muppets Take Manhattan (1984)
Night Friend (1987)
Last Action Hero (1993)

Martine **Carol**
5ft 4in
(MARIE-LOUISE MOURER)

Born: Born: May 16, 1920
St.Mandé, Val-de-Marne, France
Died: **February 6, 1967**

After meeting the future French film star, Micheline Presle, Martine decided that she was going to be an actress. She studied drama under René Simon, in Paris, and made her stage debut in 1940, in "La Route du tabac" at Le Théâtre de la Renaissance – using the name Maryse Arley. During the German occupation, French actors appeared in films financed by Germany, and her first movie, which was never distributed, was *Le Chat* – an adaptation of a novel by Colette. She made films with Pierre Fresnay and Raimu, before changing her name to Martine Carol, in 1943. After the war, she made a dozen movies – which brought popularity in France – the best of which was *Les Amants de Vérone*. After her affair with the film actor, Georges Marchal ended, she attempted suicide by throwing herself into the Seine. When rescued by a passing taxi driver – she did not thank him! In 1950, Martine became the queen of movie Art Houses around the world, when she was widely seen (in every sense of the word) in *Caroline Chérie*. She followed it with the equally popular *La Spiaggia* (The Beach) and *Lola Montès*. Up to the time Bardot arrived, Martine Carol was *the* French sex-symbol. After that it was downhill all the way. She was married four times – the last to Mike Eland – an English businessman, who was her husband for one year until her death at forty-seven. Drug abuse was suggested as the reason for Martine's fatal heart-attack at a hotel – during a visit to Monte Carlo.

Les Amants de Vérone (1949)
Caroline Chérie (1951)
Les Belles de nuit (1952)
Adorables créatures (1952)
The Beach (1954)
Secrets d'alcove (1954)
Madame du Barry (1954)
Nana (1955) **Lola Montès** (1955)
Difendo il mio amore (1957)
Austerlitz (1960)
Vanina Vanini (1961)

Leslie **Caron**
5ft 3in
(LESLIE CLAIRE MARGARET CARON)

Born: **July 1, 1931**
Boulogne-Billancourt, Seine, France

Leslie was the product of a transatlantic partnership – her father was French and her mother was American. She studied ballet at the Conservatoire National de Danse in Paris, and from 1947, she was dancing with Les Ballets des Champs-Elysées. Gene Kelly saw her there in 1951, and at it his insistence, MGM signed her to co-star with him in *An American in Paris*. Moviegoers loved it and loved Leslie, despite her buck teeth – which she had fixed. She never achieved the level of that work again, but was in charming productions, like her Best Actress Oscar-nominated role in *Lili*. She later danced with Fred Astaire, who claimed he was thoroughly impressed by her professionalism. She then did theater work in France and in London, where she was the star of the stage version of Colette's novel "Gigi". She married its director Peter Hall and in 1958, starred in the Lerner-Loewe musical film version. After she'd had a baby she fought hard to get the part in *The L-Shaped Room* for which she was Oscar-nominated – again as Best Actress. Soon after that Warren Beatty was named as the co-respondent in her divorce from Peter Hall, but the affair was short-lived. Leslie continues playing supporting roles in movies and appearing on television in Europe and America.

An American in Paris (1951)
The Man with a Cloak (1951)
The Story of Three Loves (1953)
Lili (1953)
Daddy Long Legs (1955)
The Glass Slipper (1955)
Gaby (1956) Gigi (1958)
The Doctor's Dilemma (1958)
Austerlitz (1960)
The L-Shaped Room (1962)
Father Goose (1964)
Paris brûle-t-il? (1966)
The Man who Loved Women (1977)
Dangerous Moves (1984)
Damage (1992) Funny Bones (1995)
Let It Be Me (1995)
Chocolat (2000)

David **Carradine**
6ft 0½in
(JOHN ARTHUR CARRADINE)

Born: **December 8, 1936**
Hollywood, California, USA
Died: **June 3, 2009**

The eldest son of movie legend, John, his three half-brothers became actors. After high school, he changed his first name to avoid any confusion with his dad, and studied drama at San Francisco State University. His route was the standard one – stage work coupled with some TV roles. He made his film debut in 1964, in the western, *Taggart* – starring veterans of the genre – Dan Duryea and Harry Carey Jr. That was followed by a television version of 'Shane' and the big-screen western, *The Violent Ones*. In 1969. he began a six-year relationship with Barbara Hershey. David latched on to the 'Kung Fu' craze and made a movie with that title. He was excellent in the role of Woodie Guthrie, in *Bound for Glory,* and in 1980, appeared with two members of the Carradine family in *The Long Riders*. He experienced working with Ingmar Bergman, but had a poor run during the 1990s. He's now developed a sought-after line in villains – both on TV and in big-budget movies – like *Kill Bill*. He appeared in eleven movies during 2007 – like a return to the old Hollywood studio system. David was married to his fifth wife, Annie, when he was found dead in his hotel room in Bangkok, Thailand.

The Violent Ones (1967)
Young Billy Young (1969) Kung Fu (1973)
Bound for Glory (1976)
The Serpent's Egg (1977)
Gray Lady Down (1978)
The Long Riders (1980)
Americana (1981)
Q – the Winged Serpent (1982)
Lone Wolf McQuade (1983)
Beauty and Denise (1989)
Bird on a Wire (1990)
Roadside Prophets (1992)
Kill Bill (2002) Blizhniy Boy:
The Ultimate Fighter (2002)
Dead & Breakfast (2004)
Kill Bill: Vol. 2 (2004) Camille (2007)
How to Rob a Bank (2007)
Big Stan (2007) Chatham (2008)
Richard III (2008)

John **Carradine**
6ft 2in
(RICHMOND REED CARRADINE)

Born: **February 5, 1906**
New York City, New York, USA
Died: **November 27, 1988**

John grew up in Poughkeepsie, New York, where he attended Christ Church School. When he was seventeen he went to art school to study drawing and sculpture. After a couple of years traveling around the southern states, where he paid his way by selling sketches of people, John focussed on a career in the theater. He began as a Shakespearean actor – calling himself Peter Richmond – and developing a fine voice, which was too good to be confined to the stage. He had a walk-on part as a reporter in *Bright Lights* in 1930, and two years later, played an orator in *Forgotten Commandments*. He was also heard in Cecil B. DeMille's *The Sign of the Cross*. His appearance was thought to be rather sinister and he had to wait four years, until *The Prisoner of Shark Island,* to be noticed by movie audiences. Director John Ford, liked him and used him on a regular basis. John's movie credits are impressive, he acted in *Stagecoach, The Grapes of Wrath* and *The Man Who Shot Liberty Vallance* – to name just three of his best. Despite poor horror material in later years his reputation survives. Married four times, he worked right up until the year he died of natural causes, in Milan, Italy. His four sons are all successful movie actors.

The Prisoner of Shark Island (1936)
Mary of Scotland (1936)
The Garden of Allah (1936)
Of Human Hearts (1938)
Drums along the Mohawk (1939)
Jesse James (1939) Stagecoach (1939)
The Grapes of Wrath (1940)
Western Union (1941) Manhunt (1941)
Fallen Angel (1945)
The Private Affairs of Bel Ami (1947)
Johnny Guitar (1954)
The Court Jester (1955) The Ten
Commandments (1956) The Man
Who Shot Liberty Vallance (1962)
Cheyenne Autumn (1964)
The Killer Inside Me (1976)
The Howling (1981)
House of Long Shadows (1983)

Keith **Carradine**
6ft 1in
(KEITH IAN CARRADINE)

Born: **August 8, 1949**
San Mateo, California, USA

Keith was born into a thespian family; apart from his dad, brothers, Robert and Chris, and half-brother, David are actors. He began theatrical training at Colorado State University but dropped out after one semester. In 1969, when he was in the musical "Hair" his relationship with the actress, Shelley Plimpton, resulted in Martha Plimpton, who is now a successful actress herself. Keith was twenty-one when he appeared in his first movie, the off-beat western, *A Gunfight*. In 1976, another of his talents was recognized when he won an Oscar for writing the Best Original Song, "I'm Easy" for the Robert Altman movie *Nashville*. It reached number seventeen in the U.S. charts. Keith has sustained his movie career through his choice of roles and the luck of being in the right film at the right time. He has also continued to work in Broadway shows – the "Will Rogers Follies" earning him a Tony nomination. More recently, he starred in the ABC sitcom 'Complete Savages' and was seen to good effect in Steven Spielberg's mini-series, 'Into the West'. Keith had a son, Cade, and a daughter, Sorel, with his first wife, Sandra Will. In November 2006, Keith married Hayley DuMond, in Torino, Italy.

McCabe & Mrs Miller (1971)
Emperor of the North (1973)
Nashville (1975)
The Duellists (1977)
Pretty Baby (1978)
The Long Riders (1980)
Southern Comfort (1981)
Choose Me (1984)
L'Inchiesta (1986)
The Moderns (1988)
The Bachelor (1991) Andre (1994)
Wild Bill (1995)
2 Days in the Valley (1996)
A Thousand Acres (1997)
Cahoots (2001) Fálkar (2002)
Our Very Own (2005)
Elvis and Anabelle (2007)
The Death and Life of Bobby Z (2007)
Lake City (2008)

Jim **Carrey**
6ft 2in
(JAMES EUGENE CARREY)

Born: **January 17, 1962**
Newmarket, Ontario, Canada

Jim was the youngest of four children. His father, Percy, was an accountant who aspired to be a modern jazz saxophonist. Jim performed comedy routines in front of friends, family and classmates. When he was ten, he mailed his résumé to 'The Carol Burnett Show'. After his dad lost his job, the family went to live in Toronto, where they worked eight-hour shifts in a factory. After that finished, they had to live in a camper van. The boy's school work suffered and he dropped out of high school to work as a stand-up comedian in a local club. He went to Los Angeles and got a regular gig at The Comedy Store. He married a waitress, named Melissa, with whom he had a daughter. Jim appeared in the TV sitcom 'The Duck Factory' and when it bombed, in 1985, he made his first movie, the cooly received *Once Bitten*. After success in the TV series 'In Living Color' he was in demand. *Ace Ventura: Pet Detective* and two other hits, made 1994 a very good year for him. His manic style was a regular feature in movies throughout most of the 1990s. Jim divorced two wives and also appeared in concert with Elton John. In 2000, he was engaged to his co-star in *Me, Myself & Irene*, Renée Zellweger, but he opted to remain single. In 2004, Jim became a United States citizen.

Earth Girls are Easy (1988)
Ace Ventura: Pet Detective (1994)
The Mask (1994)
Dumb & Dumber (1994)
Batman Forever (1995)
The Cable Guy (1996)
Liar Liar (1997)
The Truman Show (1998)
Man on the Moon (1999)
Me, Myself & Irene (2000)
The Majestic (2001)
Bruce Almighty (2003)
Eternal Sunshine of the
Spotless Mind (2004)
Fun with Dick and Jane (2005)
The Number 23 (2007)
Yes Man (2008)

John **Carroll**
6ft 1in
(JULIEN LAFAYE)

Born: **July 17, 1906**
New Orleans, Louisiana
Died: **April 24, 1979**

Even as a small child, John possessed a sweet and tuneful singing voice which got him a slot in the church choir. He left school in his early teens, and after a few singing lessons, was confident that he would make his fortune in the world of professional opera. A trip to Europe, and especially Italy, convinced him that this was being unrealistic. By 1926, he had settled in California, where he had various jobs including driving racing cars for prize money. With his dashing good looks, he began to get work as a film extra, starting in 1929 with *Marianne*. For five years, he was hardly noticed, as he eked out a living as an extra. In 1935, things improved. Following his appearance in the Al Jolson/Ruby Keeler musical, *Go Into Your Dance,* he appeared in the western, *Hi Gaucho!,* in which he sang three songs. It led to B-picture stardom throughout the 1940s, and supporting roles in big films. He married the actress Steffi Duna, but his off-screen philandering resulted in a quick divorce. A second marriage to Lucille Ryman was very successful. The couple were extremely kind and helpful to young Marilyn Monroe when she was starting her career in 1948. John invested in land and in the shrimping industry. He was a very rich man when he died at his Hollywood home, of leukemia.

Muss 'em Up (1936)
Murder on the Bridle Path (1936)
We Who Are About to Die (1937)
Zorro Rides Again (1937)
Only Angels Have Wings (1939)
Congo Maisie (1940) Susan and
God (1940) Phantom Raiders (1940)
Go West (1940) Lady Be Good (1941)
Rio Rita (1942) Flying Tigers (1942)
Bedside Manner (1945)
A Letter for Evie (1946)
The Fabulous Texan (1947)
Old Los Angeles (1948) Angel in
Exile (1948) Belle Le Grand (1951)
Geraldine (1953)
Decision at Sundown (1957)

Leo G. **Carroll**
5ft 11½in
(LEO G. CARROLL)

Born: **October 25, 1886**
Weedon, Northants, England
Died: **October 16, 1972**

Born into a wealthy English family, Leo was brought up as a Catholic and was in fact named after the reigning Pope. When he was fifteen, he left school to begin an apprenticeship with a company of wine merchants. In his spare time he became seriously interested in the theater. He made his English stage debut in 1911, and was on Broadway in "Rutherford & Son" a year later. He returned to England and served with the British infantry during World War I – in France, Greece, and Palestine. He was badly wounded and was only able to restart his stage career in 1920. He then continued to act in plays on both sides of the Atlantic and only moved to Hollywood in 1934. He made his film debut that year in MGM's *Sadie McKee* – a huge success for Joan Crawford. After that his face became familiar in a stream of high-powered productions, appearing in more Hitchcock films than any other actor – the first one *Rebecca,* and the last *North by Northwest.* Leo died in Hollywood of pneumonia brought on by cancer.

Sadie McKee (1934) **The Barretts of
Wimpole Street** (1934)
Clive of India (1935)
London by Night (1937)
A Christmas Carol (1938)
Wuthering Heights (1939)
Tower of London (1939)
Rebecca (1940)
Suspicion (1941)
The House on 92nd Street (1945)
Spellbound (1945)
The Paradine Case (1947)
So Evil My Love (1948)
Enchantment (1948)
Father of the Bride (1950)
Strangers on a Train (1951)
The Desert Fox (1951)
The Bad and the Beautiful (1952)
We're No Angels (1955)
Tarantula (1955)
North by Northwest (1959)
The Parent Trap (1961)
The Prize (1963)

Madeleine **Carroll**
5ft 5in
(EDITH MADELEINE CARROLL)

Born: **February 26, 1906**
West Bromwich, Staffordshire, England
Died: **October 2, 1987**

The daughter of an English-born foreign language professor and a French mother, Madeleine had brains as well as beauty. She studied for a teaching career at Birmingham University and taught for a while at Hove, in Sussex. When modeling hats in Brighton, a friend persuaded her to try her luck on the local stage. She had several small parts before making her London debut in 1927, in "The Lash". She auditioned with 150 other girls to star in the war film *The Guns of Loos,* and got the part. She made twelve films before going blonde (remaining so for the rest of her career) for *Madame Guillotine* in 1931. She then married an army officer and retired for a while. In 1933, her stage work brought film offers and *I Was a Spy* got her a role in a Hollywood movie, *The World Moves On.* It was a huge flop but she was rescued by Alfred Hitchcock, who starred her with Robert Donat in his classic, *The 39 Steps.* Her contract was sold to Walter Wanger, and she co-starred with Tyrone Power, Gary Cooper and Ronald Colman in box-office hits of the period – including *Lloyds of London* and *The Prisoner of Zenda.* In 1940, she was deeply affected by her sister's death in a German air raid. She then devoted her time to helping war victims. Active for the Red Cross, she was awarded the Legion d'Honneur in France. She made a brief film comeback in 1947 and finished her career on TV, in 1955. In 1965, after her fourth divorce, she moved to Paris and then lived in Spain until her death in Marbella of pancreatic cancer.

The 39 Steps (1935)
Secret Agent (1936)
The General Died at Dawn (1936)
Lloyds of London (1936)
On the Avenue (1937)
The Prisoner of Zenda (1937)
Blockade (1938)
One Night in Lisbon (1941)
My Favorite Blonde (1942)
An Innocent Affair (1948)
The Fan (1949)

Jack **Carson**
6ft 2in
(JOHN ELMER CARSON)

Born: **October 27, 1910**
Carman, Manitoba, Canada
Died: **January 2, 1963**

Jack went to school in Milwaukee, and military school in Wisconsin. At nineteen he established himself in vaudeville as an MC with a sense of humor. By 1935, he was a radio personality and also appeared on stage. He took a few small parts in "B" pictures before, in 1937, making his mark as a hard-boiled press agent in *Stand-In.* Working with Astaire and Rogers in *Carefree* helped him to become an in-demand freelancer. Jack was good even if the movies weren't, and Warners offered him a film with James Cagney and then gave him a contract. It lasted until 1950 – following featured roles with Errol Flynn, Bette Davis and Jane Wyman – as well as some Doris Day musicals. Jack co-starred with the young actress Lola Albright, in *The Good Humor Man,* and she became his third wife. In 1951, he was top-billed at the London Palladium before starring on Broadway in "For Thee I Sing." Along with *A Star is Born,* one of Jack's best serious roles came when his movie career was almost over – playing Paul Newman's brother – in *Cat on a Hot Tin Roof.* After four years of working on television, where in 1962, he made his last appearances, in episodes of 'Disneyland', Jack died of stomach cancer at his home in Encino, California, at the early age of fifty-two. His fourth wife, Sandra, was by his side.

Destry Rides Again (1939)
Mr Smith Goes to Washington (1939)
Gentleman Jim (1942)
The Male Animal (1942)
Arsenic and Old Lace (1943)
The Doughgirls (1944)
Mildred Pierce (1946)
Two Guys from Milwaukee (1946)
Romance on the High Seas (1948)
My Dream Is Yours (1949)
The Good Humor Man (1950)
Dangerous When Wet (1953)
A Star is Born (1954)
Phffft! (1954)
Cat on a Hot Tin Roof (1958)
The Bramble Bush (1960)

John **Cassavetes**
5ft 7in
(JOHN NICHOLAS CASSAVETES)

Born: **December 9, 1929**
New York City, New York, USA
Died: **February 3, 1989**

The son of Greek immigrants, John grew up on Long Island. His mother Katherine was an actress. When he was eighteen he went to the American Academy of Dramatic Arts in New York City. After graduating he worked mainly on television and took small movie parts – the first of any significance was *Taxi* – in 1953. John married Gena Rowlands the following year and after they started a family (their son and two daughters are actors) he began teaching method acting. An improvisation exercise in one of his workshops inspired him to make his debut as screenwriter and director with *Shadows,* in 1959. He had no luck with U.S. distributors, but it won a Critics Award at the Venice Film Festival. John was more in tune with European movie makers and audiences, but continued to direct in America and perform as an actor – being Oscar-nominated for *The Dirty Dozen.* His second independent film, *Faces,* in 1968, was nominated for three Oscars. The pioneer of American Cinema Verité, John appears on a 37 cent stamp issued in 2003. Some of his productions are considered heavy-going by viewers, but they are always interesting. His most accessible movie is arguably the last one he directed and acted in – *Love Streams.* John knew he was dying (cirrhosis of the liver) and he and Gena, (award winners in Italy) gave moving performances. He died in Los Angeles five years later.

Crime in the Streets (1956)
Edge of the City (1957)
Saddle the Wind (1959)
The Killers (1964)
The Dirty Dozen (1967)
Rosemary's Baby (1968)
Husbands (1970)
Capone (1975)
Two-Minute Warning (1976)
Opening Night (1977)
The Fury (1978)
Whose Life Is It Anyway? (1981)
Tempest (1982)
Love Streams (1984)

Jean-Pierre **Cassel**
6ft
(JEAN-PIERRE CROCHON)

Born: **October 27, 1932**
Paris, France
Died: **April 19, 2007**

After spending his teens growing up in occupied Paris, he was overjoyed when his beloved city was liberated. When he was sixteen he took acting lessons, and by 1950, was getting very small parts in stage and film productions. In 1953, he had a minor role in the Italian musical, *The Road to Happiness,* which featured jazz greats, Louis Armstrong and Sidney Bechet. Jean-Pierre's next contact with Americans was when Gene Kelly came to France to make *The Happy Road,* in 1957. He worked on it as an uncredited extra and although it wasn't a success, it was an international movie. He continued in supporting roles in French comedies until 1960, when he played the lead in *Les Jeux de l'amour,* which won a Silver Bear at the Berlin Film Festival. It was exactly the kick-start his career needed. After that, he added to his fan base with his work in English language movies. Active, until his death from cancer, in Paris, he retained his star status – up to his final appearance, in 2000 – in *Vous êtes de la police.* Jean-Pierre's son, Vincent, and his daughter Cécile, from his two marriages, continue the Cassel family tradition.

Les Jeux de l'amour (1960)
Candide (1960)
The Seven Deadly Sins (1962)
Those Magnificent Men in their Flying Machines (1965)
The Discreet Charm of the Bourgeoisie (1972)
The Three Musketeers (1973)
Murder on the Orient Express (1974)
Who Is Killing the Great Chefs of Europe? (1978)
Pétain (1993) **L'Enfer** (1994)
La Cérémonie (1995)
Sade (2000) **Narco** (2004)
Virgil (2005) **Judas** (2006)
Congorama (2006)
Fair Play (2006)
Le Scaphandre et le papillon (2007)
Astérix aux jeu olympiques (2008)

Vincent **Cassel**
6ft 2in
(VINCENT CROCHON)

Born: **November 23, 1966**
Paris, France

The son of the famous French actor, Jean-Pierre Cassel, and a mother who was a journalist, he is known to his friends as 'Vinz'. Initially he didn't want to follow in his father's footsteps so, at the age of seventeen, he went to work in a circus. Eventually he relented – making his film debut in 1991, in *Les Cis du Paradis.* He became known internationally in 1995, after his role in the explosive film, *La Haine* (The Hatred). Its theme, which focussed on social deprivation and the resulting violence, was a far cry from Vincent's own comfortable background and it was a tribute to his ability as an actor that he was able to get right inside the psyche of such people and seem like a heartless thug. In 1999, he married the Italian star, Monica Bellucci, and became a family man five years later. Apart from co-starring with his gorgeous wife in ten movies, he has worked on both sides of the Atlantic with stars such as Nicole Kidman, George Clooney, Brad Pitt and Matt Damon. He was scheduled to appear in a film with his dad (for the fourth time) before Jean-Pierre's unexpected death. It now seems probable that Vinz will outdo Jean-Pierre in terms of fame and fortune in the movie world. The Oscar-nominated film, *Eastern Promises* could be the one to provide that stepping-stone.

La Haine (1995)
L'Appartement (1996)
Dobermann (1997)
Elizabeth (1998)
Les Rivière poupres (2000)
Le Pacte des loups (2001)
Birthday Girl (2001)
Sur mes lèvres (2001)
Irréversible (2002)
The Reckoning (2003)
Blueberry (2004)
Ocean's Twelve (2004)
Derailed (2005) **Sheitan** (2006)
Ocean's Thirteen (2007)
Eastern Promises (2007)
L'Instinct de mort (2008)
L'Ennemi publi no 1 (2008)

Joanna **Cassidy**
5ft 9in
(JOANNA VIRGINIA CASSIDY)

Born: August 2, 1945
Camden, New Jersey, USA

Joanna was raised in Haddonfield, a few miles from her birthplace – in a creative family environment – both her mother and her grandfather were artists. After high school, she was an art major at Syracuse University, New York. She married a young doctor, and to help him finish his training she became a fashion model in San Francisco. When they got divorced, she moved to Los Angeles where, in 1973, she persuaded a casting director to help get her first film role, a small part in *The Laughing Policeman,* which starred Walter Matthau. She did commercials and continued modeling, but the film opportunities were increasing for her, even if married life (with two children) didn't suit her. By 1982, she could include work in Ridley Scott's *Blade Runner* and Roger Spottiswoode's *Under Fire* in her impressive portfolio. Over the next twenty-five years, the bulk of her work was as a guest-star in TV shows like 'Dallas' and 'Starsky & Hutch' and the 'Buffalo Bill' series. A four-year residency in 'Six Feet Under' got her rave notices. Since the early 1990s, she has increased her movie appearances, even if not many of them were worthwhile. One really good choice was a starring role in the quite exceptional, *Anderson's Cross.* Joanna is an avid and talented painter and sculptor and an enthusiastic collector of antiques and original art – especially American watercolorists. A dedicated animal rights activist, she lives in Los Angeles.

The Outfit (1973)
Stunts (1977)
Blade Runner (1982)
Under Fire (1983)
1969 (1988)
Who Framed Roger Rabbit (1988)
Where the Heart Is (1990)
May Wine (1990)
Vampire in Brooklyn (1995)
Chain Reaction (1996)
Dangerous Beauty (1998)
Moonglow (2000)
Intermission (2004)
Anderson's Cross (2007)

Kim **Cattrall**
5ft 9in
(KIM VICTORIA CATTRALL)

Born: August 21, 1956
Widnes, Cheshire, England

Kim is the daughter of Dennis and Shane Cattrall. Her father was a construction engineer and her mother, Shane, worked as a secretary. Kim was only three month's old when her parents made the decision to emigrate to Canada. She was raised in Courtenay, British Columbia, until she was eleven. She then returned to England to study acting at the London Academy of Music and Drama. At sixteen she went to Vancouver, where she graduated from high school and won a scholarship to the American Academy of Dramatic Arts, in New York. In 1975, in her final year, she was given her film debut by director, Otto Preminger, in *Rosebud.* For the next few years most of Kim's work was on TV. Her appearance with Jack Lemmon in *Tribute* was a turning point and by the time she co-starred with Steve Guttenberg in *Police Academy,* she had a big fan following. Her private life wasn't quite as successful – a brief marriage in 1977 was followed by a slightly better one in 1982. She has since divorced her third husband, the film sound recordist, Mark Levinson. Kim's movie career seemed to stall during the 1990s but in 1998, Kim became an international celebrity when she was perfectly cast as Samantha Jones in the hugely popular TV series 'Sex and the City'. It led to more film roles including, in 2008, the disappointing big screen version of the TV show.

Tribute (1980)
Ticket to Heaven (1981)
Porky's (1982) Police Academy (1985)
Turk 182! (1985) Hold-Up (1985)
Big Trouble in Little China (1986)
Masquarade (1988)
The Return of the Musketeers (1989)
La Famiglia Buonanotte (1989)
Star Trek: The Undiscovered
Country (1991)
Split Second (1992)
Above Suspicion (1995)
Live Nude Girls (1995)
15 Minutes (2001)
The Devil and Daniel Webster (2004)
Ice Princess (2005)

Richard **Chamberlain**
6ft 1in
(GEORGE RICHARD CHAMBERLAIN)

Born: March 31, 1934
Beverly Hills, California, USA

Richard's father, Chuck Chamberlain, used to travel extensively to lecture at Alcoholics Anonymous conventions. After Beverly Hills High School, Richard had no desire to become an alcoholic, but was more concerned about how to hide his homosexuality during those intolerant times. In 1960 he took his first steps towards stardom in a modest but effective movie, *The Secret of the Purple Reef.* His career moved forward rapidly when, the following year, he took the title role in the successful and long-running television series 'Dr. Kildare'. On the back of that fame, he embarked on a short but sweet spell as a pop singer. In 1966, despite his huge popularity, Richard's first Broadway appearance was in one of the all-time biggest flop musicals, "Breakfast at Tiffany's". But like a skilled juggler, he then switched seamlessly from stage, to television, to films – resulting in his first really good movie – *Petulia.* With co-stars of the calibre of Julie Christie and George C. Scott, the production was a winner. The 1970s were very good to him – he was even able to utilize his vocal talents in *The Slipper and the Rose.* Since the 1990s, most of his work has been on TV. In 2005, he was "Scrooge" in a Broadway national tour. In 2007, Richard appeared in two movies, and continued to act on TV – in an episode of 'Desperate Housewives'.

Petulia (1968)
The Music Lovers (1970)
Lady Caroline Lamb (1972)
The Three Musketeers (1973)
The Count of Monte Cristo (1974)
The Towering Inferno (1974)
The Last Wave (1977)
The Man in the Iron Mask (1977)
The Return of the
Musketeers (1989)
The Other Side of Murder (1991)
The Pavilion (1999)
Strength and Honor (2007)
I Now Pronounce You
Chuck & Larry (2007)
Endless Bummer (2008)

Jackie **Chan**
5ft 8½in
(KONG-SANG CHAN)

Born: April 7, 1954
Victoria Peak, Hong Kong

As refugees from the Chinese Civil War, Jackie and his family emigrated to Australia in 1960. He returned to China to attend the Peking Opera School, where he was taught acrobatics and Kung Fu skills. As one of the best students he became a member of the 'Seven Little Fortunes'. Because of the decline in Chinese Opera, Jackie worked as a stuntman on Bruce Lee movies. After Lee's death, Hong Kong action films stopped and he went back to Australia, where he worked on building sites and acquired the name "Jackie". He then accepted an offer of movie work with the director Lo Wei, who wanted a young actor he could turn into another Bruce Lee. His period with Lo did not produce the desired hits and it took a loan-out to another studio to do it. In 1978, *Snake in the Eagle's Shadow* was Jackie's first big success and that same year, he made *Drunken Master,* which got him noticed internationally. In 1981, he appeared with an American cast, in *Cannonball Run.* Jackie has continued to produce the hits into his fifties, with no apparent loss of energy. In 2004, he played Passepartout in a not very serious remake of *Around the World in 80 Days.* Still involved with many of his own stunts, Jackie injured himself on the set of *Rush Hour 3,* but was back filming again within a few days.

Drunken Master (1978)
Supercop (1992)
Legend of the Drunken
Master (1994) Thunderbolt (1995)
Rumble in the Bronx (1995)
Jackie Chan's First Strike (1996)
Rush Hour (1998)
Shanghai Noon (2000)
Rush Hour 2 (2001)
Shanghai Knights (2003)
Vampire Effect (2003)
Around the World in 80 Days (2004)
The Myth (2005)
Baby (2006)
Rob-B-Hood (2006)
Rush Hour 3 (2007)
The Forbidden Kingdom (2008)

Jeff **Chandler**
6ft 4in
(IRA GROSSEL)

Born: December 15, 1918
Brooklyn, New York City, New York, USA
Died: June 17, 1961

When Jeff left Erasmus High School, the only job he could get was in a restaurant his father was managing. So he studied art for a while until fellow students urged him to use his good looks and try acting. He enrolled at the Feagin School of Dramatic Art and began getting small roles in stage productions. He set up his own stock company, just as World War II was starting, and spent over four years in the army. In 1946, he went to Los Angeles and married actress, Marjorie Hoshell, with whom he had two daughters before they divorced in 1954. Bit parts in movies were all Jeff could get at the time – he was considered too tall for most of the leading actresses. In 1949, he was signed by Universal after he appeared in a small role in their film *Sword of the Desert.* More importantly, they loaned him to 20th-Century Fox to play Cochise, in *Broken Arrow* – for which he was nominated for a Best Supporting Actor Oscar. During his time at Universal, they were never able to give him a role of that calibre. He starred mainly in action movies and had a parallel career as a singer – making albums for Liberty Records. Then, in 1961, he injured his back playing baseball with extras on the set of *Merrill's Marauders.* He underwent surgery in hospital, but an artery was damaged during the operation. Jeff died of blood poisoning a month later, in Culver City, Los Angeles, California.

Broken Arrow (1950)
Sign of the Pagan (1954)
Foxfire (1955)
The Spoilers (1955)
Away All Boats (1956)
Pillars of the Sky (1956)
The Tattered Dress (1957)
Jeanne Eagels (1957)
Man in the Shadow (1957)
Raw Wind in Eden (1958)
Ten Seconds to Hell (1959)
The Jayhawkers! (1959)
The Plunderers (1960)
Merrill's Marauders (1962)

Lon **Chaney Jr.**
6ft 2½in
(CREIGHTON TULL CHANEY)

Born: February 10, 1906
Oklahoma City, Oklahoma, USA
Died: July 12, 1973

Lon's father, Lon Chaney Sr., the son of deaf-mute parents, was a giant of silent movies. Known as "The Man of a Thousand Faces", he was always going to be a hard act to follow. His wife, Cleva Creighton, was a singer on his road shows but, after her suicide attempt in 1913, he divorced her. Until he remarried, Lon's father sent him to boarding schools and stated firmly that he didn't want his son to follow his career path. His death in 1930, enabled Lon to go to Hollywood. He acted under his original name until 1935, when the studio saw the advantage in billing him as Lon Chaney Jr. He became famous for his roles in horror films, but his best screen performance was as the simple-minded Lennie Small, in the 1939 film *Of Mice and Men.* Two years later, Lon became *The Wolf Man* for Universal. Such roles and his presence in Dracula and Mummy films kept him employed for years. He scared Abbott and Costello almost to death, but his type-casting depressed him and he developed a very serious drink problem. He also began to suffer from throat cancer – the disease that had killed his father at the age of forty-seven. Lon died in San Clemente, California, of liver failure. As per his wishes, his body was donated for medical research.

The Most Dangerous Game (1932)
Of Mice and Men (1939)
North West Mounted Police (1940)
The Wolf Man (1941)
Son of Dracula (1943)
The Mummy's Curse (1944)
My Favorite Brunette (1947)
High Noon (1952)
A Lion Is in the Streets (1953)
Not as a Stranger (1955)
I Died a Thousand Times (1955)
The Indian Fighter (1955)
Pardners (1956)
The Defiant Ones (1958)
Witchcraft (1964)
Young Fury (1965)
Welcome to Hard Times (1967)

Stockard **Channing**
5ft 3in
(SUSAN ANTONIA WILLIAMS STOCKARD)

Born: **February 13, 1944**
New York City, New York, USA

Stockard was the daughter of a wealthy business executive and a mother of Irish ancestry. From the age of six, she travelled a lot in Europe. In New York, she attended private schools. When she was fifteen, her father died of cancer. She went to the then female-only Radcliffe College, at Harvard University, from where she graduated with a BA in American History and Literature. While there, Stockard became interested in drama through the influence of classmates such as Tommy Lee Jones. Her entry into that world was delayed when, in 1963, she married the first of four husbands – businessman Walter Channing. When they divorced in 1967, she kept his name. Her other three attempts at marriage proved equally unsuccessful – but at least she had no children to worry about. Meanwhile, following a TV appearance in 'Sesame Street', Stockard made her movie debut in *The Hospital,* in 1971. Her big break came nearly seven years later, when she played Betty Rizzo in *Grease.* It didn't result in stardom, but in view of the fact that she was thirty-four at the time, she's done rather well. In 1985, she won Broadway's Tony Award as Best Actress in "A Day in the Death of Joe Egg" and was nominated for several Emmys. Stockard received a Best Actress Oscar nomination for *Six Degrees of Separation.*

A Different Approach (1978)
Grease (1978)
The Cheap Detective (1978)
Without a Trace (1983)
Six Degrees of Separation (1993)
Smoke (1995) Moll Flanders (1996)
The First Wives Club (1996)
Twilight (1998)
Other Voices (2000)
Where the Heart Is (2000)
The Business of Strangers (2001)
Behind the Red Door (2003)
Bright Young Things (2003)
Anything Else (2003)
3 Needles (2005)
Sparkle (2007)
Multiple Sarcasms (2008)

Sir Charles **Chaplin**
5ft 6½ in
(CHARLES SPENCER CHAPLIN)

Born: **April 16, 1889**
Walworth, London, England
Died: **December 25, 1977**

Charlie grew up in south east London. His parents, who were both Music Hall stars, separated when he was three. He and his brother were brought up by their mother. When she suffered a larynx condition and was unable to work, she broke down and was committed to an asylum. Her sons survived workhouses until they formed an act and entered the Music Hall. Charlie toured the United States with Fred Karno – from 1910 to 1912 – and after a brief stay in England, returned with the troupe which included Stan Laurel. Charlie joined Mack Sennet's Keystone Studio and made his debut in the 1914 one-reel comedy, *Making a Living.* He was a great star with Sennet, but became a lot richer after he co-founded United Artists – with Pickford, Fairbanks and D.W. Griffith. His UA films were feature length and benefited from the technical advances of the time. Charlie resisted the coming of sound to the extent that the two films he made in the 1930s had little dialogue, but were enhanced by music. His first talkie, *The Great Dictator,* in 1940, was an enormous success – largely because of his impersonation of Adolf Hitler. In 1952 Charlie was forced to leave America due to the McCarthy purge of 'communists'. He was married four times – three of his wives were teenagers – and had eleven children, including actors Sydney and Geraldine. His later efforts were below par, and after acting in a cameo role in his production, *A Countess from Hong Kong,* he retired to Vevey, Switzerland – next to Lake Geneva – where he died of natural causes.

The Gold Rush (1925)
The Circus (1928)
City Lights (1931)
Modern Times (1936)
The Great Dictator (1940)
Monsieur Verdoux (1947)
Limelight (1952)
A King in New York (1957)
A Countess from
Hong Kong (1967)

Geraldine **Chaplin**
5ft 7in
(GERALDINE LEIGH CHAPLIN)

Born: **July 31, 1944**
Santa Monica, California, USA

With the legendary Charles Chaplin as a father, and the daughter of playwright Eugene O'Neil, as her mother, Geraldine was destined to express herself in a creative way. When her father was an unwanted alien in America, the family went to live in Switzerland. Geraldine went to the best private schools in the country before going to London to play a small role in her father's *Limelight.* The film and Claire Bloom's portrayal of a ballet dancer had a huge influence on the young girl. Eventually, she trained at the Royal Ballet School. An injury cut short her plans, but with her parents' encouragement she went to acting classes. In 1963, she was in a French short film called *Denier soir* and the feature *Par un beau matin été.* It gave her the confidence to get the role of Tonya, in David Lean's *Doctor Zhivago.* During the film's shooting in Spain, she met and began a long relationship with the director Carlos Saura. Geraldine has been featured in several of his films and worked with Europe's best directors during her long career. She was nominated for a Best Supporting Actress BAFTA for *Welcome to L.A.* and three times for Golden Globes – for *Doctor Zhivago* (Most Promising Newcomer), *Nashville* and *Chaplin* (both as Best Supporting Actress). Geraldine finally married, for the first time, in 2006, film-maker, Patricio Castilla. The couple have a daughter named Oona.

Doctor Zhivago (1965)
Peppermint Frappé (1967)
Nashville (1975)
Welcome to L.A. (1976)
A Wedding (1978)
Life is a Bed of Roses (1983)
Chaplin (1992)
The Age of Innocence (1993)
Home for the Holidays (1995)
Jane Eyre (1996)
Cousin Bette (1998)
Talk to Her (2002)
The Orphanage (2007)
Boxes (2007)
Imago mortis (2009)

Cyd **Charisse**
5ft 7½in
(TULA ELLICE FINKLEA)

Born: **March 8, 1921**
Amarillo, Texas, USA
Died: **June 17, 2008**

Cyd began taking ballet lessons when she was eight, and four years later she learned advance dancing with Nico Charisse, in Hollywood. He helped her get a contract with the Ballet Russe when she was fourteen. She toured with them (using the names Maria Istomina and Felia Sidorova) until the outbreak of war. After signing for MGM, she married Nico and changed her name. The studio gave her small parts, usually as a dancer, but her first starring role was in a murder mystery called *Tension,* in 1949. She was then married to the singer Tony Martin and after starting a family, did no screen work for a couple of years. Her sensational dance routine with Gene Kelly in *Singing in the Rain* had fans all over the world urging MGM to give her bigger roles. For a time they did. Sadly the musical was already in its decline and after the 1962 drama, *Two Weeks in Another Town,* when she acted with Kirk Douglas, Cyd's reign as a movie queen was over. In 1962, she was third-billed below Marilyn Monroe and Dean Martin in MM's final bow, the unfinished, *Something's Got to Give.* For several years Cyd toured in a night club act with her husband, Tony. In 1986, she starred in the London production of "Charlie's Girl" in which she showed great energy and was still very glamorous at the age of sixty-five. In 2006, Cyd Charisse was awarded the American Medal of the Arts. She died in Los Angeles of complications from a heart attack.

Till the Clouds Roll By (1946)
Words and Music (1948)
East Side, West Side (1949)
Tension (1949)
Singin' in the Rain (1952)
The Band Wagon (1953)
Brigadoon (1954)
It's Always Fair Weather (1955)
Silk Stockings (1957)
Party Girl (1958)
Black Tights (1960)
Two Weeks in Another Town (1962)
The Silencers (1966)

Ruth **Chatterton**
5ft 2½in
(RUTH CHATTERTON)

Born: **December 24, 1893**
New York City, New York, USA
Died: **November 24, 1961**

Ruth's father, an Englishman, emigrated to New York City with his French-born wife. Ruth was born there on Christmas Eve. From an early age Ruth attended ballet lessons and at fourteen, but looking much older, she took the plunge and got a job in the chorus line of a Broadway show. She established herself as an actress who could play in musical comedies. When she was dancing in one of them, she caught the eye of the English actor and movie star, Ralph Forbes, who married her. Ruth made her own film debut four years later in *Sins of the Father,* but really came into her own in *Madame X* and *Sarah and Son* – both of which earned her nominations for Best Actress Oscars. She married George Brent and moved to Warner Brothers, who were looking for talent with "class". Ruth gave it to them. Unfortunately, time caught up with her and she appeared in her last film, *A Royal Divorce,* in 1938. She had a brief new career when TV brought drama into people's homes. Ruth made her final appearance – as Gertrude – in a Hallmark Hall of Fame production of 'Hamlet', co-starring Maurice Evans. She went to live in England with her third husband, Barry Thomson, and started writing novels. She returned to the USA in 1960. After Ruth died in Norwalk, Connecticut, of a cerebral hemorrhage, Bette Davis remarked that she had been "very kind" when she first went to Warners.

Madame X (1929)
Charming Sinners (1929)
The Laughing Lady (1929)
Sarah and Son (1930)
The Lady of Scandal (1930)
Anybody's Woman (1930)
Unfaithful (1931)
The Rich Are Always with Us (1932)
Frisco Jenny (1932)
Lilly Turner (1933)
Female (1933)
Journal of Crime (1934)
Girls' Dormitory (1936)
Dodsworth (1936)

Mahima **Chaudhry**
5ft 5in
(RITU CHAUDHURY)

Born: **September 13, 1973**
New Delhi, India

Mahima's parents were totally contrasting types: her father was the easy-going sort and her mother was a strict disciplinarian. It all helped her and her older sister, Ashu, to be good students during their time at Loreto Convent in Darjeeling. Both girls were beautiful, and had ambitions of becoming models when they left school. Ashu never made it, but Mahima, as she would become known, was soon appearing in fashion magazines and had an early acting opportunity, in a Pepsi television commercial, which exposed her to a much larger audience. In 1997, she auditioned along with some 3000 other hopefuls, for the female lead in the film, *Pardes.* She got the part and was given rave reviews for her performance as the country girl who wants to hang on to her traditions. She won the 1998 Filmfare Award as Best Debut Female and the LUX Face of the Year. One of Mahima's great virtues is her flexibility and willingness to act in supporting roles, despite being recognized as a star. Her reward for this was a Best Supporting Actress Award, for *Dobara.* She's an admirer of other actresses, with a special liking for the work of Juhi Chawla. Mahima is married to Bobby Mukherjee – a top-flight architect in Mumbai. They have a daughter named Aryana.

Pardes (1997)
Dil Kya Kare (1999)
Dhadkan (2000)
Deewane (2000)
Kurukshetra (2000)
Lajja (2001)
Yeh Teraa Ghar
Yeh Meraa Ghar (2001)
Om Jai Jagadish (2002)
My Heart Is Yours (2002)
Saaya (2003)
Tere Naam (2003)
Dobara (2004)
Sehar (2005)
The Film (2005)
Souten: The Other Woman (2006)
Sandwich (2006)
Pusher (2007)

Don **Cheadle**

5ft 8¹/₂in

(DONALD FRANK CHEADLE)

Born: **November 29, 1964**
Kansas City, Missouri, USA

Of Cameroonian ancestry, Don is the son of Donald Cheadle, a clinical psychologist, and his wife Betty, who was at different times a bank manager and a psychology teacher. The family moved from Kansas to Canada – where he graduated from Nelson High School in Burlington, Ontario. After that, Don returned to the United States to study acting at the California Institute of the Arts, in Valencia. In 1984, he starred in a short film titled *3 Days,* and his feature film debut was the following year, in the comedy, *Moving Violations.* He did a few television shows before landing a good role in the powerful war drama *Hamburger Hill.* Don's breakthrough movie was *Colors,* but he really got noticed in *Devil in a Blue Dress,* which won him Supporting Actor awards from L.A. Film Critics and others. He moved fluently to a higher plane in *Traffic,* and *The United States of Leland,* before being nominated for a Best Actor Oscar, for *Hotel Rwanda.* His experiences in Africa prompted him to co-author a book about the plight of people in the Sudan. Don loves football and has made some TV commercials promoting the Super Bowl. His first love however, is his family. He has two teenaged daughters with his long-time partner, the actress Bridgid Coulter.

Hamburger Hill (1987) **Colors** (1988)
Roadside Prophets (1992) **Things to Do in Denver When You're Dead** (1995)
Devil in a Blue Dress (1995)
Rosewood (1997) **Volcano** (1997)
Boogie Nights (1997)
Bulworth (1998) **Out of Sight** (1998)
Traffic (2000)
Things Behind the Sun (2001)
Manic (2001) **Swordfish** (2001)
Ticker (2002) **The United States of Leland** (2003) **Crash** (2004)
Hotel Rwanda (2004)
After the Sunset (2004)
Talk to Me (2007)
Reign Over Me (2007)
Ocean's Thirteen (2007)
Traitor (2008)

Cher

5ft 7¹/₂in

(CHERILYN SARKISIAN LAPIERE)

Born: **May 20, 1946**
El Centro, California, USA

Cher got her exotic looks from her dad, who was Armenian, and her mother, an unsuccessful actress, who was part Cherokee. Cher went to L.A. when she was sixteen, intent on becoming a pop singer. As Bonnie Jo Mason, she made her first record, "I Love You Ringo" in 1963. She was soon famous for being half of the husband and wife pop duo, Sonny & Cher. Bono produced a couple of her early films, but they divorced in 1975 and she became the third of Gregg Allman's six wives. They split in 1979, and she was very successful as a singer and eventually, after taking acting lessons with Lee Strasberg, a movie star. Cher was Oscar-nominated as Best Supporting Actress, for *Silkwood* and four years later, won a Best Actress Oscar for *Moonstruck.* In 1998, she delivered a moving eulogy at the funeral of former husband, Sonny Bono, who had become a congressman in California. Although Cher is still active, she hasn't been seen on the big screen since the comedy drama *Stuck on You,* in 2003. It's debatable whether she's had more success as an actress or as a singer. She herself believes she is better as an actress. Who can deny that her few movie roles have nearly all been impressive? On the other hand, can the 180 million buyers of her solo albums be wrong? In 2008, she returned with live performances at the Colosseum, Caesars Palace, Las Vegas. Her son, Elijah, from her marriage to Greg Allman, is a member of the Goth Rock band, "Deadsy".

Come Back to the Five and Dime, Jimmy Dean, Jimmy Dean (1982)
Silkwood (1983)
Mask (1985)
The Witches of Eastwick (1987)
Suspect (1987)
Moonstruck (1987)
Mermaids (1990)
Faithful (1996)
Tea with Mussolini (1999)
Stuck on You (2003)

Leslie **Cheung**

5ft 9in

(CHEUNG FAT-CHEUNG)

Born: **September 12, 1956**
Hong Kong
Died: **April 1, 2003**

Leslie was the youngest of ten children. His father was a well-known tailor who made suits for film stars, Cary Grant and William Holden. Leslie began his education at Rosaryhill School in Hong Kong, but following his parents' divorce, he was sent to England to a boarding school near Norwich, called Eccles Hall. He was not happy – facing racial taunts and bullying. Leslie escaped at weekends to work in a relative's restaurant and began to develop as a singer. At Leeds University, he started studying textile management, but had to give it up when his father fell ill. In 1977, he entered the Asian Music Contest – placing second with his rendition of "American Pie". He made his film debut in 1978, in *The Erotic Dreamer,* but achieved his fame in the 1980s, in TV dramas. In 1984, he had his first top ten record with "Monica". He made music and films until emigrating to Canada, in 1989. He still acted in Hong Kong movies – voted Best Actor at their Film Awards, for *Days of Being Wild* and *Ashes of Time.* After admitting being a bi-sexual, Leslie became depressed and killed himself by leaping from the 24th floor of Hong Kong's Mandarin Oriental Hotel.

On Trial (1980) **The Drummer** (1980)
Teenage Dreamers (1982) **Nomad** (1982)
Behind the Yellow Line (1984)
For Your Heart Only (1985)
A Better Tomorrow (1986)
A Chinese Ghost Story (1987)
A Better Tomorrow II (1987)
Rouge (1987) **Fatal Love** (1988)
A Chinese Ghost Story II (1990)
Days of Being Wild (1990)
All's Well, Ends Well (1992)
Farewell My Concubine (1993)
He's a Woman, She's a Man (1994)
Ashes of Time (1994)
The Phantom Lover (1995)
The Chinese Feast (1995)
The Phantom Lover (1995)
Temptress Moon (1996) **Shanghai Grand** (1996) **Happy Together** (1997)
The Kid (1999) **Double Tap** (2000)

Maggie **Cheung**
5ft 6¼in
(MARGARET CHENG MAN YUK)

Born: **September 20, 1964**
Hong Kong

Maggie's parents were merchants, who could trace their family ancestry back to Shanghai. She began her education at the Catholic St. Paul's Convent, in Hong Kong, but while she was still a youngster, her parents emigrated to England. Maggie finished her schooling there, but in 1982, when she was on vacation in Hong Kong, she was spotted by a representative from a model agency. The following year, after a few jobs, she entered the "Miss Hong Kong" beauty contest and came second. Later that year, as Margaret Cheung Man Yuk, she was a semi-finalist in the "Miss World Pageant" at London's Royal Albert Hall. The following year, she made her film debut in *Prince Charming*. Maggie acted in around twenty decorative roles during the 1980s, but was taken more seriously after winning the Hong Kong Film Award as Best Actress, for *Fishy Story*. She won four more, and was internationally famous when she was named Best Actress at the Berlin Film Festival for *Center Stage,* and at Cannes for *Clean* – which was directed by her former husband, Olivier Assayas. In that film she performed all the songs. Hers was rated by the New York Times as one of the top 22 performances of 2006.

Behind the Yellow Line (1984) Lost Romance (1985) Jackie Chan's Police Force (1985) Heavenly Fate (1987) Jackie Chan's Project A2 (1987) Mother vs. Mother (1988) Fat Cat (1988) As Tears Go By (1988) Jackie Chan's Police Story (1988) Golden Years (1988) The Iceman Cometh (1989) A Fishy Story (1989) Farewell China (1990) Full Moon in New York (1990) Song of the Exile (1990) Days of Being Wild (1990) Dragon Inn (1992) All's Well, Ends Well (1992) Center Stage (1992) First Shot (1993) Blue Snake (1993) Ashes of Time (1994) Chinese Box (1997) In the Mood for Love (2000) Hero (2002) Clean (2004) 2046 (2004) Ashes of Time Redux (2008)

Maurice **Chevalier**
5ft 10½in
(MAURICE AUGUSTE CHEVALIER)

Born: **September 12, 1888**
Paris, France
Died: **January 1, 1972**

Maurice was the ninth of ten children – only three of whom survived. His father was a drunkard, who died when Maurice was eleven. His mother couldn't cope, so Maurice and his brother were sent to an institution. He was an acrobat until he had an accident. He then began singing outside cafes. He was heard and liked and joined the 'Folies Bergere'. He made the first of many film appearances in 1908, but when war came, he joined the army. Wounded and captured by the Germans, he had the good fortune to be taught English by one of his fellow prisoners. He made his first London appearance in 1919, in a revue called "Hullo America", and then spent three years at the Casino de Paris. Maurice formed his own film company and was signed by Paramount. He became an instant screen favorite when he co-starred in *The Love Parade,* with Jeanette MacDonald. By the late 1930s, he had become type-cast and audiences were tired of him. He returned to France where, during the war, he was accused of being a collaborator because he sang to German troops. In the 1950s, he toured again and made a triumphant return to Hollywood. For *Gigi,* he got a special Oscar, and was a celebrity until 1970. When Maurice suffered cardiac arrest and died in his Paris apartment, he was surrounded by his own memorabilia.

The Love Parade (1929) The Smiling Lieutenant (1931) One Hour with You (1932) Love Me Tonight (1932) La Veuve joyeuse (1934) The Merry Widow (1934) Folies Bergère (1935) Pièges (1939) Man About Town (1947) Ma pomme (1950) Love in the Afternoon (1957) Gigi (1958) Fanny (1961) In Search of the Castaways (1962) I'd Rather Be Rich (1964)

Julie **Christie**
5ft 2in
(JULIE FRANCES CHRISTIE)

Born: **April 14, 1941**
Chabua, Assam, India

Julie's father owned a tea plantation and could afford to send her to a boarding school in England. When Julie was sixteen she went to Paris to study art. It was a short stay but she perfected her French and got a taste for the freedom and lifestyle enjoyed by the people in post-war continental Europe. She had also made up her mind to be an actress. In London she enrolled at the Central School of Music and Drama – graduating in 1958. She spent three years with Frinton Repertory in Essex, before her television debut in 1961, in the sci-fi series 'A for Andromeda'. Her first film appearance was in that year's, *Crooks Anonymous*. In 1962, she was an instant hit after she showed that English girls (well before swinging London) could outshine continentals, in *Billy Liar.* She was the film world's *'Darling'* and won a Best Actress Oscar for that movie. It was also the year she starred as Lara, in David Lean's *Doctor Zhivago.* She worked for Truffaut, in *Fahrenheit 451* and was a Thomas Hardy heroine, in *Far from the Madding Crowd.* Never happy with stardom, a seven-year affair with Warren Beatty, and an Oscar nomination for *McCabe & Mrs Miller,* helped her to remain one. *Don't Look Now* and *Heaven Can Wait,* are true classics. Julie now appears in supporting roles, but her portrayal of a woman suffering from Alzheimer's disease in *Away from Her* was anything but that, and she was nominated for a Best Actress Oscar.

Billy Liar (1963) Darling (1965) Doctor Zhivago (1965) Fahrenheit 451 (1966) Far from the Madding Crowd (1968) Petulia (1968) The Go-Between (1970) McCabe & Mrs Miller (1971) Don't Look Now (1973) Shampoo (1973) Demon Seed (1977) Heaven Can Wait (1978) Heat and Dust (1983) Power (1986) Hamlet (1996) Afterglow (1997) Finding Neverland (2004) Away from Her (2006) New York, I Love You (2008)

Minoru **Chiaki**
5ft 10½in
(KATSUHARU SASAKI)

Born: **July 30, 1917**
Hokkaido, Japan
Died: **November 1, 1999**

During the 1930s, Minoru was the pride and joy of his parents – achieving good grades during his school years and then graduating from the University of Chuo, with degrees in Business and Economics. He'd hardly had time to consider a career when, at twenty, he decided to become an actor. He studied drama with the Shin-Tsukiji Gekikan Theater Troupe. He stayed with them until Japan entered World War II and somehow avoided military service. He served as a director and actor of the Bara-Za Theater Company and was seen in a 1947 stage production of "Dataii" by the young film director, Akira Kurosawa, who later adapted it to film. He gave Minoru his film debut in his noirish crime thriller, *Nora inu* – the first of ten movies they worked on together. He became famous through the director's growing reputation with such classics as *Rashômon, The Seven Samurai, Throne of Blood* and *The Hidden Fortress*. He had three sons with his wife, Fumie. One of them is actor Katsuhiko Sasaku. Minoru suffered a stroke in 1975, but recovered to continue his career – winning a Japanese Oscar as Best Actor for *Hana ichomonme*. He was the last surviving *Samurai* when he died of coronary and pulmonary failure.

Noru inu (1949) **Rashômon** (1950)
The Idiot (1951) **Vendetta of a**
Samurai (1952) **To Live** (1952)
The Seven Samurai (1954)
The Return of Godzilla (1955)
I Live in Fear (1955) Bushido (1956)
A Wife's Heart (1956) Throne of
Blood (1957) The Men of Tohoku (1957)
The Lower Depths (1957)
Anzukko (1958) The Hidden
Fortress (1958) The Vagabonds (1959)
Chikamutsu's Love in Osaka (1959)
The Human Condition II (1959)
Hero of the Red Light
District (1960) The Inheritance (1962)
High and Low (1963)
Stranger's Face (1966)
Hana ichimonme (1985)

Diane **Cilento**
5ft 7in
(DIANE CILENTO)

Born: **October 5, 1933**
Brisbane, Queensland, Australia

Diane's parents, Sir Raphael and Lady Phyllis, were distinguished medical practitioners. After leaving school, she went to London to study at RADA. She got bit parts in films, starting with *Captain Horatio Hornblower R.N.* in 1951, but was really discovered when she played the female lead in "Romeo and Juliet" on stage at the Library Theater, Manchester. The movie producer Sidney Cole was so impressed, he signed her to star in the title role of *The Angel Who Pawned Her Harp*. After the promise of that film, Diane appeared in some pretty disappointing efforts – the British film industry of the 1950s couldn't handle this kind of woman and she became merely decorative. She did appear on Broadway, and in 1956 she was nominated for a Tony Award, for her portrayal of Helen of Troy, in "Tiger at the Gates". Diane also made a dramatic impact in Val Guest's movie *The Full Treatment* and was next in Gary Cooper's final film, *The Naked Edge*. In 1962, she married Sean Connery and they produced a future actor, Jason. Just after his birth, Diane acted in *Tom Jones,* and was nominated for a Best Supporting Actress Oscar. *Hombre* and *The Wicker Man* are the pick of her subsequent films. Diane's sixteen-year marriage to the screen writer Anthony Shaffer ended when he died in 2001. Diane now lives in Queensland, where she runs an open-air theater.

The Angel Who Pawned
Her Harp (1957)
The Admirable Crichton (1957)
The Truth About Women (1957)
Jet Storm (1959)
The Full Treatment (1960)
The Naked Edge (1961)
Tom Jones (1963)
The Third Secret (1964)
Rattle of a Simple Man (1964)
The Agony and the Ecstasy (1965)
Hombre (1967)
Negatives (1968)
Hitler: The Last Ten Days (1973)
The Wicker Man (1973)

Dane **Clark**
5ft 10in
(BERNARD ZANVILLE)

Born: **February 26, 1912**
Brooklyn, New York City, New York, USA
Died: **September 11, 1998**

Dane was born and raised in Brooklyn and went to high school there. After graduating from Cornell University and St. John's Law School in Brooklyn, he found it hard to get a job. He became a boxer, worked in construction, and as a salesman. Finally, some work as a male model for a store led to bit parts in Broadway plays. In 1940, he made his film debut in *Money and the Woman*. Unfortunately, his scenes were deleted. After five uncredited roles he was given fourth billing in 1943, in a short U.S. Army Forces film, *The Rear Gunner,* starring Ronald Reagan. Warner Brothers signed him and cast him in *Action in the North Atlantic*. Its star, Humphrey Bogart, suggested that he change his name to Dane Clark. He didn't argue! The studio did him proud during the war years – even starring him in the Oscar-winning short – *I Won't Play*. He was also acting with Cary Grant, John Garfield and Bette Davis, and when peace returned he became a star of the studio's B-movies. In 1950, Dane starred in France with Simone Signoret, in *Gunman in the Streets*. It attempted to introduce him to a new market, but his movie career had virtually ended. For the next forty years he was employed on TV – making his final appearance in episodes of "Murder, She Wrote", in 1989. He retired to live in Santa Monica, California, with his second wife, Geraldine Zanville, until his death from natural causes.

Action in the North Atlantic (1943)
Destination Tokyo (1943)
The Very Thought of You (1944)
God Is My Co-Pilot (1945)
Pride of the Marines (1945)
A Stolen Life (1946)
That Way with Women (1947)
Deep Valley (1947)
Embraceable You (1948)
Moonrise (1948) Whiplash (1948)
Without Honor (1949)
Gunman in the Streets (1950)
Backfire (1950)
The Gambler and the Lady (1952)

Mae **Clarke**
5ft 2in
(VIOLET MARY KLOTZ)

Born: **August 16, 1910**
Philadelphia, Pennsylvania, USA
Died: **April 29, 1992**

Mae took dancing lessons from the age of three. Her dad was a motion-picture theater organist, so she got to see the shows for free. At sixteen she began her career in show business, dancing in a night club. With encouragement from star, Barbara Stanwyck, this led to parts in Broadway musicals and eventually to her movie debut, in an early talkie called *Big Time.* In 1931, she achieved screen immortality when (in an uncredited role in *The Public Enemy*) she had half a grapefruit thrust into her face by James Cagney. Her ex-husband, Lew Brice, would go to see it just to watch that scene! Cagney treated her rough in two other films, but he was a good friend in real life. Universal gave her a contract and starred her in *Waterloo Bridge* and the first sound version of *Frankenstein.* Although she wasn't a glamour girl, her friend Anita Loos used her as the model for Lorelei Lee, in her novel "Gentlemen Prefer Blondes". By the mid-thirties, Mae was in B-pictures and supporting roles in features. From the late-1940s onwards she supplemented her TV work with uncredited bit parts. She kept going into her seventies – participating in the Hollywood tours of her old studio. She then retired to the Motion Picture Country Home in Woodlands Hills, where she lived among friends until she died of cancer.

The Front Page (1931)
Waterloo Bridge (1931)
Frankenstein (1931)
Final Edition (1932)
Impatient Maiden (1932)
Night World (1932)
Penguin Pool Murder (1932)
Turn Back the Clock (1933)
Penthouse (1933)
Lady Killer (1933)
This Side of Heaven (1934)
Flying Tigers (1942)
Not as a Stranger (1955)
Ride the High Iron (1956)
Voice in the Mirror (1958)
A Big Hand for the Little Lady (1966)

Patricia **Clarkson**
5ft 5in
(PATRICIA DAVIES CLARKSON)

Born: **December 29, 1959**
New Orleans, Louisiana, USA

Patricia was the youngest of five girls born to Arthur and Jackie Clarkson. With a father who was a school administrator at Louisiana State, and a mother who was a politician and councilwoman, Patricia was always likely to be an academic, and she certainly was. After studying drama at Fordham University – at Lincoln Center, New York, (from where she graduated *summa cum laude*) she got her MFA at the Yale School of Drama. Then, in 1985, she appeared in an episode of TV's 'Spenser: For Hire' and worked in the theater. She made her film debut, playing Eliot Ness's wife, Catherine, in *The Untouchables.* Throughout the 1980s and 1990s, she landed some excellent parts. In 2002, Patricia appeared with distinction in the top-quality TV series, 'Six Feet Under'. For her role – as Sarah O'Connor – she was awarded an Emmy, in 2005. She received her one and only Oscar nomination, for Best Supporting Actress, in *Pieces of April.* Patricia cites Ingrid Bergman as being her favorite film actress and her biggest influence.

The Untouchables (1987)
The Dead Pool (1988)
Rocky Gibraltar (1988)
Everybody's All-American (1988)
Tune in Tomorrow (1990)
Pharaoh's Army (1995)
Jumanji (1995) High Art (1998)
Playing by Heart (1998)
The Green Mile (1999)
The Pledge (2001)
The Safety of Objects (2001)
Far from Heaven (2002)
All the Real Girls (2003)
Pieces of April (2003)
The Station Agent (2003)
Dogville (2003)
Miracle (2004)
Good Night, and Good Luck (2005)
All the King's Men (2006)
Lars and the Real Girl (2007)
Married Life (2007)
Elegy (2008)
Vicky Cristina Barcelona (2008)

Jill **Clayburgh**
5ft 8in
(JILL CLAYBURGH)

Born: **April 30, 1944**
New York City, New York, USA

Born into a wealthy family, Jill went to the finest schools, including Sarah Lawrence, a liberal arts college in New York City. It helped make her mind up about an acting career – she already exuded class in the way certain English people do – so she would be a leading lady. With her career path mapped out, the first step was to join the newly-opened Charles Playhouse, in Boston. It was a hotbed of young talent – providing Jill with opportunities to act with future luminaries such as Al Pacino. She made her first film appearance in 1963, in Brian De Palma's *The Wedding Party* – shot at Sarah Lawrence College – and co-starring Robert De Niro. It was finally released in 1979. She acted on Broadway in "The Rothschilds" and "Pippin", but had to wait until 'Hustling', a 1974 TV film in which she was a battered prostitute – to get noticed. Jill learned a lot from living with Al Pacino from 1970-1975. Oscar nominated performances in *An Unmarried Woman* and *Starting Over* show her at her best. She didn't seek conventional stardom during the next twenty years or so, but in 1999 'Entertainment Weekly' included her on their list of twenty-five of the greatest Hollywood Actresses. During 2007, Jill was seen in eleven episodes of the TV-series 'Dirty Sexy Money'. She is currently working on the film *Dirty Tricks,* in which she portrays Richard Nixon's wife, Pat. Her real-life husband is David Rabe, with whom she has two children – one of them is the young actress, Lily Rabe.

The Thief Who Came to Dinner (1973) Silver Streak (1976)
An Unmarried Woman (1978)
La Luna (1979)
Starting Over (1979)
First Monday in October (1981)
I'm Dancing as Fast as I Can (1982)
Hanna K. (1983)
Shy People (1987)
Rich in Love (1993)
Never Again (2001)
Vallen (2001)
Running with Scissors (2006)

John Cleese
6ft 4³/₄in
(JOHN MARWOOD CLEESE)

Born: **October 27, 1939**
Weston-Super-Mare, England

The family surname was actually "Cheese" – until his father changed it. After Clifton College, John studied Law at Cambridge University. He met writing partner, Graham Chapman, in the "Footlight Revue" which was a triumph at the Edinburgh Festival and transferred via London, to Broadway. John stayed on there to star in "Half a Sixpence" and met his future wife, Connie Booth. He became a sketch writer for the BBC which led to the series 'I'm sorry, I'll Read That Again". He made his film debut in 1968, with a small role in *Interlude*. On TV, from 1969 to 1974, 'Monty Python's Flying Circus' took Britain by storm. It was the year of the first Python movie – that, and the two sequels – are still great favorites. A year later he was starring in the classic comedy series 'Fawlty Towers'. In 1978, John guested on the 'Muppet Show', and was voted "The Funniest Man on TV". He played some serious roles, including a western. In 1987, John won an Emmy for his guest appearance in 'Cheers!' The following year, he was nominated for an Oscar when he wrote and starred in the most successful British film ever – *A Fish Called Wanda*. His voice has been used on several video games. John and his third wife, Alyce Faye Eichelberger, have recently filed for divorce .

**Monty Python and the
Holy Grail** (1975)
The Life of Brian (1979)
Silverado (1985)
Clockwise (1986)
A Fish Called Wanda (1988)
The Big Picture (1989)
Frankenstein (1994)
Fierce Creatures (1997)
The World Is Not Enough (1999)
Rat Race (2001)
**Harry Potter and the
Sorcerer's Stone** (2001)
Die Another Day (2002)
Scorched (2003)
Man About Town (2006)
The Day the Earth Stood Still (2008)
The Pink Panther 2 (2009)

Montgomery Clift
5ft 10in
(EDWARD MONTGOMERY CLIFT)

Born: **October 17, 1920**
Omaha, Nebraska, USA
Died: **July 23, 1966**

Monty had a twin-sister, Roberta. Their father made lots of money in banking, but was wiped out when Wall Street crashed. The children didn't suffer too much and when Monty was fourteen, a family friend got him a job in a summer stock production of "Fly Away Home". Its star, Thomas Mitchell saw his potential and helped him. In the years leading up to World War II, Montgomery Clift was a familiar name in New York theaters. He preferred the stage – declining several Hollywood offers until Howard Hawks persuaded him to change his mind. He made his movie debut in *Red River* and was Oscar-nominated for *The Search*. After that he was hot property and by 1953, an international star – with two more Oscar nominations – for *A Place in the Sun* and *From Here to Eternity*, in which, for his role as Private Prewitt, he deserved to win. It upset him. He turned down both *East of Eden* and *On the Waterfront,* and his drinking (possibly caused by guilt over his homosexuality) got out of hand. While making *Raintree County,* he was involved in a car crash which disfigured his face. It accelerated his drinking and he couldn't work in the afternoons. But the flame hadn't been entirely extinguished. Before he died from a heart attack, he had good movies left in him, including *Judgement at Nuremberg* – for which he received his fourth Oscar nomination – as Best Supporting Actor.

The Search (1948)
Red River (1948)
The Heiress (1949)
A Place in the Sun (1951)
I Confess (1953)
From Here to Eternity (1953)
Raintree County (1957)
Lonelyhearts (1958)
The Young Lions (1958)
Suddenly, Last Summer (1959)
Wild River (1960)
The Misfits (1961)
Judgement at Nuremberg (1961)
Freud (1962)

George Clooney
5ft 11in
(GEORGE TIMOTHY CLOONEY)

Born: **May 6, 1961**
Lexington, Kentucky, USA

Spending his early years in Columbus Ohio, George developed an interest in show business at the age of five, through visits to his father Nick's TV talk show. Other influences were his uncle, the actor Jose Ferrer, and his aunt, Rosemary Clooney, a popular singer and actress. After graduating from high school in Augusta, Kentucky, George attended a couple of universities for a short time, but his main interest was girls. Being rather handsome, he decided to become an actor. He got a part in the TV drama 'E/R' then he had a small but regular role in 'Roseanne'. He acted in his first movie, *Return to Horror High,* in 1987. From 1989 to 1993, George was married to Talia Balsam. He had his first starring role in 1996, in Quentin Tarantino's *From Dusk Till Dawn,* and within two years he was an "A-List" movie star. Nowadays, George is spending more time directing films. He was nominated for an Oscar for Best Director and Best Original Screenplay for *Good Night, and Good Luck.* He won a Best Supporting Actor Oscar for *Syriana.* Highly regarded in the film industry, George, an avid movie fan, received the American Cinematheque Award in 2006. He was nominated for a Best Actor Oscar, for *Michael Clayton.*

One Fine Day (1996)
The Peacemaker (1997)
Out of Sight (1998)
The Thin Red Line (1998)
Three Kings (1999) **O Brother
Where Art Thou?** (2000)
The Perfect Storm (2000) **Spy
Kids** (2001) **Ocean's Eleven** (2001)
Solaris (2002) **Confessions of
a Dangerous Mind** (2002)
Intolerable Cruelty (2003)
Ocean's Twelve (2004)
Good Night, and Good Luck (2005)
Syriana (2005) **The Good German** (2006)
Ocean's Thirteen (2007)
Michael Clayton (2007)
Leatherheads (2008)
Burn After Reading (2008)

Glenn **Close**
5ft 5in
(GLENN CLOSE)

Born: **March 19, 1947**
Greenwich, Connecticut, USA

One of four children, Glenn started life on a farm. Her father, who was a doctor, sold up after joining a group known as Moral Re-Armament. He then worked as a missionary and ran a clinic in the Belgian Congo. Some of Glenn's early years and schooling were spent in Africa. She also went to boarding schools in Switzerland and Connecticut. She became interested in acting at high school and at The College of William and Mary, in Williamsburg, Virginia. After she'd gained useful experience with theater work in New York, and had a brief marriage to rock guitarist, Cabot Wade, she made her movie debut in *The World According to Garp* and was nominated for a Best Supporting Actress Oscar. She was thirty-five at the time, but it was no handicap. Another four Oscar nominations – for *The Big Chill, The Natural, Fatal Attraction* and *Dangerous Liaisons* – will hopefully be added to with a future win. Meanwhile, she has starred in television productions as well as in Broadway musicals – such as "Sunset Boulevard" – for which she won a Tony Award. In 2007-2008, Glenn starred as Patty Hewes in several episodes of the TV crime drama 'Damages'. She is a life-long fan of the New York Mets baseball team. Through her relationships, she's related to the movie director Preston Sturges, and to actresses Brooke Shields and Dina Merrill. Glenn and her third husband, David Shaw, live in Maine. Her voice will be heard on the soundtrack of the a new animated film called *Hoodwinked 2: Hood vs. Evil.*

The World According to Garp (1982)
The Big Chill (1983)
The Natural (1984)
Fatal Attraction (1987)
Dangerous Liaisons (1988)
Reversal of Fortune (1990)
Hamlet (1990) **101 Dalmatians** (1996)
Air Force One (1997)
Heights (2004)
Nine Lives (2005)
The Chumscrubber (2005)
Evening (2007)

François **Cluzet**
5ft 8½in
(FRANÇOIS CLUZET)

Born: **September 21, 1955**
Paris, France

The son of a wealthy Parisian merchant, François took a keen early interest in the world of show business, when he and his brother were taken to theaters and music halls in Paris. He left school at seventeen to study drama with Jean Périmony at his Ecole d'Art Dramatique, in Paris. In 1976, he made his stage debut and during the next four years, his only screen work was on television. François made his film debut in 1980, in *Cocktail Molotov* – directed by Diane Kurys, on the subject of the 1968 student riots in Paris. During 1980, he made the first of several appearances for Claude Chabrol - in *Le cheval d'orgueil*. In 1984 François was nominated for César awards – for *L'Été meurtrier* and *Vive la sociale!* He increased his output and was seen by international audiences when he played the young fan who befriends and supports jazz musician, Dexter Gordon, in Bertrand Tavernier's *'Round Midnight*. He consolidated his position in *Une affaire des femmes, Olivier, Olivier* and *L'Enfer,* and, after six César nominations, he was voted Best Actor – for the moody and magnificent thriller, *Ne le dis à personne* (Tell No One). François had a son with the late Marie Trintignant.

Les Fantômes du chapelier (1982)
L'Été meurtrier (1983)
'Round Midnight (1986)
Association de malfaiteurs (1987)
Chocolat (1988)
Une affaire de femmes (1988)
Deux (1989)
Un tour de manège (1989)
Force majeure (1989)
Trop belle pour toi (1989)
La Révolution française (1989)
Olivier, Olivier (1992)
L'Enfer (1994)
Les Apprentis (1995)
Enfants de salaud (1996)
Rien ne va plus (1997)
L'Adversaire (2002)
Ne le dis à personne (2006)
Paris (2008)
Les Liens du sang (2008)

Lee J. **Cobb**
6ft
(LEO JACOBY)

Born: **December 8, 1911**
New York City, New York, USA
Died: **February 11, 1976**

The son of a Jewish newspaper editor, Lee was a musical prodigy as a child – mastering the violin by the age of ten. A career prospect as a violinist stopped when he broke his wrist, but his ability on the harmonica remained a source of pleasure. He left home for Hollywood when he was seventeen, but returned to New York after no success. He went to night school – studying accountancy at City College and acting in radio plays during the day. In 1931, he went back to California – making his professional stage debut at Pasadena Playhouse. Film roles in two Hopalong Cassidy features led to a role in a successful production of the play "Golden Boy" and he was in the movie version. He joined the Group Theater, and worked with Elia Kazan and John Garfield. Kazan later directed him in *Boomerang*. He starred in "Death of a Salesman" on the stage and on TV; and it is considered his greatest role. A powerful supporting actor – Lee could steal scenes from stars like Brando – as in *On the Waterfront,* for which he was Oscar nominated. He acted in the classic film, *12 Angry Men* and was also Oscar-nominated for *The Brothers Karamazov*. He was twice married – lastly to Mary Hirsch. Lee died of a heart attack in Woodland Hills, California.

The Song of Bernadette (1943)
Winged Victory (1944)
Boomerang (1947)
Call Northside 777 (1948)
Thieves' Highway (1949)
On the Waterfront (1954)
12 Angry Men (1957)
The Three Faces of Eve (1957)
The Brothers Karamazov (1958)
Man of the West (1958)
Exodus (1960)
How the West Was Won (1962)
Coogan's Bluff (1968)
Mackenna's Gold (1969)
Lawman (1971)
The Exorcist (1973)
Cross Shot (1976)

Charles **Coburn**
5ft 9½in
(CHARLES DOUVILLE COBURN)

Born: **June 19, 1877**
Savannah, Georgia, USA
Died: **August 30, 1961**

Charles was the son of Moses Douville Coburn, and his wife Emma. After doing stage-hand work he was employed as a theater manager at the age of seventeen. After making his Broadway debut in 1901, he and his wife, Ivah, formed the Coburn Players and toured the country – specializing in Shakespeare. Only when she died in 1937, did he begin his film career, which consisted of much lighter fare. He made his debut at the age of sixty-one, in *Of Human Hearts,* where he played the role of a monocled, cigar-smoking character which would be his trademark for twenty years. Due to his appearance, Charles was at his best in comedies – winning a Best Supporting Actor Oscar for his role in *The More the Merrier.* A darker side emerged in the late 1940s, when he became president of a right-wing group opposing communists in Hollywood. His last great film was with Marilyn Monroe, in *Gentlemen Prefer Blondes,* when he was sixty-six, but he kept busy on stage. He was Falstaff in "The Merry Wives of Windsor" and also worked on television. Two years before he died of a heart attack, Charles portrayed Benjamin Franklin in the movie, *John Paul Jones.* A week before he died in a New York hospital, he was in summer stock, as Grandpa Vanderhoff, in "You Can't Take It With You".

In Name Only (1939)
Stanley and Livingstone (1940)
Road to Singapore (1940)
The Lady Eve (1941)
The Devil and Miss Jones (1941)
King's Row (1942)
The More the Merrier (1943)
Heaven Can Wait (1943)
The Green Years (1946)
The Paradine Case (1947)
Impact (1949)
Louisa (1950)
Has Anybody Seen My Gal? (1952)
Gentlemen Prefer Blondes (1953)
How to Murder a Rich Uncle (1957)
John Paul Jones (1959)

James **Coburn**
6ft 2in
(JAMES COBURN)

Born: **August 31, 1928**
Laurel, Nebraska, USA
Died: **November 18, 2002**

When Jim's father's business collapsed due to the Great Depression, the Coburn family moved to Los Angeles. Jim did his military service as a radio-operator before going to Los Angeles City College. His interest in acting took him to UCLA, from where he got the opportunity to act in "Billy Budd" at the La Jolla Playhouse. After that he went to New York to study with Stella Adler, worked in shows and appeared in TV commercials. In 1958, he was newly married, when he went to Hollywood, and began getting small parts in westerns. The first one, in 1959, was *Ride Lonesome.* It was his knife-thrower in *The Magnificent Seven* that set him on the road to stardom and he twice worked with Steve McQueen after that. By 1966 Jim had shown that he could play villains too. He was given his first starring role (as a hero) in *Our Man Flint.* Five years later, he'd reached a crisis point in his career. He had to suffer until 1973 when he began to hit the target again with good movies like *Pat Garret and Billy the Kid.* Things continued to go well until he was diagnosed with rheumatoid arthritis in 1979. It affected his mental health and hampered his film-making career for several years. Through sheer determination, he made a comeback. Winning a Best Supporting Actor Oscar in 1997, for *Affliction,* gave his career a boost. He made fourteen more movies before dying of a heart attack at home in Beverly Hills, while playing a flute. His second wife, Paula, was with him.

The Magnificent Seven (1960)
The Great Escape (1963)
Our Man Flint (1966)
The President's Analyst (1967)
Pat Garret and Billy The Kid (1973)
The Last of Sheila (1973)
Bite the Bullet (1975)
Hard Times (1975)
Cross of Iron (1977)
Maverick (1994) Affliction (1997)
The Man from Elysian Fields (2001)
American Gun (2002)

Claudette **Colbert**
5ft 4½in
(LILI CLAUDETTE CHAUCHION)

Born: **September 13, 1903**
Saint-Mandé, Seine, France
Died: **July 30, 1996**

The daughter of a banker, Claudette was taken to live in New York by her parents when she was six. She grew up like an American girl, but was bi-lingual. When she was eighteen she had a part in a play called "The Wild Wescotts". For the next five years, she established herself on the New York stage. In 1927, she made her movie debut in *For the Love of Mike.* From then on she was only in leading roles. In the early 1930s, she made French versions of movies and it was apparent that she could play drama or comedy. She starred in DeMille's epic, *The Sign of the Cross* in 1932, and was an Oscar winner two years later for *It Happened One Night.* She made more 'Screwball Comedies', and by 1938, was Hollywood's highest-paid star. She insisted on using her own lighting cameraman and wasn't shown in left profile. She looked great in black and white or color and her status did not diminish until after the war. Claudette's acting ability was still intact, but in 1950 she broke her back. Most of her later work was on Broadway or TV. She made her final movie, *Parrish,* in 1961. After that there were no worthwhile film offers, so she retired to Barbados. In 1987, she reappeared on television in 'The Two Mrs. Grenvilles'. She died after a series of strokes – at her home in Speightstown.

The Sign of the Cross (1932)
Cleopatra (1934)
It Happened One Night (1934)
Private Worlds (1935)
The Gilded Lily (1935)
She Married Her Boss (1935)
I Met Him in Paris (1937)
Bluebeard's Eighth Wife (1938)
Midnight (1939) Drums Along
the Mohawk (1939) The Palm Beach
Story (1942) No Time for Love (1943)
Since You Went Away (1944)
Guest Wife (1945)
Sleep, My Love (1948)
Three Came Home (1950)
Royal Affairs in Versailles (1954)

Toni **Collette**
5ft 8in
(ANTONIA COLLETTE)

Born: **November 1, 1972**
Sydney, New South Wales, Australia

Toni was the eldest of four children born to Bob Collette, a truck driver, and his wife, Judy. After her junior schooling, she was educated at Blacktown Girls' High School, where she showed her first signs of real acting talent. While there, she attended the Australian Theater for Young People, and later studied at the National Institute of Dramatic Arts – both in Sydney. She made her film debut at the age of twenty in *Spotswood,* and two years later won an Australian Film Institute Award for her performance in *Muriel's Wedding.* Toni's fame spread far beyond Australia – leading to a starring role in *The Sixth Sense* – for which she was nominated for a Best Actress Oscar. She was then praised for her work on the Broadway stage as Queenie in "The Wild Party", for which she was nominated for a Tony Award. She turned down the lead in *Bridget Jones's Diary* because of New York commitments and lost out to Renée Zellwegger for the Roxy Hart role, in *Chicago.* But her career in films was solid. She received a Golden Globe nomination for *Little Miss Sunshine.* In 2006, Toni toured Australia to promote her vocal album titled "Beautiful Awkward Pictures". Her husband, Dave Galafass, is the drummer in her group. The couple have a daughter who was born in 2008.

Spotswood (1992) **Muriel's Wedding** (1994) **Cosi** (1996)
Emma (1996) **Clockwatchers** (1997)
Diana & Me (1997) **The Boys** (1998)
Velvet Goldmine (1998)
8½ Women (1999)
The Sixth Sense (1999)
Hotel Splendide (2000)
Changing Lanes (2002)
About a Boy (2002)
Dirty Deeds (2002) **The Hours** (2002)
Japanese Story (2003)
Connie and Carla (2004)
In Her Shoes (2005) **The Night Listener** (2006) **Little Miss Sunshine** (2006) **The Dead Girl** (2006) **Evening** (2007)
The Black Balloon (2008)

Joan **Collins**
5ft 6in
(JOAN HENRIETTA COLLINS)

Born: **May 23, 1933**
London, England

Joan and her sister, the future best-selling author, Jackie Collins, were the daughters of a Jewish South African talent agent. At the age of thirteen, while at Francis Holland School, Joan made her stage debut in "A Doll's House" – at the Arts Theater, in London. When Joan was seventeen, she went to RADA – at the same time as Roger Moore and Michael Caine. She became a J. Arthur Rank starlet and in 1951, was a beauty contest entrant in *Lady Godiva Rides Again.* In 1952, she married the actor Maxwell Reed, but divorced him four years later – claiming that he'd tried to sell her to an Arab Sheik. After ten modest film roles, she co-starred with Laurence Harvey in a successful movie, *The Good Die Young,* and was given a contract by 20th Century Fox. She was certainly beautiful, but the dozen or so films she made for the studio were not generally of a very high standard. In 1963, she quit the movies to marry the talented English singer/actor, Anthony Newley. They teamed up with Peter Sellers to record an album called "Fool Britannia", which made the UK Top 10. The marriage was over in 1970 and Joan attracted three more husbands. In 1981, she became more famous than ever when she starred in the popular soap-opera, 'Dallas'. Two years later her role as Alexis won her a Golden Globe. Her more recent television projects were episodes of 'Hotel Babylon' and 'Footballers' Wives'.

The Good Die Young (1954)
Land of the Pharaohs (1955)
The Girl in the Red Velvet Swing (1955)
The Opposite Sex (1956)
The Bravados (1958)
Seven Thieves (1960)
La Congiuntura (1965)
Warning Shot (1967)
Quest for Love (1971)
Fear in the Night (1972)
Tales from the Crypt (1972)
A Midwinter's Tale (1995)
The Clandestine Marriage (1999)

Ronald **Colman**
5ft 11in
(RONALD CHARLES COLMAN)

Born: **February 9, 1891**
Richmond, Surrey, England
Died: **May 19, 1958**

Ronald's father, a silk importer, died when he was sixteen so he was forced to miss going to Cambridge University. To help his mother, Ronald worked as a clerk for a steamship company in London. He was involved in amateur theater but the outbreak of World War I, in which he served and was badly injured, meant waiting until 1919 before his first stage role in London, as a professional actor. A year later, he set sail for America, and began a disastrous marriage. Ronald got small parts on Broadway, but struggled until a starring role in "La Tendresse" was seen by the film director, Henry King, who cast him to play opposite Lillian Gish, in *The White Sister.* It led to a contract with Sam Goldwyn. He starred in silent films before his beautiful voice was first heard on the screen in 1929, in *Bulldog Drummond.* He was nominated for two Oscars that year – for *Bulldog* and *Condemned.* In 1938, he married his second wife, Benita Hume, and enjoyed ten more years of popularity. He lost his appeal in the late 1940s, but did win an Oscar for *A Double Life* and made a cracking comedy – *Champagne for Caesar.* From 1950 onwards, Ronald worked mostly on the radio. He had a cameo role in *Around the World in Eighty Days,* but looked quite sick. In 1957, Ronald's final film, *The Story of Mankind* was very bad and a sad way to end his career. He died of a lung infection at his home in Santa Barbara, California.

Bulldog Drummond (1929)
Condemned (1929) **Arrowsmith** (1931)
Clive of India (1935)
A Tale of Two Cities (1935)
Lost Horizon (1937)
The Prisoner of Zenda (1937)
If I Were King (1938)
The Light That Failed (1939)
Lucky Partners (1940)
The Talk of the Town (1942)
Random Harvest (1942)
Kismet (1944) **A Double Life** (1947)
Champagne for Caesar (1950)

Robbie **Coltrane**
6ft 1in
(ANTHONY ROBERT MCMILLAN)

Born: **March 30, 1950**
Rutherglen, South Lanarkshire, Scotland

Robbie's father, Ian McMillan – a general medical practitioner, served as a forensic police surgeon – a fact that would be stored in Robbie's brain for a future role. His mother Jean, a teacher and pianist, would influence his love of music. Robbie attended the very exclusive, Glenalmond College, in Perthshire. He was head of the school's debating society and in the first XV at rugby. He then developed his gift for visual creativity at Glasgow School of Art. Finally, after leaving Moray House College of Education in Edinburgh, he started his career as a stand-up comic – adopting the name Robbie Coltrane – in tribute to the great jazz saxophonist, John Coltrane. He made his first appearance as an actor in a 1979 TV episode of 'Play for Today' and made his film debut with a small role in *La Mort en direct,* which was shot in Glasgow that same year. He achieved national fame in the BBC comedy series, 'A Kick Up the Eighties'. Robbie worked hard and carved himself a niche in British television history as 'Cracker' – a forensic psychologist with problems of his own. He is separated from his wife, Rhona Gemmell, with whom he has a son and a daughter.

Defense of the Realm (1985)
The Supergrass (1985)
Caravaggio (1986) **Mona Lisa** (1986)
Eat the Rich (1987) **The Fruit
Machine** (1988) **Bert Rigby, You're a
Fool** (1989) **Lenny Live and
Unleashed** (1989) **Henry V** (1989)
Nuns on the Run (1990) **Perfectly
Normal** (1991) **The Adventures of
Huck Finn** (1993) **GoldenEye** (1995)
Montana (1998)
Message in a Bottle (1999)
The World Is Not Enough (1999)
From Hell (2001)
On the Nose (2001)
**Harry Potter and the
Sorcerer's Stone** (1999)
The Chamber of Secrets (2002)
The Goblet of Fire (2005)
The Order of the Phoenix (2007)
The Half-Blood Prince (2009)

Jennifer **Connelly**
5ft 7½in
(JENNIFER LYNN CONNELLY)

Born: **December 12, 1970**
Catskills, New York, USA

Jennifer's father, Gerard, worked in the clothing industry. Her mother, Ilene, was an antiques dealer, Jennifer moved to New York City from the Catskill Mountains when she was quite young. When she was ten, a friend of her dad's suggested he sent Jennifer's photograph to a model agency. She appeared in magazine ads before working in television commercials. It was the perfect launching pad, along with a featured spot in Duran Duran's 1983 musical video "Union of the Snake". At thirteen, she made her movie debut in Sergio Leone's *Once Upon a Time in America.* During her teens, Jennifer starred in a couple of popular movies and several forgettable ones. She even made a Japanese pop record. But she wasn't neglecting her studies: she became fluent in both French and Italian. In 1991, she spent two years at Yale University studying English, and then moved to Stanford, California, before re-starting her movie career. It proceeded nicely, but arriving at the new millennium it went up a gear. Jennifer won a Best Supporting Actress Oscar in 2001, for *A Beautiful Mind,* and since then, with each passing year, her star has been in the ascendancy. Jennifer is married to English actor, Paul Bettany, with whom she has a son.

Labyrinth (1986)
The Rocketeer (1991)
The Heart of Justice (1992)
Higher Learning (1995)
Mulholland Falls (1996)
Inventing the Abbotts (1997)
Dark City (1998)
Waking the Dead (2000)
Requiem for a Dream (2000)
Pollock (2000)
A Beautiful Mind (2001) **Hulk** (2003)
House of Sand and Fog (2003)
Dark Water (2005)
Little Children (2006)
Blood Diamond (2006)
Reservation Road (2007)
The Day the Earth Stood Still (2008)
He's Just Not That Into You (2009)

Sir Sean **Connery**
6ft 2in
(THOMAS SEAN CONNERY)

Born: **August 25, 1930**
Edinburgh, Scotland

Sean's father Joseph, a Roman Catholic of Irish descent, was a factory worker. His mother Effie, a cleaning woman, was a Scottish Protestant. When he left school at fifteen, Sean worked as a milkman. He did two years in the Royal Navy and after that, worked as a bricklayer, a model at Edinburgh College of Art, and an undertaker's assistant. Not a very hopeful start for a future star! But Sean began body building, and in 1957, got a part in the chorus of "South Pacific". That led to work with a repertory company and modeling swimwear. There were small parts in movies, starting with *No Road Back.* A TV role opposite Diane Cilento, whom he married, led to his big break. The BBC wanted Jack Palance for 'Requiem for a Heavyweight'; Jack wanted too much money so Sean got the part. He signed with 20th Century Fox but, apart from being one of many actors in *The Longest Day,* he didn't get much from them. Then United Artists chose him to be the first James Bond in *Dr. No,* and the rest, as they say, is history. It gave him stardom, but little satisfaction. He needed to change his image, even though he was in the U.S. box office top ten. He dispensed with his toupee and got better parts – crowned by a Best Supporting Actor Oscar for *The Untouchables.* Since 1975, Sean has been married to Micheline Roquebrune. He was recently the narrator for the film *Scotland the Home of Golf.*

Dr. No (1962)
From Russia with Love (1963)
Marnie (1964) **Goldfinger** (1964)
The Hill (1965) **Thunderball** (1965)
You Only Live Twice (1967)
Diamonds Are Forever (1971)
The Man Who Would Be King (1975)
Time Bandits (1981)
Never Say Never Again (1983)
**Indiana Jones and the
Last Crusade** (1983) **Highlander** (1986)
The Untouchables (1987)
The Hunt for Red October (1990)
Finding Forrester (2000)

Billy **Connolly**
6ft
(WILLIAM CONNOLLY)

Born: **November 24, 1942**
Anderston, Glasgow, Scotland

Billy's father, William, was an instrument technician of Irish ancestry. He was away in the armed forces for the first three of Billy's life and by the time he came home in 1946, his wife, Mary, who worked in a hospital cafeteria, had abandoned Billy and his sister Flo, so the pair went to live with their aunt. Billy was educated at St. Peter's Primary School in Glasgow and St. Gerard's Secondary School, in Goran. He endured a terrible homelife during those years and couldn't wait to leave school and get a job. In 1958, he was a welding apprentice in the shipyard. He next joined the Territorial Army Reserve. He acquired the nickname, "Big Yin" at his local, when he grew bigger than his father. He became a folk singer, formed the "Humblebums", and for a time partnered the future star, Gerry Rafferty. In 1969, he married his first wife Iris. Billy became a comedian and in 1972, he released his first comedy album, "Billy Connolly Live!". Three years later, he appeared in 'Play for Today' on TV. His film debut in 1978's *Absolution,* was far from funny, but it did star Richard Burton. Things could only get better, and they did. He received a BAFTA Best Actor nomination for *Mrs Brown* and has since worked in several top movies – as both star and supporting actor. He's married to the Kiwi comedienne, Pamela Stephenson.

Bullshot (1983) **Water** (1985)
The Hunting of the Snark (1987)
The Big Man (1990)
Muppet Treasure Island (1996)
Mrs Brown (1997)
The Impostors (1998) **Still Crazy** (1998)
The Debt Collector (1999)
The Boondock Saints (1999)
Beautiful Joe (2000)
An Everlasting Piece (2000)
Who Is Cletis Tout? (2001)
The Man Who Sued God (2001)
White Oleander (2001)
Timeline (2003)
The Last Samurai (2003)
Lemony Snicket (2004) **Fido** (2006)
The X-Files: I Want to Believe (2008)

Richard **Conte**
5ft 8in
(RICHARD NICHOLAS PETER CONTE)

Born: **March 24, 1910**
Jersey City, New Jersey, USA
Died: **April 15, 1975**

The son of a New Jersey barber, and with an Italian family background, Richard had the ideal looks for gangster movie roles. In 1935, when he was working as an entertainer at a Connecticut resort, he was spotted by Elia Kazan and John Garfield, who helped him find stage work in New York and get a scholarship to study at the Neighborhood Playhouse. By the late-1930s, Richard had become well known as Broadway actor, Nicholas Conte, making his debut in 1939, in "Moon Over Mulberry Street". That year, he acted in his first movie, *Heaven with A Barbed Wire Fence.* He got a contract with 20th Century Fox, who called him Richard. His first movie for the studio was *Guadalcanal Diary,* in 1943 – one of several soldier roles he played during the war years. Richard became very popular during the late 1940s and early 1950s, in film noir thrillers. When they went out of fashion, he was able to get regular television work including the series 'The Four Just Men'. He also acted in, as well as directed, several movies in Europe. He returned to the USA to appear in *The Godfather,* and made eleven gangster movies in Italy after that. Richard was married to his second wife, Shirlee Garner, from 1973 until his death in Los Angeles, from a heart attack.

Guadalcanal Diary (1943)
The Purple Heart (1944)
A Walk in the Sun (1945)
Somewhere in the Night (1946)
Call Northside 777 (1948)
Cry of the City (1948)
House of Strangers (1949)
Whirlpool (1949)
The Blue Gardenia (1953)
The Big Combo (1955)
I'll Cry Tomorrow (1955)
They Came to Cordura (1959)
Ocean's Eleven (1960)
Tony Rome (1967)
The Godfather (1972)
Shoot First, Die Later (1974)
Violent City (1975)

Tom **Conti**
5ft 11in
(THOMAS CONTI)

Born: **November 22, 1941**
Paisley, Scotland

The son of an Italian father, and an Irish Catholic mother, who loved music, Tom took piano lessons from the age of four. Two years later, it was reported in the 'London Observer' newspaper that he was "threatening to be a genuine child prodigy". He was educated at Hamilton Park School, in Glasgow, where he first appeared in plays and became hooked on acting. He later graduated from that city's Royal Scottish Academy of Music and Drama. It was in 1959 that he began his stage career with the Dundee Repertory. Spells in Edinburgh and Glasgow theaters followed before he landed a starring role in the 1968 TV mini-series, 'The Flight of the Heron' – opposite that fine veteran Scottish actor, Finlay Currie. There was stage work and television roles in various shows including 'Z Cars' over the next six years. In 1975, he made his film debut in *Flame* – a drama about a rock 'n roll band. By the late 1970s, Tom was getting second or third billing below top Hollywood names. His stage career progressed to Broadway, where he won a Best Actor Tony award in 1979 for "Whose Life Is It Anyway?". After returning to London for his directorial debut, Tom built up his movie portfolio in a number of high-profile productions. In 1983, he was nominated for a Best Actor Oscar, for the comedy *Reuben, Reuben.* He has been married to the actress, Kara Wilson, for over forty years. Their daughter, Nina, is an actress. Tom has three films lined up for release – including a new version of *The Tempest.*

The Duellists (1977)
Full Circle (1977)
Reuben, Reuben (1983)
American Dreamer (1984)
Heavenly Pursuits (1985)
Djavolji raj (1989)
Shirley Valentine (1989)
Someone Else's America (1995)
Something to Believe In (1998)
Derailed (2005)
Almost Heaven (2006)
Dangerous Parking (2007)

Chris Cooper
5ft 10in
(CHRISTOPHER W. COOPER)

Born: **July 9, 1951**
Kansas City, Missouri, USA

Chris's father served as a doctor in the U.S. Air Force before running a cattle ranch. Chris and his brother, Chuck, were raised in Houston, Texas and Kansas City. He graduated from South West High School in 1969, and then majored both in agriculture and drama at the University of Missouri before moving to New York City. In 1980, he appeared on Broadway in "Of the Fields Lately" and remained on the stage and television until making his film debut in *Matewan.* In 1986 he married the actress/writer, Marianne Leone. Sadly, a son Jesse, who was born the following year, died when he was eight from causes relating to cerebral palsy. For more than twenty years, Chris Cooper has enriched a number of films with his thoughtful characterizations. His last dozen or so titles, including *Adaptation* (for which he was awarded a Best Supporting Actor Oscar), *Jarhead, Capote, The Kingdom,* and *Married Life,* have had A-list 'Gold' written all over them. In 2008, he portrayed Walt Whitman, on TV, in an episode of 'The American Experience'. He and Marianne live in Kingston, Massachusetts.

Matewan (1987)
Guilty by Suspicion (1991)
Thousand Pieces of Gold (1991)
City of Hope (1991)
This Boy's Life (1993)
Pharaoh's Army (1995)
Lone Star (1996)
Great Expectations (1998)
The Horse Whisperer (1998)
October Sky (1999)
American Beauty (1999)
Me, Myself & Irene (2000)
The Patriot (2000)
The Bourne Identity (2002)
Adaptation (2002)
Seabiscuit (2003)
Silver City (2004) Jarhead (2005)
Capote (2005)
Syriana (2005) Breach (2007)
The Kingdom (2007)
Married Life (2007)
New York, I Love You (2008)

Gary Cooper
6ft 3in
(FRANK JAMES COOPER)

Born: **May 7, 1901**
Helena, Montana, USA
Died: **May 13, 1961**

The son of Charles and Alice Cooper, Gary and his brother were sent by their father (a successful lawyer) to England for their education. They returned to the USA in 1914. Gary worked on his dad's ranch – helping with four hundred head of cattle and learning to ride. A cartoonist after leaving college, he drifted into movies – using his horsemanship as an extra in westerns. When asked to act, he looked stiff, but he improved after twenty-five 'Silents' and becoming Gary Cooper. Although a man of few words, talking parts in 1929 – in *Shopworn Angel* and *The Virginian* – set him on the road to stardom. In 1939 he was David O. Selznick's first choice for *Gone with the Wind.* He turned it down, believing it would be "the biggest flop in history". But two years later Gary won the first of his two Oscars – for *Sergeant York.* From 1945, 'Coop' was America's favorite male star. His marriage didn't stop him having affairs with several desirable women – Marlene Dietrich, Patricia Neal, and Grace Kelly. Gary kept making films – including *High Noon* (for which he won a second Oscar) up to *The Naked Edge* – the year before he died in Beverly Hills from prostate cancer. His loyal wife, Sandra Shaw, was by his side.

Morocco (1930) A Farewell to
Arms (1932) One Sunday
Afternoon (1933) Design for
Living (1933) The Lives of a Bengal
Lancer (1935) Desire (1936)
Mr. Deeds Goes to Town (1936)
The General Died at Dawn (1936)
Bluebeard's Eighth Wife (1938) Beau
Geste (1939) The Westerner (1940)
Meet John Doe (1941) Sergeant
York (1941) Ball of Fire (1941)
The Pride of the Yankees (1941)
Cloak and Dagger (1946)
The Fountainhead (1949)
High Noon (1952) Vera Cruz (1954)
Friendly Persuasion (1956)
Love in the Afternoon (1957)
Man of the West (1958)

Jackie Cooper
4ft 10in
(JOHN COOPER JR.)

Born: **September 15, 1922**
Los Angeles, California, USA

Jackie was an illegitimate child. His father John Cooper, who was Jewish, deserted the family in 1924. Jackie was raised by his mother, Mabel Polito, an Italian American, who had been a child actress. She worked as a stage pianist until she married C.J.Bigelow, a studio production manager. Other movie contacts included Mabel's actress sister, Julie Leonard, and her husband, the director, Norman Taurog. In 1931, Taurog directed Jackie in *Skippy* – winning a Best Director Oscar and coaxing a Best Actor-nominated performance out of the nine-year old boy. Prior to that Jackie appeared from 1929 in "Our Gang" comedy shorts, starting with *Boxing Gloves.* He signed for MGM, who gave him roles opposite Wallace Beery, in *The Champ, The Bowery, Treasure Island,* and *O'Shaughnessy's Boy.* The chemistry on screen between the pair completely concealed Jackie's impression that Beery was a "foul-mouthed, brutal drunkard". As an adolescent, Jackie lost most of his star appeal and after serving in World War II he was seen frequently on television. In the 1950s, he was popular as "Sock" Miller in the sitcom, 'The People's Choice' and in the 1960s, as 'Hennesey'. The experience gave him the confidence to direct for the medium. In the 1970s, Jackie re-emerged on the big screen in the *Superman* films. He was married three times and had three of his four children with his present wife, Barbara Kraus, whom he married in 1954.

Skippy (1931)
The Champ (1931)
The Bowery (1933)
Treasure Island (1934)
O'Shaughnessy's Boy (1935)
The Devil Is a Sissy (1936)
White Banners (1938)
That Certain Age (1938)
Gangster's Boy (1938)
Streets of New York (1939)
The Big Guy (1939)
The Return of Frank James (1940)
Ziegfeld Girl (1941)
Superman (1978)

Valentina **Cortese**
5ft 2in
(VALENTINA CORTESE)

Born: **January 1, 1925**
Milan, Lombardy, Italy

After leaving school at fifteen, Valentina had only one ambition – to become an actress. She was advised to study at the Academy of Dramatic Art, in Rome, and fortunately for her, one of her examiners was a film producer. When she passed a screen test, he offered her a contract and she made her debut – in a bit part in *Orizzonte dipinto* – which was released a month after her eighteenth birthday. Her first featured role was in 1941, in *Bravo di Venezia*, starring Rosanno Brazzi. She made a dozen films in Italy during the war and, following *A Yank in Rome*, in 1946, where she had a chance to practice her English, she felt ready for the international stage. Two years later, with compatriot, Tito Gobbi, she went to England to act in *The Glass Mountain*. She was signed by 20th Century Fox, and made her first film on American soil, *Thieves' Highway*. In 1951, she met Richard Basehart, when they appeared together in *The House on Telegraph Hill,* and they got married. She later helped to get him roles in Italian films including *La Strada*. In 1974, as Ingrid Bergman accepted her Best Supporting Actress Oscar, for *Murder on the Orient Express,* she conceded that it should have gone to Valentina, for *Day For Night*. Few people could argue with that. She was still acting brilliantly in her seventies, but called it a day in 1993, after playing the Mother Superior in *Storia di una capinera*.

The Glass Mountain (1949)
Thieves' Highway (1949)
The House on Telegraph Hill (1951)
The Barefoot Contessa (1954)
Le Amiche (1955)
Barabba (1961)
The Visit (1964)
Juliet of the Spirits (1965)
First Love (1970)
Brother Son, Sister Moon (1972)
Day For Night (1973)
The Adventures
of Baron Munchausen (1988)
Buster's Bedroom (1991)
Storia di una capinera (1993)

Lou **Costello**
5ft 5in
(LOUIS FRANCIS CRISTELLO)

Born: **March 6, 1906**
Paterson, New Jersey, USA
Died: **March 3, 1959**

Lou's father was Italian and his mother came from a French background. Lou was raised in the Catholic faith. He was never much interested in studying, but excelled as an athlete. He fought successfully as an amateur boxer and was a surprisingly good basketball player for his height. For a while he was a hat salesman, but at twenty-one he travelled to Hollywood where he worked as a stunt man – once doubling for Dolores Del Rio! Broke and disillusioned, he hitchhiked back East, and in the early 1930s, set himself up as a comic in vaudeville. He changed his name to Costello and became well known in New York burlesque theaters. He refused to use "off-color" material in his act – a principle he stood by for the whole of his career. His straight man fell ill one day so the theater's cashier, whose name was Bud Abbott, stood in. The two became a team officially in 1936, when they were represented by the William Morris Agency, which got them radio work. As featured performers on the 'Kate Smith Hour' they received national exposure. Universal Studios, in Hollywood, became their new home. After a few supporting roles, they were the nation's top comedy team. Their best work was in the early 1940s, when they had something fresh to offer, as in *Hold That Ghost*. As their appeal began to disappear, Lou fell out in a big way with Bud, over money. His wife, Anne, stuck with him through thick and thin – until he died of a heart attack in East Los Angeles.

Buck Privates (1941)
Hold That Ghost (1941)
Ride 'em Cowboy (1942)
Here Come the Co-Eds (1945)
The Naughty Nineties (1945)
The Time of Their Lives (1946)
Abbott and Costello Meet
Frankenstein (1948)
Mexican Hayride (1948)
Abbott and Costello Meet
The Invisible Man (1951)
Jack and the Beanstalk (1952)

Kevin **Costner**
6ft 1in
(KEVIN MICHAEL COSTNER)

Born: **January 18, 1955**
Lynwood, California, USA

Kevin was the third child born to Bill Costner, a ditch digger, and his wife Sharon. When his dad got a better job as an electric line servicer, the family were on the move regularly and Kevin never had the chance to get used to a school. He sang in Baptist church choirs and enjoyed writing poetry. Although he was quite short in his youth, Kevin was a star player at high school at football, baseball and basketball. In 1973, he was keen enough to take acting lessons while majoring in business studies at California State, at Fullerton. He married his college sweetheart, Cindy in 1978 and they raised a son and two daughters. To earn an income, Kevin took a marketing job, but on a flight from Mexico he met Richard Burton, who advised him to concentrate on acting. He quit his job and moved to Hollywood. He did all kinds of work including a soft-core sex film before he got his break in the cult Western *Silverado*. Stardom was soon his in *The Untouchables*. In 1990, he won a Best Director Oscar for his movie *Dances with Wolves,* which was also voted Best Picture. In 2006 his prints were set in concrete outside Grauman's Chinese Theater in Hollywood. Today, Kevin Costner is a true American success story!

Silverado (1985)
The Untouchables (1987)
Bull Durham (1988)
Field of Dreams (1989)
Dances with Wolves (1990)
Robin Hood: Prince of
Thieves (1991)
JFK (1991)
A Perfect World (1993)
Wyatt Earp (1994)
Message in a Bottle (1999)
For Love of the Game (1999)
Thirteen Days (2000)
Open Range (2003)
The Upside of Anger (2005)
Rumor Has It... (2005)
The Guardian (2006)
Mr. Brooks (2007)
Swing Vote (2008)

Marion **Cotillard**
5ft 6¹/₂in
(MARION COTILLARD)

Born: September 30, 1975
Paris, France

Marion was raised in Orléans, the capital of the Loire Valley, and went to school locally. Both her parents were creative people – her father, Jean-Claude, is an actor and teacher, and her mother Niseema, is a drama teacher. Apart from producing a talented actress, they have identical twin sons – Quentin, who is a sculptor/painter and Guillaume, who is a writer. Marion's first professional acting role took place in 1993 when she appeared in an episode of the TV-series 'Highlander'. Her film debut came a year later, in *The Story of a Boy Who Wanted To Be Kissed* – the French title is even longer! She became famous in France after she featured as Lily Bertineau, in writer Luc Besson's 1998 comedy-action movie, *Taxi.* Following a string of mainly good French movies, Marion impressed English-speaking audiences when she appeared in Tim Burton's film, *Big Fish,* opposite Albert Finney and Billy Crudup. She also shone in Ridley Scott's *A Good Year,* starring Russell Crowe. She beat several candidates for the role of Édith Piaf, in *La Vie en rose.* Having won five awards in her career, Marion then added a Best Actress Oscar, a César, a BAFTA and a Golden Globe – among some others – for her performance in the film. Like Charlize Theron, in *Monster,* Marion was streets ahead of any other nominated actress. A near unknown is now sitting on top of the world, but how will she follow that? The answer may be in her new film, *Public Enemies,* featuring Johnny Depp.

Les Jolies chose (2001)
Une affaire privée (2002)
Big Fish (2003)
Jeux d'enfants (2003)
Innocence (2004)
A Very Long Engagement (2004)
Ma vie en l'air (2005) **Burnt Out** (2005)
La Boîte noire (2005)
Dikkenek (2006) **Fair Play** (2006)
A Good Year (2006)
La Vie en Rose (2007)
Public Enemies (2009)

Joseph **Cotten**
6ft 2in
(JOSEPH CHESHIRE COTTEN)

Born: May 15, 1905
Petersburg, Virginia, USA
Died: February 6, 1994

After graduating from high school, Joe tried several jobs – including that of space salesman for the 'Miami Herald.' He studied acting in Washington and while there, he had an unsuccessful trial for a pro football team, and acted at a small theater. He was a theater critic in Virginia for a time and began acting in local productions. He moved to New York, where he made his Broadway debut, in 1930. Joe befriended Orson Welles and joined his Mercury Theater Company. The Welles short, *Too Much Johnson,* was his first film. More stage work followed, but *Citizen Kane* introduced him to movie audiences. His friendship with Welles culminated in his best screen performance – in *The Third Man.* He was a star for a dozen years, co-starring with many big names – his last major film role being opposite Marilyn Monroe, in *Niagara.* From the mid-fifties he was most often seen on TV, but he did make a cameo appearance in Welles' *Touch of Evil.* In 1960, after his first wife died of leukemia, he married the actress Patricia Medina. Guest spots in disaster movies and on TV kept him going. He published his autobiography, 'Vanity Will Get You Somewhere'. After completing his last film, *The Survivor,* in 1981, Joe suffered a stroke and retired from acting. He had a few peaceful years, but died of pneumonia, at Westwood, California.

Citizen Kane (1941)
The Magnificent Ambersons (1942)
Shadow of a Doubt (1943)
Gaslight (1944)
Since You Went Away (1944)
Love Letters (1945)
Duel in the Sun (1946)
The Farmer's Daughter (1947)
Portrait of Jennie (1948)
The Third Man (1949) **Niagara** (1953)
The Last Sunset (1961)
Hush...Hush, Sweet Charlotte (1964)
Tora! Tora! Tora! (1970)
Soylent Green (1973)
Heaven's Gate (1980)

George **Coulouris**
6ft
(GEORGE COULOURIS)

Born: October 1, 1903
Manchester, Lancashire, England
Died: April 25, 1989

George's mother was English, but he got his name from his Greek father. He was educated at Manchester Grammar School before deciding on an acting career. He studied with Elsie Fogerty, at the Central School of Speech and Drama in London. In 1925 he made his stage debut at the Old Vic, in "Henry V". Four years later, he was appearing on Broadway in a modern dress version of "Measure for Measure". After success on stage, in "The Late Christopher Bean" George was lured to Hollywood for the MGM film version. He befriended Orson Welles and joined his Mercury Theater Company – playing Mark Anthony in the first modern dress production of "Julius Caesar". There was a lot more stage and radio work for Mercury before he became 'immortal' by acting in one of the best films of all time, *Citizen Kane.* Although nothing else would be of that calibre, the fame attached to it launched a career that didn't slow down until he was eighty. Apart from Welles, George worked with every big star of the period – in films and on stage. He returned to live in England in the early 1950s, where he was a supporting actor in movies for another thirty years. George was living in London when he suffered a fatal heart attack, following Parkinson's disease.

Citizen Kane (1941)
Watch on the Rhine (1943)
Mr.Skeffington (1944)
Lady on a Train (1945)
Nobody Lives Forever (1946)
The Verdict (1946)
Where There's Life (1947)
Sleep, My Love (1948)
Joan of Arc (1948)
Outcast of the Islands (1952)
The Heart of the Matter (1954)
Doctor in the House (1954)
Conspiracy of Hearts (1960)
Arabesque (1966) **Papillon** (1973)
Murder on the Orient Express (1974)
Shout at the Devil (1976)
The Long Good Friday (1979)

Sir Tom **Courtenay**
5ft 8in
(THOMAS DANIEL COURTENAY)

Born: **February 25, 1937**
Hull, Humberside, England

Tom's working class background in the dock area of Hull proved no obstacle to him. After high school, he went to University College, London, where he read English. He already had a desire to be an actor, so he dropped out to study acting at RADA. He had a natural talent which manifested itself in a new breed of British actors. He could play the classics, but he could also play roles that many traditional actors found difficult. After appearing at the Old Vic and the Edinburgh Festival in "The Seagull" by Chekhov, he replaced his good pal Albert Finney, for a role that was made for him – "Billy Liar". Success in that led to his movie debut, in *Private Potter* in 1962, and more impressively, the same year, in *The Loneliness of the Long Distance Runner*. A movie version of *Billy Liar,* with Julie Christie, made Tom a star, but he is best known for his roles in *Doctor Zhivago* and *The Dresser* – where he was Oscar-nominated – as Best Supporting Actor for both. During the past twenty years he has done a lot of stage and TV work. Having been so brilliant together some fifteen years earlier, he and Albert Finney topped even that, when they demonstrated the art of acting, in the 1998 TV film, 'A Rather English Marriage'. For twenty years, Tom's second English marriage has been to Isabel Crossley.

The Loneliness of the
Long Distance Runner (1962)
Billy Liar (1963)
King & Country (1964)
King Rat (1965)
Doctor Zhivago (1965)
The Night of the Generals (1967)
A Dandy in Aspic (1968)
Otley (1968) One Day in the Life
of Ivan Denisovich (1970)
The Dresser (1983)
The Last Butterfly (1991)
Let Him Have It (1991)
The Boy from Mercury (1996)
Last Orders (2001)
Nicholas Nickleby (2001)
The Golden Compass (2007)

Sir Noël **Coward**
5ft 2in
(NOËL PEIRCE COWARD)

Born: **December 16, 1899**
Teddington, Middlesex, England
Died: **March 26, 1973**

Noël was the second of the three sons born to Arthur Sabin Coward, a piano salesman, and his wife, Violet. With enthusiastic encouragement from his mother, Noël learned to dance and attended the Italia Conti Academy, in London, which placed an emphasis on drama. His debut in the children's play, "The Goldfish" brought offers from local theaters. By the age of fourteen, he was already a practicing homosexual and the lover of a society painter. He was a soldier in the British Army for a short period towards the end of World War I, but was discharged because of ill health. In 1918, he visited America and appeared in an uncredited role in the D.W.Griffith film, *Hearts of the World.* During the 1920s and early 1930s, he starred in his own plays, which were massively popular on both sides of the Atlantic. His most famous stage partner was Gertrude Lawrence, with whom he recorded many of his amusing songs. At the outbreak of World War II, Noël came back from Paris, and began highly-publicized tours to entertain the troops. What wasn't publicized was his intelligence work for MI5. Two of his most popular songs, 'London Pride' and 'Don't Let's Be Beastly To The Germans' were in the bestselling lists of the period. He wrote, acted in and composed, the music for the British flag-waver, *In Which We Serve.* He wrote several plays which became films, including *Brief Encounter.* In the 1950s, he toured as a solo cabaret act and starred on American TV. Noël died of a heart attack in Blue Harbor, Jamaica.

The Scoundrel (1935)
In Which We Serve (1942)
The Astonished Heart (1949)
Around the World in
Eighty Days (1956)
Our Man in Havana (1959)
Surprise Package (1960)
Paris When It Sizzles (1964)
Bunny Lake is Missing (1965)
The Italian Job (1977)

Brian **Cox**
5ft 7in
(BRIAN DENIS COX)

Born: **June 1, 1946**
Dundee, Scotland

Brian was born and raised in a Roman Catholic family of Irish extraction. His parents both worked in the mills as weavers and spinners. After his father's death in 1955, and his mother's series of nervous breakdowns, he went to live with an aunt. He was a poor scholar, but a natural actor. At fourteen, Brian joined the Dundee Repertory as a cleaner and odd-job man. After a bit of stage experience, he got into the London Academy of Music and Dramatic Art, and became a pro actor at nineteen. He made several appearances in the TV series, 'The Prisoner', and in 1968, was the star of 'The Year of the Sex Olympics'. His first film role was as Leon Trotsky in *Nicholas and Alexandra.* By the early 1970s, he was known as "Scotland's answer to Marlon Brando". He had some strange coincidences in 1986: he played the role of Hannibal Lecter in *Manhunter,* when Anthony Hopkins was in "King Lear" at the National Theater. In 1990, Brian was playing King Lear at the National Theater when Hopkins was playing Lecter in *Silence of the Lambs.* Like Sir Anthony, Brian is successful, and he is even luckier with his choice of roles. He is married to Nicole Ansari. They have two sons.

Nicholas and Alexandra (1971)
In Celebration (1975)
Manhunter (1986)
Hidden Agenda (1990)
Iron Will (1994) Rob Roy (1995)
Braveheart (1995) The Long Kiss
Goodnight (1996) Rushmore (1998)
The Minus Man (1999)
A Shot at Glory (2000) Bug (2002)
The Bourne Identity (2002)
The Ring (2002) Troy (2004)
The Bourne Supremacy (2004)
Match Point (2005)
Red Eye (2005)
The Ringer (2005)
The Flying Scotsman (2006)
The Key Man (2007) Zodiac (2007)
The Water Horse: Legend of
the Deep (2007)
Red (2008)

Ronny Cox
6ft 2in
(DANIEL RONALD COX)

Born: July 23, 1938
Cloudcroft, New Mexico, USA

Ronny was the third of a big family of five children. His father was a carpenter, who also worked at a dairy. When Ronny was small they moved to Portales, where he grew up. In 1960, he married his one and only wife, Mary, with whom he had two children. They were together until her death in 2006. In 1972, Ronny made his television debut in the drama, 'Look Homeward, Angel'. That same year, he made his movie debut, in *The Happiness Cage,* and was able to utilize his musical skills when he played "Dueling Banjos" with the mountain boy, in *Deliverance.* Those skills proved useful again when four years later, Ronny co-starred with Keith Carradine in *Bound for Glory* – the story of Woodie Guthrie. There were many more movies – not all of them good ones – but his reputation remains high. TV work includes 'Apple's Way', 'Star Trek', 'The Agency' and 'Stargate SG-1'. Ronny's musical tastes cover a wide range – from jazz to country western, to blues and folk. He's released five excellent albums and performs in concerts at folk music festivals and on television. Most of Ronny's acting over the past three years has been in TV productions including an episode of 'Desperate Housewives', but he is set to reappear on the big screen – with Eddie Murphy – in the comedy, *Imagine That.*

Deliverance (1972)
Bound for Glory (1976)
Gray Lady Down (1978)
The Onion Field (1979)
Taps (1981) **Courage** (1984)
Beverly Hills Cop (1984)
Vision Quest (1985)
Beverly Hills Cop II (1987)
RoboCop (1987)
Total Recall (1990)
Murder at 1600 (1997)
Puraido: Unmei no toki (1998)
The Boys of Sunset Ridge (2001)
American Outlaws (2001)
Crazy as Hell (2002)
The L.A. Riot
Spectacular (2005)

Peter Coyote
6ft 3in
(ROBERT PETER COHON)

Born: October 10, 1941
New York City, New York, USA

Peter was the son of Morris Cohon, an investment banker, and his wife, Ruth. Having grown up in the comfort of a middle-class Jewish family, Peter graduated from Grinnell College with a BA in English Literature. In 1965, he went to San Francisco State University to study for a Master's degree in creative writing. He spent a short time at the San Francisco Actor's Workshop before becoming part of the radical "Mime Troupe". He was a founder member of "Diggers" – which sprang up during the 'Summer of Love'. Its aim being to provide free food, clothing, housing and medical care to the hordes of Flower Children. He chose his stage name Coyote, because of "a healing spiritual encounter with one". In 1978, at the Magic Theater, when Peter was playing the lead in Sam Shepard's "True West", he was contacted by a Hollywood movie agent. A deal was done and Peter made his film debut in 1980, in *Die Laughing.* It was not funny and he was relieved to find himself in *Southern Comfort* and the world-wide hit *E.T. The Extra-Terrestrial* soon afterwards. He describes himself as a "Zen Buddhist student first – actor second". His fluency in French led to work in films such as *Bon Voyage* and *Le Grand rôle.*

Southern Comfort (1981)
E.T. the Extra-Terrestrial (1982)
Endangered Species (1982)
Stranger's Kiss (1983)
Heartbreakers (1984)
Jagged Edge (1985)
A Man in Love (1987)
A Grand Arte (1991)
Bitter Moon (1992)
Kika (1993) **The Basket** (1999)
Bon Voyage (2003)
Le Grand rôle (2004)
A Little Trip to Heaven (2005)
The Sunday Man (2007)
Resurrecting the Champ (2007)
The Sunday Man (2007)
All Roads Lead Home (2008)
The Lena Baker Story (2008)
Adopt a Sailor (2008)

Daniel Craig
5ft 11in
(DANIEL WROUGHTON CRAIG)

Born: March 2, 1968
Chester, Cheshire, England

Daniel's father was a merchant seaman before becoming landlord of various pubs around Chester. He left Daniel's mother (an art teacher) in 1972, and she brought the boy and his sister up in Liverpool. Daniel's mother loved the theater and encouraged his interest by taking him to see plays. He appeared in a school production of "Oliver" and around that time, he went to see his first Bond movie, *Live and Let Die.* At Hilbre High School, he continued acting, and was good at sports – playing rugby union for the local club, Hoylake. When he was sixteen, Daniel joined the National Youth Theatre tour and then moved to London. Eventually he was accepted at the famous Guildhall School of Music and Drama, where contemporaries included Ewan McGregor, Damien Lewis and Joseph Fiennes. In 1992 he got married and also made his movie debut in *The Power of One.* He had to wait for his first role in a good film. There was plenty of TV and stage work and some dud movies before *Elizabeth,* in 1998. It was a small part but it was in the right league. From 2001, there were a series of good films leading to 'Bond'. He's already made his second in the series and is lined up for a number of others. Daniel is hot property.

Love Is the Devil (1998)
The Trench (1999)
Some Voices (2000)
Hotel Splendide (2000)
Lara Croft: Tomb Raider (2001)
Road to Perdition (2002)
The Mother (2003) **Sylvia** (2003)
Enduring Love (2004)
Layer Cake (2004)
The Jacket (2005)
Sorstalansàg (2005)
Munich (2005)
Infamous (2006)
Casino Royale (2006)
The Invasion (2007)
The Golden Compass (2007)
Flashbacks of a Fool (2008)
Quantum of Solace (2008)
Defiance (2008)

James **Craig**
5ft 9in
(JAMES HENRY MEADOR)

Born: **February 1, 1912**
Nashville, Tennessee, USA
Died: **June 28, 1985**

Jim graduated from Rice University, in Houston, Texas. With the United States economy experiencing the chill winds of recession, he decided he had the looks (if not the skills) to make a career for himself in the movies. In order to rectify his shortcomings, Jim befriended the English-born character actor, Cyril Delevanti, who was more than happy to give him acting lessons. In 1937, he began to get work as an extra – starting with an uncredited part as a waiter – in *Sophie Lang Goes West,* which included young Robert Cummings, in a small supporting role. Jim was then cast by Paramount in the B-western, *Thunder Trail* – in which he looked ideal as a cowboy – which he'd often play. It took three years before he got featured roles in high-profile productions like *Kitty Foyle* and *The Devil and Daniel Webster,* but most of his films were second-features. Jim's last role was in an episode of 'The ABC Afternoon Playbreak' in 1972. He became a real estate agent in Santa Ana, California, with his third wife, Sumie. Jim died of lung cancer, at his home in the town, thirteen years later.

Thunder Trail (1937) **Born to the West** (1937) **The Man They Could Not Hang** (1939) **Zanzibar** (1940)
Seven Sinners (1940)
Kitty Foyle (1940)
Unexpected Uncle (1941)
The Devil and Daniel Webster (1941)
Friendly Enemies (1942)
The Human Comedy (1943)
Lost Angel (1943) **The Heavenly Body** (1944) **Kismet** (1944)
Gentle Annie (1944)
Dangerous Partners (1945)
Our Vines Have Tender Grapes (1945)
Little Mister Jim (1946)
Dark Delusion (1947)
Side Street (1950) **A Lady Without a Passport** (1950) **The Strip** (1951)
Drums in the Deep South (1951)
Code Two (1953)
While the City Sleeps (1956)

Jeanne **Crain**
5ft 4in
(JEANNE CRAIN)

Born: **May 25, 1925**
Barstow, California, USA
Died: **December 14, 2003**

Jeanne moved to Los Angeles when she was a child. She was a very good ice skater during her school years and had a taste for the spotlight. She was also very good looking and was crowned "Miss Pan Pacific" at the age of sixteen. A year later, director Orson Welles tested her for *The Magnificent Ambersons.* She didn't pass the test, but she was signed by 20th Century Fox and took acting lessons at the studio school. In 1943, she had one small part, wearing a bathing suit, in *The Gang's All Here.* Darryl F. Zanuck saw her on the lot and he starred her in *Home in Indiana.* Her fan mail began pouring in and after only a couple more movies, it was reported to be second in volume to that received by Betty Grable. *State Fair,* in 1945, made her a star. On New Year's Eve 1946, Jeanne married actor Paul Brooks, with whom she had seven children. Oscar nominated for *Pinky,* she was a star for a dozen years with movies such as *A Letter to Three Wives* and *The Joker Is Wild,* among her credits. She continued working until the late 1960s – mostly on television. She re-surfaced once in a while in movies and made her final appearance in 1972's *Skyjacked.* Jeanne was a devout Roman Catholic. Despite a long-running catalog of domestic problems, she remained married until her husband's death in 2003. Jeanne followed him quickly, when she suffered a heart attack in Santa Barbara, California, two months later.

Home in Indiana (1944)
Winged Victory (1944) **State Fair** (1945)
Leave Her to Heaven (1945)
Margie (1946) **Centennial Summer** (1946)
You Were Meant for Me (1948)
Apartment for Peggy (1948)
A Letter to Three Wives (1949)
Pinky (1949) **Cheaper by the Dozen** (1950) **People Will Talk** (1951)
Man Without a Star (1955)
The Fastest Gun Alive (1956)
The Joker is Wild (1957)
The Night God Screamed (1971)

Broderick **Crawford**
6ft
(WILLIAM BRODERICK CRAWFORD)

Born: **December 9, 1911**
Philadelphia, Pennsylvania, USA
Died: **April 26, 1986**

Brod's parents were vaudeville performers and his mother, Helen Broderick, had a stage and film career, which included the Astaire and Rogers movies, *Top Hat* and *Swing Time.* Helen encouraged her son to go into show business. To begin with he was a successful radio actor, but in the early 1930s, he got roles in Broadway shows. He went to London in 1932 to appear in "She Loves Me Not" – at the Adelphi Theater. In 1937, after he had starred in "Of Mice and Men" – on Broadway, he made his movie debut – in *Woman Chases Man.* In top movies like *Beau Geste,* Brod performed well, but he had a rasping voice and was as flat-footed as a penguin. He was usually cast as a 'heavy' in westerns, Damon Runyon stories and gangster movies. In 1943, Brod joined the United States Air Force for three years. His career got back on track with *Black Angel,* but it was in 1949, with a Best Actor Oscar for *All the King's Men,* that he hit a purple patch, with a run of good films. In 1950, he starred in the classic comedy, *Born Yesterday.* From 1955 to 1959, he was on the side of law and order as Chief Dan Matthews in the hit television show 'Highway Patrol'. Brod kept on working until he was silenced forever by a series of strokes, in Rancho Mirage.

Beau Geste (1939)
When the Daltons Rode (1940)
Seven Sinners (1940)
Badlands of Dakota (1941)
Larceny, Inc. (1942) **Broadway** (1942)
The Runaround (1946) **Black Angel** (1946) **Anna Lucasta** (1949)
All the King's Men (1949)
Convicted (1950)
Born Yesterday (1950)
Human Desire (1954)
Down Three Dark Streets (1954)
Big House, U.S.A. (1955)
Not as a Stranger (1955)
The Swindle (1955)
The Fastest Gun Alive (1956)
Between Heaven and Hell (1956)

Joan **Crawford**
5ft 5in
(LUCILLE FAY LESUEUR)

Born: **March 23, 1905**
San Antonio, Texas, USA
Died: **May 10, 1977**

Joan's parents had separated before she was born, and she survived a tough childhood to make it in an even tougher world. Her mother worked in a laundry and Joan left school early to scrub floors to help keep the family afloat. When she was sixteen, she took a job as a waitress and won a Charleston competition. She changed her name to Lucille Le Suer after becoming a dancer in a nightclub. From there she joined the chorus line in the Shubert revue "Innocent Eyes". In 1925 she doubled (in long shots) for Norma Shearer and MGM ran a contest in a fan-magazine to dream up a new name for her. 'Joan Crawford' was the winner. She sang and danced in *Hollywood Revue of 1929,* but yearned for more dramatic parts. She had a tendency to overact, but in *Grand Hotel* she wasn't outshone by her illustrious co-stars. She married Franchot Tone, who had a big influence on her style. During the 1930s, her popularity came and went. It was her mature years that steadied her decline and found new audiences. She won an Oscar for *Mildred Pierce,* and the fans got the Crawford they loved, even if her fellow actors hated her. Joan was a lonely alcoholic when she died in New York of pancreatic cancer. Luckily, she didn't get to read her daughter Christina's scathing biography – "Mommie Dearest".

Grand Hotel (1932) Rain (1932)
Dancing Lady (1933) Sadie McKee (1934)
The Last of Mrs. Cheyney (1937)
Mannequin (1937) The Women (1939)
Strange Cargo (1940) Susan and
God (1940) A Woman's Face (1941)
Above Suspicion (1943)
Mildred Pierce (1945)
Humoresque (1946) Possessed (1947)
Daisy Kenyon (1947)
Flamingo Road (1949)
Sudden Fear (1952)
Johnny Guitar (1955)
Autumn Leaves (1956) The Best of
Everything (1959) What Ever Happened
to Baby Jane ? (1962)

Laird **Cregar**
6ft 3in
(SAMUEL LAIRD CREGAR)

Born: **July 28, 1913**
Philadelphia, Pennsylvania, USA
Died: **December 9, 1944**

Laird's father, Edward Matthews Cregar, was a member of the Gentleman of Philadelphia cricket team. His mother was the former Elizabeth Smith. Laird was the youngest of six brothers of whom, when fully grown, he was the shortest. At eight years of age he was sent by his parents to be educated in England and attended Winchester College. After returning home he had difficulty settling down and at one point, ran away from home. To his father's annoyance, he dropped out of high school to work as a theater bouncer, and took acting lessons during the day. That led to a scholarship at the Pasadena Community Playhouse, but without his parents' support he soon ran out of money. He was forced to sleep in a friend's car and depended on fellow students for food. He was grossly overweight by the time he got bit parts in two movies, in 1940, but he used it to his advantage. He played Oscar Wilde on stage in L.A. and not only did he get rave reviews, he was signed by 20th Century Fox. He was twenty-seven when he made his movie debut, in *Hudson's Bay.* Laird's final film, *Hangover Square,* was released eight months after he died of heart failure, in Los Angeles, at the age of thirty – following a crash diet. Based on all the evidence of his all too short career, there is little doubt that, had Laird lived, he would have become a movie giant in every sense of the word.

Hudson's Bay (1941)
Blood and Sand (1941)
Charlie's Aunt (1941)
I Wake Up Screaming (1941)
Joan of Paris (1942)
Rings on Her Fingers (1942)
This Gun for Hire (1942)
Ten Gentlemen from
West Point (1942)
Heaven Can Wait (1943)
Hello Frisco, Hello (1943)
Holy Matrimony (1943)
The Lodger (1944)
Hangover Square (1945)

Richard **Crenna**
6ft 1in
(RICHARD DONALD CRENNA)

Born: **November 30, 1926**
Los Angeles, California, USA
Died: **January 17, 2003**

Although Dick's parents were uneducated Italian immigrants, his mother bought and ran a small hotel to pay for his education. He responded magnificently. After graduating from Belmont High School, he majored in Theater Arts at the University of Southern California, where he was a member of the Kappa Sigma Fraternity. Dick's first acting assignment was when he appeared on the radio show, 'A Date With Judy'. In 1946 he transferred to 'Our Miss Brooks' – continuing to play the role of a teenager, after it became a television show, in 1952 – and a movie four years later! His film debut is believed to have been an uncredited one in the 1950 musical, *Let's Dance,* but he was certainly in a 1952 western, *Red Skies of Montana.* He did an episode of 'I Love Lucy' and his career was dominated by long-running TV series such as 'The Real McCoys' and 'Slattery's People'. But he appeared in more than sixty movies – good, bad, and indifferent. He was nominated for three Golden Globes. His star on the Hollywood Walk of Fame is two away from that of Sly Stallone. Dick was married to Penni Sweeney, for forty-four years. He died in Los Angeles of pancreatic cancer.

The Pride of St. Louis (1952)
It Grows on Trees (1952)
Our Miss Brooks (1956)
The Sand Pebbles (1966)
Wait Until Dark (1967)
Marooned (1970)
Red Sky at Morning (1970)
Doctors' Wives (1970)
The Deserter (1971)
Red Sky in the Morning (1971)
Catlow (1971)
Un Flic (1972)
Breakheart Pass (1975)
Stone Cold Dead (1980)
Body Heat (1981)
The Flamingo Kid (1984)
First Blood Part II (1985)
Hot Shots! Part Deux (1993)
Sabrina (1995)

Donald Crisp
5ft 8½in
(GEORGE WILLIAM CRISP)

Born: **July 27, 1882**
Bow, London, England
Died: **May 25, 1974**

Donald grew up and went to school in the East End of London, but claimed, in his Hollywood days, that he was an Old Etonian. He served as a trooper in the 10th Hussars during the Boer War, in South Africa. Then in 1906, he sailed to America. On board the ship was an impresario, who was so taken by Donald's singing during a ship's concert, that he offered him employment with his Opera Company. In 1910, Donald was stage manager for George M. Cohen, and through his job, got to know D.W. Griffith. They went to Los Angeles together, with Donald serving as D.W.'s assistant director as well as appearing in such notable films as *Birth of a Nation* and *Broken Blossoms*. Directing Buster Keaton and Fairbanks wasn't as appealing as acting, and by 1930, he was a top character actor. He won an Oscar for his supporting role in *How Green Was My Valley,* but there were many other good films in which he shone. Donald was an influential figure in Hollywood and was – at different times, an adviser and chairman of the Bank of America. He died in Van Nuys, California, following a series of strokes, at the age of ninety-one.

Red Dust (1932)
The Little Minister (1934)
Mutiny on the Bounty (1935)
The Charge of the Light
Brigade (1936) Confession (1937)
The Life of Emile Zola (1937)
The Amazing Dr. Clitterhouse (1938)
The Dawn Patrol (1938) Jezebel (1938)
Wuthering Heights (1939)
The Sea Hawk (1940)
How Green Was My Valley (1941)
Lassie Come Home (1943)
The Valley of Decision (1945)
Ramrod (1947)
Bright Leaf (1950)
The Long Gray Line (1955)
The Man from Laramie (1955)
The Last Hurrah (1958)
Pollyanna (1960)

James Cromwell
6ft 7in
(JAMES OLIVER CROMWELL)

Born: **January 27, 1940**
Los Angeles, California, USA

Jim's pedigree has movies written all over it. His mother was the actress, Kay Johnson, and his father was film director and film producer, John Cromwell. *The Prisoner of Zenda* and *Algiers* being just two of the top Hollywood titles he worked on before being blacklisted during the McCarthy era. Jim was brought up in Manhattan. After The Hill School, he attended Middlebury College, in Vermont and Carnegie Mellon University, in Pittsburgh, where he studied engineering. Jim began his acting career on TV in 1974, in an episode of the 'Rockford Files'. His first film role was in Neil Simon's *Murder by Death* in 1976 – the year he married his first wife – Anne Ulvestad. His career jogged along for the next fifteen years or so – mostly on television and in some supporting roles in movies. He stepped up a gear following his Best Supporting Oscar nomination for *Babe* and, two years later, impressed in one of the best movies of the 1990s – *L.A. Confidential*. In recent years, his career as a first-class character actor has kept him busy in roles as diverse as President Lyndon Johnson, in the TV drama, 'RFK' and Prince Philip, in the film, *The Queen.*

The Man with Two Brains (1983)
Revenge of the Nerds (1984)
Explorers (1985)
Romeo Is Bleeding (1993)
Babe (1995)
Eraser (1996)
Owd Bob (1997)
L.A. Confidential (1997)
The Deep Impact (1998)
The General's Daughter (1999)
Snow Falling on Cedars (1999)
The Green Mile (1999)
Space Cowboys (2000)
The Sum of All Fears (2002)
The Snow Walker (2003)
I, Robot (2004) The Queen (2006)
Dante's Inferno (2007)
Becoming Jane (2007)
Spider-Man 3 (2007)
Tortured (2008) W. (2008)

Richard Cromwell
5ft 10in
(LEROY MELVIN RADABAUGH)

Born: **January 8, 1910**
Long Beach, California, USA
Died: **October 11, 1960**

Dick was the eldest of five children born to Hobart and Faye Radabaugh. His father died young – a victim of the influenza pandemic. Dick was only in grade school at the time but he did what he could to support his mother, by taking on odd-jobs. In his mid-teens, he won a scholarship to the Chouinard Art School, in Los Angeles. He had a talent for oil-painting – among his sitters for portraits were Joan Crawford, Tallulah Bankhead and Greta Garbo. He worked as a movie extra starting with *King of Jazz* in 1930, and he auditioned for and won the title role in the remake of the silent film *Tol'able David.* He had established a lasting friendship with Mary Dressler in his days as an art student and she insisted that he was cast opposite her in *Emma*. It helped make 1932 a very good year for Dick. A few months later he was acting with Clara Bow, in her final movie, *Hoop-La*. It didn't exactly boost his career but *The Lives of a Bengal Lancer,* with Gary Cooper, most certainly did. Dick also co-starred with the legendary Will Rogers, in *Life Begins at Forty* and with comedian W.C.Fields, in *Poppy.* That year saw him debut on Broadway in "So Proudly We Hail" and in 1938, he was on the radio. As World War II got under way, Dick's star faded and he worked in Bs until joining the U.S. Coast Guards in 1944. In 1945, he was married to Angela Lansbury for nine months and was believed to be gay. He studied ceramics and designed decorative tiles. He was also a good cook. Dick died in Hollywood of liver cancer.

Tol'able David (1930) Maker of
Men (1931) Emma (1932) The Strange
Love of Molly Louvain (1932) Tom Brown
of Culver (1932) The Age of
Consent (1932) That's My Boy (1932)
This Day and Age (1933)
The Most Precious Thing in Life (1934)
The Lives of a Bengal Lancer (1935)
Life Begins at Forty (1935) Poppy (1936)
The Road Back (1937) Jezebel (1938)
Young Mr. Lincoln (1939)

Hume **Cronyn**
5ft 6in
(HUME BLAKE CRONYN)

Born: **July 18, 1911**
London, Ontario, Canada
Died: **June 15, 2003**

One of five children of a politician and local businessman, and an heiress from the Labatt brewing company, Hume attended the prestigious Ridley College, in St. Catherines, Ontario. By the time he began law studies at McGill University, he was a good enough boxer to be short-listed to represent Canada at the 1932 Olympic Games. He didn't make the team, so he switched to drama studies under Max Reinhardt, at the American Academy of Dramatic Arts. He made his Broadway debut in 1934, in "Hipper's Holiday" and had nine successful years on stage before appearing in his first movie, Hitchcock's *Shadow of a Doubt*. A year earlier, he married the actress Jessica Tandy – his wife and frequent co-star on stage, TV, radio and in films, until her death in 1994. An excellent character actor, he was nominated for a Best Supporting Actor Oscar for *The Seventh Cross*. He won a Tony in 1964, for his performance as Polonius, in the Broadway production of "Hamlet" – starring Richard Burton. In 1996, Hume married the English screenwriter, Susan Cooper. He was ninety-one when he died of prostate cancer at his home in Fairfield, Connecticut.

Shadow of a Doubt (1943)
The Cross of Lorraine (1943)
Lifeboat (1944)
The Seventh Cross (1944)
The Green Years (1946)
The Postman Always
Rings Twice (1946)
Brute Force (1947)
Sunrise at Campobello (1960)
Cleopatra (1963)
The Arrangement (1969)
There Was a Crooked Man (1970)
The Parallax View (1974)
The World According to Garp (1982)
Impulse (1984)
Brewster's Millions (1985)
Cocoon (1985)
The Pelican Brief (1993)
Marvin's Room (1996)

Bing **Crosby**
5ft 7in
(HARRY LILLIS CROSBY)

Born: **May 2, 1903**
Tacoma, Washington, USA
Died: **October 14, 1977**

The fourth of seven children born to a bookkeeper at a brewery, Bing studied law at Gonzaga University in Spokane. With his friend Al Rinker, he formed a singing duo, which was hired by Paul Whiteman and absorbed into his 'Rhythm Boys'. He started making solo recordings and was hired by Mack Sennett to appear in 'shorts' built around songs. Bing made his feature movie debut, in *King of Jazz*, in 1930. A year later, he was given his own radio show and had a season at the Paramount Theater, in New York. His records were best-sellers and he was offered a movie contract by Paramount. He was soon a mega-star who was never out of the top-ten box-office draws. In the 1930s, his movies were dependent on the songs and it took him a while to get more dramatic material. Teaming up with Bob Hope did help him play comedy, but it was the hit movie *Going My Way* which established him as a dramatic actor to be reckoned with and won him an Oscar. He was nominated for both *The Bells of St. Mary's* and *The Country Girl*. Bing continued making movies and records until the late 1960s. When he died from a heart attack, he was playing his beloved game of golf – on a course near Madrid, Spain.

The Big Broadcast (1932)
Pennies from Heaven (1936)
Sing You Sinners (1938) **Road to**
Singapore (1940) **Road to**
Zanzibar (1941) **Birth of the**
Blues (1941) **Holiday Inn** (1942)
Going My Way (1944)
The Bells of St. Mary's (1945)
Road to Utopia (1946)
Road to Rio (1947)
A Connecticut Yankee in
King Arthur's Court (1949)
White Christmas (1954)
The Country Girl (1954)
High Society (1956)
Man on Fire (1957)
High Time (1960)
Robin and the 7 Hoods (1964)

Russell **Crowe**
5ft 11in
(RUSSELL IRA CROWE)

Born: **April 7, 1964**
Wellington, New Zealand

Rusty has lived in Australia since he was a little boy. His parents were movie set caterers and it was only natural that he developed the acting bug early. He spoke a line of dialogue in an Australian television series called 'Spyforce' when he was six. Its star, Jack Thompson, played Rusty's father in the 1994 movie, *The Sum of Us*. Rusty and his family moved back to New Zealand when he was fourteen. He went to school in Auckland with cousins Jeff and Martin Crowe – future Test cricketers. Rusty became famous as a rock 'n' roll singer in NZ – releasing a single "I Wanna Be Marlon Brando" under the name Russ Le Roq. When he was twenty-one, he returned to Australia. After a tough couple of years he got a part in the TV series 'Neighbours'. His first movie appearance was in 1990's *Prisoners of the Sun*. In 1993, Sharon Stone saw him in *Romper Stomper* and asked for him to appear with her in *The Quick and the Dead*. Two years later he was highly praised for his work in *L.A. Confidential*. Rusty was Oscar-nominated for *The Insider*, in 1999, and won one, for *Gladiator*. When that was finished, he rode with a group of friends on motorbikes for 4,000 miles around Australia. He and his wife, singer/actress, Dani Spencer, have two sons – Charlie and Tennyson.

The Quick and the Dead (1995)
Rough Magic (1995)
L.A. Confidential (1997)
Heaven's Burning (1997)
Mystery, Alaska (1999)
The Insider (1999)
Gladiator (2000)
Proof of Life (2000)
A Beautiful Mind (2001)
Master and Commander:
The Far Side of the World (2003)
Cinderella Man (2005)
A Good Year (2006)
3:10 to Yuma (2007)
American Gangster (2007)
Tenderness (2008)
Body of Lies (2008)
State of Play (2009)

Marie-Josée **Croze**
5ft 6¼in
(MARIE-JOSÉE CROZE)

Born: **February 23, 1970**
Montréal, Québec, Canada

Marie-Josée was adopted when she was three years old. She was a difficult child to handle as she was growing up. Her stepmother suffered depression, due to the combined stress of Marie-Josée's behavior and her husband's alcoholism. At sixteen, Marie-Josée was a sullen punk, with no idea about her future. Looking back, she thinks her stepmother must have been a tolerant saint, because it was with her encouragement, Marie-Josée began studying fine arts. When she was twenty, her interest switched to acting. She joined the Montréal-based, La Veillée-Prospero Theater workshop. In 1989, she began appearing on Canadian television – starting with an episode of 'Chambres en ville'. In 1992, she made her film debut, in a comedy, *La Postière*. She continued to work in French and English language TV films, in Canada, until an appearance in her first Hollywood movie, *Battlefield Earth* almost killed her career at its birth. Denis Villeneuve, a Canadian director, rescued Marie-Josée later that year, when he cast her in his film, *Maelström.* It won her Best Actress Genie and Jutra Awards as well as the vote from the Vancouver Film Critics Circle. She worked with the top directors in Canada and after her Best Actress Award at the Cannes Film Festival for *Les Invasions barbares,* she received offers from France. Her international break came in Steven Spielberg's *Munich.* Marie-Josée was seen recently in the Oscar-nominated, *Le Scaphandre et le papillon.*

Maelström (2000)
Wolves in the Snow (2002)
Ararat (2002) **Les Invasion barbares** (2003) **Mensonges et trahisons** (2004) **La Petite Chartreuse** (2005) **Munich** (2005)
Birds of Heaven (2006)
Moon on the Snow (2006)
Tell No One (2006)
Jacquou le croquant (2007)
Le Scaphandre et le papillon (2007)
Love Me No More (2008)
The New Protocol (2008)

Billy **Crudup**
5ft 8½in
(WILLIAM GAITHER CRUDUP)

Born: **July 8, 1968**
Manhasset, New York, USA

The second of three sons, Billy was already entertaining his family and friends with celebrity impressions when growing up in Florida and Texas. Billy was awarded an undergraduate degree at the University of North Carolina – where he developed a keen interest in acting. He went on to get a Masters in Fine Arts from the Tisch School of the Arts at New York University. In New York City, he became a member of a theater troupe known as 'The Lab'. In 1995, Billy appeared on Broadway in "Arcadia" by Tom Stoppard – earning the Outer Critics Circle Award as 'Outstanding Newcomer'. A year earlier, he made his first movie appearance, in an independent film titled *Grind,* which wasn't released until 1997. Movie audiences first saw Billy in *Sleepers,* starring Brad Pitt, and he was soon getting more good roles on a regular basis. Despite not wanting to be a star, he was heading in that direction. He began to look stardom firmly in the eye – winning the Best Actor Award – for *Jesus' Son* at the Paris Film Festival, and going on to appear in hit movies including *Almost Famous, Mission Impossible* and *The Good Shepherd.* He was living with the actress, Marie-Louise Parker, but he left her in 2003, when she was expecting their son, William. From 2004-2006, Billy was dating his former co-star, the young actress, Claire Danes.

Sleepers (1996)
Everyone Says I Love You (1996)
Inventing the Abbotts (1997)
Snitch (1998)
Without Limits (1998)
The Hi-Lo Country (1998)
Jesus' Son (1999)
Waking the Dead (2000)
Almost Famous (2000)
Charlotte Gray (2001)
Big Fish (2003) **Stage Beauty** (2004)
Mission Impossible III (2006)
The Good Shepherd (2006)
Dedication (2007)
Pretty Bird (2008)
Public Enemies (2009)

Tom **Cruise**
5ft 7in
(THOMAS CRUISE MAPOTHER IV)

Born: **July 3, 1962**
Syracuse, New York, USA

Because of their nomadic parents, Tom and his three sisters were constantly on the move. By the age of fourteen he had attended fifteen different schools in the United States and Canada – including a Franciscan seminary – where he began training as a priest. After high school, where he had played a leading role in "Guys and Dolls", he decided to pursue an acting career in New York. He made his movie debut in 1981, with a small part in *Endless Love.* Tom's first leading role came two years later, in *Risky Business.* After initially turning down the part in *Top Gun,* he took it when he was allowed to help alter the script. It was the highest grossing movie of 1986 and it made him a star all across the world. Currently he and Tom Hanks are the only actors to have had seven consecutive $100 million plus blockbusters. Tom's private life has been extremely public – with several high-profile wives and girlfriends. Tom has been a Best Actor Oscar nominee three times – for *Born on the Fourth of July, Jerry Maguire,* and *Magnolia.* It is said that his first wife, Mimi Rogers introduced him to Scientology – for which he renounced his Catholic faith. Since 2006, he has been married to his third wife, the actress Katie Holmes. They have a baby daughter.

Risky Business (1983)
Top Gun (1986) **The Color of Money** (1986) **Rain Man** (1988)
Born on the Fourth of July (1989)
A Few Good Men (1992)
The Firm (1993)
Mission Impossible (1996)
Jerry Maguire (1996)
Magnolia (1999)
Vanilla Sky (2001)
Minority Report (2002)
The Last Samurai (2003)
Collateral (2004)
War of the Worlds (2005)
Mission Impossible III (2006)
Lions for Lambs (2007)
Tropic Thunder (2008)
Valkyrie (2008)

Penélope **Cruz**
5ft 5½in
(PENÉLOPE CRUZ SANCHEZ)

Born: April 28, 1974
Madrid, Spain

Penélope's father, Eduardo Cruz, was an auto mechanic. Being a hairdresser, her mother, Encarna, managed to make her beautiful little girl look extra special. As a child, Penélope spent nine years studying ballet at the Conservatorio National. When she was fifteen she won a fashion agency audition in competition against three hundred young hopefuls and it resulted in a lot of work in commercials and music videos. The pressure caused Penélope to have a nervous breakdown, but she soon got back on track. In 1992, she made her movie debut, in *Jamón, Jamón.* But it was her second film that year, the Best Foreign Language Oscar winner, *Belle Epoque,* that made people sit up and take notice. She averaged three films a year after that, and in 1998, she was voted Best Actress at Spain's Goya Awards, for *La Niña de tus ojos.* That film and a first international hit, *Todo sobre mi madre,* in 1999, combined to give her a chance in Hollywood as the co-star to big names like Johnny Depp and Matt Damon. Her relationship with Tom Cruise and modeling for Ralph Lauren helped fuel her fame and she is now securely in the major league on both sides of the Atlantic. Penélope's work with Pedro Almodóvar in *Volver* – for which she was nominated for an Oscar – almost put the icing on the cake. Her turn came when she won a Best Supporting Actress Oscar for *Vicky Cristina Barcelona.*

Belle Epoque (1992)
Abre los ojos (1997)
The Hi-Lo Country (1998)
Todo sobre mi madre (1999)
Blow (2001) **Captain**
Corelli's Mandolin (2001)
No News from God (2001)
Vanilla Sky (2001)
Non ti muovere (2004)
Head in the Clouds (2004)
Noel (2004) **Sahara** (2005)
Volver (2006) **Manolete** (2007)
The Good Night (2007)
Elegy (2008) **Vicky Cristina**
Barcelona (2008)

Billy **Crystal**
5ft 7in
(WILLIAM JACOB CRYSTAL)

Born: March 14, 1948
Long Island, New York, USA

Billy's dad, Jack, was a well-known concert promoter and co-founder of the jazz record label, Commodore. From an early age, he and his two brothers were familiar with stars like Billie Holiday, who used to visit their home. Sadly Jack Crystal died of a heart attack when Billy was fifteen, but with the help of her sons, his mother kept the family going. Meanwhile, with inspiration from comics like Ernie Kovacs and Jonathan Winters, Billy began doing stand-up comedy at the age of sixteen. His real ambition was to play baseball for his favorite team, the New York Yankees. At eighteen he earned a baseball scholarship from Marshall University, but the program was suspended and he returned to New York. At Nassau Community College he met a girl called Janice Goldfinger, whom he later married. He then studied under Martin Scorsese, at New York University. Until 1976, when he left for Hollywood, Billy worked as a stand-up comic. His first big break was playing a gay guy in the ABC TV sitcom 'Soap'. His movie debut, *Rabbit Test,* was not a success, nor was his own variety show, in 1982. It took four years for Billy to get his ideal movie role, in *Running Scared.* He turned his hand to writing and directing – *Mr. Saturday Night, Forget Paris* and *American Sweethearts.* Billy's been married to Janice since 1970. They have two actress daughters. He is currently working on the movie *Tooth Fairy* – which features Julie Andrews.

Running Scared (1986)
The Princess Bride (1987)
Throw Momma from the Train (1987)
Memories of Me (1988)
When Harry Met Sally (1989)
City Slickers (1991)
Mr. Saturday Night (1992)
Forget Paris (1995)
Hamlet (1996)
Deconstructing Harry (1997)
Analyze This (1999)
America's Sweethearts (2001)
Analyze That (2002)

Robert **Culp**
6ft 2in
(ROBERT MARTIN CULP)

Born: August 16, 1930
Oakland, California, USA

After beginning his teenage years in the middle of World War II, Bob graduated from Berkeley High School, in 1947. He took a few acting classes and journeyed to New York. At twenty-one, he made his Broadway debut, in "He Who Gets Slapped". In 1953, he appeared in an episode about Socrates, in the Walter Cronkite TV-series, 'You Are There'. For four years, Bob acted in the western series, 'Trackdown'. He appeared in his first movie in 1963, and made two more that year, but he specialized in TV work and enjoyed his biggest success in the medium, beginning in 1965, when he co-starred with Bill Cosby, in 'I Spy'. Bob played the role of a murderer in three 'Columbo' TV movies, and in 1971, with Peter Falk and others, he was in 'The Name of the Game'. In 1969, he was 'Bob' in *Bob & Carol & Ted & Alice.* It was ahead of the thinking of many of its audiences in showing that mature married people could happily change partners just for the night. There were many movies to come, but none of them had quite as much impact on Bob's career. Since 1981, he's been with his fifth wife, Candace Faulkner, with whom he has a daughter, Samantha. He has four grown-up offspring from his first wife, Nancy – one of whom is the actor, Joseph Culp. Bob's voice was recently featured in the popular video game, "Half-Life 2". He will be seen again on the big screen during 2009, in *The Assignment.*

PT 109 (1963)
Sunday in New York (1963)
Bob & Carol & Ted & Alice (1969)
Hannie Caulder (1971)
Hickey and Bogs (1971)
The Castaway Cowboy (1974)
Inside Out (1975)
Calendar Girl Murders (1984)
Turk 182! (1985)
The Pelican Brief (1993)
Panther (1995)
Most Wanted (1997)
The Almost Guys (2004)

Robert **Cummings**
5ft 10in
(CHARLES CLARENCE ROBERT CUMMINGS)

Born: **June 10, 1908**
Joplin, Missouri, USA
Died: **December 2, 1990**

Bob was at Joplin High School when he was taught to fly by his godfather, the famous aviator, Orville Wright. After he had attended the American Academy of Dramatic Arts in New York, he began a Broadway career using the stage name Blade Stanhope Conway – passing himself off as British. Using the name Bruce Hutchens, he went to Hollywood. One of his first movie appearances was in the 1933 Laurel and Hardy comedy, *Sons of the Desert.* But he had to wait six years before achieving stardom. His success in the CBS Radio series, 'Those We Love' kept his name in the spotlight until *Three Smart Girls Grow Up,* with Deanna Durbin. After that, he co-starred with Jean Arthur, Barbara Stanwyck, and Ronald Reagan, and was twice directed by Alfred Hitchcock. During World War II he was a pilot in the United States Air Force Reserve. In 1952, he started a career on American television with 'The Bob Cummings Show', which ran (including a follow-up) from 1955 to 1962. Married five times, he was the father of seven children, none of whom went into show business. An advocate of health foods, Bob suffered from Parkinson's Disease, before dying of kidney fever, at Woodland Hills.

Three Smart Girls Grow Up (1939)
Spring Parade (1940)
The Devil and Miss Jones (1941)
Moon Over Miami (1941)
It Started with Eve (1941)
King's Row (1942)
Saboteur (1942)
You Came Along (1945)
The Lost Moment (1947)
Sleep My Love (1948)
The Accused (1949)
Reign of Terror (1949)
Paid in Full (1950)
Lucky Me (1954)
Dial M for Murder (1954)
My Geisha (1962)
The Carpetbaggers (1964)
What a Way to Go! (1964)

Peggy **Cummins**
5ft 2in
(PEGGY CUMMINS)

Born: **December 18, 1925**
Prestatyn, Wales

Peggy's parents had moved from Ireland and settled in the popular holiday resort of Prestatyn, on the coast of North Wales. During the summer season, Britain's best entertainers would appear at the town's theaters. Peggy was fascinated by show business from a very young age. At school, she acted in plays and by the time she was twelve, she was with a local drama group. She was a keen filmgoer and, after leaving school at fifteen, she moved to London. Warner Brothers-First National were financing the making of movies there, so in 1940, the pretty teenager was given a starring role as the daughter of *Dr. O'Dowd.* It took four years for her to mature into a reasonable actress – in a romantic comedy – *English Without Tears.* She caught the eye of Darryl F. Zanuck, in Hollywood. He signed her to star in *Forever Amber,* but she wasn't experienced enough to play a woman like Amber and was replaced by Linda Darnell, who was. Peggy starred in more suitable movies, and just before returning to England, she acted in her most famous role – as Annie Laurie Starr, in the cult-classic *Gun Crazy.* The pick of her other films is *Night of the Demon.* She retired in the early 1960s, and devoted her time to working for charities. Her husband of fifty-one years, Derek Dunnett, died in 2001.

English Without Tears (1944)
The Late George Apley (1947)
Moss Rose (1947)
Escape (1948)
Green Grass of Wyoming (1948)
That Dangerous Age (1949)
Gun Crazy (1950)
My Daughter Joy (1950)
Street Corner (1953)
Always a Bride (1953)
Meet Mr. Lucifer (1953)
The Love Lottery (1954)
To Dorothy a Son (1954)
Carry On Admiral (1957)
Hell Drivers (1957)
Night of the Demon (1957)
The Captain's Table (1959)

Tim **Curry**
5ft 9in
(TIMOTHY JAMES CURRY)

Born: **Born: April 19, 1946**
Grappenhall, Cheshire, England

Tim's father was a Methodist chaplain who served in the Royal Navy. After he died in 1958, Tim moved to London and went to Kingswood School, where he shone as a boy soprano. He studied English and drama at Birmingham University, and worked with the famous Guild Theater Group, before switching to Cambridge University. Although his first major musical influence was jazz singer Billie Holiday, his first stage role was in the rock musical "Hair" in 1968. Since then, Tim's made several albums under his own name. His film debut was also his most famous stage characterization – as Dr. Frank. N. Furter – in *The Rocky Horror Picture Show.* His later movie roles have been generally unusual and interesting – if not always successful. He was a good Bill Sykes, in a 1982 TV-movie version of 'Oliver Twist' and as the 'Lord of Darkness' in *Legend,* Tim was almost unrecognizable under the make-up. In 1990, he performed the role of 'prosecutor' in Berlin, in Roger Waters' "The Wall". In 2007, Tim finally won an award – the 'What's On Theatergoers' Choice' as Best Actor in a Musical – for his role as King Arthur, in "Monty Python's Spamalot". He hasn't been seen in any worthwhile films during the last four years, but Tim's voice can be heard in animated films like *Queer Duck: The Movie* and *Garfield: A Tail of Two Kitties,* as well as in video games such as 'Nicktoons: Attack on the Toybots'.

The Rocky Horror Picture Show (1972)
The Shout (1978)
The Ploughman's Lunch (1983)
The Hunt for Red October (1990)
Oscar (1991)
The Shadow (1994)
Muppet Treasure Island (1996)
Four Dogs Playing Poker (2000)
Sorted (2000)
Charlie's Angels (2000)
The Scoundrel's Wife (2002)
Kinsey (2004)
The Secret of Moonacre (2008)

Jamie Leigh **Curtis**
5ft 9in
(JAMIE LEIGH CURTIS)

Born: **November 22, 1958**
Los Angeles, California, USA

Jamie Leigh and her older sister, Kelly, are the daughters of movie stars, Tony Curtis and Janet Leigh. Jamie Leigh went to schools in Los Angeles and Beverly Hills and graduated from Choate Rosemary Hall, a private school in Connecticut. In 1976, she started at the University of the Pacific, but dropped out when Universal Studios put her under contract. Having made her television debut in an episode of 'Columbo', she became well known in the 1978 horror classic, *Halloween.* After several movies in that genre, she was known as the "scream queen". *Trading Places* in 1983, established her as an actress with much more to offer and five years later, she showed her ability as a comedienne in *A Fish Called Wanda.* Jamie Leigh has written a number of critically-acclaimed children's books in collaboration with the illustrator, Laura Cornell. Ever since her husband, Christopher, inherited the title of Baron, in 1996, Jamie Leigh Curtis has been known as Lady Haden-Guest. In her spare time she has increasingly supported a number of philanthropic groups. Nobody goes on forever, so it made sense when in 2006, after a run of several fairly mediocre movies, Jamie Leigh Curtis announced her retirement from acting. Unfortunately for her, she returned in 2008, in the truly mediocre, *Beverly Hills Chihuahua.*

Halloween (1978) **The Fog** (1980)
Terror Train (1980)
Road Games (1981)
Halloween II (1983)
Trading Places (1984)
Love Letters (1984)
Dominick and Eugene (1988)
A Fish Called Wanda (1988)
Blue Steel (1990)
Queen's Logic (1991)
My Girl (1991)
Forever Young (1991)
True Lies (1994)
House Arrest (1996)
Fierce Creatures (1997)
The Tailor of Panama (2001)
Freaky Friday (2003)

Tony **Curtis**
5ft 11in
(BERNARD SCHWARTZ)

Born: **June 3, 1925**
The Bronx, New York City, New York, USA

As a kid, Tony lived with his parents – Hungarian Jewish immigrants – in one room at the back of a tailor's shop. It was a great childhood – his mother was a schizophrenic who regularly beat him up and when he was eight, Tony lived in an orphanage because his parents couldn't afford to feed him! With such harsh reality in his life it wasn't surprising that he sought escape in the movie theater. In 1942, he did escape: he served in the United States Navy and actually witnessed the Japanese surrender, in Tokyo Bay. After the war he studied acting along with Walter Matthau. His handsome face got him a contract with Universal, who changed his name to Anthony Curtis. He took riding and fencing classes, which came in useful in westerns and swashbuckling roles. But from 1955, he proved to be an exceptionally good actor in more serious movies. His first wife, Janet Leigh, broke his heart, but he has remarried five times. In 1959, he starred with Marilyn Monroe and Jack Lemmon in the greatest comedy of all time – *Some Like It Hot.* His big passion nowadays is painting – one of his works, 'Red Table', is on display in the Metropolitan Museum, in Manhattan.

Houdini (1953)
The Black Shield of Falworth (1954)
Six Bridges to Cross (1955)
Trapeze (1956)
Sweet Smell of Success (1957)
The Midnight Story (1957)
Kings Go Forth (1958)
The Defiant Ones (1958)
The Vikings (1958)
Operation Petticoat (1959)
Some Like it Hot (1959)
Who Was That Lady? (1960)
The Rat Race (1960) Spartacus (1960)
Sex and the Single Girl (1964)
The Great Race (1965)
The Boston Strangler (1968)
The Last Tycoon (1976)
The Mirror Crack'd (1980)
Insignificance (1985)
Naked in New York (1993)

Joan **Cusack**
5ft 9in
(JOAN MAY CUSACK)

Born: **October 11, 1962**
New York City, New York, USA

Joan was the second child born to an Irish Catholic couple, who started an acting dynasty. They also produced Joan's older sister, Ann, her brothers Bill and John, and her younger sister, Susie. Joan's father was the late Dick Cusack – an actor and documentary filmmaker – who ran his own film production company. Her mother, Nancy, was a mathematics teacher, who was described as a political activist. After leaving high school, Joan attended the University of Wisconsin at Madison, and was trained as an actress at the Piven Theater Workshop, in Evanston, Illinois. An appearance as an extra in the 1980 film *Cutting Loose,* was followed by a featured role in *My Bodyguard.* She then appeared for the first of ten times with her brother John, in *Sixteen Candles,* and became a regular on the TV show, 'Saturday Night Live'. She was nominated for a Best Supporting Actress Oscar, for *Working Girl,* which won her the first of three Comedy Awards. In 1993, she married a Chicago attorney, Richard Burke. They have two sons – Dylan and Miles. By the mid-1990s, Joan's was a regular face in excellent comedies and tense dramas. She was again nominated for a Best Supporting Actress Oscar – for *In & Out.* It won her a second American Comedy Award and a NY Film Critics Circle Award.

My Bodyguard (1980)
Class (1983) Sixteen Candles (1984)
Broadcast News (1987) Married to the Mob (1988) Working Girl (1988)
Men Don't Leave (1990) My Blue Heaven (1990) The Cabinet of Dr. Ramirez (1991) Hero (1992)
Addams Family Values (1993)
Corrina, Corrina (1994) Nine Months (1995) Two Much (1995) Grosse Pointe Blank (1997) In & Out (1997) Arlington Road (1999) Cradle Will Rock (1999)
Where the Heart Is (2000) The School of Rock (2003) Raising Helen (2004)
Ice Princess (2005) Friends with Money (2006) War, Inc. (2008)
Kit Kittredge: An American Girl (2008)

John **Cusack**
6ft 2½in
(JOHN PAUL CUSACK)

Born: **June 28, 1966**
Evanston, Illinois, USA

The son of an actor, Dick Cusack, and a mother who had been a political activist, John certainly inherited some dramatic genes. At twelve years of age, he got voice-over jobs. He participated in the Piven Workshop in his home town, before spending a year at New York University. After a supporting role in the film *Class,* in 1983, John achieved fame in several teen movies – the best of which was *Say Anything,* in 1989. For his part in that movie he trained as a kick boxer – a sport he has continued with ever since. An avid fan of 'The Clash', John often appears in his movies wearing a 'Clash' T-shirt. From 1990 onwards he began to take on serious adult roles. In 1992, he learned a lot from Woody Allen, when he had a small part in *Shadows and Fog.* In 1994, John starred in *Bullets Over Broadway.* By the end of that decade, he'd proved himself at the box office and had been nominated for awards for *Being John Malkovich* and *High Fidelity.* He is known to be a man who firmly believes in keeping his private life private, even though he has been very public in his opposition to the Iraq war and the Bush administration in particular.

The Sure Thing (1985)
Stand by Me (1986)
Broadcast News (1987)
Eight Men Out (1988)
Say Anything (1989) **The Grifters** (1990)
True Colors (1991)
Map of the Human Heart (1993)
Bullets Over Broadway (1994)
City Hall (1996) **Con Air** (1997)
Grosse Pointe Blank (1997)
The Thin Red Line (1998)
Being John Malkovich (1999)
High Fidelity (2000)
Serendipity (2001) **Max** (2002)
Identity (2003)
Runaway Jury (2003)
Must Love Dogs (2005)
The Ice Harvest (2005)
Grace Is Gone (2007)
Martian Child (2007)
1408 (2007) **War, Inc.** (2008)

Peter **Cushing**
5ft 11½in
(PETER WILTON CUSHING)

Born: **May 26, 1913**
Kenley, Surrey, England
Died: **August 11, 1994**

Peter spent his early years in Dulwich, south London. After leaving school he worked for two years as a surveyor's assistant. He got a scholarship to the Guildhall School of Music and Drama and began his early career in repertory theater. In 1939, he went to Hollywood, where he made his film debut in *The Man in the Iron Mask* and also appeared in Laurel and Hardy's *A Chump at Oxford.* During World War II he was an entertainer with ENSA. At thirty-five, he got the important role of Osric, in Laurence Olivier's *Hamlet,* but for the next eight years he was only known to British TV audiences. Terence Fisher, who worked as a director for Hammer Films, changed all that. He picked Peter to star in *The Curse of Frankenstein,* in 1956, and Cushing's name became synonymous with juicy horror films filled with blood – in brilliant color. He was actually a gentle shy man, whose hobbies were country walks and bird-watching. When he began playing Sherlock Holmes, his image was softened. In 1971, when Peter's beloved wife Helen died, he attempted suicide. Happily he was unsuccessful and movies such as *Star Wars* introduced him to new audiences. From 1985 onwards, Peter limited both his film and public appearances after being diagnosed with prostate cancer. He died in Canterbury, Kent.

The Curse of Frankenstein (1956)
Dracula (1958)
The Hound of the
Baskervilles (1959)
The Flesh and the Fiends (1960)
Cash on Demand (1961)
Frankenstein Must
Be Destroyed (1969) **Horror**
Express (1973) **The Beast Must**
Die (1974) **Frankenstein and**
the Monster from Hell (1974)
Star Wars (1977)
Shock Waves (1977)
House of the Long Shadows (1983)
Top Secret (1984)
Biggles: Adventures in Time (1986)

Zbyszek **Cybulski**
5ft 9½in
(ZBIGNIEW CYBULSKI)

Born: **November 3, 1927**
Kniaze, Poland
Died: **January 8, 1967**

Zbyszek, as he was always known, was born in a tiny Polish village which is now part of the Ukraine. His father, Alexander, worked in the Ministry of Foreign Affairs and his mother, Eve, looked after their home. After graduating from the Jana Sniadeckiego High School, he made up his mind to be an actor. As a fail-safe, Zbyszek learned journalism at the same time as he was studying at the Higher State School of Acting in Cracow. Happily he didn't need it. After graduating he found theater work in Gdansk – making his stage debut at the Wybrzeze Theater in 1953. Later, with his friend, Bogumil Kobiela, he founded the student theater which they called "Bim-Bom". Zbyszek's first movie, as an extra, was *Kariera* in 1954, but it was Andrzej Wajda's *A Generation,* in which Roman Polanski made his debut, that really set his mind on making movies. By 1958, when he had starred in Wajda's classic film, *Ashes and Diamonds,* Zbyszek was a huge star in Poland and famous in the art-houses of the world. In the early sixties he went to work in Warsaw, where he joined the 'Wagabunda' experimental theater. He was described at the time as Poland's James Dean. There was a similarity in terms of rebellious behavior which was fairly obvious, but very little in physical appearance. What really gave them something in common was Zbyszek's tragically early death. In 1967, when he was on his way home to Warsaw from a film shoot, he was killed after slipping on the icy platform at Wroclaw railway station and falling under a moving train. Forty years after his death, he is still regarded as the best Polish actor ever.

A Generation (1954)
Ashes and Diamonds (1958)
Night Train (1959) **See you**
Tomorrow (1960) **How to be**
Loved (1962) **Att Älska** (1964)
The Saragossa Manuscript (1965)
Salto (1966)

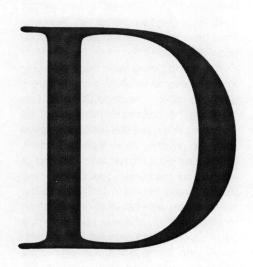

Willem Dafoe
5ft 9½in
(WILLIAM DAFOE JR.)

Born: **July 22, 1955**
Appleton, Wisconsin, USA

He was the seventh of eight children born to Dr. William Dafoe and his wife, Muriel. As a kid, he adopted the name Willem because he hated being called "Billy". After high school, Willem went to the University of Wisconsin to study drama, but left before graduation to join the avant-garde group "Theater X", which toured the United States and Europe. Four years later he moved to New York City, where he became a founding member of the "Wooster Group". He had a son with the director, Elizabeth LeCompte, but twenty years later, he married Giada Colagrande. Willem started his movie career in 1981, with what ended up as an invisible role, in *Heaven's Gate*. In 1982 he starred in *The Loveless* and was considered for the "The Joker" role in *Batman*. His fifty films since then have seen him in a diversity of roles. In 1988 Willem played 'Jesus' – working with Martin Scorsese for the first time. He is very athletic – doing most of his own stunts in the *Spider-Man* series. Many of his performances have received rave reviews. Willem is the only actor in movie history (for playing the part of a vampire) to be nominated for a Best Supporting Actor Oscar – for *Shadow of the Vampire*.

Platoon (1986)
The Last Temptation of Christ (1988)
Mississippi Burning (1988)
Wild at Heart (1990)
Clear and Present Danger (1994)
The English Patient (1996)
Affliction (1997) eXistenZ (1999)
American Psycho (2000)
Shadow of the Vampire (2000)
Spider-Man (2002)
The Life Aquatic with Steve Zissou (2004)
Spider-Man 2 (2004) Control (2004)
The Aviator (2005) Manderlay (2005)
Ripley Under Ground (2005)
American Dreamz (2006)
Inside Man (2006)
Mr. Bean's Holiday (2007)
Spider-Man 3 (2007)
Go Go Tales (2007) Anamorph (2007)
Fireflies in the Garden (2008)

Arlene Dahl
5ft 6in
(ARLENE DAHL)

Born: **August 11, 1928**
Minneapolis, Minnesota, USA

Of Norwegian ancestry, Arlene was a beautiful child – with red hair and perfect skin. As soon as she'd graduated from Washburn High School, in Minneapolis, she took her first step towards a movie career with a series of appearances in local theater productions and modeling for departmental stores. She moved to Hollywood at the end of World War II, after being voted the "Rheingold Beer Girl" of 1946 and signed a contract with Warners. They gave Arlene her film debut, with an uncredited role in the comedy, *Life With Father,* the following year, but it was only after she moved to MGM that her career began to move. *The Bride Goes Wild,* in 1948, was her first film for the studio. It led to starring roles, but she was rarely asked to do do anything more than look lovely. Which was great for her fans. The first of Arlene's six husbands, Lex Barker, who played Tarzan, arrived in 1951, but he ran out of steam with her after only eighteen months. More durable was number two, a Latin Lover called Fernando Lamas, with whom she produced a son, the actor Lorenzo Lamas. She actually guested in his film *Night of the Warrior,* in 1991. Arlene retired from mainstream movies in 1959, after the very successful *Journey to the Center of the Earth,* to become a beauty columnist. She made the occasional movie in France, did television work, and marketed her own brand of Arlene Dahl products, including lingerie and cosmetics. Since 1984, she's been married to her sixth husband, Marc Rosen.

The Bride Goes Wild (1948)
A Southern Yankee (1948)
Ambush (1949)
Reign of Terror (1949)
Three Little Words (1950)
No Questions Asked (1951)
Here Come the Girls (1953)
Woman's World (1954)
Slightly Scarlet (1956)
Journey to the Center of
the Earth (1959)
The Pleasure Pit (1969)

Eva Dahlbeck
5ft 7½in
(EVA DAHLBECK)

Born: **March 8, 1920**
Saltsjö-Duvnäs, Stockholms län, Sweden
Died: **February 8, 2008**

After high school, Eva studied at the Royal Dramatic Theater in Stockholm. She made her professional stage debut in 1941, and a year later, her film debut, in *Rid i Natt!* Throughout the 1940s she continued to work on the stage and in Swedish films. In 1944, she married Colonel Sven Lampell, of the Swedish Air Force. Eva met Ingmar Bergman through her theater work and acted in one of his early film projects – he wrote the story and screenplay for *Eva*. She became well known outside Sweden in the 1950s – beginning with Bergman's *Waiting Women* – one of six of his films she acted in. The others being *A Lesson in Love, Dreams, Smiles of a Summer Night* and *Brink of Life* – for which at Cannes, she shared the Best Actress Award, and *All These Women.* In 1961, she won the Eugene O'Neill Award for her stage work. She spoke good English but made only two appearances in American productions. She was in several episodes of a TV series, 'Foreign Intrigue' and the film, *The Counterfeit Traitor.* In 1970, she retired to start writing – publishing ten novels before the onset of Alzheimer's disease. After her husband Sven died in 2007, Eva's health deteriorated. She died of an infection at Hässelby, Stockholm.

Love Goes Up and Down (1946)
Meeting in the Night (1946)
Eva (1948) Defiance (1952)
Waiting Women (1952)
The Village (1953)
Barabbas (1953)
A Lesson in Love (1954)
Dreams (1955)
Smiles of a Summer Night (1955)
Tarps Elin (1956)
The Last Pair Out (1956)
Möten i skymningen (1957)
Brink of Life (1958)
Tre önskningar (1960)
The Counterfeit Traitor (1962)
All These Women (1964)
Loving Couples (1964)
A Day at the Beach (1970)

Dan **Dailey**
6ft 3in
(DANIEL JAMES DAILEY)

Born: **December 14, 1913**
New York City, New York, USA
Died: **October 16, 1978**

His father, a hotel manager, paid for Dan's dancing lessons until he lost his job at the start of the Great Depression. Luckily for the Daileys, their son had talent and by the time he was sixteen, he was working in minstrel shows and vaudeville. It was the perfect grooming for Broadway and a role in the 1937 production of "Babes in Arms". His easy going style was recognized by Hollywood. MGM signed him and Dan made his movie debut (as a Nazi) in the 1940 drama, *The Mortal Storm*. After that, he was used for what he did best – singing and dancing. He served in the United States Army from 1942 until the end of World War II and his first movie was very appropriately, with the armed forces' favorite pin-up, Betty Grable. He was Oscar-nominated for *When My Baby Smiles at Me*. Dan was a natural light comedian – mixing musicals with comedy for about ten years. From the late 1950s he was seen on television – winning a Golden Globe award in 1969, for 'The Governor & J.J'. His only child, Dan Dailey III, who was born to the third of his four wives, Elizabeth Hofert, committed suicide in 1975. Two years later, Dan made his last film, *The Private Files of J. Edgar Hoover*, and retired. Dan lasted another year before dying of anemia, in New York. His sister is the award-winning actress, Irene Dailey.

Ziegfeld Girl (1941)
Mother Wore Tights (1947)
Give My Regards to Broadway (1948)
When My Baby Smiles At Me (1948)
A Ticket to Tomahawk (1950)
Call Me Mister (1951)
I Can Get It for you Wholesale (1951)
The Girl Next Door (1953)
There's No Business Like
Show Business (1954)
It's Always Fair Weather (1956)
The Best Things in Life are Free (1957)
The Wayward Bus (1957) Hemingway's
Adventures of a Young Man (1962)
The Private Files of
J. Edgar Hoover (1977)

Timothy **Dalton**
6ft 2in
(TIMOTHY PETER DALTON)

Born: **March 21, 1944**
Colwyn Bay, Wales

Tim was the oldest of five children, whose English father – who later worked as an advertising executive, had been stationed in Wales during World War II, with his American-born wife. His dad moved the family to Belper, Derbyshire, after the war, and worked in the advertising industry in Manchester. Tim attended the Herbert Strutt Grammar school, where he was keenly interested in the sciences and was good at sports. Both his grandparents had worked in the old music halls, and their stories sparked an urge to pursue a theatrical career. At sixteen, Tim saw a performance of "Macbeth" and his mind was made up. On leaving secondary school, Tim joined the National Youth Theater and toured with it. From 1964 he studied at the Royal Academy of Dramatic Art in London, which he did not enjoy. Within two years, he had quit to take up the offer of a job with the Birmingham Repertory Theater. He became a professional actor, and played the lead in several of their productions. He first TV role was a starring one, in 1967's drama, 'Saturday While Sunday'. The following year, his film career got off to a flying start when he played King Philip of France, in *The Lion in Winter*. After his Heathcliff in *Wuthering Heights,* Tim was a movie star. His first disaster was with Mae West, in *Sextette,* but he bounced back as James Bond. Unmarried, he has a son with a Ukrainian girl, Oksana Grigorieva.

The Lion in Winter (1968)
Wuthering Heights (1970)
Cromwell (1970)
Giochi particolari (1970)
Mary Queen of Scots (1972)
Permission to Kill (1975)
Agatha (1979)
Flash Gordon (1980)
The Living Daylights (1987)
Hawks (1988) Licence to Kill (1989)
The Informant (1997)
American Outlaws (2001)
Looney Tunes: Back in Action (2003)
Hot Fuzz (2007)

Matt **Damon**
5ft 10in
(MATTHEW PAIGE DAMON)

Born: **October 8, 1970**
Cambridge, Massachusetts, USA

Matt's father, Kent Damon, was a tax preparer. His mother Nancy, was a college professor. Matt and his older brother, Kyle, showed creative talent from an early age. Kyle pursued an artistic career and is now a successful sculptor. In 1989, the year after he had graduated from high school in Cambridge, Matt went on to Harvard University. He interrupted his classes because of his involvement with outside acting projects, which included the 1992 film, *School Ties,* and eventually dropped out. His first big movie appearance was the following year, with a role in Walter Hill's *Geronimo: An American Legend.* With his close friend, Ben Affleck, Matt worked on the script for the 1997 movie *Good Will Hunting,* for which they both received Oscars for the Best Original Screenplay. The two pals then founded "Project Green Light" which was set up to find and fund worthwhile projects by novice filmmakers. Matt is now on the A-list of Hollywood actors and has had a great run of success with the action-packed and hugely popular, 'Bourne' movies. In 2003, while filming *Stuck on You,* Matt first met his wife, Luciana, in Miami – where they now live. A daughter, Isabella, was born in 2005. Matt has only a cameo role in *Che: Part Two,* but there are around half-a-dozen Matt Damon movies awaiting release.

Good Will Hunting (1997)
Saving Private Ryan (1998)
Rounders (1998) Dogma (1999)
The Talented Mr. Ripley (1999)
Ocean's Eleven (2001) Gerry (2002)
The Bourne Identity (2002)
Stuck on You (2003)
EuroTrip (2004)
The Bourne Supremacy (2004)
The Brothers Grimm (2005)
Syriana (2005)
The Departed (2006)
The Good Shepherd (2006)
Ocean's Thirteen (2007)
The Bourne Ultimatum (2007)
Che: Part Two (2008)

Charles **Dance**
6ft 3in
(WALTER CHARLES DANCE)

Born: **October 10, 1946**
Redditch, Worcester, England

Charles dropped the name Walter (his engineer father's name) at an early age. When he was four, his father died and his mother Eleanor took the family to live in Devon. Shortly after he left school, Charles studied graphic design at the Plymouth College of Art. He switched to drama after meeting and being coached by a couple of retired former actors who lived locally. When he was twenty-four, he got married to a girl named Joanna. They had two children and remained together until their divorce in 2004. She saw his career take off with a first outing on television in 1974 – an episode of the series, 'Father Brown'. In tandem with this was a short period of stage activity with the Royal Shakespeare Company. A small part as a German in the 1981 Roger Moore, Bond film, *For Your Eyes Only,* was Charles' movie debut. It was followed by more television, including his starring role in a 1984 mini-series, 'The Jewel in the Crown' – for which he was nominated for a Best Actor BAFTA – and it introduced him to a wider audience. Since the late 1980s, Charles has been seen a lot more regularly on the big screen in top films such as *Gosford Park.*

Plenty (1985)
White Mischief (1987)
Good Morning, Babylon (1987)
Pascali's Island (1988)
Hidden City (1988)
La Valle di pietra (1992)
Alien 3 (1992)
Century (1993)
Kabloonak (1995)
Michael Collins (1996)
What Rats Won't Do (1998)
Hilary and Jackie (1998)
Chrono-Perambulator (1999)
Dark Blue World (2001)
Gosford Park (2001)
Black and White (2002)
Swimming Pool (2003)
Labyrinth (2003)
Scoop (2006)
Twice Upon a Time (2006)
Intervention (2007)

Hugh **Dancy**
5ft 11in
(HUGH DANCY)

Born: **June 19, 1975**
Stoke-on-Trent, Staffs, England

Hugh was the eldest of three children. His father Jonathan Dancy, is both a writer and a philosophy professor, at Reading University and the University of Texas, at Austin. His mother Sarah, is a book publisher. He was educated at Winchester College, in Hampshire, and at St. Peter's College Oxford, from where he graduated with degrees in English and English Literature. After that, he moved down to London to seek work as an actor. His first role was in the TV dramatization of Lynda La Plante's crime drama, 'Trial and Retribution' in 1998. While keeping himself alive with jobs as a barman or a waiter, he had parts in TV series such as 'Kavanagh Q.C.' and 'Dangerfield'. What got his career moving faster was a role in the costume drama, 'Madame Bovary' in 2000. Hugh not only looked the part – he followed up with 'David Copperfield'. Hugh's film debut was in 2001, as D'Artagnan, in the cooly received, *Young Blades.* Later that year, he was praised for his work in a supporting role, in Ridley Scott's powerful war movie, *Black Hawk Down.* From then on he's had star billing in popular movies such as *Ella Enchanted* and *Shooting Dogs.* He's even found the time to feature with the supermodel Kate Moss, in Burberry's advertising campaign. He met Claire Danes when they were making the movie, *Evening,* and the chemistry was right – both on and off screen. Hugh now chooses to live in New York, where he recently appeared as Captain Dennis Stanhope, in "Journey's End" at Broadway's Belasco Theater.

Black Hawk Down (2001)
The Sleeping Dictionary (2003)
Tempo (2003)
Ella Enchanted (2004)
King Arthur (2004)
Shooting Dogs (2005)
Blood and Chocolate (2007)
Savage Grace (2007)
Evening (2007)
The Jane Austin
Book Club (2007) **Adam** (2009)

Dorothy **Dandridge**
5ft 5in
(DOROTHY JEAN DANDRIDGE)

Born: **November 9, 1922**
Cleveland, Ohio, USA
Died: **September 8, 1965**

Dorothy's father, Cyril Dandridge, was a minister. Her mother, Ruby, was an aspiring dancer. After she and Cyril parted, she formed a group with her daughters – known as "The Dandridge Sisters". They performed with great success at both the Cotton Club and the Apollo Theater. At the start of the Great Depression gigs became scarce and Ruby took her family to Los Angeles. Her intention was to make a new career in Hollywood for herself and her children. She got small parts on the radio and in films while her children, who had missed out on education, went to school. In 1935, Dorothy had a bit part in an 'Our Gang' short, called *Teacher's Beau,* and in 1937, she appeared in the Marx Brothers' *A day at the Races.* It was difficult for a black woman to get decent parts and her next acting opportunity was in 1940, when she played a murderess in a 'race film' titled *Four Shall Die.* She supported big stars for ten years. Dorothy married in 1942, but her only child was mentally handicapped. At that time she was appearing in poverty row musicals and booked to sing at hotels where she wasn't allowed to stay. In 1954, Dorothy starred in the all-black, *Carmen Jones,* and was nominated for an Oscar, but life wasn't good. Her second husband (a white restaurant owner) took her money. She made her last screen appearance in 1962 – on TV – an episode of the crime drama series,'Cain's Hundred'. One year later, she declared bankruptcy. She was drinking heavily and after fracturing her foot she committed suicide in her West Hollywood apartment with an overdose of an antidepressant. Dorothy was born forty years too soon – today she would be a big star.

Sundown (1941)
Bright Road (1953)
Carmen Jones (1954)
Island in the Sun (1957)
Tamango (1958)
The Decks Ran Red (1958)
Porgy and Bess (1959)

Claire **Danes**
5ft 5½in
(CLAIRE CATHERINE DANES)

Born: **April 12, 1979**
Manhattan, New York City, New York, USA

Claire is the product of a creative home, where her father Chris was a computer expert who had been an architectural photographer. He met her mother Carla – a painter and textile designer, at the Rhode Island School of Design. So it was natural that the couple should recognize and encourage their daughter's potential. Claire was six when she began modern dance classes and nine when she was enrolled at the Lee Strasberg Theater Institute. Conventional schooling was very difficult as she was often out working as an actress, but she did attend Dalton School, on New York's Upper East Side. She made her film debut in 1990, in an independent production called *Dreams of Love* and continued to get TV work as well as important film roles like Beth March in *Little Women*. She won a Golden Globe for playing Angela Chase in the TV series 'My So-Called Life' and landed the title role in *Romeo + Juliet*. At eighteen, she went to Yale as a psychology major, but dropped out after two years to concentrate on acting. Her career is now very much in the ascendancy and she's not limiting it to movies. Claire will soon be making her Broadway debut, as Eliza Doolittle, in George Bernard Shaw's "Pygmalion". A cockney accent should prove no problem, as her current flame is the English actor, Hugh Dancy.

Little Women (1994)
The Pesky Suitor (1995)
Home for the Holidays (1995)
Romeo + Juliet (1996)
U Turn (1997)
The Rainmaker (1997)
Les Misérables (1998)
Brokedown Palace (1999)
Igby Goes Down (2002)
The Hours (2002)
Stage Beauty (2004)
Shopgirl (2005)
The Family Stone (2005)
Evening (2007) The Flock (2007)
Stardust (2007)
Me and Orson Welles (2008)

Beverly **D'Angelo**
5ft 2in
(BEVERLY HEATHER D'ANGELO)

Born: **November 15, 1951**
Columbus, Ohio, USA

Beverly's father Gene, who was of Italian descent, was a bass player in a band, and the General Manager of WBNS-TV, in Columbus. Beverly's mother Priscilla, was a violinist. As a child, Beverly showed sufficient talent to study visual arts. When she finished her studies she got a job as a cartoonist at Hanna-Barbera Studios, in Hollywood. She spent some time as a folk singer in Canada, and was good enough to tour with a rock band called "Elephant". It was a skill she would use in one of her early movies. She'd begun acting in regional theaters and by the early 1970s, had made her Broadway debut, playing Ophelia, in the rock musical "Rockabye Hamlet". Beverly made her film debut in 1976, in Michael Winner's *The Sentinel* and she appeared briefly in Woody Allen's *Annie Hall* that same year. But it was her portrayal of Patsy Cline, in *Coal Miner's Daughter*, which earned her much critical praise. In 1981, her romance with film director, Milos Forman, ended, and she began a short marriage to an economics student – Italian Duke – Lorenzo de Medici. She lived with Irish director, Neil Jordan, from 1985 until 1991. For twenty-five years Beverly's been seen regularly in a mixture of good and bad films and television roles. She became seriously involved with Al Pacino, and in 2001, she gave birth to their twins. Unfortunately, they broke up shortly after that and have been battling over custody ever since.

Hair (1979)
Coal Miner's Daughter (1980)
Maid to Order (1987)
Christmas Vacation (1989)
Miracle (1991)
Eye for an Eye (1996)
Illuminata (1998)
American History X (1998)
King of the Corner (2004)
Gamers (2006)
Relative Strangers (2006)
Harold & Kumar Escape from
Guantanamo Bay (2008)
The House Bunny (2008)

Henry **Daniell**
6ft
(CHARLES HENRY DANIELL)

Born: **March 5, 1894**
London, England
Died: **October 31, 1963**

Henry was educated as a day boy at St. Paul's School, in Hammersmith, West London, before boarding at Gresham's School, in Norfolk. After small roles in provincial theaters he made his London stage debut in 1914, in "Kismet". World War I had started, so he joined the 2nd Battalion Norfolk Regiment. In 1915, he was wounded and invalided out. He spent the rest of the war establishing himself on the London stage. Henry first went to New York in 1921, and he was commuting between there and London for the next ten years. In 1929, he made his film debut in the comedy, *The Awful Truth,* which was shot in America. Henry's first major movie was in Greta Garbo's *Camille.* The actor had struck a rich vein – appearing in strong supporting roles in hit after hit. His duel with Errol Flynn in *The Sea Hawk* was one of the best ever filmed. He transferred to television work with ease. Henry died from a heart attack after shooting a scene in *My Fair Lady,* in which he appeared in a small role, as a foreign Ambassador.

Camille (1936) The Firefly (1937)
Madame X (1937)
Holiday (1938)
Marie Antoinette (1938)
The Private Lives of Elizabeth
and Essex (1939)
We Are Not Alone (1939)
The Sea Hawk (1940)
All This, and Heaven Too (1940)
The Great Dictator (1940)
The Philadelphia Story (1940)
A Woman's Face (1941)
Sherlock Holmes and the
Voice of Terror (1942)
Sherlock Holmes in Washington (1943)
Watch on the Rhine (1943)
Jane Eyre (1944)
The Body Snatcher (1945)
The Exile (1947)
The Egyptian (1954)
Lust for Life (1956)
Witness for the Prosecution (1957)
The Comancheros (1961)

Bebe **Daniels**
5ft 3in
(PHYLLIS VIRGINIA DANIELS)

Born: **January 14, 1901**
Dallas, Texas, USA
Died: **March 16, 1971**

Bebe's father was a theater manager and her mother was a stage actress. It wasn't long before she made her first appearance (aged four) in a stage production of "The Squaw Man". By the time her family had moved to Los Angeles, she was so used to acting she had no problem facing the lights and cameras for her first movie, a short, *The Courtship of Miss Standish*. In March 1922, when Bebe celebrated her twenty-first birthday, she was a veteran of over 200 films. Admittedly, most of them were 2-reelers, but that kid was certainly busy! It didn't change in the run-up to her first talkie – the musical, *Rio Rita*. In 1930, Bebe married her second big love (her first was Harold Lloyd) – film actor Ben Lyon. They co-starred in that year's *Alias French Gertie* and were together for forty-one years. In five years until the Lyons moved to England, Bebe saw her popularity as a movie star decline. She starred in some good movies – most famous of them was the classic 1930s musical – *42nd Street*, when co-stars included Warner Baxter, George Brent and Ruby Keeler. After her Warner Brothers contract lapsed, Bebe played opposite John Barrymore in one of his most powerful dramas, *Counsellor at Law*. She bowed out from the American screen with the new star Alice Faye, in *Music Is Magic*. In 1936, she and Ben made a BBC TV pilot in an episode of 'Starlight'. They would later be famous in Britain for their radio show, 'Life with the Lyons' – which featured their two children – Richard and Barbara. Bebe died in London, of a cerebral hemorrhage.

Rio Rita (1929)
Dixiana (1930)
Reaching for the Moon (1930)
My Past (1931)
The Maltese Falcon (1931)
Silver Dollar (1932) **A Southern
Maid** (1933) **42nd Street** (1933)
Cocktail Hour (1933)
Counsellor at Law (1933)
Music Is Magic (1935)

Jeff **Daniels**
6ft 3in
(CHARLES HENRY DANIEL)

Born: **February 19, 1955**
Athens, Georgia, USA

Jeff grew up as a Methodist in Chelsea, Michigan, where his father, Robert Lee Daniels, ran a lumber yard. He attended Central Michigan University, where he showed promise as an actor. In 1979, he appeared in New York's Second Stage Theater's inaugural season – in "The Shortchanged Review". It was also the year he married his high school sweetheart, Kathleen Treado. They had three children and still live in Chelsea, where Jeff founded the Purple Rose Theater. Since making his first film appearance – in *Ragtime,* in 1981 – Jeff has had a steady career in the movies, making a very high percentage of good films. He was Golden Globe-nominated three times – for *The Purple Rose of Cairo, Something Wild* and *The Squid and the Whale*. Two of his recent efforts – *Infamous* and *The Lookout* – are well worth your time. If his film career ever stops, he has thirty years experience of writing songs to draw on. If you want to hear Jeff sing and play his guitar, get the recent CD *'Grandfather's Hat'* or catch him at a live gig. Jeff's not superstitious – he got married on Friday the 13th and wore number 13 when he played baseball. He supports the Detroit Tigers.

Terms of Endearment (1983)
The Purple Rose of Cairo (1985)
Something Wild (1986)
Radio Days (1987)
The House on Carroll Street (1988)
Arachnophobia (1990)
Grand Tour: Disaster in Time (1992)
Gettysburg (1993) **Speed** (1994)
Dumb & Dumber (1994)
Fly Away Home (1996)
Pleasantville (1998)
Chasing Sleep (2000)
Blood Work (2002) **The Hours** (2002)
Imaginary Heroes (2004)
The Squid and the Whale (2005)
Good Night and Good Luck (2005)
Infamous (2006)
The Lookout (2007)
Traitor (2008)
State of Play (2009)

Paul **Dano**
6ft 1in
(PAUL FRANKLIN DANO)

Born: **June 19, 1984**
New York City, New York, USA

Paul's father was a businessman in New York. For the first few years of his education, Paul went to the Browning School in the heart of the city's Upper East Side. After the Dano family transferred to New Canaan, Connecticut, he attended Wilton High School, which fired his ambition to be an actor. He graduated from Wilton in 2002. He had been involved with the local community theater for some time and had attended casting sessions in New York before landing his first film role in 2000, a weak family drama, *The Newcomers*, with the saving grace of involving future talent Kate Bosworth, Billy Kay and Chris Evans. Paul's next project, *L.I.E.* was, by contrast, a real winner – earning him awards as far away as Stockholm. Paul's other talent – the musical one – wasn't neglected. He played lead guitar and sang vocals with the Wilton-based band, "Mook". He continued with his education – studying English and literature at Pace University, in downtown Manhattan, and going on to study literature at Eugene Lang College – the new School for Liberal Arts – in Greenwich Village. Paul's film career has taken off since *Little Miss Sunshine* – for which he shared two 'cast' awards. His big breakthrough was in *There Will Be Blood,* in which he had the chance to put his acting skills to the test in the company of Best Actor Oscar winner, Daniel Day-Lewis. Paul learned a hell of a lot from that experience, and for his truly exceptional performance he was nominated for a BAFTA Best Supporting Actor Award.

L.I.E. (2001)
The Emperor's Club (2002)
Light and the Sufferer (2004)
Taking Lives (2004)
The Ballad of Jack
and Rose (2005)
The King (2005)
Fast Food Nation (2006)
Little Miss Sunshine (2006)
There Will Be Blood (2007)
Explicit Ills (2008)
Gigantic (2008)

Ted **Danson**
6ft 2½in
(EDWARD BRIDGE DANSON III)

Born: **December 29, 1947**
San Diego, California, USA

He is the son of Edward Bridge Danson Jr., an archaeologist and museum director, and his wife Jessica. Ted, who is of British ancestry, grew up in Flagstaff, Arizona. When he was twelve, he was sent to Kent School, a boarding school in Connecticut, where he became the star basketball player. At Stanford University, he first became seriously interested in acting. He transferred to Carnegie Institute of Technology, where he gained a bachelor's degree. Ted married his first wife, Randy, in 1970. They were divorced in the very year his career was getting started. In 1975, following TV-commercial work, he began his television acting career in the soap opera, 'Somerset'. Four years later, he made his movie debut in the excellent *The Onion Field*. It led in 1982, to the TV show that made him a household name – 'Cheers'. After that popular series, he would always be remembered as the bartender, Sam Malone. Ted has appeared in a large number of films – several of which were not very good. Recently, he seems to have hit a purple patch with strong roles in movies such as the superb, *Nobel Son*. There are a couple more in the pipeline waiting for release. Ted is currently married to his third wife, that fine experienced actress, Mary Steenburgen – with whom he first worked in the film *Pontiac Moon*. They live in Oxford, Mississippi.

The Onion Field (1979)
Body Heat (1981)
Creepshow (1982)
3 Men and a Baby (1987)
Cousins (1989)
Dad (1989)
Pontiac Moon (1994)
Loch Ness (1996)
Jerry and Tom (1998)
Homegrown (1998)
Saving Private Ryan (1998)
Mumford (1999)
The Moguls (2005)
Nobel Son (2007)
Mad Money (2008)
The Human Contract (2008)

Helmut **Dantine**
6ft
(HELMUT GUTTMAN)

Born: **October 7, 1917**
Vienna, Austro-Hungary
Died: **May 2, 1982**

When the threat to Europe by Hitler's Germany became a real concern, he was outspoken enough to be arrested by the Nazis and imprisoned in a concentration camp for three months. Helmut's parents urged him to leave and arranged for him to stay with a friend in California. In 1939 he started his acting career at the Pasadena Playhouse. His personality and looks were exactly what the Hollywood studios were after. Helmut had a small uncredited role in the 1940 film, *Escape,* before signing a contract with Warner Bros. His first credited role was as a German pilot, in *Mrs. Miniver,* and there was an even stronger part for him in *Edge of Darkness,* with Errol Flynn. During the war, apart from a small and sympathetic role in *Casablanca,* he greatly helped the propaganda effort by portraying nasty Germans. He appeared on television during the 1950s, but still got decent movie roles. After his acting career slowed down, Helmut tried his hand at directing and later, producing movies. His second wife Niki, was the daughter of Loew's president, Nicholas Schenk and Helmut became the president of Schenk Enterprises in 1970 – producing two Sam Peckinpah movies – including *Bring Me the Head of Alfred Garcia,* both of which he acted in. Helmut died of heart failure at his home in Beverly Hills.

Mrs. Miniver (1942)
Edge of Darkness (1943)
Mission to Moscow (1943)
Watch on the Rhine (1943)
Northern Pusuit (1943)
Passage to Marseille (1944)
Hotel Berlin (1945)
Whispering City (1947)
Call Me Madam (1953)
War and Peace (1956)
Fräulein (1958) **La Tempesta** (1958)
Operation Crossbow (1965)
**Bring Me the Head of
Alfred Garcia** (1974)
The Wilby Conspiracy (1975)
The Killer Elite (1975)

Ray **Danton**
6ft 1in
(RAYMOND KAPLAN)

Born: **September 19, 1931**
New York City, New York, USA
Died: **February 11, 1992**

Ray's first exposure to the world of show business was at the age of four, when his voice was heard on NBC's radio show, 'Let's Pretend'. He attended the Horace Mann School and then studied acting at Carnegie Tech, in Pittsburgh. His first role was in an episode of the television science fiction series, 'Out There', in 1951. After a few more TV roles in New York, he got a Hollywood contract with Universal. In 1954, he married one of the studio's stars, Julie Adams, and made his movie debut in 1955, as 'Little Big Man' in *Chief Crazy Horse.* That same year, Ray appeared with Rory Calhoun in a couple of westerns. In 1956, he shared the "Most Promising Newcomer" Golden Globe, with Russ Tamblyn. With parallel careers in films and TV, he was able to remain fully employed for the next twenty years. A 1960 biographical movie, *The Rise and Fall of Legs Diamond,* featured his most memorable performance, in the title role. During the 1960s, he made a number of unmemorable films in Italy and Spain. Back in the USA, Ray turned his hand to directing movies with limited success but had much better luck with popular TV series such as 'Quincy', 'The Incredible Hulk', 'Dallas' and 'Cagney & Lacey'. His last screen appearance was on television, in an episode of 'Barnaby Jones' in 1977. Ray died of kidney disease in Los Angeles.

The Looters (1955) **The Spoilers** (1955)
I'll Cry Tomorrow (1955)
Too Much Too Soon (1958)
Tarawa Beachhead (1958)
The Big Operator (1959)
Yellowstone Kelly (1959)
Ice Palace (1960)
**The Rise and Fall of
Legs Diamond** (1960)
A Fever in the Blood (1961)
Portrait of a Mobster (1961)
The George Raft Story (1961)
A Majority of One (1961)
The Longest Day (1962)
The Chapman Report (1962)

Linda **Darnell**
5ft 4in
(MONETTA ELOYSE DARNELL)

Born: **October 16, 1923**
Dallas, Texas, USA
Born: **April 10, 1965**

Because Linda's mother was obsessed with making money from her pretty daughter, she sent her to dancing lessons when she was five. At eleven, she was modeling – giving her age as sixteen – and doing amateur theater work. When she was really sixteen, she went to Hollywood for a screen test, and was signed by 20th Century-Fox. Linda was given the lead in *Hotel for Women* and Darryl Zanuck was impressed. By the time she was twenty she'd starred in nine movies, but hadn't really caught on with audiences. After Linda married the studio's cameraman, Peverell Marley, she was freed from her mother's clutches and her career began to move forward. She decorated horror films, musicals and comedies; starred in one of John Ford's finest westerns; and the critically panned, box office success, *Forever Amber* – both films increased her standing at the studio and kept her on top for a further three years. When filming *A Letter to Three Wives,* Linda fell in love with its director Joe Mankiewicz, who was married. She contemplated suicide, but took friendly therapy from Norman Rockwell, who taught her to paint. In the 1950s, her popularity waned and she became an alcoholic, put on weight, married twice more, did TV guest spots, and acted in poor films. She was sleeping on the couch in a friend's apartment when her cigarette caused a fire and she was burnt alive.

The Mark of Zorro (1940)
Blood and Sand (1941)
It Happened Tomorrow (1944)
Summer Storm (1944)
Hangover Square (1945)
Fallen Angel (1945)
My Darling Clementine (1947)
Forever Amber (1947)
Unfaithfully Yours (1948)
A Letter to Three Wives (1949)
Everybody Does It (1949)
No Way Out (1950)
Second Chance (1953)
Zero Hour! (1957)

Danielle **Darrieux**
5ft 4¹/₂in
(YVONNE MARIE ANTIONETTE DARRIEUX)

Born: **May 1, 1917**
Bordeaux, Gironde, Aquitaine, France

Danielle's birthplace was a rich source of talented people who were successful in music, theater and cinema during the twentieth century. Her father, an army doctor, moved the family to Paris in 1919, but he died five years later. Her mother was wealthy enough for Danielle to study cello at the Paris Conservatoire. In 1931, with mother's encouragement, Danielle (who was a natural actress) auditioned for a film called *Le Bal,* and got the part. She had supporting roles in half a dozen films before her international breakthrough, in *Mayerling.* In Paris in 1937, she made her stage debut in "Jeux Dangereux". Danielle went to Hollywood that same year and signed a nine-year contract with Universal. In the event she made only one movie for them – *The Rage of Paris,* which was a big success. The studio wanted more, but she was homesick and threatened to sue. World War II intervened and she made movies for the Germans in occupied Paris. In 1942 she married the playboy, Porfirio Rubirosa. After the war, she remained the biggest female star in France – on stage – as well as in films and on records. She even returned to Hollywood in the 1950s, for *Rich, Young and Pretty,* and outshone the film's cast. She continues to delight audiences right up to her 92nd year.

Mauvaise graine (1934)
La Crise est finie (1934)
Mayerling (1936)
Club des femmes (1936)
Abus de confiance (1938)
The Rage of Paris (1938)
Battement de coeur (1940)
Adieu Chérie (1946)
Ruy Blas (1948) La Ronde (1950)
Rich, Young and Pretty (1951)
5 Fingers (1952)
Madame de...(1953)
Le Rouge et le noir (1954)
Le Salaire du péché (1956)
Pot-Bouille (1957)
La Vie à deux (1958)
Marie-Octobre (1959)
The Greengage Summer (1961)

Jane **Darwell**
5ft 6in
(PATTI WOODWARD)

Born: **October 15, 1879**
Palmyra, Missori, USA
Died: **August 13, 1967**

Jane was the daughter of a wealthy railroad executive. She was raised on a sprawling ranch in Missouri. When she was little, she demonstrated a fine singing voice, but her ambitions to be an opera singer were quashed by her disciplinarian father. She never married and took a long time to leave home. When she did, she changed her name to Darwell. She made her stage debut in Chicago, in 1912, and the following year, she was in a short silent film called *The Capture of Aguinaldo.* She'd been in a dozen films when, in 1915, she decided to concentrate on the stage for the next several years. Director, John Cromwell lured her back to the screen in 1930, not just by offering her a small role in his film, *Tom Sawyer,* but because she was keen to play in a talkie. She enjoyed it so much, she became a familiar face in movies throughout the next two decades. In 1933, Jane signed a contract with 20th Century Fox. She was in popular Shirley Temple films, including *Bright Eyes* and *Captain January* and was in the cast of *Gone with the Wind.* Her performance in *The Grapes of Wrath* won her a Best Supporting Actress Oscar. She was a respected professional – working up to her 85th year – when she acted in *Mary Poppins.* Jane died of a heart attack.

Design for Living (1933)
Poor Little Rich Girl (1936)
Craig's Wife (1936)
Slave Ship (1937)
Little Miss Broadway (1938)
Jesse James (1939)
Gone with the Wind (1939)
The Grapes of Wrath (1940)
The Devil and Daniel Webster (1941)
All Through the Night (1941)
The Ox-Bow Incident (1943)
Sunday Dinner for a Soldier (1944)
My Darling Clementine (1946)
3 Godfathers (1948)
Wagon Master (1950)
Caged (1950) The Bigamist (1953)
There's Always Tomorrow (1956)

Claude **Dauphin**
5ft 8in
(CLAUDE MARIE EUGÉNE LEGRAND)

Born: **August 19, 1903**
Corbeil-Essonnes, France
Died: **November 16, 1978**

Although both his parents were French music hall performers, Claude decided to start his theatrical career as a set designer. With a front row view of stage productions, he soon decided to give acting a try and made his first appearance in "Tristan Bernard". After doing a voice-over commentary for an animated movie called *Le Roman du Renard* (The Story of a Fox) in 1930, he made his film debut in *Figuration* the following year. Throughout the 1930s and into the 40s, he was unknown outside France. He had acted in almost forty films when he came to England for a so-so British Comedy, *English Without Tears,* which starred one of Elizabeth Taylor's future husbands – Michael Wilding. What did make him known and sought after was a wonderful film with Simone Signoret, titled *Casque d'Or.* After that, he was in a few English language films including *The Quiet American* and *Grand Prix.* Claude worked in films and on television right up until his death in Paris – from intestinal occlusion. Claude's son, Jean-Claude, is a successful actor.

Jean de la Lune (1949)
Le Plaisir (1952)
Casque d'or (1952)
Innocents in Paris (1953)
Little Boy Lost (1953)
Phantom of the
Rue Morgue (1954)
Les Mauvaises rencontres (1955)
The Quiet American (1958)
Le Diable et les dix
commandements (1962)
Symphonie pour un
massacre (1963)
La Bonne soupe (1964)
The Visit (1964)
Paris brule-t-il? (1966)
Grand Prix (1966)
Two for the Road (1967)
Barbarella (1968)
Églantine (1971)
L'Important c'est d'aimer (1975)
The Tenant (1976)

Jack **Davenport**
6ft 2in
(JACK DAVENPORT)

Born: **March 1, 1973**
Suffolk, England

The son of actors, Nigel Davenport and Maria Aitken, Jack lived with his parents on the Mediterranean island of Ibiza for the first seven years of his life. At that point, his parents got divorced and he was sent to board at the Dragon School, in Oxford. He completed his early education (like his dad) at Cheltenham College. After that, he attended a drama course and was invited by a director from the Welsh National Theater to go and work in Wales. Jack acted in a lot of classic plays including Shakespeare's "Hamlet" and he became a close friend of the actor, Rhys Ifans. A year or so after that, he went to the University of East Anglia, in Norwich, for film studies coupled with English Literature. While he was there he did some acting, but felt more inclined towards a future as a member of a film crew. With this in mind, his mother suggested that he should write to John Cleese to ask if he could work on the set of John's film, *Fierce Creatures.* He wound up in the cast – as an assistant zoo keeper – and knew immediately that acting was his future. He found an agent and in 1996, was in the BBC TV drama, "This Life'. Reaction was good – leading to a number of roles in films – including *The Talented Mr. Ripley* and the box-office hit, *Pirates of the Caribbean: The Curse of the Black Pearl,* and its sequels. Jack has also provided the voice over for Mastercard TV commercials. He's been married to the actress, Michelle Gomez, since 2000.

The Talented Mr. Ripley (1999)
Sunterrain (2001)
Gypsy Woman (2001)
Not Afraid, Not Afraid (2001)
The Bunker (2001)
Pirates of the Caribbean:
The Curse of the Black Pearl (2003)
The Libertine (2004)
The Wedding Date (2005)
Pirates 2 (2006)
The Key Man (2007)
Pirates of the Caribbean:
At World's End (2007)
The Boat That Rocked (2009)

Nigel **Davenport**
5ft 10½in
(NIGEL DAVENPORT)

Born: **May 23, 1928**
Shelford, Cambridgeshire, England

The son of a Cambridge University Don, Nigel was at Cheltenham College at the same time as Lindsay Anderson. He then went to Oxford University, where he was an enthusiastic member of the Dramatic Society. After spending several years with various repertory companies and at Stratford, he went to work for the newly-formed Independent Television Network and for four years had a lot of fun in 'The Adventures of Robin Hood'. In 1959, he began his film career with a small role in *Look Back in Anger.* While continuing to do film work, Nigel's next step was to join the English Stage Company at London's Royal Court Theater. His first important role was in "A Taste of Honey", which later transferred to Broadway. His first telling film role was as the Duke of Norfolk, in Fred Zinnemann's *A Man for All Seasons.* Throughout the thirty years that followed, Nigel was in many good movies and had a string of hits at the end of the 1960s. On television, he was praised for his acting in the 1974 dramatization of 'South Riding' as well as for his portrayal of the mad King George III, in the 1979 BBC series 'Prince Regent'. Nigel retired in 2000, but his two actor children – his daughter Laura, and his son Jack – are doing their best to keep the Davenport name famous.

The Third Secret (1964)
Sands of the Kalahari (1965)
Life at the Top (1965)
A Man for All Seasons (1966)
Play Dirty (1968)
Sebastian (1968)
The Strange Affair (1968)
Sinful Davey (1969)
The Royal Hunt of the Sun (1969)
The Virgin Soldiers (1969)
No Blade of Grass (1970)
The Last Valley (1970) Villain (1971)
Mary, Queen of Scots (1971)
Phase IV (1974) Zulu Dawn (1979)
Chariots of Fire (1981)
Nighthawks (1981)
Caravaggio (1986)
Without a Clue (1988)

Lolita **Davidovich**
5ft 8in
(LOLITA DAVIDOVIAE)

Born: **July 15, 1961**
London, Ontario, Canada

Lolly was the daughter of immigrants from what was then known as the Socialist Federal Republic of Yugoslavia. Her father was from Belgrade – now the capital of Serbia – and her mother was from what is now known as Slovenia. Because of her parents Lolly spoke nothing but their common language, Serbian, until, at five years of age, she was introduced to the Canadian school system. Apart the fact that she was a tall, good-looking redhead, she didn't do much more than appear in a few plays during her high school years. In 1974, she'd made up her mind – heading for New York City, where she enrolled as a drama student at the Herbert Berghof Studio. After she'd graduated, Lolly did the rounds of the casting agents and in 1981, got her first television assignment, in an episode of 'Three's Company'. Two years later, she made her film debut, with a small role in the comedy/drama, *Class*. It was her title role in *Blaze,* opposite Paul Newman, which first established her as a movie actress. Her only award so far was at the 1993 Tokyo Film Festival, for one of her least appealing movies, *Younger and Younger.* But she has plenty of good films on her c.v. My personal favorites are *Gods and Monsters, Mystery Alaska* and *Dark Blue.* She has a daughter, Valentina, with her writer/director husband, Ron Shelton. Lolly is currently working on a film called *Antique,* set in Echo Park, Los Angeles.

Adventures in Babysitting (1987)
Blaze (1989)
The Object of Beauty (1991)
JFK (1991)
The Inner Circle (1991)
Raising Cain (1992)
Leap of Faith (1992)
Cobb (1994)
Now and Then (1995)
Salt Water Moose (1996)
Gods and Monsters (1998)
Play It to the Bone (1999)
Mystery Alaska (1999)
Dark Blue (2002)
September Dawn (2006)

Marion **Davies**
5ft 5in
(MARION CECELIA DOURAS)

Born: **January 3, 1897**
Brooklyn, New York City, New York, USA
Died: **September 22, 1961**

Marion was the youngest of five children born to a Judge – Bernard J. Douras and his wife, Rose Reilly. They changed their name to Davies in the belief that it was more acceptable in the melting pot of new immigrants which represented New York City. Marion attended a Roman Catholic school, the Convent of the Sacred Heart in Hastings, N.Y., but her brother-in-law, theatrical producer, George Lederer, got her a job in the chorus of one of his shows when she was seventeen. After Broadway productions including "Ziegfeld Follies", Marion made her film debut in 1917's *Runaway Romany,* which Lederer directed. William Randolph Hearst saw it, fell madly in love with her and began to promote her throughout his newspaper empire. Hearst master-minded her first starring role, in *Cecilia of the Pink Roses,* in 1918, and he made sure it got rave reviews. Under his guidance, she enjoyed ten years of silent stardom and became a fine comedienne. The problem with sound was her stutter. Even the lovestruck Hearst approached her first talkie *The Five O'Clock Girl* with trepidation. Her stutter proved a plus – especially in her next film *The Patsy,* and in several comedies she made for Warner Bros. Age was the thing that finished her. After her final film *Ever Since Eve,* Hearst's business collapsed and she gave him money and creature comforts until his death in 1951. Marion married Horace Brown and died of cancer, in Hollywood, ten years later.

The Patsy (1928) **The Cardboard Lover** (1928) **Show People** (1928) **Marianne** (1929) **Not So Dumb** (1930) **The Florodora Girl** (1930) **The Bachelor Father** (1931) **It's a Wise Child** (1931) **Five and Ten** (1931) **Polly of the Circus** (1932) **Blondie of the Follies** (1932) **Peg o' My Heart** (1933) **Operator 13** (1934) **Page Miss Glory** (1935) **Cain and Mabel** (1936) **Ever Since Eve** (1937)

Bette **Davis**
5ft 3in
(RUTH ELIZABETH DAVIS)

Born: **April 5, 1908**
Lowell, Massachusetts, USA
Died: **October 6, 1989**

Bette's parents, Harlow Davis, and his wife Ruthie, got divorced when she was seven, and she and her sister were raised by their mother. She attended Cushing Academy, a boarding school, and while there, she went to see a production of Ibsen's "The Wild Duck". It inspired Bette to become an actress, but her application to the Manhattan Civic Repertory was turned down. Unfazed, she enrolled at John Murray Anderson's Dramatic School and became its star pupil. In 1923, she got a part in the off-Broadway play, "The Earth Between", but it was six more years before she made her Broadway debut, in "Broken Dishes". In 1930, she signed a contract with Universal. It was doomed to failure after her first film, *The Bad Sister* bombed. Luckily *The Man Who Played God,* made her a star. She won Oscars for *Dangerous* and *Jezebel,* and was nominated for eight others, including *The Letter, Now, Voyager,* and *All About Eve.* As four failed marriages may suggest, Bette's career always came first. She died in France, of metastasized breast cancer.

The Man Who Played God (1932)
Of Human Bondage (1934)
Dangerous (1935) **The Petrified Forest** (1936) **Jezebel** (1938)
The Private Lives of Elizabeth and Essex (1939)
Dark Victory (1939) **Juarez** (1939)
The Old Maid (1939) **The Letter** (1940)
All This and Heaven Too (1940)
The Little Foxes (1941)
The Man Who Came To Dinner (1941)
Now Voyager (1942)
Mr.Skeffington (1944)
All About Eve (1950)
The Star (1952) **The Catered Affair** (1956) **The Scapegoat** (1959)
Whatever Happened to Baby Jane? (1962)
The Anniversary (1968)
Death on the Nile (1978)
The Watcher in the Woods (1980)
The Whales of August (1987)

Geena **Davis**
6ft
(VIRGINIA ELIZABETH DAVIS)

Born: **January 21, 1956**
Wareham, Massachusetts, USA

Geena was the daughter of William Morris, a civil engineer, and his wife Lucille, who was a teacher's assistant. As a child, she showed a talent for music and by her early teens Geena could play piano, flute and drums, and was the organist at her local church. At school, her height caused her serious embarrassment, but by the time she'd graduated with a degree in drama from Boston University, it enabled her to take the first steps to stardom. She joined the Zoli agency and modeled for the fashion chain, Ann Taylor. In 1982, the movie director Sidney Pollack saw her and gave her a role in *Tootsie*. She was then in a short-lived television series 'Buffalo Bill', but made her breakthrough four years later, in *The Fly* – co-starring with one of her husbands – Jeff Goldblum. She won a Best Supporting Actress Oscar for *The Accidental Tourist*. In 1999, she reached the semi-finals in the U.S. trials for the Olympic Archery team. Geena is also an exceptionally bright woman – with an American Mensa IQ of 140. Apart from her movie credits, on television she hosted 'The Geena Davis Show.' In 2006, she was playing what now seems a somewhat optimistic role as the first female President of the United States, in 'Commander in Chief'. For the latter, she won the 2005 Golden Globe Award as Best Actress. Apart from acting, she promotes equality for women in sport. Geena's latest film *Accidents Happen* – was shot in Australia.

Tootsie (1982)
The Fly (1986)
Beetle Juice (1988)
Earth Girls are Easy (1988)
The Accidental Tourist (1988)
Quick Change (1990)
Thelma & Louise (1991)
A League of Their Own (1992)
Hero (1992) Angie (1994)
Cutthroat Island (1995)
The Long Kiss Goodnight (1996)
Stuart Little (1999)
Stuart Little 2 (2002)
Accidents Happen (2009)

Judy **Davis**
5ft 5in
(JUDY DAVIS)

Born: **April 23, 1955**
Perth, Western Australia, Australia

Judy was educated at Loreto Convent, in Perth. Her parents were so strict they forbade her to go to the movies as a child, but she eventually went her own way. She graduated from Sydney's National Institute of Dramatic Art in 1977. One of her fellow students there, with whom she acted in "Romeo and Juliet", was Mel Gibson. In 1977, Judy appeared in her first movie – an independent production called *High Rolling* – but her big break came two years later in a film she dislikes intensely – *My Brilliant Career*. She did her own piano playing in it and there is no denying that it helped her on the road to international stardom. In 1982, she made the American TV movie 'A Woman Called Golda', in which Ingrid Bergman made her final bow. Since 1984 she has been married to the actor Colin Friels, whom she met at drama school. For more than twenty years, Judy was as good in comedies as she was in dramas – giving her best whether starring or supporting. She was one of the cast of *Dark Blood* – which was unfinished when River Phoenix died. Her portrayal of 'Judy Garland' in the 2001 TV-movie earned her a second Emmy. In 2008, Judy, who lives on Sydney waterfront, won a defamation suit against a Rupert Murdoch controlled Australian newspaper.

My Brilliant Career (1979)
A Passage to India (1984)
Kangaroo (1986)
High Tide (1987)
Georgia (1988) Alice (1990)
Impromptu (1991)
Barton Fink (1991)
Where Angels Fear to Tread (1991)
On My Own (1992)
Husbands and Wives (1992)
The Ref (1994)
The New Age (1994)
Blood and Wine (1996)
Deconstructing Harry (1997)
The Man Who Sued God (2001)
Swimming Upstream (2003)
Marie Antoinette (2006)
The Break-Up (2006)

Ossie **Davis**
6ft 3in
(RAIFORD CHATMAN DAVIS)

Born: **December 18, 1917**
Cogdell, Georgia, USA
Died: **February 4, 2005**

The name Ossie came from his mother's mispronunciation of his initials, "R.C." – when she registered his birth with the County clerk. It stuck. After leaving school Ossie bowed to his parents wishes and attended Howard University. In 1939, he dropped out to pursue an acting career with the Rose McClendon Players, in Harlem. As a black actor in those days, it was hard to get roles in major productions other than those of porters, servants or slaves. He just about made a living and in 1946, he had a short-lived stage role, in "Jeb". In 1948, he married Ruby Dee, who had had similar experiences and with the moral support they gave each other, they began to make (slow) progress. In 1950, Ossie made his film debut with an uncredited role in *No Way Out*. It was another fourteen years before he had his first role of any significance in *The Hill*. But the times were changing. Ossie and Rubee were Civil rights activists – not always very popular – because of their involvement in the 1963 march on Washington and links with Martin Luther King and Malcolm X. In the late 1970s, he was getting film work from Hollywood while retaining his ties with Sidney Potier, and Spike Lee. Ossie died of natural causes in Miami, Florida.

The Hill (1965)
The Scalphunters (1968)
Sam Whiskey (1969) Let's Do It
Again (1975) Hot Stuff (1979)
Harry & Son (1984)
School Daze (1988)
Do the Right Thing (1989)
Joe Versus the Volcano (1990)
Jungle Fever (1991) Gladiator (1992)
Grumpy Old Men (1993)
The Client (1994)
Get on the Bus (1996)
I'm Not Rappaport (1996)
Doctor Doolittle (1998)
Here's to Life! (2000)
How to Get the Man's Foot
Outta Your Ass (2003)
She Hate Me (2004) Proud (2004)

Bruce **Davison**
6ft 1in
(BRUCE DAVISON)

Born: **June 28, 1946**
Philadelphia, Pennsylvania, USA

Bruce's parents divorced when he was three years old and he went to live with his mother, Clair, who worked as a secretary. While still at high school, Bruce had dreams of becoming a painter and was earmarked to study art at Pennsylvania State University. After he had successfully auditioned for a school play, he decided to become an actor. He made his Broadway debut in 1968, in "Tiger at the Gates". It was followed by much admired stage work in "The Elephant Man" and playing opposite Jessica Tandy, in Tennessee Williams' "The Glass Menagerie". In 1969, Bruce made his film debut in *Last Summer*. He worked hard for twenty more years before his breakthrough, playing a gay man whose partner is dying of AIDS, in *Longtime Companion*. He received an Oscar nomination for Best Supporting Actor. Since then Bruce has enjoyed a twenty year period of success in films as well as getting plenty of challenging roles on television. He's been married for twelve years to his third wife, Michele Corey. They have a daughter, Sophia Lucinda, and live in Los Angeles.

Last Summer (1969)
The Strawberry Statement (1970)
Ulzana's Raid (1972)
Short Eyes (1977) Lies (1983)
Crimes of Passion (1984)
Longtime Companion (1990)
Short Cuts (1993)
Six Degrees of Separation (1993)
Yellow Dog (1995)
The Cure (1995)
It's My Party (1996)
The Crucible (1996)
Apt Pupil (1998)
At First Sight (1999) X-Men (2000)
Crazy/Beautiful (2001)
High Crimes (2002)
Dahmer (2002) X2 (2003)
Runaway Jury (2003)
Hate Crime (2005)
Confession (2005)
Breach (2007)
La Linea (2008)

Doris **Day**
5ft 7in
(DORIS ANN KAPPELHOF)

Born: **April 3, 1924**
Cincinnati, Ohio, USA

Doris was the only daughter of a Roman Catholic couple – William and Sophia Kappelhoff – whose own parents originated from Germany. As a young girl she longed to be a dancer when she left school, but her dream was shattered when she was injured in an automobile accident. Her recovery took a year, but it enabled her to concentrate on her other talent – singing. She got work at a local radio station. In 1939, she had a brief spell with Les Brown's Band and after an awful marriage, rejoined him. In 1946, they had a hit record with 'Sentimental Journey'. It was the start of a journey to movie stardom. In 1948, Doris landed a role in *Romance on the High Seas.* One of its songs 'It's Magic' was a massive hit. She didn't need to prove that she could act because she was usually in musicals. From 1952, she was the most popular female star in the USA. Her comedies with Rock Hudson and James Garner, were made just before the 'sixties started to swing and she was nominated for an Oscar for *Pillow Talk.* She then looked out-of-date, and couldn't hide the fact that she was forty. In 1968, she did 'The Doris Day Show' on TV, after discovering that she was bankrupt, when her husband and crooked agent, Marty Melcher, died. After that she has devoted her life to the only creatures she could trust – her animals.

Romance on the High Seas (1948)
It's a Great Feeling (1949)
My Dream is Yours (1949)
Young Man with a Horn (1950)
Tea for Two (1950)
I'll See You in My Dreams (1951)
On Moonlight Bay (1951)
Calamity Jane (1953)
Young at Heart (1954)
Love Me or Leave Me (1955)
The Man Who Knew Too Much (1956)
The Pajama Game (1957)
Teacher's Pet (1958) Pillow Talk (1959)
Please Don't Eat the Daisies (1960)
Move Over, Darling (1963)
Send Me No Flowers (1964)

Laraine **Day**
5ft 5in
(LARAINE JOHNSON)

Born: **October 13, 1920**
Roosevelt, Utah, USA
Died: **November 10, 2007**

Laraine and her twin brother, Lamar, were born into a family of prominent Mormons. After her parents relocated to California, she finished high school, joined the Long Beach Players and took a serious interest in an acting career. She made her first steps to stardom by contacting Hollywood studios and after a screen-test, made her first film appearance (uncredited) in a good 1937 Barbara Stanwyck tear-jerker, *Stella Dallas.* As Laraine Johnson, she had a few more small roles before she made her entrance as Nurse Mary Lamont in 1939, in *Calling Doctor Kildare.* The influence of it's stars Lionel Barrymore and Lew Ayres, could not be over-estimated. Her acting improved from that point on. To ring the changes, Laraine appeared with Johnny Weissmuller and Maureen O'Sullivan in a Tarzan film, *Tarzan Finds a Son!* before continuing with her *Dr. Kildare* 'nursing career'. There was other work too: Alfred Hitchcock liked her pretty face enough to co-star her with Joel McCrea in *Foreign Correspondent* and throughout the 1940s she was in some high profile movies, including *Journey for Margaret,* and *The Locket.* She became known as "The First Lady of Baseball" after marrying Leo Durocher, who was the manager (among others), of the Brooklyn Dodgers and the New York Giants. Laraine died of cancer in Utah, eight months after the death of her third husband, Michael Grilikhes.

Calling Doctor Kildare (1939)
And One Was Beautiful (1940)
Foreign Correspondent (1940)
Unholy Partners (1941)
Kathleen (1941)
Fingers at the Window (1942)
Journey for Margaret (1942)
The Story of Dr. Wassell (1944)
Bride by Mistake (1944)
Keep Your Powder Dry (1945)
The Locket (1946)
The Woman on Pier 13 (1949)
Without Honor (1949)
The High and the Mighty (1954)

Daniel **Day-Lewis**
6ft 1½in
(DANIEL MICHAEL BLAKE DAY-LEWIS)

Born: **April 29, 1957**
London, England

Daniel is the son of English Poet Laureate, Cecil Day-Lewis. On his mother's side, his grandfather was Sir Michael Balcon – the former head of Ealing Studios. Daniel was miserable at Sevenoaks school, but began acting there and had a small film role in *Sunday, Bloody Sunday* when he was fourteen. He transferred to Bedales School in Petersfield, where he enjoyed life. He studied at the Bristol Old Vic School and appeared in a number of their productions. In 1982, he had a bit part in *Gandhi* and was in several television films before getting a featured role in *The Bounty*, in 1984. Daniel joined the Royal Shakespeare Company and played Romeo, and Count Dracula, for them. His film career accelerated from then on and he was soon demonstrating his remarkable range and star quality. In 1989, playing the part of Christy Brown, the Irish painter, poet and cerebral palsy sufferer, in *My Left Foot*, he won a Best Actor Oscar. He returned to the theater in "Hamlet" but he withdrew because of sheer physical exhaustion and hasn't been seen on stage since. He had time off from film-making and is extremely selective when taking on movie roles – a policy which has paid off handsomely – with his second Best Actor Oscar, for his portrayal of Daniel Plainview, in Paul Thomas Anderson's powerful drama, *There Will Be Blood*. Daniel is now married (with two young sons) to Arthur Miller's daughter, Rebecca. He is filming the star-studded drama *Nine*.

My Beautiful Launderette (1985)
A Room with a View (1985)
**The Unbearable Lightness
of Being** (1988)
My Left Foot (1989)
The Last of the Mohicans (1992)
The Age of Innocence (1993)
In the Name of the Father (1993)
The Crucible (1996)
The Boxer (1997)
Gangs of New York (2002)
The Ballad of Jack and Rose (2005)
There Will Be Blood (2007)

James **Dean**
5ft 8in
(JAMES BYRON DEAN)

Born: **February 8, 1931**
Marion, Indiana, USA
Died: **September 30, 1955**

Jimmy was the son of Winton and Mildred Dean. After his mother died when he was nine years old, Jimmy was raised by his uncle and aunt on a farm in Fairmount, Indiana. He was always a loner and as a boy, a very studious youngster. During his years at Brentwood High School, Jimmy began to develop his passion for acting – winning the Indiana State Dramatic prize for his efforts. He then went to UCLA, where he joined a drama group run by the actor, James Whitmore. Through that he began getting television work and bit parts in movies starting with Samuel Fuller's war film, *Fixed Bayonets* in 1951, and followed by the Martin and Lewis comedy, *Sailor Beware*. For the next two years Jimmy was in New York City – acting in television dramas – and appearing on Broadway, in "See The Jaguar" and Andre Gide's "The Immoralist". When Elia Kazan saw him in the latter, he knew he'd be ideal to play Cal in his planned film of John Steinbeck's absorbing novel, *East of Eden*. Jimmy was more than just ideal – his personality shone from the screen like a beacon and audiences and critics hailed a new star. He did a couple of television dramas before entering his final twelve months in the sun. Jimmy's next movie was the iconic *Rebel Without A Cause*. Although he was more than twenty-three years of age at the time, Jimmy spoke for many teenagers – who as part of the post-war generation, didn't want to follow in their parents' footsteps. He himself was a rebel – described by all three directors of his movies – as "difficult". He could also be reckless: following the completion of work on his final film, *Giant*, he was driving his brand new Porsche 550 Spyder at over 115 miles an hour, along Highway 46, when just outside Cholame, California, he collided with a Ford Tudor. Jimmy died before reaching the nearest hospital in the town.

East of Eden (1955)
Rebel Without a Cause (1955)
Giant (1956)

Yvonne **De Carlo**
5ft 4in
(PEGGY YVONNE MIDDLETON)

Born: **September 1, 1922**
Vancouver, Canada
Died: **January 8, 2007**

Her mother had been frustrated by the fact that she got married early and never had the chance to become an actress. Her husband felt the bad vibes and left when Yvonne was three. From then on, her main aim in life was to get Yvonne, (who took her maiden name) into the movies. It began with dancing lessons and in 1937 they made the first of several very fruitless trips to Hollywood. It improved in 1940, when Yvonne was second in a "Miss Venice Beach" contest and was hired as a showgirl at the Florentine Gardens. Following a small part in the film *I Look at You,* she had to wait four years before anything substantial was offered. That was in 1945, when Universal starred her in *Salome Where She Danced*. The critics panned it, but it was certainly an opportunity to show off her curvaceous figure and audiences loved her. Leading roles in two movies with Burt Lancaster followed, and in the 1950s, she remained popular. In 1955, Yvonne married the stunt man, Bob Morgan, but when he was injured, she was forced to make a comeback in 'The Munsters' TV series, in 1964. Her role as Lily made her famous again and led to more good television work but several poor movies. At least it paid for Bob's medical bills. Her generous efforts were not enough to keep them together. Yvonne died of natural causes, at Woodland Hills, California.

Brute Force (1947)
Black Bart (1948)
Casbah (1948)
Criss Cross (1949)
Hotel Sahara (1951)
Scarlet Angel (1953)
The Captain's Paradise (1953)
Happy Ever After (1954)
The Ten Commandments (1956)
Death of a Scoundrel (1956)
Band of Angels (1957)
McLintock! (1963)
The Power (1968)
Oscar (1991)

Frances **Dee**
5ft 4¹/₂in
(FRANCES MARION DEE)

Born: **November 26, 1909**
Los Angeles, California, USA
Died: **March 6, 2004**

As a child, because her father was an army officer, Frances moved around the country a lot. She received her education at the aptly named Shakespeare Grammar School and Hyde Park High School, in Chicago. When she graduated from the latter, Frances had little idea of what she wanted to do. She attended UCLA for two years then looked for work. There were some jobs available as movie extras in Hollywood and it was as an extra that she made her screen debut in 1929 in an early sound film, *Words and Music*. Maurice Chevalier liked her in it and he insisted on featuring her in *The Playboy of Paris,* the following year. She met Joel McCrea on the set of *The Silver Cord* in 1933, and the "Made in Heaven" couple were happily married for fifty-seven years. Both Frances and Joel were extremely successful in the movies and amassed a large fortune from the business. In 1953, Frances retired to concentrate on bringing up her three sons and devoted more time to developing the impressive McCrea family ranch in Thousand Oaks, California. She will be remembered for making several poor movies a lot better than they would have been without her, and for never being outplayed by any of the great names she acted with in the good ones. Frances died aged ninety-four, in Norwalk, Connecticut, fourteen years after husband Joel, from complications following a stroke.

Crime of the Century (1933)
Blood Money (1933)
Little Women (1933)
Of Human Bondage (1934)
Becky Sharp (1935)
The Gay Deception (1935)
Souls at Sea (1937)
Wells Fargo (1937)
If I Were King (1938)
Coast Guard (1939)
So Ends Our Night (1941)
Meet the Stewarts (1942)
I Walked with a Zombie (1943)
Payment on Demand (1951)

Ruby **Dee**
5ft 2¹/₂in
(RUBY ANN WALLACE)

Born: **October 27, 1924**
Cleveland, Ohio

Ruby started her life in humble and rather unsettling circumstances. Her poor father, Marshall, worked hard but he earned little from jobs as a waiter, porter, and cook. Her mother Gladys Hightower, left him and remarried, but Marshall's second wife, Emily Benson, who was a schoolteacher, proved a very positive influence on young Ruby's life. She encouraged her to read and study hard at school. Her moral support pushed Ruby forward and she graduated from Hunter College, with degrees in French and Spanish. She married the blues singer Frankie Dee, and after they divorced Ruby used his surname for the rest of her career – starting in the early 1940s – with small parts on Broadway. There were no big parts for African Americans back then. In 1946 she was in 'The First Year' on TV and made her film debut in 1947, with an all black cast in *That Man of Mine*. She married second husband, Ossie Davis in 1948. They had three children and became civil rights activists. Ruby co-starred with Joe Louis in *The Fight Never Ends* and then acted with another sporting hero, in *The Jackie Robinson Story*. Her early roles in mainstream films were confined to maids, but as actors such as Sidney Poitier gained acceptance, Ruby benefited – co-starring with him in *A Raisin in the Sun*. She won an Emmy in 1990 for 'Decoration Day' and was nominated for a Best Supporting Actress Oscar, for *American Gangster*.

The Jackie Robinson Story (1950)
The Tall Target (1951)
Edge of the City (1957)
Virgin Island (1958)
St. Louis Blues (1958)
Take a Giant Step (1959)
A Raisin in the Sun (1961)
The Balcony (1963)
The Incident (1967)
Buck and the Preacher (1972)
Black Girl (1972) **Do the Right Thing** (1989) **Just Cause** (1995)
The Way Back Home (2006)
American Gangster (2007)

Sandra **Dee**
5ft 4in
(ALEXANDRE CYMBOLIAK ZUCK)

Born: **April 23, 1942**
Bayonne, New Jersey, USA
Died: **February 20, 2005**

The daughter of John and Mary Zuck, Sandy was pretty as a picture from early childhood. Her mother gave her age differently depending on what the situation required. By the age of twelve she was not only a successful model with the Harry Conover agency – her face was on many magazine covers and she appeared in TV commercials. She was only fourteen when she signed a personal contract with the producer Ross Hunter and made her film debut, in *Until They Sail*. Sandy won a Golden Globe Award for one of the "Most Promising Newcomers" of 1958. She was a genuine American teenager of the 1950s, who appealed to kids in other parts of the world as well. When she married Bobby Darin, in 1960, her looks and his music were still in fashion. They made three movies together, but the quality began to deteriorate after the first one *Come September* – for which she won a huge following among young girls and a seven year contract with Universal. By 1967, her marriage was over and so was her film career. Her style was no longer acceptable and she could do nothing to change it. Sandy appeared in episodes of various television series in the 1970s and made her last film, a poor drama titled *Lost,* in 1983. She was beset with drug and alcohol problems for her remaining years and died of kidney disease.

Until They Sail (1957)
The Reluctant Debutante (1958)
The Restless Years (1958)
Gidget (1959)
Imitation of Life (1959)
The Wild and the Innocent (1959)
A Summer Place (1959)
Portrait in Black (1960)
Romanoff and Juliet (1961)
Tammy Tell Me True (1961)
Come September (1961)
Take her, She's Mine (1963)
That Funny Feeling (1965)
A Man Could Get Killed (1966)
Rosie! (1967)

Don **Defore**
6ft 1in
(DONALD JOHN DEFORE)

Born: **August 25, 1913**
Cedar Rapids, Iowa, USA
Died: **December 22, 1993**

The son of a locomotive engineer and a mother who loved theater, Don acted in church plays she directed, from the age of three. At junior school and all through his time at Washington High School in Cedar Rapids, he dreamed of a career as an actor. He'd go regularly to the local movie theater to watch screen greats – George Arliss and John Barrymore. When he was awarded a scholarship to the University of Iowa, he opted instead to study drama at the Pasadena playhouse. Being so near Hollywood gave him opportunities for film work - he made his debut in 1937 – with an uncredited role – in *Kid Galahad*. He had three more bit parts while he toured the country with various stock companies. His Broadway debut was in 1938 and after appearing in a successful play "The Male Animal", Don repeated his role in the film version. He had a good marriage and five children with Marion Holmes, and was a character actor for forty-five years. He became the first honorary mayor of Brentwood, where he made his home in 1948. He also ran his own restaurant in Disneyland. Don died of a heart attack in Los Angeles.

The Male Animal (1942)
Men of the Sky (1942)
A Guy Named Joe (1943)
Thirty Seconds Over Tokyo (1944)
The Affairs of Susan (1945)
You Came Along (1945)
The Stork Club (1945)
Without Reservations (1946)
It Happened on 5th Avenue (1947)
Ramrod (1947)
Romance on the High Seas (1948)
One Sunday Afternoon (1948)
Too Late for Tears (1949)
My Friend Irma (1949) **Dark City** (1950)
The Guy Who Came Back (1951)
Jumping Jacks (1952)
Battle Hymn (1957)
**A Time to Love and
a Time to Die** (1958)
The Facts of Life (1960)

Cécile **De France**
5ft 8½in
(CÉCILE DE FRANCE)

Born: **July 17, 1975**
Namur, Belgium

Cécile grew up and went to school in the French-speaking city of Namur, which is in the south of Belgium. With the looks and desire to become an actress, she left for France when she was seventeen. In Paris, she studied for two years with the drama coach, Jean Paul Denizon, in preparation for the École National Superior des Arts et Techniques du Théâtre. Once accepted, she attended Département Comédie, in Paris and went to further classes in Lyon – graduating in 1998. In 1996, Cécile made her stage debut in "Dormez je le veux" and appeared in two other plays that year, including "A Midsummer Night's Dream" by William Shakespeare. The following year, she was first seen on the screen – on TV – in an episode of 'Cas de divorce', and in a short film titled *Tous nos vœux de bonheur*. After she was seen acting in a school production of "Electra", she was taken on by Artmedia, under the wing of the actor and well-known casting agent, Dominique Besnehard – who's responsible for most of the biggest names in French Cinema and Theater. She returned to Belgium in 2000, to act in another short, *Le Dernier rêve*. Cécile's first successful feature was *Toutes les nuits* (in the role of a prostitute), which was shot in Paris. She then made a short film, *A Paper Marriage,* with a mainly Arab cast. Her international breakthrough was in the horror thriller, *Haute tension*. She was named one of European films' Shooting Stars, but was in the ill-advised remake of *Around the World in 80 Days*. Cécile has a baby boy, Lino, with her boyfriend, Guillaume.

Toutes les nuits (2001)
L'Auberge Espagnole (2002)
Irène (2002)
I, Caesar (2003)
Haute tension (2003)
The Russian Dolls (2005)
Orchestra Seats (2006)
Quand j'étais chanteur (2006)
Mon Colonel (2006)
Bad Faith (2006) **Un secret** (2007)
L'Instinct de mort (2008)

Louis **De Funès**
5ft 4½in
(LOUIS GERMAIN DAVID DE FUNÈS DE GALARZA)

Born: **July 31, 1914**
Courbevoie, Seine, France
Died: **January 27, 1983**

In 1904, Louis' parents came from Seville, in Spain, to settle in France. His father Carlos, was a young lawyer who married Leonar, Louis' mother, against her parents wishes – so they ran away. Carlos did well in Paris, where Louis was educated at the Lycée Sondorcet. After graduating, he took time to get a job, so, as he'd learned to play the piano as a child, he ended up tinkling the ivories in bars all over the city. He was frequently fired for trying his ideas for comedy on the audiences, but when he eventually transferred to bigger venues, his unique facial mannerisms were better appreciated. Louis took acting lessons at Cours Simon, where he met Daniel Gelin, who helped him to make his film debut in 1946 in *La Tentation de Barbizon*. For the next dozen or so years, Louis acted in dramas, fantasies, crime films, and when possible – comedy. In his late forties, he became a big favorite in France, working in the genre he was best at. He died of a heart attack two years after his final film. His second wife, Jeanne de Maupassant, was the grand-niece of the novelist, Guy de Maupassant.

La Belle Américaine (1961)
Pouic-Pouic (1963)
Faites sauter la banque! (1964)
Le Gendarme de Saint-Tropez (1964)
Fantômas (1964)
Le Corniaud (1965)
Les Bons vivants (1965)
Fantômas se déchaine (1965)
Le Grand restaurant (1966)
La Grande Vadrouille (1966)
Fantômas contre Scotland Yard (1967)
Oscar (1967)
Le Gendarme se marie (1968)
L'homme orchestra (1970)
Le Gendarme en balade (1970)
Delusions of Grandeur (1971)
The Adventures of Rabbi Jacob (1973)
L'aile ou la cuisse (1976)
**Le gendarme et les extra-
terrestres** (1978) **The Miser** (1980)
La soupe aux choux (1981)

Gloria **DeHaven**
5ft 2½in
(GLORIA MILDRED DEHAVEN)

Born: **July 23, 1925**
Los Angeles, California, USA

Gloria's parents were actor-director Carter DeHaven, and Flora Parker – both former vaudeville stars – who had appeared in some silent films and were friendly with Charlie Chaplin. When she was ten, she appeared as an extra (playing Paulette Goddard's little sister) in Chaplin's film, *Modern Times.* Her father was assistant director on the movie. Gloria continued her education (including acting and singing classes) at the Mar-Ken School, in Hollywood. It wasn't long before she was ready to launch her show business career. Gloria had a nice voice as well as being pretty and at sixteen she was hired by bandleader Muzzy Marcellino to sing with his band on the West Coast. She later joined the Jan Savitt Orchestra. While there, she appeared in another Chaplin movie, *The Great Dictator.* Jan Savitt had good Hollywood contacts and it led to more film work for Gloria. During the war years, she was in Greta Garbo's final movie *Two-Faced Woman,* and musicals including Frank Sinatra's *Step Lively.* In 1944 she married John Payne, and was suspended by MGM in 1947, when she preferred to take care of her family rather than act in *Good News.* She was seen mostly on TV from 1957, but forty years later, appeared with Jack Lemmon and Walter Matthau in the movie, *Out to Sea.*

Susan and God (1940)
Best Foot Forward (1943)
Broadway Rhythm (1944)
Two Girls and a Sailor (1944)
Step Lively (1944)
The Thin Man
Goes Home (1944)
Scene of the Crime (1949)
Yes Sir That's My
Baby (1949)
Three Little Words (1950)
Summer Stock (1950)
I'll Get By (1950)
The Yellow Cab Man (1950)
Two Tickets to Broadway (1951)
The Girl Rush (1955)
Out to Sea (1997)

Olivia **De Havilland**
5ft 3½in
(OLIVIA MARY DE HAVILLAND)

Born: **July 1, 1916**
Tokyo, Japan

Olivia's father, a British patent attorney, had a practice in Japan. He was related to Sir Geoffrey de Havilland, the aviation pioneer. Her mother had been an actress whose stage name was Lilian Fontaine. Olivia and her sister (later Joan Fontaine) lived in Japan until her parents parted when she was five. Her mother took them to California, where they settled in Saratoga, and Olivia later attended the Notre Dame Convent School, in Belmont. While still at college, she played Puck in Shakespeare's "A Midsummer Night's Dream". A talent scout saw it and recommended her to Max Reinhardt, who was planning a film version. She played Hermia so well she was given a seven-year contract with Warners, and a starring role with Joe E. Brown in *Alibi Ike.* They teamed her with Errol Flynn and the recipe worked on a total of eight occasions. She had a Best Supporting Actress Oscar nomination for *Gone with the Wind,* and in 1941, she became a US citizen. Olivia won her first Oscar for *To Each His Own* and did it again in *The Heiress.* She worked on Broadway, but film was her medium. Later roles couldn't match the quality of her earlier material, but she did make a couple of good 1970s horror movies to finish with.

Captain Blood (1935)
The Charge of the Light
Brigade (1936)
The Adventures of
Robin Hood (1938)
Gone with the Wind (1939)
Hold Back the Dawn(1941)
They Died with Their
Boots On (1941)
To Each His Own (1946)
The Dark Mirror (1946)
The Snake Pit (1948)
The Heiress (1949)
My Cousin Rachel (1952)
Not as a Stranger (1955)
Libel (1959)
Light in the Piazza (1962)
Lady in a Cage (1964)
Hush...Hush, Sweet Charlotte (1964)

Albert **Dekker**
6ft 3in
(ALBERT ECKE)

Born: **December 20, 1905**
Brooklyn, New York City, New York, USA
Died: **May 5, 1968**

After graduating from Bowdoin College, in Maine, where he had intended to become a psychologist, Albert, on the urging of a fellow student who had seen him act, joined a Cincinnati-based stock company. He did so well that in 1927 he was cast in the Broadway production of Eugene O'Neill's "Marco Millions". For ten years, Albert was a solid performer on the stage. Appropriately, he made his film debut in 1937, in the biopic, *The Great Garrick.* He appeared in good movies such as *Beau Geste, The Killers* and *East of Eden* during a long career. In 1944, he won a seat on the California State Assembly. He didn't last very long in politics, mainly because of his outspoken criticism of Senator Joseph McCarthy. In the early 1950s, he returned to Broadway, but went back to Hollywood to complete nearly seventy films. After he finished work on *The Wild Bunch* and had planned his wedding to the glamour model Geraldine Saunders, Albert died a horrible death. His naked body was discovered at his home in Hollywood, bound hand and foot, with hypodermic needles jammed into both arms. The ruling of accidental asphyxiation was unsatisfactory.

Beau Geste (1939)
Strange Cargo (1940)
Dr. Cyclops (1940)
Seven Sinners (1940)
Honky Tonk (1941)
Once Upon a Honeymoon (1942)
War of the Wildcats (1943)
Experiment Perilous (1944)
Incendiary Blonde (1945)
Two Years Before
the Mast (1946)
The Killers (1946)
Gentleman's Agreement (1947)
As Young as You Feel (1951)
East of Eden (1955)
Kiss Me Deadly (1955)
Middle of the Night (1959)
The Wonderful Country (1959)
Suddenly, Last Summer (1959)
The Wild Bunch (1969)

Alain **Delon**
5ft 11³/₄in
(ALAIN DELON)

Born: November 8, 1935
Sceaux, Seine, France

Alain's parents divorced when he was four. He was adopted by foster parents, who sent him to boarding school. After being expelled from several schools he worked in his step-father's butchery. At seventeen, he joined the French Marines as a parachutist – serving in Indo-China. He settled in Paris, doing various menial jobs until he became friendly with Jean-Claude Brialy. The actor invited him to the 1957 Cannes Film Festival, where he made good contacts. His film debut was later that year in *Quand la femme s'en mêle*. Within two years he'd co-starred with, and romanced Romy Schneider, and was famous after *Plein Soleil*, an adaptation of 'The Talented Mr. Ripley'. Alain's good looks overcame any limitations he may have had as an actor, and working with the great Visconti – on stage as well as on the screen – soon improved his skills. By the mid-sixties he was a super-star in Europe and attempted unsuccessfully to do the same in America. In 1969, his bodyguard was shot and left to die on a garbage site. The scandal reignited his career – appropriately with a series of very popular French gangster movies. Alain has kept busy for over thirty years, as a director, writer, and actor. In 1998, he was re-united with his old friend Jean-Paul Belmondo, in their all-action movie, *Une chance sur deux.*

Plein Soleil (1960)
Rocco e i suoi fratelli (1960)
L'Eclipse (1962)
The Leopard (1963)
Le Samurai (1967)
Borsalino (1970)
Le Cercle Rouge (1970)
The Professor (1972)
Un flic (1972)
Scorpio (1973)
Les Grange brulées (1973)
Flic Story (1975)
Monsieur Klein (1976)
Mort d'un pourri (1977)
Swann in Love (1984)
Un Crime (1993)
Une chance sur deux (1998)

Julie **Delpy**
5ft 6¹/₂in
(JULIE DELPY)

Born: December 21, 1969
Paris, France

Julie's parents acted in films and were supporters of the avant-garde theater in Paris. They encouraged her to follow a similar path. In 1985, aged fourteen, and following three earlier experiences as an extra, she landed a small role in Jean-Luc Godard's *Détective*. Two years later, Julie funded her first visit to New York with her earnings from the title role in the movie, *Beatrice*. She perfected her English over the next few years and studied filmmaking at New York University's Tisch School of the Arts, where she was totally involved in the production of around thirty films. She acted in the trilogy by the Polish director, Krzysztof Kieslowski beginning with *Three Colors Blue*, in 1993. In 1995, Julie wrote, produced and directed the short film, *Looking for Jimmy*. Since then she has enhanced her reputation as an actress internationally, in films like *Broken Flowers* – shot in New Jersey – and she covered other disciplines with total success. The recent *2 Days in Paris,* is a Delpy one-woman production. She not only starred in it, she wrote the script, directed it, co-produced it, edited it and she composed the music! What more can I say? Nowadays, Julie makes her home in Los Angeles. Her next multi-skill project is *The Countess.*

Mauvais sang (1986)
La Passion Béatrice (1987)
L'Autre nuit (1988)
Europa Europa (1990)
Warszaw Année 5703 (1992)
Three Colors Blue (1993)
The Three Musketeers (1993)
Three Colors White (1994)
Three Colors Red (1994)
Killing Zoe (1994)
Before Sunrise (1995)
CinéMagique (2002)
Before Sunset (2004)
Broken Flowers (2005)
3 & 3 (2005)
The Hoax (2006)
The Air I Breathe (2007)
2 Days in Paris (2007)
The Countess (2009)

Dolores **Del Rio**
5ft 3¹/₂in
(DOLORES ASÚNSOLO LÓPEZ NEGRETE)

Born: August 3, 1905
Durango, Mexico
Died: April 11, 1983

After her wealthy family lost all its assets during the Mexican Revolution, this second cousin of Ramón Navarro, decided to follow his route to fame and fortune in Hollywood. She was only sixteen when she married writer, Jaime Martinez del Rio and they emigrated to the USA, intending to work as a team. In the event, they did not and they were soon divorced. Dolores retained her married name – making her first film appearance in *Joanna*, in 1925. Along with Joan Crawford and Mary Astor, she was one of the thirteen WAMPAS Baby Stars of 1926. Her looks alone won her roles in several successful silent movies. When she married the MGM art director, Cedric Gibbons, in 1930, she hoped her talking picture career would take off. But she mostly got bit parts as exotic-looking beauties who outshone the female stars. After a second divorce she had a passionate affair with the ten-year younger Orson Welles, and starred in his *Journey Into Fear*. She returned home to be a major part of the 'Golden Age of Mexican Cinema'. In 1978, she starred in her final film, *The Children of Sanchez,* which was made in Mexico. Dolores died of liver failure in Long Beach, California.

Bird of Paradise (1932)
Flying Down to Rio (1933)
Madame DuBarry (1934)
Accused (1936)
Lancer Spy (1937)
Journey into Fear (1943)
Flor silvestre (1943)
María Candelaria (1944)
Las Abandonadas (1945)
Bugambilia (1945)
La Otra (1946)
The Fugitive (1947)
La Malquerida (1949)
Dona Perfecta (1951)
El Nino y la niebla (1953)
La Cucaracha (1959)
Cheyenne Autumn (1964)
More Than a Miracle (1967)
The Children of Sanchez (1978)

Benicio **Del Toro**
6ft 2in
(BENITO MONSERRATE RAFAEL DEL TORO SANCHEZ)

Born: **February 19, 1967**
San Germán, Puerto Rico

The son of two lawyers, Gustavo Adolfo del Toro Bermúdez and Fausta Sánchez Rivera, Beno grew up in Santurce – a district of San Juan. He was educated at a Roman Catholic school – Academia del Perpetuo Socorro, in Miramar. His mother died of hepatitis when he was nine, and his father moved with Beno and his older brother, to Mercersburg, Pennsylvania, where they both attended Mercersburg Academy. After graduating, Beno began studying for a degree in business at the University of California, San Diego, but he dropped out after being successful in an elective drama course. He moved to Los Angeles, where he studied with drama teachers Stella Adler and Arthur Mendoza before enrolling at the Circle in the Square Theater School, in New York. He made his first appearance on television in 1987, in an episode of 'Miami Vice'. The following year, he made his film debut in a light-weight family comedy called *Big Top Pee-wee.* That was followed by the Bond film, *Licence to Kill.* Beno began to get plenty of work in supporting roles. He traveled to Spain to work with Javier Bardem in *Golden Balls,* and by the time he acted in *Fearless,* he was moving up the cast list. Beno's breakthrough came with *The Usual Suspects* and he was soon getting into the habit of featuring in major hits. He won a Best Supporting Actor Oscar, for *Traffic* and was nominated for *21 Grams.*

Money for Nothing (1993)
Fearless (1993) **China Moon** (1994)
Swimming with Sharks (1994)
The Usual Suspects (1995)
Basquiat (1996) **The Funeral** (1996)
**Fear and Loathing
in Las Vegas** (1998)
Snatch (2000)
The Way of the Gun (2000)
Traffic (2000) **The Pledge** (2001)
The Hunted (2003) **21 Grams** (2003)
Sin City (2005)
Things We Lost in the Fire (2007)
The Argentine (2008)
Guerrilla (2008)

Dom **Deluise**
5ft 11½in
(DOM DELUISE)

Born: **August 1, 1933**
Brooklyn, New York City, New York, USA

The son of Italian American parents – John and Vincenza DeLuise – Dom was outgoing and confident as a youngster, and was able to make his friends and family laugh. He graduated from the High School of Performing Arts, in Manhattan. His first professional gig was in a children's play – when he performed the title role of "Bernie the Dog". In 1964, he made his film debut in the independent comedy, *Diary of a Bachelor,* and showed a rare serious side that same year, in *Fail-Safe,* as a nervous airman. During that time, he was a regular guest on the television show, 'The Entertainers'. In 1965 he married actress Carol Arthur, with whom he has three sons. Dom starred in the 1968 Broadway production of Neil Simon's "Last of the Red Hot Lovers". Among his many talents is his voice – he sang in the opera 'Die Fledermaus' at the New York Met. He appeared with Burt Reynolds in six of his movies. He's hosted his own TV show, 'Cooking with Dom Deluise' and he's already published two books – titled 'Eat This' and 'Eat This Too'. In 1984, Dom was named "King of Brooklyn" by local civic leaders. Dom's voice-over work includes the recent animated film, *Bongee Bear and the Kingdom of Rhythm.* Dom will next be seen on the big screen in the the 3-D horror comedy, *Horrorween.*

Fail-Safe (1964)
The Glass Bottom Boat (1966)
**What's So Bad About
Feeling Good?** (1968)
The Twelve Chairs (1970)
Blazing Saddles (1974)
Silent Movie (1976)
The End (1978)
The Muppet Movie (1979)
History of the World: Part I (1981)
The Cannonball Run (1981)
**The Best Little Whorehouse
in Texas** (1982)
Robin Hood: Men in Tights (1993)
**My X-Girlfriend's Wedding
Reception** (2001)
Breaking the Fifth (2004)

William **Demarest**
5ft 9½in
(CARL WILLIAM DEMAREST)

Born: **February 27, 1892**
St. Paul, Minnesota, USA
Died: **December 28, 1983**

Bill was convinced from an early age, that it would be an entertainer's life for him. He left school at thirteen – to form a song and dance act with his brother. They began in vaudeville and county fairs, where beefy Bill would earn extra money through prize-fighting. In seven years, he established himself as an all-round actor, dancer and singer, as well as a comic, and was hired for the Broadway show, "Earl Carroll's Sketch Book". In 1926, Bill signed a contract with Warner Bros., and made his film debut that year in *When the Wife's Away.* He appeared in several silent films before an uncredited role in *The Jazz Singer.* His first all-talking picture was *Seeing Things,* in 1930. By 1935, he began to feature in films like *Diamond Jim,* but it was the Preston Sturges movies, starting with *The Lady Eve,* which gave him fame. Bill had appeared with the real Al Jolson in 1927, so it was appropriate that he was nominated for a Best Supporting Actor Oscar for *The Jolson Story* – twenty years later. He acted in films until 1976 and achieved great popularity on TV, as Uncle Charley, in 'My Three Sons'. Bill died from prostate cancer and pneumonia at his home in Palm Springs.

Diamond Jim (1935)
Easy Living (1937)
Big City (1937)
Romance on the Run (1938)
The Great McGinty (1940)
The Lady Eve (1941)
All Through the Night (1941)
Sullivan's Travels (1941)
The Palm Beach Story (1942)
**The Miracle of Morgan's
Creek** (1944)
**Hail the Conquering
Hero** (1944)
The Jolson Story (1946)
Night Has a Thousand Eyes (1948)
Jolson Sings Again (1949)
Excuse My Dust (1951)
Escape from Fort Bravo (1953)
Lucy Gallant (1955)

Mylène **Demongeot**
5ft 7¼in
(MARIE-HÉLÈNE DEMONGEOT)

Born: **September 29, 1935**
Nice, France

She grew up in a family of amateur actors and theater enthusiasts. After leaving school at sixteen, Mylène studied drama in Paris, with Maria Ventura, a Rumanian-born stage and film actress, who had started teaching when she was in her sixties. With the required looks of the French "Futures vedettes" of the period, Mylène soon caught the eye of a casting director, who in 1953, gave her a small role in the film *Les Enfants de l'amour*. Appropriately enough, her next film, two years later, was titled *Futures vedettes*. Mylène became a star after playing the role of Abigail Williams, in *Les Sorcières de Salem* from the Arthur Miller play "The Crucible". It also starred those fine French actors, Simone Signoret and Yves Montand. Mylène had earlier appeared in a British musical comedy called *It's a Wonderful World,* but her true international debut was in Otto Preminger's film of Françoise Sagan's best-selling novel, *Bonjour Tristesse*. After co-starring with the young Alain Delon, in *Faibles femmes*, Mylène went to England to star in *Upstairs and Downstairs* and to Italy to make *La Notte Brava* and a Steve Reeves movie, *Giant of Marathon*. Mylène was married to director, Marc Simenon, until his death in 1999. She lives in Nice.

Les Sorcières de Salem (1957)
A Kiss for a Killer (1957)
Bonjour Tristesse (1958)
Sois belle et tais-toi (1958)
Night Heat (1958)
Faibles femmes (1959)
Upstairs and Downstairs (1959)
La Notte Brava (1959)
Under Ten Flags (1960)
Love in Rome (1960)
**The Singer Not the
Song** (1961)
The Fighting Musketeers (1961)
**Vengeance of the
Musketeers** (1961)
Fantômas (1964)
Fantômas Strikes Back (1965)
**Fantômas Against
Scotland Yard** (1967)

Rebecca **De Mornay**
5ft 5½in
(REBECCA JANE PEARCH)

Born: **August 29, 1959**
Santa Rosa, California, USA

Rebecca is the daughter of the TV talk show host, Wally George, but was raised by her mother, Julie, and her stepfather, Richard De Mornay – who gave her his name. Richard died when she was five and her mother took Rebecca and her half-brother, Peter, to Europe – where, when they lived in England, she attended the Summerhill boarding school. After she graduated from high school in Austria, Rebecca spoke fluent German. When she returned to the USA, she lived in Los Angeles, where she was trained as an actress at Lee Strasberg's Institute before her apprenticeship at Francis Ford Coppola's Zoetrope Film Studio. She made her film debut in Coppola's *One from the Heart* in 1982, and a year later, starred in *Risky Business,* with Tom Cruise. They lived together for two years after that film. An ill-advised remake of the Brigitte Bardot movie, *And God Created Woman* – directed by BB's former husband, Roger Vadim, didn't accelerate Rebecca's road to stardom. It took the 1990s to do it. *The Hand That Rocks the Cradle* is generally considered her key movie. In 1999, her performance as a cancer survivor in TV's 'ER', added to her standing as an actress. Recently, she was good, in *Music Within*. She lives in Los Angeles with her husband Patrick O'Neal, and their two daughters. Rebecca played Cissy Yost in several episodes of the 2007 TV drama, 'John from Cincinnati'.

Risky Business (1983)
Runaway Train (1985)
The Trip to the Bountiful (1985)
By Dawn's Early Light (1990)
Backdraft (1991)
**The Hand That Rocks
the Cradle** (1992)
Guilty as Sin (1993)
Thick as Thieves (1998)
Identity (2003)
**Lords of
Dogtown** (2005)
Wedding Crashers (2005)
Music Within (2007)

Dame Judi **Dench**
5ft 3½in
(JUDITH OLIVIA DENCH)

Born: **December 9, 1934**
York, North Yorkshire, England

Judi was raised as a Quaker and attended Mount School, in York. At the Central School of Speech and Drama, in London she was in the same class as Vanessa Redgrave. Judi made her professional debut in 1957, when she appeared in Liverpool – playing the role of Ophelia, in "Hamlet". Four years later she joined the Royal Shakespeare Company and concentrated on stage work in London and Stratford – collecting six Olivier awards in the process. Judi did very little film work after her bit part debut in 1964's *The Third Secret*. She chose her roles carefully when she did and she'd passed her fiftieth birthday before *A Room with a View* heralded the start of an important movie career. In 1998, she was Oscar nominated for playing Queen Victoria, in *Mrs. Brown*. The following year, she was Best Supporting Actress for her eight minute impersonation of Queen Elizabeth I, in *Shakespeare in Love*. That same year, she won a Tony for her role in "Amie's View", on Broadway. From 1971 until his death in 2001, Judi was married to actor, Michael Williams. Their daughter is the young actress, Finty Williams. Since *Golden Eye,* Judi's been enjoying the key role of 'M' in the James Bond movies and was recently seen in *Quantum of Solace.*

A Room with a View (1985)
84 Charing Cross Road (1987)
A Handful of Dust (1988) **Henry V** (1989)
Jack & Sarah (1995)
Golden Eye (1995) **Hamlet** (1996)
Mrs. Brown (1997)
Shakespeare in Love (1997)
Tea with Mussolini (1999)
Chocolat (2000) **Iris** (2001)
The Shipping News (2001)
Die Another Day (2002)
The Chronicles of Riddick (2004)
Ladies in Lavender (2004)
Pride and Prejudice (2005)
Mrs. Henderson Presents (2005)
Casino Royale (2006)
Notes on a Scandal (2006)
Quantum of Solace (2008)

Catherine **Deneuve**
5ft 6in
(CATHERINE FABIENNE DORLÉAC)

Born: **October 22, 1943**
Paris, France

Catherine's father was theatrical in the sense that he dubbed foreign movies into French. Her older sister, Françoise Dorléac was only slightly ahead of her in starting a movie career and when Catherine was still at school she began getting small parts in films – starting with *Les Collégiennes,* in 1957. When, in 1960, Catherine portrayed her sister's sister, in *Les Portes claquent,* Françoise was already a very successful actress. Two years later, Catherine met Roger Vadim, who turned her blonde and directed her in *Le Vice et la vertu.* His efforts to make her erotic didn't work, but Jacques Demy had a role for her. She was beautiful in *Les Parapluies de Cherbourg,* which made her famous in France and her next wise decision was to work with Roman Polanski. That film *Repulsion* was seen internationally and by the mid-sixties, she was a star. In 1967, Françoise was killed in a car crash near Nice and that sad event was said to be a factor in Catherine's marriage to David Bailey turning sour. She soon got back on course and after several impressive roles, she was nominated for a Best Actress Oscar for *Indochine.* She has remained hugely popular and is still acting in films. She had a son with Vadim and a daughter with Marcello Mastroianni. When she's not busy filming, Catherine designs shoes, jewelry and spectacles.

Les Parapluies de Cherbourg (1964)
Repulsion (1965) La Vie de
Château (1966) Belle du Jour (1968)
Benjamin (1968) La Chamade (1968)
Tristana (1970) Fatti di Gente
Perbene (1975) Anima Persa (1977)
L'Argent des Autres (1978)
Le Dernier Metro (1980) L'Africain (1983)
Indochine (1992) My Favorite
Season (1993) Les Voleurs (1996)
Le Temps retrouvé (1999)
Dancer in the Dark (2000)
8 femmes (2002)
A Talking Picture (2003)
Rois et reine (2004)
Un conte de Noël (2008)

Robert **De Niro**
5ft 10in
(ROBERT MARIO DE NIRO JR.)

Born: **August 17, 1943**
New York City, New York, USA

Bob's parents met in an art class. His father became an abstract painter and also a sculptor. They divorced when he was two and he was raised by his mother in New York's 'Little Italy', where he was known as "Bobby Milk", due to his complexion. He enrolled at the High School of Music and Art, but at thirteen, he dropped out to join a street gang. He eventually saw the light and joined the Stella Adler Conservatory and later, Lee Strasberg's Actor's Studio. By the time he was eighteen he had several stage roles under his belt and had reconciled with his father. Bob did stage work until what is regarded as his official movie debut in *Greetings,* in 1968. Martin Scorsese's *Mean Streets* was his breakthrough, the start of many fruitful collaborations. Six Oscar nominations – two of them wins – as Best Supporting Actor, for *The Godfather: Part II, and* Best Actor, in *Raging Bull,* cover fifteen years of quality screen work, and demonstrate his consistency. Bob doesn't stop making films, and he directed *The Good Shepherd.* Many people consider him to be the greatest screen actor of the modern era. Few would argue, but some judge his recent work too harshly because of the high standards he has set himself.

Mean Streets (1973)
The Godfather: Part II (1974)
Taxi Driver (1976)
New York, New York (1977
The Deerhunter (1978)
Raging Bull (1980)
The Untouchables (1987)
Goodfellas (1990)
Backdraft (1991)
Cape Fear (1991)
This Boy's Life (1993)
A Bronx Tale (1993)
Casino (1995) Heat (1995)
Jackie Brown (1997) Ronin (1998)
Men of Honor (2000)
Meet the Fockers (2004)
The Good Shepherd (2006)
Stardust (2007)
What Just Happened? (2008)

Brian **Dennehy**
6ft 2in
(BRIAN MANNION DENNEHY)

Born: **July 9, 1938**
Bridgeport, Connecticut, USA

Brian was the son of Edward Dennehy, a wire service correspondent for Associated Press. His mother's name was Hannah. When they were kids, Brian and his two brothers were taken by their parents to live in Long Island. He attended Chaminade High School, in Mineola, before going to Columbia University on a football scholarship and majoring in history. After that, he studied drama at Yale. From 1959, after getting married and starting a family, he served four years in the United States Marine Corps. Following that, Brian appeared in summer stock productions and Off-Broadway shows, while working as a stockbroker. He took time to get his acting career on track – making his first screen appearance in an episode of TV's 'Kojak' in 1977. His film debut was that same year, in *Looking for Mr. Goodbar.* His imposing presence soon led to regular work, both in films – *First Blood, Gorky Park, Cocoon, Tommy Boy* and *Silverado* – as well as plenty of TV appearances. For his stage work, Brian won two Tony Awards for Best Actor from his only two nominations – for "Death of a Salesman" in 1999, and "Long Day's Journey into Night" in 2003. He currently lives with his second wife, Jennifer, in Woodstock, Connecticut. His daughters, Elizabeth and Kathleen Dennehy, are both actresses.

Semi-Tough (1977)
Foul Play (1978)
Split Image (1982)
First Blood (1983)
Never Cry Wolf (1983)
Gorky Park (1983)
The River Rat (1984)
Cocoon (1985)
Silverado (1985)
Twice in a Lifetime (1985)
F/X (1986) Legal Eagles (1986)
Best Seller (1987)
Presumed Innocent (1990)
Tommy Boy (1995)
The Ultimate Gift (2006)
War Eagle, Arkansas (2007)
Righteous Kill (2008)

Sandy **Dennis**
5ft 2in
(SANDRA HALE DENNIS)

Born: **April 27, 1937**
Hastings, Nebraska, USA
Died: **March 2, 1992**

Sandy was the daughter of Jack Dennis, a postal clerk, and his wife, Yvonne – who was a secretary. Sandy and her brother Frank grew up in Keneshaw and Lincoln, in Nebraska. At high school, she was a classmate of the Talk Show host, Dick Cavett. In Lincoln, she attended both the Nebraska Wesleyan University and University of Nebraska. She performed in a few plays with the Lincoln Community Theater Group before heading for New York City at the age of nineteen. Sandy had immediate success, appearing that same year in the television drama 'The Guiding Light' and in several off-Broadway productions. She concentrated on stage work until her big screen debut, in *Splendor in the Grass*. She was a true 'method' actress who used to display a rather neurotic technique when delivering her lines. Nevertheless, she was highly regarded, winning Tony Awards for her theater work and a Best Supporting Actress Oscar for *Who's Afraid of Virginia Woolf?* – in which she more than matched Richard Burton and Liz Taylor. After she played a lesbian, in *The Fox,* there were rumors about her sexual leanings, but although she never married she had a long lasting love affair with the modern jazz giant – the baritone saxophonist, Gerry Mulligan. Sandy died from ovarian cancer in Westport, Connecticut, at the age of fifty-four. It was a year after the release of her final movie, *The Indian Runner.*

Who's Afraid of Virginia
Woolf? (1966)
Up the Down Staircase (1967)
The Fox (1967)
Sweet November (1968)
The Out of Towners (1970)
The Four Seasons (1981)
Come Back to the
Five and Dime, Jimmy Dean,
Jimmy Dean (1982)
Another Woman (1988)
Parents (1989)
The Indian Runner (1991)

Reginald **Denny**
5ft 11in
(REGINALD LEIGH DUGMORE)

Born: **November 20, 1891**
Richmond, Surrey, England
Died: **June 16, 1967**

Reginald appeared on stage at three, as the Infant Prince, in "A Royal Family". He was educated at St. Francis Xavier School in Sussex. Although he served as a pilot in the Royal Flying Corps, during World War I, Reginald was able to continue his stage career. In the early 1920s, he went to America where his flying experience got him work as a stunt pilot in silent films. He'd appeared in more than fifty before starring in the part-talkie *Red Hot Speed,* in 1929. Apart from acting in films during a fifty year career, Reginald ran his own company specializing in the manufacture of model plane kits. Later, he and his firm helped provide U.S. Army anti-aircraft gunners with target practice during World War II, by producing radio-controlled target drones. The young Marilyn Monroe was believed to have been discovered when she worked at his Radioplane plant. Reginald's best films are *Of Human Bondage, Anna Karenina* and *Rebecca.* The twice married actor worked on TV and in movies into his late-seventies. He died of cancer only a few months after completing his last film, *Batman,* a 1966 spin-off from the television series.

Private Lives (1931)
Only Yesterday (1933)
The Lost Patrol (1934)
Of Human Bondage (1934)
The Richest Girl in
the World (1934)
Anna Karenina (1935)
Rebecca (1940)
One Night in Lisbon (1941)
Sherlock Holmes and the
Voice of Terror (1942)
The Locket (1946)
My Favorite Brunette (1947)
The Secret Life of
Walter Mitty (1947)
Mr. Blandings Builds His
Dream House (1948)
Around the World in
Eighty Days (1956)
Cat Ballou (1965)

Gérard **Depardieu**
5ft 10¾in
(GÉRARD XVAVIER MARCEL DEPARDIEU)

Born: **December 27, 1948**
Châteauroux, Indre, France

Gérard's father – who was employed as a sheet-metal worker – was reported to be an illiterate alcoholic. The actor may not be illiterate, but he's done his best on several occasions to emulate his father on the drinking front. He didn't make much of an effort to get an education either. Dropping out of school at the age of twelve – he hitchhiked across Europe – funding his existence by stealing cars and selling them on the black market. As luck would have it, Gérard had a friend he respected who was attending drama school in Paris. Through his influence, the young reprobate enrolled at the Theatre National Populaire. His film debut was in *Le Beatnik et le Minet.* Despite his lack of education and unorthodox upbringing, he learnt quickly. He got work in French TV dramas, but his first movie success was in *Going Places* in 1974. Gérard became an icon of French cinema without being pretty. He looks like a giant even though he is only of average height. Despite having undergone quintuple heart surgery in 2001, it didn't slow down his work rate or destroy his zest for life. On the subject of work rate, Gérard has no fewer than a dozen film projects in production at this time.

La Dernier Métro (1980)
Le Retour de Martin Guerre (1982)
Jean de Florette (1986)
Camille Claudel (1988)
Cyrano de Bergerac (1990)
Green Card (1990) Germinal (1993)
Le Colonel Chabert (1994)
Hamlet (1996)
The Man in the Iron Mask (1998)
Un pont entre deux rives (1999)
Le Placard (2001)
Bon Voyage (2003)
Tais-tois! (2003)
36 Quai des Orfères (2004)
Last Holiday (2006)
La Vie en rose (2007)
Michou d'Auber (2007)
Bouquet final (2008)
Hello Goodbye (2008)
Diamant 13 (2009)

Guillaume **Depardieu**
6ft 1in
(GUILLAUME JEAN MAXIME ANTOINE DEPARDIEU)

Born: **April 7, 1971**
Paris, France
Died: **October 13, 2008**

When he was three years old, Guillaume was taken to visit the film sets where his father, Gérard, was working. In 1974, he made his first screen appearance, in *Pas si méchant que ça.* It was another sixteen years before his next movie and a great deal happened in between. As busy actors, his father and mother were not ideal parents. When Guillaume reached his teens, their lack of affection sent him off the rails. He sought solace in alcohol and drugs and was expelled from several schools. There were periods when he spent more time in police custody than in the classroom. His father disowned him when, in 1988, he was sent to prison for trafficking heroin. Somehow he overcame the demons and acted in *Tous les matins du monde,* (with Gérard playing his older character). Guillaume was building a career of his own – he won a César as Most Promising Actor for *Les Apprentis.* Things looked good, or so he must have thought. Then, in 1996, he was riding his motorbike through the St. Cloud tunnel in Paris when he was hit by a suitcase which fell off a vehicle. He was left with a serious knee injury. For the next eight years, he lived in constant pain due to botched operations and treatment. In 2002, he co-starred with Gérard in the moving 'father and son' movie *Aime ton père,* but within a year, they were at each others throats. Reliance on morphine and antibiotics affected Guillaume's life and in 2003, he had his leg amputated and wore a prosthesis. He died in Garches of complications from pneumonia – leaving a wife, Elise Ventre, and a daughter, Louise.

Tous les matins du monde (1991)
Wild Target (1993)
L'Histoire du garçon qui voulait qu'on l'embrasse (1994)
Les Apprentis (1995) Marthe (1997)
White Lies (1998) The Sandmen (2000)
Aime ton père (2002) Process (2004)
La France (2007) De la guerre (2008)
Versailles (2008)

Julie **Depardieu**
5ft 7in
(JULIE DEPARDIEU)

Born: **June 18, 1973**
Paris, France

The younger sister of Guillaume, Julie has movies in her blood. Her father, Gérard, was already a star when she was born. Her mother, Elisabeth Guignot, has acted in a dozen or so films including *Jean de Florette* and *Manon des Sources.* Even so, when she was at college, Julie first focussed on the non-showbusiness subject of philosophy. She began her film career in 1994, with a small role in *Le Colonel Chabert* – which starred her father. Two years later, she was cast in the TV-film, 'La Passion du docteur Bergh' – which was directed by Josée Dayon, who would use Julie's talents several times in the future. She was a junior player in a number of films until getting her first award – a Best Supporting Actress César for *La Petite Lili* and also being named Most Promising Actress. She was nominated for *Podium* - directed by Yann Moix – who like other young directors – has benefited from Julie's support. She also works with the more experienced directors – a good example being André Téchiné – for whom she acted in the highly-rated film, *Les Témoins.* She has reached the point of an international breakthrough with her role in *Un secret,* and *Les femmes de l'ombres* (Female Agents).

Midnight Exam (1998)
Peut-être (1999)
Love Me (2000) Les Destinées sentimentales (2000)
Veloma (2001)
Fool's Song (2003)
La Petite Lili (2003)
Podium (2004)
A Very Long Engagement (2004)
La Febbre (2005)
Essaye-moi (2006)
Moon on the Snow (2006)
If You Love Me, Follow (2006)
Blame it on Fidel! (2006)
Poltergay (2006)
Les Témoins (2007)
Rush Hour 3 (2007)
Un secret (2007)
Female Agents (2008)

Johnny **Depp**
5ft 10in
(JOHN CHRISTOPHER DEPP)

Born: **June 9, 1963**
Owensboro, Kentucky, USA

Johnny was raised – along with his two sisters and a brother – in twenty different locations, until the family settled in Miramar, Florida. He was a disturbed child who engaged in self-harm, but when he was twelve, his mother bought him an electric guitar and he played in garage bands. At sixteen, he dropped out of high school and was eventually part of a group known as "The Kids". On Christmas Eve 1983, Johnny married the drummer's sister. It caused friction, so he then recorded with "Rock City Angels". His wife introduced him to Nicolas Cage, who advised him to take up acting. In 1984, Johnny was in *A Nightmare on Elm Street,* and shortly after that, he got divorced. He (unwillingly) became a teen idol during his appearance in the TV series, '21 Jump Street' but shed that image from *Edward Scissorhands* onwards. He still appeals to young audiences, but he has branched out into darker roles, playing complex types, whose behavior fascinates adults. Johnny was Oscar-nominated three times – for *Pirates of the Caribbean, Finding Neverland,* and *Sweeney Todd.* After divorce from his wife Lori, he dated a series of beautiful women before settling down and having two children with French actress/singer, Vanessa Paradis. Johnny still retains his interest in music. His next screen role will be in Terry Gilliam's *The Imaginarium of Doctor Parnassus,* which was Heath Ledger's final movie.

Edward Scissorhands (1990)
Ed Wood (1994) Donnie Brasco (1997)
Fear and Loathing in Las Vegas (1998)
The Ninth Gate (1999) Sleepy Hollow (1999) Chocolat (2000) Blow (2001)
From Hell (2001) Pirates of the Caribbean (2003) Once Upon a Time in Mexico (2003) Secret Window (2004)
Finding Neverland (2004)
The Libertine (2005) Charlie and the Chocolate Factory (2005)
Pirates 2 (2006) Pirates 3 (2007)
Sweeney Todd (2007)
Public Enemies (2009)

John **Derek**
6ft 1in
(DEREK DELEVAN HARRIS)

Born: **August 12, 1926**
Hollywood, California, USA
Died: **May 22, 1998**

Born into a show business family, John was the son of Lawson Harris, a writer-director of silent movies, and an actress called Dolores Johnson. When he was about eighteen, John was described as impossibly handsome. He was living close enough to the studios to get noticed and as Derek Harris, he made his film debut with a walk-on role in the 1944 tearjerker *Since You Went Away.* After service with the U.S. Army, he changed his name to John Derek, and in 1948, landed a contract with Columbia Pictures. There were two important films the following year and at one time, it looked as if he would have a big future. In 1951, he married the first of his four wives, Pati Behrs – a grand-niece of Leo Tolstoy. Columbia released him and in 1953, he became a freelance actor with immediate success. He played a priest who became a boxer, in *The Leather Saint* and kept to the religious theme as Joshua in Cecil B. DeMille's biblical epic *The Ten Commandments.* His mainstream movie career ended in 1960, in the appropriately named, *Exodus.* He had a minor directing career, but he married and photographed his wives – Ursula Andress, Linda Evans and Bo Derek for Playboy and co-directed Ursula in his last film appearance – in *Nightmare in the Sun.* No wonder it was from heart problems that he died at his home in Santa Maria, California!

Knock on Any Door (1949)
All the King's Men (1949)
Saturday's Hero (1951)
The Family Secret (1951)
Scandal Sheet (1952)
The Last Posse (1953)
The Outcast (1954)
Prince of Players (1955)
Run for Cover (1955)
The Leather Saint (1956)
The Ten Commandments (1956)
Fury at Sundown (1957)
Omar Khayyam (1957)
Exodus (1960)
Nightmare in the Sun (1965)

Bruce **Dern**
6ft
(BRUCE MACLEISH DERN)

Born: **June 4, 1936**
Chicago, Illinois, USA

The son of John and Jean Dern, it was surprising that Bruce decided to take up acting rather than politics – his grandfather had been Governor of Utah – his godfather was Adlai Stevenson! Following his early education, Bruce was set to attend the University of Pennsylvania, but the urge to act was so strong, he opted for Lee Strasberg's Actors' Studio in New York. He was a contemporary of Jane Fonda's, but as Bruce wasn't such obvious star material, he worked extra hard. In 1958 he made his Broadway debut in "A Touch of the Poet" – an apt title, considering that his uncle is the poet Archibald MacLeish. He made his first movie in 1960 – Elia Kazan's *Wild River* – and appeared regularly in the TV western series 'Stoney Burke'. He also acted on television for Alfred Hitchcock as well as in his movie, *Marnie.* Bruce built a reputation as a 'heavy' and through his contact with Jack Nicholson, he got parts in Roger Corman movies. In the 1970s, he climbed the ladder to leading roles, only to stutter during the 1980s. The past fifteen years have seen a resurgence. Bruce is the father of Laura Dern.

Will Penny (1968)
They Shoot Horses,
Don't They? (1969)
The Cowboys (1972)
The King of Marvin Gardens (1972)
The Great Gatsby (1974)
Posse (1975)
Black Sunday (1977)
Coming Home (1978)
The Driver (1978)
The 'burbs (1989)
Wild Bill (1995)
Last Man Standing (1996)
Madison (2001) Monster (2003)
The Hard Easy (2005)
Down in the Valley (2005)
Believe in Me (2006)
Walker Payne (2006)
The Astronaut Farmer (2006)
The Cake Eaters (2007)
Chatham (2008)

Laura **Dern**
5ft 10in
(LAURA ELIZABETH DERN)

Born: **February 10, 1967**
Los Angeles, California, USA

Laura is the daughter of film stars, Bruce Dern and Diane Ladd. They lost their first child in a swimming pool tragedy and for a while, they took great care of their new daughter – even taking her on to the set when they were filming the TV show 'Castle Keep'. They split up when she was two and Laura stayed with her mother. Her pedigree gave her early access to the world of movies. She was six years old when she played a scene with Burt Reynolds, in *White Lightning.* After she'd attended a private Catholic school and high school, Laura started appearing in films. The 1980s was a good beginning for her. While still a teenager, she could look older than her years because of her height. She had made two David Lynch films by the time she consolidated her star status in the 1990s – the first was *Blue Velvet* – and then for the second, *Rambling Rose,* Laura was nominated for a Best Actress Oscar. Into the present century, she has done well – both professionally and privately. Following engagements to Billy Bob Thornton, and Jeff Goldblum, Laura made her choice – after two years of getting to know him she married singer/songwriter Ben Harper, in 2005. They now have two children.

Teachers (1984) Mask (1985)
Smooth Talk (1985)
Blue Velvet (1986)
Wild at Heart (1990)
Rambling Rose (1991)
A Perfect World (1993)
Citizen Ruth (1996)
October Sky (1999)
Novocaine (1993)
Focus (2001) I Am Sam (2001)
We Don't Live Here
Anymore (2004)
Happy Endings (2005)
The Prize Winner
of Defiance, Ohio (2005)
Lonely Hearts (2006)
Inland Empire (2006)
Year of the Dog (2007)
Tenderness (2008)

Vittorio De Sica
5ft 9¼in
(VITTORIO DE SICA)

Born: **July 7, 1902**
Sora, Latium, Italy
Died: **November 13, 1974**

Vittorio was raised by his parents in extreme poverty, in Naples. By a quirk of nature, he was blessed with intelligence and good looks. He was also fired with a determination to get away from the squalor and began working at the age of fourteen. Vittorio became interested in acting and his first taste of movie making was when he played a small part in *The Clemenceau Affair,* in 1917. Three years later he joined Tatiana Pavlova's stage company and became a matinee idol of the Italian Theater circuit. His big talent for light comedy was projected to a wider audience when he starred in his first sound film *La Vecchia Signora,* in 1932. It made him a huge star in Italy and kept him employed as an actor right up to the start of World War II. He began directing, but after 1942's superb *Bambini ci guardano* conditions in Italy made it impossible. He resurfaced as a director in 1946, with *Sciuscià.* His classic movies are *Ladri di biciclette, Miracolo di Milano* and *Umberto D.* In the 1950s, some commercial failures took him back to acting. But Vittorio directed Sophia Loren's Oscar winning performance in *Two Women* in 1961, and was on top form with the beautiful film, *Una breve vacanza,* only a year before he died after an operation. The movies listed below prove what a fine actor he was too.

I'll Give a Million (1936)
I Grandi magazzini (1939)
Maddalena, zero in condotta (1940)
Teresa Venerdì (1941)
Un Garibaldino al convento (1942)
Abbasso la ricchezza! (1948)
Cuore (1948)
Domani è troppo tardi (1950)
Pane, amore e fantasia (1953)
Secrets d'alcove (1954)
Il Segno di Venere (1955)
Bread, love and... (1955)
Il Bigamo (1956)
Padre e figli (1957)
A Farewell to Arms (1957)
Il Generale della Rovere (1959)

Danny DeVito
4ft 11in
(DANIEL MICHAEL DEVITO JR.)

Born: **November 17, 1944**
Asbury Park, New Jersey, USA

Danny spent his formative years at the Catholic Oratory Preparatory School, as a boarder. When he graduated in 1961, he had no profession in mind, so he spent a couple of years employed as a cosmetician in a beauty parlor run by his sister. It appears to have been all he could expect from life, because he then entered the American Academy of Dramatic Arts with the express purpose of improving his skills as a make-up artist. The atmosphere soon seduced him and he transferred to studying acting. He had a small part in a very small film called *Dreams of Glass,* in 1968, but the studios weren't exactly clamoring for his services. For a period of about four years Danny had little choice other than to concentrate on stage work. In the early 1970s, he started to get a few movie roles – the best of which was when he played the mental patient, Martini, in *One Flew Over the Cuckoo's Nest.* Danny then worked regularly as Louie De Palma, in the TV series, 'Taxi'. His big break came with his pal, Mike Douglas, in *Romancing the Stone.* Despite a quality drought during recent years, Danny's been involved as an actor and director (his best was *Death to Smoochie*), and producer, in all kinds of movies – some of them are excellent. He is a much-loved Hollywood character.

Romancing the Stone (1984)
Twins (1988) The War of the
Roses (1989) Other People's
Money (1991) Get Shorty (1995)
Matilda (1996)
L.A. Confidential (1997)
Man on the Moon (1999)
Heist (2001) Death to
Smoochy (2002)
Anything Else (2003)
Big Fish (2003) Be Cool (2005)
The Oh in Ohio (2006)
10 Items or Less (2006)
The Good Night (2007)
Reno 911: Miami (2007)
Just add Water (2007)
Nobel Son (2007)
Just Add Water (2008)

Cameron Diaz
5ft 8½in
(CAMERON MICHELLE DIAZ)

Born: **August 30, 1972**
San Diego, California, USA

Cameron is an interesting mixture – in terms of her personality, character, and physique. She has some Cuban, English, German, and Native American blood in her veins, but she is, at the end of the day, an All-American girl. She attended the same high school in Long Beach as the rapper, Snoopy Dogg. During those years, she was known as 'Skeleton' by her classmates because she was so thin. She left home at sixteen to travel round the world – returning in 1992 to look for a job. Being tall and skinny she joined the *Elite model agency,* working on products like Calvin Klein, Levi's, and Coca Cola. Without any previous movie acting experience, she returned to California in 1994 for a co-starring role in *The Mask.* After that, she took acting lessons and gained good experience in independent movies – *The Last Supper* and *Feeling Minnesota.* Cameron's first major movie, *There's Something About Mary,* earned her a Golden Globe nomination. *Being John Malkovich, Vanilla Sky* and *Gangs of New York* – were all near misses for the same prize. But Cameron has plenty of talent to combine with her obvious beauty, and her time will come. After a three year relationship with the actor, Matt Dillon, Cameron dated singers, Jared Leto, and Justin Timberlake. At the time of writing she is a free agent once more.

Fear and Loathing in
Las Vegas (1998)
There's Something
About Mary (1998)
Being John Malkovich (1999)
Any Given Sunday (1999)
Things You Can Tell Just by
Looking at Her (2000)
Charlie's Angels (2000)
Vanilla Sky (2001)
My Father's House (2002)
Gangs of New York (2002)
In Her Shoes (2005)
The Holiday (2006)
What Happens in Vegas (2008)
My Sister's Keeper (2009)

Leonardo **DiCaprio**
5ft 11in
(LEONARDO WILHELM DICAPRIO)

Born: November 11, 1974
Hollywood, California, USA

An Italian father and a German mother who loved da Vinci paintings, will tell you how Leonardo got his name. Following his parents' divorce he spent some of his early childhood with his mother, living in Germany, and is fluent in the language. Their eventual return to L.A. resulted in some hard times, but he saw a way out of it after watching his step-brother acting in commercials. He attended Marshall High School and got a role in a television series 'Parenthood'. He acted in TV commercials and appeared in the soap opera, 'Santa Barbara'. He was seventeen when making his film debut, in *Critters 3*. While working in the TV sitcom, 'Growing Pains' he beat four hundred other young hopefuls for the plum role of Toby, in *This Boy's Life*. He was then Oscar-nominated for playing a mentally handicapped boy in that same year's *What's Eating Gilbert Grape*. Leo's star status was confirmed and his promotion from star to superstar arrived in 1997 – in the worldwide blockbuster, *Titanic*. Since then he has enjoyed ten years at the top. A toughening of his image has added to his popularity with male moviegoers and resulted in another Oscar-nomination, for *Blood Diamond*. Leo's current girlfriend is Israeli supermodel, Bar Refaeli.

This Boy's Life (1993)
What's Eating Gilbert Grape? (1993)
The Quick and the Dead (1995)
The Basketball Diaries (1995)
Total Eclipse (1995)
Romeo and Juliet (1996)
Marvin's Room (1996)
Titanic (1997)
The Man in the Iron Mask (1998)
Celebrity (1998)
The Beach (2000)
Don's Plum (2001)
Catch Me if you Can (2002)
Gangs of New York (2002)
The Aviator (2004)
The Departed (2006)
Blood Diamond (2006)
Body of Lies (2008)
Revolutionary Road (2008)

Angie **Dickinson**
5ft 5in
(ANGELINE BROWN)

Born: September 30, 1931
Kulm, North Dakota, USA

Angie's father was publisher of The Kulm Messenger newspaper until the family moved to Burbank, in 1942. Angie won a beauty contest when she was a senior at Bellamarine Jefferson High School. She briefly dreamed of a stage or screen career, but in reality became a secretary in an airplane parts factory. At twenty-one, she was a stunning looking girl. She then married a former football player, Gene Dickinson. In 1953, she entered beauty pageants whilst working for a degree in business at the Immaculate Heart College in Los Angeles. From her dad, Angie inherited a love of the written word , but any idea of a writing career vanished when she got a small part in the 1954 Doris Day film, *Lucky Me*. Initially it only led to a series of walk on parts in movies and TV shows, but two years later, she had the female lead in a western titled *Hidden Guns*. Although magazines used to focus on her fabulous legs, another cowboy film, the popular, *Rio Bravo* – in which she wore long skirts – made her famous. Co-star Dean Martin was part of the Rat Pack and Angie became the ideal choice to appear in *Ocean's Eleven,* with former lover, Frank Sinatra. Angie was still looking fabulous in her fifties, but she was mainly to be seen on television – the last time being in 2004 – in an episode of 'Judging Amy'.

Cry Terror! (1958)
Rio Bravo (1959)
Ocean's Eleven (1960)
Rome Adventure (1962)
Captain Newman M.D. (1963)
The Killers (1964)
The Art of Love (1965)
The Chase (1966)
Cast a Giant Shadow (1966)
Point Blank (1967)
Pretty Maids All in a Row (1971)
Big Bad Mama (1974)
Dressed to Kill (1980)
Death Hunt (1981)
Sabrina (1995)
Pay It Forward (2000)
Big Bad Love (2001)

August **Diehl**
5ft 10½in
(AUGUST DIEHL)

Born: January 4, 1976
Berlin, Germany

August is the son of Hans Diehl, an actor who has done most of his work on TV. His mother is a costume designer, and his brother, with whom he shares a passion for music, is a composer. Both boys have benefited from their parents' creative genes and early on, because of their father's work, they enjoyed the pleasure of living in some of Europe's most inspiring cities – including Hamburg, Vienna and Munich. At high school in Bavaria, August displayed a talent for acting which was best demonstrated by his performance as Franz Mohr, in a production of Friedrich Schiller's play "Die Räuber". After passing his Abitur exams, his parents sent him to Berlin to study acting at the Hochschule für Schauspielkunst Ernst Busch. August graduated in 1998, and had his first movie making experience that year, in the short subject, *Poppen*. His next film role, in the excellent drama *23,* won him the Bavarian Film Award as Best Young Actor, as well as a German Film Award Gold. August has since been further recognized for his performances in *Love in Thoughts* and *The Ninth Day*. Unlike his dad, he has chosen to concentrate on film. His only venture on to the small screen was a 2004 telefilm called 'Feuer in der Nacht'. He is married to actress, Julia Malik and lives in Berlin. In his leisure moments, he plays the guitar. He is fluent in both French and English.

23 (1998) **Entering Reality** (1999)
Der Atemkünstler (2000)
Cold Is the Breath of Evening (2000)
Tattoo (2002) **Anatomie 2** (2003)
Distant Lights (2003)
The Birch-Tree Meadow (2003)
Love in Thoughts (2004)
The Ninth Day (2004)
Mouth to Mouth (2005)
Slumming (2006)
I Am the Other Woman (2006)
Nothing But Ghosts (2006)
The Counterfeiters (2007)
Freischwimmer (2007)
Dr. Alemán (2008)
A Woman in Berlin (2008)

Marlene **Dietrich**
5ft 6in
(MARIA MAGDALANA DIETRICH)

Born: **December 27, 1901**
Berlin-Schöneberg, Germany
Died: **May 6, 1992**

Marlene was the daughter of a Royal Prussian Police officer. She studied the violin briefly before joining The Deutsche Theaterschule in Berlin. Her first stage role was in "Der Kleine Napoleon" in 1923. She married casting director, Rudolf Sieber, who helped her career. In 1930 she was signed by Paramount along with her 'Svengali' – Josef von Sternberg. He set about changing her image from the plump Marlene of *The Blue Angel* into one of the twentieth century's most glamorous icons. Over in Hollywood she acted and had affairs with, Cary Grant and Gary Cooper. With Josef's help (and a great lighting cameraman) she was beautiful to look at, but it was often style over substance – which is the best way to enjoy her. Von Sternberg's wife sued her for the alienation of his affections and lost the case. Hitler ordered her to return to Germany, but she said "Nein!" By 1937, due to Josef's outdated influence, Marlene was box-office poison in America. Once rid of him, she made the hit movie, *Destry Rides Again* and did herself a power of good during World War II, by entertaining US troops. In 1948, although lying about her true date of birth, Marlene became "The World's Most Glamorous Grandmother". Around that time she began demanding more money than studios were willing to pay. After 1952, she was a touring cabaret star, who made an occasional movie. Marlene died of kidney failure, at her home in Paris.

The Blue Angel (1930) Morocco (1930)
Shanghai Express (1932)
The Scarlet Empress (1934) The Devil
is a Woman (1935) Desire (1936)
Knight Without Armour (1937)
Destry Rides Again (1939)
Manpower (1941) The Spoilers (1942)
A Foreign Affair (1948)
Stage Fright (1950) No Highway (1951)
Rancho Notorious (1952)
The Monte Carlo Story (1957)
Witness for the Prosecution (1957)
Judgement at Nuremberg (1961)

Anton **Diffring**
5ft 11½in
(ALFRED POLLACK)

Born: **October 20, 1918**
Koblenz, Germany
Died: **May 20, 1989**

Anton's family belonged to one of the most famous theatrical dynasties in pre-World War II Europe. After he'd finished his standard education, he went to Vienna to train for the stage. He later transferred to Berlin, where he attended the Academy of Drama. In his late teens, through mixing with Jewish actors, he developed a strong anti-Nazi stance and in 1939, he decided to leave Germany and go to Canada. He was probably surprised when he was put into an internment camp, where he was forced to stay for the duration of the war. He continued acting in productions staged with other prisoners and when he was released in 1946, he had improved his English enough to make his Canadian stage debut in Toronto, in "The Tempest". He appeared on Broadway, in "Winners and Losers", "The Deputy of Paris", and "Faust". But his European roots were still strong enough to take him to England in 1950. Anton made his film debut in 1950, in *State Secret,* and with British studios crying out for real Germans to act in their war movies, he was type-cast as a Nazi for much of his career, but it kept him employed. Anton died at Chateauneuf-de-Grasse, in France.

The Red Beret (1953)
Albert R.N. (1953) Betrayed (1954)
The Colditz Story (1955) I Am a
Camera (1955) The Crooked
Sky (1957) The Traitor (1957)
Seven Thunders (1957)
A Question of Adultery (1958)
The Man Who Could Cheat Death (1959)
Circus of Horrors (1960)
The Heroes of Telemark (1965)
The Blue Max (1966)
Fahrenheit 451 (1966) The Double
Man (1967) Counterpoint (1967)
Where Eagles Dare (1968)
Zeppelin (1971)
The Beast Must Die (1974)
Operation Daybreak (1975)
The Accuser (1977) Victory (1981)
Faceless (1988)

Matt **Dillon**
6ft
(MATTHEW RAYMOND DILLON)

Born: **February 18, 1964**
New Rochelle, New York, USA

The son of Paul Dillon and his wife Mary Ellen, Matt was raised with four brothers and a sister in Mamaroneck, New York, in an Irish Catholic family environment. Brother Kevin is also an actor. Matt went to Hommocks School in Larchmont and Mamaroneck High School. He was spotted by a casting director and he was just fourteen when he made his screen debut in *Over the Edge*. He got roles in two good 1980 productions, *Little Darlings* and *My Bodyguard*. Both those films appealed strongly to the teenage market, so he was cast in more of the same until he began to look for something with a bit more beef in it. He then found it to some degree in 1983, in Francis Coppola's *Rumble Fish,* but it was the very adult *Drugstore Cowboy,* in 1989, which made the critics sit up and take notice. Frustratingly for his fans, he started slowly in the early 1990s, but by the end of the decade he was scoring hit after hit. During the past five years he has continued to grow in stature. He made his directorial debut in 2002, with *City of Ghosts* and received his first Oscar nomination – as Best Supporting Actor – in the very successful movie *Crash*. In 1998, he ended a serious two-year relationship with Cameron Diaz – his co-star in *There's Something about Mary*. In 2007 he married supermodel, Adriana Johnson. They have a son named Liam.

Rumble Fish (1983)
The Flamingo Kid (1984)
The Big Town (1987)
Drugstore Cowboy (1989)
Singles (1992) To Die For (1995)
Frankie Starlight (1995)
Beautiful Girls (1996)
Grace of My Heart (1996)
In & Out (1997) Wild Things (1998)
There's Something
About Mary (1998)
One Night at McCool's (2001)
City of Ghosts (2002)
Employee of the Month (2004)
Crash (2004) Factotum (2005)
Nothing But the Truth (2008)

Troy **Donahue**
6ft 3in
(MERLE JOHNSON JR.)

Born: **January 27, 1936**
New York City, New York, USA
Died: **September 2, 2001**

Troy's father was a vice-president of General Motors. His mother, Edith, had appeared on stage in amateur theatrical productions. When Troy was thirteen, his father fell ill and he began drinking alcohol. After his dad died a year later, Troy was sent to the New York Military Academy at Cornwallon-Hudson. It was there, as a young cadet, that he befriended Francis Ford Coppola – who would remember him years later when he needed work – and cast him in *The Godfather: Part II*. In 1955, Troy studied journalism at Columbia University, but he was spotted by a talent scout from Hollywood and signed up with Rock Hudson's agent, Henry Willson. It was Willson who gave him his new name, and as Troy Donahue, he made his film debut for Universal in 1957 – an uncredited role in *Man Afraid*. In 1958, he established himself as a teenage heartthrob in films like *Summer Love* and seven others. *A Summer Place* made him a star and he was signed by Warners. When it ended in 1965, he became dependent on alcohol. He survived with TV work and small roles in films for thirty-five years. Divorced four times, he lived with opera singer, Zheng Cao, until he died of a heart attack.

The Tarnished Angels (1958)
Summer Love (1958)
Live Fast, Die Young (1958)
This Happy Feeling (1958)
Voice in the Mirror (1958)
Wild Heritage (1958)
The Perfect Furlough (1958)
Monster On the
Campus (1958)
Imitation of Life (1959)
A Summer Place (1959)
The Crowded Sky (1960)
Parrish (1961)
Susan Slade (1961)
Rome Adventure (1962)
Palm Springs Weekend (1963)
A Distant Trumpet (1964)
My Blood Runs Cold (1965)
The Godfather: Part II (1974)

Robert **Donat**
6ft
(FRIEDRICH ROBERT DONATH)

Born: **March 18, 1905**
Withington, Lancashire, England
Died: **June 9, 1958**

Despite having a Polish-born father and German ancestry on his mother's side, Robert grew up to epitomize the gentle, old-fashioned, upper-class Englishman. When he was a small boy he suffered from a terrible stammer. His mother persuaded him to take elocution lessons. He developed into a confident youngster and while still at school, he began to reveal acting ability. He made his stage debut in Birmingham, in "Julius Caesar" when he was fifteen, and after a few more stage roles, joined Sir Frank Benson's touring Company. He got married and went to London in 1930. Some plays were flops, but he persevered with the stage to the extent that he turned down an offer from Thalberg to go to Hollywood. He was signed by Korda to work in Britain, but after *The Private Life of Henry VIII*, he was loaned out for his first Hollywood venture, in *The Count of Monte Cristo*. Robert had no time for Hollywood money and glamour and stayed at home to work in his preferred medium, the stage. He made a handful of British classics – one with Alfred Hitchcock – but the pinnacle was when he beat off the challenge of Gable's Rhett Butler, to win an Oscar for *Goodbye, Mr. Chips*. His career had been dogged by asthma, and it was no surprise when he died in London of a massive attack, aged fifty-three – after completing his final movie, *The Inn of the Sixth Happiness*. Robert left his estate to his three children and left nothing at all to his second wife, Renee Asherson.

The Count of Monte Cristo (1934)
The 39 Steps (1935)
The Ghost Goes West (1935)
Knight Without Armour (1937)
The Citadel (1938)
Goodbye, Mr. Chips (1939)
The Young Mr. Pitt (1942)
Perfect Strangers (1945)
The Winslow Boy (1948) The Magic
Box (1951) Lease of Life (1954)
The Inn of the Sixth Happiness (1958)

Brian **Donlevy**
5ft 8in
(WALDO BRIAN DONLEVY)

Born: **February 9, 1901**
Portadown, County Armagh, Northern Ireland
Died: **April 5, 1972**

The Hollywood machine created the myth that Brian was born in Ireland. Some years before that, he had already lied about his age (when he was fifteen) so he could join American troops pursuing Pancho Villa, in Mexico. Later, he became a pilot during World War I with the Lafayette Escadrille, in France. Apart from the Irish blarney, he was "Mister Personality". He managed to get work as a stage hand in New York and then, through careful observation, he became an actor. It was a natural progression into silent films – his first bit part was in *Jamestown,* in 1923. His talking picture debut was in *Gentlemen of the Press,* in 1929, but he had no lines. Primarily a stage actor until 1935, when he had a featured role in *Barbary Coast,* he became in demand as a tough, dynamic second lead. In 1939, his vintage year, he made six films. He was Oscar-nominated for his portrayal of the sadistic Sergeant Markoff, in *Beau Geste*. It consolidated his career – he was still getting top billing in 1955 – in *The Quatermass Xperiment.* Years later, he co-starred with Jerry Lewis. He said his farewell in the very entertaining *Pit Stop*. A life-long smoker, he died of throat cancer.

Crack-Up (1936)
In Old Chicago (1937)
This Is My Affair (1937)
Jesse James (1939)
Union Pacific (1939)
Beau Geste (1939)
Destry Rides Again (1939)
The Great McGinty (1940)
When the Daltons Rode (1940)
Birth of the Blues (1941)
The Remarkable Andrew (1942)
The Miracle of Morgan's Creek (1944)
Two Years Before the Mast (1946)
Kiss of Death (1947)
Impact (1949) Shakedown (1950)
The Big Combo (1955)
The Quatermas Xperiment (1955)
A Cry in the Night (1956)
Cowboy (1958) The Errand Boy (1961)
Pit Stop (1969)

Françoise **Dorléac**
5ft 6in
(FRANÇOISE DORLÉAC)

Born: **March 21, 1942**
Paris, France
Died: **June 26, 1967**

Françoise was from a theatrical family. Maurice Dorléac, a film actor, and his wife, Renée Deneuve, couldn't have had two more beautiful little girls than Françoise and Catherine. Born eighteen months before her sister, Françoise was always the more confident and outgoing. In 1952, she appeared on stage for the first time and at fifteen years of age, was in the short movie called *Mensonges*. Françoise studied at the Conservatoire National Supérieur d'Art Dramatique, in Paris, for two years and modeled for Christian Dior. Her first starring role in *Les Loups dans la bergerie,* was in 1960. Her breakthrough film was the 1964 adventure movie – *L'Homme de Rio,* starring Jean-Paul Belmondo. She then worked with top directors, François Truffaut and Roman Polanski. It was in the latter's bizarre *Cul de sac,* where she played a flighty young girl living in an isolated house with the very weird, bald-headed, middle-aged English owner, Donald Pleasance, that she first struck a chord outside France. It is still modern after forty-five years. By the time she and her sister co-starred in *The Young Girls of Rochefort,* both had become big names. Sadly for Françoise, that fame was taken away by the cruelest possible fate. She was driving to Nice airport, on her way to the London premiere of *Young Girls* when she lost control of her car and hit a sign post. The car flipped right over and quickly burst into flames. Françoise didn't have enough strength to open the door and she died soon afterwards.

Ce soir ou jamais (1961)
Arsène Lupin contre
Arsène Lupin (1962)
L'Homme de Rio (1964)
La Peau douce (1964)
La Chasse à l'homme (1964)
Where the Spies Are (1965)
Cul de sac (1966)
The Young Girls of
Rochefort (1967)
Billion Dollar Brain (1967)

Diana **Dors**
5ft 5½in
(DIANA MARY FLUCK)

Born: **October 23, 1931**
Swindon, Wiltshire, England
Died: **May 4, 1984**

With encouragement from her parents – especially her mother, Diana began her stage career when she was in junior school. She took dancing lessons, and by the age of fourteen – during World War II – she was performing in variety shows at theaters, to entertain servicemen. In 1946, she went to London, where she stayed with relatives until she was accepted as a student at the Royal Academy of Dramatic Art. In 1947, Diana went with some girlfriends to Worton Hall Studios in Isleworth. She was given an uncredited role in *The Shop at Sly Corner.* Later that year, she had an opportunity to show off her figure in *Holiday Camp,* which was shot in Filey, North Yorkshire. Her first good role was as Charlotte, in David Lean's *Oliver Twist.* It led to more work, but few acting opportunities. Diana didn't fight the system – she adapted to it – even becoming a peroxide blonde and allowing herself to believe the studio hype, that she was Britain's answer to Marilyn Monroe – she wasn't! In *Yield to the Night* she had one of her few chances to show that she could really act. Diana went to Hollywood in 1957 – making three forgettable movies. She returned home, where she worked regularly in films and TV until her death at her home in Windsor, from stomach cancer.

Oliver Twist (1948)
Here Come the Huggetts (1948)
A Boy, a Girl and a Bike (1949)
Diamond City (1949)
Dance Hall (1950)
The Last Page (1952)
The Saint's Return (1953)
A Kid for Two Farthings (1955)
Value for Money (1955)
Yield to the Night (1956)
Tread Softly Stranger (1958)
On the Double (1961)
There's a Girl in My Soup (1970)
Deep End (1971)
Hannie Caulder (1971)
The Pied-Piper (1972)
Steaming (1985)

Kirk **Douglas**
5ft 9in
(ISSUR DANIELOVITCH DEMSKY)

Born: **December 9, 1916**
Amsterdam, New York, USA

Kirk grew up in a ghetto, but he was brainy and brawny, and at St. Lawrence University he was the inter-collegiate wrestling champ. At twenty he was a soda-jerk, parking attendant, and theater usher – which made him determined to be an actor. After the American Academy of Dramatic Arts, he landed his first role in the Broadway show, "Spring Again". In 1942, he joined the US Navy. When the hostilities ceased he did radio work until Lauren Bacall recommended him to Hal Wallis. In 1946, Kirk had a featured role in *The Strange Loves of Martha Ivers,* and shortly after that was loaned to RKO for the classic film-noir, *Out of the Past.* He was the new star of 1950, following his leading role in the movie, *Champion.* Why he never won an Oscar in the years that followed remains a mystery. At least three performances were better than those of the winners, but the ultimate reward was denied him. In 1996, Kirk suffered a stroke which impaired his speech. Determined as some of the characters he'd played in movies, Kirk kept on going into his late eighties – delivering yet another powerful performance in 2004 – in *Illusion*.

The Strange Love of Martha Ivers (1946)
Out of the Past (1947) Mourning
Becomes Electra (1947)
Champion (1949) Young Man with a
Horn (1950) The Glass Menagerie (1950)
Ace in the Hole (1951) Detective
Story (1951) The Big Sky (1952) The Bad
and the Beautiful (1952) Act of
Love (1953) Ulysses (1954) Man Without
a Star (1955) Lust for Life (1956) Gunfight
at the O.K. Corral (1957) Paths of
Glory (1957) The Vikings (1958) Last
Train from Gun Hill (1959) The Devil's
Disciple (1959) Strangers When We
Meet (1960) Spartacus (1960)
The Last Sunset (1961) Lonely are the
Brave (1962) Two Weeks in Another
Town (1962) Seven Days in May (1964)
The War Wagon (1967) A Gunfight (1971)
The Final Countdown (1980) Eddie
Macon's Run (1983) Illusion (2004)

Melvyn **Douglas**
6ft 1¹/₂in
(MELVYN EDOUARD HESSELBERG)

Born: **April 5, 1901**
Macon, Georgia, USA
Died: **August 4, 1981**

Although his father was concert pianist, Edouard Hesselbeg, Melvyn had none of his musical talent. He wasn't enough of a scholar to get through high school, but he shone in school plays. He then honed his skills with stock companies in Michigan – where he made his debut at eighteen, in Chicago. He then worked in Indiana, Wisconsin, and New York. A Broadway hit, "Tonight or Never" ended in marriage to Helen Gahagan, and a Hollywood offer. Gloria Swanson loved him in it, and when it was made into a film, Melvyn was her co-star. He was then chosen by Garbo to act with her in *As You Desire Me*. It was followed by less desirable, mediocre material – causing his career to stall until 1935 – when he had a hit with *She Married Her Boss*. Columbia signed him and he did well opposite stars like Dunne, Rainer, and Crawford. He even went out on loan to act with Deanna Durbin. He joined the US Army in 1942 and served until 1945. He struggled on his return and after 1950, he acted mainly on Broadway and on TV. Melvyn's comeback in the early 1960s, produced top performances and two Best Supporting Actor Oscars – for *Hud* and *Being There*. After completing work on *The Hot Touch* Melvyn died of pneumonia and cardiac complications.

She Married Her Boss (1935)
Annie Oakley (1935)
Theodora Goes Wild (1936)
I Met Him in Paris (1937)
There's Always a Woman (1938)
Ninotchka (1939)
This Thing Called Love (1940)
A Woman's Face (1941)
Mr. Blandings Builds His Dream
House (1948) A Woman's
Secret (1949) Hud (1963)
The Americanization of Emily (1964)
I Never Sang for My Father (1970)
The Candidate (1972)
Being There (1979)
The Changeling (1980)
Tell Me a Riddle (1980)

Michael **Douglas**
5ft 10in
(MICHAEL KIRK DOUGLAS)

Born: **September 25, 1944**
New Brunswick, New Jersey, USA

Kirk's son lived with his mother after his parents divorced, when he was six years old. Mike went to school in Deerfield, Massachusetts, and because his dad opposed the idea, he was set on being an actor. After graduating from UCSB with a B.A. in drama, he cut his teeth in the TV series, 'The Streets of San Francisco' – learning a lot from playing Karl Malden's partner. With his growing fame it was even possible for him to produce and win an Oscar for, *One Flew Over the Cuckoo's Nest*, in 1975. After a supporting role in *Coma*, Mike's next movie landmarks were *The China Syndrome* and *Romancing the Stone* (both of which he produced). But it was the dark, violent, and sexy thrillers of the 1980s and 90s that turned him into a Hollywood super-star. He won a Best Actor Oscar in 1987, for *Wall Street*, and his success continued up to the turn of the century. Since his second marriage – to actress Catherine Zeta-Jones – he has become a family man with two children. He and his wife seem to manage both careers successfully. His dad may have acted in more great movies than he did, but Mike does have two gold statuettes on his mantelpiece! After a couple of years away, Mike has three movies scheduled for release during 2009.

Napoleon and Samantha (1972)
Coma (1978) The China
Syndrome (1979) It's My Turn (1980)
The Star Chamber (1983)
Romancing the Stone (1984)
Wall Street (1987)
Fatal Attraction (1987)
Black Rain (1989)
The War of the Roses (1989)
Basic Instinct (1992)
Falling Down (1993) Disclosure (1994)
The American President (1995)
The Ghost and the Darkness (1996)
The Game (1997) A Perfect
Murder (1998) Traffic (2000)
Don't Say A Word (2001)
The Sentinel (2006)
King of California (2007)

Paul **Douglas**
5ft 11in
(PAUL DOUGLAS)

Born: **April 11, 1907**
Philadelphia, Pennsylvania, USA
Died: **September 11, 1959**

His father was a physician and Paul grew up enjoying the good things in life. He was academically bright as well as being a good athlete. After West Philadelphia High School, he went to Yale. Paul left before graduating to become a professional foot-baller with the Philadelphia Yellow Jackets. A bad injury turned him into a sports commentator and broadcasting gave him the chance to act. Through using the show business contacts he'd made, he worked as a straight man for both Jack Benny and Burns and Allen. Garson Kanin, who was casting for his play, "Born Yesterday" had witnessed Paul slapping one of his five wives around in public. He realized that the big ape would be ideal in the role of the loud-mouthed junk tycoon, Harry Brock, opposite Judy Holliday. It's success on Broadway sparked interest from movie studios, but he turned them down. It may explain why Broderick Crawford got the movie role. Paul's film debut was *A Letter to Three Wives*. He was given a Fox contract and his Runyonesque acting style remained popular throughout the 1950s. Paul died in Hollywood of a heart attack shortly before filming began on Billy Wilder's *The Apartment* – he would have played the Fred MacMurray role.

Everybody Does It (1949)
A Letter to Three Wives (1949)
It Happens Every Spring (1949)
Everybody Does It (1949)
Love That Brute (1950)
Panic in the Streets (1950)
Fourteen Hours (1951)
Angels in the Outfield (1951)
Clash By Night (1952)
We're Not Married! (1952)
Forever Female (1953)
The Maggie (1954)
Executive Suite (1954)
Joe MacBeth (1955)
The Solid Gold Cadillac (1956)
Beau James (1957)
Fortunella (1958)
The Mating Game (1959)

Robert **Downey Jr.**
5ft 9in
(ROBERT JOHN DOWNEY JR.)

Born: **April 4, 1965**
New York City, New York, USA

Bob is the son of the Golden Gloves boxer, minor-league baseball star, and later, the underground filmmaker, Robert Downey Senior. Bob began his life in Greenwich Village. He was surrounded by creative people including his mother – a dancer and singer. As a five-year-old, he played a puppy in his dad's off-the-wall movie *Pound,* and he was the star of *Greaser's Palace,* when he was seven. Moving to California with his dad after his parents split, he dropped out of high school to start his adult career. He had one season on the TV show, 'Saturday Night Live' before, in 1983, landing a small part in a movie his dad wasn't involved in, *Baby It's You.* His first leading role was in the following year's, *Firstborn.* By the 1990s, Bob was getting some high profile parts and was chosen to star in Richard Attenborough's *Chaplin.* Sadly for him, he had become addicted to heroin – which threatened to destroy his career. After serving time in jail, he fought off the demons and nowadays – practicing Wing Chun Kung Fu, he is back on the movie road with a bang. His third wife, producer Susan Levin, will certainly help to keep him on the straight and narrow. In 2005, Bob released an album called *"The Futurist"* – showcases his singing talent. For his role in *Tropic Thunder,* Bob received a Best Supporting Actor Oscar nomination.

Chaplin (1992) **Short Cuts** (1993)
Natural Born Killers (1994)
Richard III (1995)
The Gingerbread Man (1998)
Bowfinger (1999) **Wonder Boys** (2000)
The Singing Detective (2003)
Kiss Kiss Bang Bang (2005)
Goodnight, and Good Luck (2005)
A Scanner Darkly (2006)
**Fur: An Imaginary Portrait of
Diane Arbus** (2006) **A Guide to
Recognizing Your Saints** (2006)
Zodiac (2007) **Charlie Bartlett** (2007)
Lucky You (2007) **Iron Man** (2008)
Tropic Thunder (2008)
The Soloist (2009)

Tom **Drake**
5ft 10½in
(ALFRED ALDERDICE)

Born: **August 5, 1918**
Brooklyn, New York City, New York, USA
Died: **August 11, 1982**

Tom was the only son of Scottish-born, Alfred Alderdice, and his wife, Gertrude, who hailed from Norway. After the family moved to New Rochelle, in Westchester County, Tom attended Iona School and was a member of the local church choir. From Iona, he went to the Mersburg Academy, in Pennsylvania, where he had the opportunity to act in plays. He got his diploma in 1936, and having decided on an acting career, joined Poughkeepsie Stock Company. Both his parents passed away within a year of each other and with money they'd inherited, he and his sister, Claire, moved to New York. Tom made his Broadway debut in 1937, in "June Night", which folded quickly. In 1940, he went to Hollywood – using a stage name, Richard Alden. He made his film debut with an uncredited role in 1940's *Our Town,* and took drama classes from Alice B. Young. He toured in summer stock and played the juvenile lead in a hit Broadway show, "Janie". Tom was signed by MGM, who gave him a role in *Two Girls and a Sailor.* Tom was declared unfit for service during World War II so his film career continued – most famously with Judy Garland – in *Meet Me in St, Louis.* Active until 1978 Tom died of lung cancer at his home in Torrance, California.

Two Girls and a Sailor (1944)
Maisie Goes to Rio (1944)
Mrs. Parkington (1944) **Meet Me in
St. Louis** (1944) **The Green Years** (1946)
Courage of Lassie (1946)
I'll Be Yours (1947)
The Beginning or the End (1947)
Cass Timberlane (1947)
Alias a Gentleman (1948)
Hills of Home (1948)
Words and Music (1948)
Mr. Belvedere Goes to College (1949)
Scene of the Crime (1949)
The Great Rupert (1950)
FBI Girl (1951) **Sangaree** (1953)
Raintree County (1957) **Warlock** (1959)
The Sandpiper (1965)

Marie **Dressler**
5ft 7in
(LEILA MARIE DRESSLER)

Born: **November 9, 1868**
Cobourg, Ontario, Canada
Died: **July 28, 1934**

There are several theories about Marie's actual date of birth, but nobody argues about the fact that she was quite old when she became a movie star. It is believed that she joined a theater troupe when she was fourteen – continuing with a private education for a further two years. She also worked in a circus, where she was able to perfect her comedic talent. To complete her showbusiness education Marie performed in operettas. In 1892, she began appearing in Broadway shows as a singer and actress. By the turn of the century she was a famous comedienne in vaudeville. In 1910, Marie starred on the stage in "Tillie's Nightmare". Mack Sennett turned it into the film, *Tillie's Punctured Romance* in 1914, and Marie was billed above the young Charles Chaplin. She was blacklisted by theaters in 1917, when she was involved in the chorus girls' strike. For ten years she struggled, until MGM cast her in *The Callahans and the Murphys.* After protests from Irish-American groups, it was withdrawn and Marie lived in near poverty until there was renewed interest in her with the advent of sound films. *Anna Christie* with Greta Garbo, made her more famous than she'd ever been. For three consecutive years, she was the exhibitors' most popular actress. Marie won a Best Actress Oscar for *Min and Bill,* and was nominated for *Emma.* Marriage to George Hoppert, in 1900, resulted in a daughter who died in infancy. From 1914, she lived with James Dalton. Marie died of cancer in Santa Barbara, California.

Anna Christie (1930)
Girl Said No (1930)
One Romantic Night (1930)
Let Us Be Gay (1930)
Min and Bill (1930)
Reducing (1931)
Politics (1931) **Emma** (1932)
Prosperity (1932)
Tugboat Annie (1933)
Dinner at Eight (1933)
Christopher Bean (1933)

Ellen **Drew**
5ft 3½in
(ESTHER LORETTA RAY)

Born: **November 23, 1915**
Kansas City, Missouri, USA
Died: **December 3, 2003**

The daughter of an Irish, canine-loving barber, father, Ellen grew up to love dogs too. When she was four, her parents moved to Chicago, but in 1931, during the Great Depression, her father left her and her mother to struggle on alone. To help her, Ellen got a job in a department store. In 1934, her employers entered her for the "Miss Englewood" beauty contest – which she won. With strong encouragement from her mother, she headed for Los Angeles. Working as a waitress near Grauman's Chinese Theater, she caught the eye of the actor, William Demarest. He helped her get a contract with Paramount – as Terry Ray. In 1936 she made seven uncredited appearances in films, but after lightening her hair she began to get better parts. Her big break was in the 1938 Bing Crosby film, *Sing You Sinners* and the next – *If I Were King* – starring Ronald Colman, gave her a hint of stardom. She was in several films during the 1940s, but only *Christmas in July* and *Johnny O'Clock* stood out as special. Apart from an appearance in a 1957 B-western *Outlaw's Son,* Ellen did television work from the early 1950s and retired after marrying for the fourth time, in 1971. She died of a liver ailment, at her home in Palm Desert.

Sing You Sinners (1938)
If I Were King (1938)
Geronimo(1939)
French Without Tears (1940)
Buck Benny Rides Again (1940)
Christmas in July (1940)
The Monster and the Girl (1941)
The Remarkable Andrew (1942)
My Favorite Spy (1942)
The Impostor (1944)
Isle of the Dead (1945)
Crime Doctor's Man Hunt (1946)
Johnny O'Clock (1947)
The Swordsman (1948)
The Crooked Way (1949)
Stars in My Crown (1950)
The Great Missouri Raid (1951)
Man in the Saddle (1951)

Richard **Dreyfuss**
5ft 5in
(RICHARD STEPHEN DREYFUSS)

Born: **October 29, 1947**
Brooklyn, New York City, New York, USA

Richard's father, Norman Dreyfuss, was an attorney who owned a restaurant. His mother Geraldine, was described as a peace activist. They left New York for Los Angeles when he was nine. His acting career began at the Beverly Hills Jewish Center. His TV debut was in 'Mama's House' when he was fifteen. After San Fernando State College, Richard became a conscientious objector on being called up for military service during the Vietnam conflict. He served instead as a clerk in a hospital and continued getting small television roles in shows like 'Peyton Place' and 'Bewitched'. During the mid-1960s, he acted on Broadway, and made his film debut in *Valley of the Dolls.* A good role in the 1973 hit, *American Graffiti,* and an Oscar (youngest ever Best Actor winner at that time) for *The Goodbye Girl,* looked to have opened the door to movie stardom, but it wasn't to be. From 1978-1983, he couldn't make a hit for love or money. It brought about manic depression and a dependency on drugs. After rehab, he came back strongly as a top actor and has continued into his sixties. His third wife is Russian-born, Svetlana Erokhin.

American Graffiti (1973)
Dillinger (1973)
The Apprenticeship of Duddy
Kravitz (1974) Jaws (1975)
Close Encounters of
the Third Kind (1977)
The Goodbye Girl (1977)
Down and Out in Beverly Hills (1986)
Stand By Me (1986)
Stakeout (1987) Nuts (1987)
Always (1989)
Postcards from the Edge (1990)
What About Bob? (1991)
Lost in Yonkers (1993)
Mr. Holland's Opus (1996)
Night Falls on Manhattan (1997)
The Old Man Who Read
Love Stories (2001)
Who Is Cletis Tout? (2001)
Silver City (2004)
Poseidon (2006) W. (2008)

Bobby **Driscoll**
4ft 10in
(ROBERT CLETUS DRISCOLL)

Born: **March 3, 1937**
Cedar Rapids, Iowa, USA
Died: **March 30, 1968**

Bobby's father worked as an installer of asbestos insulation and his mother was a school teacher. In 1943, the Driscolls moved to Altadena, in California. When Bobby was taken for a haircut, a barber suggested that the boy should be in the movies. Within months he'd made his debut, in *Lost Angel.* He was quoted as saying "I'm going to save my money and go to college and then become a G-man". Starting with *Song of the South,* he made four movies for Walt Disney – including *Treasure Island.* At the Academy Awards, in 1950, the twelve-year-old received a special Oscar for his role in the film noir, *The Window.* The following year he played Jim Hawkins, in the classic version of *Treasure Island.* Bobby was on top of the world for two years, but as soon as he reached puberty, his voice changed and he developed a severe case of acne. He did the voice of *Peter Pan* in Walt Disney's animated film, but wasn't given anything else by the studio. From 1954, apart from *The Scarlet Coat,* which is his only decent adult film, most of his work was on television. Bobby got married in 1956, but even with the responsibility of three children, he had become addicted to drugs. After serving three months in Chino State Penitentiary, in California, Bobby simply disappeared. He eventually moved to New York in an attempt to revive his career, but nothing came of it. He died of a heart attack and his body was found by some kids in an old building. He lay in a pauper's grave at Potter's Field, until his mother used the FBI and Disney Studios to find his grave – more than a year later.

Song of the South (1946)
Pecos Bill (1948)
So Dear to
My Heart (1948)
The Window (1949)
Treasure Island (1950)
When I Grow Up (1951)
The Happy Time (1952)
The Scarlet Coat (1955)

Minnie **Driver**
5ft 10in
(AMELIA FIONA J. DRIVER)

Born: **January 31, 1970**
London, England

Minnie was the daughter of businessman Ronnie Driver. and his wife Gaynor, who was a designer and former model. Minnie was raised in Barbados, before receiving her education at Bedale's School, near Petersfield, in Hampshire, and at finishing schools in Paris and Grenoble. After being impressed by Meryl Streep's performance in *Sophie's Choice,* she made up her mind to be an actress. Eventually she studied at the famous Webber Douglas Academy of Dramatic Arts, in London – whose alumni includes Angela Lansbury and Terence Stamp. Minnie worked as a singer and guitarist with a band called "Puff Rocks and Brown" until she got television work beginning with 'God on the Rocks', in 1990. Her first film appearance was in the short subject, *The Zebra Man,* in 1992, and her first feature film was *Circle of Friends,* three years later. By the 1990s she was working almost exclusively in movies. She was Oscar-nominated for a Best Supporting Actress Award, in *Good Will Hunting.* Still a busy actress, she has somehow found the time to return to music – signing with EMI and releasing two singles – 'Everything I've Got in My Pocket' which was also the title of an album - and 'Invisible Girl'. A lifelong fan of Chelsea Football Club, Minnie watches their matches on a television in her trailer on a beach in California. Minnie portrays Dahlia Malloy on TV in 'The Riches'.

Big Night (1996)
Sleepers (1996)
Grosse Pointe Blank (1997)
Good Will Hunting (1997)
At Sachem Farm (1998)
An Ideal Husband (1999)
Return to Me (2000)
High Heels and Low Lifes (2001)
Owning Mahowney (2003)
Hope Springs (2003)
Ella Enchanted (2004)
The Phantom of the Opera (2004)
Delirious (2006)
Take (2007)
Motherhood (2009)

Joanne **Dru**
5ft 7in
(JOANNE LETITIA LACOCK)

Born: **January 31, 1922**
Logan, West Virginia, USA
Died: **September 10, 1996**

Joanne was the daughter of a West Virginia druggist. Soon after high school, she sensibly changed her name to Dru in order to find work as a fashion model in New York. While she was working, she was seen by Al Jolson, who cast her in his Broadway show, "Hold Onto Your Hats". In 1941, she met and married, crooner Dick Haymes, and shortly after that she went with him to Hollywood, where he began to carve out a career in movies. It took Joanne a bit longer (because she had three children) to get her break in films. Around 1946, she was working on the Los Angeles theater scene, when she was spotted by a talent scout. She made her debut that year in the poor, *Abie's Irish Rose,* and had to wait until *Red River* for something of quality. On the set, she met her second husband, John Ireland, and also appeared with him in *All The King's Men.* Although she always believed that too many westerns typecast her, she would have to admit that they were among the best handful of films she ever made. Unfortunately, John Ireland didn't make much difference to either the quality of her future work or her ability as an actress – which relied too much on her beauty. When they divorced in 1956, her career was heading downhill. She did get TV work and finally retired after making a film in Italy – *Super Fuzz* – was popular among lovers of action. She died at her home in Beverly Hills, of lymphedema.

Red River (1948)
She Wore a Yellow Ribbon (1949)
All The King's Men (1950)
Wagon Master (1950)
711 Ocean Drive (1950)
Vengeance Valley (1951)
The Pride of St. Louis (1952)
Hell on Frisco Bay (1955)
The Light in the Forest (1958)
The Wild and the Innocent (1959)
Sylvia (1965)
Super Fuzz (1980)

David **Duchovny**
6ft 0½in
(DAVID WILLIAM DUCHOVNY)

Born: **August 7, 1960**
Brooklyn, New York City, New York, USA

David's father Amran, who worked as a writer and publicist, was Jewish. His mother, Margaret, an immigrant from Scotland, who worked as a school administrator, was Lutheran. David, had an older brother, Daniel, and a younger sister, Laurie. When he was eleven, his parents split up and the kids remained with their mother. It upset him so much that when he won a scholarship to the Collegiate School for Boys, in Manhattan, he was known as a quiet, serious child. He was very good at sports, but when playing baseball he was hit in the eye, which caused him to need a contact lens on one side. He later graduated from Princetown. David traveled in South-East Asia before going to Yale, where he earned a Masters degree in English Literature. In 1987, while taking acting classes and looking for work, he appeared in an advertisement for Löwenbrau beer and had small parts in off-Broadway plays. He made his film debut in 1988, as a party guest in *Working Girl.* More film work, and his appearance in the 'Twin Peaks' TV series, led to his breakthrough film role, as journalist, Brian Kessler, in *Kalifornia.* 'The X-Files' brought him wider fame. He quit that in 2002, and since then, he has been concentrating on films. In 1997, he married Téa Leoni, with whom he has two young children. David appeared in several episodes of the TV series, 'Californication' and was re-united with Gillian Anderson for *The X-Files: I Want to Believe.*

The Rapture (1991) **Ruby** (1992)
Chaplin (1992) **Kalifornia** (1993)
Playing God (1997)
The X Files (1998)
Return to Me (2000)
Evolution (2001)
Zoolander (2001)
Connie and Carla (2004)
House of D (2004)
The TV Set (2006)
Things We Lost in the Fire (2007)
Si j'étais toi (2007)
The X Files: I Want to Believe (2008)

Keir **Dullea**
6ft 1in
(KEIR DULLEA)

Born: **May 30, 1936**
Cleveland, Ohio, USA

Keir's parents were Robert and Margaret Dullea. When he was small they moved to New York City, where they bought a bookshop in Greenwich Village. They raised their son in that stimulating environment until he was nine. They next sent him to board at George School, in Middletown, Pennsylvania and several years later, Keir attended Rutgers, in New Jersey and San Francisco State. Keir studied acting at the Neighborhood Playhouse in New York City before his first stage work in summer stock. He made his New York debut in 1956, in "Sticks and Bones". There were roles in TV dramas such as 'Route 66' which in 1961, brought him a choice role on his film debut, in *Hoodlum Priest* – opposite Don Murray. In 1962, he won a Golden Globe award for *Davis and Lisa,* as "Most Promising Male Newcomer". There were several good roles for Keir during the 1960s, but none as important to his career as when he portrayed astronaut David Bowman in Stanley Kubrick's *2001: A Space Odyssey.* The previous year, he'd made his Broadway debut in "Dr. Cook's Garden" with Burl Ives. The signs were good, but that momentum wasn't maintained. Keir was laid back. He and his wife Susan Fuller, ran the Theater Artists Workshop in Westport, from 1983 until her death in 1998. In 1999 he married the actress, Mia Dillon, with whom he has acted on stage in "Death Trap".

Hoodlum Priest (1961)
David and Lisa (1962)
Mail Order Bride (1964)
The Thin Red Line (1964)
Bunny Lake Is Missing (1965)
Madame X (1966)
The Fox (1967)
2001: A Space Odyssey (1968)
Il Diavolo nel cervello (1972)
Paperback Hero (1973)
Black Christmas (1974)
Full Circle (1977)
Three Days of Rain (2003)
The Good Shepherd (2006)
The Accidental Husband (2008)

Margaret **Dumont**
5ft 5in
(DAISY JULIETTE BAKER)

Born: **October 20, 1882**
Brooklyn, New York City, New York, USA
Died: **March 6, 1965**

Margaret was brought up in the home of her god-father, the author, Joel Chandler Harris – creator of "Uncle Remus" and "Brer Rabbit". She trained as an opera singer before, as Daisy Dumont, working as a show girl in English and French music halls. She then became an actress and while appearing in a musical, "The Summer Widowers" she met John Moller Jr., whom she married in 1910 and then retired from the stage until his death on Christmas Eve, 1918. Not long after her return to the stage, was seen by the producer of "The Cocoanuts". She made her screen debut in in 1929, in the movie version. Margaret became Groucho Marx's favorite leading lady – he romanced her then insulted her in equal measures. She was given a Paramount contract at the same time as the Marx Brothers and appeared in seven of their films – the last being *The Big Store.* She supported W.C. Fields, Jack Benny, Danny Kaye, Laurel and Hardy *and* Abbott and Costello, but they didn't have Groucho. She made her final movie bow in *What a Way to Go!* She did go – a year later, when she died of a massive heart attack, in Hollywood.

The Cocoanuts (1929)
Animal Crackers (1929)
Duck Soup (1933)
A Night at the Opera (1935)
Anything Goes (1936)
A Day at the Races (1937)
Wise Girl (1937)
At the Circus (1939)
The Big Store (1941)
Never Give a Sucker an
Even Break (1941)
Rhythm Parade (1942)
The Dancing Masters (1943)
Up in Arms (1944)
The Horn Blows at
Midnight (1945)
Diamond Horseshoe (1945)
Little Giant (1946)
Stop, You're Killing Me (1951)
What a Way to Go! (1964)

Faye **Dunaway**
5ft 7in
(DOROTHY FAYE DUNAWAY)

Born: **January 14, 1941**
Bascom, Florida, USA

When Faye was thirteen her parents got divorced. She was a lonely and miserable girl until she found escape in school plays. She then studied Theater Arts at Boston University. After an audition for the Lincoln Center Repertory Company, she was taken on by Elia Kazan. Her first success, in "Hogan's Goat" resulted in a contract with Otto Preminger, who directed her film debut, *Hurry Sundown,* in 1967. Faye was an international star within twelve months, when she played Bonnie Parker. She alternated between films and stage – and was highly praised for her acting in Harold Pinter's "Old Times" and for her television portrayal of Mrs. Simpson, in 'The Woman I Love'. She hit the movie jackpot again in Roman Polanski's *Chinatown,* and won a Best Actress Oscar for the outstanding *Network.* During the 1980s, her private life and career seemed to hit a low ebb. Foreign movies didn't help, but a film with Johnny Depp and one with Depp *and* Brando did. Faye was in the remake of *The Thomas Crown Affair* in 1999. She made her directorial debut and also acted in *Yellow Bird,* two years later.

Bonnie and Clyde (1967)
The Thomas Crown Affair (1969)
Little Big Man (1970)
Oklahoma Crude (1973)
The Three Musketeers (1973)
Chinatown (1974)
The Towering Inferno (1974)
Three Days of the Condor (1975)
Network (1976)
Voyage of the Damned (1976)
The Champ (1979)
Barfly (1987)
Arizona Dream (1993)
Don Juan DeMarco (1995)
Albino Alligator (1996)
The Yards (2000)
Yellow Bird (2001)
Mid-Century (2002)
Changing Hearts (2002)
Blind Horizon (2003)
Love Hollywood Style (2007)
Say It in Russian (2007)

James **Dunn**
6ft
(JAMES HOWARD DUNN)

Born: **November 2, 1901**
New York City, New York, USA
Died: **September 3, 1967**

Of Irish descent, Jimmy was the son of a Wall Street stockbroker, who went through the ups and downs associated with his very risky profession. After finishing high school, Jimmy took a safer route when he began his career in vaudeville. In 1929, he appeared in the short film, *In the Nick of Time,* and made his feature debut in *Bad Girl,* two years later. Other than five films, including roles in Shirley Temple's first three pictures, Jimmy's forty-odd movies during that decade, were undistinguished. To add to his feelings of professional insecurity, he was battling with alcoholism. In 1938, married his second wife, Frances Gifford. Her career was on an upward path at the time, and three years later, they divorced. Jimmy found it hard to get good film parts, but in 1945, he won the Best Supporting Actor Oscar, for his moving portrayal of Johnny Nolan, in *A Tree Grows in Brooklyn.* It was a once in a lifetime role and Jimmy felt that it heralded great things. That same year, he married his third wife, Edna Rush, who remained with him until his death. The comeback he was desperate for could not be sustained and most of his future employment was on television. Jimmy died in Santa Monica following abdominal surgery.

Bad Girl (1931)
Take a Chance (1933)
Bright Eyes (1934)
George White's Scandals (1935)
Hearts in Bondage (1936)
Son of the Navy (1940)
Hold That Woman! (1940)
The Living Ghost (1942)
Government Girl (1943)
Leave it to the Irish (1944)
A Tree Grows in Brooklyn (1945)
The Caribbean Mystery (1945)
That Brennan Girl (1946)
Killer McCoy (1947) Texas, Brooklyn
and Heaven (1948)
The Bramble Bush (1960)
Hemingway's Adventures of
a Young Man (1962)

Irene **Dunne**
5ft 5in
(IRENE MARIE DUNN)

Born: **December 20, 1898**
Louisville, Kentucky, USA
Died: **September 4, 1990**

Irene, whose father was a United States government officer, was educated locally at the Loretto Academy. She had a beautiful singing voice which she was able to use to good effect after graduating from the Chicago College of Music. She went on tour playing "Irene" in the musical. By the time she came home, she was sought after for Broadway shows. After touring in "Showboat" she was signed by RKO Studios. Irene's film debut, in 1930, was *Leathernecking.* On the strength of that, Richard Dix chose her to be his co-star in *Cimarron.* Irene was nominated for an Oscar and quickly became a big star. She was perfect in the 'weepies' of the early thirties, but after she returned to musicals with Astaire and Rogers, in *Roberta* and the 1936 film version of *Showboat,* she revealed fine comedic talent. At RKO, she was great with Cary Grant. In 1943, she went to MGM, where for several years she remained very popular. Around 1950, she faded away as her career suddenly nose-dived, following a brave but only partially successful attempt to portray Queen Victoria, in *The Mudlark.* After one television drama in 1956, she became an alternative delegate at the United Nations.

Cimarron (1930)
Bachelor Apartment (1931)
Symphony of Six Million (1932)
Back Street (1932)
Roberta (1935)
Showboat (1936)
The Awful Truth (1937)
Love Affair (1939)
When Tomorrow
Comes (1939)
My Favorite Wife (1940)
Penny Serenade (1941)
A Guy Named Joe (1943)
The White Cliffs of Dover (1943)
Anna and the King
of Siam (1946)
I Remember Mama (1948)
Life With Father (1948)
The Mudlark (1950)

Kirsten **Dunst**
5ft 5½in
(KIRSTEN CAROLINE DUNST)

Born: **April 30, 1982**
Point Pleasant, New Jersey, USA

Kiki's father, Klaus, was a German medical services executive from Hamburg. Her mother Inez, was a Swedish lady, who at one time ran her own art gallery. Kiki has a younger brother named Christian. She was a lovely child who started modeling when she was three, and was represented by both Ford and Elite management. Kiki appeared in a number of TV commercials and by the time of her first acting assignment, in 1988, she was a seasoned pro. It was an episode of 'Saturday Night Live' in which she played President George H.W. Bush's granddaughter. One year later, she made her film debut – an uncredited role in Woody Allen's, *New York Stories.* Kiki's first really important movie roles were in *Interview with the Vampire* – in which she received her first screen kiss – from Brad Pitt - and as the younger Amy March, in *Little Women.* For those two roles she won a Best Supporting Actress Award from Boston Society of Film Critics and Most Promising Actress, from the Chicago equivalent. She was soon enjoying great success and popularity in *Spider-Man* and its sequels. In early 2008, Kiki was treated for depression, but the glowing reviews of her latest movie, *How to Lose Friends & Alienate People* should cheer her up.

Interview with the Vampire (1994)
Little Women (1994) Jumanji (1995)
Mother Night (1996)
Wag the Dog (1997)
Small Soldiers (1998) Strike! (1998)
The Virgin Suicides (1999)
Drop Dead Gorgeous (1999)
Dick (1999) Bring It On (2000)
Deeply (2000) Get Over It (2001)
Crazy/Beautiful (2001) The Cat's
Meow (2001) Spider-Man (2002)
Levity (2003) Mona Lisa
Smile (2003) Spider-Man 2 (2004)
Wimbledon (2004)
Elizabethtown (2005)
Marie Antoinette (2006)
Spider-Man 3 (2007)
How to Lose Friends &
Alienate People (2008)

June **Duprez**
5ft 4in
(JUNE DUPREZ.)

Born: May 14, 1918
Teddington, Middlesex, England
Died: October 30, 1984

June was born during an air raid over Teddington in the last few weeks of World War I. She was the only daughter of an American vaudeville performer and bit-part movie actor by the name of Fred Duprez. Touring in a show towards the end of World War I, Fred met and married June's mother. With her parents' blessing, she left school at fourteen to pursue an acting career with Coventry Repertory Company. Three years later she made her film debut (as an extra) in *The Crimson Circle* and was put under contract by Alexander Korda. June was just nineteen when she married a Harley Street doctor. At first he encouraged her ambitions, but as soon as she achieved movie stardom in *The Four Feathers* – which meant screen kisses – he became jealous. After *The Thief of Bagdad,* June went to Hollywood without him and they were divorced. It was an escape from the war in Europe, but her battle to be paid what she and Korda thought she was worth, proved a losing one. Her first American film was a poverty row effort called *They Raid by Night.* During her five years in Hollywood she was in only three films of any merit – *None But the Lonely Heart* and the superb, *And Then There Were None* being the pick. She left to settle in New York where she was in a couple of Broadway shows before her second marriage to a wealthy sportsman. June made one final film, in 1961, in *One Plus One.* Then after her marriage ended in 1965, she lived mainly in Rome but returned to London in her final months up until her death.

The Four Feathers (1939)
The Spy in Black (1939)
The Lion Has Wings (1939)
The Thief of Bagdad (1940)
Forever and a Day 1943)
None But the Lonely Heart (1944)
The Brighton Strangler (1945)
And Then There Were None (1945)
The Brennan Girl (1946)
Calcutta (1947)

Jimmy **Durante**
5ft 7in
(JAMES FRANCIS DURANTE)

Born: February 10, 1893
Brooklyn, New York City, New York, USA
Died: January 29, 1980

The third of five children born to an Italian American couple, Mitchell and Margaret Durante, Jimmy grew up with a nose as his big physical asset. He was immensely talented in other ways, having mastered the piano by the age of nine. He dropped out of school in the eighth grade – calling himself "Ragtime Jimmy" and entertained customers in bars. It wasn't long before he was invited to join the "The Original New Orleans Jazz Band", but with so many other guys stealing the limelight he soon opted for his own trio, which became a hit in vaudeville and transferred successfully to radio. That national fame resulted in his film debut in 1929, in *Roadhouse Nights.* He played "Schnozzle" in *New Adventures of Get Rich Quick Wallingford* and that name stuck for the rest of his life. He was comic relief to the handsome leading men in films – Including Ricardo Montalban and Frank Sinatra. From 1950 he guested on TV – a highlight being Tallulah Bankhead's 'The Big Show'. When Carmen Miranda collapsed during his TV show in 1964 Jimmy was shocked. He was confined to a wheelchair after a stroke in 1972 and died of pneumonia in Santa Monica.

New Adventures of Get
Rich Quick Wallingford (1931)
Speak Easily (1932) **Hell Below** (1933)
Palooka (1934) **George White's**
Scandals (1934) **Strictly Dynamite** (1934)
Forbidden Music (1936)
Sally, Irene and Mary (1938)
Little Miss Broadway (1938)
You're in the Army Now (1941)
The Man Who Came to Dinner (1942)
Two Girls and a Sailor (1944)
Music for Millions (1944)
Two Sisters from Boston (1946)
It Happened in Brooklyn (1947)
On an Island with You (1948)
The Great Rupert (1950)
The Milkman (1950)
Billy Rose's Jumbo (1962)
It's a Mad Mad
Mad Mad World (1963)

Deanna **Durbin**
5ft 3½in
(EDNA MAE DURBIN)

Born: December 4, 1921
Winnipeg, Manitoba, Canada

Her parents emigrated from Lancashire to Canada in 1920. Shortly after she was born they settled in Los Angeles. By the time she was thirteen, Deanna's voice had attracted an MGM talent scout to her school. They put her in a short with Judy Garland called *Every Sunday,* but after that film, they dropped her. Universal signed her just as she'd started singing on the Eddie Cantor Radio Show. It was a stroke of luck for the struggling studio: when her first film *Three Smart Girls* was released, she was already famous nationwide. They gave her a highbrow musical with Leopold Stokowski – which brought culture to the masses and with each new film, Deanna's popularity grew. She was awarded a juvenile Oscar and in Britain she was by far the top female box-office star – from 1939 until 1942. At that point, she grew up, and after her first screen kiss (from Robert Stack) Deanna got married. She even attempted a more dramatic style of film which her fans found hard to accept. After a run of musicals she retired at the age of twenty-seven. In 1950, Deanna married her third husband, French film producer, Charles David. She settled down with him outside Paris, and they remained together until his death in 1999.

Three Smart Girls (1937)
One Hundred Men and a Girl (1937)
Mad About Music (1938)
That Certain Age (1938)
Three Smart Girls Grow Up (1939)
First Love (1939)
It's a Date (1940)
Spring Parade (1941)
Nice Girl? (1941)
It Started With Eve (1941)
His Butler's Sister (1943)
Christmas Holiday (1944)
Can't Help Singing (1944)
Lady on a Train (1945)
Because of Him (1946)
I'll Be Yours (1947)
Something in the Wind (1947)
Up in Central Park (1948)
For the Love of Mary (1948)

Dan **Duryea**
6ft 1in
(DANIEL DURYEA)

Born: **January 23, 1907**
White Plains, New York, USA
Died: **June 7, 1968**

Dan was the son of a textile salesman. He demonstrated an early talent as an actor, at White Plains High School, where he was involved with theatrical productions. His enthusiasm continued when he went to Cornell University, where he majored in English. In his senior year there, he succeeded Franchot Tone as President of the Drama Society. After graduation in 1930, he bowed to parental pressure by taking a "practical job" at the N.W.Ayer advertising agency. It was so stressful, he suffered a mild heart attack and returned to acting. He got parts in off-Broadway plays. Four years later, he was in the successful play, "Dead End". By the end of the decade, he had made his name as the irritating weakling, Leo Hubbard, in the Broadway production of "The Little Foxes". Dan played the same role in the movie version. For the next quarter of a century there wasn't a year when Dan didn't add one of his memorable characterizations to a movie. He was especially good as the villain in gangster films and westerns – the best of which were *Criss Cross* and *Winchester '73*. Unlike his screen persona, Dan was a loving husband to Helen Bryan, his wife of 35 years, and was a good father to his two children. He made spaghetti westerns and was often in TV series. He completed his final film, *The Bamboo Saucer,* the year he died of cancer, in Hollywood.

Ball of Fire (1941)
Sahara (1943)
Ministry of Fear (1944)
The Woman in the Window (1944)
The Valley of Decision (1945)
Along Came Jones (1945)
Lady on a Train (1945)
Scarlet Street (1945) Black Bart (1948)
Another Part of the Forest (1948)
Criss Cross (1949)
One Way Street (1950)
Winchester '73 (1950)
Silver Lode (1954) Battle Hymn (1957)
Night Passage (1957)
Slaughter on Tenth Avenue (1957)

Robert **Duval**
5ft 9½in
(ROBERT SELDEN DUVALL)

Born: **January 5, 1931**
San Diego, California, USA

Robert's father, William Howard Duvall, was a U.S. Navy admiral, and his mother, Mildred Hart, had dabbled in amateur dramatics. Because of her, Robert was raised in the Christian Science religion. He was educated at Severn School, in Maryland and majored in drama at Principia College, in Illinois, before serving in the United States Army from 1953 until 1954. On the G.I. Bill, he studied acting with Dustin Hoffman, at The Neighborhood Playhouse under Sanford Meisner. He was cast in Horton Foote's play, "The Midnight Caller" and it was on Foote's recommendation that Robert made his film debut in 1962's *To Kill a Mockingbird*. By the mid-1960s, Robert had made a name for himself on the New York stage – in the off-Broadway production of Arthur Miller's "A View from the Bridge".Television work and supporting roles in movies followed thick and fast. In 1972, Robert's career breakthrough came, when he played Tom Hagen, in *The Godfather*. He got the first of six Oscar nominations for that role – eventually won one for *Tender Mercies.* Following that, Robert suffered the curse of many Oscar winners, but by the early 1990s he was back at the top of his form.

The Rain People (1969)
True Grit (1969)
M*A*S*H (1970)
The Godfather (1972)
The Godfather: Part II (1974)
The Killer Elite (1975)
Network (1976)
Apocalypse Now (1979)
The Great Santini (1979)
Tender Mercies (1983)
Falling Down (1993)
The Paper (1994)
The Apostle (1997)
A Civil Action (1997)
The 6th Day (2000)
Gods and Generals (2003)
Open Range (2003)
Secondhand Lions (2003)
Thank You For Smoking (2005)
We Own the Night (2007)

Ann **Dvorak**
5ft 4½in
(ANNA MCKIM)

Born: **August 2, 1912**
New York City, New York, USA
Died: **December 10, 1979**

Ann's father, Sam McKim, was employed by the Biograph Film Studios in the Bronx. Her mother, Anna Lehr, starred in silents and acted in many supporting roles, up until the coming of sound. In 1916, the four-year-old Ann made her film debut in *Ramona*. After three very junior roles she concentrated on her education at St. Catherine's Convent in New York. In 1920 her parents split up, so she lived with her mother in Los Angeles, where she studied at the Page School for Girls and trained as a dancer. This led to movie chorus work in *The Hollywood Revue of 1929* and a job at MGM, as dancing instructor and bit-part actress. She was introduced to Howard Hawks by the MGM star, Joan Crawford, and when she returned from England with her new husband, Leslie Fenton, she got her big chance, in Howard Hawks's classic gangster movie *Scarface*. It was given a Warners contract and within a golden three-year period, she starred in twenty-two more films – most notably – *Love Is a Racket* and *Three on a Match*. Ann made films and worked on TV until 1951, when she retired to Hawaii with her third husband, Nicholas Wade. She died of natural causes, in Honolulu.

Scarface (1932)
The Crowd Roars (1932) The Strange
Love of Molly Louvain (1932)
Love is a Racket (1932)
Three on a Match (1932)
The Way to Love (1933)
College Coach (1933)
Midnight Alibi (1934)
Side Streets (1934)
Murder in the Clouds (1934)
'G' Men (1935)
Bright Lights (1935)
Dr. Socrates (1935)
Thanks a Million (1935)
We Who Are About to Die (1937)
Merrily We Live (1938)
Abilene Town (1946)
The Private Affairs of Bel Ami (1947)
The Secret of Convict Lake (1951)

E

Clint **Eastwood**
6ft 2in

(CLINTON EASTWOOD JR.)

Born: **May 31, 1930**
San Francisco, California, USA

The son of a steelworker, Clint worked as a lifeguard after graduating from Oakland Technical High School. In the US Army in 1950, he was a swimming instructor. He met his first wife in 1952 and pursued an acting career. He had a screen test at Universal which resulted in a dozen or so small parts in horror films – beginning with an uncredited part in *Revenge of the Creature,* in 1955. Clint was given small roles in comedies, war movies, and westerns. It was the TV-western, 'Rawhide' that made Eastwood a household name. In 1964, Sergio Leone liked him enough to cast him as 'The Man With No Name' in three of the category known as Spaghetti westerns, starting with *A Fistful of Dollars.* He was already an international star when he was called to Hollywood. By 1968, after making his first movie – with Don Siegel – *Coogan's Bluff,* Clint was also number one at the box-office. *Dirty Harry* made him an American icon. Cops and cowboys have kept Clint at the top. He has been directing with great success since 1971 – with Oscars for *Unforgiven,* and *Million Dollar Baby* and many plaudits for *Flags of our Fathers* and *Letters from Iwo Jima,* in 2006. A jazz lover for many years, Clint's employed some great talents on his movie soundtracks. His son, Kyle Eastwood, is a double bass player and the leader of a modern jazz combo.

The Good, the Bad and the Ugly (1966)
Hang 'Em High (1968)
Coogan's Bluff (1968)
Where Eagles Dare (1968)
Kelly's Heroes (1970)
Play Misty for Me (1971)
Dirty Harry (1971)
The Outlaw Josey Wales (1976)
The Guantlet (1977)
Escape from Alcatraz (1979)
Sudden Impact (1983) **Pale Rider** (1985)
Unforgiven (1992) **A Perfect World** (1993)
In the Line of Fire (1993)
The Bridges of Madison County (1995)
Space Cowboys (2000)
Million Dollar Baby (2004)

Aaron **Eckhart**
5ft 11in

(AARON E. ECKHART)

Born: **March 12, 1968**
Cupertino, California, USA

His father is an executive in the computer business and his mother writes children's books. Aaron and his two brothers lived in England and Australia during their teenage years. After finishing high school, he took three years off – first to surf in Hawaii, and secondly to work for The Church of Latter-day Saints, in Switzerland and France. After that, he enrolled as a film major at Brigham Young University, in Utah, where he met the future director, Neil LaBute, who has been a good friend as well as an employer. In 1992, Aaron had a small role in the TV thriller, 'Double Jeopardy'. His movie debut was two years later, in *Slaughter of the Innocents.* For his first starring role, as Chad, in Neil's directorial debut, *The Company of Men,* Aaron won a couple of awards as best new talent and a Filmmakers Trophy at the Sundance Film Festival. He has since played leading and supporting roles in some excellent films. Being athletic often helps. For his role in *Erin Brockovich* he learned to ride a motorcycle – he had so much fun doing it, he now owns one. He was nominated for a Golden Globe Best Actor Award, for *Thank You for Smoking.* Aaron's pair of rather disappointing movies in 2006, did not stop his march to the top. The trio of films he starred in the following year, with special mention of *Bill,* confirm this.

In the Company of Men (1997)
Your Friends & Neighbors (1998)
Any Given Sunday (1999)
Erin Brockovich (2000)
Nurse Betty (2000)
The Pledge (2001)
Possession (2002) **The Core** (2003)
The Missing (2003)
Paycheck (2003)
Conversations with
Other Women (2005)
Neverwas (2005)
Thank You for Smoking (2005)
The Black Dahlia (2006)
No Reservations (2007) **Bill** (2007)
Nothing Is Private (2007)
The Dark Knight (2008)

Nelson **Eddy**
6ft

(NELSON ACKERMAN EDDY)

Born: **June 29, 1901**
Providence, Rhode Island, USA
Died: **March 6, 1967**

Nelson's parents were singers, and as a boy soprano, he was the star of his church choir. His nickname, because of his mop of red hair, was "Bricktop". When he was fifteen, he went to Philadelphia where he worked on a switchboard while taking a course in journalism. He continued singing while writing obituaries for a local paper, but when he joined an advertising agency he was fired for singing on the job. In 1922, he was in an amateur production of the musical, "The Marriage Tax". He then did some Gilbert and Sullivan, which gave him the confidence to enter a contest. The prize (which he won) was an opportunity to perform with the Philadelphia Opera Society. He sang in "Aïda" and "Pagliacci" but it was his last minute substitution for the diva, Lotte Lehmann (he had eighteen curtain calls) at a concert in Los Angeles, in February 1933, which resulted in an MGM contract. They didn't know what to do with him until they had a problem finding a leading man to play opposite Jeannette MacDonald, in a film version of *Naughty Marietta.* The pair's teaming was box-office dynamite and they made six more – their last one, *I Married an Angel,* in 1942, was disappointing, but without her, Nelson was never the same. In the 1950s, he appeared on TV in 'The Desert Song' and toured for a time in a night-club act. He collapsed during one of his shows at a hotel in Miami, and died of a stroke.

Naughty Marietta (1935)
Rose Marie (1936)
Maytime (1937)
Rosalie (1937)
The Girl of the
Golden West (1938)
Sweethearts (1938)
Let Freedom Ring (1939)
Balalaika (1939)
New Moon (1940)
Bitter Sweet (1940)
The Chocolate Soldier (1941)
Phantom of the Opera (1943)
Knickerbocker Holiday (1944)

Samantha **Eggar**
5ft 5in
(VICTORIA LOUISE SAMANTHA MARIE EGGAR)

Born: March 5, 1939
Hampstead, London, England

Sam inherited her strong character from her father Ralph – who was a major in the British Army. Her beauty came from her mother Muriel – who was of Dutch and Portuguese descent. Sam spent eleven years at a convent school, but her rebellious nature and quick temper, proved poor material for the Sisterhood. She left school with the idea of becoming an actress, but her parents were dead set against it. Instead, she took a two year course in fashion design. Sam lived in Chelsea before London began to swing – but she did. In 1959, a playboy lover paid for lessons at Webber Douglas Dramatic School. She got a small part in a play where she was seen by Cecil Beaton, who put her in his "Landscape with Figures" at the Royal Court Theatre. In 1962, she made her debut, in the independent horror film, *Dr.Crippen,* but it was *The Collector,* with Terence Stamp, which gave her a first early taste of stardom and won her a Golden Globe Award. For the rest of the decade she was hot – and once, in *Walk, Don't Run* – she even got to co-star with Cary Grant! The 1970s weren't so kind, and co-starring with Kirk Douglas and Yul Brynner in the disastrous, *The Light at the Edge of the World,* didn't help. For the past twenty years, Sam has worked in TV plays more often than films. Six years of marriage to producer/director/writer, Tom Stern, produced two children – Jenna Stern, who is also a professional actress, and Nicolas Stern, who is a production supervisor. Both live and work in the USA.

Psyche 59 (1964)
The Collector (1965)
Return from the Ashes (1965)
Walk Don't Run (1966)
Doctor Doolittle (1967)
The Molly Maguires (1970)
The Walking Stick (1970)
The Seven-Per-Cent
Solution (1976)
Why Shoot the
Teacher? (1977)
The Brood (1979)

Chiwetel **Ejiofor**
5ft 10in
(CHIWETEL EJIOFOR)

Born: July 10, 1974
Forest Gate, London, England

"Chewy" as his many friends – and people who can't pronounce his name – call him, was born in London to Nigerian parents, who belonged to the Igbo ethnic group. His father, Arinze, was a doctor, and his mother, Obiajulu, was a pharmacist. They were comfortably off and Chewy was sent to the fee-paying Dulwich College to receive his English education. When he was thirteen, he began acting in school plays and had soon developed a passion for dramatic art. He was given a thorough grounding in all aspects of his chosen career after he was accepted at the National Youth Theater, in North London. In 1995, Chewy played "Othello" at the Bloomsbury Theater and again, at the Arts Theater, a year later. He made his screen debut in a 1996 television movie, 'Deadly Voyage'. He alternated between stage and TV until making his film debut, in *Dirty Pretty Things* – which won him a British Independent Film and American Black Film Festival Award, as Best Actor. It was only a short time later when he starred opposite Hilary Swank, in the South Africa filmed *Red Dust.* He added to his status and list of credits all the time. Chewy had a featured role in *Inside Man* – starring Denzel Washington, Clive Owen and Jodie Foster – and he was right up there with the big guns, in *American Gangster.* He plays South African President, Thabo Mbeki, in a recent political drama, *Endgame.*

Dirty Pretty Things (2002)
Love Actually (2003)
She Hate Me (2004)
Red Dust (2004)
Melinda and Melinda (2004)
Four Brothers (2005)
Serenity (2005)
Slow Burn (2005)
Kinky Boots (2005)
Inside Man (2006)
Children of Men (2006)
Talk to Me (2007)
American Gangster (2007)
Redbelt (2008)
Endgame (2009)

Anita **Ekberg**
5ft 6½in
(KERSTIN ANITA MARIANNE EKBERG)

Born: September 29, 1931
Malmö, Skåne län, Sweden

One of eight children born to a working-class Swedish family during the worldwide recession, Anita endured a very tough life, including the hardship which came to her country despite Sweden's neutrality during World War II. At eighteen, she possessed a winning smile and a statuesque beauty which was well-developed by the time she left secondary school. She was crowned "Miss Sweden" in 1950, but she didn't win the "Miss Universe" contest in the United States, partly because she didn't speak a word of English. As one of the prizes for all six contestants, she was given a starlet's contract at Universal. Anita then attended drama and elocution lessons at the studio and she had soon learned enough English to tell Howard Hughes where to go, when he suggested making some structural changes to her body. After some bit parts for Universal, she appeared for Paramount in *Artists and Models* and the aptly named *Hollywood or Bust* – both of which starred Martin and Lewis. In 1956, she married the British actor Anthony Steel – who was able to survive for three years. Anita's love life was sometimes more interesting than her films, but in 1960, she was selected by the Italian director, Federico Fellini, for *La Dolce Vita.* The scene of Anita frolicking in La Fontana di Trevi in Rome, is as much of an iconic image as Marilyn Monroe's in *The Seven Year Itch.* In the 1960s, Anita made her home in Italy. Most of her later films were poor, but she will be remembered for a few good ones – made during the ten years she was in the spotlight.

Artists and Models (1955)
War And Peace (1956)
Back from Eternity (1956)
Hollywood or Bust (1956)
Interpol (1957)
Valerie (1957)
Screaming Mimi (1958)
La Dolce Vita (1960)
Boccaccio '70 (1962)
4 For Texas (1963)
Cicciabomba (1982)
The Red Dwarf (1998)

Jack **Elam**
6ft
(WILLIAM SCOTT ELAM)

Born: **November 13, 1920**
Miami, Gila, Arizona, USA
Died: **October 20, 2003**

After his mother passed away when he was approaching his fourth birthday, young Jack spent six unhappy years being raised by various relatives. His father remarried, so Jack and his older sister went back to live with him. To earn extra money during the Great Depression, he picked cotton in the company of dozens of black folk. When he was eleven, he joined the American Boy Scouts. One evening at a troop meeting he was hit in the left eye by a pencil hurled by another scout, and blinded. At the time it was a tragedy, but when he began his career in films, it became his trademark. After graduating from Phoenix Union High School, he attended Junior College in Santa Monica, California. He was an accountant for a while, then manager of the Bel Air Hotel in Los Angeles. He had made a few contacts in Hollywood and in 1949 he got a small role in the anti-marijuana film, *She Shoulda Said No!* It was the first of more than forty movie appearances – mostly westerns – some of which – *Vera Cruz, The Man from Laramie, Gunfight at the O.K. Corral* and *Once Upon a Time in the West* – are considered classics of the genre. Two years before he died of congestive heart failure, Jack acted out his last role, in the television documentary, 'Dobe and the Company of Heroes'.

Rawhide (1951)
Rancho Notorious (1952)
The Far Country (1954)
Vera Cruz (1954)
The Man from Laramie (1955)
Jubal (1956) Gunfight at the O.K.
Corral (1957) The Comancheros (1961)
The Way West (1967)
Once Upon a Time in
the West (1968)
Support Your Local Sheriff! (1969)
Rio Lobo (1970)
Hannie Caulder (1971)
The Cannonball Run (1981)
Sacred Ground (1983)
The Giant of Thunder Mountain (1991)

Hector **Elizondo**
6ft 2¹/₂in
(HECTOR ELIZONDO)

Born: **December 22, 1936**
New York City, New York, USA

Hector's parents emigrated to the USA from Puerto Rico. His father, Martin, had been born on a boat bound for Argentina from Spain. His mother, Carmen, was from a land-owning family. He and his younger brother were raised as Catholics and Hector shone in his church choir and at ten years of age he performed with the Frank Murray Boy's Choir. He excelled at sports and after graduating from junior high school, he was invited for trials by the New York Giants. In 1954, he began studying to be a history teacher, but dropped out when his wife gave birth and he needed to support his family. Hector did various jobs until he studied dance at the Ballet Arts Company. In 1963, he got his acting career started with roles in off-Broadway productions of "Kill the One-Eyed Man" and "The Great White Hope". He made his movie debut in *The Fat Black Pussycat.* Hector was awarded an Obie for his performance as a Puerto Rican attendant, in "Steam Bath". He was in demand from then on. In the 1980s, he made several films with Garry Marshall, including *Pretty Woman* – for which he was nominated for a Golden Globe. Hector is married to Emmy award-winning actress Carolee Campbell.

The Landlord (1970) Valdez Is
Coming (1971) Born to Win (1971)
Pocket Money (1972) Taking of
Pelham One Two Three (1974)
Report to the Commissioner (1975)
Cuba (1979) American Gigolo (1980)
The Flamingo Kid (1984)
Leviathan (1989)
Pretty Woman (1990)
Taking Care of Business (1990)
Frankie and Johnny (1991)
Samantha (1992)
Safe House (1998) The Other
Sister (1999) Runaway Bride (1999)
The Princess Diaries (2001)
The Princess Diaries 2 (2004)
I-See-You.Com (2006)
Music Within (2007)
Georgia Rule (2007)

Denholm **Elliott**
5ft 10³/₄in
(DENHOLM MITCHELL ELLIOTT)

Born: **Born: May 31, 1922**
Ealing, London, England
Died: **October 6, 1992**

After Malvern College, Denholm served as a radio operator and gunner in the RAF. In 1942, his aircraft was shot down over Denmark and he spent the next three years as a P.O.W. at a camp in Silesia, on the river Oder. He went to RADA shortly after the war and made his stage debut at the Playhouse Theater, in Amersham. He worked on the stage in London until 1949, when he made his first film, *Dear Mr. Prohack.* He never sought real stardom – preferring instead to become a reliable character actor. His first major screen role was in 1952, when he got good notices for his part in *The Sound Barrier,* directed by David Lean. He was married for a few months during 1954, to English actress, Virginia McKenna. Plenty of good movie roles followed but he didn't challenge the stars until he was excellent opposite Alan Bates, in *Nothing But the Best.* In 1961 he married the actress, Susan Robinson, with whom he had two children. He was at his peak during the 1970s and 1980s and he won a Best Supporting Actor Oscar, for his role as Colman, the English butler, in *Trading Places.* From 1970, Denholm was living on the Mediterranean island of Ibiza. He was then openly bi-sexual and in 1987 he tested HIV positive. He was appointed CBE in 1988, but died of AIDS at his island home a few months after completing work on his final film, *Noises Off...*

The Sound Barrier (1952) The Cruel
Sea (1953) The Heart of the
Matter (1953) The Night My
Number Came Up (1955)
Nothing But the Best (1964)
King Rat (1965) Alfie (1966)
The Sea Gull (1968) The Vault of
Horror (1973) Saint Jack (1979) Zulu
Dawn (1979) Trading Places (1983)
Defence of the Realm (1985)
A Room with a View (1985)
September (1987)
Indiana Jones and the
Last Crusade (1989)
Noises Off... (1992)

Sam **Elliott**
6ft 2in
(SAMUEL PACK ELLIOTT)

Born: **Born: August 9, 1944**
Sacramento, California, USA

In his early teens, Sam's parents took him to live in Portland, Oregon, where he graduated from the David Douglas High School. He'd been bitten by the acting bug as a kid, so he went to live in Los Angeles, where he worked on construction sites to pay for acting classes. While he was still a student at the University of Oregon, he did film extra work. Sam's screen career started in 1968, when he appeared on television in three episodes of 'Felony Squad'. In 1969 he had a small role in the movie *Butch Cassidy and the Sundance Kid,* which was where he first saw his future wife, Katherine Ross. They became soul-mates in London, in 1978, and have been together ever since. Their daughter was named Cleo Rose. Sam's appearance made him an ideal cowboy, but because there were very few western movies being made at that time, he had to be content with the television variety. His first real break was when he starred with Cher, in *Mask,* but it would be another three years before he would put together a run of worthwhile films, with *Shakedown* starting things off. Meanwhile, Sam was twice nominated for Golden Globes – for his performances in television movies – 'Conagher' and 'Buffalo Girls'. He had a good role as the cancer-riddled cowboy in the excellent satirical comedy, *Thank You for Smoking.*

Lifeguard (1976)
Mask (1985)
Shakedown (1988)
Roadhouse (1989)
Prancer (1989) Rush (1991)
Gettysburg (1993)
Tombstone (1993)
The Big Lebowski (1998)
The Hi-Lo Country (1998)
The Contender (2000)
We Were Soldiers (2002)
Off the Map (2003)
Hulk (2003)
Thank You for Smoking (2005)
The Alibi (2006)
The Golden Compass (2007)

Chris **Evans**
6ft
(CHRISTOPHER ROBERT EVANS)

Born: **June 13, 1981**
Sudbury, Massachusetts, USA

Chris's father, Bob Evans, was a dentist. His mother, Lisa, had been a dancer. His parents were of Italian and Irish descent and they raised young Chris as a Roman Catholic. His older sister Carly had started acting when Chris was in the first grade and he was soon appearing in school plays. During the summer vacations he attended theater and all-year-round, he acted in community theater productions. In 1999, Chris graduated from Lincoln-Sudbury Regional High School, where his drama teacher had encouraged him to make acting his career. Chris then went to work in a casting office in Brooklyn, while attending the Lee Strasberg Theater Institute. He soon acquired an agent, who in 2000, got him his first film role – aptly titled *The Newcomers* and the role of Cary Baston, in eight episodes of the TV series "Opposite Sex". Chris scored with younger audiences in *Not Another Teen Movie.* There were some less than ideal vehicles for a couple of years, but he has made rapid progress after his breakthrough film, *Cellular,* and has become a cult figure, as Johnny Storm (a.k.a. The Human Torch) in the *Fantastic Four* series. For two years Chris was in a serious relationship with the actress, Jessica Biel, but in 2006, the couple went their separate ways. For his acting in his most recent films, *The Nanny Diaries* and *Street Kings,* Chris has received much critical praise.

Not Another Teen Movie (2001)
The Perfect Score (2004)
Cellular (2004)
The Orphan King (2005)
Fierce People (2005)
Fantastic Four (2005)
London (2005)
Sunshine (2007)
4: Rise of the Silver
Surfer (2007)
The Nanny Diaries (2007)
Street Kings (2008)
The Loss of a
Teardrop Diamond (2008)
Push (2009)

Dame Edith **Evans**
5ft 6in
(EDITH MARY EVANS)

Born: **February 8, 1888**
London, England
Died: **October 14, 1976**

The daughter of a civil servant, Edith left St. Michael's Church of England School in Pimlico at fifteen, to begin an apprenticeship as a milliner. Six years later, she was in an amateur production of "Twelfth Night" with the Streatham Shakespeare Players – and the die was cast. She made her professional debut, in a little known sixth-century Hindu classic "Sakuntala" and followed that by playing Cressida, in "Troilus and Cressida" on the London stage and at Stratford Upon Avon. Apart from three silent films, beginning with *Honeymoon for Three* in 1915, Edith concentrated all her efforts on becoming the finest stage actress in British theater. Her portrait was painted by Walter Sickert as Katharine, in "The Taming of the Shrew", but she also created definitive roles for the characters of Ibsen, Wilde, Coward and George Bernard Shaw. In 1925, she married George Booth, who died exactly ten years later. Edith was knighted in 1946. She had achieved just about everything in the theater when she returned to films, opposite Richard Burton, in *The Last Days of Dolwyn,* in 1949. All of Edith's movie performances were special and she had three nominations for Best Supporting Actress Oscars – for *Tom Jones, The Chalk Garden* and *The Whisperers.* She was a Christian Scientist who had no time for doctors or medicines. She completed *Nasty Habits* before dying peacefully in her sleep, at her home in Cranbrook, Kent.

The Queen of Spades (1948)
The Importance of
Being Earnest (1952)
Look Back in Anger (1958)
The Nun's Story (1959)
Tom Jones (1963)
The Chalk Garden (1964)
Young Cassidy (1965)
The Whisperers (1966)
Crooks and Coronets (1969)
Scrooge (1970)
A Doll's House (1973)
Nasty Habits (1977)

Madge **Evans**
5ft 4¹⁄₂in
(MARGHERITA EVANS)

Born: **July 1, 1909**
New York City, New York, USA
Died: **April 26, 1981**

Madge was a beautiful baby. By the age of three months, she earned extra money for her family by posing for soap advertisements. When she was four, she started her acting career in a series of children's plays. She proved a little gold mine for her mother, who took her to the New York Movie Studio on Long Island, where in 1914, Madge was given her film debut, as Mildred, in *Shore Acres*. She became so popular as a child actress, she was soon endorsing beauty products and ladies hats and her photos even appeared in a calender – it was published by a brewing company! She was thirteen when she co-starred with John Barrymore in the film *Peter Ibbetson*, and appeared in several plays on the New York stage. In 1925, her mother used some of Madge's earnings to embark on an eighteen month tour of Europe. Back on Broadway, Madge was given a contract by MGM. She had a good speaking voice and the talkies extended her popularity. In 1939 she married playwright, Sidney Kingsley, and retired to his fifty-acre estate in New Jersey. Sidney's plays, "Dead End" and "Detective Story" would earn him big money when they became films. Madge reappeared on radio and TV in the 1950s. She died of cancer in Oakland, New Jersey.

Son of India (1931) Guilty Hands (1931)
West of Broadway (1931)
The Greeks Had a Word for Them (1932)
Are You Listening? (1932)
Fast Life (1932) Hallelujah I'm a
Bum (1933) Made on Broadway (1933)
The Nuisance (1933)
The Mayor of Hell (1933) Dinner at
Eight (1933) Day of Reckoning (1933)
Paris Interlude (1934)
Death on the Diamond (1934)
David Copperfield (1935)
Age of Indiscretion (1935)
The Tunnel (1935) Piccadilly Jim (1936)
Pennies from Heaven (1936)
The Thirteenth Chair (1937)
Sinners in Paradise (1938)

Rupert **Everett**
6ft 4in
(RUPERT JAMES HECTOR EVERETT)

Born: **May 29, 1959**
Norfolk, England

The son of an army major, Rupert is a great-nephew of the infamous British spy, Donald Maclean. From the age of seven he was educated by Benedictine monks at Ampleforth College, in Yorkshire, but at fifteen he ran away – with the purpose of becoming an actor in London. The only acting he did in order to support himself was as a male escort, but he did spend some time at London's Central School of Speech and Drama. He was expelled before graduating – for arguing with his teachers. He ended up in Scotland, at the Citizen's Theater in Glasgow. While there, he acted in productions of "Don Juan" and "Heartbreak House". In 1982, he made his film debut in the award winning short, *A Shocking Accident*. He acted in the West End production of "Another Country" and two years later, was in the film version. Things went well until his first flop, *Hearts of Fire*. In 1989 he went to live in Paris and 'came out' as gay. Playing Julia Roberts' homosexual chum, in *My Best Friend's Wedding*, he proved he could portray men of either persuasion with equal facility and it won him an American Comedy Award. Recent efforts contain credits any actor would be proud to have. His next appearance will be in *Wild Target*.

Another Country (1984)
Dance With a Stranger (1985)
Duet For One (1986)
Chronicle of a Death Foretold (1987)
Tolérance (1989)
The Comfort of Strangers (1990)
Dellamorte Dellamore (1994)
The Madness of King George (1994)
My Best Friend's Wedding (1997)
B. Monkey (1998)
An Ideal Husband (1999)
The Importance of
Being Ernest (2002)
Unconditional Love (2002)
Stage Beauty (2004)
Separate Lies (2005)
Quiet Flows the Don (2006)
Stardust (2007) St. Trinian's (2007)
Wild Target (2009)

Tom **Ewell**
5ft 10³⁄₄in
(SAMUEL YEWELL TOMPKINS)

Born: **April 29, 1909**
Owensboro, Kentucky, USA
Died: **September 12, 1994**

When Tommy graduated from Owensboro High School, where he was a charter member of the 'Rose Curtain Players', his parents wanted him to study to be a lawyer. He defied them by opting to major in Liberal Arts at the University of Wisconsin. He became a professional actor in 1928 when he went on tour with a stock company, but on returning to New York at the start of the Great Depression he had to endure several years of hardship. He enrolled at the Actor's Studio at the same time as Karl Malden and Montgomery Clift, but after his Broadway debut in 1934, he was in a series of flops. His film debut, in *They Knew What They Wanted* wasn't of any consequence. Four years in the US Navy during World War II interrupted his career and he had to wait until 1947 for a part in the Broadway hit show "John Loves Mary". Two years later he made a big impression with Spencer Tracy and Katherine Hepburn, in *Adam's Rib*. In 1952, on Broadway, Tommy began the first of 750 performances in the role he would be most famous for – Richard Sherman – in "The Seven Year Itch". 20th Century Fox transferred it to the screen – with the key addition of Marilyn Monroe, and Tommy briefly became a star. His funny face went out of style by 1960 and his film roles were rare. He worked on TV and in 1986, after his final appearance in an episode of 'Murder, She Wrote', retired to Woodlands Hills with his second wife, Marjorie. He died there of natural causes.

Adam's Rib (1949)
A Life of Her Own (1950)
Mr. Music (1950)
Finders Keepers (1951)
Up Front (1951)
Back at the Front (1952)
The Seven Year Itch (1955)
The Girl Can't Help It (1956)
State Fair (1962)
They Only Kill Their Masters (1972)
To Find a Man (1972)
Easy Money (1983)

F

Jeff **Fahey**
5ft 10¾in
(JEFFREY FAHEY)

Born: **November 29, 1952**
Orlean, New York, USA

One of thirteen children, Jeff moved with his family to Buffalo when he was ten years old. He attended Father Baker's High School and after he graduated, in 1972, he went traveling around the world as a backpacker and doing a variety of jobs to pay his way, including driving an ambulance and working on a trawler. On his return, he won a scholarship to the Joffrey Ballet which resulted in work as a dancer and in Broadway shows. As an actor, he got his first major role as Gary Corelli in the television soap opera 'One Life to Live'. He made his film debut in 1985 in *Silverado*. There were some lesser movies including one which took Jeff to Australia. In 1990, he acted in a thriller called *Impulse*, directed by Sondra Locke. It was a turning point in his career. His next role was opposite Sondra's lover, Clint Eastwood, in the exciting *White Hunter Black Heart*. For three years or so, he appeared in a mixed bag of film and TV productions – some of them quite bad. One of the good ones was the western, *Wyatt Earp*, but it was the TV-western 'The Marshall', which kept him in the public eye. Considering the unevenness of his early career, Jeff has since been lucky with many roles given to him – especially over the past ten years or so. Look at his list of credits – he was even in the monster hit *Grindhouse!* Currently, Jeff plays Frank Lapidus, in the TV series 'Lost'.

Silverado (1985) Backfire (1987)
Minnamurra (1989) Impulse (1990)
White Hunter Black Heart (1990)
The Lawnmower Man (1992)
Wyatt Earp (1994)
Small Time (1996) Dazzle (1999)
Spin Cycle (2000)
Choosing Matthias (2001)
Maniacts (2001)
Day of Redemption (2004)
Split Second (2005)
Only the Brave (2005)
Grindhouse (2007)
Planet Terror (2007)
Matchmaker Mary (2008)

Douglas **Fairbanks Jr.**
6ft 1in
(DOUGLAS ELTON ULMAN FAIRBANKS)

Born: **December 9, 1909**
New York City, New York, USA
Died: **May 7, 2000**

Doug was the son of the swashbuckling hero of the silent screen, and Anna Beth Sully. After his parents divorced when he was ten years old, Doug lived with his mother. His famous father was opposed to the idea of his son following him into films, but when he was thirteen, Doug did just that. He starred in a poor picture called *Stephen Steps Out,* and went on to act in fifteen more silent films, including *A Woman of Affairs,* which starred Greta Garbo. He was married to Joan Crawford for four years and that helped his career. Doug had an ideal voice for the talkies which led to a Warner Brothers contract. He split with them and set up his own production company. It was a disaster so he went with his father to England to lick his wounds and to act on the stage. When he returned to Hollywood, he signed a contract with David O. Selznick. It resulted in four golden years before he joined the US Navy, in 1942. He was decorated by the French and British as well as by the USA. In 1947, he made *Sinbad the Sailor,* which was his most financially successful film, but his career was waning. He went to live in London, where he was made an honorary Knight. In his last film, *Ghost Story,* Doug co-starred with Fred Astaire. From 1991, until he died of a heart attack in New York, Doug was married to his third wife, Vera Shelton.

The Dawn Patrol (1930)
Little Caesar (1931)
Union Depot (1932)
The Life of Jimmy Dolan (1933)
Morning Glory (1933)
The Amateur Gentleman (1936)
The Joy of Living (1938)
The Rage of Paris (1938)
The Young In Heart (1938)
Gunga Din (1939) Safari (1940)
Angels Over Broadway (1940)
The Corsican Brothers (1941)
Sinbad the Sailor (1947)
State Secret (1950)
Mister Drake's Duck (1951)

Peter **Falk**
5ft 6in
(PETER MICHAEL FALK)

Born: **September 16, 1927**
New York City, New York, USA

His father, Michael, owned a clothing and dry goods store. His mother Madeleine, was an accountant. Both were descended from Eastern European Jews, but they were not religious. At the age of three, Peter had his right eye surgically removed because of a malignant tumor. It didn't hinder his progress in life. He was a bright boy during his time at Ossining High School in Westchester County, where he was president of his class. After graduation, he joined the U.S. Merchant Marines as a cook. In 1951, he completed a B.A. at the New School for Social Research and went on to Syracuse University, where he gained a Masters in Public Admin. His first job was as a management analyst in Hartford. He left the job in 1956, after deciding to become an actor. He gained experience at the White Barn Theater in Westport before making his off-Broadway debut, in Molière's "Don Juan". He made his TV debut in an episode of 'Robert Montgomery Presents' in 1957. His film debut was in *Wind Across the Everglades* the following year. He was nominated for Best Supporting Actor Oscars – for *Murder Inc.,* in 1960, and *Pocketful of Miracles,* in 1961. He is most famous for playing the shabby detective 'Columbo' in the TV-series, which began in 1971 and ran for over thirty years. He's still working.

Murder Inc. (1960)
Pocketful of Miracles (1961)
Pressure Point (1962)
Robin and the 7 Hoods (1964)
The Great Race (1965)
Husbands (1970)
A Woman Under the Influence (1974)
The Cheap Detective (1978)
The Brinks Job (1978)
Wings of Desire (1987)
The Princess Bride (1987)
Roommates (1995)
Made (2001)
Three Days of Rain (2003)
Checking Out (2005)
The Thing About My Folks (2005)
Next (2007)

Frances **Farmer**
5ft 6in
(FRANCES ELENA FARMER)

Born: **September 19, 1913**
Seattle, Washington, USA
Died: **August 1, 1970**

Frances was the daughter of a Seattle lawyer, Ernest Farmer - the second husband of her mother, Lillian Van Ornum. While Ernest was a gentle character, Lillian was outspoken and ambitious – often getting involved in political issues and supporting feminine causes. Frances was most like her. She made her stage debut at fourteen, in "The Pirate's Daughter". At West Seattle High School, she was good at sports, debating and writing. Her essay, "God Dies", provoked an uproar in Seattle. She studied Journalism and Drama at the University of Washington – paying her way by working as a singing waitress. In 1935, she won a theater trip to the Soviet Union. It so upset her mother, Frances remained in New York after she came back. An agent got her a screen test and she signed with Paramount. Frances' film debut, in 1936, was in *Too Many Parents.* She first got noticed – as Bing Crosby's leading lady, in *Rhythm on the Range* and was brilliant when loaned out to MGM for *Come and Get It.* Unfortunately, Frances was like her mother – difficult to work with. She hated the studio system, so in 1938, after marrying the actor, Leif Erickson, she went to New York to star on stage, in "Golden Boy". Her marriage ended and her relationship soured with Paramount – who forced her to act in B-pictures. A traumatic relationship with the playwright, Clifford Odets, turned Frances to alcohol. Hollywood disowned her and she suffered several nervous breakdowns and was in and out of mental institutions. She died of cancer, in Indianapolis, Indiana.

Rhythm on the Range (1936)
Come and Get It (1936)
Exclusive (1937) **The Toast of New York** (1937) **Ebb Tide** (1937)
Ride a Crooked Mile (1938)
South of Pago Pago (1940)
Flowing Gold (1940)
Badlands of Dakota (1941)
Among the Living (1941)
Son of Fury (1942)

Richard **Farnsworth**
6ft
(RICHARD FARNSWORTH)

Born: **September 1, 1920**
Los Angeles, California, USA
Died: **October 6, 2000**

Dick had a tough early life growing up at the beginning of the Great Depression. His father, who was a qualified engineer, worked as a poorly paid stable hand and died when Dick was seven years old. His job had at least given the boy an opportunity to learn to ride – a skill which came in useful later in life. From then on he lived with his mother and two sisters in downtown Los Angeles. Dick started his film career as a stuntman – riding horses in films beginning with the Gary Cooper epic, *Marco Polo,* in 1937, and driving a chariot in *The Ten Commandments,* in 1956. He happily continued in such supporting roles until 1966, when he was given his first film credit – as Dick Farnsworth, in *Texas Across the River.* In 1961, Dick co-founded the Stuntsmen's Association. During his 'second career' – which built up to meatier parts after several small roles, he was twice nominated for Oscars – as Best Supporting Actor for *Comes a Horseman,* and Best Actor in his superb final movie, *The Straight Story.* In 1947, he married Margaret Hill with whom he had two kids and was with until her death in 1985. He lived alone – dying of a self-inflicted gunshot wound, in Lincoln, New Mexico. He'd been diagnosed with terminal cancer.

Monte Walsh (1970)
The Cowboys (1972)
Ulzana's Raid (1972)
The Life and Times of Judge Roy Bean (1972)
The Duchess and the Dirtwater Fox (1976)
Comes a Horseman (1978)
Tom Horn (1980)
Resurrection (1980)
Waltz Across Texas (1982)
The Grey Fox (1982)
Independence Day (1983)
The Natural (1984)
Misery (1990)
The Getaway (1994)
Lassie (1994)
The Straight Story (1999)

David **Farrar**
5ft 11in
(DAVID FARRAR)

Born: **August 21, 1908**
Forest Gate, London, England
Died: **August 31, 1995**

David began his interest in acting when he played Shakespearean roles at school. He gained experience with a repertory company before becoming actor/manager of his own company in 1930. That year, he took the leading role in "The Wandering Jew" in London's West End and established a reputation with his virile good looks. He exploited them even further by taking over the Grafton Theater and starring in many of its productions. He made his film debut in 1937, in *The Face Behind the Scar.* A bomb hit the Grafton in 1940 and he was commissioned by the Ministry of War to make propaganda films. He also acted in poor movies which did little for his reputation. This all changed in 1947, when he starred in two films which struck a chord with U.S. audiences. One of them, Powell and Pressburger's, *The Black Narcissus,* is quite rightly regarded as a classic, and the other one, *Frieda,* was pretty good. David appeared in a number of good movies until, in his early fifties, following *The 300 Spartans,* he decided to retire and live quietly with his wife, Irene. When she died in 1976, he went to South Africa to be near his daughter. He lived a pleasant family life there for the next nineteen years before dying of natural causes.

Went the Day Well? (1942)
They Met in the Dark (1943)
The Black Narcissus (1947)
Frieda (1947)
Mr. Perrin and Mr. Traill (1948)
The Small Back Room (1949)
Gone to Earth (1950)
The Late Edwina Black (1951)
The Golden Horde (1951)
I Vinti (1953)
Duel in the Jungle (1954)
The Black Shield of Falworth (1954)
Escape to Burma (1955)
The Sea Chase (1955) **Lost** (1956)
I Accuse! (1958)
John Paul Jones (1959)
Solomon and Sheba (1959)
Beat Girl (1960)

Colin **Farrell**
5ft 10in
(COLIN JAMES FARRELL)

Born: **May 31, 1976**
Castleknock, Dublin, Ireland

Colin is the son of the ex-Shamrock Rovers soccer player, Eamon Farrell, and his wife Rita. He has a brother and two sisters. Colin was educated at St. Brigid's National School, Castleknock College, and the fee-paying, Catholic secondary school, Gormanston College, which is about twenty miles north of Dublin. In his teens, Colin was a promising goalkeeper with Castleknock Celtic. Before Colin became an actor, he auditioned for an early version of the Irish band, "Boyzone", but was turned down due to being tone-deaf. He made his movie debut in 1996, with an uncredited role in a mediocre drama – the Irish, Swedish and British co-production, *The Disappearance.* He then concentrated on Drama, at The Gaiety School of Acting, in Dublin, but dropped out in 1998, when he secured the role of Danny Byrne, in the popular TV-series, 'Ballykissangel'. A year later, Colin made his first good film appearance, in *The War Zone,* made in England. He followed that with *Ordinary Decent Criminal,* which was shot in Dublin and starred Kevin Spacey and Linda Fiorentino. Farrell was hot and the movies, *Tigerland* and *Hart's War,* were even hotter. He was paired with Al Pacino, in *The Recruit,* and returned home to make the excellent *Intermission.* Colin has now become a top Hollywood star in films like *Miami Vice,* and internationally, in both Woody Allen's *Cassandra's Dream,* and *In Bruges.* A four-month marriage to Amelia Warner, is Colin's only real failure.

The War Zone (1999)
Ordinary Decent Criminal (2000)
Tigerland (2000)
Hart's War (2002) **Phone Booth** (2002)
The Recruit (2003) **Daredevil** (2003)
Veronica Guerin (2003)
Intermission (2003) **A Home at
the End of the World** (2004)
Alexander (2004)
Ask the Dust (2006) **Miami Vice** (2006)
Cassandra's Dream (2007)
In Bruges (2008)
Pride and Glory (2008)

Glenda **Farrell**
5ft 3in
(GLENDA FARRELL)

Born: **June 30, 1904**
Enid, Oklahoma, USA
Died: **May 1, 1971**

From the age of seven, Glenda acted on stage – playing little Eva, in "Uncle Tom's Cabin". By the time she reached her teens, she was a Broadway veteran. In 1925 she appeared in "Cobra" at the Morosco Theater, in Los Angeles. She was starring in "Life Begins", when First National Pictures decided to transfer it to the screen. They gave her a contract and co-starred her with Edward G. Robinson in the gangster movie, *Little Caesar.* Glenda's wise-cracking personality was used to good effect opposite stars like Paul Muni and Joan Blondell. From 1933 to 1935 she appeared in a dozen worth-while movies. When her career dipped in 1937, she was given her own series – playing *Torchy Blane, Girl Reporter* – and uttering 390 words a minute! In 1941, she married Dr. Henry Ross. Their son was club entertainer, Tommy Farrell. Glenda worked on TV during the 1950s, and in 1963, won an Emmy for 'Ben Casey'. She was acting in the Broadway production, "Forty Carats" when she was diagnosed with lung cancer and forced to retire. She died in New York the following spring.

Little Caesar (1931) **I Am a
Fugitive from a Chain Gang** (1932)
The Match King (1932)
Mystery of the Wax Museum (1933)
Grand Slam (1933)
Girl Missing (1933) **The Keyhole** (1933)
Mary Stevens, M.D. (1933)
Lady for a Day (1933)
Bureau of Missing Persons (1933)
Man's Castle (1933)
The Big Shakedown (1934)
Hi, Nellie! (1934) **I've Got Your
Number** (1934) **Dark Hazard** (1934)
Heat Lightning (1934)
Gold Diggers of 1935 (1935)
Traveling Saleslady (1935)
Go Into Your Dance (1935)
Smart Blonde (1937)
Breakfast for Two (1937) **Prison
Break** (1938) **Johnny Eager** (1942)
The Talk of the Town (1942)

Mia **Farrow**
5ft 4¼in
(MARIA DE LOURDES VILLIERS FARROW)

Born: **February 9, 1945**
Los Angeles, California, USA

Mia's father was Australian film director, John Farrow, an Oscar winner in 1956, for his screenplay for *Around the World in Eighty Days.* Her mother was the Irish movie actress, Maureen O'Sullivan, who had played Jane in early Tarzan films. Mia was two when she appeared with her mother in a short about famous mothers and their kids. In the early 1950s, Mia was stricken with polio and spent a year in an iron lung. When she was fourteen, she had a small role in *John Paul Jones,* which was directed by her father. Her adult career really began in 1964, in the TV soap, 'Peyton Place'. In 1965, Mia was a Golden Globe Most Promising Newcomer. She married Frank Sinatra, but after four years, he served her with divorce papers – on the set of *Rosemary's Baby.* Their divorce got the headlines, but the film made Mia Farrow a name to remember. She was able to consolidate her position after she met Woody Allen and starred in his nod towards Ingmar Bergman – *A Midsummer Night's Sex Comedy.* Their key relationship resulted in thirteen movies and it was clearly beneficial to both. Since they parted, few of her films have been anywhere near as stimulating. Mia has 15 children – eleven of them are adopted.

Rosemary's Baby (1968)
John and Mary (1969)
Blind Terror (1971)
The Great Gatsby (1974)
A Wedding (1978)
Death on the Nile (1978)
**A Midsummer Night's
Sex Comedy** (1982)
Zelig (1983)
Broadway Danny Rose (1984)
The Purple Rose of Cairo (1985)
Hannah and Her Sisters (1986)
Radio Days (1987)
Another Woman (1988) **Alice** (1990)
Shadows and Fog (1992)
Husbands and Wives (1992)
Arthur et les Minimoys (2006)
Fast Track (2006)
Be Kind Rewind (2008)

Alice **Faye**
5ft 5in
(ALICE JEANNE LEPPERT)

Born: **May 5, 1915**
New York City, New York, USA
Died: **May 9, 1998**

Alice was the daughter of a New York police officer, Charley Leppert, and his wife Alice. After being raised in Hell's Kitchen, escape to the world of showbusiness was a must for Alice. She was fourteen when she joined the group of dancers managed by a choreographer called Chester Hale. He had started to work in movies, and was the stepping stone to her film debut, in 1934, in *George White's Scandals.* In 1936, she supported Shirley Temple in two films, and met her first husband, Tony Martin, when they appeared in *Sing Baby Sing.* By 1937, she was a big star in her own right – appearing in consecutive hits at 20th Century Fox, with Ty Power and Don Ameche. In 1938, she was in Hollywood's top ten stars at the box office. Many of Alice's best films like *On the Avenue* and *Alexander's Ragtime Band,* were musicals, but when she had the chance to do some serious acting, as in *Little Old New York,* she was good. From 1940, she was married to Phil Harris. Most of Alice's movies were pure escapism. Her final film was *The Magic of Lassie,* in 1978. Alice retired to Rancho Mirage, California, in 1980. She died there of stomach cancer, eighteen years later.

Poor Little Rich Girl (1936)
In Old Chicago (1937)
On the Avenue (1937)
You Can't Have Everything (1937)
Wake Up and Live (1937)
You're a Sweetheart (1937)
Sally, Irene and Mary (1938)
Alexander's Ragtime Band (1938)
Rose of Washington Square (1939)
Hollywood Cavalcade (1939)
Little Old New York (1940)
Tin Pan Alley (1940)
That Night in Rio (1941)
Weekend in Havana (1941)
Hello Frisco, Hello (1943)
The Gang's All Here (1943)
Fallen Angel (1945)
State Fair (1962)
The Magic of Lassie (1978)

Fernandel
5ft 7in
(FERNAND JOSEPH DÉSIRE CONSTANDIN)

Born: **May 8, 1903**
Marseille, Bouches-du-Rhône, France
Died: **February 26, 1971**

As a boy, Fernandel would take round the collection hat, in cafés, where his father worked as a singer. His mother had been an amateur actress and his parents encouraged their son to leave school at twelve to enter show business. He started out as a singer and comic – his horse-like features being a big draw in the music-hall revues. In 1925, he married the sister of his best friend and immediately started a family. He made his feature film debut, as a very shy groom, in *Le blanc et le noir,* in 1931. During the 1930s, he was hugely popular in France – working with such noted directors as Jean Renoir (son of the French Impressionist) – and the great Marcel Pagnol. He continued to perform in musicals, several of which became films. His work during the 1940s (partly because of the German occupation) wasn't especially good, but his fame had spread abroad. In 1948, photographer, Phillipe Halsman, met him in Paris and produced a book featuring his remarkable facial reactions – entitled "The Frenchman". In 1950, he made the first of six films as an Italian village priest, Don Camillo. His Hollywood efforts only proved that he was at his best in France – where he made around one hundred and fifty films in forty years. He died of lung cancer, in Paris.

Topaze (1951)
The Red Inn (1951)
The Little World of
Don Camillo (1952)
Forbidden Fruit (1952)
The Return of Don Camillo (1953)
The Sheep Has Five Legs (1955)
Don Camillo's Last Round (1955)
Le Chômeur de Clochemerle (1957)
La Legge è legge (1958)
La Vie à deux (1958)
The Cow and I (1959)
Don Camillo: Monsignor (1961)
Il Giudizio universale (1961)
The Devil and the Ten
Commandments (1962)
La Cuisine au beurre (1963)

José **Ferrer**
5ft 9¼in
(JOSÉ VICENTE FERRER DE OTERO Y CINTRÓN)

Born: **January 8, 1912**
Santurce, Puerto Rico
Died: **January 28, 1992**

Joe moved to the United States in the early 1930s, and in 1933, he graduated from Princeton University. He made his Broadway debut in 1935 and after a lot of supporting roles, became famous five years later, with his first starring role, in "Charley's Aunt". With his wife, Uta Hagen and Paul Robeson, Joe acted in the 1943 production of "Othello", but his greatest stage triumph came in 1946, when he played the title role in "Cyrano de Bergerac" and won a Tony Award. On his film debut, in *Joan of Arc,* in 1948, he was nominated for an Oscar. He won a Best Actor Oscar, in 1950, for the film version of *Cyrano de Bergerac.* Before it was released, Joe had been subpoenaed to appear before the McCarthy hearings, charged with being a Communist. His award-winning portrayal was so brilliant, even a conviction wouldn't have stopped him. He was equally impressive as Henri de Toulouse-Lautrec in *Moulin Rouge,* and received another Oscar nomination. He continued making films, but would return to the stage as often as possible. Joe's eight year marriage to Rosemary Clooney produced four children. He was George Clooney's uncle. He died of colon cancer, in Coral Cables, Florida.

Whirlpool (1949)
Joan of Arc (1950) Crisis (1950)
Cyrano de Bergerac (1950)
Anything Can Happen (1952)
Moulin Rouge (1952)
The Caine Mutiny (1954)
Deep in My Heart (1954)
The Shrike (1955)
The Cockleshell Heroes (1955)
I Accuse! (1958)
Lawrence of Arabia (1961)
Ship of Fools (1965)
Who Has Seen the Wind (1977)
Fedora (1977) A Midsummer
Night's Sex Comedy (1982)
To Be or Not to Be (1983)
The Evil That Men Do (1984)
Dune (1984)

Mel **Ferrer**

6ft 3in

(MEL CHOR GASTON FERRER)

Born: **August 25, 1917**
Elberon, New Jersey, USA
Died: **June 2, 2008**

Mel grew up in a wealthy family environment. His father, José, was a Cuban-born surgeon and his mother, Mary, was a New York socialite. He was sent to private schools and overcame polio before going to Princeton University. In his sophomore year, Mel dropped out of University to concentrate on acting. He had already worked in summer stock and he first appeared on Broadway, as a dancer, when he was just twenty-one, and gained experience as a radio DJ, at several stations in Texas and Arkansas. In 1946 he managed to persuade Columbia to let him direct a short black and white film called *The Girl of the Limberlost*. Mel went back to Broadway to star in "Strange Fruit". His debut as a film actor was in 1949, in *Lost Boundaries* – about a doctor who passes for white in a segregated community. Mel was never a conventional leading man, but starred in several movies during the 1950s. In 1954, he married the screen icon, Audrey Hepburn, with whom he had a son. They appeared together in *War and Peace,* and lived in Switzerland until their divorce in 1968. He began directing – including the TV-series 'The Farmer's Daughter' – and married his fifth wife, Elizabeth, in 1971. He acted in European films including working for Fassbinder and appeared in television plays until retiring in 1995. Mel died of heart failure, in Santa Barbara.

Lost Boundaries (1949)
Born to Be Bad (1950)
The Brave Bulls (1951)
Rancho Notorious (1952)
Scaramouche (1952)
Knights of the Round Table (1953)
Lili (1953) Oh...Rosalinda!! (1955)
War and Peace (1956)
The Sun Also Rises (1957)
The World, the Flesh and
the Devil (1959) The Fall of
the Roman Empire (1964)
Sex and the Single Girl (1964)
El Greco (1966)
Lili Marleen (1981)

America **Ferrera**

5ft 1in

(AMERICA GEORGINE FERRERA)

Born: **April 18, 1984**
Los Angeles, California, USA

Georgina as she is known as by her friends, was the youngest of six children. Following her birth to Honduran parents, her father and mother separated and she was raised by her mother (who stressed the importance of an education to all her children) in the largely Jewish area of Woodland Hills, California. She started acting in plays at George Ellery Hale Middle School, when she was eight years old and appeared in several community theater productions. Georgina later attended El Camino High School, in Woodlands Hills and after her professional career had started, she went to the University of Southern California – where she majored in Theater and International Relations. She made her film debut in *Real Women Have Curves* – but for the next couple of years was only seen in TV productions. By 2005, she was gaining early fame in movies such as the comedy, *The Sisterhood of the Traveling Pants*. The following year, America "Georgina" Ferrera became an international household name (and face) when she boldly accepted the challenging title role – and dental braces – in the smash-hit TV-series, 'Ugly Betty' – which, in its second season, won her an Emmy as Outstanding Lead Actress and a Golden Globe. Luckily for Georgina, she hasn't become completely type-cast. During the show's run, her winning smile and curvaceous figure have been enjoyed in some far from ugly film roles. Next year her voice will be heard in the animated film *How to Train Your Dragon*.

Real Women Have
Curves (2002)
How the Garcia Girls Spent
Their Summer (2005)
The Sisterhood of the
Traveling Pants (2005)
Lords of Dogtown (2005)
3:52 (2005)
Steel City (2006)
La Misma luna (2007)
The Sisterhood of the
Traveling Pants 2 (2008)

Gabriele **Ferzetti**

5ft 9¼in

(PASQUALE FERZETTI)

Born: **March 17, 1925**
Rome, Italy

By the time Gabriele left school, World War II was in full swing and Italian leader, Benito Mussolini, had taken sides with Hitler's Germany. As in any time of hardship, people sought to escape by going to the cinema. The film industry in Rome was operating as usual, even though much of its output had a fascist slant. Gabriele, who was at that time, a very good-looking seventeen-year-old, was starting studies at the Accademia d'Arte Drammatica. When he seized the opportunity to earn some money, by making his film debut, in 1942 – in a romantic drama, *Via delle cinque lune,* the academy, which had a very low opinion of film acting, expelled him. He wasn't put off and he appeared in two more movies that year. After military service, he actually concentrated on the theater until, in 1948, he reappeared in an uncredited role in an Italian version of *Les Miserables*. His first featured role was two years later, in *The Counterfeiters*. He reached stardom when Antonioni cast him opposite Eleonora Rossi Drago, in the hit film, *The Girlfriends – Le Amiche*. Another of the director's movies – the classic, *L'Avventura,* got Gabriele an international reputation. He acted in several English language films including *On Her Majesty's Secret Service,* but his heavily-accented voice was dubbed. Gabriele appeared in films and on television until 2006.

Camilla (1954)
The Girlfriends (1955) Donatella (1956)
Honor Among Thieves (1957)
Girls for the Summer (1958)
It Happened in '43 (1960)
L'Avventura (1960) Crime Does Not
Pay (1962) Beach Casanova (1962)
La Calda vita (1963) Three Rooms in
Manhattan (1965) The Devil in
Love (1966) The Bible (1966)
Once Upon a Time in the West (1968)
Machine Gun McCain (1969)
On Her Majesty's Secret Service (1969)
The Confession (1970)
Hitler: The Last Ten Days (1973)
The Night Porter (1974)

Edwige **Feuillière**
5ft 6¼in
(EDWIGE LOUISE CAROLINE CUNATI)

Born: **October 29, 1907**
Vesoul, Haute-Saone, France
Died: **November 13, 1998**

After her secondary education, Edwige decided to pursue an acting career and began her studies at the Conservatory of Dramatic Art, in Dijon. She made her stage debut in 1928 in a provincial theater production. In December 1930, following her two-year marriage to the future French film actor, Pierre Feuillère, she continued to use her stage name, Cora Lynn. Edwige made her film debut in 1931, in a short starring Fernandel, titled *La Fine combine*. Her name began to creep up the cast lists but the quality of her material was poor and confined to comedies. By 1933, she had adopted Feuillère as a her stage name and it resulted in both an improvement in quality and the status of co-starring with Raimu, in *Ces messieurs de la santé* and in the witty comedy, *Topaze*. By 1935, she was a star of the famous director, Abel Gance's rather disappointing film, *Lucrèce Borgia*. Nevertheless, she had become very popular with the French audiences, who were also aware of her work on the Paris stage. Edwige starred in dramas such as Max Ophüls' *Sans lendemain* and *De Mayerling à Sarajevo* – in which her co-star was the future US congressman, John Lodge. She stayed in France and began her post-war career in *The Idiot*, with Gérard Philipe, and made her only English-language movie, *Woman Hater*, with Stewart Granger. Edwige acted in films, on the stage, and on television until her death from natural causes at her home in Boulogne-Billancourt, France.

Ces Messieurs de la santé (1933)
Topaze (1933) Stradivarius (1935)
Golgotha (1935) Mister Flow (1936)
Sans lendemain (1939)
De Mayerling à Sarajevo (1940)
Wicked Duchess (1942)
The Honorable Catherine (1943)
The Idiot (1946)
Woman Hater (1949) Olivia (1951)
The Game of Love (1954)
Love Is My Profession (1958)
Flesh and the Orchid (1975)

Betty **Field**
5ft 2¾in
(BETTY FIELD)

Born: **February 8, 1913**
Boston, Massachusetts, USA
Died: **September 13, 1973**

Betty was descended from the original "Mayflower" Colonists. After her parents divorced, she went with her mother to South America and became fluent in Spanish. When she was a girl, her mother referred to her as the "ugly duckling". She wore spectacles, braces on her teeth and even pads in her shoes to correct her feet. Somehow, her desire to act helped her overcome. When at high school, she wrote several times to the local theater for a chance, and they gave her a few lines in several plays. At nineteen she enrolled at the American Academy of Dramatic Arts in New York, and made her stage debut, when the leading lady she was understudying in "The First Mrs. Fraser" fell ill. In 1934, she was on Broadway, in "Page Miss Glory". In 1937, for the impresario George Abbott, she starred in "What a Life". Paramount saw it and transferred it to the screen. After that, she worked with stars like John Wayne and Frederic March, but by far her best film performance was as the repressed daughter of Claude Rains, in *King's Row*. In the 1940s, her film career was virtually over, but she did well in three big 1950s productions – *Picnic, Bus Stop* and *Peyton Place*. In 1968, she made her movie bow, in *Coogan's Bluff* with Clint Eastwood, and appeared in a couple of TV plays. She retired and died of a cerebral hemorrhage, five years later, in Hyannis, Massachusetts.

What a Life (1939)
Of Mice and Men (1939)
Victory (1940)
The Shepherd of the Hills (1941)
Blues in the Night (1941)
King's Row (1942)
Flesh and Fantasy (1943)
Tomorrow the World (1944)
The Southerner (1945)
Picnic (1955) Bus Stop (1956)
Peyton Place (1957)
Birdman of Alcatraz (1962)
7 Women (1966)
Coogan's Bluff (1968)

Sally **Field**
5ft 2½in
(SALLY MARGARET FIELD)

Born: **November 6, 1946**
Pasadena, California, USA

Sally's father was a salesman named Richard Field. When Sally was four, her parents got divorced and her mother, the actress Margaret Field, married stuntman turned actor, Jock Mahoney. After she'd graduated from Van Nuys High School in California, where she'd appeared in plays, Sally was encouraged by her stepfather to pursue an acting career. She enrolled in an acting workshop at Columbia Studios. Her determination to succeed enabled her to beat all opposition for the television role of 'Gidget' in 1965. A second TV sitcom, 'The Flying Nun' (during the run of which she got married) secured her popularity with young audiences. In 1967 Sally made her film debut, in *The Way West* – starring Douglas, Mitchum and Widmark – but not very good. Other than divorce and sitcom roles, nothing much happened until her outstanding performance in the 1976 TV-movie 'Sybil', won her an Emmy *and* Burt Reynolds. The films they did together were fun to make but were never going to win awards, then, in 1979, she won an Oscar for her powerful acting in *Norma Rae*. She was also nominated for a Golden Globe in 1982. Two years later, after splitting from Burt and marrying for a second time, she also enjoyed her second Oscar triumph, for *Places in the Heart*. Much of her work since the mid-1990s has been on television – most recently as Nora Walker, in the series 'Brothers & Sisters'.

Stay Hungry (1976)
Smokey and the Bandit (1977)
Hooper (1978)
Norma Rae (1979)
Absence of Malice (1981)
Places in the Heart (1984)
Murphy's Romance (1985)
Surrender (1987)
Punchline (1988)
Steel Magnolias (1989)
Mrs. Doubtfire (1993)
Forrest Gump (1994)
Eye for an Eye (1996)
Where the Heart Is (2000)
Two Weeks (2006)

Shirley Anne **Field**
5ft 4in
(SHIRLEY BROADBENT)

Born: **June 27, 1938**
Bolton, Lancashire, England

Because their mother was unable to care for them, Shirley and her brother were raised in the Edgeworth Children's Home and Orphanage. By the age of seventeen she was appearing in magazines with very little on – and she was crowned "Miss London". Her tough early life made her determined to be a success. She sent her photos to all the studios in England and began getting extra work and small parts – beginning with *Simon and Laura,* in 1955. Shirley made her first real impression in 1960. The year began with a leading role in Michael Powell's classic film, *Peeping Tom.* She was then featured in the cool *Beat Girl* and Laurence Olivier's star vehicle, *The Entertainer,* before rounding off a vintage year by playing Albert Finney's girlfriend, in *Saturday Night and Sunday Morning.* Shirley co-starred with Steve McQueen and Robert Wagner in *The War Lover* and until the mid-1960s, she continued to get roles worthy of her obvious talents. After that, the choice parts dried up and she concentrated on the theater – being especially praised for her performance in the South African production of "Wait Until Dark". Her movie comeback in 1985, was in the acclaimed British-made box office hit – *My Beautiful Launderette.* Shirley has kept on working right up to 2009. Her autobiography, "A Time For Love" is well worth reading.

Horrors of the Black
Museum (1959)
Peeping Tom (1960)
The Entertainer (1960)
Beat Girl (1960)
Saturday Night and
Sunday Morning (1960)
The War Lover (1962)
The Damned (1963) Alfie (1966)
My Beautiful Launderette (1985)
Shag (1989) Getting It Right (1989)
The Rachel Papers (1989)
Hear My Song (1991)
At Risk (1994) Christie Malry's Own
Double-Entry (2000)
The Gift: At Risk (2007)

W.C. **Fields**
5ft 8in
(WILLIAM CLAUDE DUKENFIELD)

Born: **January 29, 1880**
Darby, Pennsylvania, USA
Died: **December 25, 1946**

Bill endured a childhood of exceptional hardship at the hands of a brutal, alcoholic father. Because of his father's drunken singing he had a hatred for music which lasted throughout his life. Bill ran away from home when he was eleven and lived rough for the next few years. During that time, he became a skilled pool player and took up juggling, which enabled him to get a job in an amusement park in Norristown, Pennsylvania. Bill moved on to Atlantic City, and by the tender age of nineteen, was promoted as "The Distinguished Comedian". When he turned twenty, he married Harriet Hughes. They remained together until he died forty-six years later. She accompanied him on a successful tour of Europe, South Africa and Australia. After his return, he joined the 'Ziegfeld Follies' and he remained with them until 1921. Four years later his first starring film role was in *Sally of the Sawdust.* His silent films were popular, but it was the advent of sound and hearing Bill's unique rasping voice that made him a star. His 1930s films are masterpieces of comic chaos. He became ill through drink, but its effect and the resultant red bulbous-nose, was an essential part of his screen personality, although it would kill him eventually. He duly died in Pasadena from a stomach hemorrhage, on Christmas day – a holiday he claimed to loathe.

Million Dollar Legs (1932)
If I Had a Million (1932)
International House (1933)
Six of a Kind (1934)
You're Telling Me (1934)
The Old Fashioned Way (1934)
It's a Gift (1934)
David Copperfield (1935)
Man on the Flying Trapeze (1935)
You Can't Cheat an
Honest Man (1939)
My Little Chickadee (1940)
The Bank Dick (1940)
Never Give a Sucker an
Even Break (1941)

Joseph **Fiennes**
6ft
(JOSEPH ALBERIC TWISLETON-WYKEHAM-FIENNES)

Born: **May 27, 1970**
Salisbury, Wiltshire, England

Joseph, the youngest of six children is the son of a professional photographer, Mark Fiennes, and the novelist, Jenny Lash. His brother, Ralph, and two sisters are also in the film industry. He moved around a lot during his childhood, but mainly grew up in West Cork, Ireland – where he became a skilled horseman and also excelled at swimming and tennis. After attending art college, in Suffolk, he joined the Young Vic Youth Theater to begin his acting career, but didn't give up the idea of becoming a painter. He was usually seen carrying a sketch book. Joseph studied acting at the Guildhall School of Music and Drama, in London. Top stage work in the West End theaters, in "The Woman in Black" and "A Month in the Country" – when he acted opposite Helen Mirren, led to a two-year spell with famous Royal Shakespeare Company. In 1995, Joseph made his first appearance on TV in 'The Vacillations of Poppy Carew'. A year later, he made his film debut, in the romantic drama directed by the Italian master, Bernardo Bertolucci, titled *Stealing Beauty.* An excellent trio of films including *Shakespeare in Love* – for which he was nominated for a Best Actor BAFTA – were followed by a pair of duds, but *Enemy at the Gates* got him back on track and quality abounded. One highlight was *The Merchant of Venice* - in which he was able to flex his acting muscles in the company of Al Pacino and Jeremy Irons. Joseph has continued to progress.

Stealing Beauty (1996)
Elizabeth (1998)
Shakespeare in Love (1998)
Enemy at the Gates (2001)
Dust (2001)
Leo (2002)
Luther (2003)
The Merchant of Venice (2004)
Man to Man (2005)
Running with Scissors (2006)
Goodbye Bafana (2007)
The Escapist (2008)
The Red Baron (2008)
Spring 1941 (2008)

Ralph **Fiennes**
6ft
(RALPH NATHANIEL FIENNES)

Born: **December 22, 1962**
Ipswich, Suffolk, England

Ralph was the eldest of the six children of a photographer and a lady novelist. The Fiennes family moved to Ireland when he was he was eleven, and for one year he attended Saint Kieran's College. After returning to England to live in Salisbury, Ralph finished his education at Bishop Wordsworth' School in the city center. As his first ambition had always been to become a painter, he then enrolled at the Chelsea Art College. At twenty-two, he transferred his energies to acting – at the Royal Academy of Dramatic Art. After graduating he joined the National Theater and a year or so later, he acted in various classic plays with the Royal Shakespeare Company. Ralph first got wider recognition in 1991 – when starring in "A Dangerous Man: Lawrence After Arabia". His film debut came when he co-starred with Juliette Binoche, in *Wuthering Heights.* An Oscar nomination for his role as a psychotic Nazi, in Spielberg's *Schindler's List* kept the momentum going and three years later, he received another Oscar nomination, for *The English Patient.* Each year since then has usually produced one pretty good performance from the actor and it can only be a question of *when* he will win an Oscar. Ralph's sisters, Martha and Sophie, are both filmmakers and his youngest brother, Joseph Fiennes, is also a movie actor of some note.

Wuthering Heights (1992)
Schindler's List (1993)
Quiz Show (1994) Strange Days (1995)
The English Patient (1996)
Oscar and Lucinda (1997)
Sunshine (1999) Onegin (1999)
The End of the Affair (1999)
Spider (2002) Red Dragon (2002)
The Chumscrubber (2005)
The Constant Gardener (2005)
Land of the Blind (2006)
The Order of the Phoenix (2007)
Bernard and Doris (2007)
In Bruges (2008) The Duchess (2008)
The Hurt Locker (2008)
The Reader (2008)

Jon **Finch**
6ft 2¹/₂in
(JONATHAN FINCH)

Born: **March 2, 1941**
Caterham, Surrey, England

Jon was the son of a merchant banker who worked in the City of London. At school, he was a regular in plays. His first stage role was playing a Roman 'lady' at the age of thirteen. When he was eighteen, he qualified for the London School of Economics, but chose instead to serve in the Parachute Regiment for nearly two years. After that, he was an assistant stage manager with Croydon Repertory Theater. When he was promoted to Stage Manager, he was thrust into a situation where he had to act, and soon realized what he'd been missing. He moved to the Chesterfield Repertory company, in Derbyshire, with whom he appeared in over fifty plays. Seven years experience as an actor in Shakespearian productions as well as contemporary works, brought his name to the attention of filmmakers, but for a while, he filled in with jobs as a night-club bouncer, and motor mechanic. In 1967, he appeared in an episode of the TV-series, 'Z Cars' and in 1970, he was playing supporting roles in horror films – starting with *The Vampire Lovers.* In 1971, Jon made a cameo appearance in the John Schlesinger movie, *Sunday Bloody Sunday.* Jon continued to enjoy his stage career and starred in Hitchcock's last film, *Frenzy.* Jon has had many love affairs – probably most seriously, with the actress Francesca Annis, but he never married.

The Vampire Lovers (1970)
Sunday Bloody Sunday (1971)
Macbeth (1971)
Lady Caroline Lamb (1972)
Frenzy (1972)
The Final Program (1973)
Diagnosis: Murder (1975)
Death on the Nile (1978)
La Sabina (1979)
Breaking Glass (1980)
Doktor Faustus (1982)
Streets of Yesterday (1989)
Bloodlines:
Legacy of a Lord (1997)
Anazapta (2001)
Kingdom of Heaven (2005)

Peter **Finch**
5ft 11in
(FREDERICK GEORGE PETER INGLE-FINCH)

Born: **September 28, 1912**
South Kensington, London, England
Died: **January 14, 1977**

Peter's parents – who were Australians, divorced when he was still a toddler. He went to live in France and then India with his mother. At the age of ten, when she remarried, he moved to Australia to be raised by his relatives. After leaving school in Sydney he tried several badly-paid jobs before he appeared in vaudeville and on the local radio. Peter was twenty when he acted in his first film, *Dad and Dave Come to Town,* in 1938. Apart his first marriage in 1943, nothing of great consequence occurred until in the late 1940s, Laurence Olivier and Vivien Leigh toured Australia. Peter was taken under Larry's wing and worked with him in London, while Vivien fell in love with him. He had a small role in the Hollywood film, *The Miniver Story,* in 1950, and made several films before his movie career began to take off in 1954, with a role opposite Elizabeth Taylor, in *Elephant Walk.* He was a leading actor in Britain for a few years, but not very highly regarded in the Unites States. That all changed after his appearance with Audrey Hepburn, in *The Nun's Story.* Peter had first been nominated for an Oscar for his performance in the movie *Sunday Bloody Sunday.* His Best Actor Oscar for *Network* was the only time it had been awarded posthumously. Peter died in Beverly Hills, just six weeks before the Academy Awards. His third wife, Eletha, accepted the Oscar on his behalf.

The Heart of the Matter (1953)
Father Brown (1954)
A Town Like Alice (1956)
The Battle of the River Plate (1956)
The Nun's Story (1959)
Kidnapped (1960)
The Trials of Oscar Wilde (1960)
The Pumpkin Eater (1964)
The Flight of the Phoenix (1965)
Far From the
Madding Crowd (1967)
Sunday Bloody Sunday (1971)
The Abdication (1974)
Network (1976)

Frank **Finlay**
5ft 8in
(FRANK FINLAY)

Born: August 6, 1926
Farnworth, Lancashire, England

Frank was the son of Josiah and Margaret Finlay, who raised him as a Catholic. He was educated accordingly, at St. Gregory the Great School, but left at fourteen and did a variety of jobs, including butcher's assistant, to pay for his evening classes, where he studied English and Art. He began his stage career in 1951, when he worked with repertory companies. He won a Sir James Knott's scholarship to RADA and made his stage debut at Guildford, in "The Queen and the Welshman" in 1957. Frank made his Broadway debut the following year in "Epitaph for George Dillon". From 1960, he worked on television as well as on the stage. Frank then made his film debut, in *The Loneliness of the Long Distance Runner* and enjoyed it. A great performance as Iago in Laurence Olivier's "Othello" at the National Theater in 1964 was repeated in the movie version, the following year – earning him a Best Supporting Actor Oscar nomination. He is best remembered for playing Porthos, in *The Three Musketeers* and its sequels. He was married to actress Doreen Shepherd until her death in 2005. He's still active in 2008, despite being erroneously reported to have died in 1986 – in the 9th edition of "Halliwell's Filmgoer's Companion".

The Comedy Man (1964)
A Study in Terror (1965)
Othello (1965) **Robbery** (1967)
I'll Never Forget What's'isname (1967)
The Molly Maguires (1970)
Cromwell (1970) **Gumshoe** (1971)
Sitting Target (1972)
The Three Musketeers (1973)
The Four Musketeers (1974)
The Wild Geese (1978)
Murder by Decree (1979)
The Return of the Soldier (1982)
Enigma (1983)
The Ploughman's Lunch (1983)
Stiff Upper Lips (1997)
The Pianist (2002)
The Statement (2003)
Lighthouse Hill (2004)
The Waiting Room (2007)

Albert **Finney**
5ft 9in
(ALBERT FINNEY)

Born: May 9, 1936
Salford, Manchester, England

The son of a bookmaker, Albert Finney Sr., and his wife, Alice, young Albert was streetwise forty years before the term was used. Along with other Northern actors, he took the British theater world by storm when it badly needed a fresh approach and new blood. Albert stuck with tradition by getting married to the actress, Jane Wenham, when he was twenty-one, but was divorced shortly after his first starring role – in *Saturday Night and Sunday Morning*, had helped change the face of british acting forever. He earned the first of his Oscar nominations in 1963, when after turning down the lead in *Lawrence of Arabia* he starred in *Tom Jones.* From then on, Albert selected his roles carefully, which tended to leave large gaps in his film career. In 1968, he tried his hand at directing (and also acted in) *Charlie Bubbles.* He married the actress, Anouk Aimée, and after 1975, was hardly seen on the big screen for seven years. During the 1980s, he was Oscar-nominated twice more – for *The Dresser,* and *Under the Volcano.* A third marriage produced his second child. In 1998, Albert co-starred with Tom Courtnay in a brilliant TV-film 'A Rather English Marriage' and in 2001, he was nominated for a Best Supporting Actor Oscar, for *Erin Brokovich.* In 2002, his portrayal of Churchill in 'The Gathering Storm' won him a BAFTA and an Emmy.

Saturday Night and Sunday Morning (1960) **Tom Jones** (1963)
The Victors (1963) **Two for the Road** (1967) **Charlie Bubbles** (1967)
Scrooge (1970) **Murder on the Orient Express** (1974) **Shoot the Moon** (1982) **The Dresser** (1983)
Under the Volcano (1984)
The Browning Version (1994)
Erin Brokovich (2000)
Traffic (2000) **Big Fish** (2003)
Aspects of Love (2005)
A Good Year (2006)
The Bourne Ultimatum (2007)
Before the Devil Knows You're Dead (2007)

Linda **Fiorentino**
5ft 7in
(CLORINDA FIORENTINO)

Born: March 9, 1958
Philadelphia, Pennsylvania, USA

The daughter of a steel contractor and his wife. Her parents were Italian American Catholics who produced two sons and six daughters. Her mother was also called Clorinda, so becoming Linda was a way to avoid any confusion. She was raised in Turnersville, New Jersey, where, when she was a student at Washington Township High School, in Sewell, she was tall enough to excel at basketball. She then studied political science and pre-law at Rosemount College, outside Philadelphia, but dropped the idea of becoming a lawyer to go to New York City, where she studied drama at Circle in The Square Acting School. During that time she worked alongside Bruce Willis, as a bartender, at the 'Kamikaze Club'. Since studying at the International Center of Photography in New York, she has been actively involved in taking pictures. In 1985, Linda made her film debut, in the sports drama, *Vision Quest,* but it took nine years for her to be taken seriously, when she starred in *The Last Seduction.* Her performance was considered to be Oscar potential, but because the film had been shown on HBO television, Linda was ineligible, but did get a BAFTA nomination. Her brief marriage to the film director John Byrum ended in divorce in 1993. Although Linda was described by *Dogma* director, Kevin Smith, as "difficult to work with" her six-year absence from the screen was a big loss to her many fans, but she's back!

Gotcha! (1985)
After Hours (1985)
The Moderns (1988)
Queen's Logic (1991)
Beyond the Law (1992)
The Last Seduction (1994)
Unforgettable (1996)
Men in Black (1997)
Dogma (1999)
What Planet Are You From? (2000)
Ordinary Decent Criminal (2000)
Where the Money Is (2000)
Liberty Stands Still (2002)
Once More with Feeling (2009)

Colin **Firth**
6ft 1¹/₂in
(COLIN ANDREW FIRTH)

Born: September 10, 1960
Grayshott, Hampshire, England

Colin's parents were both born and raised in India, where their own parents had been missionaries. His father, David Firth, who was a teacher, moved the family to Nigeria when he took up a post with the Nigerian government. Colin's mother, Shirley, was a comparative religion lecturer in Lagos, but when he was eleven, the Firths moved to St. Louis, Missouri. Back in England, he attended the Montgomery of Alamein School, in Winchester, and the Barton Peveril College at Eastleigh, in Hampshire. Colin took his acting lessons at The Drama Center, in Clerkenwell, London and his career started on the London stage in 1981, when he starred in "Another Country" and reprised that role for his film debut, in 1984. During the making of *Valmont,* he became involved with his co-star, Meg Tilley, and their relationship resulted in a son, Will Firth. Although he received a lot of praise for his acting, it was only after his portrayal of Fitzwilliam Darcy, in the 1995 BBC TV production of 'Pride and Prejudice' that he was considered star material. After that, Colin was written into the *Bridget Jones* scripts and appeared in the films as Mark Darcy. In 1997, Colin married the Italian documentary filmmaker, Livia Giuggioli. They live with their two sons in London and Italy. 2007 was his bumper year.

A Month in the Country (1987)
Apartment Zero (1988)
Valmont (1989) Wings of Fame (1990)
The English Patient (1996)
Shakespeare in Love (1998)
My Life So Far (1999)
Relative Values (2000)
Bridget Jones's Diary (2001)
The Importance of Being Earnest (2002)
Love Actually (2003)
Where the Truth Lies (2005)
Nanny McPhee (2005)
And When Did You Last See
Your Father? (2007)
Then She Found Me (2007)
St.Trinian's (2007)
Mamma Mia! (2008)

Laurence **Fishburne**
6ft 0¹/₂in
(LAWRENCE FISHBURNE III)

Born: July 30, 1961
Augusta, Georgia, USA

Larry's dad, Laurence John Fishburne Jr., worked as a corrections officer with problem juveniles. His mother, Hattie, was a mathematics and science teacher at a junior high school Following their divorce, the boy lived with his mother in Brooklyn. Without any training, and calling himself Larry Fishburne, he began acting in 1971, in a play titled "In My Many Names and Days". In 1972, he played Fish in the TV-drama, 'If You Give a Dance, You Gotta Pay the Band' and from 1973, he was Joshua Hall in the soap opera 'One Life to Live'. He made his movie debut in 1975, in *Cornbread, Earl and Me.* Later in that decade, after graduating from Lincoln Square Academy, in New York, he was given the first of four roles in Francis Ford Coppola movies, with a cameo part in *Apocalypse Now.* Larry worked steadily in films and as Ike Turner, he earned a Best Actor Oscar nomination, for *What's Love Got to Do with It.* On stage, Larry then won several awards for his powerful performance in the August Wilson play, "Two Trains Running". He had two children with his first wife, the actress Hajna O. Moss. Since 2002, Larry has been married to Cuban-American actress, Gina Torres.

Rumble Fish (1983) The Cotton
Club (1984) The Color Purple (1985)
A Nightmare on Elm Street:
Dream Warriors (1987)
Gardens of Stone (1987)
Red Heat (1988)
King of New York (1990)
Cadence (1990) Class Action (1991)
Boyz n the Hood (1991)
Deep Cover (1992) What's Love
Got to Do with It (1993) Searching for
Bobby Fischer (1993)
Just Cause (1995) Othello (1995)
Event Horizon (1997) The Matrix (1999)
The Matrix Reloaded (2003)
Mystic River (2003)
Assault on Precinct 13 (2005)
Akeelah and the Bee (2006)
Bobby(2006) 21 (2008)
Tortured (2008)

Carrie **Fisher**
5ft 1in
(CARRIE FRANCES FISHER)

Born: October 21, 1956
Los Angeles, California, USA

Carrie's parents were both big stars in show business – her dad was the popular 1950s singer, Eddie Fisher, whose parents were Jewish immigrants from Russia. Her mother was the talented movie star, Debbie Reynolds. They were divorced by the time Carrie was three, after her dad fell in love with Liz Taylor and married her. For several years, Carrie lived with her mother. She was just twelve years old when they appeared together in a Las Vegas show. There was no way she was going to lead a conventional life after that. At sixteen, while at Beverly Hills High School, she dropped out to make her Broadway debut with her mother in a revival of "Irene". She then spent eighteen months in London, studying acting at the Central School of Speech and Drama. In 1975, Carrie made her film debut, in *Shampoo.* Two years after that she became world famous for her role as Princess Leia, in *Star Wars.* She reprised the role in the TV-movie 'Star Wars Holiday Special' in 1978 – also that year – she hosted 'Saturday Night Live' when Dan Aykroyd and John Belushi first performed their Blues Brothers routine. She had a cameo role in the movie and then starred on Broadway in "Censored Scenes from King Kong". Carrie's only marriage – to the singer/songwriter, Paul Simon, lasted less than a year. In 1987, she published the first of five novels – the semi-autobiographical "Postcards from the Edge". It became a best seller and was turned into a movie in 1990.

Star Wars (1977)
The Empire Strikes Back (1980)
The Blues Brothers (1980)
Return of the Jedi (1983)
The Man with One Red Shoe (1985)
Hannah and Her Sisters (1986)
Appointment with Death (1988)
The 'burbs (1989)
When Harry Met Sally (1989)
Soapdish (1991)
This Is My Life (1992) Scream 3 (2000)
Wonderland (2003) Stateside (2004)
Fanboys (2008)

Barry **Fitzgerald**
5ft 4in
(WILLIAM JOSEPH SHIELDS)

Born: **March 10, 1888**
Dublin, Ireland
Died: **January 14, 1961**

Barry started work at the Board of Trade Unemployment Insurance Division. It was dull, but it allowed him time off to appear in amateur stage productions. In 1915 he changed his name and joined the Abbey Players in Dublin – along with his younger brother, Arthur Shields. Slowly he established himself and in 1929, Sean O'Casey wrote "The Silver Tassle" for him. He was over forty when he starred in another O'Casey play, "Juno and the Paycock'. Hitchcock saw it and gave him his film debut in the screen version. Barry first appeared on Broadway with the Abbey Theater Company in 1932 and three years later, he and Arthur went to Hollywood to co-star in John Ford's *The Plough and the Stars.* It was no masterpiece, but it established Barry as an ideal character for any film which required a 'touch of the Blarney' – although he did play a Welshman in *How Green was My Valley.* When Barry won an Oscar as Best Supporting Actor in *Going My Way,* it was a unique occasion in the Academy's history; He'd been nominated for both 'Best Actor' and 'Best Supporting Actor' for the same role. Barry returned to Ireland to make his final film, *Broth of a Boy,* in 1959. He died of a heart attack in Dublin, two years later.

The Plough and the Stars (1936)
Bringing Up Baby (1938)
Four Men and a Prayer (1938)
The Dawn Patrol (1938)
The Long Voyage Home (1940)
The Sea Wolf (1941)
How Green Was My Valley (1941)
Going My Way (1944)
None But the Lonely Heart (1944)
Incendiary Blonde (1945)
And Then There Were None (1945)
The Stork Club (1945)
Two Years Before the Mast (1946)
The Naked City (1948)
Miss Tatlock's Millions (1948)
Union Station (1950) **The Quiet Man** (1952) **Happy Ever After** (1954)
The Catered Affair (1956)

Geraldine **Fitzgerald**
5ft 3in
(GERALDINE FITZGERALD)

Born: **November 24, 1913**
Greystones, County Wicklow, Ireland
Died: **July 17, 2005**

Geraldine's mother converted to her husband's faith, Catholicism, and they sent their daughter to a Dublin convent school. When she was eighteen she joined the Gate Theater and made her debut there in 1932. Her first film appearance was in 1934, in a dull British film, *Blind Justice.* Three years later, Geraldine emigrated to the USA. She made her Broadway debut soon after, in the Orson Welles' Mercury Theater production of George Bernard Shaw's "Heartbreak House". Warner Brothers took her to Hollywood, where in her first film, *Wuthering Heights,* she was nominated for a Best Supporting Actress Oscar. During the 1940s she appeared in prestigious films – acting opposite stars like Bette Davis and Olivia de Havilland. Geraldine's problem was that she was strong-willed and unable to accept every film role they offered her. The resulting suspension meant a five year period with few films. She became a TV actress and in 1960 she founded the Everyman Theater. Geraldine's Broadway work included an acclaimed 1971 performance opposite Robert Ryan, in "Long Day's Journey into Night". She suffered from Alzheimer's Disease and died in New York.

Wuthering Heights (1939)
Dark Victory (1939) **A Child is Born** (1939) **Shining Victory** (1941)
The Gay Sisters (1942)
Watch on the Rhine (1943)
Wilson (1944) **The Strange Affair of Uncle Harry** (1945)
Three Strangers (1946)
O.S.S. (1946)
Nobody Lives Forever (1946)
So Evil My Love (1948)
The Late Edwina Black (1951)
Ten North Frederick (1958)
The Fiercest Heart (1961)
The Pawnbroker (1964)
Rachel, Rachel (1968)
Harry and Tonto (1974)
Arthur (1981)
Easy Money (1983)

Tara **Fitzgerald**
5ft 5in
(TARA FITZGERALD)

Born: **September 18, 1967**
Cuckfield, Sussex, England

Tara was the daughter of Michael Callaby – who was of Italian descent, and Sarah Fitzgerald – who is related to the famous Irish movie actress, Geraldine Fitzgerald. Tara spent the first three years of her life living in Freeport, Barbados, where her grandfather had a law practice. After her parents separated when she was four years old, Tara, her sister, Arabella, and their mother, returned to England to live in a basement flat in the London suburb of Clapham. Her mother's life was unsettled and she briefly remarried. Tara attended five different primary schools before her secondary education, at Walsingham Comprehensive. She then decided to study drama, but was unsuccessful when applying to both RADA and the Guildhall School. At seventeen, she traveled around Europe and on her return – in 1987, was accepted at The Drama Center, in North London. She worked as a waitress to pay her tuition fees, and after graduating, in 1991, she secured her first film role, in *Hear My Song.* Tara gained experience in television dramas and on the West End stage, where she co-starred with Peter O'Toole in "Our Song". For the film *Sirens,* she was nominated for a Best Actress Award by the Australian Film Institute. She was re-united with its star, Hugh Grant, in 1995, and played Ophelia on Broadway to Ralph Fiennes' "Hamlet". She was named Best Actress by the New York Critics Circle. Tara is separated from her husband, John Sharian. She's recently been seen in the TV series, 'Waking the Dead'.

Hear My Song (1991)
Sirens (1994)
A Man of No Importance (1995)
The Englishman Who Went Up a Hill But Came Down a Mountain (1995)
Brassed Off (1996)
Conquest (1998)
Childhood (1999)
Dark Blue World (2001)
I Capture the Castle (2003)
Secret Passage (2004)
Five Children and It (2004)

Rhonda **Fleming**
5ft 4in
(MARILYN LOUIS)

Born: **August 10, 1923**
Hollywood, California, USA

A popular local girl, Rhonda completed her schooling at Beverly Hills High School. She was beautiful enough to get in the fast lane to a movie career. She was a lyrical soprano who idolized Deanna Durbin. In 1943, she had a role as a dance-hall girl in the John Wayne film, *In Old Oklahoma*. Two years later, she was fifth-billed in Hitchcock's *Spellbound*. She looked even better in color, proof of which came in 1946, when she starred in *Adventure Island*. She married the first of her six husbands, Thomas Lane, and had her only child, a son. Rhonda remained popular for fifteen years, with a big fan following. She was always extremely approachable and never refused to sign autographs. Having sung with Crosby in *A Connecticut Yankee in King Arthur's Court,* Rhonda was on the 78rpm release of "When is Sometime".Ten years later, she made an album of standards, titled simply, "Rhonda". During the 1960s and 70s, she did a lot of television work and also made her Broadway debut in Clare Boothe Luce's "The Women". Her fifth husband, Ted Mann, helped her to set up the Rhonda Fleming Ted Mann Clinic, at the UCLA Medical Center.

Spellbound (1945)
The Spiral Staircase (1945)
Abilene Town (1946)
Out of the Past (1947)
A Connecticut Yankee in
King Arthur's Court (1949)
The Great Lover (1949)
The Eagle and the Hawk (1950)
Cry Danger (1951)
The Redhead and
the Cowboy (1951)
Pony Express (1953)
Inferno (1953)
Yankee Pasha (1954)
Slightly Scarlet (1956)
While the City Sleeps (1956)
Gunfight at the O.K. Corral (1957)
Home Before Dark (1958)
Alias Jesse James (1959)
The Crowded Sky (1960)
Run for Your Wife (1965)

Louise **Fletcher**
5ft 9½in
(LOUISE FLETCHER)

Born: **July 22, 1934**
Birmingham, Alabama, USA

Louise and her brother and two sisters were born to parents who were both deaf. Her father was an episcopal minister, who devoted his life to founding over forty churches in Alabama for the hearing impaired. Louise and her three siblings were born with regular hearing. She was taught to speak and introduced to acting by an aunt. She took acting lessons in Los Angeles after graduating from the University of North Carolina – working as a secretary to pay for them. Louise began getting plenty of television work in the late 1950s, most notably in the western series 'Maverick'. In 1960, she married Jerry Bick and put her career on hold to raise two children. She was almost forty when she returned to acting. In 1974, she had a good small role in the film *Thieves Like Us* and the following year, she featured in *Russian Roulette*. She was selected by Milos Forman to play Nurse Mildred Ratched, in *One Flew over the Cuckoo's Nest*. Louise won the Best Actress Oscar as well as Golden Globe and BAFTA awards. Like many Oscar winners, she has never managed to find that level again, but has kept busy. If you want to see the best of Louise's recent film work, get hold of *The Last Sin Eater*.

Thieves Like Us (1974)
One Flew Over the
Cuckoo's Nest (1976)
The Cheap Detective (1978)
The Lucky Star (1980)
Brainstorm (1983)
The Best of the Best (1989)
Giorgino (1994)
Virtuosity (1995)
2 Days in the Valley (1996)
Cruel Intentions (1999)
A Map of the World (1999)
Big Eden (2000)
Very Mean Men (2000)
Dial 9 for Love (2001)
Finding Home (2003)
Dancing in Twilight (2005)
Aurora Borealis (2005)
The Last Sin Eater (2007)

Errol **Flynn**
6ft 2½in
(ERROL LESLIE THOMSON FLYNN)

Born: **June 20, 1909**
Hobart, Tasmania, Australia
Died: **October 14, 1959**

Errol's father was a biologist. His mother was a descendent of an officer on "HMS Bounty" and a Tahitian woman. When he was twelve, the family moved to England. Errol was expelled three times during his schooldays, so he sought adventure overseas instead. He joined the Northampton Repertory Company on his return to England, but after convincing himself that he knew everything about acting, he went to Australia in 1933 to make a movie titled *In the Wake of the Bounty*. A Hollywood mogul saw it and, with the Australian taxman on his trail, Errol signed a contract with Warners. When Robert Donat fell ill, he took his place, in *Captain Blood*. He became the world's favorite swashbuckler in classic films such as *The Adventures of Robin Hood* and *The Sea Hawk*. He was heroic, in *They Died with Their Boots On,* and he won the war, in *Objective Burma*. Errol's affairs and heavy drinking sessions were legendary. He used his luxury yacht, the "Zaca" for many of his conquests and by the early 1950s, the effects of his excesses began to show in his screen appearances. After he died from a heart attack in Vancouver, the autopsy stated that "he had the body of a seventy-five year-old man". Errol was barely fifty.

Captain Blood (1935)
The Charge of the
Light Brigade (1936) The Prince and
the Pauper (1937)
The Adventures of Robin Hood (1938)
The Dawn Patrol (1938)
Dodge City (1939)
The Private Lives of
Elizabeth and Essex (1939)
The Sea Hawk (1940)
Dive Bomber (1941)
They Died with Their Boots On (1941)
Gentleman Jim (1942)
Edge of Darkness (1943)
Objective Burma! (1945)
Adventures of Don Juan (1948)
Kim (1950) Against All Flags (1952)
The Sun Also Rises (1957)

Nina **Foch**
5ft 9in
(NINA CONSUELO MAUD FOCK)

Born: **April 20, 1924**
Leiden, Holland
Died: **December 5, 2008**

Nina's mother was the American actress, Consuelo Flowerton, who went to Holland after marrying the Dutch conductor/composer, Dirk Fock. Following her divorce, she took her daughter back to the USA. Nina tried to forge a career as a concert pianist, but soon switched to acting and enrolled at the American Academy of Dramatic Arts, in New York. She gained experience on stage and soon became a contract starlet at Columbia Pictures. After she appeared in a short, called *Wagon Wheels,* she made her feature movie debut, in 1943, in *Return of the Vampire.* There were several B-pictures before she was given the chance to play supporting roles in first-features, including *A Song to Remember* and *Johnny O'Clock.* One of her most notable and moving roles was as the chic patroness of the Arts, spurned by Gene Kelly, in *An American in Paris.* In 1954, Nina was nominated for an Oscar when she appeared in the sophisticated movie *Executive Suite.* The following year, she was in a Martin and Lewis comedy. Nina bowed out of the movie mainstream after playing Helena, in the blockbuster, *Spartacus.* After that most of Nina's roles had been on television. She was teaching 'Directing the Actor' at the University of Southern California Cinema Department, up to her death in Los Angeles, caused by complications of myelodysplasia.

Nine Girls (1944) Shadows in the
Night (1944) A Song to
Remember (1945) I Love a
Mystery (1945) Escape in the Fog (1945)
My Name Is Julia Ross (1945)
Johnny O'Clock (1947)
The Guilt of Janet Ames (1947)
The Undercover Man (1949)
Johnny Allegro (1949)
An American in Paris (1951)
Young Man with Ideas (1952)
Scaramouche (1952)
Executive Suite (1954) Illegal (1955)
The Ten Commandments (1956)
Spartacus (1960)

Bridget **Fonda**
5ft 6in
(BRIDGET JANE FONDA)

Born: **January 27, 1964**
Los Angeles, California, USA

Bridget is the daughter of the actor/filmmaker, Peter Fonda, and an artist by the name of Sarah Jane Brewer. The couple got divorced when she was twelve years old. Bridget and her brother, Justin, were raised in the Coldwater Canyon section of Los Angeles by their dad's second wife, Portia Crockett. While she attended the Westlake School for Girls, neither she nor her brother were in contact with the famous Fonda family. After appearing in a school production of "Harvey", Bridget studied method acting at New York University's Tisch School of the Arts, and at the Lee Strasberg Theater Institute, but suffered from severe stage fright. She made her film debut, in 1982, when she had a non-speaking role in *Partners.* Six years later, she played Mandy Rice-Davies in the film *Scandal* and was nominated for a Golden Globe. During the 1990s Bridget was in twenty-seven movies, but few of them – apart from *City Hall,* and *Jackie Brown* – did her justice. In 1997 she was nominated as outstanding actress in a mini series or special, for 'In the Gloaming'. In 2002, Bridget was praised for her acting in the TV mini series 'After Amy' . She married the film music composer, Danny Elfman, in 2003, and for the past five years or so, she has devoted her time to raising their little son, Oliver.

Scandal (1989) Shag (1989)
The Godfather: Part III (1990)
Single White Female (1992)
Army of Darkness (1992)
It Could Happen to You (1994)
Camilla (1994)
Rough Magic (1995)
City Hall (1996)
Grace of My Heart (1996)
Mr. Jealousy (1997)
Jackie Brown (1997)
Finding Graceland (1998)
A Simple Plan (1998)
Lake Placid (1999)
Delivering Milo (2001)
Kiss of the Dragon (2001)
The Whole Shebang (2001)

Henry **Fonda**
6ft 1½in
(HENRY JAYNES FONDA)

Born: **May 16, 1905**
Grand Island, Nebraska, USA
Died: **August 12, 1982**

Hank's father was from an Italian background. His mother's ancestors were Dutch. After he witnessed the result of a lynching he developed a social awareness and fought against prejudice. Majoring in Journalism at the University of Minnesota, he dropped out to begin his acting career in 1925, with a leading role in "You and I" at the Omaha Community Playhouse. He then joined the Provincetown Players, where he befriended James Stewart, and met his future wife, Margaret Sullavan. Hank's film debut was in *The Farmer Takes A Wife,* in 1935. His movies up to the start of World War II were examples of the best in American film making. In 1942, he enlisted in the United States Navy – serving on the destroyer, USS Satterlee, in the central Pacific. When peace returned, Hank continued to make excellent movies such as *My Darling Clementine, Mister Roberts, 12 Angry Men* and *The Best Man* – up until a year before he died of heart disease in Los Angeles – when he won his Best Actor Oscar, for *On Golden Pond.*

You Only Live Once (1937)
Jezebel (1938) Jesse James (1939)
Young Mr. Lincoln (1939)
Drums Along the Mohawk (1939)
The Grapes of Wrath (1940) The Return
of Frank James (1940) The Lady
Eve (1941) The Male Animal (1942)
The Ox-Bow Incident (1943)
My Darling Clementine (1946)
The Fugitive (1947) Daisy Kenyon (1947)
Fort Apache (1948)
Mister Roberts (1955)
War and Peace (1956)
The Wrong Man (1956)
12 Angry Men (1957) Warlock (1959)
Advise and Consent (1962)
How the West Was Won (1962)
The Best Man (1964) Fail-Safe (1964)
The Boston Strangler (1968)
Once Upon a Time in the West (1968)
The Cheyenne Social Club (1970)
The Serpent (1973)
On Golden Pond (1981)

Jane **Fonda**
5ft 8in
(LADY JAYNE SEYMOUR FONDA)

Born: December 21, 1937
New York City, New York, USA

Jane and her brother Peter were raised by Henry Fonda's second wife, Susan Blanchard. Jane was educated at Emma Willard School in Troy, New York. In 1954, Jane acted with her father in a charity performance of "The Country Girl". After she left Vassar College, she joined the Actors Studio and appeared on stage – playing a role in "Tall Story" which became her film debut, in 1960. She averaged two movies a year and achieved star status in the Oscar-nominated comedy western, *Cat Ballou*. It was also the year she began an eight year marriage to Roger Vadim, whose attempt to turn her into another Bardot was a failure. Jane won her first Oscar for *Klute*, but because of her political views, she was rarely seen for the next six years. Her second Oscar was for the Vietnam War themed, *Coming Home*. When she announced her retirement from acting, she was almost as well known for her exercise videos. She published her autobiography "My Life so Far" and after fifteen years returned to the screen, in *Monster in Law*. Following her divorce from third husband Ted Turner, in 2001, she became a born-again Christian. Jane hasn't lost her interest in politics and isn't afraid to speak out against the Iraq war.

Walk on the Wild Side (1962)
Period of Adjustment (1962)
Sunday in New York (1963)
Cat Ballou (1965)
The Chase (1966)
Barefoot in the Park (1967)
They Shoot Horses,
Don't They? (1969) Klute (1971)
Fun with Dick and Jane (1977)
Julia (1977)
Coming Home (1978)
The China Syndrome (1979)
Nine to Five (1980)
On Golden Pond (1981)
Agnes of God (1985)
The Morning After (1986)
Stanley & Iris (1990)
Monster in Law (2005)
Georgia Rule (2007)

Peter **Fonda**
6ft 3in
(PETER HENRY FONDA)

Born: February 23, 1940
New York City, New York, USA

When he was ten, Peter's mother, Frances committed suicide. His father was a top movie star at the time, and his sister Jane became one within a dozen or so years. Peter studied acting in Omaha before attending the University of Nebraska. He also joined the Omaha Community Playhouse, where actors such as Brando started out. In the early 1960s, he was on Broadway – getting wide recognition for his work in "Blood, Sweat and Stanley Poole". He then went to Hollywood and made his film debut in 1963 in *Tammy and the Doctor*. It was a poor movie, but he did enough to impress director Robert Rossen, who cast him in a good one, *Lilith*. Peter became increasingly nonconformist as far as the Hollywood establishment was concerned. Turning to the pop scene for his pleasures he was close to the Byrds and the Beatles. In 1966, he was arrested when taking part in an anti-war demonstration on Sunset Strip. He starred in Roger Corman's *Wild Angels* and *The Trip,* and later made one of the most important movies of the 1960s – *Easy Rider*. He was Oscar-nominated for the screenplay and although he's never been able to repeat that success, Peter has gone on working. He was nominated for a Best Actor Oscar, for *Ulee's Gold*. He's been married to his second wife, Portia Rebecca Crockett, since 1975.

The Victors (1963) Lilith (1964)
The Wild Angels (1966) The Trip (1967)
Easy Rider (1969) The Hired Hand (1971)
Two People (1973) Dirty Mary Crazy
Larry (1974) Open Season (1974)
Race with the Devil (1975) 92 in the
Shade (1975) Futureworld (1976)
Fighting Mad (1976)
Outlaw Blues (1977) Split Image (1982)
Peppermint-Frieden (1983)
The Rosegarden (1989)
Love and a .45 (1994)
Nadja (1994) Ulee's Gold (1997)
The Limey (1999) The Laramie
Project (2002) 3:10 to Yuma (2007)
Japan (2008)

Joan **Fontaine**
5ft 3in
(JOAN DE BEAUVOIR DE HAVILLAND)

Born: October 22, 1917
Tokyo, Japan

After starting life in Japan, Joan and her sister went with their mother to live in Saratoga. As Olivia started her acting career, Joan returned to Tokyo to attend the American School. In 1934, she went back to California, where she attended Oak Street School in Saratoga, before joining a theater group in San Jose. In 1935, as Joan Burfield, she tried her luck in Hollywood and got a small part in *No More Ladies*. Rooming with Olivia, the magic started to work and by the time Joan got her first Oscar nomination, in 1941, for *Rebecca,* the two sisters were neck-and-neck in the stardom stakes. A year later, Joan became the only actress ever to win a Best Actress Oscar in a Hitchcock movie – *Suspicion*. The sibling rivalry continued amicably throughout the 1940s and beyond, but eventually some ill-feeling developed between them and they didn't talk to each other. Joan starred in several Broadway plays including "Forty Carats" and "Lion in Winter". Her final big screen appearance was in *The Witches* in 1966. Joan has remained single since her fourth divorce in 1969. Second husband William Dozier, said her autobiography, "No Bed of Roses" (1979), would have been better titled "No Shred of Truth".

Music for Madame (1937)
A Damsel in Distress (1937)
Gunga Din (1939)
Rebecca (1940)
Suspicion (1941)
This Above All (1942)
Jane Eyre (1944)
The Affairs of Susan (1945)
From This Day Forward (1946)
Ivy (1947) Letter from an
Unknown Woman (1948)
The Emperor Waltz (1948)
September Affair (1950)
Born to Be Bad (1950)
Something to Live For (1952)
Ivanhoe (1952) The Bigamist (1953)
Island in the Sun (1957)
Until They Sail (1957)
A Certain Smile (1958)

Glenn **Ford**
5ft 11in
(GWYLLYN SAMUEL NEWTON FORD)

Born: **May 1, 1916**
Sainte-Christine, Quebec, Canada
Died: **August 30, 2006**

Glenn's parents were Newton Ford, a railroad executive, and his wife, Hannah. He was born in the English section of Quebec and was a grand-nephew of Canada's first Prime Minister, Sir John MacDonald. In 1922, his family moved to California. After high school, he heeded a warning from his father to consider an alternative to an acting career – Glenn learned plumbing and wiring – just in case. He appeared in local stage productions before his film debut, in 1939 – in *Heaven with a Barbed Wire Fence.* That year, he became a US citizen and when the war started he volunteered for duty with the United States Marine Corps. In 1944, he broadcast the radio program, 'Halls of Montezuma'. On his return to civilian life he quickly achieved star status when he played opposite Rita Hayworth, in *Gilda*. His career flourished with *The Big Heat, Blackboard Jungle* and the original *3:10 to Yuma* and by 1958, he was Number One on Quigley's top ten box office champions. Glenn won a Golden Globe in 1961, for *Pocketful of Miracles.* His four wives included dancer/film star, Eleanor Powell. He continued working for another thirty years, but after developing blood clots in his legs in the early 1990s, he had to retire. Glenn died in Beverly Hills, of complications from strokes.

So Ends Our Night (1941)
Texas (1941) The Desperadoes (1943)
Gilda (1946) A Stolen Life (1946)
Framed (1947) The Undercover
Man (1949) Lust for Gold (1949)
Convicted (1950) The Big Heat (1953)
Human Desire (1954)
The Violent Men (1955)
Blackboard Jungle (1955)
Trial (1955) Jubal (1956)
The Fastest Gun Alive (1956)
The Teahouse of the August
Moon (1956) 3.10 to Yuma (1957)
The Sheepman (1958)
Experiment in Terror (1962)
The Rounders (1965)
Superman (1978)

Harrison **Ford**
6ft 1in
(HARRISON FORD)

Born: **July 13, 1942**
Chicago, Illinois, USA

The son of an advertising man who had dabbled in amateur dramatics, and a radio actress, young Harrison had no interest in acting, but he was a keen Boy Scout. He was a victim of bullying at Maine East High School, and wasn't popular with girls. After a spell at Ripon College in Wisconsin Harrison took drama classes as a means of meeting women. Even though he never graduated, he became a success in both pursuits. In 1964, Harrison moved to Los Angeles, where he signed a contract with Columbia Pictures to play bit parts, like a bellhop in his first film, *Dead Heat on a Merry-Go-Round.* Moving to Universal, he was given minor roles in TV series. Married, with two young sons, he did carpentry, and was a stage hand and a camera-operator for "The Doors" rock band. In 1973 he was cast by George Lucas in *American Graffiti.* While working at the Lucas family residence, the director used Harrison to read lines for his upcoming movie, *Star Wars.* By the time he'd finished erecting the shelves, Harrison had was Han Solo, and very soon he had become a megastar – in hit after hit – *Raiders of the Lost Ark, Witness* and *The Fugitive,* among others. His 2004 divorce from Melissa Mathison, was the most expensive in Hollywood's history. The new *Indiana Jones* film is very different from the others and much better than expected.

Star Wars (1977)
The Empire Strikes Back (1980)
Raiders of the Lost Ark (1981)
Blade Runner (1982) Return of the
Jedi (1983) Indiana Jones and
the Temple of Doom (1984)
Witness (1985)
The Mosquito Coast (1986)
Frantic (1988) Presumed
Innocent (1990) Patriot Games (1992)
The Fugitive (1993)
Clear and Present Danger (1994)
What Lies Beneath (2000)
Firewall (2006)
Indiana Jones and the Kingdom of
the Crystal Skull (2008)

Wallace **Ford**
5ft 9½in
(SAMUEL JONES GRUNDY)

Born: **February 12, 1898**
Bolton, Lancashire, England
Died: **June 11, 1966**

Wally was born into extreme poverty. He was four when he was sent to live at Dr. Barnardo's home for orphans, at Birkdale, on the Lancashire coast – about twenty miles from his birthplace. Three years later, he went to the Barnardo's in Toronto, Canada, prior to a foster home being found. There was little control over the suitability of foster parents and the poor boy was treated like a slave. When he was eleven, he ran away from a farming family who were ill-treating him and he joined a vaudeville troupe called "The Winnipeg Kiddies" and stayed with them until he was sixteen. With a pal called Wallace Ford he traveled across the United States. His friend was crushed to death by a railroad car, and 'Wallace Ford' became his stage name. He worked with repertory companies and eventually made his name on Broadway. After acting in a couple of Vitaphone shorts, Wally was third-billed below Joan Crawford and Clark Gable, in *Possessed.* Throughout the 1930s he acted in several good movies. He was in two Hitchcock films and also supported Cagney and Bogart. His final film was *A Patch of Blue,* in 1965. Early the following summer, Wally died of a heart attack, at Woodland Hills, California.

Possessed (1931) Freaks (1932)
Are You Listening? (1932)
Skyscraper Souls (1932)
Employee's Entrance (1933)
Three Cornered Moon (1933)
The Whole Town's Talking (1935)
The Informer (1935) Jericho (1937)
Back Door to Heaven (1939)
The Mummy's Hand (1940) Murder By
Invitation (1941) Blues in the Night (1941)
All Through the Night (1941)
Shadow of a Doubt (1943)
Blood on the Sun (1945)
The Great John L. (1945)
Spellbound (1945) Crack-Up (1946)
Dead Reckoning (1947) T-Men (1947)
The Set-Up (1949) Harvey (1950)
The Man from Laramie (1955)

Frederic **Forrest**
6ft 1in
(FREDERIC FENIMORE FORREST JR.)

Born: December 23, 1936
Waxahachie, Texas, USA

When Frederic first auditioned for school plays he was shy and flunked every time. At Texas Christian University, he overcame the nerves and got a minor in Theater Arts and a major in Radio and TV studies. He studied with Sanford Meisner in New York while supporting himself as a page at NBC Studios. Frederic made his off-Broadway debut in the anti-war musical, "Viet Rock" and then joined Tom O'Horgan's stock company at La Mama. In 1968, he made his film debut (uncredited) in *The Filthy Five* and featured in O'Horgan's film, *Futz*, about a farmer who falls for a pig. Moving to Los Angeles in 1971, he earned a Golden Globe nomination for a good western, opposite Richard Widmark – *When the Legends Die.* His experience with Francis Ford Coppola, in *The Conversation,* paid dividends four years later, when the director used him in *Apocalypse Now* – his second movie with Marlon Brando. It was also the year he was nominated for a Best Supporting Actor Oscar, for *The Rose.* In 1981, he played the romantic lead in one of Coppola's few financial disasters, *One from the Heart.* In the last few years, he's had supporting roles and has done TV work. Frederic hasn't been seen on the big screen since *All The King's Men.* He was twice married and divorced. His second wife was the actress, Marilu Henner.

When the Legends Die (1972)
The Conversation (1974)
The Gravy Train (1974)
Permission to Kill (1975)
The Missouri Breaks (1976)
Apocalypse Now (1975)
The Rose (1979) **Hammett** (1982)
Valley Girl (1983)
**Tucker: The Man
and His Dreams** (1988)
Music Box (1989) **Falling Down** (1993)
Trauma (1993) **The Brave** (1997)
The End of Violence (1997)
Whatever (1998)
A Piece of Eden (2000)
All the King's Men (2006)

Sally **Forrest**
5ft 3in
(SALLY FEENEY)

Born: May 28, 1928
San Diego, California, USA

Sally's parents, Michael and Agnes Feeney, were ballroom dancers, who encouraged her to take dancing lessons. By the time she finished her high school education she was qualified enough to set up her own business as a dancing instructor. It only lasted three years – because in 1945, her parents took her to live in Los Angeles. Sally approached Hollywood studios and in 1946, following her graduation from high school, Sally signed a contract with MGM. The studio used her talent as a dancer in four uncredited roles, which began with *Till the Clouds Roll By,* in 1946. It was followed by the disastrous Sinatra movie, *The Kissing Bandit,* and a good Gene Kelly film, *Take Me Out to the Ball Game.* MGM then fired her, and it was only through a chance meeting with actress Ida Lupino, that she remained in Hollywood. Ida was branching out as a producer and she needed a beautiful girl to play opposite Keefe Brasselle, in her movie about an unmarried mother – *Not Wanted.* On Ida's directorial debut *Never Fear* she used the same actors and again engaged Sally for *Hard Fast and Beautiful,* made two years later. Sally had been enjoying a romance with the former child-star Roddy McDowall, but in 1951 she married her agent Milo Frank, and it lasted (through a few storms) until his death in 2004. Sally's last movie was in a western *Ride the High Iron,* in 1956. Her final TV role was in 1967, in an episode of 'Family Affair'. After that, she has lived a quiet existence in Beverly Hills.

Not Wanted (1949)
Never Fear (1949)
Mystery Street (1950)
Vengeance Valley (1951)
Hard Fast and Beautiful (1951)
Excuse My Dust (1951)
The Strip (1951)
Bannerline (1951)
The Strange Door (1951)
Code Two (1953)
While the City Sleeps (1956)
Ride the High Iron (1956)

Jodie **Foster**
5ft 3½in
(ALICIA CHRISTIAN FOSTER)

Born: November 19, 1962
Los Angeles, California, USA

When Jodie's father left a few months before she was born, it only took a little while before she contributed to the family income. She was three when she did a TV commercial for Coppertone and six when she had a leading role in an episode of 'The Doris Day Show'. After that, there was plenty of television work on shows like 'Disneyland', 'Mayberry R.F.D.' and 'Gunsmoke'. Her mother, who worked as a film producer sent Jodie to the exclusive prep school, the Lycée Français de Los Angeles, from where she was able to keep working. 1976 was a special year – she hosted 'Saturday Night Live' and for her role as a teenage prostitute, in *Taxi Driver,* was nominated for a Best Supporting Actress Oscar. She spent part of 1977 in France, where she starred in *Moi, fleur bleue* and recorded two vocals for the film's soundtrack. In 1981, while at Yale University, she was stalked by John Hinckley jr., who shot President Reagan in a sick attempt to impress her. In 1985, she graduated from Yale with a BA in Literature. Jodie won two Best Actress Oscars – for *The Accused* and *The Silence of the Lambs,* and has appeared regularly in quality productions. She's also directed with some success. Jodie is described as an extremely private person – she has never married and she refuses to name the father(s) of her two children.

**Alice Doesn't Live Here
Anymore** (1974) **Taxi Driver** (1976)
Bugsy Malone (1976) **Carny** (1980)
The Hotel New Hampshire (1984)
The Accused (1988)
The Silence of the Lambs (1991)
Little Man Tate (1991)
Shadows and Fog (1992)
Sommersby (1993) **Maverick** (1994)
Nell (1994) **Contact** (1997)
Anna and the King (1999) **Dangerous
Lives of Altar Boys** (2002)
A Very Long Engagement (2004)
Flightplan (2005) **Inside Man** (2006)
The Brave One (2007)
Nim's Island (2008)

Preston **Foster**
6ft 2in
(PRESTON S. FOSTER)

Born: **August 24, 1900**
Ocean City, New Jersey, USA
Died: **July 14, 1970**

Growing up in a music-loving home, Preston sang in his church choir. During his high school years his voice deepened to a rich baritone. To pay for his singing lessons he sold papers, drove a bus and did several other odd jobs. From 1925, he performed with Pittsburgh Grand Opera Company. His operatic career was put on hold after he married the actress Gertrude Warren. Operettas and musical shows were much more popular than highbrow music. Gertrude introduced him to the British actor Lionel Atwill, who at that time was appearing on Broadway. With his help, Preston was soon in musicals and eventually, more dramatic roles, on stage and in movies. In 1931, he was in a play called "Two Seconds", which persuaded Warners to cast him in the screen version with Edward G. Robinson. The studio made good use of his powerful presence in a string of movies including *The Last Mile* as "Killer Mears". Serving with the U.S. Coast Guard during World War II (he held the honorary rank of Commodore) enabled him to continue making films – *Guadalcanal Diary* being the best. By the 1950s, he was seen on TV. His last film was *Chubasco,* in 1968. His second wife, Sheila Darcy was with him when he died, in La Jolla, California.

Doctor X (1932) **The Last Mile** (1932)
Life Begins (1932) **I Am a Fugitive from a Chain Gang** (1932)
Elmer the Great (1933)
Annie Oakley (1935) **The Informer** (1935)
The Last Days of Pompeii (1935)
Muss "Em Up (1936) **We Who Are About to Die** (1937) **First Lady** (1937)
20,000 Men a Year (1939)
North West Mounted Police (1940)
Secret Agent of Japan (1942)
Thunder Birds (1942) **My Friend Flicka** (1943) **Guadalcanal Diary** (1943)
The Valley of Decision (1945) **The Harvey Girls** (1946) **The Hunted** (1948)
Ramrod (1947) **Tomahawk** (1951)
Kansas City Confidential (1952)

Edward **Fox**
5ft 8in
(EDWARD CHARLES MORRICE FOX)

Born: **April 13, 1937**
Chelsea, London, England

The senior member of the Fox Dynasty, Edward was the son of a theatrical agent and an actress whose father was the dramatist, Frederick Lonsdale. Edward was educated at Harrow and then served as a Lieutenant in the Coldstream Guards. He first appeared on stage in 1958 and continued in that medium until 1963, when he was an extra in *This Sporting Life*. Initially, he was outshone by his brother as a film actor. Edward came into his own in 1970, at the very point where James turned to religion. *The Go Between* was a big step forward, but it was the title role in 1973's *The Day of the Jackal,* which really established him as a movie actor internationally. From that point on he has been in demand, both in leading roles and as a fine supporting actor in all mediums. He was highly-praised for his portrayal of the Duke of Windsor in the expensive and well-researched television production of 'Edward and Mrs. Simpson'. His work in London's West End theaters is always of the top quality and his festival renditions of T.S.Eliot's "Four Quartets" – accompanied by the keyboard music of J.S.Bach, prove especially memorable. Edward had been married before and divorced in 1961, so he was very cautious the second time around. A long-standing relationship with the actress Joanna David, eventually resulted in their marriage in 2005.

I'll Never Forget
What'isname (1967)
Journey to Midnight (1968)
The Go-Between (1970)
The Day of the Jackal (1973)
A Bridge Too Far (1977)
The Duellists (1977)
Soldier of Orange (1977)
Gandhi (1982)
The Dresser (1983)
The Bounty (1984)
The Shooting Party (1985)
A Month by the Lake (1995)
Nicholas Nickleby (2002)
Stage Beauty (2004)
Lassie (2006)

James **Fox**
6ft 1in
(WILLIAM FOX)

Born: **May 19, 1939**
London, England

William (now James) and his two brothers, Edward and Robert are the sons of the-atrical agent Robin Fox, and the stage actress, Angela Worthington. In 1950 – at the age of ten, James made his first film appearance, in the *Miniver Story*. It was a dozen more years until he next acted in a film, but this time it was something rather better – Harold Pinter's fascinating *The Servant* – with Dirk Bogarde and Sarah Miles. In 1970, James starred with Mick Jagger and Anita Pallenberg in the film *Performance,* and in the eyes of British moviegoers at least, was a star. Following his father's death, James was moved to give up the material world and he became an evangelical Christian. For fourteen years he devoted himself to the Ministry – appearing in only one film, in 1978 - *No Longer Alone* – an inspiring story of a sui-cidal woman saved by Christianity. His return to mainstream movies was in *Greystoke: The Legend of Tarzan, Lord of the Apes*. Since then he's often played character roles in TV dramas – he was a perfect Anthony Eden, in 'Suez: A Very British Crisis' – and acted in stage plays and in several Hollywood movies.

The Servant (1963)
Those Magnificent Men in their Flying Machines (1965) **King Rat** (1965)
The Chase (1966) **Thoroughly Modern Millie** (1967) **Isadora** (1968)
Performance (1970) **Greystoke: The Legend of Tarzan, Lord of the Apes** (1984) **A Passage to India** (1984)
The Mighty Quinn (1984)
The Russia House (1990)
Patriot Games (1992)
The Remains of the Day (1993)
Jinnah (1998)
Mickey Blue Eyes (1999)
Up at the Villa (2000)
The Golden Bowl (2000)
Sexy Beast (2000)
The Mystic Masseur (2001)
Charlie and the Chocolate Factory (2005)
Mister Lonely (2007)

Michael J. **Fox**
5ft 4½in
(MICHAEL ANDREW FOX)

Born: June 9, 1961
Edmonton, Alberta, Canada

Michael's family settled in Vancouver, which is where he made his film debut at the age of fifteen, in *Leo and Me*. Three years later, he moved to Los Los Angeles where he began getting small roles on television. His breakthrough was in a popular TV-series 'Family Ties' – which ran from 1982 to1989, and won him three Emmy Awards. It gave him the exposure he needed to launch a movie career and he achieved this through his appearance as Marty McFly, in *Back to the Future*. Before the sequels – which were both hits, Michael starred in a terrific anti-war film *Casualties of War*. He has been married since 1988 – to the actress Tracy Pollan, whom he first met when they were acting in the television series, 'Family Ties'. The clincher came when they both appeared in the movie *Bright Lights, Big City*. They have four children. Michael continued to appear regularly in movies up until 1996, when Parkinson's disease, which was first diagnosed five years earlier, worsened. He was in the 'Spin City' TV sitcom, until 2001, and in 'Boston Legal' during 2006. Apart from voice-over work on TV, Michael has now virtually retired from full-time acting. At present, much of his energy is spent on running the Michael J. Fox Foundation – which is dedicated to raising money to fight Parkinson's disease.

Class of 1984 (1982)
Back to the Future (1985)
Casualties of War (1985)
The Secret of My Succe$s (1987)
Back to the Future Part II (1989)
Back to the Future Part III (1990)
The Hard Way (1991)
Doc Hollywood (1991)
For Love or Money (1993)
Where the River
Flows North (1994)
Greedy (1994)
Blue in the Face (1995)
Coldblooded (1995)
The American President (1995)
The Frighteners (1996)
Mars Attacks (1996)

Vivica A. **Fox**
5ft 7in
(VIVICA ANJANNETTA FOX)

Born: July 30, 1964
South Bend, Indiana, USA

The youngest of four children born to William and Everlyena Fox. Vivica was a bright child. She did well at Arlington High School – good academically and great as an athlete – at volleyball and track. She was a member of the 1982 "Girls City Basketball" championship team. Vivica then attended Golden West College, Huntingdon Beach, California, until she moved to Los Angeles. There, as Vivica Fox, she worked as a model before being discovered by producer Trevor Walton, while she was eating lunch at a restaurant on Sunset Boulevard in Hollywood. Vivica made her television debut in 1988, in episodes of 'China Beach'. By 1989, she was well known enough on the small screen to make her movie debut (as a hooker) in the blockbuster, *Born on the Fourth of July*. It was a very significant title, because her first important role, for which she received a Saturn nomination as Best Supporting Actress) – seven years later, was in *Independence Day*. In 1996, she was in one of the longest-titled films ever made. In 1998, she married singer Christopher Harvest (aka Sixx-Nine), but the couple divorced four years later. Her 2004-6 series 'Missing' – on the Lifetime Television Network, was highly rated. She is prolific in terms of quantity, but has recently hit a low-quality patch. In 2007, she was an unsuccessful contestant on the TV show, 'Dancing with the Stars'. Hopefully her bad run is about to end. Vivica lives in the San Fernando Valley.

Don't Be a Menace to South
Central While Drinking Your Juice
in the Hood (1996)
Independence Day (1996)
Set It Off (1996)
Soul Food (1997)
Why Do Fools Fall in Love (1998)
Little Secrets (2001)
Kill Bill: Vol.1 (2003)
Ella Enchanted (2004)
The Hard Corps (2006)
Three Can Play That Game (2007)
Junkyard Dog (2009)

Jamie **Foxx**
5ft 9in
(ERIC MARLON BISHOP)

Born: December 13, 1967
Terrell, Texas, USA

Due to his parents' divorce, Jamie was adopted at seven months old by the same couple who had adopted his mother. So his grandparents became his father and mother and his birth mother became his sister! He had a strict upbringing. He was a member of the Boy Scouts and sang in the church choir. He also played quarterback for his high school. When he was a three-year-old he'd been encouraged to play the piano by his grandmother and he has been crazy about music ever since. Jamie attended the Alliant International University, in California, before moving to Los Angeles to start his musical career. He also studied classical piano at Juilliard College. In 1988, he had a small role in the Eddie Murphy movie, *Coming to America* – so why not two careers he thought? In 1989, a girlfriend persuaded him to go up on stage at the Comedy Store, in L.A. Two years later, he enhanced his reputation on a TV show, 'In Living Color' – his celebrity impressions winning him many new fans. In 1994, he released his first R&B album "Peep This", and acted in movies. The door to stardom opened for him in 2001, with the biopic *Ali,* but 2004 was his year – with two nominations – and a Best Actor Oscar for his blistering portrayal of the music legend, *Ray* Charles. It was also the year he featured on the Billboard Hot 100 number one, with "Slow Jamz". Jamie's portrayal of the hostage cab driver, Max, in the thriller *Collateral,* provided him with an opportunity to show another side of his considerable acting talent. Jamie's latest movie, *The Soloist,* could be a winner.

The Great White Hype (1996)
Any Given Sunday (1999)
Bait (2000) **Ali** (2001)
Shade (2003)
Breakin' All the Rules (2004)
Collateral (2004)
Ray (2004) **Jarhead** (2005)
Miami Vice (2006)
Dreamgirls (2006)
The Kingdom (2007)
The Soloist (2009)

Anthony **Franciosa**
6ft 1in
(ANTHONY PAPALEO)

Born: **October 25, 1928**
New York City, New York, USA
Died: **January 19, 2006**

Tony never really got to know his father – his parents divorced shortly after he was born. Not long after he left high school, he experienced an incredible stroke of luck which led to an acting career. He went to the local Y.M.C.A. to take advantage of a free dancing lesson. There was an audition for a play taking place. He went in and was given the part! He took his mother's maiden name and after studying at the Actor's Studio, he became a professional with the Cherry Lane Theater Group, off Broadway. His breakthrough came in a stage production of "End as a Man" in 1955 – in which he co-starred with Ben Gazzara. Only Ben reappeared in the movie version. After that stage triumph, and rave reviews for his work in "A Hatful of Rain", Tony made his film debut in 1957 in *This Could Be the Night*. He married Shelley Winters and was Oscar nominated as Best Supporting Actor, when he reprised his role for the film *A Hatful of Rain*. He became a busy and popular actor, with good roles in top movies, for about ten years. One of them, *Senilità*, was made in Italy with a very young Claudia Cardinale. Tony retired in 1996 – enjoying ten more years of life before his death in Los Angeles, from a massive stroke. His fourth wife – the former fashion model, Rita Thiel, was with him.

This Could Be the Night (1957)
A Face in the Crowd (1957)
A Hatful of Rain (1957)
Wild is the Wind (1957)
The Long, Hot Summer (1958)
Career (1959)
The Story on Page One (1959)
Senilità (1962)
Period of Adjustment (1962)
Rio Conchos (1964)
A Man Could Get Killed (1966)
Fathom (1967)
In Enemy Country (1968)
The Drowning Pool (1975)
Tenebre (1982)
City Hall (1996)

Anne **Francis**
5ft 8in
(ANNE FRANCIS)

Born: **September 16, 1930**
Ossining, New York, USA

During the Great Depression, Anne was able to help her family by earning money as a child model with the Powers Agency. She was only eleven when she made her Broadway debut, with Gertrude Lawrence in "Lady in the Dark". She was signed by MGM and made her film debut in 1947, with an uncredited role in the Esther Williams film, *This Time for Keeps*. Anne's first credited role in a movie was in 1948, when she appeared in *Summer Holiday.* To begin with, her movie opportunities were few, but she made the most of them. In 1952, she got married and the following year starred in *A Lion is in the Streets* with James Cagney. By 1955, she had worked with top actors Dick Powell, Robert Taylor, and Spencer Tracy. She was a star by the time she made the groundbreaking drama *Blackboard Jungle,* and the Sci-Fi classic, *Forbidden Planet.* Anne's movie career may have slowed down in the 1960s, but her workload did not. In 1965, she won new fans with her portrayal of 'Honey West' on television. After that, she was a welcome regular in a long list of TV-movies and television shows such as 'My Three Sons', 'Columbo', 'Ironside' and 'Dallas'. Anne was diagnosed with cancer in 2007 and had part of her right lung removed.

So Young So Bad (1950)
Lydia Bailey (1952)
Dreamboat (1952)
A Lion Is in the Streets (1953)
Susan Slept Here (1954)
Rogue Cop (1954)
Bad Day at Black Rock (1955)
Battle Cry (1955)
Blackboard Jungle (1955)
The Scarlet Coat (1955)
Forbidden Planet (1956)
The Rack (1956)
Don't Go Near the Water (1957)
The Crowded Sky (1960)
The Satan Bug (1965)
Brainstorm (1965)
Funny Girl (1968)
More Dead Than Alive (1968)
The Love God? (1969)

Kay **Francis**
5ft 9in
(KATHERINE EDWINA GIBBS)

Born: **January 13, 1905**
Oklahoma City, Oklahoma, USA
Died: **August 26, 1968**

Kay's mother, Katherine Clinton Franks, was a vaudeville artist and nice woman, but her father, Joseph Gibbs, was a brutal drunk – who deserted the pair of them. Kay was raised by her mother and in her early teens, attended Miss Fuller's School for Young Ladies, followed by Cathedral School. She then enrolled at Katherine Gibbs' Secretarial School, in New York, where she experienced her first mistake. After a two-year marriage at seventeen, to James Francis, Kay kept his name and focussed on an acting career. She made her professional debut in 1919, in a modern dress version of "Hamlet" and continued to work on the stage. An important role in "Elmer the Great" – with Walter Huston, led to her film debut with him, in *Gentlemen of the Press,* in 1929. It got her a Paramount contract and a small part in the Marx Brothers movie, *The Coconuts.* Kay bounced back with MGM after some poor films. Warners finally signed her and William Powell, and Kay's career took off with him in – *Jewel Robbery* and *One Way Passage.* Up until the early1940s, she was getting star billing. Kay joined the USO during the war and toured with Martha Raye and Carole Landis. By 1945, she was working for the Poverty Row studio, Monogram, and drinking heavily. In 1948, she was rushed to hospital after over-dosing on pills, but lived twenty more years before dying of cancer, in New York.

Raffles (1930) Scandal Sheet (1931)
Guilty Hands (1931) Girls About
Town (1931) Jewel Robbery (1931)
One Way Passage (1931)
Trouble in Paradise (1932)
I Loved a Woman (1933)
The House on 56th Street (1934)
Doctor Monica (1934)
I Found Stella Parrish (1935)
Confession (1937)
First Lady (1937)
In Name Only (1939)
It's a Date (1940)
When the Daltons Rode (1940)

Déborah **François**
5ft 5in
(DEBORAH FRANÇOIS)

Born: May 24, 1987
Liège, Belgium

Belgium may not be in the front line when it comes to producing film stars, but in recent years, there have been a number of actresses like Cécile de France – ideally named to move to that country, and a girl from near Liege – Marie Gillain. Nowadays, there is Déborah François – one of three children of a policeman and his social worker wife. Déborah was at school, studying for her Bacalaureat, when the film-maker brothers, Jean-Pierre and Luc Dardenne visited Liege. They were holding open casting sessions to find an unknown to act in their film, *L'Enfant* – the story of a teenage single mother, whose boyfriend sells her baby. Déborah beat off competition from around one hundred and fifty young hopefuls. Without any training or previous experience she played the role of Sonia perfectly. She won the Joseph Plateau Award for Best Belgian Actress and helped to win the Dardenne brothers their second Palm D'Or, at the Cannes Film Festival. After promoting the film in Argentina, Déborah went home to complete her schooling and on the strength of that one film, she moved to Paris, where she set up home with her two cats. Meanwhile, she starred in the French movie, *La Tourneuse de pages* (The Page Turner) for which she was nominated for a César, as Most Promising Actress. Her career looks certain to take off now that she has six movies to her name. *Les Femmes de l'ombres* (Female Agents), was widely released during 2008, and received positive reviews. In the illustrious company of three movie actresses with proven pedigrees – Sophie Marceau, Julie Depardieu and Marie Gillain, Déborah isn't outshone and has gone on from there.

L'Enfant (2005)
La Tourneuse de pages (2006)
Les Fourmis rouges (2007)
L'Été indien (2007)
Female Agents (2008)
The First Day of the Rest of
Your Life (2008)
Unmade Beds (2009)

Arthur **Franz**
6ft
(ARTHUR FRANZ)

Born: February 29, 1920
Perth Amboy, New Jersey, USA
Died: June 17, 2006

When Arthur, known as "Turo" was attending Blue Ridge College, he developed a keen interest in the theater. His career began on the Broadway stage, but it was interrupted by the outbreak of World War II. He served as a navigator in the United States Army Air Force. He was shot down over Rumania and taken prisoner, but was able to escape and fight on. At the end of the war, he married his first wife Anna Minot, who bore him a child. They divorced in 1946 and he married Adele Longmire, with whom he had two children and stayed with for over eleven years. Turo worked on the stage until 1947, when his strong Broadway performance in "Command Decision" aroused interest from MGM, who wanted him for the film version. He never reprised his stage role, but in 1948, he made his film debut, in *Jungle Patrol*, a low-budget film with a war theme. By 1949, he was getting good supporting parts – one of them was the classic *Sands of Iwo Jima*. Director Edward Dmytryk gave him his best ever role – as Eddie Miller, in the gripping film noir, *The Sniper*. He appeared in seven more of Dmytryk's movies – including *The Caine Mutiny* and *The Young Lions*. He retired after acting in *That Championship Season*. Turo later lived in New Zealand with his fourth wife, Sharon, but returned to the United States when he became seriously ill. He died of emphysema, in Oxnard, California.

Red Light (1949)
Sands of Iwo Jima (1949)
Three Secrets (1950) Abbott and Costello
Meet The Invisible Man (1951)
Submarine Command (1951)
The Sniper (1952)
Invaders from Mars (1953)
The Caine Mutiny (1954)
The Young Lions (1958)
The Carpetbaggers (1964)
Alvarez Kelly (1966)
The 'Human' Factor (1975)
That Championship Season (1982)

Mona **Freeman**
5ft 3½in
(MONICA FREEMAN)

Born: June 9, 1926
Baltimore, Maryland, USA

Mona was the daughter of Stuart Freeman and his wife. Of Irish and French descent, she was raised in Pelham, New York, where she attended Pelham High School. She became a model for the Powers Agency and was voted "Miss Subway" after her face appeared on posters. A magazine cover portrait was seen by Howard Hughes, who sent her a personal two-year contract without having met her. Mona started at Maryland Institute of Art, but dropped out to go for a screen test. Hughes wasn't around, so she ended up at Paramount. In 1944, she made her debut for the studio, in a war drama, *Till We Meet Again*. It was a small role, but she was sweet in it and made three more that year, including a loan out to MGM for an uncredited bit part, in *National Velvet*, and to Columbia, when she was fourth-billed below Irene Dunne and Charles Boyer, in *Together Again*. The following year, she married her first husband, Pat Nerney, and was pregnant with their daughter by the time she filmed *Mother Wore Tights*. After that, the studio gave her several good films including *The Heiress*, and two good westerns, *Streets of Laredo* and *Branded* – in which she co-starred with Alan Ladd. Mona married Los Angeles businessman, Jack Ellis, and did a bit of TV work before retiring in 1972, to spend her time painting portraits and landscapes. She and Jack are the parents of actress, Monie Ellis.

Till We Meet Again (1944)
Together Again (1944)
Junior Miss (1945)
Danger Signal (1945)
Dear Ruth (1947)
Mother Wore Tights (1947)
Streets of Laredo (1949)
The Heiress (1949)
Dear Wife (1949) Branded (1950)
Dear Brat (1951)
Flesh and Fury (1952)
Jumping Jacks (1952)
Angel Face (1952)
Battle Cry (1955)

Morgan **Freeman**
6ft 2½in
(MORGAN FREEMAN)

Born: **June 1, 1937**
Memphis, Tennessee, USA

Morgan was the youngest of four children. His parents weren't wealthy – his father was a barber and his mother worked as a cleaner, but they did their best to give their kids a good start in life. At around the age of eight, Morgan first revealed his acting talent when he played the lead in a school play. Four years later, he won a state-wide drama competition. While at high school, he performed on a radio show in Nashville, but turned down a partial drama scholarship to become a mechanic in the U.S. Airforce. During the early 1960s, he tried show business again – this time as a dancer in New York. In 1965 he made his professional acting debut – on stage in "The Royal Hunt of the Sun" and was also a film extra, in *The Pawnbroker*. He first became more widely known through TV appearances starting in 1971, in 'Another World' and 'The Electric Company'. He was in his mid-forties by the time he began to get strong supporting roles in movies. He earned the first of his four Oscar nominations for *Street Smart* – he finally won seventeen years later, when he was Best Supporting Actor in *Million Dollar Baby*. By the 1990s, he was an A-list actor and has continued to be one well after he celebrated his 70th birthday.

Street Smart (1987)
Driving Miss Daisy (1989)
Unforgiven (1992)
The Shawshank Redemption (1994)
Se7en (1995)
Deep Impact (1998)
Under Suspicion (2000)
Along Came a Spider (2001)
Levity (2003)
Bruce Almighty (2003)
Million Dollar Baby (2004)
An Unfinished Life (2005)
Lucky Number Slevin (2006)
10 Items or Less (2006)
Gone Baby Gone (2007)
Feast of Love (2007)
The Bucket List (2007)
Wanted (2008)
The Dark Knight (2008)

Anna **Friel**
5ft 2in
(ANNA LOUISE FRIEL)

Born: **July 12, 1976**
Rochdale, Lancashire, England

Anna's parents were schoolteachers who were both of Irish descent. She finished her own education, at Crompton House Secondary School, in Shaw, about four miles away from her home. During her schooldays, Anna became interested in an acting career and was successful in local talent shows. At the age of thirteen, she was cast as the daughter of the Michael Palin character, in the Channel 4 television series, 'G.B.H.' It led to more TV roles – in popular soaps such as 'Emmerdale' and 'Brookside'. For the latter, in 1995, Anna received the National Television Award for Most Popular Actress. She made her film debut in 1998, in *The Stringer,* and that same year, went to New York, where she acted in the original Broadway production of "Closer" at the Music Box Theater. Her portrayal of 'Alice' won her Drama Desk and Theater World awards. It proved to be a very good year for her – she also had two good movie releases to her credit – *The Tribe* and *St. Ives*. A year later, she was Hermia, in a star-studded film version of *A Midsummer Night's Dream* and acted with Ewan McGregor, in *Rogue Trader*. In 2008, Anna was nominated for a Golden Globe as Best Actress, for her role as 'Chuck' Charles, in the TV Series 'Pushing Daisies'. She met her partner, the English actor, David Thewlis, on a flight to Cannes in France. They have a daughter named Gracie, who was born in 2005.

The Tribe (1998)
St. Ives (1998)
A Midsummer Night's
Dream (1999)
Rogue Trader (1999)
Sunset Strip (2000)
An Everlasting Piece (2000)
The War Bride (2001)
Me Without You (2001)
Timeline (2003)
Goal! (2005)
Irish Jam (2006)
Niagara Motel (2006)
Goal II: Living the Dream (2007)
Bathory (2008)

Kyôko **Fukada**
5ft 4¼in
(KYÔKO FUKADA)

Born: **November 2, 1982**
Tokyo, Japan

"Fuya-kyon" – as she is known in her own country, was a prodigious talent – with a sweet voice and piano skills. In 1995, she became a big fan of the new Japanese pop singing sensation, Kahala Tomomi and she made up her mind to follow in her footsteps. In 1996, aged fourteen, she won the local talent agency, Horipro's splendidly-named "21st Talent Scout Caravan Grand Prix" – as part of the "Pure Girl Audition". In 1998, she was one of the agency's "HIP" group. Fuya-kyon was then on radio and in television programs and special events, before graduating in 1998. In no time at all she was being acclaimed for her role as a girl who contracts HIV, in the TV-drama, 'Kamisama mousukoshi dake' in which she played opposite famous actor, Takeshi Kaneshiro. Later that year, she was given her own radio program, 'In My Room', which ran until 2002. She made her movie debut in the horror film sequel, *Ringu 2*. Since then, apart from films and TV shows, Fuya-kyon has enjoyed dipping into several careers – including modeling in fashion magazines such as "Kera" during 2003, and releasing singles and albums featuring her vocals as well as her piano playing. On the movie front, her biggest hit to date was in *Shimotsuma Monogatari* – released internationally as *Kamikaze Girls*. Her performance as Momoko in the movie won her Best Actress Awards at the Yokohama Film Festival, the Mainichi Film Contest and the Nippon Academy. After a three-year gap away from the big screen, Fuya-kyon has recently finished filming an action comedy titled *Yattâman,* which is due to be released during 2009.

Ringu 2 (1999)
Shisha no gakuensai (2000)
Dolls (2002)
Ashuru no gotoku (2003)
Onmyoji 2 (2003)
Kamikaze Girls (2004)
Angel (2006)
The Inugamis (2006)
Yattâman (2009)

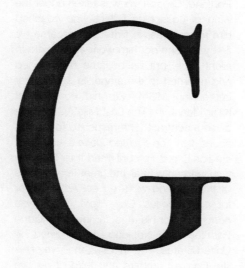

Jean **Gabin**
5ft 7in
(JEAN-ALEXIS MONCORGÉ)

Born: **May 17, 1904**
Paris, France
Died: **November 15, 1976**

The seventh son of a cabaret duo, Jean's first job after leaving school at fifteen, was with a construction firm. The hard physical work soon made up his mind to follow his parents into show business. After World War I, France took the precaution of building its armed forces, and at eighteen, Jean did military service. In his early twenties, he traveled with a company specializing in operettas which toured South America. In Paris, he secured a job at the 'Moulin Rouge' and adopted his father's name, Gabin. In 1928, he married Gaby Basset and they both made their film debuts in *Chacun sa Chance,* in 1930. Jean was in films with comic, Fernandel, and went to Germany, to act with Brigitte Helm. In 1932, he co-starred with Marcelle Romée in *Coeur de Lilas.* She committed suicide after filming finished. By the mid-1930s. Jean Gabin was a star of the French cinema. His fame was spreading abroad, but he turned down offers from Hollywood. In 1940, he did go on a 20th Century Fox contract. It proved unfruitful, so in 1943 he joined his compatriots in North Africa and with a *Croix de Guerre* on his chest, he marched through liberated Paris. His post-war comeback saw him appear with all the new young French stars in a string of hit movies. He died of a heart attack at his home in Neuilly-sur-Seine, France.

La Bandera (1935) La Belle
équipe (1936) Les Bas-fonds (1936)
Pépé le Moko (1937) La Grande
Illusion (1937) Le Quai des
brumes (1938) La Bête humaine (1938)
Le Jour se lève (1939) Moontide (1942)
Martin Roumagnac (1946)
Le Plaisir (1951) Grisbi (1954)
French Cancan (1954) Razzia (1955)
People of No Importance (1956)
Maigret tend in piège (1958)
Les Misérables (1958)
Le Président (1961)
The Sicilian Clan (1969)
Le Chat (1971) Deux hommes
dans la ville (1973)

Clark **Gable**
6ft 1in
(WILLIAM CLARK GABLE)

Born: **February 1, 1901**
Cadiz, Ohio, USA
Died: **November 16, 1960**

Clark was the son of an oil-well driller and a German mother, who had him baptized Roman Catholic – before passing away when he was ten months old. Within a year, his father had remarried and they went to live near Akron. Clark went to work in a tire factory. At twenty-one, he started acting with stock companies. In Portland, Oregon, he was taken under the wing of Josephine Dillon, who coached him for a career in films and became his first wife. She got him work as an extra in silent films, but he became disillusioned and returned to the stage. In 1930, after impressing MGM with his portrayal of Killer Mears, in "The Last Mile", Clark was given a contract. The response to his first sound film *The Painted Desert* – a Pathé studios B-picture confirmed their faith. He was teamed with all the great female stars of the day and won a Best Actor Oscar for *It Happened One Night.* Clark was nominated for his most famous film, *Gone With the Wind.* Not long after he joined the United States Army in 1942, the love of his life, Carole Lombard (the third of his five wives) died in a plane crash. A star until the end – his final film role, in *The Misfits,* resulted in the best reviews of his career – only he didn't live to read them. Clark died from a heart attack, in Los Angles.

Red Dust (1932)
It Happened One Night (1934)
China Seas (1935)
Mutiny on the Bounty (1935)
San Francisco (1936)
Cain and Mabel (1936)
Test Pilot (1938)
Too Hot to Handle (1938)
Gone with the Wind (1939)
Boom Town (1940)
Command Decision (1948)
Mogambo (1953)
The Tall Men (1955)
Band of Angels (1957)
Run Silent Run Deep (1958)
Teacher's Pet (1958)
The Misfits (1961)

Charlotte **Gainsbourg**
5ft 8in
(CHARLOTTE LUCY GAINSBOURG)

Born: **July 21, 1971**
London, England

Charlotte was raised in Paris by her very talented, but infamously alcoholic father, Serge Gainsbourg, and her mother, the actress, Jane Birkin. Because of her dad's notoriety, young Charlotte was often ostracized by the other pupils at her school. There was also the envy factor: at twelve, she acted in her first film, playing Catherine Deneuve's daughter, in *Paroles et Musique.* She was thirteen when she recorded a duet with Serge, called 'Lemon Incest'. It was featured on his 1984 album 'Love on the Beat' and caused much controversy. As good an actress as she's proved to be, Charlotte cannot get over her belief that she has inherited the worst physical aspects from each of her parents. I'd argue that they've also given her their adventurous spirit – which has been an essential ingredient in her remarkable career so far. In 1986, she won a César Award as 'Most Promising Actress' for *L'Effrontée* and in 2000, was voted 'Best Supporting Actress' for *La Bûche.* She sang the title songs on three of her films and has released two albums so far. She has two young children with her longtime boyfriend, the actor/director, Yvan Attal, with whom she co-starred in *And They Lived Happily Ever After.* Charlotte's next film is *Antichrist,* in which she co-stars with Willem Dafoe.

L'Effrontée (1985)
La Petite voleuse (1988)
In the Eyes of the World (1990)
The Cement Garden (1993)
La Bûche (1999)
My Wife is an Actress (2001)
21 Grams (2003)
And They Lived
Happily Ever After (2004)
L'Un reste, l'autre part (2005)
Lemming (2005)
The Science of Sleep (2006)
Nuovomondo (2006)
Prête-moi ta main (2006)
I'm Not There (2007)
The City of Your Final
Destination (2007)

Anna **Galiena**
5ft 7in
(ANNA GALIENA)

Born: **December 22, 1954**
Rome, Italy

After leaving school in Rome, Anna set out with a passionate desire to become an actress. It took her to the United States, where she attended drama lessons and perfected her English – she already had fluent French. She made her stage debut off-Broadway in "Romeo and Juliet". After she'd shown her potential in a variety of roles, she stepped up to a higher level, in 1978, when she entered Elia Kazan's Actors' Studio. Three years later, she returned to Italy to make her film debut with a bit part in *I Carabbinieri.* Her first featured role was in *Nothing Underneath,* in 1985. Anna didn't neglect the theater – she was especially praised when she played Natasha in Chekhov's "Three Sisters" at the Teatro Stabile in Genoa. Her first big success in movies was in the French film, The *Hairdresser's Husband.* That film and *Jamòn, jamòn,* brought her international attention, but her Hollywood debut in 1993's *Being Human,* starring Robin Williams was a disaster. Since then she's appeared regularly in Italian, French and Spanish movies and is a big star of European cinema. Anna's two marriages – to an American writer, and a French film producer, ended in divorce.

Mosca addio (1987) **Willy Signori**
e vengo da lontano (1990)
The Hairdresser's Husband (1990)
Captain Estrada's Widow (1991)
Jamón, jamón(1992) **Old Rascal** (1992)
The Great Pumpkin (1993)
No Skin(1994) **La Scuola** (1995)
Cervellini fritti impanati(1996)
A Question of Luck (1996)
Les Caprices d'un fleuve (1996)
The Leading Man (1996)
Come te nessuno mai (1999)
Excellent Cadavers (1999)
Off Key (2001) **Oltre il confine** (2002)
Les Parrains (2005)
Un Amore su misera (2007)
Flying Lessons (2007)
Guido che sfidiò
le Brigate Rosse (2007)
Sans état d'âme (2008)

Peter **Gallagher**
5ft 9in
(PETER GALLAGHER)

Born: **August 19, 1955**
New York City, New York, USA

Peter's grandfather was a coal miner, but his father had a university education, and he made his living in Advertising. Peter's mother became a bacteriologist. Peter was raised in Armonk, New York, where he appeared in plays and musicals during his years at Byram Hills High School. After graduating from Tufts University, where he worked with the Boston Shakespeare Company, Peter sang with the *a capella* group the 'Beelzebubs' he made his professional debut in the 1977 revival of the rock-musical "Hair" on Broadway. Peter was over the moon at the time. After that, came "Grease" and six more top stage shows. Peter worked on some television productions before his film debut, in *The Idolmaker.* In 1983, Peter married Paula Harwood and is the proud father of two children – Jamey and Kathryn. In 1986 he was nominated for a Best Actor Tony Award for "Long Day's Journey into Night". By that point, his movie career had taken off with a number of high-profile roles in big productions. He shared a Golden Globe with a cast of hundreds for his work in Robert Altman's *Short Cuts,* but is still waiting to win something as an individual. Although he's not been in a hit movie during the past seven years, Peter's role as Sandy Cohen, in the current TV series, 'The O.C.', is highly rated.

The Idolmaker (1980)
Police Academy (1984)
DreamChild (1985)
Sex, Lies, and Videotape (1989)
The Player (1992)
Watch It (1993)
Short Cuts (1993)
Malice (1993)
Mrs. Parker and the
Vicious Circle (1994)
While You Were Sleeping (1995)
Underneath (1995)
American Beauty (1999)
Center Stage (2000)
Protection (2001) **Mr. Deeds** (2002)
Center Stage: Turn It Up (2008)
Adam (2009)

Sir Michael **Gambon**
6ft
(MICHAEL GAMBON)

Born: **October 19, 1940**
Dublin, Ireland

After Michael started school, his father, Edward, took the family to London, where he could find work as a builder after the war. With his wife, Mary, they moved to Mornington Crescent, where as a Catholic boy, he attended St. Aloysius Boys School and later its college, in Highgate. At nineteen, he joined the Unity Theater, in Kings Cross. Michael made his film debut in Laurence Olivier's *Othello,* in 1964. It was six years before his next movie, *Eyeless in Gaza,* and he made little impression until *The Beast Must Die,* in 1974. His breakthrough role was twelve years after that, when he starred as Philip E. Marlow, in Dennis Potter's TV-series 'The Singing Detective'. His first major movie success was in *The Cook the Thief His Wife & Her Lover.* Unlike other 'character actors' Michael's roles grew bigger as the years passed and by the early part of the new century, he was firmly established as a regular in Hollywood films. He is currently separated from his only wife, Anne Miller.

The Rachel Papers (1989) **A Dry White**
Season (1989) **The Cook the Thief His**
Wife & Her Lover (1989) **Mobsters** (1991)
The Browning Version (1994) **A Man of**
No Importance (1994) **Squanto: A**
Warrior's Tale (1994) **Two Deaths** (1995)
Nothing Personal (1995)
Mary Reilly (1996) **The Wings of the**
Dove (1997) **The Gambler** (1997)
Dancing Lughnasa (1998) **Plunkett &**
Macleane (1999) **The Last**
September (1999) **The Insider** (1999) **High**
Heels and Low Lifes (2001) **Gosford**
Park (2001) **Charlotte Gray** (2001) **Open**
Range (2003) **Sylvia** (2003) **Standing**
Room Only (2004) **The Prisoner of**
Azkaban (2004) **Being Julia** (2004)
Sky Captain and the World of
Tomorrow (2004) **Layer Cake** (2004) **The**
Life Aquatic with Steve Zissou (2004)
The Goblet of Fire (2005) **Amazing**
Grace (2006) **The Good Shepherd** (2006)
The Order of the Phoenix (2007)
Brideshead Revisited (2008)
The Half-Blood Prince (2009)

Greta **Garbo**
5ft 7½in
(GRETA LOVISA GUSTAFSSON)

Born: **September 18, 1905**
Stockholm, Stockholms län, Sweden
Died: **April 15, 1990**

The daughter of a humble laborer, Greta started work in a barber's shop when she was fourteen. Two years later, she was working in the "PUB" department store, when she was chosen to appear in their movie theater commercial. Greta got a scholarship to the Royal Theater School in Stockholm, from where she was recommended to Mauritz Stiller. He directed her debut, *The Atonement of Gösta Berling.* Louis B. Mayer was keen to sign Stiller, and although he considered Garbo too fat, he took her as part of the package. MGM gave her the role of a peasant girl in *The Torrent,* but it was in 1927, when she showed star potential, in *Flesh and the Devil* – thrilling audiences with her passion for John Gilbert. They co-starred in *Queen Christina,* but Hollywood had taken a dislike to his high-pitched voice and he would hardly be heard from again. Greta's career continued – creating more legend with each film. She was four times an Oscar nominee – for *Anna Christie, Romance, Camille* and *Ninotchka.* As she neared her forties, she made her final film, the comedy, *Two-faced Woman.* For the next ten years rumors about a come-back persisted. It never happened and her fans had to be content with fuzzy photos of her wearing dark glasses. She was awarded a special Oscar in 1954, but she wanted to be alone! And that was how she died – in New York, from cardiac arrest after treatment for kidney trouble.

Romance (1930)
Anna Christie (1931)
Susan Lennox –
Her Fall and Rise (1931)
Mata Hari (1931)
Grand Hotel (1932)
Queen Christina (1933)
The Painted Veil (1934)
Anna Karenina (1935)
Camille (1936)
Conquest (1937)
Ninotchka (1939)
Two-Faced Woman (1941)

Andy **Garcia**
5ft 11in
(ANDRÉS ARTURO GARCIA MENÉNDEZ)

Born: **April 12, 1956**
Havana, Cuba

Andy's father René, was an attorney in Havana, who also farmed avocados. His mother Amelie, was an English teacher. When he was five, the aftermath of the disastrous Bay of Pigs invasion forced his family to relocate to Miami. There, over the years, they established and built up a thriving perfume business. Andy was in the basketball squad at Miami Beach Senior High School. Hepatitis ended his sporting activity and when he was at Florida International University, he turned his attention to acting. He left and went to Hollywood – working as a waiter, while getting bit parts in TV shows. In 1983, he made his film debut in a comedy about baseball, called *Blue Skies Again.* Three years after that, Brian de Palma was so impressed by his work in *8 Million Ways to Die,* he offered him the featured role as Agent George Stone, in his superb gangster movie, *The Untouchables.* It made Andy a bankable star – leading to featured roles in important movies such as *The Godfather: Part III,* which earned him a Best Supporting Actor Oscar nomination. After a slow spell during the late 1990s, he hit the spot again in *Ocean's Eleven.* Andy is very protective of his family's right to privacy. He's been married for twenty-five years to Maria Lorido. The couple have three daughters and a son.

The Untouchables (1987)
Black Rain (1989)
Internal Affairs (1990)
The Godfather: Part III (1990)
Dead Again (1991)
Accidental Hero (1992)
When a Man Loves a Woman (1994)
Things to Do in Denver When
You're Dead (1995)
Night Falls on Manhattan (1996)
The Unsaid (2001)
Ocean's Eleven (2001)
Modigliani (2004)
The Lost City (2005)
The Air I Breathe (2007)
New York, I Love You (2008)
La Linea (2008)

Vincent **Gardenia**
5ft 5in
(VINCENZO SCOGNAMIGLIO)

Born: **January 7, 1922**
Naples, Italy
Died: **December 9, 1992**

In 1924, Vince's parents set sail for the New World with their two-year-old son. They settled in New York City, where his father, Gennaro Gardenia Scognamiglio, founded a theater troupe among the Italian immigrant community. Vince acted there in his mother tongue while still at school, but when he was fourteen, he left full-time education to become a member of the troupe. After four years of good experience, World War II interrupted his career and he left to serve in the United States Army. When peace returned in 1945, he went back to New York. Just by chance, the movie *The House on 92nd Street,* was being shot near his home in Manhattan, and he made his debut in a small uncredited role. Until 1957, he was perfectly happy to work with his father. He made his Broadway debut in "Volpone" and appeared in an episode of 'Studio One' on television. Branching out further, he played his first featured film role, as Danny Gimp, in *Cop Hater.* More stage and television work led to a key role, as the barman, in *The Hustler.* In 1972, he won an Emmy for Neil Simon's play, "The Prisoner of Second Avenue". Vince was twice nominated for Best Supporting Actor Oscars – for *Bang the Drum Slowly* and *Moonstruck.* He died of heart failure in Philadelphia, less than two years after his final film, *The Super.*

Murder, Inc. (1960) **View from the Bridge** (1961) **The Hustler** (1961) **Where's Poppa?** (1970)
Little Murders (1971) **Cold Turkey** (1971) **Bang the Drum Slowly** (1973) **Death Wish** (1974) **The Front Page** (1974) **The Manchu Eagle Murder Caper Mystery** (1975) **The Big Racket** (1976) **Greased Lightning** (1977) **Heaven Can Wait** (1978) **The Last Flight of Noah's Ark** (1980) **Little Shop of Horrors** (1986) **Moonstruck** (1987) **Skin Deep** (1989)

Ava **Gardner**
5ft 6in
(AVA LAVINIA GARDNER)

Born: December 24, 1922
Grabtown, North Carolina, USA
Died: **January 25, 1990**

Ava was the seventh child of a couple of poor sharecroppers, who lived in a small wooden house on a tenant farm. At her local school, Ava developed her love for dancing. The 1929 stockmarket crash brought more hardship and her father's early death, in 1935. After finishing high school, Ava went to New York to visit a sister. Her photographer husband sent pictures of her to MGM, and a screen test secured her a 7-year contract. Her early years were frustrating – in her first 24 films starting with *Fancy Answers,* in 1941, she had two credited appearances. Even her short marriage to Mickey Rooney did little to further her career. But then everything changed. She married bandleader, Artie Shaw, and was absolutely stunning in *Whistle Stop,* with George Raft. Because of that, she was loaned out to Universal for their classic thriller, *The Killers.* For twenty years, she was a huge star. She had an Oscar nomination for *Mogambo,* and played 'The World's Most Beautiful Animal', in *The Barefoot Contessa.* Ava expressed her complete dissatisfaction with her movie career, but the reality is that she's left us with an impressive selection of good films. Her final years were spent as a recluse in her London apartment. She died of bronchial pneumonia following a stroke, which left her partially paralyzed.

The Killers (1946) **One Touch of Venus** (1948) **The Bribe** (1949) **Pandora and the Flying Dutchman** (1951) **Showboat** (1951) **Snows of Kilimanjaro** (1952) **Knights of the Round Table** (1953) **Mogambo** (1953) **The Barefoot Contessa** (1954) **Bhowani Junction** (1956) **The Sun Also Rises** (1957) **On the Beach** (1959) **55 Days at Peking** (1963) **Seven Days in May** (1964) **The Night of the Iguana** (1964) **The Sentinel** (1977) **Priest of Love** (1981)

John **Garfield**
5ft 7in
(JACOB JULIUS GARFINKLE)

Born: March 4, 1913
New York City, New York, USA
Died: **May 21, 1952**

John was the son of Russian Jewish immigrants, David and Hannah Garfinkle. After his mother died when he was seven, John was raised by his father on New York's Lower East Side. Later, he was sent to a special school for problem children, where he was taught boxing skills to help him overcome a damaged heart, caused by a childhood illness. While there, he became interested in drama. He was never short of something to say – he came first in a state-wide debating contest sponsored by the N.Y. Times. He won a scholarship to the Maria Ouspenskaya Drama School and went on to work with Eva La Gallienne's repertory company, in a lot of plays. John married Roberta Seidman in 1935. Two of their three children became actors. He was so angry at being overlooked for the lead in "Golden Boy" in 1937, he signed with Warner Bros., who named him John Garfield. His first film, *Four Daughters* earned him an Oscar nomination, but later films were even better – including a Best Actor Oscar-nominated role in *Body and Soul*. The Communist witch-hunts of the late-1940s hurt his career. In 1952, he was in the Broadway revival of "Golden Boy" but his career was over. The stress got to him and he succumbed to the long-term heart trouble which finally killed him.

Four Daughters (1938) **They Made Me a Criminal** (1939) **Jaurez** (1939) **Castle on the Hudson** (1940) **The Sea Wolf** (1941) **Out of the Fog** (1941) **Tortilla Flat** (1942) **Air Force** (1943) **Destination Tokyo** (1943) **Pride of the Marines** (1945) **The Postman Always Rings Twice** (1946) **Nobody Lives Forever** (1946) **Humoresque**(1946) **Body and Soul** (1947) **Gentleman's Agreement** (1947) **Force of Evil** (1948) **We Were Strangers** (1949) **The Breaking Point** (1950) **He Ran All the Way** (1951)

William **Gargan**
6ft
(WILLIAM DENNIS GARGAN)

Born: **July 17, 1905**
Brooklyn, New York City, New York, USA
Died: **February 17, 1979**

Bill was one of two Gargan brothers who became actors. After he graduated from high school, in 1923, his dad, who was a bookmaker, gave him a job. It was the beginning of a life-long passion for horse-racing. His brother was singing in the chorus of the Metropolitan Opera, and through that contact, Bill, complete with brown make-up, made his professional stage debut in "Aloma of the South Seas". He enjoyed a long career on Broadway, but after his success in "The Animal Kingdom", he was approached by several studios in Hollywood. In 1929, he was given a bit part in a musical/comedy starring George Jessel, called *Lucky Boy*. Two years later, he was eighth-billed – below Claudette Colbert, in *Misleading Lady*. His career after that was impressive – both as star and supporting player. He was nominated for a Best Supporting Actor Oscar for *They Knew What They Wanted*. His career ended in 1958, when he developed throat cancer and doctors removed his larynx. He was fitted with an artificial voice box. Bill was happily married to Mary Kenny from 1928 until his death from a heart attack, on board a flight from New York to San Diego.

Rain (1932) **The Animal Kingdom** (1932) **Sweepings** (1933) **The Story of Temple Drake** (1933) **Headline Shooter** (1933) **Strictly Dynamite** (1934) **Traveling Saleslady** (1935) **Black Fury** (1935) **Don't Bet on Blondes** (1935) **Bright Lights** (1935) **The Milky Way** (1936) **You Only Live Once** (1937) **The Devil's Party** (1938) **The Crowd Roars** (1938) **Star Dust** (1940) **Turnabout** (1940) **They Knew What They Wanted** (1940) **Cheers for Miss Bishop** (1941) **I Wake Up Screaming** (1941) **The Canterville Ghost** (1944) **The Bells of St. Mary's** (1945) **Miracle in the Rain** (1956)

Judy **Garland**
4ft 11½in
(FRANCES ETHEL GUMM)

Born: **June 10, 1922**
Grand Rapids, Minnesota, USA
Died: **June 22, 1969**

Baby Judy was baptized Episcopalian. Her parents, Frank and Ethel Gumm, were vaudevillians who pushed her at every opportunity. Her dad ran a theater where, at the age of three she sang 'Jingle Bells'. A trio known as the Gumm Sisters was unsuccessful, but she went solo with mother's urging. After failing a test at Columbia she got an MGM contract. They changed her name to Judy Garland and put her in a short, where she sang 'You Made Me Love You' to a photo of Clark Gable. He and MGM, adored it, and used it in *Broadway Melody of 1938.* They then starred Judy with Mickey Rooney in *Thoroughbreds Don't Cry* and in 1939, she was Dorothy, in *The Wizard of Oz.* It made her a star and gave her the hit-song, 'Over the Rainbow'. She married Vincente Minnelli, who directed her in the charming *Meet Me in St. Louis.* She was a top box-office star, but three years later, the pills she used to fuel her incredible energy, took their toll – physically and emotionally. She was in and out of hospital until MGM released her from her contract. Personal appearances in sell-out concerts restored her confidence and she gave two Oscar-nominated film performances with later films, *A Star is Born* and *Judgement at Nuremburg.* Judy continued touring until 1969, when she performed her final concert in Copenhagen. She died in London from an overdose of barbiturates.

The Wizard of Oz (1939) **Babes in Arms** (1939) **Strike Up the Band** (1940) **Ziegfeld Girl** (1941) **Babes on Broadway** (1941) **For Me and My Gal** (1942) **Presenting Lily Mars** (1943) **Girl Crazy** (1943) **Meet Me in St. Louis** (1945) **The Clock** (1945) **The Harvey Girls** (1946) **The Pirate** (1948) **Easter Parade** (1948) **Summer Stock** (1950) **A Star is Born** (1954) **Judgement at Nuremberg** (1961)

James **Garner**
6ft 1in
(JAMES SCOTT BAUMGARNER)

Born: **April 7, 1928**
Norman, Oklahoma, USA

Jim was the youngest of three children. His father, Warren Baumgarner, worked as a carpet layer. His mother, Mildred, who was of Cherokee ancestry, died when he was four. He and his two brothers lived with relatives until their father remarried in 1934. Their stepmother was so cruel, the boys hated her. Jim joined the Merchant Marines at sixteen but did not enjoy going to sea. A year later, he moved in with his father in L.A. and went to Hollywood High School. He modeled Jantzen swimwear, then returned to his home town and Norman High School, to play football and basketball. He served in the Army in Korea. In 1954, Jim got a small role in the Broadway production of "The Caine Mutiny". After acting on TV, his name was changed to James Garner for his 1956 film debut, in *Toward the Unknown.* Warners then starred him in the popular western series 'Maverick' and for three years it helped support Lois – the girl he married in 1956, and their children. The 1960s was a good period in his film career and later on television – which in 1974, provided him with the starring role of Jim Rockford, in the hit series, 'The Rockford Files'. Jim was re-united with Julie Andrews in *Victor Victoria* – and hasn't stopped working – despite heart bypass surgery and two knee replacements.

The Children's Hour (1961)
The Thrill of it All (1963)
The Americanization of Emily (1964)
36 Hours (1964) **Duel at Diablo** (1966)
Grand Prix (1966) **Hour of the Gun** (1967)
Support Your Local Sheriff! (1969)
Marlowe (1969)
Support Your Local Gunfighter (1971)
Skin Game (1971)
The Castaway Cowboy (1974)
Victor Victoria (1982) **Murphy's Romance** (1985) **Sunset** (1988)
Fire in the Sky (1993)
Maverick (1994)
My Fellow Americans (1996)
Space Cowboys (2000)
The Note Book (2004)

Jennifer **Garner**
5ft 9in
(JENNIFER ANNE GARNER)

Born: **April 17, 1972**
Houston, Texas, USA

Jennifer's parents are Methodists. Her father, William Garner, was a chemical engineer, at Union Carbide, and her mother, Patricia, an English teacher. Jennifer, who has two sisters, was only three years old when she began to take ballet lessons. She continued to do so after the family relocated first to Princeton, and then Charleston, West Virginia, but she never had the ambition to become a dancer. After graduating from George Washington High School, where, in the school band she played the saxophone, she enrolled at Denison University, in Ohio. To start with, she studied chemistry, but soon switched to drama. Following her graduation, she took a serious step by continuing learning at the National Theater Institute. In 1995, Jennifer moved to New York, where she understudied for the play, "A Month in the Country" prior to making a TV movie, Danielle Steele's 'Zoya'. in 1997, Jennifer appeared in a short film, *In Harm's Way,* and that year, had a tiny role in Woody Allen's *Deconstructing Harry.* In 2001, she won a Golden Globe for Best Actress in a TV series – 'Alias'. Jennifer's break was in the critically panned, *Pearl Harbor,* when, more importantly, she met her future husband, Ben Affleck. They starred together in *Daredevil* and after their baby daughter, Violet Anne was born in December 2005, Jennifer's film career took an upswing. She has been involved as a producer and directed one episode of the TV-series, 'Alias'. In 2007, she was in two excellent movies – *The Kingdom* and *Juno.* A year after that, she played the role of Roxane, in the television adaptation of Edmond Rostand's classic French stage play, "Cyrano de Bergerac".

Washington Square (1997)
1999 (1998) **Pearl Harbor** (2001)
Rennie's Landing (2001)
Catch Me If You Can (2002)
Daredevil (2003)
13 Going on 30 (2004)
Catch and Release (2006)
The Kingdom (2007) **Juno** (2007)

Terri **Garr**
5ft 7in
(TERRY ANN GARR)

Born: **December 11, 1947**
Lakewood, Ohio, USA

Terri got her good-humored looks from her father, the actor and comedian Eddie Garr, who appeared in a few films and television series before his early death in 1956. Like her mother, Phyllis, Terri trained as a dancer and in her teens performed with the San Francisco Ballet. After Phyllis became a wardrobe mistress for films and television, young Terri aimed her sights at a career in show business. In the early 1960s, she danced in prime television variety shows like 'Shindig'. Her first movie role was in the 1963 independent film, *A Swingin' Affair.* That was quickly followed by a number of uncredited dancing roles in Elvis Presley films, beginning with *Fun in Acapulco.* During that decade she had a small role in the Monkees film, *Head,* but was making more of a name for herself on TV, with appearances in episodes of 'McCloud' and 'Star Trek'. Then, in 1974, Terri had a strong featured role in the *The Conversation,* starring Gene Hackman. She was taken seriously as an actress, with roles in high-profile movies – in *Tootsie* she was nominated for a Best Supporting Actress Oscar – and she was impressive in Martin Scorsese's comedy thriller, *After Hours.* She was married to actor John O'Neil from 1993 until 1996. They adopted a daughter. Terri's career has continued with plenty of film and television work, despite the fact that she was diagnosed with multiple sclerosis in 1983. She is an Ambassador for the MS Society.

The Conversation (1974)
Close Encounters of the
Third Kind (1977)
The Black Stallion (1979)
One from the Heart (1982)
Tootsie (1982)
Mr. Mom (1983)
After Hours (1985)
Let it Ride (1989)
Waiting for the Light (1990)
Dumb and Dumber (1994)
The Sky is Falling (2000)
Expired (2007)
Kabluey (2007)

Betty **Garrett**
5ft 5in
(BETTY GARRETT)

Born: **May 23, 1919**
St. Joseph, Missouri, USA

Betty graduated from The Annie Wright School in Tacoma, Washington. She then studied acting under Sanford Meisner, at the Neighborhood Playhouse in New York. She began her acting career at Orson Welles' Mercury Theater. During that same period, she was performing with Martha Graham's dance company. The combination of the two disciplines pushed her towards specializing in musical comedy. Mike Todd saw her at the American Youth Theater and signed her to understudy Ethel Merman in the show, "Something for the Boys". She was then in several Broadway shows including "Call Me Mister" in which her rendition of "South America, Take It Away" won her the forerunner of a Tony – the Donaldson Award. In 1944 – Betty married Larry Parks, and they became a great couple - both on and off stage. In 1948, she was signed by MGM and got off to a good start with her debut in the Margaret O'Brien movie, *Big City.* A trio of very good musicals followed before her great one – *On The Town.* Unfortunately, it virtually spelt the end of her movie career. Larry was black-listed for his Communist connections and she was tarred with the same brush – which made getting film work impossible. The couple toured the United States and England in stage shows and cabaret, but movie fans were prevented from seeing Betty on the screen until 1955, when she appeared in *My Sister Eileen.* Most of her work since then has been on television but she has recently acted in two movies. Her son, Andy Parks, is an actor.

Big City (1948)
Words and Music (1948)
Take Me Out to the
Ball Game (1949)
Neptune's Daughter (1949)
On the Town (1949)
My Sister Eileen (1955)
The Shadow on the
Window (1957)
Trail of the Screaming
Forehead (2007)

Greer **Garson**
5ft 6in
(EILEEN EVELYN GREER GARSON)

Born: **September 29, 1904**
London, England
Died: **April 6, 1996**

In her teens, Greer was set on being a schoolteacher. Instead, she took a job in Advertising, where she found time to join an amateur drama group. Through a friend, she was able to move up to the Birmingham Repertory Company, and in 1934, appeared in Regent's Park Open Air Theater. Laurence Olivier saw her and featured her in several productions including "Twelfth Night" and "A School for Scandal". Louis B. Mayer was in the audience one night and he went back home with her signature on a contract. Things moved rather too slowly until the director, Sam Wood needed just her kind of Englishness for his film *Goodbye Mr. Chips.* Her part was short and sweet – she dies after twenty minutes, but the film's success led to her being in demand. A reunion with Olivier was even better for her image and she even out-acted Crawford before, in 1942, her most famous role as *Mrs Miniver* won her a Best Actress Oscar. She married Richard Ney, who played her son in the film. She remained in the Box Office Top Ten until 1946 and had other Oscar nominations for *Madame Curie, Mrs. Parkington, The Valley of Decision* and *Sunrise at Campobello* – in which she portrayed Eleanor Roosevelt. One of the first big stars to work on early TV, Greer was in her nineties when she died of heart failure in Dallas, Texas.

Goodbye Mr. Chips (1939)
Pride and Prejudice (1940)
Blossoms in the Dust (1941)
Mrs. Miniver (1942)
Random Harvest (1942)
Madame Curie (1943)
Mrs. Parkington (1944)
The Valley of Decision (1945)
Julia Misbehaves (1948)
That Forsyte Woman (1949)
The Law and the Lady (1951)
Julius Caesar (1953)
Her Twelve Men (1954)
Sunrise at Campobello (1960)
The Happiest Millionaire (1967)

Vittorio **Gassman**
6ft 1½in
(VITTORIO GASSMAN)

Born: **September 1, 1922**
Genoa, Liguria, Italy
Died: **June 29, 2000**

His mother Luisa, was Italian, but he got his surname from his father, Heinrich Gassman who was an Austrian. At school, Vittorio was a fine athlete who represented his country at basketball. He was such a handsome young man, his mother registered him with the Accademia Nazionale d'Arte Drammatica, in Rome. He met a girl called Nora, who was the daughter of the actor, Renzo Ricci. After his stage debut in "La Nemica" in 1943, he married her. In 1946, when he made his first movie, *Preludio d'Amore,* Vittorio was a veteran of more than thirty plays. He took time to develop his screen technique, but it was worth the wait. In 1948, he was Silvana Mangano's lover in *Bitter Rice* – which did more for his long-term career than it did hers. His stage work got him a reputation as "Italy's Olivier" but marriage to the Hollywood star, Shelley Winters, got him an MGM contract, which allowed him to spend six months a year in Italy. After four flops, and a good role in *War and Peace,* he returned home. Vittorio soon revealed a talent for comedy in the international smash-hit *I Soliti Ignoti.* He toured the USA in a one-man show "Via Vittorio" and was busy until his fatal heart attack, in Rome. All three of Vittorio's wives were actresses. His son Alessandro – from his affair with Juliette Mayniel, is an actor.

War and Peace (1956) **I Soliti Ignoti** (1958) **Il Mattatore** (1960) Crimen (1961) **Barabbas** (1962) I Briganti Italiani (1962) Il Successo (1963) **Parliamo di Donne** (1964) **Profumo di Donne** (1974) C'eravamo tanti amati (1974) I Telefoni bianchi (1976) **Anima Persa** (1977) **La Terrazza** (1980) Sharkey's Machine (1981) Tempest (1982) Life is a Bed of Roses (1983) Count Tacchia (1983) La Famiglia (1987) **Motacci** (1989) The Sleazy Uncle (1989) Sleepers (1996) **The Dinner** (1998)

John **Gavin**
6ft 4in
(JOHN ANTHONY GOLENOR)

Born: **April 8, 1931**
Los Angeles, California, USA

Jack was the son of Herald Gavin and his wife Delia. Descended on his father's side, from Irish landowners, in old Spanish California, the boy had Mexican blood from his mother and he was completely bi-lingual from his early childhood. After Stanford University, Jack was an air intelligence officer with the U.S. Navy until 1956. A friend arranged a screen test and he was signed by Universal. Jack made his film debut in the western, *Raw Edge,* later that year, and by 1960, when he was cast as Sam Loomis, in the Hitchcock classic, *Psycho,* he had already starred in two good movies for his studio. After he appeared in *Thoroughly Modern Millie,* his screen roles dropped sharply in quality and quantity. Jack was president of the Screen Actors Guild from 1971-1973 and by coincidence, during that period, he was twice signed to play Bond – in *Diamonds Are Forever* and *Live* and *Let Die.* On both occasions the return to the role by Connery and Moore stopped it. He continued to work in films, on television and and on the stage but retired in 1981. A Republican, Jack was appointed U.S. Ambassador to Mexico in June of that year, by Ronald Reagan and served until 1986. He has been married to his second wife, the actress Constance Towers, since 1974. They each had two children from their previous marriages. Jack's own daughter Christina Gavin, from his first marriage to Cecily Evans, is an actress.

Four Girls in Town (1957) Quantez (1957) A Time to Love and a Time to Die (1958) Imitation of Life (1959) Psycho (1960) Spartacus (1960) Midnight Lace (1960) Romanoff and Juliet (1961) Tammy Tell Me True (1961) Back Street (1961) Pedro Páramo (1967) Thoroughly Modern Millie (1967) Keep It in the Family (1973)

Janet **Gaynor**
5ft
(LAURA AUGUSTA GAINOR)

Born: **October 6, 1906**
Philadelphia, Pennsylvania, USA
Died: **September 14, 1984**

Janet's family moved around the country and her schoolwork suffered. After a brief stop in San Francisco, they finally settled in Los Angeles, where Janet was happy to take a job as an usherette in a theater. She was petite and pretty. Very soon she was earning extra money as a film extra. In 1925, she had small parts in two reelers for Roach, and a western at Universal. The following year, Fox gave her the lead in *The Johnstown Flood* and a five-year contract. F.W. Murnau's *Sunrise,* was released after *Seventh Heaven,* which made her a star. Janet and her co-star in the latter, Charles Farrell, were dubbed "America's Sweethearts" and rushed into *Street Angel.* At the 1928 Academy Awards, she had the unique experience of receiving a Best Actress Oscar for all three. Gaynor and Farrell made the singing talkie, *Sunny Side Up* and she begged Fox not to put her in any more musicals. After another huge success, in *Daddy Long Legs,* she was teamed with her screen sweetheart twice more. As she reached thirty, her little girl personality began to grate. After a final Oscar nomination, for *A Star is Born,* she married the MGM dress designer, Adrian, and retired. She died largely due to the aftermath of a traffic accident, when the taxicab she was in was hit by a speeding car. Her husband and her friend, Mary Martin, were injured and Mary's manager was killed. Janet suffered broken ribs, a fractured collarbone and internal injuries. She died in Palm Springs, California, after several operations.

Sunnyside Up (1929) Daddy Long Legs (1931) State Fair (1933) Change of Heart (1935) One More Spring (1935) The Farmer Takes a Wife (1935) Small Town Girl (1936) Ladies in Love (1936) A Star is Born (1937) The Young in Heart (1938) Bernardine (1957)

Mitzi **Gaynor**
5ft 6in
(FRANCESCA MARLENE VON GERBER)

Born: **September 4, 1931**
Chicago, Illinois, USA

Of Austrian-Hungarian ancestry, Mitzi's father was a musician as well as a director of stage musicals, and her mother was a dancer. It was she who encouraged her daughter to follow in her footsteps. Mitzi's Carmen Miranda impression was so good, she toured the U.S. Army camps as a speciality act, when she was fourteen. Two years later, she was discovered by Edwin Lester and hired as a dancer by the Los Angeles Light Opera Company. The company gave her the opportunity to perform in such popular shows as "Roberta" and "Naughty Marietta" and when she was starring in "The Great Waltz" an agent of 20th Century Fox approached her. It resulted in her film debut, in 1950, in *My Blue Heaven* – for which she was given better notices than its star, Betty Grable. She appeared in some pleasant musicals before marrying Jack Bean, in 1954. He became her manager and worked hard to make her a real star. He succeeded on four occasions, one of which was her last big screen role, as Nellie Forbush in *South Pacific,* for which she was nominated for a Golden Globe as Best Actress in a Comedy/Musical. From the early 1960s, she concentrated on the nightclub circuit. Her marriage endured until Jack's death in 2006. In 1966, at the Academy Awards, Mitzi's sparkling dancing and singing of the hit song "Georgy Girl" received a standing ovation, but there were to be no movie come-backs for this talented kid.

My Blue Heaven (1950)
Take Care of My
Little Girl (1951)
We're Not Married! (1952)
Bloodhounds of Broadway (1952)
The I Don't Care Girl (1953)
There's No Business Like
Show Business (1954)
Anything Goes (1956)
The Joker Is Wild (1957)
Les Girls (1957)
South Pacific (1958)
Happy Anniversary (1959)
For Love or Money (1963)

Ben **Gazzara**
5ft 10½in
(BIAGIO ANTHONY GAZZARA)

Born: **August 28, 1930**
New York City, New York, USA

The son of Italian immigrants, Ben grew up on New York's tough lower East Side. After Stuyvesant High School, he joined a theater company which, he claims helped to save him from a life of crime. He began his higher education by studying electrical engineering, but he soon got back on the drama track at the Actors Studio. Ben first achieved a reputation with his dynamic playing of Jocko de Paris, in "End as a Man" which would provide him with his film debut, in 1957, when re-titled *The Strange One.* Despite his powerful performance, it was surprisingly overlooked for an Oscar. Although he starred on Broadway in "Cat On A Hot Tin Roof", directed by Elia Kazan, Ben missed out on the film role to the better known, Paul Newman. After 1962, most of his work was on TV until he began working with his good friend, John Cassavetes. After they appeared in *Bloodline,* Ben and Audrey Hepburn, who were both experiencing marital problems, had a brief affair. During the 1980s, he made several European films, which varied in quality, but he had the knack of bouncing back in some good Hollywood productions. Although nearing eighty, Ben is still acting – in the feel-good movie *Paris, je t'aime* and recently starred in the comedy, *Looking for Palladin.*

The Strange One (1957)
Anatomy of a Murder (1959)
The Young Doctors (1961)
Convicts 4 (1962) Husbands (1970)
The Killing of a Chinese Bookie (1976)
Opening Night (1977)
Saint Jack (1979)
They All Laughed (1981)
Il Camorrista (1986)
Road House (1989) Buffalo '66 (1998)
The Big Lebowski (1998)
Happiness (1998)
Summer of Sam (1999)
The Thomas Crown Affair (1999)
Very Mean Men (2000)
Dogville (2003)
Paris, je t'aime (2006)
Looking for Palladin (2008)

Martina **Gedeck**
5ft 9in
(MARTINA GEDECK)

Born: **September 14, 1961**
Munich, Bavaria, Germany

The eldest of three daughters born to a businessman, Karl-Heinz Gedeck, and his wife, Helga, Martina spent her early years in the Bavarian city of Landshut. In 1971, the family moved to Berlin, where she appeared in the TV drama, 'Die Sendung mit der Maus'. Martina attended the Schadow-Oberschule and completed her Abitur. She then read German and History at the Free University of Berlin, before studying drama at Berlin's University of the Arts. In 1986, Martina made her film debut in *In the Cold of the Sun,* but by the early 1990s, most of her work had been on television. Then, in 1993, after setting up home with the actor Ulrich Wildgruber, she appeared in a movie titled *Krücke,* which set the standard for a career which would lead to international recognition, through releases like *Talk of the Town* and *Harald,* which were enjoyed overseas. In 1999, Martina had to endure the pain of losing her partner when Wildgruber committed suicide by drowning. Martina continued with her life and career – and after acting in several successful German productions, she appeared in her first Hollywood movie, *The Good Shepherd* – the year she was voted Germany's most important actress by "Gala" Magazine. Martina is the companion of Swiss writer/director, Markus Imboden. She lives in Berlin.

Krücke (1993)
Maybe, Maybe Not (1994)
Talk of the Town (1995)
Harald (1997) Rossini (1997)
Frau Rettich, de
Czerni und ich (1998)
Jew Boy (1999)
Alles Bob! (1999)
The Green Desert (1999)
Bella Martha (2001)
Elementarteilchen (2006)
The Lives of Others (2006)
Sommer '04 (2006)
The Good Shepherd (2006)
Meine schöne Bescherung (2007)
The Baader Meinhof
Complex (2008)

Judy **Geeson**
5ft 3in
(JUDITH AMANDA GEESON)

Born: **September 10, 1948**
Arundel, West Sussex, England

Judy's father, the editor of the enticingly titled, "National Coal Board Magazine", moved his family to London when she was ten. She and her sister, Sally, who also became an actress, attended the Corona Stage School, in Chiswick. Judy's ambition was to become a ballet dancer, but serious headaches suffered because of the strenuous moves, changed her mind. After making her stage debut in 1957, she concentrated on acting. In 1960, at the age of twelve, she made her first appearance on television in an episode of 'Dixon of Dock Green'. She made her screen debut in 1963, in a short family film called *Wings of Mystery*. Four years later, she was elevated to a higher level when she starred opposite Sydney Potier, in *To Sir, With Love*. She enjoyed a ten year spell of making high-profile movies. Judy has many fond memories of *Brannigan* – the film she made in London with screen icon, John Wayne. Judy's last big movie was *The Eagle Has Landed,* which was shot around the time she appeared regularly on television – as Caroline, in the highly-rated drama series, 'Poldark'. In 1985, Judy married Kristoffer Tabori, the actor son of Viveca Lindfors and Don Siegel, and went to live in California. Following their divorce five years later, Judy chose to remain in the United States. In the 1990s, she starred in the popular television series, 'Mad About You'. She now lives in Los Angeles, where she runs her own antique store, called Blanche and Co.

**Here We Go Round the
Mulberry Bush** (1967)
To Sir, With Love (1967
Three Into Two Won't Go (1969)
10 Rillington Place (1970)
Fear in the Night (1972)
Brannigan (1975)
The Eagle Has Landed (1976)
**The Secret Life of
Kathy McCormick** (1988)
The Duke (1999)
Everything Put Together (2000)
Spanish Fly (2003)

Leo **Genn**
5ft 10in
(LEO JOHN GENN)

Born: **August 9, 1905**
London, England
Died: **January 26, 1978**

Leo grew up in the East End of London where his father Woolfe Genn, worked as a jewelry salesman. His mother, Rachel didn't work so the family struggled. Luckily for Leo, he was accepted at the City of London School, which educated children from poorer backgrounds. Many of them would go on to study at Oxford or Cambridge Universities. At Cambridge, in 1928, Leo qualified as a barrister. Agent Leon M. Lion took him on as an actor and his attorney. So that was how, in 1930, without any previous acting experience, Leo began to get work on the London stage. Three years later, he married Marguerite van Praag, who worked as a casting director at Ealing Studios. In 1935, she got him his film debut, as Shylock, in *Immortal Gentleman*. He was an active member of the Old Vic Company and got regular small roles in films until the war. Leo served in the Royal Artillery and was awarded the *Croix de Guerre* in 1945. Leo appeared in *The Way Ahead,* and Olivier's *Henry V,* towards the end of the war. When peace returned, he was in many good British and American films, such as *The Snake Pit, Quo Vadis* and *Moby Dick.* Other than screen roles, Leo used his fine voice as narrator for the film of Queen Elizabeth's Coronation, in 1953, and it was used in feature films such as *Khartoum*. Leo died of a heart attack in London.

The Way Ahead (1944)
Henry V (1944)
Green for Danger (1946)
**Mourning Becomes
Electra** (1947)
The Velvet Touch (1948)
The Snake Pit (1948)
The Miniver Story (1950)
The Wooden Horse (1950)
Quo Vadis (1951)
Moby Dick (1956)
I Accuse (1958)
Too Hot to Handle (1960)
The Longest Day (1962)
55 Days at Peking (1963)

Gladys **George**
5ft 2½in
(GLADYS ANNA CLARE)

Born: **September 13, 1900**
Patten, Maine, USA
Died: **December 8, 1954**

Gladys was born to English actors, when they were on a tour of America with a Shakespearian company. They settled there, and by the time Gladys was three, she was working in vaudeville as one of "The Three Clares". Due to the touring, her schooling was intermittent, but she was a bright, observant child – learning all she needed to know, quickly. She worked in stock, until, at the age of eighteen, she made her Broadway debut, in "The Betrothal" – starring Isadora Duncan. A good friend, actress Pauline Frederick, persuaded Gladys to start her film career in *Red Hot Dollars,* in 1919, but after an accident in 1921, when she was burned, she retired from the screen and married the first of four husbands – the millionaire, Edward Fowler. She returned in 1934, in the gangster film, *Straight Is The Way,* and was Oscar-nominated as Best Actress, for *Valiant is the Word for Carrie.* She was a star until a drinking habit forced her into supporting roles and acting on television in shows like 'Hopalong Cassidy'. Whatever the roles, Gladys made the most of them – which usually meant something special, but she was sad and worn out by the time she died from a cerebral hemorrhage at her home in Los Angeles.

**Valiant is the Word for
Carrie** (1936) **Madame X** (1937)
They Gave Him a Gun (1937)
Love Is a Headache (1938)
Marie Antoinette (1938)
The Roaring Twenties (1939)
A Child Is Born (1939)
The Maltese Falcon (1941)
The Hard Way (1942)
Christmas Holiday (1944)
The Best Years of Our Lives (1946)
Flamingo Road (1949)
Undercover Girl (1950)
Lullaby of Broadway (1951)
He Ran All the Way (1951)
Detective Story (1951)
Silver City (1951)
It Happens Every Thursday (1953)

Susan George
5ft 5in
(SUSAN MELODY GEORGE)

Born: July 26, 1950
London, England

Susan, whose mother was the actress and dancer, 'Bubbles Percival', started acting at the age of four, and studied at the Corona Stage School. During that time she worked in several TV commercials. She made her first dramatic screen appearance, in 1963, in an episode of the children's television-series, 'Swallows and Amazons'. Susan's film debut was a small role in the 1965 soccer drama, *Cup Fever*, which featured a number of Manchester City and Manchester United players, including George Best, Denis Law and Bobby Charlton. She acted in a number of British movie productions including the swinging 1960s drama, *Up the Junction*, before her breakthrough film opposite Dustin Hoffman – Sam Peckinpah's violent drama, *Straw Dogs*. The film certainly aroused attention but typecast her as a sexy young thing in a run of mainly lesser pictures. Susan worked on TV, and in 2001, featured in eleven episodes of the popular BBC soap series 'Eastenders'. Nowadays, with occasional help from her husband, actor, Simon MacCorkindale, she runs the "Georgian Arabians Stud Farm" with twenty Arab horses, in the Exmoor National Park. Through this hands-on experience, Susan has been able to perfect a wide range of equine therapeutic treatments. She takes really beautiful photographs of her horses and their progeny. Look up her website!

Up the Junction (1968)
The Strange affair (1968)
The Looking Glass War (1969)
Spring and Port Wine (1970)
Eyewitness (1970)
Fright (1971)
Straw Dogs (1971)
Bandera Bandits (1972)
Dirty Mary Crazy Larry (1974)
Mandingo (1975)
Out of Season (1975)
A Small Town in Texas (1976)
The Jigsaw Man (1983)
Djavolji raj (1989)
In Your Dreams (2007)

Richard Gere
5ft 11in
(RICHARD TIFFANY GERE)

Born: August 31, 1939
Philadelphia, Pennsylvania, USA

The second of five children of Homer George Gere, an insurance salesman, and his wife Doris, Richard showed early ability as a musician. At North Syracuse Central High School, he played several instruments – most notably, trumpet, and wrote music for school productions. He graduated in 1967 – winning a scholarship to the University of Massachusetts, where he majored in philosophy. He left to pursue an acting career – landing a role in the London stage production of "Grease" in 1973. That year, he did some television work and made his film debut, in *Report to the Commissioner*. After *Looking for Mr. Goodbar*, Richard enjoyed star status. He traveled to Nepal in 1978, to meet with monks and lamas. He is now a practicing Buddhist. On his return he starred on Broadway, in "Bent" and won the 1980 Theater World Award for his powerful portrayal of a concentration camp prisoner. He was in several massive hits over the next quarter of a century – including *An Officer and a Gentleman, Pretty Woman,* and *Chicago*. Richard's humanitarian efforts include the preservation of cultures and establishing an AIDS care home. Since 2002, he has been married to Carey Lowell, with whom he has a son.

Looking for Mr, Goodbar (1977)
Days of Heaven (1978)
Bloodbrothers (1978) Yanks (1979)
American Gigolo (1980)
An Officer and a Gentleman (1982)
The Cotton Club (1984)
Internal Affairs (1990)
Pretty Woman (1990)
Primal Fear (1996)
Runaway Bride (1999)
The Mothman Prophecies (2002)
Unfaithful (2002) Chicago (2002)
Shall We Dance (2004)
The Hoax (2006)
The Hunting Party (2007)
I'm Not There (2007)
The Flock (2007)
Nights in Rodanthe (2008)
Brooklyn's Finest (2009)

Gina Gershon
5ft 5¾in
(GINA L. GERSHON)

Born: June 10, 1962
Los Angeles, California, USA

The youngest of Stanley and Mickey Gershon's five children, Gina's distinctive looks are the result of her ethnic background – a mixture of Dutch, Russian and French. When she was quite young, Gina's family moved to California. She attended Beverly Hills High School at the same time as Lenny Kravitz. While there, she starred in a production of "The Music Man". She attended Emerson College in Boston before transferring to New York University from where she graduated with a BFA in Drama in 1983. After dancing in a couple of movies without a credit, Gina appeared in the 1984 pop video for "Hello Again" by The Cars. Her first significant appearance on film was in *Pretty in Pink*. She kept plugging away in a steady stream of movies such as *Face/Off*, and in TV series such as 'Snoops', 'Spiderman', 'Tripping the Rift' and 'Ugly Betty'. In 2003, she co-wrote the songs for *Prey for Rock and Roll,* with the recording artist, Linda Perry. Gina's career in movies has remained strong for more than twenty years, so she is obviously doing something right. Something very right is her sexy new CD, "In Search of Cleo". Gina will next be seen on the big screen in *Love Ranch* – with Helen Mirren and Joe Pesci.

Pretty in Pink (1986)
Red Heat (1988)
City of Hope (1991)
The Player (1992)
Bound (1996)
Touch (1997)
Face/Off (1997)
Lulu on the Bridge (1998)
Prague Duet (1998)
Guinevere (1999)
Picture Claire (2001)
Prey for Rock and Roll (2003)
One Last Thing (2005)
Dreamland (2006)
I Want Someone to Eat
Cheese With (2006)
Delirious (2006)
P.S. I Love You (2007)
Love Ranch (2009)

Paul **Giamatti**
5ft 8¹/₂in
(PAUL EDWARD VALENTINE GIAMATTI)

Born: **June 6, 1967**
New Haven, Connecticut, USA

As his father, A. Bartlett Giamatti, was a professor of Renaissance Literature, at Yale, Paul was bound to follow an academic path. His mother, Toni Smith, had been an actress before becoming a teacher of English at Hopkins School, in New Haven. With regard to Paul's academic progress, the combination worked out well. After Choate Rosemary prep school, Paul majored in English at Yale and obtained a Fine Arts degree at the Yale School of Drama. After his graduation, he had a small role in a 1990 television comedy, 'She'll Take Romance' and two years later, he appeared in a featured role in a Rutger Hauer horror film, *Past Midnight*. He began to be taken seriously after appearing in Howard Stern's screen adaptation of *Private Parts*. It took him up another rung on the ladder and he was playing good supporting roles in big movies such as *Saving Private Ryan, Storytelling,* and *American Splendor*. After not even being considered for Oscar honors in 2004 for the excellent *Sideways,* he was nominated as Best Supporting Actor the following year for *Cinderella Man,* but was pipped by George Clooney. Paul Giamatti has a six-year-old son, Samuel, with Elizabeth Cohen, who has been his wife since 1997. Paul's brother, Marcus, is also an actor.

Private Parts (1997)
The Truman Show (1998)
Saving Private Ryan (1998)
The Negotiator (1998)
Safe Men (1998)
Cradle Will Rock (1999)
Storytelling (2001)
American Splendor (2003)
Confidence (2003)
Paycheck (2003) Sideways (2004)
Cinderella Man (2005)
The Illusionist (2006)
Lady in the Water (2006)
Shoot 'Em Up (2007)
The Nanny Diaries (2007)
Cold Souls (2008)
Pretty Bird (2008)

Giancarlo **Giannini**
5ft 8¹/₂in
(GIANCARLO GIANNINI)

Born: **August 1, 1942**
La Spezia, Italy

When he was ten years old, Giancarlo and his family moved to Naples. From 1958, he studied at the Accademia Nazionale d'Arte Drammatica Silvio D'Amica. He made his stage debut in "In memoria di una signora amica" when he was eighteen. He did Shakespeare and contemporary Italian works and appeared with Anna Magnani at London's Old Vic. In 1965, he made his movie debut – a starring one, in the Giallo crime thriller, *Libido*. He kept busy in films and television and also dubbed the voices of stars like Pacino, Hoffman, and Depardieu into Italian. In 1966, he began his long collaboration with director Lina Wertmüller in the musical *Rita la zanzara*. A year later, he married Livia Giampalmo, a writer/director. They had two children, but got divorced in 1975 – the year he was nominated for a Best Actor Oscar – in Lina Wertmüller's *Seven Beauties*. He has also impressed English-speaking audiences in Hollywood productions such as *A Walk in the Clouds, Man on Fire,* and the recent Bond films, *Casino Royale* and *Quantum of Solace*. Giancarlo has another talent: He has a total mastery of several foreign languages.

Jealousy Italian Style (1970)
The Seduction of Mimi (1972)
Swept Away (1974) Seven
Beauties (1975) L'Innocente (1976)
Life is Beautiful (1979)
Lili Marleen (1980) Picone Sent
Me (1984) American Dreamer (1984)
Saving Grace (1985)
Ternosecco (1987) Lo Zio
Indegno (1989) Giovanni Falcone (1993)
Like Two Crocodiles (1994)
A Walk in the Clouds (1995)
Celluloide (1996)
La Stanza dello scirocco (1998)
Hannibal (2001) CQ (2001)
I Love You Eugenio (2002)
Incantato (2003)
Man on Fire (2004)
The Shadow Dancer (2005)
Casino Royale (2006)
Quantum of Solace (2008)

Mel **Gibson**
5ft 9in
(MEL COLUMCILLE GERARD GIBSON)

Born: **January 3, 1956**
Peekskill, New York, USA

The sixth of eleven children of American railroad worker, Hutton Gibson, and an Australian mother, Mel went to live in New South Wales when he was a boy. He attended University in Sydney, and at the National Institute of Dramatic Arts, he performed with future film stars, Judy Davis and Geoffrey Rush. In 1976, he had a small role in the TV-series 'The Sullivans' and an even smaller one in the film *I Never Promised You a Rose Garden*. Back in Australia, his second movie there, *Mad Max,* turned him into an international star. This was consolidated in 1981, by his role in the great war film, *Gallipoli*. The previous year, he married Robyn Moore with whom he has seven children. His American film debut came in 1984, when he played Fletcher Christian, in *The Bounty,* in the illustrious company of Sir Laurence Olivier and Anthony Hopkins. *Mad Max*, the *Lethal Weapon* series – *Maverick,* and *Payback* kept the money pouring in while he tackled more serious parts, including the title role in *Hamlet,* and Sir William Wallace in *Braveheart* – the film for which he won two Oscars – for Best Picture and Best Director. Mel is still a superstar even after a few years' absence. His marriage is on the rocks, but he returns to the movie screen in *Edge of Darkness*.

Mad Max (1979) Gallipoli (1981)
Mad Max 2 (1981) The Year of
Living Dangerously (1982)
The Bounty (1984)
Lethal Weapon (1987)
Tequila Sunrise (1988)
Lethal Weapon 2 (1989)
Hamlet (1990)
Lethal Weapon 3 (1992)
The Man Without a
Face (1993) Maverick (1994)
Braveheart (1995) Ransom (1996)
Conspiracy Theory (1997)
Lethal Weapon 4 (1998)
Payback (1999) The Patriot (2000)
What Women Want (2000)
We Were Soldiers (2002) Signs (2002)
The Singing Detective (2003)

Sir John **Gielgud**
5ft 11in
(ARTHUR JOHN GIELGUD)

Born: **April 14, 1904**
Kensington, London, England
Died: **May 21, 2000**

John's mother, Kate, was a sister-in-law of the famous English stage actress, Ellen Terry. There were also several thespians on his father's side. Young John attended the exclusive Westminster School, before he studied with Lady Benson and went on to RADA. His first film was *Who Is the Man?* in 1924, but he had little interest in the medium especially as nobody could hear his superb voice. His route to becoming one of the great British actors included two seasons at the Old Vic, beginning in 1929. John's performances as Richard II and Hamlet were highly acclaimed and after he had performed the latter on Broadway with Lillian Gish as Ophelia in 1936, he was a star on both sides of the Atlantic. Alfred Hitchcock persuaded him to star in *Secret Agent,* but John's heart was firmly on the stage. Only when he'd achieved all he wanted to do did he work on three film versions of Shakespeare's plays, starting in 1953. Much of his film work was of a serious nature, but in 1981, he showed a great feel for comedy when he played Dudley Moore's Valet, Hobson, in *Arthur.* His performance won him a Best Supporting Actor Oscar. John's final film – the year he died, was Samuel Beckett's, *Catastrophe.*

The Good Companions (1933) **Secret Agent** (1936) **The Prime Minister** (1941)
Julius Caesar (1953) **Romeo and Juliet** (1954) **Richard III** (1955)
The Barretts of Wimpole Street (1957)
Beckett (1964) **Sebastian** (1968)
The Charge of the Light Brigade (1968)
Murder on the Orient Express (1974)
Murder By Decree (1979)
Dyrygent (1980) **The Elephant Man** (1980)
Chariots of Fire (1981) **Arthur** (1981)
Gandhi (1982) **Time After Time** (1986)
Getting It Right (1989)
Prospero's Books (1991)
The Power of One (1992)
Haunted (1995) **Shine** (1996)
The Tichborne Claimant (1998)
Elizabeth (1998)

Marie **Gillain**
5ft 7in
(MARIE GILLAIN)

Born: **June 18, 1975**
Liège, Belgium

Marie was very close to her younger sister, Céline, and the pair would delight their family and friends by performing little comic sketches. When she was fourteen, Marie responded to a newspaper advert – inviting girls to audition for a role in an upcoming movie called *L'Amant.* Marie didn't get the part, but she made a good impression with the casting director. He gave her a part in *Mon père ce Héros* (My father the hero) as the teenage daughter of Gérard Depardieu. After graduating from Saint-Louis College, in Liege, Marie began to act in television plays, including a locally produced drama for French TV, 'Un Homme à la mer'. She was aware of her limited experience and acting technique, so she went to Brussels to attend L'Ecole du Cirque. For several months, she was coached in acting, singing, dancing and acrobatics. In 1995, she made her stage debut, in Lyon, in the title role of "The Diary of Anne Frank" – which transferred to Paris after fifty performances. At around that time, she made her film debut, for Bertrand Tavernier, in *L'Appât,* which was greeted with critical acclaim. The director would employ her again in his film, *Safe Conduct.* In 1998, Marie became the face of Lancôme. In 2004, she gave birth to a daughter she christened Dune. She is in the recent hit, *Les Femmes de l'ombre.* – known in English as *Female Agents.*

My Father, the Hero (1991)
Marie (1994) **L'Appât** (1995)
Le Affinità elettive (1996)
Un air si pur... (1997)
Le Bossu (1997)
The Dinner (1998)
Harem suaré (1999)
Barnie et ses petites contrariétés (2001)
Safe Conduct (2002)
Not For or Against (2002)
L'Enfer (2005)
Ma vie n'est pas une comédie romantique (2007)
La Clef (2007)
Les Femmes de l'ombre (2008)

Annie **Girardot**
5ft 5in
(ANNIE SUZANNE GIRARDOT)

Born: **October 25, 1931**
Paris, France

After she left school in the late 1940s, Annie began training for a nursing career. After a short time, friends and members of her own family remarked on her natural flair for comedy, and told her to consider a career as an actress. In 1949, she became a student at the Conservatoire de la rue Blanche and in the evenings, using the name Annie Girard, appeared in cabaret at La Rose Rouge in Montmartre. Annie then joined the famous Comédie-Française and was highly praised by Jean Cocteau for her 1956 performance in "La Machine à écrire". A year earlier, Annie had made her film debut in *Treize à table* but her appearances in later films, especially two with screen icon, Jean Gabin, led to employment for Luchino Visconti, in her breakthrough movie, *Rocco and his Brothers.* One of her co-stars in that film, the Italian actor, Renato Salvatori, became her husband in 1962, and they remained together until his death in 1988. Their daughter, Giulia is an actress. In 1965, Annie was voted Best Actress at the Venice Film Festival, for *Trois chambres à Manhattan.* For the next forty years, Annie was an important force in the French cinema – acting in nearly one hundred movies. Sadly, that might now be halted: In 2006, the French magazine "Paris Match" revealed that she is suffering from Alzheimer's disease. Her last appearance was in the 2007 release, *Christian.*

Rocco e i suoi fratelli (1960)
The Organizer (1963)
Shock Treatment (1973)
Doctor Françoise Gailland (1975)
Cours après moi que je t'attrape (1976)
Hit List (1984)
Comédie d'amour (1989)
Les Miserables (1995)
La Pianiste (2001)
This Is My Body (2001)
Epstein's Night (2002)
Je préfère qu'on reste amis (2005)
Caché (2005)

Lillian **Gish**
5ft 5¹/₂in
(LILLIAN DIANA DE GUICHE)

Born: October 14, 1893
Springfield, Ohio, USA
Died: February 27, 1993

Lillian, her sister, Dorothy, and their mother, Mary, were abandoned by their father when they were small girls. In order to support them, Mary became a stage actress. When they were in their teens, they all began to appear in theaters and Lillian once played a supporting role to the legendary Sarah Bernhardt. In 1912, they were introduced to the director, D.W. Griffith, by Mary Pickford. Both girls made their film debuts with her, in *An Unseen Enemy.* Within two years, Lillian was known as "The First Lady of the Screen". Her silent credits included *Birth of a Nation, Broken Blossoms, Way Down East, Orphans of the Storm, The Scarlet Letter* and *The Wind.* In 1920, she tried directing for the only time, and decided that it was a job for men. Lillian made her talkie debut in 1930, in *One Romantic Night,* but she wasn't overly impressed by the medium and she acted on the stage for most of that decade. It wasn't until she neared her fifties that she established herself as a film actress. She was nominated for a Best Supporting Actress Oscar, for *Duel in the Sun,* and was superb in *Night of the Hunter.* Lillian retired after making her final film, *The Whales of August.* She was eight months short of one hundred, when dying of heart failure.

One Romantic Night (1930)
His Double Life (1933)
Commandos Strike at Dawn (1942)
Top Man (1943)
Miss Susie Slagle's (1946)
Duel in the Sun (1946)
Portrait of Jennie (1948)
The Cobweb (1955)
The Night of the Hunter (1955)
Orders to Kill (1958)
The Unforgiven (1960)
Follow Me, Boys! (1966)
Warning Shot (1967)
The Comedians (1967)
A Wedding (1978)
Sweet Liberty (1986)
The Whales of August (1987)

Jackie **Gleason**
5ft 10¹/₂in
(HERBERT JOHN GLEASON)

Born: Febuary 26, 1916
Brooklyn, New York City, New York, USA
Died: June 24, 1987

His father, Herb Gleason, an immigrant from Ireland, who worked as an insurance auditor, abandoned his wife Mae, and their two sons early on. Jackie's brother died young and he was raised by his mother, who died when he was nineteen. He had a somewhat sketchy education in New York, but showed a natural gift as a master of ceremonies and later as a radio disc jockey. In the 1930s. Jackie was a nightclub comedian, whose talents first gained wider recognition when he appeared on Broadway, in the show, "Follow the Girls". In 1936, he married the first of three wives, Genevieve Halford. He made his film debut in 1941, in a musical comedy, *Navy Blues,* but his film output during the 1940s and 50s was small. He was best known from 1952, for the 'Jackie Gleason Show' on television – which ran, with a couple of breaks – until 1970. He was also popular at that time for the series of lush, best-selling musical albums he recorded for Capitol, beginning in 1953, with "Music for Lovers Only" and including "Music, Martinis and Memories" and "Champagne Candlelight and Kisses". His excessive drinking and womanizing were legendary, but his hour of movie fame came in *The Hustler,* when he was absolutely outstanding as the great pool player, "Minnesota Fats". He was nominated for a Best Supporting Actor Oscar. After his final movie *Nothing in Common,* he died in Fort Lauderdale, Florida – of colon and liver cancer. His daughter, Linda, is an actress.

Navy Blues (1941)
All Through the Night (1941)
Lady Gangster (1942)
Larceny Inc. (1942)
The Hustler (1961) Gigot (1962)
Requiem for a Heavyweight (1962)
Papa's Delicate Condition (1963)
Soldier in the Rain (1963)
How to Commit Marriage (1969)
Smokey and the Bandit (1977)
The Toy (1982)
Nothing in Common (1986)

James **Gleason**
5ft 10in
(JAMES AUSTIN GLEASON)

Born: May 23, 1882
New York City, New York, USA
Died: April 12, 1959

The son of theatrical folk, William and Mina Gleason, Jim was only sixteen when he left home to fight in the Spanish-American War. On his return in 1898, he joined his parents' stock company in Oakland, California. In 1905, he married childhood sweetheart, Lucile Webster – remaining with her until her death in 1947. A fifteen year stage career was interrupted by army service during World War I. In 1919, he began to appear on Broadway, and three years later, he made his film debut, in *Polly of the Follies.* Jim was primarily a stage actor, who had a voice worth hearing. Silent movies didn't convey that power and he waited until the 'talkies' before getting very seriously involved, in both by co-writing the screenplay and acting in, the Academy Award-winning movie, *The Broadway Melody* of 1929. Jim became a prominent character actor – nominated for a Best Supporting Actor Oscar, in *Here Comes Mr. Jordan.* His son Russell – who was making a living in Hollywood, had just been drafted into the army when he fell to his death from a hotel window. Russell's wife, Cynthia Lindsay wrote a biography of screen legend, Boris Karloff. Jim died of Asthma in Woodland Hills.

The Ex-Mrs. Bradford (1936)
Meet John Doe (1941)
Here Comes Mr. Jordan (1941)
My Gal Sal (1942)
Manila Calling (1942)
Crash Dive (1943)
A Guy Named Joe (1943)
Arsenic and Old Lace (1944)
A Tree Grows in Brooklyn (1945)
The Clock (1945)
The Bishop's Wife (1947)
The Dude Goes West (1948)
The Life of Riley (1949)
I'll See You in My Dreams (1951)
Suddenly (1954)
The Night of the Hunter (1955)
Loving You (1957)
Man or Gun (1958)
The Last Hurrah (1958)

Brendan **Gleeson**
6ft 2in
(BRENDAN GLEESON)

Born: **March 29, 1955**
Dublin, Ireland

When he was a child, Brendan was fond of the Irish playwrights, and loved reading and play-acting. During his teenage years, he began performing – at school in plays like "Waiting for Godot" – and in local stage productions. After two years with the Dublin Shakespeare Festival, he studied acting at RADA in London. He returned to Dublin intent on a stage career, but as it took a while to get going, and he needed an income (he'd got married and started a family) Brendan became a teacher of English and drama – which helped to keep his interest alive. Eventually, he auditioned for the Royal Shakespeare Company, at Stratford Upon Avon – spending two years performing in the classics. In 1989, he had his first TV role, in 'Dear Sarah. He made his film debut in 1990, in *The Field,* which starred Richard Harris. In 1997, he was given his first starring role – in *I Went Down.* For his work in *The General,* he won a Best Actor Award from Boston Society of Film Critics, and won an Irish Film and TV Award and a London Critics Circle. Since then, he's been a busy actor – working in Europe as well as Hollywood. He's a *Harry Potter* regular and co-starred with Colin Farrell, in the excellent black comedy, *In Bruges.* His next movie, *Into the Storm,* sees him as Winston Churchill.

Into the West (1992) Braveheart (1995)
Michael Collins (1996)
Trojan Eddie (1996) Before I Sleep (1997)
I Went Down (1997)
The General (1998) Harrison's
Flowers (2000) Saltwater (2000)
Artificial Intelligence: AI (2001)
28 Days Later (2002) Gangs of New
York (2002) Dark Blue (2002)
Cold Mountain (2003) Country of My
Skull (2004) The Village (2004)
Kingdom of Heaven (2005)
Breakfast on Pluto (2005)
The Goblet of Fire (2005)
The Tiger's Tale (2006) Black Irish (2007)
The Order of the Phoenix (2007)
Beowulf (2007) In Bruges (2008)

Scott **Glenn**
6ft
(THEODORE SCOTT GLENN)

Born: **January 26, 1941**
Pittsburgh, Pennsylvania, USA

Scott's parents were business executive, Theodore Glenn, and his wife, Elizabeth. Growing up in Appalachia proved a very tough period for Scott, who because of childhood illnesses, was bedridden for a year, and threatened with the prospect of limping for the rest of his life. Through sheer determination, he underwent hard training programs and cured it. Scott majored in English at the William and Mary College, before doing three years service in the Marines. He spent a few months as a crime reporter, and planned to become an author. A problem with dialogue led him to take acting classes in New York, with George Morrison. Scott had walk on parts in a couple of TV shows, starting in 1965. He made his Broadway debut that year, in "The Impossible Years". In 1968, he joined the Actors Studio, and landed his first film role two years later, in *The Baby Maker.* The fifteen years after *Urban Cowboy,* was a rollercoaster, but following the vintage Glenn years of 1990 and 1991, there was a slump. Since then, several good movies, starting with *Training Day* and *Buffalo Soldiers,* have proved the old adage that you can't keep a good man down.

Nashville (1975)
Apocalypse Now (1979)
Urban Cowboy (1980)
Personal Best (1982)
The Right Stuff (1983)
The River (1984) Silverado (1985)
Miss Firecracker (1989)
The Hunt for Red October (1990)
The Silence of the Lambs (1991)
My Heroes Have Always
Been Cowboys (1991)
Backdraft (1991)
Carla's Song (1996)
Training Day (2001)
Buffalo Soldiers (2001)
The Shipping News (2001)
Freedom Writers (2007)
Camille (2007)
The Bourne Ultimatum (2007)
Nights in Rodanthe (2008)
W. (2008)

Danny **Glover**
6ft 3½in
(DANNY LEBERN GLOVER)

Born: **July 22, 1946**
San Francisco, California, USA

Both of Danny's parents, James and Carrie Glover, were postal workers. After graduating from George Washington High School, he attended American University and matriculated at San Francisco State University. It was there, that he met his future wife, Asake Bomani. Danny got a job with the city administration and was in his late twenties when he enrolled in the Black Actors Workshop, at the American Conservatory Theater. He also trained with Jean Shelton at his Actors Lab. In 1979, he had his first professional assignment, in Clint Eastwood's, *Escape from Alcatraz.* His first featured role in a movie, was as Loomis, in the 1984 Sci-Fi drama, *Iceman.* In 1987, Danny played the title role in the TV drama 'Mandela'. There was a flurry of good pictures in the 1980s and 1990s, which included the entertaining, *Lethal Weapon* series, with Mel Gibson. In more recent years, he has proved his staying power with a mixture of serious and fun roles as seen in *Manderlay,* and *Be Kind Rewind.* Danny has also used his voice for children's animated films, *The Adventures of Brer Rabbit* and *Barnyard.*

Iceman (1984)
Places in the Heart (1984)
Witness (1985)
Silverado (1985)
The Color Purple (1985)
Lethal Weapon (1987)
Lethal Weapon 2 (1989)
Grand Canyon (1991)
Lethal Weapon 3 (1992)
Bopha! (1993)
Switchback (1997)
Lethal Weapon 4 (1998)
The Royal Tenenbaums (2001)
Saw (2004) Manderlay (2005)
Missing in America (2005)
Dreamgirls (2006)
Poor Boy's Game (2007)
Shooter (2007)
Honeydripper (2007)
Be Kind Rewind (2008)
Blindness (2008)
Night Train (2009)

Paulette **Goddard**
5ft 4in
(MARION GODDARD LEVY)

Born: **June 3, 1910**
Long Island, New York, USA
Died: **April 23, 1990**

When she was twelve, her parents split up, so she was forced to quit school and go out to work. She was blessed with a pretty face and with the help of a little subtle padding, she was able to pass as older than her fourteen years and become a Ziegfeld Girl. Four years later, she married a timber magnate, but when that turned sour, she went off with her mother, to Hollywood. Her first film appearance was as a train passenger, in Laurel and Hardy's *Berth Marks,* a 1929 silent. She was in the chorus of Eddie Cantor's, *The Kid from Spain,* in 1931, when she met her mentor and later, her husband, Charlie Chaplin. He coached her and starred her in his 1936 silent film, *Modern Times,* and she progressed to featured roles where she talked – most notably in the classic Bob Hope picture, *The Cat and the Canary.* Her confidence was so high in 1939, she even tested for the role of Scarlett O'Hara. There was another Chaplin movie, *The Great Dictator,* but they divorced shortly afterwards. A Bob Hope comedy, *Nothing But the Truth,* began six years of stardom. She was nominated for a Best Supporting Actress Oscar for *So Proudly We Hail!* In 1959, she married author, Erich Remarque and retired to enjoy her big collection of jewelry. The Italian film *Gli Indifferenti,* was her last. Paulette died of heart failure at her home in Ronco, Switzerland.

Modern Times (1936)
The Young In Heart (1938)
The Cat and the Canary (1939)
The Ghostbreakers (1940)
The Great Dictator (1940)
Nothing But the Truth (1941)
Reap the Wild Wind (1942)
So Proudly We Hail! (1943)
Kitty (1945)
Diary of a Chambermaid (1946)
Unconquered (1947
An Ideal Husband (1947)
On Our Merry Way (1948)
Vice Squad (1953)
Time of Indifference (1964)

Whoopi **Goldberg**
5ft 5in
(CARYN ELAINE JOHNSON)

Born: **November 13, 1955**
New York City, New York, USA

Whoopi was the daughter of a preacher, Robert James Johnson, and his wife, Emma, who was a nurse and a teacher. Whoopi began performing in children's theaters when she was eight. She would later adopt the second name Goldberg, in response to her mother's observation that Johnson was not Jewish enough to make her rich. After dropping out of high school, she became addicted to heroin – marrying her drug counselor – who was the first of three husbands. She then worked in a mortuary applying make-up to corpses, and for a time, as a bricklayer. Moving to California, Whoopi made her screen debut in 1982, in *Citizen.* A one-woman series of monologues – "The Spook Show" was so successful it transferred to Broadway. Steven Spielberg saw her performance one evening and cast her in his film *The Color Purple.* She won a Golden Globe for her portrayal of Celie Johnson and was also nominated for a Best Actress Oscar. There were a few comedy films, starting with the modestly successful *Jumpin' Jack Flash,* but Whoopi shone in a good dramatic role, in *Clara's Heart.* She won a Best Supporting Actress Oscar and a Golden Globe for *Ghost.* Up until the late 1990s, her movie career went smoothly. Since then, Whoopi's best work has been on television, but *If I Had Known I Was A Genius* is a pretty good comedy.

The Color Purple (1985)
Clara's Heart (1988)
Ghost (1990)
The Long Walk Home (1990)
Soapdish (1991)
The Player (1992)
Sister Act (1992)
Sarafina! (1992)
Corrina, Corrina (1994)
Boys on the Side (1995)
Ghosts of Mississippi (1996)
Girl, Interrupted (1999)
Golden Dreams (2001)
Rat Race (2001)
If I Had Known I Was
A Genius (2007)

Jeff **Goldblum**
6ft 4½in
(JEFFREY LYNN GOLDBLUM)

Born: **October 22, 1952**
Pittsburgh, Pennsylvania, USA

Jeff was one of four children born to a Jewish doctor, Harold Goldblum, and his wife, Shirley, who had experience as a radio broadcaster. Jeff moved to New York when he was seventeen – determined to pursue an acting career. His first step was to fine tune his skills at Sanford Meisner's Neighborhood Playhouse. In the early 1970s, he began acting regularly in both on and off-Broadway productions. He made his film debut in 1974, in a small but telling role – as a rapist, in Michael Winner's violent revenge movie, *Death Wish.* For the next few years, Jeff was a busy supporting actor in a variety of films – one of the most notable being *Annie Hall.* In 1980, he tried his hand at television, in the short-lived comedy series, 'Tenspeed and Brown Shoe'. He first got the attention he deserved, for his work as a magazine reporter in *The Big Chill.* For thirteen years, from 1987, Jeff was married to Geena Davis, who co-starred with him three times during a period when both were at their creative peaks. In 1995, Jeff's only directorial effort to date, was the Oscar-nominated, short comedy – *Little Surprises.* Jeff has done voice overs for TV commercials for Apple as well as the recent spots for the National Lottery on Irish TV. He's currently starring in the U.S television detective series, 'Raines'.

The Big Chill (1983)
Silverado (1985)
The Fly (1986) Earth Girls Are
Easy (1988) The Tall Guy (1989)
Deep Cover (1992)
Jurassic Park (1993) Powder (1995)
Independence Day (1996)
Chain of Fools (2000)
One of the Hollywood Ten (2000)
Igby Goes Down (2002)
Dallas 362 (2003)
Spinning Boris (2003)
The Life Aquatic with
Steve Zissou (2004)
Fay Grim (2006)
Man of the Year (2006)
Adam Resurrected (2008)

Matthew **Goode**
6ft 2in
(MATTHEW WILLIAM GOODE)

Born: April 3, 1978
Exeter, Devon, England

The youngest of five children, Matthew grew up in the little Devon village of Clyst St. Mary. His father is a geologist and his mother a nurse, who also got involved in local amateur theater. She was the one who encouraged her son's early interest in acting, and whenever possible, featured him in her productions. After leaving school, Matthew studied drama at the University of Birmingham, and in London, classical theater, at the Webber Douglas Academy of Dramatic Art. He appeared on the London stage in a number of plays, most notably as Ariel, in Shakespeare's "The Tempest". In 2002, Matthew had a supporting role in the TV production, 'Confessions of an Ugly Stepsister'. It was followed by his film debut, starring in the Spanish *Al sur de Granada* (South from Granada) and a higher profile movie for Warner Bros. – *Chasing Liberty*. In 2005, Matthew featured in the Emmy-nominated biography of naturalist Gerald Durrell, 'My Family and Other Animals'. During that year, his work in Woody Allen's, *Match Point,* received good notices and Matthew followed up with an equally impressive performance in the romantic comedy, *Imagine Me and You*. Like any actor, he needs some luck in selecting the right parts. He's in a couple of big movies which certainly fit the bill, including a film version of Evelyn Waugh's famous 1945 novel, *Brideshead Revisited*. Anyone who saw the 1981 television miniseries will certainly remember what a dramatic story it is. The new movie version is terrific, and should be enjoyed by a whole new generation. One can confidently predict that the future for Matthew is looking good! His latest film, *Watchmen,* confirms it.

South from Granada (2003)
Chasing Liberty (2004)
Match Point (2005)
Imagine Me & You (2005)
Copying Beethoven (2006)
The Lookout (2007)
Brideshead Revisited (2008)
Watchmen (2009)

Cuba **Gooding Jr.**
5ft 10in
(CUBA M. GOODING JR.)

Born: January 2, 1968
The Bronx, New York City, New York, USA

Cuba and his brother Omar, were the sons of Cuba Gooding Sr., lead vocalist with the soul group, "The Main Ingredient" and his wife, Shirley, who was also a singer with the "Sweethearts". None of that musical talent rubbed off on Cuba, who, after his dad abandoned the family, became a born-again Christian in 1972. He was then raised by his mother who had to struggle to support the two boys and their sister. He attended four different schools during those years – at one of which, he was a classmate of Janet Jackson. In his teens Cuba did a bit of fashion modeling and performed as a breakdancer with singer Lionel Richie. He eventually graduated from the John F. Kennedy High School, in Los Angeles. In 1986, he got his first TV role, in an episode of 'Hill Street Blues'. Two years later, he made his film debut with a small part in the Eddie Murphy movie, *Coming to America*. In 1991, he was on the list – as one of John Willis' Promising New Actors. After several years together, he married his high school sweetheart, Sara, in 1994. The couple now have three children. Cuba's big breakthrough was in *Jerry Maguire,* for which he received an Oscar as Best Supporting Actor. The pick of his recent work is in *American Gangster.*

Boyz n the Hood (1991)
Gladiator (1992)
A Few Good Men (1992)
Judgement Night (1993)
Outbreak (1995)
Losing Isiah (1995)
Jerry Maguire (1996)
As Good as It Gets (1997)
What Dreams May Come (1998)
Instinct (1999)
Men of Honor (2000)
Rat Race (2001)
Radio (2003)
Shadowboxer (2005)
American Gangster (2007)
Hero Wanted (2008)
Harold (2008) Linewatch (2008)
Lies & Illusions (2009)

John **Goodman**
6ft 2in
(JOHN STEPHEN GOODMAN)

Born: June 20, 1952
St. Louis, Missouri, USA

John was the son of postal worker, Leslie Goodman, and his wife, Virginia. After his father died from a heart attack just before John's second birthday, his seventeen-year-old brother Leslie stepped in and became a surrogate father to him and his baby sister. His mother worked hard to make sure that they all had a future and gave them every encouragement. John attended Affton High School, before graduating from Southwest Missouri State University with a drama degree. It wasn't a passport into show business – before his career got started, he was a night club bouncer and a waiter. In 1975, he hosted 'Saturday Night Live' – the first of eleven such appearances. His movie debut was in the 1977 drama, *Jailbait Babysitter,* and another early screen role was in a Burger King commercial, where all he had to do was bite into one and look as if he was enjoying it. In 1985, John was in the Broadway cast of "Big River" – a musical based on Huckleberry Finn's adventures. From 1988 to 1997, John starred as Dan Conner, in the TV sitcom, 'Roseanne'. In New Orleans, when filming *Everybody's All American,* he met his wife Annabeth. The couple now live there with their daughter Molly. John is now busier than ever.

Sweet Dreams (1985)
True Stories (1986)
Raising Arizona (1987)
The Big Easy (1987)
Everybody's All American (1988)
Sea of Love (1989)
Always (1989)
Arachnophobia (1990)
Barton Fink (1991)
Matinee (1993) Fallen (1998)
Bringing Out the Dead (1999)
O Brother, Where Art Thou? (2000)
My First Mister (2001)
One Night at McCool's (2001)
Dirty Deeds (2002) Beyond the
Sea (2004) Evan Almighty (2007)
Speed Racer (2007)
Gigantic (2008) Confessions of
a Shopaholic (2009)

Ruth **Gordon**
5ft 1in
(RUTH GORDON JONES)

Born: **October 30, 1896**
Quincy, Massachusetts, USA
Died: **August 28, 1985**

Ruth was brought up in an extremely strict family environment. Her father Clinton Jones, who was the softer of her parents, was captain on board a merchant ship, so in his absence, much of her early childhood was spent with her mother, Annie, who ruled with a very firm hand. Ruth was educated at Quincy High School. It was while she was there, that she got seriously interested in the theater. She started collecting the autographs of her favorite stage actresses, and by the time she graduated, she persuaded her father to allow her to make it her career. In 1914, he took Ruth to New York, where he enrolled her at the American Academy of Dramatic Art. A year later, she was an extra in the film, *The Whirl of Life,* but more importantly, she made her Broadway debut, in "Peter Pan". The stage was her world until, at the age of forty-four, she was persuaded to appear with the fine actor, Raymond Massey, in the movie *Abe Lincoln in Illinois.* Ruth enjoyed the new experience and was soon supporting Greta Garbo, and acting with Humphrey Bogart. But she returned in 1944, to more triumphs on Broadway in "The Strings, My Lord, Are False" and "Three Sisters". She and her husband, Garson Kanin, were nominated for Best Screenplay Oscars – for *A Double Life, Adam's Rib* and *Pat and Mike.* An Oscar nomination for her movie comeback role, in *Inside Daisy Clover,* was followed by an Oscar as Best Supporting Actress, for *Rosemary's Baby.* Ruth died of a stroke in Edgartown, Massachusetts.

Abe Lincoln in Illinois (1940)
Dr, Ehrlich's Magic Bullet (1940)
Two-Faced Woman (1941) Edge of
Darkness (1943) Action in the North
Atlantic (1943) Inside Daisy Clover (1965)
Lord Love a Duck (1966) Rosemary's
Baby (1968) Whatever Happened to
Aunt Alice? (1969) Where's
Poppa? (1970) Harold and Maude (1971)
Scavenger Hunt (1979) Any Which Way
You Can (1980) Maxie (1985)

Marius **Goring**
5ft 10in
(MARIUS BLACKMAN GORING)

Born: **May 23, 1912**
Newport, Isle of Wight, England
Died: **September 30, 1998**

The son of Doctor Charles Buckman Goring M.D. and Kate MacDonald, Marius was educated on the Isle of Wight until he was eleven. He was then sent to board at The Perse School, in Cambridge. He became a key performer in school plays and made his London stage debut when he was fifteen. He went on to study at the Universities of Paris, Frankfurt, Munich and Vienna, before attending the Old Vic Dramatic School, in London. In 1929, he was a founding member of the actors union, 'UK Equity'. He married the first of his three wives, in 1931. By 1934, Marius had a string of theater credits under his belt, including the Old Vic, Sadler's Wells, and a West End debut, at the Shaftesbury Theater, in "The Voysey Inheritance". Two years later, he made his film debut with a bit part in *The Amateur Gentleman.* At the outbreak of World War II, he began army duty after appearing in the first Powell-Pressburger collaboration, *The Spy in Black* – the first of four appearances for them. After his last screen appearance, in *Strike It Rich,* Marius was awarded a CBE in 1991. He died of cancer at his home in Heathfield, East Sussex.

The Spy in Black (1939)
Pastor Hall (1940)
The Case of the
Frightened Lady (1940)
A Matter of Life and Death (1946)
The Red Shoes (1948)
Odette (1950) Pandora and the
Flying Dutchman (1951)
Circle of Danger (1951)
The Magic Box (1951)
So Little Time (1952)
The Man Who Watched the
Trains Go By (1952)
The Barefoot Contessa (1954)
Quentin Durward (1955)
I Was Monty's Double (1958)
Up from the Beach (1965)
First Love (1970)
Zeppelin (1971) Little Girl in
Blue Velvet (1978)

Ryan **Gosling**
6ft 1in
(RYAN THOMAS GOSLING)

Born: **November 12, 1980**
London, Ontario, Canada

He was the youngest of two children born to Mormon parents – Thomas Gosling, a paper mill employee, and his wife, Donna. Because he was the victim of bullying at his elementary school, Ryan was taught his school lessons at home by his mother until the family moved to Burlington, Ontario, where he attended the Lester B. Pearson High School. It was during that time, that he and his sister Mandi, began to enter talent contests as singers. When he was thirteen, Ryan beat over 17,000 aspiring young actors in an open audition for a spot on the 'Mickey Mouse Club' television show. For two years he lived with the family of one of his co-stars, Justin Timberlake. With no formal training as an actor, Ryan was able to charm his way into TV roles – beginning in 1995, with the series, 'Are You Afraid of the Dark?'. The following year, he made his film debut, in *Frankenstein and Me,* which was shot in Montreal. There were three more years of television work before his first Hollywood film, *Remember the Titans.* It was only a small part, but the movie was a huge hit. Later that year, he was highly praised for his work in the *The Believer.* Ryan kept improving with each role and it was no surprise when he was nominated for a Best Actor Oscar, for *The Notebook.* In the recent *Lars and the Real Girl,* he shows his funny side and was nominated for a Golden Globe Award. Apart from his fine acting ability, Ryan is also an outstanding modern jazz guitarist. He's also executive producer on the upcoming film, *Broken Kingdom.*

Remember the Titans (2000)
The Believer (2001)
The Slaughter Rule (2002)
The United States of
Leland (2003)
The Notebook (2004)
Stay (2005)
Half Nelson (2006)
Fracture (2007)
Lars and the Real Girl (2007)
All Good Things (2009)

Louis **Gossett Jr.**
6ft 4in
(LOUIS CAMERON GOSSETT JR.)

Born: May 27, 1936
Brooklyn, New York City, New York, USA

Louis grew up in the Coney Island area of Brooklyn, where his dad, Louis Gossett Sr., worked as a porter, and his mother, Rebecca, was a nurse. He attended Abraham Lincoln High School, where he was a success both academically and as an athlete. It was in fact a sports injury that forced him to turn his attention to acting. At sixteen, he was in the school version of "You Can't Take It With You" and then auditioned successfully for the Broadway production of "Take a Giant Step". His performance in that won him the 1954 Donaldson Award, for most promising newcomer to the theater. He went to New York University on an athletic scholarship, where he was a star basketball player, but a chance to play for the New York Kicks wasn't enough to lure him away from a career as an actor. He appeared in the Broadway play, "A Raisin in the Sun" in 1959, and following television work, Louis made his film debut, in 1961, in the highly regarded Sidney Poitier movie version. Throughout the 1960s Louis concentrated on stage work and was frequently seen on television. In 1977, he won an Emmy for his acting in 'Roots'. In the 1980s, his film career picked up pace again and he won a Best Supporting Actor Oscar, for *An Officer and a Gentleman*. Since the early 1990s, a large proportion of Louis's best roles have been in television productions. He has been married three times.

A Raisin in the Sun (1961)
Leo the Last (1970)
The Landlord (1970)
Skin Game (1971)
Travels with My Aunt (1972)
The White Dawn (1974)
The River Niger (1976)
The Deep (1977)
An Officer and a Gentleman (1982)
Finders Keepers (1984)
Enemy Mine (1985)
The Punisher (1989)
Digtown (1992)
Club Soda (2006)
The Perfect Game (2008)

Betty **Grable**
5ft 4in
(ELIZABETH RUTH GRABLE)

Born: December 18, 1916
St. Louis, Missouri, USA
Died: **July 2, 1973**

Betty was the daughter of John Grable, and his wife, Lillian Rose. On each family vacation, Betty's father would take the family to a different part of the United States. After one trip, her mother liked California so much, she decided to stay. In Los Angeles, when she was twelve, Betty began dancing classes. In 1929, she had a small part as a dancer on her film debut, in a Fox musical *Let's Go Places*. The following year, she quit school and worked in burlesque shows. She then became a Goldwyn Girl and changed her name to Frances Dean, but was known as Betty Grable, when she took a job as a singer with Ted Fiorito's Band. Betty sang in an Astaire and Rogers musical and toured as well as making a film with Wheeler and Woolsey. In 1937, she had her first leading role, in *This Way Please,* for Paramount. Switching to 20th Century Fox made her a star in Technicolor musicals throughout World War II. She (her shapely legs were insured for more than Dietrich's) was the G.I.'s favorite pin-up. In 1944 she married Harry James and it lasted until 1965. As the 1940's drew to a close, so did Betty's career. In 1955, her last film, *How to Be Very, Very Popular,* simply proved that she no longer was. Betty retired in 1958, after appearing on the 'Chrysler Shower of Stars' TV show. In later years, she suffered from demophobia (fear of crowds). She died of lung cancer, in Santa Monica.

Down Argentine Way (1940)
I Wake Up Screaming (1941)
Song of the Islands (1942)
Springtime in the Rockies (1942)
Coney Island (1943)
Diamond Horseshoe (1945)
The Dolly Sisters (1945)
Mother Wore Tights (1947)
That Lady in Ermine (1948)
When My Baby Smiles at Me (1948)
Wabash Avenue (1950)
My Blue Heaven (1950)
Meet Me After the Show (1951)
How to Marry a Millionaire (1953)

Heather **Graham**
5ft 8in
(HEATHER JOAN GRAHAM)

Born: January 29, 1970
Milwaukee, Wisconson, USA

Heather's parents are a former FBI man, James Graham, and his wife, Joan, who is an author of children's books. Joan had earlier been a schoolteacher. Heather and her sister Aimee (who would also become an actress and a writer), grew up in a strict Catholic home environment. Heather was a shy little girl who found the frequent moves due to her father's work, unsettling. Even so, she developed a love for acting and in her early teens, her mother would drive her to auditions, which in 1984, resulted in her first movie role – a small one, in *Mrs. Soffel*. By the time Heather attended Agoura High School, she was considered by her classmates to be a "theater geek" and voted "Most Talented" by her senior class. She went to live in Los Angeles and got small roles in films and on TV. It was a slow process, so in 1989, she enrolled at UCLA, to study drama. After two years her career started to move again when James Woods cast her in his film, *Diggstown*. She then concentrated on acting – supplementing her income by modeling for Emanuel Ungaro Liberte. Heather has already won ensemble awards, for *Boogie Nights* and *Bobby* and a Blockbuster Entertainment Award for *Austin Powers: The Spy Who Shagged Me,* but her true star status has yet to be achieved. In 2008, she was Emily Sanders in TV's 'Emily's Reasons Why Not'.

The Ballad of Little Jo (1993)
Six Degrees of Separation (1993)
Desert Wind (1994) Mrs. Parker
and the Vicious Circle (1994)
Swingers (1996)
Entertaining Angels (1996)
Boogie Nights (1997)
Austin Powers: The Spy Who
Shagged Me (1999)
Bowfinger (1999)
Committed (2000)
Sidewalks of New York (2001)
From Hell (2001) The Guru (2002)
Bobby (2006)
Gray Matters (2006) Broken (2006)
Miss Conception (2008)

Gloria **Grahame**
5ft 6in
(GLORIA HALLWARD)

Born: **November 28, 1923**
Los Angeles, California, USA
Died: **October 5, 1981**

Gloria's father, Reginald Hallward, was an industrial designer. Her mother was the British-born actress and acting coach, whose stage-name was Jean Grahame. She provided Gloria with her movie name. Gloria was discovered acting in a high school play which was seen by a theatrical agent. He got her a job as an understudy to Miriam Hopkins, in the Broadway play "The Skin of Our Teeth". She was twenty-one when she landed a contract with MGM, who gave her a debut in a little comedy called *Blonde Fever.* A loan-out to RKO in 1946, was lucky for her – it happened to be in the all-time favorite – *It's a Wonderful Life.* Only a few of the movies she made after that were as wonderful, but there were some good ones. In 1949, she married the young director, Nicholas Ray. She was just okay when he directed her in *A Woman's Secret,* but superb in his *In a Lonely Place,* a year later – when she more than matched Humphrey Bogart. Her best period was the 1950s – which included a Supporting Actress Oscar for *The Bad and the Beautiful.* Highly-rated films were *The Big Heat* and *Oklahoma.* She had four children from four marriages – the last was with her former stepson, Anthony Ray. Gloria died in New York from a combination of cancer and peritonitis.

It's a Wonderful Life (1946)
It Happened in Brooklyn (1947)
Crossfire (1947)
Song of the Thin Man (1947)
In a Lonely Place (1950)
The Greatest Show on Earth (1952)
The Bad and the Beautiful (1952)
The Big Heat (1953)
Human Desire (1954)
The Cobweb (1955)
Not as a Stranger (1955)
Oklahoma (1955)
The Man Who Never Was (1956)
Odds Against Tomorrow (1959)
A Nightingale Sang in
Berkeley Square (1979)
Melvin and Howard (1980)

Farley **Granger**
6ft 1in
(FARLEY EARLE GRANGER II)

Born: **July 1, 1925**
San Jose, California, USA

The son of Farley Earle Granger Sr. and his wife, Eva Mae, Farley lived a comfortable childhood up until the stock market crash of 1929. His parents lost almost everything but they moved to a small apartment in San Jose, where his father ran an automobile dealership. Always a good-looking and popular boy at his high school, Farley was destined to find fame in the film industry. His father then worked as a clerk in a Hollywood unemployment office and got friendly with actors who came in to cash their checks. One of them, the silent screen comedian, Harry Langdon, gave him advice about his son's future and they were able to arrange for two of Sam Goldwyn's men to see Farley perform in "The Wookie" at a local theater. From that one viewing he got a small role in *The North Star.* Following a bigger part, in *The Purple Heart,* he joined the US Army. On his release, in 1946, he had a tough time getting his career re-started. Nicholas Ray's low-budget classic, *They Live by Night* earned him a recall from Goldwyn and a starring role in Hitchcock's *Rope.* Not much was offered by his studio, but in 1951, Farley had his best ever role in *Strangers on a Train.* From then on his Broadway work was usually superior to his later films. In 2001, Farley appeared in a comedy movie, *The Next Big Thing.* In 2007, he published his autobiography "Include Me Out" – written in collaboration with long-time partner, Robert Calhoun.

The North Star (1943)
The Purple Heart (1944)
They Live By Night (1948)
Rope (1948)
Enchantment (1948)
Side Street (1949)
Our Very Own (1950)
Strangers on a Train (1951)
I Want You (1951)
Hans Christian Andersen (1952)
The Story of Three Loves (1953)
Senso (1954)
The Serpent (1973)
The Prowler (1981)

Stewart **Granger**
6ft 3in
(JAMES LEBLANCHE STEWART)

Born: **May 6, 1913**
London, England
Died: **August 16, 1993**

Stewart was the grandson of a Victorian actor, Luigi Leblanche. After his education at Epsom College, he enrolled in an acting course at the Webber-Douglas School of Dramatic Art. He worked at the Old Vic in small roles as a film extra in *A Southern Maid,* in 1933. He spent three years with provincial repertory companies before hitting London with small parts in plays, starring Flora Robson – "Autumn" and Vivien Leigh – "Serena Blandish". After changing his name to avoid confusion with the American star, he played the romantic lead in *So This is London.* He then joined the Black Watch Regiment at the outbreak of war, but was invalided out after two years and continued with his film career with Gainsborough Studios. In 1949, he co-starred with Jean Simmons, in *Adam and Evelyne,* and she became his second wife. They went to Hollywood where he was given a seven-year contract with MGM. Stewart soon became Hollywood's most unpopular Englishman, but he made some good films there. Jean's career had taken off and by 1958, he couldn't cope with being second best, so they divorced. In 1968, he expressed the view that he'd never made a film that he was proud of. Most of the titles listed below will prove that he was wrong to say that. Stewart died of prostate cancer, at his home in Santa Monica, California.

The Man in Grey (1943)
Waterloo Road (1944)
Caesar and Cleopatra (1945)
Blanche Fury (1948)
Saraband for Dead Lovers (1948)
King Solomon's Mines (1950)
The Light Touch (1952)
Scaramouche (1952) **The Prisoner of
Zenda** (1952) **Moonfleet** (1955)
Footeps in the Fog (1955)
Bhowani Junction (1956)
The Last Hunt (1956)
North to Alaska (1960)
The Trygon Factor (1966)
The Wild Geese (1978)

Cary **Grant**
6ft 1¹/₂in
(ARCHIBALD ALEXANDER LEACH)

Born: **January 18, 1904**
Horfield, Bristol, England
Died: **November 29, 1986**

Following an unhappy childhood, when his mother, Elsie, was committed to a mental institution by his father, Elias Leach, Cary was expelled from Fairfield Grammar School at fourteen. He then became a stilt walker with a troupe which took him on a tour of the USA. He stayed there and performed small roles in musical comedies and supplemented his income by working as a male escort for wealthy socialites. In 1931, he went to Hollywood, where his name was changed to Cary Grant. He made his film debut the following year in the successful comedy, *This Is the Night*. With little training, he revealed a natural flair for that genre, and in the early 1930s, was not outshone by such established stars as Marlene Dietrich and Mae West. It was when he began playing in "Screwball Comedies" that his career took off. Cary used his suave sense of humor in other types of movies and he became a great favorite of Hitchcock's – in *Suspicion, Notorious, To Catch a Thief* and *North By North West*. He was loved by audiences all over the world. In the 1980s, he toured in "A Conversation with Cary Grant". Just before one such show – at the Adler Theater in Davenport, Iowa – he suffered a cerebral hemorrhage, and died.

The Eagle and the Hawk (1933)
She Done Him Wrong (1933)
Sylvia Scarlett (1935) **Topper** (1937)
The Awful Truth (1937)
Bringing Up Baby (1938)
Holiday (1938) **Gunga Din** (1939)
Only Angels Have Wings (1939)
His Girl Friday (1940) **My Favorite
Wife** (1940) **The Philadelphia Story** (1940)
Suspicion (1941) **Arsenic and
Old Lace** (1944) **Notorious** (1946)
I Was a Male War Bride (1949)
Monkey Business (1952)
To Catch a Thief (1955)
An Affair to Remember (1957)
Houseboat (1958) **Indiscreet** (1958)
North By North West (1959)
Charade (1963)

Hugh **Grant**
5ft 11in
(HUGH JOHN MUNGO GRANT)

Born: **September 9, 1960**
Hammersmith, London, England

Hugh's father, Captain James Grant, ran a carpet business after leaving the Seaforth Highlanders. In his spare time, he liked to paint. His mother, Fynvola, was a teacher, who taught Latin, French, and music during her thirty-year career. When he was a small boy, Hugh was taught to play the piano by Andrew Lloyd Webber's mother. After Latymer Upper School, where he excelled at rugby, cricket and soccer, he studied English at New College Oxford. While he was there, in 1982, he made his film debut, in *Privileged*. Hugh made his mind up to concentrate on an acting career after leaving Oxford – the early years were on television. Things began to move forward in 1987, when he shared the Best Actor Award at the Venice Film Festival, with his co-star in *Maurice* – James Wilby. It was a dozen films after that before he became an international name, following *Four Weddings and a Funeral*. Offers from America included a starring role opposite Julia Roberts, in *Notting Hill*. He has since been Renée Zellweger's love interest in the *Bridget Jones* series. His own love interest, with Liz Hurley, ended in 2000. Despite his arrest in Hollywood five years earlier, for lewd conduct with a prostitute, he and Liz remain good friends. In 2004 he began a three year relationship with Jemima Khan – the ex-wife of the Pakistani Test cricketer and politician, Imran Khan. Hugh is still single at the time of writing.

Maurice (1987)
The Dawning (1988)
La Nuit Bengali (1988)
Impromptu (1991)
Bitter Moon (1992)
The Remains of the Day (1993)
**Four Weddings and
a Funeral** (1994)
Sense and Sensibility (1995)
Notting Hill (1999)
Bridget Jones's Diary (2001)
About a Boy (2002)
American Dreamz (2006)
Music and Lyrics (2007)

Lee **Grant**
5ft 4in
(LYOVA HASKELL ROSENTHAL)

Born: **October 31, 1927**
New York City, New York, USA

Lee was the daughter of two Eastern European Jewish immigrants, Abraham and Witia Rosenthal. Both parents had a strong tradition of culture, and they gave every encouragement to Lee, who was actually performing as a ballerina, with the Metropolitan Opera in New York, at the age of four. She was eleven when she joined the American Ballet Theater, and later, studied music at Juilliard. After focussing on an acting career she established herself as a potential Broadway star – and got good notices for her performance as a shoplifter, in the stage play "Detective Story". When it was turned into a film, she made her screen debut and was nominated for a Best Supporting Actress Oscar. At that year's Cannes Film Festival, she won the Best Actress Award. Lee's path to fame stalled when she refused to testify against her husband Arnold Manhoff, before a House Un-American Activities Committee, and she was blacklisted in Hollywood for a time. There was no question about her acting ability - she continued working on stage and television. She returned to films in the 1960s – winning a Best Supporting Actress Oscar, for *Shampoo*. Apart from her film roles, since 1980, Lee's been directing films for the AFI and she won an Academy Award for her outstanding documentary – *Down and Out in America*.

Detective Story (1949)
Storm Fear (1955)
The Balcony (1963)
Divorce American Style (1967)
In the Heat of the Night (1967)
Buona Sera, Mrs. Campbell (1968)
Marooned (1969)
The Landlord (1970)
There Was a Crooked Man (1970)
Plaza Suite (1971) **Shampoo** (1975)
Voyage of the Damned (1976)
Little Miss Marker (1980)
Defending Your Life (1991)
The Substance of Fire (1996)
Mulholland Drive (2001)
Going Shopping (2005)

Richard E. **Grant**
6ft 2in
(RICHARD GRANT ESTERHUYSEN)

Born: **May 5, 1957**
Mbabane, Swaziland

Richard's father, an Afrikaaner, called Henrik Esterhuysen, was a head of education for the British government's administration in Swaziland, a landlocked country bordered by South Africa (on three sides) and Mozambique. His mother, who was of German stock, taught ballet in the capital, Mbabane. He began his education at the local school, St. Mark's, and went outside the city for his secondary schooling, at Waterford Kamhlaba. When he was in his early teens his parents split up. In the 1970s, Richard attended the University of Cape Town, in South Africa, where he studied English and Drama. In 1982, with a little bit of stage experience under his belt, he moved to London. The first thing he had to work on was his accent, which to English ears, sounded old-fashioned 'colonial'. In 1986, Richard married Joan Washington, with whom he would have two children. His first acting job was that year in a teleplay, 'Honest, Decent & True'. He made his film debut in *Withnail and I*. It required him to play a drunk and as he was a teetotaler, he had extra coaching from the director, Bruce Robinson, in the form of a bottle of Vodka which he drank in one sitting. His subsequent films didn't require such sacrifice and he was soon acting in Hollywood productions, including *The Player*. In 2008, Richard appeared in Madonna's directorial debut, *Filth and Wisdom*. In October, in Sydney, Australia, he made his musical theater debut, as Professor Henry Higgins in "My Fair Lady".

Withnail and I (1987)
Hidden City (1988) **How to Get Ahead in Advertising** (1989)
L.A. Story (1991 **The Player** (1992)
Dracula (1992) **The Age of Innocence** (1993) **Jack & Sarah** (1995)
The Cold Light of Day (1996)
Twelfth Night (1996)
The Serpent's Kiss (1997) **Keep the Aspidistra Flying** (1997) **St. Ives** (1998)
The Match (1999) **Gosford Park** (2001)
Monsieur N. (2003) **Penelope** (2006)
Filth and Wisdom (2008)

Bonita **Granville**
5ft
(BONITA GRANVILLE)

Born: **February 2, 1923**
Chicago, Illinois, USA
Died: **October 11, 2000**

Bonita was born into a show business family – both parents, Bernard 'Bunny' Granville and his wife Dorothy, were on the stage and her father was a Ziegfeld Follies star. Bonita herself took her first steps to fame when she was three-years-old. She was only nine when she made her film debut in *Westward Passage,* and ten when she appeared in the award-winning movie, *Cavalcade.* Bonita was a talented child actress, who progressed seamlessly into adulthood – via roles – often as spoilt kids, in such pictures as *Ah, Wilderness!, Merrily We Live,* and the very misleadingly titled, *The Beloved Brat.* From 1938, she began to grow up in a series of Nancy Drew movies and co-starred in some excellent features. In 1947, she married the oil millionaire and producer, Jack Wrather, with whom she had two daughters and two sons. Bonita's film career slowed after that, but she and her husband co-produced the "Lassie" TV series in 1954. They owned a hotel within sight of Disneyland, in Anaheim, California. Bonita died of cancer at her home in Santa Monica, California.

Ah, Wilderness! (1935)
These Three (1936)
It's Love I'm After (1937)
White Banners (1938)
The Beloved Brat (1938)
My Bill (1938) **Hard to Get** (1938)
**Nancy Drew -
Private Detective** (1938)
Reporter (1939)
Troubleshooter (1939)
The Mortal Storm (1940)
Third Finger, Left Hand (1940)
Gallant Sons (1940)
H.M.Pelham, Esq. (1941)
Syncopation (1942) **The Glass Key** (1942) **Now Voyager** (1942)
Hitler's Children (1943)
Song of the Open Road (1944)
Suspense (1946) **The Guilty** (1947)
Guilty of Treason (1950)
The Lone Ranger (1956)

Coleen **Gray**
5ft 3½in
(DORIS BERNICE JENSEN)

Born: **October 23, 1922**
Staplehurst, Nebraska, USA

Although the daughter of a Nebraskan corn farmer and his wife, Coleen grew up with a natural sophistication and a kind of beauty that would look right in the big cities. After graduating from high school, where she shone in stage presentations, Coleen went to study drama at Hamline University in Red Wing, Minnesota. She left with a bachelor of arts degree. She then moved to California – first to La Jolla, where she worked as a waitress – then on to Los Angeles, where she attended acting classes. She soon got stage roles in local presentations such as "Letters to Lucerne" and "Brief Music", which led, in 1944, to a contract with 20th Century-Fox. They changed her name to Colleen Gray, and sent her to the studio's "starlet school". A bit part later that year, in the Betty Grable musical, *Pin Up Girl,* was her modest debut, but after marriage to the producer/director, Rodney Amateau, and a couple of uncredited film appearances, she registered strongly in the film-noir classics, *Kiss of Death,* with Victor Mature and Richard Widmark, and the same year's *Nightmare Alley* – co-starring Tyrone Power. From the late 1950s until 1986, Coleen was seen regularly on TV. With her third husband, Fritz Zeiser, she is involved in the non-profit Prison Fellowship.

Kiss of Death (1947)
Nightmare Alley (1947)
Fury at Furnace Creek (1948)
Red River (1948)
Sand (1949)
I'll Get You For This (1950)
Father is a Bachelor (1950)
Riding High (1950)
The Sleeping City (1950)
Kansas City Confidential (1952)
The Fake (1953)
The Killing (1956)
Star in the Dust (1956)
Death of a Scoundrel (1956)
The Vampire (1957)
Hell's Five Hours (1958)
P.J. (1968) **The Late Liz** (1971)
Cry from the Mountain (1985)

Kathryn **Grayson**
5ft 2in
(ZELMA KATHRYN ELISABETH HEDRICK)

Born: **February 9, 1922**
Winston-Salem, North Carolina, USA

Kate received her vocal training as a child in St. Louis, then studied with Frances Marshall of the Chicago Civic Opera. She was still at high school when she was approached by MGM scouts. The studio had lost Deanna Durbin to Universal and were desperate to find a replacement. Having already proven herself on Eddie Cantor's radio show, Kate was signed without a screen test, in 1939. She spent the next two years being groomed for stardom. She made her film debut in 1941, in the title role of *Andy Hardy's Private Secretary* – and sang "Voices of Spring" by Johann Strauss. She supported Abbott and Costello in *Rio Rita,* before being given her first starring role, in *Seven Sweethearts. Thousands Cheer* became her launching pad. She co-starred with Gene Kelly and Frank Sinatra in *Anchors Aweigh* and had a dress rehearsal for the future *Show Boat* in *Till the Clouds Roll By.* Kate's teaming with Mario Lanza, in *That Midnight Kiss* and *The Toast of New Orleans,* did wonders for her – MGM was doubtful after *The Kissing Bandit* bombed. The superb *Show Boat* and two more with Howard Keel, secured it. Her films are of another age, but are charming because of the music. Kate made her operatic debut in 1960, and was on stage and TV until 1989. In the 1990s, Kate gave private classes in voice training. Twice divorced, she has a daughter named Patricia.

Thousands Cheer (1943)
Anchors Aweigh (1945)
Till the Clouds Roll By (1946)
Two Sisters from Boston (1946)
It Happened in Brooklyn (1947)
That Midnight Kiss (1949)
The Toast of
New Orleans (1950)
Grounds for Marriage (1951)
Show Boat (1951)
Lovely to Look at (1952)
The Desert Song (1953)
So This Is Love (1953)
Kiss Me Kate (1953)
The Vagabond King (1956)

Richard **Greene**
6ft
(RICHARD GREENE)

Born: **August 25, 1918**
Plymouth, Devon, England
Died: **June 1, 1985**

His parents were a couple of Plymouth-based repertory company actors, Richard Abraham Greene and Kathleen Gerrard. His aunt – was actress, Evie Greene, and his grandfather was the motion-picture inventor, William Friese-Greene. Following junior school, Richard went to Cardinal Vaughan Memorial School, in London. His first acting role was in a production of "Julius Caesar". In 1934, he had a bit part in the Gracie Fields musical film, *Sing As We Go.* In 1936, he joined the Brandon Thomas Repertory Company, and made his breakthrough in "French Without Tears". Richard was pursued by Zanuck and signed a contract with Fox. He went to Hollywood to co-star with Loretta Young, in *Four Men and a Prayer.* He was touted as a rival to MGM's Robert Taylor, but didn't reach that level of stardom. His first wife, from 1941 to 1951 was the English actress, Patricia Medina. After his film career, which faded around the time he appeared in *Forever Amber,* Richard became famous in the title role of TV's 'The Adventures of Robin Hood' and he bred horses. He was in poor health from 1982, when he suffered injuries from a fall. He died of cardiac arrest, at his home in Norfolk, England.

Four Men and a Prayer (1938)
My Lucky Star (1938)
Submarine Patrol (1938)
Kentucky (1938)
The Hound of the Baskervilles (1939)
Stanley and Livingstone (1939)
Little Old New York (1940)
I Was an Adventuress (1940)
Unpublished Story (1942)
Yellow Canary (1943)
Don't Take It to Heart (1944)
Forever Amber (1947)
The Fighting O'Flynn (1949)
The Fan (1949)
My Daughter Joy (1950)
The Black Castle (1952)
Beyond the Curtain (1960)
Tales from the Crypt (1972)

Sydney **Greenstreet**
6ft
(SYDNEY HUGHES GREENSTREET)

Born: **December 27, 1879**
Sandwich, Kent, England
Died: **January 18, 1954**

One of eight children born to a leather merchant and his wife, Sydney left home at eighteen to become a tea planter in Ceylon. He was forced out of business and had to return home because of a prolonged drought. In England, he got a job as the manager of a brewery. In his spare time he took acting lessons, and progressed enough to make his stage debut in Ramsgate, in 1902, as the murderer in a Sherlock Holmes play. After touring the UK with a Shakespearian company, he made his New York debut, in 1905. He appeared in numerous plays over more than thirty years and refused all offers to appear in films. In 1918, Sydney married Dorothy Marie Ogden and they had a son. For some reason, he changed his mind about movies aged sixty-two, when he began working for Warner Brothers, in Hollywood. He made up for lost time by appearing in twenty-four films from a 1941 debut in *The Maltese Falcon* – in which he was first teamed with Peter Lorre and was nominated for a Best Supporting Actor Oscar. He made his last film *Malaya* – with Spencer Tracy, James Stewart and Lionel Barrymore. Sydney's health deteriorated and he retired as he reached the age of seventy. He battled with diabetes and Bright's disease and died in Hollywood.

The Maltese Falcon (1941)
They Died with Their
Boots On (1941)
Across the Pacific (1942)
Casablanca (1942)
Background to Danger (1943)
Between Two Worlds (1944)
The Mask of Dimitrios (1944)
Christmas in Connecticut (1945)
Three Strangers (1946)
The Verdict (1946)
The Hucksters (1947)
The Woman in White (1947)
Ruthless (1948)
The Velvet Touch (1948)
Flamingo Road (1949)
Malaya (1949)

Joan **Greenwood**
5ft 2in
(JOAN GREENWOOD)

Born: **March 4, 1921**
Chelsea, London, England
Died: **February 27, 1987**

Joan was the daughter of the British artist, Sydney Earnshaw Greenwood. She was educated at St. Catherine's School, at Bramley, in Surrey. Joan studied acting at RADA before making her stage debut in "Le Malade Imaginaire" in 1938 – at the Apollo Theater, in London. Her film debut was in *John Smith Wakes Up* – In 1940. She had a small role in Leslie Howard's *The Gentle Sex* then joined Donald Wolfit's theater company. Joan's first starring role in a film was in 1946, as an artist's model in *Latin Quarter*. In 1947 she signed for J. Arthur Rank, but after The *October Man* with John Mills, she appeared in three flops including the very bad, *The Bad Lord Byron*. In 1949, Joan was rescued by Ealing Studios, who borrowed her for two of their classic comedies, and re-united her with Alec Guinness, in *The Man in the White Suit*. Her unique sexy voice became popular with audiences and she used it to maximum effect in Oscar Wilde's farce, *The Importance of Being Earnest*. In 1954, the year of her first appearance on the Broadway stage, in "The Confidential Clerk", she was at her best on film, with the French star, Gerard Philipe, in *Knave of Hearts*. She married André Morell in 1959. Their son, Jason is an actor. Joan died from a heart attack at her home in London after completing her final film *Little Dorrit*.

The October Man (1947)
Saraband for Dead Lovers (1948)
Whiskey Galore (1949)
Kind Hearts and Coronets (1949)
Whiskey Galore (1949)
The Man in the White Suit (1951)
The Importance of Being
Earnest (1952)
Knave of Hearts (1954)
Father Brown (1954)
Moonfleet (1955)
Stage Struck (1958)
Mysterious Island (1961)
Tom Jones (1963)
The Moon-Spinners (1964)
Little Dorrit (1988)

Jane **Greer**
5ft 5in
(BETTEJANE GREER)

Born: **September 9, 1924**
Washington, DC., USA
Died: **August 24, 2001**

Jane was outstandingly beautiful as a little girl. By the time she was in her mid-teens, she had won a beauty-contest and had become a professional model. Around that time, she worked as a singer, with Enrico Madriguera's Orchestra, at the Latin Club Del Rio, in Washington. She began her film career after her photo on the cover of Life magazine was spotted by the ever-watchful, Howard Hughes. In 1942, she arrived in Hollywood and to escape Howard's clutches, that same year, she married the forty-year-old crooner, Rudy Vallee, whom she had first met on a radio show. It lasted eight months due to some extent to Hughes's jealousy. He punished her by starving her of good opportunities until he loaned her out for what was her greatest role – Kathie Moffatt, in the 1947 film noir classic, *Out of the Past*. Jane married the movie producer and racehorse breeder, Edward Lasker, and they were together until after her film roles had virtually dried up, in 1963. During those sixteen years, apart from another film with Mitchum, *The Big Steal,* there was little else of "classic" quality. In 1984, she was in the re-make, called *Against All Odds* – playing the mother of her original character, Kathie Moffat. She retired after her final film, *Perfect Mate*. She died of cancer in Los Angeles. Jane's two sons, Alex and Lawrence Lasker, are writer/producers.

Sinbad the Sailor (1947)
They Won't Believe Me (1947)
Out of the Past (1947)
Station West (1948) **The Big Steal** (1949)
The Company She Keeps (1951)
The Prisoner of Zenda (1952)
The Clown (1953)
Run for the Sun (1956)
Man of a Thousand Faces (1957)
Where Love Has Gone (1964)
Billie (1965)
The Outfit (1973)
Immediate Family (1989)
Perfect Mate (1996)

Judy **Greer**
5ft 10in
(JUDITH LAURA EVANS)

Born: **July 20, 1975**
Livonia, Michigan, USA

As a little girl, Judy showed great potential as a dancer. For ten years, she trained in classical Russian ballet at Bunny Sanford's School of Dance, in Livonia. Judy was educated at the Winston Churchill High School, where she participated in the Creative and Performing Arts Program and eventually showed a preference for acting as a career. At De Paul University, in Chicago, Judy starred in plays such as "Insignificance" and "Yellow Boat", before graduating in 1997. That same year, Judy made her television debut in an episode of 'Early Edition'. Shortly after that, she made her film debut, in an independent production, a thriller titled, *Stricken*. Judy quickly proved to have a natural gift for comedy, and it is in those kind of movie roles with which she has had most success – good examples being *13 Going on 30, The Great New Wonderful, American Dreamz*, and *The Grand*. At the start of her career she had taken acting lessons from Jeffrey Tambor. In 2003 she played the role of his mistress, in the television drama, 'Arrested Development'. In recent times, Judy has starred as Becky Freeley, in the television comedy series, 'Miss Guided'.

Kissing a Fool (1998)
Three Kings (1999)
The Big Split (1999)
What Planet Are
You From? (2000)
The Specials (2000)
What Women Want (2000)
Rules of Love (2002)
The Hebrew Hammer (2003)
13 Going on 30 (2004)
The Village (2004)
LolliLove (2004)
The Great New Wonderful (2005)
In Memory of
My Father (2005)
Elizabethtown (2005)
American Dreamz (2006)
The TV Set (2006)
The Go-Better (2007)
The Grand (2007)
27 Dresses (2008)

John Gregson
5ft 10in
(HAROLD THOMAS GREGSON)

Born: **March 15, 1919**
Liverpool, Lancashire, England
Died: **January 8, 1975**

Of Scottish descent, John attended the St. Francis Xavier School, in Liverpool. When he was seventeen, he hitch-hiked to Denham Studios looking for work as an extra. Robert Donat told him to learn to act first. He joined an amateur group, but the war started and he spent six years on a minesweeper. He worked for a year with the Liverpool Old Vic, then in 1946, when he was acting with the Perth Repertory Company, he met his future wife, Thea. He made his film debut in 1948, with a small role in Stewart Granger's, *Saraband for Dead Lovers*. There were over forty movies in the next twenty-three years, including some classic Ealing comedies and the hugely popular *Genevieve*. He acted in several war films – usually as an army or navy officer – which kept his screen career going well into the 1960s. From 1965, he worked mainly on television – being best-known for his role as Commander George Gideon, in the police series, 'Gideon C.I.D'. During the 1970s, John appeared in films as a supporting player. His last film was a horror comedy, *Fright*. When he died suddenly of a heart attack at the early age of fifty-five, he left a widow and six children.

Scott of the Antarctic (1948)
Whiskey Galore (1949)
Treasure Island (1950)
The Lavender Hill Mob (1951)
Angels One Five (1952)
The Holly and the Ivy (1952)
Genevieve (1953)
The Titfield Thunderbolt (1953)
Three Cases of Murder (1954)
Above Us the Waves (1955)
Jacqueline (1956) Rooney (1958)
Sea of Sand (1958)
The Captain's Table (1959)
The Frightened City (1961)
The Longest Day (1962)
Live Now – Pay Later (1962)
Tomorrow at Ten (1962)
The Night of the Generals (1967)
Fright (1971)

Virginia Grey
5ft 5in
(VIRGINIA GREY)

Born: **March 22, 1917**
Los Angeles, California, USA
Died: **July 31, 2004**

The daughter of the silent film actor, Ray Grey, one of Virginia's earliest baby-sitters was Gloria Swanson. When she was ten she made her movie debut, as Little Eva in *Uncle Tom's Cabin*. She had three more small roles in silents, before concentrating on her schooling. Her first talking picture was in 1931, in *Misbehaving Ladies,* and there was plenty of work as an extra. She signed a contract with MGM who gave her small parts in big films such as *The Great Ziegfeld* and *Rosalie*. In between she had an uncredited role in Laurel and Hardy's *Our Relations*. In 1936, there was a big part in a small film (a short) called *Violets in Spring*. Averaging six films a year, some of them opposite cowboy stars, Roy Rogers and Gene Autry, Virginia kept her face and lovely figure up there on the screen. She did her quota of B-movies and in one of them, *Swamp Fire,* she had what must be the unique experience of acting with two former Tarzans – Johnny Weissmuller and Buster Crabbe – in one picture. Virginia made her final movie appearance in *Airport,* and was last seen on television in 1976. A hopeless love affair with Clark Gable, during the 1940s, is believed to be the reason why she never got married. Virginia retired to Woodland Hills, where she died from heart failure.

The Captain is a Lady (1940)
The Big Store (1941)
Whistling in the Dark (1941)
Grand Central Murder (1942)
Tarzan's New York
Adventure (1942)
Sweet Rosie O'Grady (1943)
Swamp Fire (1946)
So This Is New York (1948)
The Bullfighter and
the Lady (1951)
The Rose Tattoo (1955)
All That Heaven Allows (1955)
No Name on the Bullet (1959)
The Naked Kiss (1964)
Rosie! (1967)
Airport (1970)

Hugh Griffith
5ft 9in
(HUGH EMRYS GRIFFITH)

Born: **May 30, 1912**
Marian Glas, Anglesey, Wales
Died: **May 14, 1980**

The son of William and Mary Griffith, Hugh was educated at his village school, and at Llangefni Grammar School, but failed his university entrance exams. He became a bank clerk – working for the National Provincial, in four different locations. Because of his interest in the theater, in his spare time Hugh taught drama at the national Welsh youth movement. After being transferred to London by the bank he began his own acting career with the St. Pancras People's Theater. He gained a place at RADA – being the top applicant out of a total intake of 300. That quality soon showed when Hugh gained a Bancroft Gold Medal, as Shakespearean actor of his year. He'd only had time for two television roles when World War II interrupted his plans. He served in India and Burma before re-starting his career in 1946. Hugh joined the Royal Shakespeare Company and had small roles in films. His first major picture was *So Evil My Love*. His movie career highlights were a Best Supporting Actor Oscar, for *Ben-Hur* and a nomination, for *Tom Jones*. Hugh died of a heart attack in London.

So Evil My Love (1948)
The Last Days of Dolwyn (1949)
Kind Hearts and Coronets (1949)
Gone to Earth (1950)
The Titfield Thunderbolt (1953)
The Sleeping Tiger (1954)
Lucky Jim (1957) Ben Hur (1959)
The Story on Page One (1959)
Exodus (1960)
The Counterfeit Traitor (1962)
Lisa (1962) Term of Trial (1962)
Mutiny on the Bounty (1962)
Tom Jones (1963)
How to Steal a Million (1966)
Oliver! (1968) The Fixer (1968)
The Canterbury Tales (1972)
The Final Programme (1973)
Luther (1973) The Last Remake of
Beau Geste (1977)
A Nightingale Sang in
Berkeley Square (1979)

Melanie **Griffith**
5ft 9¼in
(MELANIE GRIFFITH)

Born: August 9, 1957
New York City, New York, USA

Melanie is the only child of one of Alfred Hitchcock's favorite actresses, the former model, Tippi Hedren, who divorced her father – an advertising executive, Peter Griffith, when she was four. When she was only nine months old, Melanie starred in her first TV commercial. Tippi married the agent, Noel Marshall, who brought with him three stepbrothers for her daughter. Melanie appeared as an extra in *Smith!* when she was twelve. By the time she was fourteen, she had fallen in love with Don Johnson, and moved in with him. Two years later, she played her first featured role in the 1975 Gene Hackman film, *Night Moves*. Sadly, drug problems plagued her for the remainder of the 1970s, until she made her comeback, in Brian De Palma's *Body Double*. The next twenty years were a mixture of good and bad for her. Not only was she nominated for a Best Actress Oscar, for *Working Girl,* 1996 was the year of her second divorce from Don Johnson, and also the year she married the Spanish actor and director, Antonio Banderas. In 1999, Melanie made her stage debut at London's Old Vic Theater, in "The Vagina Monologues". Four years later, she got rave reviews when making her Broadway debut, as Roxie Hart, in "Chicago". Most of her recent work has been on television.

Night Moves (1975)
The Drowning Pool (1975)
Smile (1975)
Body Double (1984)
Something Wild (1986)
Stormy Monday (1988)
Working Girl (1988)
Pacific Heights (1990)
Paradise (1991)
Nobody's Fool (1994)
Mulholland Falls (1996)
Another day in Paradise (1997)
Lolita (1997)
Celebrity (1998)
Forever Lulu (2000)
The Night We Called It a Day (2003)
Shade (2003)

Charles **Grodin**
6ft
(CHARLES GRODINSKY)

Born: April 21, 1935
Pittsburgh, Pennsylvania, USA

The son of Orthodox Jewish parents, Theodore and Lena Grodin, who owned and ran a wholesale business, Chuck made an early (and very brief) first screen appearance at the age of nineteen, in Walt Disney's, *20000 Leagues Under the Sea*. After graduating from high school, Chuck attended the University of Miami, in Coral Gables, Florida, but didn't graduate. He switched his attention instead to studying acting with Uta Hagen and Lee Strasberg in New York. Chuck made his Broadway debut in 1962, opposite Anthony Quinn, in "Tchin Tchin". That same year, he was seen on television in an episode of 'The Defenders'. Two years later, he made his 'official' film debut in *Sex and the College Girl*. Chuck, who felt he was too old for the part, turned down the lead (played by Dustin Hoffman) in *The Graduate*. He did however, score high marks for a small but effective role in *Rosemary's Baby*. His first big opportunity came in the film of Neil Simon's *The Heartbreak Kid*. Although he is a pal of go-getter, Gene Wilder, he has shown little ambition to be more than a supporting actor in many of his films. In 1985, Chuck married his second wife, Elissa Durwood. They have two children and live in Wilton, Connecticut. At present, Chuck's big screen appearances are confined to family movies. He is a best-selling author of several books. His new one is expected in the stores in Spring 2009.

Rosemary's Baby (1968)
Catch-22 (1970)
The Heartbreak Kid (1972)
11 Harrowhouse (1974)
Heaven Can Wait (1978)
Real Life (1979)
Midnight Run (1988)
Cranium Command (1989)
Dave (1993)
So I Married an
Axe Murderer (1993)
Heart and Souls (1993)
It Runs in the
Family (1994)
Fast Track (2006)

Ioan **Gruffudd**
5ft 11in
(IOAN GRUFFUDD)

Born: October 6, 1973
Llwydcoed, Mid-Glamorgan, Wales

Ioan's parents, Peter Griffiths, and his wife Gillian, were teachers. Peter became a headmaster at two Welsh comprehensive schools. Ioan has a younger brother, Alun and a younger sister named Siwan. Ioan was educated at Ysgol Gymraeg Melin Gruffyd and Ysgol Gyfun Gymraeg Glantaf – where he sat his GCSE and A-Level exams and developed considerable ability as an oboist – appearing with the South Glamorgan Youth Orchestra. He also won prizes for his singing. Ioan made his acting debut in 1986, in a Welsh TV film called 'Austin' – then moved into a soap opera, 'Pobol y Cwm' (People of the Valley). At eighteen, Ioan won a scholarship to London's Royal Academy of Dramatic Art. In 1995, Ioan acted in his first English TV role, in 'A Relative Stranger' and two years after that, made his English language film debut, as John Gray, in *Wilde*. It was soon followed by a part in the Hollywood blockbuster, *Titanic*. From 1998, he became famous as Captain Horatio Hornblower, in the highly rated British television films of C.S. Forester's novels. In 2000, Ioan lit the National Millennium beacon in Cardiff. His big breakthrough internationally came in the *Fantastic Four* and its sequel – as the comic book character, 'Mister Fantastic'. Since September 2007, Ioan has been married to the British actress, Alice Evans. They live in Los Angeles.

Wilde (1997)
Titanic (1997)
Solomon and Gaenor (1999)
Happy Now (2001)
Black Hawk Down (2001)
The Gathering (2002)
This Girl's Life (2003)
King Arthur (2004)
Fantastic Four (2005)
The TV Set (2006)
Amazing Grace (2006)
4: Rise of the Silver Surfer (2007)
Fireflies in the Garden (2008)
The Secret of
Moonacre (2008)
W. (2008)

Harry **Guardino**
5ft 10in
(HAROLD GUARDINO)

Born: **December 23, 1925**
New York City, New York, USA
Died: **July 17, 1995**

Harry grew up in an Italian environment in Brooklyn. By the age of twelve he was already acting mad and getting juvenile roles in local stage productions. He was fifteen when World War II began and he couldn't wait to get into uniform. As soon as he was old enough he enlisted in the United States Navy and experienced action in the Pacific. When peace returned, Harry took a variety of jobs to boost his meagre income from acting. In 1951, he landed his first film roles – uncredited in *Sirocco,* and way down the cast list as Lt. Roberts in *Purple Heart Diaries.* There was plenty of TV work after that, but he had to wait until 1958 for movie recognition, when he was nominated for a Golden Globe and awarded the Foreign Critics Prize for Best Supporting Actor – in the film, *Houseboat* – starring Cary Grant and Sophia Loren. He had further nominations after that – including a Tony, in 1960, for "One More River" – but he remained primarily a character actor in films. He acted in several television series including 'The Reporter' and 'Perry Mason' but his face became well-known after *Dirty Harry.* He appeared three times with Clint Eastwood and in 1981, co-starred with Lauren Bacall on Broadway in the musical version of "Woman of the Year". Harry's later work was mainly on television. His final movie, in 1993, was the poor *Fist of Honor.* In 1985, he married Elyssa Patermoster. Harry died of bone cancer – in Palm Springs, California.

Houseboat (1958) **Pork Chop Hill** (1959)
The Five Pennies (1959)
King of Kings (1961)
The Pigeon That Took Rome (1962)
Hell is for Heroes (1962)
Madigan (1968)
Lovers and Other Strangers (1970)
Red Sky at Morning (1971)
Dirty Harry (1971) **St. Ives** (1976)
The Enforcer (1976)
Rollercoaster (1977)
Any Which Way You Can (1980)

Sir Alec **Guiness**
5ft 10in
(ALEC GUINESS DE CUFFE)

Born: **April 2, 1914**
Marylebone, London, England
Died: **August 5, 2000**

The name of Alec's biological father has never been identified, but it is known that his benefactor was a Scottish banker named Andrew Geddes. His mother was Agnes Cuff. When Alec first left school, he intended to conquer the world of advertising, as a copywriter. By the time he was 19, he'd begun studying at a school run by the actress Fay Compton. He had a walk-on part in "Libel" in 1934, and later that year, he was seen briefly in the film "Evensong". His career went to another level after he joined John Gielgud's company the following year. By 1938, he was in leading roles at the Old Vic – most notably in a modern-dress version of "Hamlet". After getting married, he joined the Royal Navy in 1941, but was given time off to appear on Broadway in "Flare Path". Rejecting Hollywood offers he appeared in a number of British films which are regarded as classics – including *Great Expectations, Oliver Twist, Kind Hearts and Coronets, The Lavender Hill Mob* and *The Ladykillers.* His Best Actor Oscar for *Bridge on the River Kwai,* was the beginning of a busy period internationally. He returned to the stage during the 1960s, but within a few years, he was an incredibly rich mega-star after appearing in *Star Wars* and its sequels. In 1985, he published his very amusing autobiography titled "Blessings in Disguise".

Great Expectations (1946)
Oliver Twist (1948)
Kind Hearts and Coronets (1949)
The Lavender Hill Mob (1951)
The Man in the White Suit (1951)
The Card (1952)
Father Brown (1954)
The Ladykillers (1955)
The Bridge on the River Kwai (1957)
The Horse's Mouth (1958)
Our Man in Havana (1959)
Tunes of Glory (1960)
The Fall of the Roman Empire (1964)
Doctor Zhivago (1965)
Cromwell (1970) **Star Wars** (1977)

Steve **Guttenberg**
6ft
(STEVEN ROBERT GUTTENBERG)

Born: **August 24, 1958**
Brooklyn, New York City, New York, USA

Steve is the son of Jerome Guttenberg, an electrical engineer, and his wife, Ann, who worked as a surgical assistant. After his parents moved out of Brooklyn when he was young. Steve grew up in a traditional Jewish household in North Massapequa, Long Island. He attended the local Plainedge High School from where he graduated in 1976. He then studied at The Juilliard School, State University of New York and UCLA. To prepare himself for an acting career Steve studied with the renowned Herbert Berghof. When he was nineteen, he made an uncredited appearance in the film *Rollercoaster.* It was also the year of Steve's first featured role on television – in ' Something for Joey'. He became a member of "The Groundlings", an improvisational comedy group which performed at the Helen Hayes Theater on Broadway and in London's West End. In 1980, Steve starred in a famous commercial for Coca-Cola, in which he helps a woman who can't speak English, but loves his Coke. During the 1980s, he starred in about eighteen movies of varying quality – especially his *Police Academy* films. in 1988, he married the actress Denise Bixler, but the couple divorced four years later. He was off the big screen for five years and until the new millennium, his film output was very disappointing. Steve's recent movie-acting efforts have indicated a welcome return to form.

The Boys from Brazil (1978)
Diner (1982)
Police Academy (1984)
Cocoon (1985)
Short Circuit (1986)
The Bedroom Window (1987)
Surrender (1987)
3 Men and a Baby (1987)
High Spirits (1988)
Home for the Holidays (1995)
The Stranger (2003)
Domino One (2005)
Mojave Phone Booth (2006)
Cornered! (2008)
Jackson (2008)

Edmund **Gwenn**
5ft 5½in
(EDMUND KELLAWAY)

Born: September 26, 1877
Wandsworth, London, England
Died: **September 6, 1959**

When Teddy was seventeen, his father kicked him out of the house for having the affront to suggest that he wished to become an actor. After traveling around the British Empire with various theatrical companies, Teddy married Minnie Terry and filed for divorce the following day. He settled in London in 1902 and the great George Bernard Shaw selected him for a role in "Man and Superman" which firmly established him as a character actor of some repute. The only interruption to his career was a two year period of military service during World War I. Teddy was exclusively a stage actor at that time, but in 1916, he made a one off appearance as Rupert K. Thunder, in a J.M.Barrie satire of Macbeth, *The Real Thing at Last.* It was one of only three films he made until *How He Lied to Her Husband,* in 1931, which began a love affair with the big screen that endured for over a quarter of a century. Teddy brightened dozens of movies during that period, *Pride and Prejudice* and *Lassie Come Home* are good examples, but none more so than when he won an Oscar for playing Kris Kringle in *Miracle on 34th Street.* From 1950, he suffered from severe arthritis. Teddy died of pneumonia in Woodland Hills – after a stroke.

The Bishop Misbehaves (1935)
Sylvia Scarlett (1935)
The Walking Dead (1936)
Anthony Adverse (1936)
A Yank at Oxford (1938)
Pride and Prejudice (1940)
Foreign Correspondent (1940)
The Devil and Miss Jones (1941)
One Night in Lisbon (1941)
Charley's Aunt (1941)
Lassie Come Home (1943)
Between Two Worlds (1944)
The Keys of the Kingdom (1944)
Miracle on 34th Street (1947)
Life with Father (1947)
Mister 880 (1950)
The Trouble with Harry (1955)
Calabuch (1956)

Jake **Gyllenhaal**
6ft
(JACOB BENJAMIN GYLLENHAAL)

Born: December 19, 1980
Los Angeles, California, USA

The son of the film and TV director Stephen Gyllenhaal and the producer and screenwriter, Naomi Foner, Jake didn't wait long to make his presence felt on the big screen. In 1991, on his screen debut, he had the role of Billy Crystal's son in the comedy *City Slickers.* He worked as a lifeguard before getting regular work as an actor. On a family note, he played the screen brother of his sister Maggie – in *Donnie Darko.* In 2002, he gave up his studies at Columbia University to allow him to concentrate on his acting career. Jake went to London for two months that year to star in "This is Our Youth" at The Garrick Theater. His fine performance won him a London Evening Standard Award as 2002's 'Outstanding Newcomer'. He made three films during that busy time, and was clearly much more than another promising actor when he co-starred with Dennis Quaid, in the blockbuster, *The Day After Tomorrow* . The following year, Jake was faced with one of the most challenging roles of his career. Initially, he was hesitant about playing a cowboy who succumbs to a homosexual relationship in *Brokeback Mountain.* In the event, the movie proved to be a landmark. He was nominated for a Best Supporting Actor Oscar and won a BAFTA in the same category. Jake's recent work – in *Zodiac* and *Rendition* – have been an indication of his rapid progress as an actor.

City Slickers (1991)
October Sky (1999)
Bubble Boy (2001)
Donnie Darko (2001)
Lovely & Amazing (2001)
The Good Girl (2002)
Highway (2002)
Moonlight Mile (2002)
The Day after
Tomorrow (2004)
Brokeback Mountain (2005)
Proof (2005)
Jarhead (2005)
Zodiac (2007)
Rendition (2007)

Maggie **Gyllenhaal**
5ft 9in
(MAGGIE RUTH GYLLENHAAL)

Born: November 16, 1977
New York City, New York, USA

Like her brother Jake, Maggie is the daughter of the film director Stephen Gyllenhaal, who is of Swedish descent. Her mother, Naomi Achs, is a producer and screenwriter from a New York Jewish family. Maggie was raised in Los Angeles. She was educated at the Harvard-Westlake preparatory school and The Mountain School in Vershire, Vermont. In 1999, she graduated from Columbia University with a BA in literature and Eastern religions. Maggie then went to London, England, where she spent the summer months studying acting at the Royal Academy of Dramatic Art. She made her film debut in 1992, in her father's *Waterland.* She acted in several small supporting roles before playing Darko's sister Elizabeth, opposite her real-life brother Jake, in *Donnie Darko.* A year later, Maggie's breakthrough role was as Lee Holloway, in *Secretary* – for which she received a Golden Globe nomination. She has a two-year-old daughter, Ramona with the actor Peter Sasgaard and they live in Brooklyn. If you can find it, catch Maggie in the short 2007 movie, *High Falls.* Apart from film work Maggie has modeled underwear for the famous British lingerie company, 'Agent Provocateur'.

The Photographer (2000)
Cecil B. DeMented (2000)
Donnie Darko (2001)
Secretary (2002)
Adaptation (2002)
Confessions of a
Dangerous Mind (2002)
Mona Lisa Smile (2003)
Criminal (2004)
Happy Endings (2005)
The Great New
Wonderful (2005)
Trust the Man (2005)
SherryBaby (2006)
Paris, je t'aime (2006)
World Trade Center (2006)
Stranger Than Fiction (2006)
The Dark Knight (2008)
Away We Go (2009)

H

Joan **Hackett**
5ft 7in
(JOAN ANN HACKETT)

Born: **March 1, 1934**
New York City, New York, USA
Died: **October 8, 1983**

Joan was raised in East Harlem, by strict Catholic parents. After she left high school, she attended New York University and earned extra money as a part-time model. She received acting training from Lee Strasberg. Following that training, she made her television debut in 1959, in the series 'Young Doctor Malone' and did one season in the law drama, 'The Defenders'. Joan got stage roles off-Broadway, where she came to prominence following her Obie-winning work in "Call Me by My Rightful Name", in 1961. She was given plenty of television work after that and was especially good in the small screen adaptation of 'Rebecca', in 1962. She was then Emmy-nominated for a 1964 episode of 'Ben Casey' Joan made her movie debut in the Sidney Lumet-directed, *The Group.* She was nominated for a BAFTA as Best Foreign Actress and consolidated her reputation in the excellent western, *Will Penny,* where she co-starred with Charlton Heston. In 1967, she married the actor, Richard Mulligan, whom she'd met while working on *The Group,* a year earlier. They were divorced in 1973. *Support Your Local Sheriff* proved that she could play comedy. *Mackintosh and T.J.* gave her the rare opportunity of acting with Roy Rogers. Joan's final film, *Only When I Laugh,* won her a Golden Globe Award for Best Supporting Actress and an Oscar-nomination in the same category. She made her final appearance in the 1987 movie, *Flicks.* Joan died of ovarian cancer, in Encino, California, at the age of forty-nine.

The Group (1966)
Will Penny (1968)
Assignment to Kill (1968)
Support Your Local Sheriff! (1969)
The Last of Sheila (1973)
Mackintosh and T.J. (1975)
Treasure of Matecumbe (1976)
One Trick Pony (1980)
Only When I Laugh (1981)
The Escape Artist (1982)

Gene **Hackman**
6ft 2in
(EUGENE ALLEN HACKMAN)

Born: **January 30, 1930**
San Bernardino, California, USA

Gene was the son of Eugene Ezra Hackman, who worked for a newspaper. His mother's name was Lyda. His parents split up when he was a child and he was raised by his maternal grandmother, Beatrice, in Danville, Illinois. When he was sixteen, Gene joined the United States Marine Corps and served three years as a field radio operator. Later, he used the G.I.Bill, to study television production and journalism at the University of Illinois. He was thirty when he decided to become an actor. He joined the Pasadena Playhouse, where he he befriended Dustin Hoffman. In New York, Gene worked as a doorman before getting parts in off-Broadway plays. He made his film debut, in 1964, in *Lilith* and earned a Best Supporting Actor Oscar nomination for *Bonnie and Clyde.* Gene was hot. After another nomination in 1970, he won his a Best Actor Oscar for the *The French Connection.* In 1986, after thirty years of marriage, Gene and his wife Faye, divorced. In 1991, he married Betsy Arakawa. A year after that, he won a Supporting Actor Oscar for *Unforgiven.* Gene continued to be a major screen presence up until 2004. He and Betsy are now living in Santa Fe, New Mexico.

Bonnie and Clyde (1967)
I Never Sang for
My Father (1970)
The French Connection (1971)
The Conversation (1974)
Bite the Bullet (1975)
Superman (1978)
Under Fire (1983)
No Way Out (1987)
Mississippi Burning (1988)
Narrow Margin (1990)
Unforgiven (1992)
The Firm (1993)
Geronimo (1993)
Crimson Tide (1995)
Get Shorty (1995)
Enemy of the State (1998)
The Royal Tenenbaums (2001)
Runaway Jury (2003)
Welcome to Mooseport (2004)

Jean **Hagen**
5ft 6in
(JEAN SHIRLEY VERHAGEN)

Born: **August 3, 1923**
Chicago, Illinois, USA
Died: **August 29, 1977**

Jean was the daughter of an immigrant from Holland, Christian Verhagen, and his Chicago-born wife, Marie. The family moved to Indiana when Jean was twelve. She was a graduate of Elkhart High School before majoring in drama at Northwestern University. She then headed for New York. She did day-shifts as an usherette in a movie theater, and in the evenings, acted in radio plays. In 1947, she married the character actor, Tom Seidel, with whom she had two children. Jean made her film debut in the Robert Taylor western, *Ambush,* in 1949, and that same year, she appeared in the Katherine Hepburn and Spencer Tracy comedy, *Adam's Rib.* In 1950, she got good notices for her first starring role, in the classic film noir, *The Asphalt Jungle.* A Best Supporting Actress Oscar nomination two years later for *Singing' in the Rain* failed to make her a star, but she will always be remembered for that role, as the silent screen star whose voice isn't quite right for the 'Talkies'. From 1953, she was Danny Thomas's wife, in the TV series, 'Make Room for Daddy'. It was to earn her two Emmy Award nominations, but she left after three seasons. She continued to work on television. One of her rare films, was the excellent, *Panic in the Year Zero!* In the mid-1960s, Jean began to suffer from ill-health which was a major cause of her divorce from Seidel, in 1965. After her final appearances in episodes of 'Starsky and Hutch', 'The Streets of San Francisco', and a TV movie, 'Alexander: The Other Side of Dawn', Jean died of throat cancer, in Los Angeles.

Ambush (1949)
Adam's Rib (1949)
The Asphalt Jungle (1950)
Singing' in the Rain (1952)
The Big Knife (1955)
The Shaggy Dog (1959)
Sunrise at Campobello (1960)
Panic in the Year Zero! (1962)
Dead Ringer (1964)

Julie **Hagerty**
5ft 7in
(JULIE HAGERTY)

Born: **June 15, 1955**
Cincinnatti, Ohio, USA

Both of Julie's parents were musical. Her father, Jerry Hagerty, was a musician and her mother, Harriet was a singer and a model. Apart from her good looks, Julie showed little sign of inheriting their talent herself. While she was attending Indian Hill High School, in her home town, she spent her summer vacations in New York, where she signed with Ford Models at the age of fifteen. She took some acting lessons in Cincinnatti and at Julliard, before settling in New York. She continued studying with the actor William Hickey. In Greenwich Village, she co-founded (with her brother Mike) a theatre troupe – The Production Company. It was to provide her with a nice variety of roles and eventually led to a starring role on Broadway, in "The House of Blue Leaves". Julie's first film scenes, in *All That Jazz,* were cut from the finished print, but a year later, she made a big impression in the successful parody, *Airplane!* What followed was a mixed bag in terms of quality, and the 1990s saw her get a divorce from husband, Peter Burkin. She appeared in supporting roles and made television movies. In 1996, Julie won the Los Angeles Drama Critics Award, for her outstanding performance, in "Raised in Captivity". In 2002 she hit a rich vein of form – on the Broadway stage, in the play, "Mornings at Seven" as well as several good roles in high-profile films.

Airplane! (1980)
**A Midsummer
Night's Sex Comedy** (1982)
Lost in America (1985)
What About Bob? (1991)
Noises Off (1992)
The Wife (1995)
Bridget (2002)
The Badge (2002)
Pizza (2005)
A Host of Trouble (2005)
Just Friends (2005)
She's the Man (2006)
Pope Dreams (2006)
**If I Had Known I Was
A Genius** (2007)

Barbara **Hale**
5ft 5½in
(BARBARA HALE)

Born: **April 18, 1922**
DeKalb, Illinois, USA

Barbara's father, Luther, was a landscape gardener. Her mother's name was Willa. Shortly after she was born, the family moved to Rockford, Illinois. When she was twelve, Barbara began taking lessons in both classical ballet and tap dancing. At high school, she revealed a talent for painting, so she enrolled at the Chicago Academy of Fine Arts. She pursued a career in advertising, but soon ended up working as a model. The boss of the Chicago Model Bureau sent her photos to RKO, and Barbara's successful screen test resulted in a contract. Her first screen appearance was a very brief one, in *The 7th Victim,* in 1943, but led to a decent supporting role, in Sinatra's debut movie, *Higher and Higher,* and a trio of westerns. In one of then, *West of the Pecos,* Barbara met and fell in love with future husband, the actor, Bill Williams. By 1953, she'd had three children. The marriage was a happy one – lasting forty-six years – until Bill's death. Barbara received an Emmy in 1959, for her role in the first Perry Mason television series. At Raymond Burr's insistence, Barbara was essential, when he was asked to make some TV-movies of the stories during the 1980s and 1990s. She continued to do so for two years after Ray's death, in 1993.

Higher and Higher (1943)
The Falcon Out West (1944)
The Falcon in Hollywood (1944)
West of the Pecos (1945)
Lady Luck (1946)
The Boy with Green Hair (1948)
The Clay Pigeon (1949)
The Window (1949)
Jolson Sings Again (1949)
The Jackpot (1950)
Emergency Wedding (1950)
The First Time (1952)
Last of the Comanches (1953)
A Lion is in the Streets (1953)
The Oklahoman (1957)
Slim Carter (1957)
Desert Hell (1958) **Airport** (1970)
Big Wednesday (1978)

Irma P. **Hall**
5ft 0½in
(IRMA DOLORES PLAYER HALL)

Born: **June 3, 1935**
Beaumont, Texas, USA

Irma's father was a jazz saxophone player. She was still a young child when her mother, Josephine, took her to live in Chicago. She attended the local Chicago elementary and high school before, in her teens, spending two years at Briar Cliff College, in Sioux City, Iowa. A few years after that, Irma graduated from Texas College, in Tyler, Texas, and for over thirty years, was a teacher of English and Foreign languages - Spanish and French – at various schools throughout the State – including four in Dallas. She also did work for the "Dallas Express" as Editor of the Entertainment and Sports sections. In 1972, Irma was employed as the interim publicist for the film, *Book of Numbers,* which starred its producer, Raymond St. Jacques. Raymond heard her reciting some of her poems and he gave Irma her film debut as 'Georgia Brown' in the film. At that time, Irma was a single mother with two children, and even in her wildest dreams she'd never considered becoming an actress. Two years later, her infectious enthusiasm helped found The Dallas Minority Repertory Theater. Irma's next experience was performing on stage for three years, before making her first TV appearances, in 'Dallas' – as Tilly, the housekeeper. She played small roles in films such as *Backdraft* and eventually became a highly respected character actress. Sadly, at the peak of her career in 2004, she was badly injured in a car crash. Irma is a very determined lady and was soon working again. Barely a year later, she was in two good short films.

A Family Thing (1996)
Soul Food (1997)
**Midnight in the
Garden of Evil** (1997)
Beloved (1998)
Patch Adams (1998)
A Slipping-Down Life (1999)
Don't Let Go (2002)
Bad Company (2002)
The Ladykillers (2004)
Collateral (2004) **Rain** (2008)

Mark **Hamill**
5ft 9in
(MARK RICHARD HAMILL)

Born: September 25, 1951
Concord, California, USA

Because Mark's father, William Thomas Hamill, a Unites States Navy captain, was frequently away on duty, Mark's mother, Virginia, raised seven children virtually on her own. Mark lived in several places as a child. He eventually graduated from Nile C. Kinnick High School, in Japan, before returning to America and majoring in drama, at Los Angeles City College. In 1970, he made his dramatic entrance, on 'The Bill Cosby Show' and among other early work, he voiced the character Corey Anders, for a TV cartoon series, 'Jeannie'. It was only his voice which was heard on his movie debut, in *Wizards,* but he shot to fame that year, when he became Luke Skywalker, in the blockbuster *Star Wars.* In 1978, he married Marilon York, a dental hygienist. They have three children. He fell into a bit of a rut from 1980 onwards, but he wasn't just sitting back. Mark's original childhood ambition was to be a cartoonist and his enthusiasm for the medium led to him co-writing the mini-series 'Black Pearl', then, in 2004, directing and starring in *Comic Book: The Movie,* which won the 2005 DVD Premiere Award. Mark's forty or so theater and TV films since *Star Wars* have included a number of voice assignments. He can be heard as 'The Joker' in the animated version of 'Batman' among others. He has also used his talents for video and computer games. Up until 2008, Mark's has been a familiar voice as Fire Lord Ozai, in the animated television-series, 'Avatar: The Last Airbender', and Senator Stampingston, in 'Metalocalypse'. Mark has plenty of other work at present.

Star Wars (1977)
The Empire Strikes Back (1980)
The Big Red One (1980)
Star Wars VI:
Return of the Jedi (1983)
Village of the Damned (1995)
Hamilton (1998)
Walking Across Egypt (1999)
Jay and Silent Bob
Strike Back (2001)
Reeseville (2003)

George **Hamilton**
6ft 1in
(GEORGE STEVENS HAMILTON)

Born: August 12, 1939
Memphis, Tennessee, USA

George's father, George "Spike" Hamilton, was a band leader, who encouraged his son's love of music. From his mother, Ann, he got his sophistication. Although not a great scholar, George went to some good schools, including Hackley, an exclusive private school, in Tarrytown, New York. At Palm Beach High School, in Florida, he was active in plays. When he was thirteen, George made his first appearance on the silver screen in a Clark Gable, Ava Gardner western, *Lone Star.* Before he left Palm Beach High School, he won the award for Best Actor – as Tommy Albright, in the musical "Brigadoon". In 1957, George arrived in Hollywood with style – borrowing a battered old Rolls Royce to drive to auditions. He made his featured-role movie debut as the law student, Robert, in a modern version of Dostoevsky – *Crime and Punishment USA.* From 1960, when he shared a Golden Globe Award as Best Newcomer, the handsome actor was a regular feature of films and TV. In 1965, he co-starred with the French icons, Brigitte Bardot and Jeanne Moreau, in *Viva Maria!* George never seemed to age and one endearing trait was his willingness to send himself up, as in *Love at First Bite, Zorro The Gay Blade* and *Doc Hollywood.*

Crime and Punishment (1959)
Home from the Hill (1960)
All the Fine Young Cannibals (1960)
Where the Boys Are (1960)
Angel Baby (1961)
By Love Possessed (1961)
Light in the Piazza (1962)
Two weeks in Another Town (1962)
The Victors (1963)
Your Cheatin' Heart (1964)
Viva Maria! (1965)
Jack of Diamonds (1967)
The Power (1968)
Love at First Bite (1979)
Zorro, the Gay Blade (1979)
The Godfather: Part III (1990)
Doc Hollywood (1991)
Off Key (2001)
The L.A. Riot Spectacular (2005)

Neil **Hamilton**
5ft 11in
(JAMES NEIL HAMILTON)

Born: September 9, 1899
Lynn, Massachusetts, USA
Died: **September 24, 1984**

Neil was an only child. A distant cousin of Margaret Hamilton, he was raised in a devoutly Catholic family environment and educated at West Haven High School, in Connecticut. He began his working life modeling Arrow shirts for magazine ads and then became interested in acting. He played small roles in stock company productions before, in 1923, being signed by D.W. Griffith, to play the John White, in *White Rose.* He appeared in several films directed by Griffith and had amassed a big list of credits by the time he moved to Paramount in the late 1920s – and had a new career in talking pictures. 1932 was a vintage year for Neil, but as the decade wore on, his film roles were confined more and more to B-pictures and later, working for Poverty Row studios. At one period, in the mid-1940s, Neil felt so negative and unhappy, he actually contemplated the idea of suicide. A priest changed his mind, and after nine days of prayer, he was offered a part in a movie for Universal. His TV career lasted until 1971 – his role in the movie, *Batman,* led to one hundred and twenty episodes of the television series – in the role of Commissioner Gordon. Neil was married for sixty-two years to Elsa Whitmer, with whom he had one child. His last role was in 1971, in a television drama called 'Vanished'. Neil died after suffering a severe asthma attack, at his home in Escondido, California.

The Dawn Patrol (1930)
Strangers May Kiss (1931)
The Sins of Madelon Claudet (1931)
Tarzan the Ape Man (1932)
The Animal Kingdom (1932)
Payment Deferred (1932)
What Price Hollywood? (1932)
Tarzan and His Mate (1932)
Hollywood Stadium Mystery (1938)
The Saint Strikes Back (1939)
Father Takes a Wife (1941)
King of the Texas Rangers (1941)
When Strangers Marry (1944)
Batman (1966)

Tom **Hanks**
6ft
(THOMAS JEFFREY HANKS)

Born: July 9, 1956
Concord, California, USA

Tom (the third of four children) was the son of Amos Hanks, who was a professional chef and a distant relation to Abraham Lincoln. His mother, Janet Frager, was a Portuguese American. Tom's parents got divorced when he was four, and he stayed with his dad. He was a shy and rather unpopular boy during his early years, but improved after going to Skyline High School in Oakland, where he appeared in school plays including "South Pacific". He studied acting at Chabot College before attending Sacramento State University. Tom then spent three years working in Cleveland, where he learned everything from lighting to stage management. While there, he won the Cleveland Critics Circle Award, for his portrayal of Proteus, in "The Two Gentlemen of Verona". In 1979, after he moved to New York, Tom made his film debut in *He Knows You're Alone*. After TV work, including guesting on 'Happy Days', Ron Howard starred him in the comedy, *Splash!* Following that promising start he couldn't buy a hit for nearly four years. When it happened, with *Big*, Tom was nominated for a Best Actor Oscar. From the 1990s, he was a winner – with Oscars for *Philadelphia* and *Forrest Gump*. In 2002, he and his wife Rita Wilson produced the hit movie, *My Big Fat Greek Wedding*. Tom and Rita have two children.

Big (1988) The 'burbs (1989)
Sleepless in Seattle (1993)
Philadelphia (1993)
Forrest Gump (1994)
Apollo 13 (1995)
Saving Private Ryan (1998)
You've Got Mail (1998)
The Green Mile (1999)
Cast Away (2000)
The Road to Perdition (2002)
Catch Me if You Can (2002)
The Terminal (2003)
The Polar Express (2004)
The Da Vinci Code (2006)
Charlie Wilson's War (2007)
The Great Buck Howard (2008)
Angels & Demons (2009)

Marcia Gay **Harden**
5ft 4in
(MARCIA GAY HARDEN)

Born: August 14, 1959
La Jolla, California, USA

Marcia was one of a family of five children born to a Texan, Thaddeus Harden, and his wife Beverly. Because her dad moved frequently due to his work, Marcia had first-hand knowledge of living and going to school overseas, including Germany, Greece and Japan. Eventually, the family settled in Maryland, where she attended Surrattsville High School, in Clinton. She had acting aspirations and gained a BA in theater from the University of Texas at Austin and completed a graduate theater program at New York University – from where she came away with a Master of Fine Arts. She had her first taste of film acting in 1979, when she appeared in a twenty-three minute short titled *Not Only Strangers*. Her feature film debut was in 1986, when she had a small role in *The Imagemaker*. She gained experience in TV dramas before co-starring with Gabriel Byrne, in her first big film, *Miller's Crossing* and was named one of twelve "Promising New Actors of 1990". There were more successful pictures and a chance to play Ava Gardner, in the TV film, 'Sinatra'. In 1993, Marcia made her Broadway debut in Tony Kushner's play "Angels in America" Marcia won a Best Supporting Actress Oscar for *Pollock* and was nominated for *Mystic River*. She is married to Thaddaeus Scheel, with whom she has three children.

Miller's Crossing (1990)
Late for Dinner (1991)
Crush (1992) Used People (1992)
Safe Passage (1994)
The Spitfire Grill (1996)
The First Wives Club (1996)
Desperate Measures (1998)
Meet Joe Black (1998)
Curtain Call (1999) Space
Cowboys (2000) Pollock (2000)
Gaudi Afternoon (2001)
Mystic River (2003)
Mona Lisa Smile (2003)
American Gun (2005) American
Dreamz (2006) The Hoax (2006)
Canvas (2006) Rails & Ties (2007)
Into the Wild (2007) The Mist (2007)

Ann **Harding**
5ft 2in
(DOROTHY WALTON GATLEY)

Born: August 7, 1901
Fort Sam Houston, Texas, USA
Died: **September 1, 1981**

Ann was the daughter of an army career officer, George C. Gatley, who served in the American Expeditionary Force during World War I. He moved his family all around the country before he retired and settled in New York City. Ann attended Bryn Mawr College, outside Philadelphia, before working as a script reader for a theatrical agent. Through the connections she made, Ann got small roles in Broadway plays, beginning with "Like a King" in 1921. After several years on the stage, she signed for Pathé in 1929, and made her film debut opposite Frederic March, in *Paris Bound*. To begin with, she was criticized for her theatrical mannerisms, but she improved her screen acting technique so quickly, by 1930, she was one of Hollywood's highest-paid stars. She had a Best Actress Oscar nomination for *Holiday,* and stayed at the top of the cast list throughout the first half of the decade. She co-starred with such luminaries as Cary Grant, Ronald Colman and Leslie Howard, but retired in 1937 after marrying conductor Werner Janssen. Five years later, Ann resurfaced and played supporting roles in movies like *Mission to Moscow, The North Star* and *The Man in the Gray Flannel Suit.* A return to Broadway in 1962 ended after only three performances. She died of natural causes at her home in Sherman Oaks, California.

The Animal Kingdom (1932)
The Life of Vergie Winters (1934)
Peter Ibbetson (1935)
Love from a Stranger (1937)
Eyes in the Night (1942)
Mission to Moscow (1943)
The North Star (1943)
Those Endearing Young
Charms (1945) It Happened on
5th Avenue (1947)
The Magnificent Yankee (1950)
Two Weeks with Love (1950)
The Unknown Man (1951)
The Man in the Gray
Flannel Suit (1956)

Sir Cedric **Hardwicke**
5ft 6in
(CEDRIC WEBSTER HARDWICKE)

Born: **February 19, 1893**
Lye, Worcestershire, England
Died: **August 6, 1964**

Cedric's father, a physician, had hoped his son would follow in his career path, but when the youngster enrolled at RADA in London, he gave him every support. After making his stage debut in 1912, he interrupted his career to serve in the army during World War I. In 1918, Cedric joined a repertory company in Birmingham. He was soon a famous figure on the British stage and was said to be George Bernard Shaw's favorite actor. He made his film debut in 1926, in *Nelson,* but resisted offers from MGM to go to Hollywood. He was knighted by King George V, in 1934, while appearing in "The Late Christopher Bean", in London. In 1935, he accepted a film role in *Becky Sharp,* and also made his Broadway debut, in "The Promise". He settled in Hollywood, and played what he considered his finest film role – Mr. Brink, in *On Borrowed Time.* He acted for Hitchcock and sang with Bing Crosby. He wrote his biography, "A Victorian in Orbit". He kept working up to the year he died of a lung ailment, in New York. Cedric was married twice and had two children.

Jew Süss (1934) Les Misérables (1935)
Things to Come (1936)
Tudor Rose (1936) Green Light (1937)
King Solomon's Mines (1937)
On Borrowed Time (1939)
Stanley and Livingstone (1939)
The Hunchback of Notre Dame (1939)
The Invisible Man Returns (1940)
Tom Brown's Schooldays (1940)
Suspicion (1941)
The Lodger (1944)
Sentimental Journey (1946)
I Remember Mama (1948)
Rope (1948)
The Winslow Boy (1948)
A Connecticut Yankee in King
Arthur's Court (1949)
The Desert Fox (1951)
Richard III (1955)
The Ten Commandments (1956)
Baby Face Nelson (1957)
The Pumpkin Eater (1964)

Oliver **Hardy**
6ft 1in
(OLIVER NORVELL HARDY)

Born: **January 18, 1892**
Harlem, Georgia, USA
Died: **August 7, 1957**

His father, (also named Oliver Hardy) was a Confederate veteran, who died when Oliver was only a few months old. The boy had a fine voice, and when he was eight, his mother Emily, who ran a small hotel, permitted him to spend his summer vacation touring with a troupe called Coburn's Minstrels. When he was fourteen, he took on the name Oliver in his father's honor, when he went to military school. He then studied Law at the University of Georgia, but gave it up to open and run the first movie theater in the little town of Milledgeville. He gave it up in 1913, when he went to work for Lubin Motion Pictures in Florida. Five years later, he moved to California, where he was put under contract by Hal Roach. He first met Stan Laurel in 1917, when he was a heavy in Stan's film *Lucky Dog.* They began working as a team in 1927, and when they appeared in the all-talking *Unaccustomed As We Are,* in 1929, they'd starred as a duo in thirty two-reelers. Their first feature length film, *Pardon Us,* in 1931, proved so successful, they had to make more. Despite a rumor that they were splitting up, they worked as a team until 1939, when Ollie made *Zenobia.* They broke away from Roach, but the great days were over. In the late 1940s, Oliver acted in two supporting roles and the pair made their final film – the truly dreadful – *Atoll K,* in 1951. Ollie was attempting to lose weight when he suffered fatal strokes at his home in North Hollywood. He had three wives.

Pardon Us (1931)
The Devil's Brother (1933)
Sons of the Desert (1933)
Babes in Toyland (1934)
Bonnie Scotland (1935)
The Bohemian Girl (1936)
Our Relations (1936)
Way Out West (1937)
Swiss Miss (1938)
Blockheads (1938)
A Chump at Oxford (1940)
The Fighting Kentuckian (1949)

Jean **Harlow**
5ft 2in
(HARLEAN HARLOW CARPENTER)

Born: **March 3, 1911**
Kansas City, Missouri, USA
Died: **June 7, 1937**

Jean's parents divorced when she was a youngster, and at sixteen, she eloped with a rich young man from Chicago. It didn't last, so she joined her mother and stepfather, in Los Angeles. She got work as a film extra and was featured in Laurel and Hardy two-reelers. Jean's success in *Hell's Angels* earned her a contract with Howard Hughes, who loaned her out to various studios. She shone in the company of stars like Cagney, Tracy, Crawford and Shearer. In 1932, her second husband, MGM executive, Paul Bern, killed himself. His suicide note cited his impotency as the reason. Within a year Jean began a third marriage, which was over inside six months. The scandals didn't affect her rise to stardom. In *Red Dust,* she was sensational opposite Clark Gable. After co-starring with William Powell in *Reckless,* she added further spice to her reputation by eloping with him without getting married. It was to be a short rollercoaster life for Jean. During the shooting of the horse-racing movie, *Saratoga,* she suddenly became seriously ill. She was rushed to hospital, where despite her mother's Christian Science beliefs, she was given medical treatment. Jean died of acute nephritis. A double (who looked nothing like her) was used to finish the film. But then Jean Harlow was utterly unique.

Hell's Angels (1930)
The Secret Six (1931)
The Public Enemy (1931)
Platinum Blonde (1931)
The Beast of the City (1932)
Red-Headed Woman (1932)
Red Dust (1933)
Dinner at Eight (1933)
Bombshell (1933)
The Girl from Missouri (1934)
Reckless (1935)
China Seas (1935)
Riff Raff (1935)
Wife vs. Secretary (1936)
Libeled Lady (1936)
Personal Property (1937)

Woody **Harrelson**
5ft 10in
(WOODROW TRACY HARRELSON)

Born: **July 23, 1961**
Midland, Texas, USA

Woody's parents divorced when he was three-years old. His father, Charles Voyde Harrelson, was sentenced to two life terms for the 1979 assassination of a U.S. District Judge. He died in maximum security prison. Woody's mother took him to live in Lebanon, Ohio, where he went to Lebanon High School. He later received a BA in Theater Arts and English at Hanover College, in Indiana. After moving to New York, he began an eight-year run as the bartender, Woody Boyd, in the TV series, 'Cheers'. His first credited movie role was in the 1986 comedy, *Wildcats,* and his first starring role – opposite Wesley Snipes – was in *White Men Can't Jump.* He was the lead in the successful *Natural Born Killers.* Woody was nominated for a Best Actor Oscar for his portrayal of Larry Flint in *The People vs. Larry Flint.* Following another ten years of great acting, he was voted Best Actor, for *The Walker,* at the Verona Love Screens Film Festival in Italy. It's small reward for a man who rarely puts a foot wrong. After a first marriage, to Neil Simon's daughter, didn't work out, Woody has enjoyed ten years and three children with his second wife, Laura Louie.

White Men Can't Jump (1992)
Natural Born Killers (1994)
The Sunchaser (1996) **Kingpin** (1996)
The People vs. Larry Flint (1996)
Welcome to Sarajevo (1997)
Wag the Dog (1997) **Palmetto** (1998)
The Thin Red Line (1998)
The Hi-Lo Country (1998) **EdTv** (1999)
Scorched (2003) **Anger
Management** (2003) **After the
Sunset** (2004) **The Big White** (2005)
North Country (2005)
**The Prize Winner of Defiance,
Ohio** (2005) **A Prairie
Home Companion** (2006)
A Scanner Darkly (2006)
The Walker (2007)
No Country for Old Men (2007)
The Grand (2007)
Battle in Seattle (2007)
Transsiberian (2008)

Barbara **Harris**
5ft 7in
(BARBARA HARRIS)

Born: **July 25, 1935**
Evanston, Illinois, USA

Barbara grew up with a combination of creative talent and a level head – from her father Oscar Harris – who worked as a tree-surgeon, but was later a successful businessman, and her mother, Natalie, who was an accomplished classical pianist. After she'd graduated from Wright Junior College, in Chicago, Barbara enrolled at the Goodman Theater School. While there, she began getting small parts in stage productions at the Playwrights Theater Club. Later, she joined The Compass Players – the first ongoing improvisational theater troupe in America, which was founded by her first husband, Paul Sills. It evolved into the Second City Company, which, when performing on Broadway, resulted in a Tony nomination for the young actress in 1962. She went on to win one for "The Apple Tree", in 1967 – two years after making her film debut in *A Thousand Clowns.* The 1970s and 80s proved a fertile period in terms of Barbara's ability to pick the right vehicles. In 1971, she was nominated for a Best Supporting Actress Oscar, for what is probably the longest film title ever to be up for an Academy Award: *Who is Harry Kellerman and Why Is He Saying Those Terrible Things About Me?* It was a fairly mediocre film, and Barbara didn't win. Following a nine-year absence from the screen, she reappeared in *Gross Pointe Blank.* Nowadays Barbara teaches acting and directs stage productions.

A Thousand Clowns (1965)
Plaza Suite (1971)
**The War Between Men
and Women** (1972)
Mixed Company (1974)
Nashville (1975)
Family Plot (1976)
Freaky Friday (1976)
Movie Movie (1978)
**The Seduction of
Joe Tynan** (1979)
Peggy Sue Got Married (1986)
Dirty Rotten Scoundrels (1988)
Grosse Pointe Blank (1997)

Ed **Harris**
5ft 9in
(EDWARD ALLEN HARRIS)

Born: **November 28, 1950**
Tenafly, New Jersey, USA

Ed's father was a member of a vocal group in Fred Waring's band, but young Ed showed little musical talent. After Tenafly High School, he went to Columbia University. It was there that he decided to pursue an acting career. Because his parents were living there, Ed enrolled at the University of Oklahoma's Theater department. He then moved to the California Institute of the Arts, from where he graduated. It didn't take him long to get TV work, starting with an episode of 'Gibbsville' – in 1976. Ed made his film debut five years later, in *Knightriders,* and after his portrayal of the astronaut, John Glenn, in *The Right Stuff,* he was in demand. That was also the year he made his New York stage debut, in "Fool for Love" – which won him an Obie. In 1983, during the filming of *Places in the Heart,* Ed and co-star Amy Madigan, fell in love and were married. So far, he's been an Oscar nominee four times – for *Apollo 13, The Truman Show, The Hours,* and when he directed and acted in the superb film about the alcoholic American abstract painter, Jackson *Pollock.*

The Right Stuff (1983)
Under Fire (1983)
Places in the Heart (1984)
Sweet Dreams (1985)
Jacknife (1989)
The Abyss (1989)
State of Grace (1990)
Paris Trout (1991)
Glengarry Glen Ross (1992)
Apollo 13 (1995) **Nixon** (1995)
The Truman Show (1998)
Pollock (2000)
Enemy at the Gates (2001)
Buffalo Soldiers (2001)
A Beautiful Mind (2001)
The Hours (2002)
A History of Violence (2005)
Copying Beethoven (2006)
Gone Baby Gone (2007)
**National Treasure: Book of
Secrets** (2007)
Touching Home (2008)

Julie **Harris**
5ft 4in
(JULIE ANNE HARRIS)

Born: **December 2, 1925**
Grosse Pointe Park, Michigan, USA

Julie studied at the Yale Drama School, before making her New York stage debut, in "It's A Gift". Time spent at the Actors' Studio proved rewarding. She was praised for her acting in Michael Redgrave's "Macbeth" in 1948, and her success in "Member of the Wedding" led to her debut in the screen version, in 1952, for which she was nominated for a Best Actress Oscar. In 1955, the stage to screen link was repeated when she starred in the film version of her 1951 hit, "I Am a Camera". That was also the year she co-starred with James Dean, in his debut film, *East of Eden*. At that time, Julie's heart was really in the theater and during the 1950s, she made little effort to build a film career. There were often plenty of good television dramas to keep her face in front of a wider audience, but from the 1960s onwards, she made some important contributions to the art of movie-acting, in *Requiem for a Heavyweight, Reflections in a Golden Eye* and *The Haunting*. As far as her stage career goes, Julie's had ten Tony nominations and five wins – that's more than any other performer. She has been married and divorced three times. In 2001, Julie suffered a stroke, but she recovered and has made two further movies.

**The Member of the
Wedding** (1952)
East of Eden (1955)
I Am a Camera (1955)
**Requiem for a
Heavyweight** (1962)
The Haunting (1963)
Harper (1966)
You're a Big Boy Now (1966)
**Reflections in a
Golden Eye** (1967)
The Split (1968)
The Hiding Place (1975)
Voyage of the Damned (1976)
Gorillas in the Mist (1988)
Carried Away (1996)
The First of May (1999)
The Way Back Home (2006)
Chatham (2008)

Richard **Harris**
6ft 1in
(RICHARD ST.JOHN HARRIS)

Born: **October 1, 1930**
Limerick, Ireland
Died: **October 25, 2002**

One of a farming couple's nine children, Richard displayed an insatiable love of literature from an early age. He was also fanatical about rugby – especially when it involved Munster. A promising player himself, any hopes of a career were dashed when he suffered a bout of tuberculosis in his teens. He turned his attention to acting after seeing a performance of "Henry IV" at a local theater, and moved to London, where after being turned down by RADA, he studied at the Academy of Music and Dramatic Art. Richard made his movie debut in *Alive and Kicking,* in 1959, but had to wait four years before becoming an international name (portraying a rugby player) in *This Sporting Life,* for which he won the Best Actor award at Cannes, and was Oscar-nominated. In 1968, his debut recording of Jim Webb's 'MacArthur Park' got to number two in the U.S. charts. Despite getting the thumbs down from the critics, more often than not, he enjoyed star status for over thirty years – his best screen work being in *The Molly Maguires, Cassandra Crossing* and his second Best Actor Oscar-nominated role, in *The Field.* Two *Harry Potter* films provided late exposure, but Richard's final appearance was in a TV version of 'Julius Caesar' in the year he died in London. He had three children from his first marriage – one of whom is a film director. The other two are actors.

Mutiny on the Bounty (1962)
This Sporting Life (1963) **The Heroes of
Telemark** (1965) **Camelot** (1967)
The Molly Maguires (1970) **A Man
Called Horse** (1970) **Cromwell** (1970)
Juggernaut (1974) **The Cassandra
Crossing** (1976) **The Wild Geese** (1978)
The Field (1990) **Patriot Games** (1992)
Unforgiven (1992)
Wrestling Ernest Hemingway (1993)
Cry the Beloved Country (1995)
Trojan Eddie (1996)
Gladiator (2000)
**Harry Potter and
the Sorcerer's Stone** (2001)

Sir Rex **Harrison**
6ft 1in
(REGINALD CAREY HARRISON)

Born: **March 5, 1908**
Huyton, Lancashire, England
Died: **June 2, 1990**

Rex's father was employed at a local steel works – a career his rather sensitive son had no desire to follow. When Rex left Liverpool College at sixteen, he took a job with the Liverpool Repertory company. After three years, he went to London in 1930. His first role was in "Getting George Married" at the Everyman Theater. Film studios liked him and gave him small parts beginning with *The Great Game* that year. His roles in films and on the stage got bigger in the 1930s, and after success in "French Without Tears" Rex was put under contract by Alexander Korda . After featuring in *Men Are Not Gods,* he made two films with Vivien Leigh, before arousing the interest of Hollywood, in *Night Train to Munich* and *Major Barbara.* Unfortunately, the war had started. He joined the RAF and wasn't seen on the screen again until 1945. He finally went to Hollywood on a Fox contract. His first film, *Anna and the King of Siam* proved he was no Yul Brynner. There were better parts until Carole Landis committed suicide, in 1948, because Rex wouldn't leave his wife, Lilli Palmer. His contract with Fox was terminated. He eventually left Lilli for Kay Kendall. In 1956, he triumphed on the New York stage, as Professor Higgins, in "My Fair Lady". Eight years later the film version won him an Oscar. Nothing had quite that quality afterwards and he was last seen in a 1986 TV play, 'Anastasia: The Mystery of Anna'. Four years later, Rex died in New York, of pancreatic cancer.

Night Train to Munich (1940)
Major Barbara (1941)
Blithe Spirit (1945)
The Ghost and Mrs. Muir (1947)
Unfaithfully Yours (1948)
The Constant Husband (1955)
The Reluctant Debutante (1958)
Cleopatra (1963)
My Fair Lady (1964)
The Agony and the Ecstasy (1965)
The Honey Pot (1967)
Doctor Doolittle (1967)

Laurence **Harvey**
6ft 1in
(ZVI MOSHEH SKIKNE)

Born: **October 1, 1928**
Jonischkis, Lithuania
Died: **November 25, 1973**

Larry was the youngest of three boys born to a Jewish couple, who emigrated to South Africa when he was five. He grew up in Johannesburg and served in the South African Army during World War II. His experience in the forces' entertainment unit, in Egypt and Italy, during that period encouraged him to pursue an acting career. He went to London, where he studied at RADA and then acted in regional theaters. His film debut was in 1948, when he starred in the independent production *House of Darkness*. For six years, he didn't do anything of note, but in 1954, he made it – in *The Good Die Young*. Larry was billed above three Americans and the young Joan Collins, and also met the first of his three wives, Margaret Leighton. That same year, he scored in what is now considered the best screen version of *Romeo and Juliet*. For ten years or so, he was lucky with the opportunities offered to him and became a big star in Britain as well as Hollywood. In 1959, he was Oscar-nominated for *Room at the Top*. He was known to live an extravagant life-style and it was his need to earn money that kept him acting in films until his last movie, in 1974, *Welcome to Arrow Beach* – which he also directed. He died from stomach cancer at his home in London. In 2005, Larry's only child – his daughter, Domino, died after taking an overdose of the painkiller, Fentanyl.

The Good Die Young (1954)
Romeo and Juliet (1954)
Three Men in a Boat (1956)
Room at the Top (1959)
Expresso Bongo (1960)
The Alamo (1960)
BUtterfield 8 (1960)
Walk on the Wild Side (1962)
The Wonderful World of the Brothers Grimm (1962)
The Manchurian Candidate (1962)
The Running Man (1963)
The Outrage (1965) **Darling** (1965)
Life at the Top (1965)

Signe **Hasso**
5ft 4in
(SIGNE ELEONORA CECILIA LARSSON)

Born: **August 15, 1910**
Stockholm, Sweden
Died: **June 7, 2002**

Signe's father died when she was very young, so she lived with her two brothers, her mother and grandmother, in a one-bedroom apartment, in Stockholm. She was a bright imaginative child who, at the age of twelve, began to get work as an extra at the Royal Dramatic Theater. When she was sixteen, Signe became their youngest ever full-time actress. In 1933, she made her film debut, in *Tystadens Hus,* but after a pact was signed with Nazi Germany, she and her husband Harry Hasso, fled to America, in 1941. When she arrived in Hollywood, the studio cut her age by five years. Her first good role was when she played a French maid in the classic Ernst Lubitsch comedy, *Heaven Can Wait.* Her seven good years included co-starring with Spencer Tracy, George Raft and Cary Grant. Signe's own favorite work was as Brita – opposite the Oscar-winner, Ronald Colman – in *A Double Life.* After her only son was killed in a car crash, Signe went back to Sweden, where she started a national repertory theater. On her return to the United States she did very little movie work, but she appeared on Broadway, and on television, and worked at translating Swedish songs into English. Her last screen role was in a straight to video film, in 1998, titled *One Hell of a Guy.* She died in Los Angeles, of pneumonia, which resulted from lung cancer.

Karriär (1938)
Assignment in Brittany (1943)
Heaven Can Wait (1943)
The Story of Dr. Wassell (1944)
The Seventh Cross (1944)
The House on 92nd Street (1945)
Johnny Angel (1945)
Strange Triangle (1946)
A Scandal in Paris (1946)
Where There's Life (1947)
A Double Life (1947)
To the Ends of the Earth (1948)
Outside the Wall (1950)
I Never Promised You a Rose Garden (1977)

Hurd **Hatfield**
6ft 0½in
(WILLIAM RUKARD HURD HATFIELD)

Born: **December 7, 1917**
New York City, New York, USA
Died: **December 26, 1998**

Hurd was the son of an attorney, William Hatfield, and his wife, Adele. After finishing high school, Hurd went to Columbia University. Deciding to become an actor and having a great admiration for the British classical theater, he journeyed to England, where he studied at the Michael Chekhov Drama School, in Devon. Before the outbreak of World War II, he made his debut in London's West End. When he returned to the United States, he had had enough experience to begin his career on the Broadway stage. He was a success and his reputation was being noted in Hollywood. In 1944, Hurd made his film debut in support of Walter Huston and Katherine Hepburn, in the drama, *Dragon Seed,* set in China. The following year, Hurd guaranteed himself a place in movie history after his simply extraordinary performance in the title role, in Oscar Wilde's *The Picture of Dorian Gray*. His subsequent movies never matched it, and he made a living as a supporting actor until 1991. He came out as gay in the 1960s, and had many affairs with younger men. During the making of *Dorian Gray,* he became a life-long friend of actress Angela Lansbury. When he retired, he moved to a home he bought on her recommendation, at Monkstown, County Cork, in Ireland. He died there of a heart attack in his sleep, seven years later – a few hours after he'd been enjoying a Christmas Day dinner celebration with some friends.

Dragon Seed (1944)
The Picture of Dorian Gray (1945)
The Diary of a Chambermaid (1946)
The Beginning or the End (1947)
The Unsuspected (1947)
Chinatown at Midnight (1949)
The Left Handed Gun (1958)
King of Kings (1961)
El Cid (1961) **Mickey One** (1965)
The Boston Strangler (1968)
Waiting to Act (1985)
Crimes of the Heart (1986)

Anne **Hathaway**
5ft 8in
(ANNE JACQUELINE HATHAWAY)

Born: November 12, 1982
Brooklyn, New York City, New York, USA

The product of a Catholic family upbring-ing, in Milburn, New Jersey, Anne, whose father was a lawyer, was given plenty of encouragement with regards her future career, by her actress mother, Kate McCauley. Anne started on stage as a child and by her teens, acted regularly in plays performed at Milburn High School. She later became the first-ever teenager to participate in the Barrow Group Theater Company's acting program. Another big talent was her singing voice. In 1998, she was in the All-Eastern U.S. High Schools Honors Chorus, at New York's Carnegie Hall. The following year, she starred for one season in the TV series 'Get Real'. In 2001, Anne made her movie debut, in the Disney family comedy, *The Princess Diaries,* which was well received. Also that year, she acted in the New Zealand-made *The Other Side of Heaven,* which wasn't bad. To begin with, she was specializing in comedy roles in movies aimed at young people – which she was herself . She only started to get away from that limiting straitjacket in 2005, when she made a couple of adult-themed movies – one of which was *Havoc* – where she appeared in nude scenes. A year later, she acted with her idol, Meryl Streep, in *The Devil Wears Prada,* which raised her profile to a new level. She then did a 'voice-over' job on the good animated film, *Hoodwinked!* From 2004, Anne and former boyfriend, Raffaello Follieri, ran a foundation which provides medical assistance to children in third-world nations. Anne's film career has continued to flourish – she was nominated for an Oscar, for *Rachel Getting Married.*

The Princess Diaries (2001)
The Other Side of Heaven (2001)
Nicholas Nickleby (2002)
Ella Enchanted (2004)
Brokeback Mountain (2005)
The Devil Wears Prada (2006)
Becoming Jane (2007)
Get Smart (2008)
Rachel Getting Married (2008)
Passengers (2008)

Rutger **Hauer**
6ft 1in
(RUTGER OELSEN HAUER)

Born: January 23, 1944
Breukelen, Utecht, Holland

The son of actor parents, Arend and Teunke Hauer, who taught drama in Amsterdam, Rutger and his three sisters were mainly raised by nannies. He made his stage debut at eleven and was acting in a television play a year later. When he was fifteen, he left home to join the Dutch Merchant Navy. It sharpened his language skills which he used at acting school until spending a few miserable months in the army in 1962. He then toured Holland with a company devoted to bringing theater to small villages. In 1968, he met the love of his life – a painter and sculptress, called Ineke. The following year should have been his film debut but his scenes were deleted. Meanwhile, while acting in the TV series 'Floris', he befriended the director, Paul Verhoeven, who in 1973, provided his first film credit, *Turkish Delight.* The film was Oscar-nominated, and led to Rutger's name spreading far beyond the Dutch borders. He made his Hollywood debut in *Nighthawks,* which was soon followed by a leading role in the Ridley Scott classic, *Bladerunner.* An eight-year run of good material, including *The Hitcher* was fol-lowed by an eight year period when little seemed to work for him. Thankfully, he now seems to be back on track again. His daughter, Ayesha, is an actress.

Nighthawks (1981)
Blade Runner (1982)
Ladyhawke (1985)
Flesh+Blood(1985)
The Hitcher (1986)
**The Legend of the
Holy Drinker** (1988)
The Blood of Heroes (1989)
**Knocking on
Heaven's Door** (1997)
Simon Magus (1999)
I Banchieri di Dio (2002)
Sin City (2005)
Batman Begins (2005)
Mentor (2006)
7eventy 5ive (2007)
Moving McAllister (2007)
Bride Flight (2008)

June **Haver**
5ft 2in
(JUNE STOVENOUR)

Born: June 10, 1926
Rock Island, Illinois, USA
Died: July 4, 2005

June's stage name was decided shortly after her parents divorced when she was a toddler, and her mother married Bert Haver. The family moved to Cincinnati, Ohio, where she was first heard singing in public at six years of age, in a local theater production of "Midnight in a Toyshop". In 1936, following an unsuccessful screen test, she and her mother returned to her birthplace in Illinois, where June began appearing in local radio shows. They then went to Los Angeles, and at high school, she began to act in plays. While awaiting a contract from 20th Century Fox (she was only sixteen) June was hired by the Ted Fio Rito Orchestra – a Chicago band, whose list of vocalists included Betty Grable. June made her film debut, with a tiny role, in the 1943 musical, *The Gang's All Here.* She was nicknamed "The Pocket Grable" and appeared with Betty in *The Dolly Sisters.* A disastrous first marriage to a trumpeter named Jimmy Zito, in 1947, took a lot of the focus from June's career. By the early 1950s, she'd decided to become a nun. Luckily for her, she was rescued from life in a convent by the actor, Fred MacMurray, who married her in 1954. They were a happy couple until his death in 1991. June died of respiratory failure, fourteen years later, at her home in Brentwood, California.

Home in Indiana (1944)
Irish Eyes Are Smiling (1944)
**Where Do We Go
From Here?** (1945)
The Dolly Sisters (1945)
Three Little Girls in Blue (1946)
Wake Up and Dream (1946)
**I Wonder Who's Kissing
Her Now** (1947) **Look for
the Silver Lining** (1949)
Oh, You Beautiful Doll (1949)
**The Daughter of
Rosie O'Grady** (1950)
I'll Get By (1950)
Love Nest (1951)
The Girl Next Door (1953)

June **Havoc**
5ft 6in
(ELLEN EVANGELINE HOVICK)

Born: November 8, 1913
Vancouver, British Columbia, Canada

June was the daughter of the notorious stage mother, Rose Thompson Hovick – who had married at fifteen and was the mother of Gypsy Rose Lee – who was two years older than June. Her father, John Hovick, a newspaper reporter, didn't approve of Rose's obsession with turning the girls into stars and eventually left her. Meanwhile, little June was pushed into performing as "Baby June" and made her screen debut in 1918, in *Hey There!* Both sisters went into vaudeville and in 1929, June's eagerness to escape her mother's clutches resulted in the sixteen year old marrying the first of her three husbands, Bobby Reed. Rose still took a slice of her earnings. When the Great Depression loomed and the economy collapsed, so did June's marriage. She then competed in dance marathons to make ends meet. In 1936, June made her Broadway debut in a musical called "Forbidden Melody", but it was "Pal Joey", with Van Johnson and Gene Kelly, in 1940, which got her career moving. She made her film debut as an adult, in the 1942 wartime musical, *Four Jacks and a Jill,* and then appeared on Broadway, in "Mexican Hayride". After her film career finished in the 1950s, she did TV work and appeared on Broadway. Rose died in 1954 and June told the truth about her in her memoirs. June tried playwriting and in 1964 she was nominated for a Best Director Tony Award for "Marathon '33". June lives in Connecticut.

My Sister Eileen (1942)
Hello Frisco, Hello (1943)
No Time for Love (1943)
Hi Diddle Diddle (1943)
Timber Queen (1944)
Casanova in Burlesque (1944)
Brewster's Millions (1945)
Gentleman's Agreement (1947)
The Iron Curtain (1948)
When My Baby Smiles at Me (1948)
Chicago Deadline (1949)
Red, Hot and Blue (1949)
Once a Thief (1950)
Follow the Sun (1951)

Jack **Hawkins**
5ft 11in
(JOHN EDWARD HAWKINS)

Born: September 14, 1910
Wood Green, London, England
Died: July 18, 1973

Jack was the son of a master builder, Tom Hawkins, and his wife, Phoebe. His early education at Trinity School, in Middlesex was followed by the Italia Conti Academy. He made his London stage debut in 1922, when he played the Elf King, in "Where the Rainbow Ends". At the age of eighteen, he appeared on Broadway, in "Journey's End". He made his screen debut in 1930 in *Birds of Prey.* In 1932, he married the actress, Jessica Tandy, and although he continued to act in films, his stage work took precedence until after he'd served in the Royal Welsh Fusiliers, during World War II. Jack's first high-profile movie was *The Fallen Idol,* but his recognition on a global scale only occurred after he had starred in *The Cruel Sea.* Jack had an unbroken run of excellent movies up to and beyond 1960, when the first signs of the throat cancer which killed him were apparent. He cut down his smoking to five a day from sixty, but by 1965, it had taken hold and he was forced to use a mechanical larynx. His voice was dubbed by other actors. Jack retained his sense of humor during the ordeal and died in London. His autobiography "Anything For a Quiet Life" was published posthumously.

The Fallen Idol (1948)
State Secret (1950)
Home at Seven (1952)
Angels One Five (1952)
Mandy (1952)
The Cruel Sea (1953)
The Intruder (1953)
The Prisoner (1955)
Land of the Pharaohs (1955)
The Long Arm (1956)
The Bridge on the River Kwai (1957)
Gideon's Day (1958)
The Two-Headed Spy (1958)
Ben-Hur (1959)
The League of Gentlemen (1960)
Lawrence of Arabia (1962)
Zulu (1964)
The Third Secret (1964)
Guns at Batasi (1964)

Sally **Hawkins**
5ft 5in
(SALLY HAWKINS)

Born: April 27, 1976
London, England

Sally's parents, Colin and Jacqui Hawkins, are creative people. They both write and illustrate children's books. Sally grew up in Dulwich, south-east London and was educated at James Allen's Girls' School. After graduating in 1994, she went on to study acting at London's Royal Academy of Dramatic Art. Sally graduated in 1998 and started her career soon after that. In 1999, she made her television debut in an episode of 'Casualty'. In 2000, Sally made a further TV appearance and was seen on stage in two of William Shakespeare's plays - "Much Ado About Nothing" and "A Midsummer Night's Dream". Two years later, she made her first real impact – in Mike Leigh's film drama – *All or Nothing* and that same year, impressed as Zena Blake, in the controversial television film, 'Tipping the Velvet'. Her career has progressed rapidly since then – with good roles in some excellent movies including *Vera Drake, Layer Cake* – with Daniel Craig, and a fine production of Somerset Maugham's novel, *The Painted Veil.* Sally's performance in the television version of Jane Austen's 'Persuasion' was of a high standard, but it was her recent film work which really brought her name to the fore. Woody Allen's *Cassandra's Dream,* might not have been one of his very best, but it is a Woody Allen movie – which can be added to her list of credits. The Mike Leigh comedy, *Happy-Go-Lucky,* is in another league. It won Sally a Silver Bear as Best Actress, at the Berlin International Film Festival and as early as summer 2008, she was being touted for an Oscar. She's already won a Golden Globe for the film – as Best Actress – Comedy or Musical.

All or Nothing (2002)
Vera Drake (2004)
Layer Cake (2004)
The Painted Veil (2006)
W Delta Z (2007)
Cassandra's Dream (2007)
Happy-Go-Lucky (2008)
An Education (2008)
Happy Ever Afters (2009)

Goldie **Hawn**
5ft 6in
(GOLDIE JEAN HAWN)

Born: **November 21, 1945**
Washington, D.C., USA

Goldie's father, Edward Rutledge Hawn, was a musician, and her mother, Laura, owned a jewelry shop and a dance studio. Goldie and her sister were raised in the Jewish religion, in Takoma Park, Maryland. When she was three years old, Goldie began ballet and tap dance lessons. At ten years old she danced in the chorus of 'The Nutcracker' by Tchaikovsky. In 1961, she made her stage debut, as Juliet in "Romeo and Juliet". After graduating from Montgomery Blair High School, in Silver Spring, Maryland, she started majoring in drama at the American University, in Washington, but dropped out to manage a ballet school. Her professional dancing debut was in 1964, in "Can-Can" – at the New York World's Fair. Goldie's acting career began in the television sit-com, 'Good Morning, World', in 1967. Even though the show didn't last long, she had the good fortune to be part of the hugely successful, "Rowan and Martin's Laugh-In'. Her film debut in Cactus Flower, with Walter Matthau and Ingrid Bergman, earned her a Best Supporting Actress Oscar. Although she was in many films during the 1970s and 1980s, few were of the standard of Private Benjamin, which earned a Best Actress Oscar nomination. Goldie married Bill Hudson of the Hudson Brothers pop group, in 1976. They were divorced in 1980. Their children, Oliver and Kate, are film actors. Goldie hasn't been in a movie since The Banger Sisters – nearly seven years ago.

Cactus Flower (1969)
Butterflies Are Free (1972)
The Sugarland Express (1974)
Shampoo (1975) The Duchess and
the Dirtwater Fox (1976)
Foul Play (1978)
Private Benjamin (1980)
Seems Like Old Times (1980)
Overboard (1987)
Death Becomes Her (1992)
The First Wives Club (1996)
Everyone Says I Love You (1996)
The Banger Sisters (2002)

Nigel **Hawthorne**
5ft 11½in
(NIGEL BARNARD HAWTHORNE)

Born: **April 5, 1929**
Coventry, Warwickshire, England
Died: **December 26, 2001**

Nigel's parents, Dr. Charles Hawthorne, and his wife Agnes, emigrated to South Africa when he was three. They settled in Cape Town, where Nigel, whose family were Catholic, attended the Christian Brothers College. He was eighteen when he went to Cape Town University intending to get a BA in Broadcasting. After making his stage debut on his twenty-first birthday, in 1950, in a production of "The Shop at Sly Corner" he was encouraged by one of the actors to try his luck in England. He became an assistant stage manager at Buxton, getting small roles in plays, but his strange accent and plain appearance proved a barrier. He returned to Cape Town thoroughly chastened and worked very hard until making his name in Johannesburg, in 1961. He got his break in England, with Joan Littlwood's Theater Workshop, and he progressed to a high rating as a stage actor. After several TV roles, Nigel made his movie debut in 1972 (uncredited) in Young Winston. In 1980, he began to portray Sir Humphrey Appleby in 'Yes, Prime Minister'. His first serious stab at film acting was in the Julie Christie Sci-Fi film, Memoirs of a Survivor. Eventually he acted in both English and American movies. He was nominated for a Best Actor Oscar for The Madness of King George. Towards the end of his life, he had the pleasure of working on a good South African film – A Reasonable Man. Nigel died of a heart attack at his 15th-century manor house in Hertfordshire, and was survived by his long-term partner, Trevor Bentham.

The Hiding Place (1975)
Memoirs of a Survivor (1981)
King of the Wind (1990)
Demolition Man (1993)
The Madness of King George (1994)
Twelfth Night (1996) Amistad (1997)
The Object of My Affection (1998)
At Sachem Farm (1998)
The Winslow Boy (1999)
A Reasonable Man (1999)

Will **Hay**
5ft 9½in
(WILLIAM THOMSON HAY)

Born: **December 6, 1888**
Stockton-on-Tees, Durham, England
Died: **April 18, 1949**

After his family moved to Lowestoft, in Suffolk, young Will began to develop a keen interest in the night sky, and before he left secondary school, was an expert on astronomy. He began his working life as an apprentice printer, and was only nineteen when he married Gladys Perkins. They had three children. Will began his career in music halls, in 1909, but in 1914, he toured Australia, South Africa, and the United States, with the Fred Karno troupe. After World War I, he had qualified as a pilot and gave Amy Johnson her first flying lessons. In 1925, he was a big hit at the Royal Variety Performance. Will worked on BBC radio for many years and even after enjoying a successful tour of America in 1927 – his show, 'St. Michael's School' was still listened to by millions. In 1933, he was made a Fellow of the Royal Astronomical Society, after he discovered a white spot on Saturn. Will didn't make his first feature film, Those Were the Days, until he was forty-six. The first important picture in which he was able to demonstrate his unique brand of comedy, was Boys Will Be Boys. From then until the end of World War II, he was immensely popular with the British public and much of the English-speaking world – apart from the United States. In 1940, Will contributed to the war effort, by teaching astronomy and navigation to the Royal Navy Reserve Special Branch. In 1944, after his final film, My Learned Friend, Will underwent an operation for cancer. For much of the following five years he struggled on with radio work, until a stroke finally silenced him at his home in Chelsea.

Boys Will Be Boys (1935)
Windbag the Sailor (1936)
Oh, Mr. Porter! (1937)
Good Morning, Boys (1937)
Ask a Policeman (1938)
The Ghost of St. Michael's (1941)
The Black Sheep of Whitehall (1941)
The Goose Steps Out (1942)
My Learned Friend (1943)

Sessue **Hayakawa**
5ft 7½in
(KINTARO HAYAKAWA)

Born: **June 10, 1889**
Nanaura, Chiba, Japan
Died: **November 23, 1973**

Sessue was from an aristocratic family of the Samurai class. His father was a provincial governor who had served in the Japanese Navy. It was to his eternal shame, when a hearing problem prevented him from following in his father's footsteps. To get way from home, he joined a theatrical company which left for a tour of the United States, in 1913. He was seen by the film producer, Thomas Ince, who gave him his debut, in *The Wrath of the Gods*. In 1914, he married the Japanese actress, Tsuru Aoki, and a year later, became a favorite with American audiences after starring with Fannie Ward, in Cecil B. DeMille's, *The Cheat*. It caused outrage among the Japanese-American community, who objected to racial mixing, but made Sessue a big star. He formed a production company and together with his wife, Tsuru, he appeared in Asian-themed movies. A rise in anti-Asian sentiment made him go home to Japan and then to France, where he made several films. A return to Hollywood in 1931, for his first talkie, *Daughter of the Dragon*, with Anna May Wong, led to criticism of his accent. The next eighteen years were spent in France where the best film he made was titled *Gambling Hell*. Sessue re-launched his Hollywood career in 1949, in *Tokyo Joe*, and made a big impact in movies – most notably *The House of Bamboo* and *The Bridge on the River Kwai*. After his wife died in 1970, he returned to Japan and became a Zen master. He died in Tokyo of cerebral thrombosis.

Daughter of the Dragon (1931)
The Cheat (1937)
Gambling Hell (1942)
Tokyo Joe (1949)
Three Came Home (1950)
The House of Bamboo (1955)
The Bridge on the
River Kwai (1957)
The Geisha Boy (1958)
Hell to Eternity (1960)
Swiss Family Robinson (1960)

Sterling **Hayden**
6ft 5in
(STERLING RELYEA WALTER)

Born: **March 26, 1916**
Upper Montclair, New Jersey, USA
Died: **May 23, 1986**

After his father died when he was nine, he was adopted by James Hayden. Sterling attended Wassookeag School, in Dexter, Maine. When he was seventeen, he ran away to sea – firstly working as a ship's boy and later sailing round the world as a master. Back on dry land, he worked as a photographic model for men's outdoor clothing. He was signed by Paramount and made his film debut, in *Virginia,* with Madeleine Carroll, who became his first wife. After only two movies, he became a commando and later, a U.S. marine. He was awarded a Silver Star by Tito of Yugoslavia, and briefly took Communist membership, which to his eternal shame, led to his cooperation with the HUAC. It interrupted his post-war career, but he needed the work to pay for his boats and his alimony. After his first marriage ended in 1946, he went through three divorces with Betty Ann de Noon, who bore him four of his six children. His film career took off again when he starred in *The Asphalt Jungle*. His film legacy is impressive, but he surprisingly, was only once nominated for an award – for a "Best Foreign Actor" BAFTA, for *Dr. Strangelove*. Sterling died of prostate cancer in Sausalito, California.

Virginia (1941)
The Asphalt Jungle (1950)
The Star (1952) **So Big** (1953)
Crime Wave (1954)
Prince Valiant (1954)
Johnny Guitar (1954) **Suddenly** (1954)
The Eternal Sea (1955)
The Last Command (1955)
The Killing (1956) **Crime of**
Passion (1957) **Valerie** (1957)
Terror in a Texas Town (1958)
Dr. Strangelove (1964)
Loving (1970)
The Godfather (1972)
Deadly Strangers (1974)
Novecento (1976)
Winter Kills (1979)
The Outsider (1979)
Nine to Five (1980)

Salma **Hayek**
5ft 2in
(SALMA VALGARMA HAYEK-JIMENEZ)

Born: **September 2, 1966**
Coatzacoalcos, Veracruz, Mexico

Salma and her brother Sami, grew up in the lap of luxury. Her father, Sami Hayek, who was of Lebanese descent, was a rich oil company executive. Her mother, Diana Jiménez, was an opera singer. Selma was five when she decided she wanted to be an actress. She went to a convent school – the Academy of the Sacred Heart, in Grand Couteau, Louisiana – where she was an outstanding gymnast. She then studied International Relations at the Universidad Iberoamericana, in Mexico City. In 1989, she landed a role in the popular TV soap opera, 'Teresa' which gave her star status in her own country. In 1991, she left Mexico to study with Stella Adler, in Los Angeles, but found the going tough and getting decent roles even tougher. In 1993, she had a very small movie debut, in *Mi vida loca*. She publicly expressed her frustration with the lack of opportunities on a Spanish-language chat show, which was seen by director, Robert Rodriguez. He cast Salma in *Desperado* opposite Antonio Banderas. Fans adored it and Hollywood started to show some interest. Securing her future even further, Robert starred her in *From Dusk Till Dawn,* with George Clooney. She was nominated for a Best Actress Oscar, for *Frida,* and has made films and TV projects for her production company called Ventanarosa. With her appearances in TV's 'Ugly Betty', Salma's popularity has spread all over the world – and there's more to come.

Midaq Alley (1995)
Desperado (1995)
Follow Me Home (1996)
From Dusk Till Dawn (1996)
The Faculty (1998) **Dogma** (1999)
No One Writes to
the Colonel (1999)
Chain of Fools (2000)
La Gran Vida (2000)
Frida (2002)
Once Upon a Time in Mexico (2003)
After the Sunset (2004)
Lonely Hearts (2006)
Across the Universe (2007)

Helen **Hayes**
5ft
(HELEN HAYES BROWN)

Born: **October 10, 1900**
Washington, D.C., USA
Died: **March 17, 1993**

Helen's father, Francis Brown, worked as a clerk and later as a salesman. Her mother, Catherine Hayes, was from Irish stock and had worked as an actress with touring companies. When Helen was barely five years old, she made her stage debut, as the young Prince Charles, in "The Royal Family", in Washington. Her Broadway debut came only four years later. Helen enjoyed a successful career as a child actress, and made her movie debut, in 1910, in the Vitagraph two-reeler, *Calico Doll.* A year later, she was banned from touring in stage productions because she was under age. When she was eighteen, she started again, as "Pollyanna", and made a name for herself on Broadway. In 1930, she somewhat reluctantly signed a contract with MGM, but the move to Hollywood proved helpful to her husband, the dramatist, Charles MacArthur. Helen won a Best Actress Oscar for her first film, *The Sin of Madelon Claudet,* and she continued getting good screen roles – usually based on best-selling novels – until 1935, when she told the studio she no longer wished to appear in pictures. Shortly after that, she and Charles adopted a baby they named James MacArthur. Helen spent the next few years raising him. He had a brief career as a film actor. Jim was a fixture on the TV show. 'Hawaii Five-O'. Helen's return to the screen was on TV. She was 'The First Lady of the American Theater' but she won a second Oscar, for *Airport.* She retired in 1985, and died eight years later of congestive heart failure.

The Sin of Madelon Claudet (1931)
Arrowsmith (1931)
A Farewell to Arms (1932)
The Son-Daughter (1932)
The White Sister (1933)
Another Language (1933)
Night Flight (1933)
Another Language (1933)
What Every Woman Knows (1934)
Anastasia (1956) Airport (1970)
Candleshoe (1977)

Louis **Hayward**
5ft 10¹/₂in
(LOUIS CHARLES HAYWARD)

Born: **March 19, 1909**
Johannesburg, South Africa
Died: **February 21, 1985**

Young Louis left South Africa in 1922, when his parents sent him to a boarding school in France. Five years later, he went to England to study for an acting career and by the early thirties, while managing a London nightclub, he started getting small parts on the West End stage. In 1932, he made his film debut, when he was fifth-billed in *Self Made Lady*. He continued in British film and stage productions until Noel Coward was so impressed by his performance in one of his plays, he encouraged the young actor to try his luck in Hollywood. Coward then wrote a part especially for him, in his new play, "Point Valaine" and Louis was in the original cast when it ran for three months at the Ethel Barrymore Theater, on Broadway, in 1935. His film career moved a step forward when supporting Frederic March and Olivia de Havilland, in the very successful, *Anthony Adverse.* Louis was popular in swashbucklers such as *The Return of Monte Cristo* and *Pirates of Capri,* in the 1940s and early 1950s, and remained a film and television actor for over twenty-five years. His last acting assignment was in a 1974 episode of the TV series, 'The Magician'. His heavy smoking led to his death from lung cancer, at his home in Palm Springs, California.

Anthony Adverse (1936)
Condemned Women (1938)
The Saint in New York (1938)
The Rage of Paris (1938)
The Duke of West Point (1938)
The Man in the Iron Mask (1939)
My Son, My Son! (1940)
The Son of Monte Cristo (1940)
Ladies in Retirement (1941)
And Then There Were None (1945)
The Strange Woman (1946)
The Return of Monte Cristo (1946)
Repeat Performance (1947)
Ruthless (1948) Walk a Crooked
Mile (1948) House by the River (1950)
The Search for Bridey Murphy (1956)
Chuka (1967)

Susan **Hayward**
5ft 3¹/₂in
(EDYTHE MARRENNER)

Born: **June 30, 1917**
Brooklyn, New York City, New York, USA
Died: **March 14, 1975**

Susan's parents were Walter Marrenner, and his wife Ellen, whose parents were from Sweden. Raised in a tenement block in Brooklyn, the very pretty young Susan dreamed of becoming a movie star. As soon as she'd left school, she studied dress design and then worked as a model. Her photograph on the cover of a magazine was seen by David O. Selznick, who tested her for *Gone With the Wind.* Despite losing out to Vivien Leigh, the test footage proved useful in getting a contract with Paramount. The studio did little for her, and even after a good independent film, *The Hairy Ape,* in 1944, they didn't renew her contract. She married Jess Barker, and then had twins before her next assignment, *Canyon Passage.* Susan's roles got better and by 1950, she was a major star. *With a Song in My Heart,* a biopic of the singer, Jane Froman, and *The Snows of Kilimanjaro,* with Gregory Peck, placed her in the top-ten at the box office, but the cost to her health due to stress resulted in a pill overdose. After a rest, she bounced back with *I'll Cry Tomorrow,* a film about the alcoholic singer, Lilian Roth, and won a Best Actress Oscar, for *I Want to Live!* Her career slumped around 1968, when her health deteriorated. She had a small role in her final film, *The Avengers,* in 1972. After a brave struggle, Susan died of brain cancer, in Hollywood.

Adam Had Four Sons (1941)
The Canyon Passage (1946)
Smash-Up: The Story of
a Woman (1947) They Won't
Believe Me (1947) The Lost
Moment (1947) My Foolish
Heart(1949) I'd Climb the Highest
Mountain (1951) Rawhide (1951)
With a Song in My Heart (1952)
The Lusty Men (1952)
I'll Cry Tomorrow (1955)
I Want to Live! (1958)
Woman Obsessed (1959)
Back Street (1961) The Honey Pot (1967)

Rita **Hayworth**
5ft 6in
(MARGARITA CARMEN CANSINO)

Born: **October 17, 1918**
Brooklyn, New York City, New York, USA
Died: **May 14, 1987**

Rita was born to dance. Her father was the Latin-American dancer, Eduardo Cansino, and her cousin was Ginger Rogers. As a teenager, she danced at the 'Agua Caliente', a nightclub in downtown Tijuana, frequented by film people. Her beauty and talent was appreciated by Fox, who gave her a contract and her film debut, in 1935, (as a dancer) in *Under the Pampas Moon*. Two years after that, she married Ed Judson, who became her manager and persuaded Columbia to give her a seven-year contract. Following loan-outs, the studio put her in *Blood and Sand,* filmed in color, which her appearance deserved. She was soon dancing with Fred Astaire and, in 1944, with Gene Kelly, in *Cover Girl* – a film which raised her profile several notches. The film noir, *Gilda* made Rita a true Hollywood star, but after going blonde in *The Lady from Shanghai,* with ex-husband, Orson Welles, she married Prince Aly Khan, and went to live in Europe. When that marriage ended, she returned to Hollywood, but in the 1950s, apart from *Pal Joey,* her old magic was rarely seen. From 1960, the early signs of Alzheimer's disease led to a dependence on alcohol. The last ten years in the life of one the screen's most beautiful stars were sad indeed, but we can remember Rita at her loveliest by watching any of this list.

The Shadow (1937)
Only Angels Have Wings (1939)
Susan and God (1940)
Strawberry Blonde (1941)
Affectionately Yours (1941)
Blood and Sand (1941)
You Were Never Lovelier (1942)
Cover Girl (1944) **Tonight and Every Night** (1945) **Gilda** (1946)
The Lady from Shanghai (1948)
Affair in Trinidad (1952)
Fire Down Below (1957)
Pal Joey (1957)
Separate Tables (1958)
They Came to Cordura (1959)
The Story on Page One (1959)

John **Heard**
5ft 9½in
(JOHN HEARD)

Born: **March 7, 1945**
Washington, D.C., USA

His father (also John Heard) worked at the Pentagon. His mother Helen, took care of the family and entertained guests. Young John starred in plays at Gonzaga College High School, from where he graduated in 1964. He went on to graduate from Clark University, in Worcester, Massachusetts. He began his career at the Organic Theater, in Chicago, where he won a Theater World Award in 1976, and a year earlier, made his TV debut with a small part in the war drama, 'Valley Forge'. He then went to New York City, where he won Obie Awards for his Off-Broadway work, in "Othello" and "Split". His film debut was in *Rush It,* an independent production made in 1976, starring Tom Berenger. In 1979, after his film career had started to move he spent a few months as the husband of the actress, Margot Kidder. He has a son who was the result of a relationship with Melissa Leo. In 1997, after they split up, he was charged with stalking her. Unpleasant things aside, from the 1990s onwards, John's career has been a roller-coaster ride – a true American success story. His films and television appearances number well over one hundred, and he's currently busier than ever.

Between the Lines (1977)
Heaven Help Us (1985)
After Hours (1985)
The Trip to Bountiful (1985)
The Milagro Beanfield War (1988)
Big (1988) **Beaches** (1988)
Home Alone (1990)
Awakenings (1990)
Rambling Rose (1991)
The Pelican Brief (1993)
Before and After (1996)
My Fellow Americans (1996)
One Eight Seven (1997)
Desert Blue (1998) **Pollock** (2000)
O (2001) **Under the City** (2004)
Steel City (2006) **The Guardian** (2006)
Brothers Three: An American Gothic (2007) **The Great Debaters** (2007) **P.J.** (2008)
The Lucky Ones (2008)

Tippi **Hedren**
5ft 5in
(NATHALIE KAY HEDREN)

Born: **January 19, 1930**
New Ulm, Minnesota, USA

The daughter of Scandinavians who ran a general store, Tippi's name was given to her by her Swedish father, Bernard Carl Hedren, who first used it when she was a baby. Her mother Dorothea Eckhardt, was of German and Norwegian ancestry. When she was a teenager, Tippi took part in fashion shows at a department store. After her family relocated to California, she began to think about an acting career, but when she was eighteen, she became a professional model, in New York. In 1950, she had a brief moment on screen as a model, in a comedy titled *The Petty Girl*. Tippi married her first husband, Peter Griffith, in 1952, and she became the mother of the future film star, Melanie Griffith. In the late 1950s she was seen by Alfred Hitchcock in a television commercial for a diet drink . Always on the lookout for cool blondes, he took her under his wing. When she was thirty-three, she made her featured role debut, as Melanie Daniels, in his film, *The Birds.* That, and *Marnie,* the following year opposite Sean Connery, appeared to have set Tippi on the road to movie stardom. To make other movies, she had to have the approval of Mr. Hitchcock who had taken control. Any director who wished to use her, had to speak to him first. When she ended their agreement following three years of virtual inactivity, he said he "would ruin her career". He more or less did. Chaplin's *The Countess from Hong Kong,* in 1967, did her no favors, and after that it was a struggle to get good starring parts. Since 2002, Tippi has been married to her fourth husband, Martin Dinnes. She is a tireless supporter of charitable causes and relief programs around the world.

The Birds (1963)
Marnie (1964) **Roar** (1981)
Pacific Heights (1990)
Citizen Ruth (1996)
I Woke Up Early the Day I Died (1998)
Rose's Garden (2003)
Strike the Tent (2005)
Her Morbid Desires (2008)

Van **Heflin**
6ft
(EMMETT EVAN HEFLIN JR.)

Born: **December 13, 1910**
Walters, Oklahoma, USA
Died: **July 23, 1971**

Van was the son of a dentist, Dr. Emmett Heflin, and his wife, Fannie. When he was in the seventh grade, his family moved to California. Van enrolled at Long Beach Polytechnic High School and during summer vacations, worked as a crew member on schooners sailing to South America. He went to Liverpool on a tramp steamer. His next port of call was Oklahoma University, but he interrupted his studies, in 1928, to make his stage debut in "Mr. Moneypenny". After graduating in 1931, he decided to have another go at acting – at the Hedgerow Theater, in Philadelphia – where Katherine Hepburn saw him in a play. He made his film debut with her in *A Woman Rebels*. B-pictures followed its failure, and he turned to radio work before getting back to acting with Hepburn, in the stage version of "Philadelphia Story". It was enough to re-kindle Hollywood interest and he was soon acting in *Santa Fe Trail*, with Errol Flynn. Van was signed by MGM in 1941, after winning a Best Supporting Actor Oscar for *Johnny Eager*. In the 1950s, he was perfect in two outstanding westerns – *Shane* and *3:10 to Yuma*. His final film role was in *Airport*. A year later, he suffered a heart attack in the swimming pool at his Hollywood home. He died without ever regaining consciousness. Van's cremated remains were scattered into the Pacific Ocean.

Santa Fe Trail (1940)
The Feminine Touch (1941)
Johnny Eager (1942) **Kid Glove**
Killer (1942) **Tennessee Johnson** (1942)
The Strange Love of
Martha Ivers (1946) **Possessed** (1947)
Green Dolphin Street (1947)
The Three Musketeers (1948)
Act of Violence (1948)
Madame Bovary (1949)
The Prowler (1951) **Shane** (1953)
The Raid (1954) **Battle Cry** (1955)
Count Three and Pray (1955)
Patterns (1956) **3:10 to Yuma** (1957)
They Came to Cordura (1959)

David **Hemmings**
5ft 9in
(DAVID LESLIE EDWARD HEMMINGS)

Born: **November 18, 1941**
Guildford, Surrey, England
Died: **December 3, 2003**

David's father, a cookie merchant who had been a dance band pianist, encouraged his son to sing. While at Glyn College, in Epsom, he displayed an exceptional talent as a boy soprano. He performed with the English Opera Group and was admired by the composer, Benjamin Britten, who wrote the part of Miles, in his "Turn of the Screw", especially for him. In 1953, David began his acting career with brief appearances in the TV series 'Billy Bunter of Greyfriars School'. The following year he had a small part in the racing drama, *The Rainbow Jacket*. When he was fifteen, David studied painting at Epsom School of Art before going to live in London and surviving the 1950s, with supporting roles in the television series, 'Dixon of Dock Green', singing in night clubs, and acting in undistinguished films. Once the 'sixties began to swing, so did David's career. He had exactly the type of looks for the era, and was selected by Antonioni, to play the photographer, Thomas, in his landmark film, *Blowup*. The second of his four wives was Gayle Hunnicutt. David worked as movie actor and director, for the next twenty-five years. He died of a heart attack while he was on location, shooting *Samantha's Child*, in Bucharest, Rumania.

Blowup (1966)
The Charge of the Light
Brigade (1968)
The Long Day's Dying (1968)
Only When I Larf (1968)
The Walking Stick (1970)
Unman, Wittering and
Zigo (1971)
Juggernaut (1974)
Profondo rosso (1975)
La Via della droga (1977)
Murder by Decree (1979)
Beyond Reasonable Doubt (1980)
Gladiator (2000)
Last Orders (2001)
Gangs of New York (2002
The Night We Called
It a Day (2003)

Sonja **Henie**
5ft 3in
(SONJA HENIE)

Born: **April 8, 1912**
Kristiania, Norway
Died: **October 12, 1969**

Born in the city which became Oslo in 1924, Sonja was the daughter of a wealthy fur trader, Wilhelm Henie, and his wife, Selma. After sending her to dancing classes from the age of four, her parents switched her to ice-skating after she showed exceptional natural ability on the local outdoor rink. She was only eleven when she easily won the Norwegian Figure Skating Championships and two years later, she was placed second in the European Championships – winning it the following year. She was then World Champion for ten consecutive years. After her third Olympic Gold medal, in 1936, she decided to turn professional and after appearing in ice shows, she considered the prospect of a film career. She was no great actress, but she pushed herself onto the Hollywood scene by hiring a rink in Los Angeles, and projecting her bubbly personality towards the film moguls who had been invited. It got her a contract and resulted in her first movie that same year – *One in a Million* – with Don Ameche. Its success led to a series of films with other top leading men including Tyrone Power. By 1939, Sonja was the highest paid star in Hollywood. To begin with, nobody seemed to care that each film was a carbon copy of the same formula – romance at a winter-sports resort – followed by a skating climax. After the success of *Sun Valley Serenade*, which was considerably helped by the great Glenn Miller and his Orchestra and its several hit songs, Sonja's career began to crumble. She made her final film in 1948, and died of leukemia, during a flight to Oslo.

One in a Million (1936)
Thin Ice (1937)
Happy Landing (1938)
My Lucky Star (1938)
Second Fiddle (1939)
Everything Happens at Night (1939)
Sun Valley Serenade (1941)
Wintertime (1943)
It's a Pleasure (1945)

Paul **Henreid**
6ft 3in
(PAUL GEORG JULIUS HERNREID)

Born: **January 10, 1905**
Trieste, Austro-Hungary
Died: **March 29, 1992**

Paul grew up in an area which was part of the Austro-Hungarian Empire. His father was a banker from Vienna, and when Paul finished his schooling, he went there to study acting. He made his stage debut under the direction of Max Reinhardt. In 1933, he made his film debut in Germany as Paul von Hernreid, in the excellent submarine drama *Morgenrot*. He made a few more films there, but in 1936, with the threat of Hitler growing by the day, he decided to go to England. Through his contact with the Austrian actor, Anton Walbrook, Paul got a small part in the film he was starring in, *Victoria the Great*. Paul played supporting roles in British films until *Night Train to Munich*, where he featured strongly. He moved to Hollywood in 1941 and acted opposite Bette Davis, in his first film there, *Now Voyager*. Paul's most memorable role was that same year, as the anti-Nazi leader, Victor Laszlo, in *Casablanca*. Paul became a U.S. citizen in 1946, and was in a number of successful films during the next few years. In 1952, he was blacklisted as an actor by HUAC, so he directed films, beginning with *For Men Only*. He directed 'Alfred Hitchcock Presents' and several other TV dramas until he retired in 1971. Paul's marriage to Elizabeth Gluck was an enduring success – lasting over fifty-six years. He died of pneumonia in Santa Monica, California.

Morgenrot (1933)
Goodbye Mr.Chips (1939)
Night Train to Munich (1940)
Now Voyager (1942) **Casablanca** (1942)
Between Two Worlds (1944)
The Conspirators (1944)
The Spanish Main (1945)
Devotion (1946)
Of Human Bondage (1946)
Deception (1946)
Song of Love (1947)
Hollow Triumph (1948)
Deep in My Heart (1954)
Holiday for Lovers (1959)
Operation Crossbow (1965)

Taraji P. **Henson**
5ft 5in
(TARAJI PENDA HENSON)

Born: **September 11, 1970**
Washington, D.C., USA

Taraji was the daughter of Boris Henson and Bernice Gordon. Bernice was a lively, ambitious lady, who eventually achieved the position of corporate manager, at the department store, Woodwards Lothrop. A famous ancestor of Taraji's on her father's side of the family, was a distant relative, Matthew Henson. He was one of the team of explorers who first discovered the Geographic North Pole, in 1909. Taraji began her education at Oxon Hill School, in Maryland. She later attempted to major in Electrical Engineering at North Carolina and Technical State University. It wasn't for her. She left and transferred to Howard University, from where she graduated in 1995. Taraji paid her way through school by working part-time at the Pentagon and in the evenings, entertaining diners on the cruise ship, "The Spirit of Washington", by singing and dancing. After graduating, she had her son, Marcel, with her boyfriend, William Johnson. With the need to keep her child, she had to earn money. After a year or so, she began attending casting sessions. In 1997, she made her television debut, in an episode of the family comedy series, 'Sister, Sister'. Taraji's movie debut was a year later, when she landed a small supporting role, in *Streetwise*, which was filmed in Washington. She worked hard and had her first recognition, at Locarno International Film Festival, in Switzerland – sharing the ensemble prize, for *Baby Boy*. She won a Black Reel Award as Best Supporting Actress, for *Hustle & Flow*, and was nominated for a Best Supporting Actress Oscar, for *The Curious Case of Benjamin Button*. Taraji stars with Forest Whitaker, in *Hurricane Season*.

Streetwise (1998)
Baby Boy (2001)
Hustle & Flow (2005)
Four Brothers (2005)
Something New (2006)
Smoking Aces (2006)
Talk to Me (2007)
**The Curious Case of
Benjamin Button** (2008)

Audrey **Hepburn**
5ft 7in
(AUDREY KATHLEEN RUSTON)

Born: **May 4, 1929**
Brussels, Belgium
Died: **January 20, 1993**

She was the only child of an Englishman, Joseph Ruston, who represented a British insurance company. Her mother, Ella van Heemstra, was a Dutch aristocrat. Audrey went to junior school in Belgium and in 1935, was sent to a boarding school in England. Her father, who was a Fascist sympathizer, was interned in England during the war. Audrey studied at Arnhem Conservatory and in 1947, she moved to London to study classical ballet – returning to Holland the following year – for her movie debut, in *Netherlands in 7 Lessen*. That same year, she made her stage debut in London's West End, in *"High Button Shoes"*. Her first English film (uttering three short lines) was a comedy, *Laughter in Paradise*. She was then tested for *Quo Vadis*, but MGM were not very impressed. Much more enlightened was the novelist, Colette, who saw her in Monte Carlo, and said she would be perfect to star in "Gigi" on Broadway. She was. It brought her to the attention of William Wyler, who wanted a fresh face to appear in *Roman Holiday*. It not only made her a star it won her a Best Actress Oscar. She was just as good in epics, dramas and musicals. From 1954 until 1968, she was married to Mel Ferrer. Although her stardust faded by 1970, Audrey had become a movie icon. From 1988 until her death from appendicular cancer, she was a UNICEF Goodwill Ambassador. She left us a legacy of fine movies and her photo images are still among the most popular with generations of fans.

The Secret People (1952)
Roman Holiday (1953)
Sabrina (1954)
War and Peace (1956)
Funny Face (1957)
Love in the Afternoon (1957)
The Nun's Story (1959)
Breakfast at Tiffany's (1961)
Charade (1963) **My Fair Lady** (1964)
Two for the Road (1967)
Wait Until Dark (1967)

Katharine **Hepburn**
5ft 7½in
(KATHARINE HOUGHTON HEPBURN)

Born: **May 12, 1907**
Hartford, Connecticut, USA
Died: **June 29, 2003**

Kate was from a wealthy New England family background. Her father was Doctor Thomas Hepburn, a successful urologist. Her mother, Katherine Houghton, was an heiress to the Corning Glass fortune. Kate went to Bryn Mawr College – earning degrees in History and Philosophy in 1928. That year, she made her professional stage debut in "The Czarina" and married. Kate wasn't an instant success, but through intelligent adjustment to her style she was a Broadway star by 1932. RKO cast her in *Bill of Divorcement* and gave her a five-year contract. Kate won her first Best Actress Oscar, for *Morning Glory* and although she was great in dramatic roles, she was even better acting in screwball comedies with Cary Grant and James Stewart. Her love affair with Spencer Tracy began after they appeared in *Woman of the Year* – the first of ten films they made together. In 1951, she returned to Broadway in "As You Like It" – and then portrayed George Bernard Shaw's, "The Millionairess" – in New York and London. Her next screen appearance was with Bogart in *The African Queen*. As she grew older, she thrived, and won Oscars for *Guess Who's Coming to Dinner, The Lion in Winter* and *On Golden Pond*. Despite the onset of Parkinson's disease Kate continued acting until 1994. She died of natural causes at her Connecticut home.

Little Women (1933)
Morning Glory (1933)
Alice Adams (1935) Stage Door (1937)
Bringing Up Baby (1938) Holiday (1938)
The Philadelphia Story (1940)
Woman of the Year (1941)
State of the Union (1948)
Adam's Rib (1949)
The African Queen (1951)
Pat and Mike (1952) Summertime (1955)
Suddenly, Last Summer (1959)
Guess Who's Coming to Dinner (1967)
The Lion in Winter (1968)
Rooster Cogburn (1975)
On Golden Pond (1981)

Barbara **Hershey**
5ft 5in
(BARBARA LYNN HERZSTEIN)

Born: **February 5, 1948**
Hollywood, California, USA

Barbara was the daughter of a Jewish journalist, Arnold Herzstein, who was a horse-racing columnist. Her mother was Irish. She first got interested in acting while at Hollywood High School. In 1965, she made her television debut in 'Gidget'. She then worked on 'The Monroes' series, which she hated. Barbara's film debut was in Doris Day's final movie, *With Six you get Eggroll,* in 1968. A year after that, she met David Carradine, when they were both working on *Heaven with a Gun*. It was the beginning of a long relationship. They soon became parents and in true hippie fashion, they called the child 'Free'. Barbara's next movie, *Last Summer,* was traumatic. A seagull was killed during the filming, and she felt so guilty – that she changed her name to Barbara Seagull. By 1975, her 'way out' reputation had become a handicap and for a while she only acted in television movies. The 1980s, starting with *The Stunt Man,* and back-to-back wins at Cannes*,* for *Shy People* and *A World Apart,* resurrected her movie career. In 1990, she won an Emmy for 'A Killing in a Small Town' and in 1996, earned a Best Supporting Actress Oscar nomination, in Henry James's *The Portrait of a Lady*. After a brief marriage in 1992, Barbara lives with actor, Naveen Andrews, who is twenty-one years her junior.

The Liberation of L.B.Jones (1970)
The Stunt Man (1980)
The Entity (1981)
The Right Stuff (1983)
The Natural (1984)
Hannah and Her Sisters (1986)
Hoosiers (1986) Tin Men (1987)
Shy People (1987)
A World Apart (1988) The Last
Temptation of Christ (1988)
Beaches (1988) Paris Trout (1991)
Defenseless (1991)
Falling Down (1991)
The Portrait of a Lady (1996)
Lantana (2001)
Riding the Bullet (2004)
Love Comes Lately (2007)

Jean **Hersholt**
5ft 11in
(JEAN HERSHOLT)

Born: **July 12, 1886**
Copenhagen, Denmark
Died: **June 2, 1956**

A member of a well-known Danish acting family, Jean was educated at grammar and high schools in Copenhagen. He made his first film, *Konfirmanden,* when he was twenty. In 1914, he was married for the one and only time, to Via Andersen. His reputation was by then so high, he was chosen by the Danish government to stage its Fair, at the 1915 San Francisco Exhibition. He went there with his young wife, Via, and met the producer, Thomas Ince, who gave him his first American film role, later that year, in *Never Again*. With war raging in Europe, Jean didn't take much persuading to stay. He never regretted it; appearing as he did in some silent classics such as *The Four Horseman of the Apocalypse,* which made Rudolph Valentino a star, in 1921. Three years later, Jean had a featured role in Erich von Stroheim's *Greed.* By the advent of sound, he was a veteran of seventy-five films. His talkies, starting with *The Climax,* in 1930, didn't diminish his reputation at all. His rather Germanic-sounding voice was in fact an asset, and he became popular on the radio. A film titled *The Country Doctor,* in 1936, prolonged his career after he persuaded RKO to finance six Dr. Christian movies, from 1939 until 1941. In 1949 he published his translations of the Hans Christian Anderson fairy tales. The uncle of actor Leslie Nielsen, he died of cancer at his home in Hollywood.

Susan Lenox – Her
Fall and Rise (1931)
The Sin of Madelon Claudet (1931)
Emma (1932)
The Beast of the City (1932)
Grand Hotel (1932)
Unashamed (1932)
Flesh (1932)
The Crime of the Century (1933)
The Painted Veil (1934)
Seventh Heaven (1937)
Heidi (1937)
Alexander's Ragtime Band (1938)
Happy Landing (1938)

Charlton **Heston**
6ft 3in
(JOHN CHARLES CARTER)

Born: **October 4, 1923**
Evanston, Illinois, USA
Died: **April 5, 2008**

At New Trier High School, in Chicago, Chuck was crazy about acting. Later, at Northwestern University, he majored in speech and used that skill in his first jobs with Chicago radio stations. His dramatic progress was interrupted by World War II, when he served as a radio operator in the U.S. Air Force. In 1944, he married the actress, Lydia Clarke, and they were together until his death. After the war, they managed the Asheville Playhouse, in North Carolina, until 1948. They moved to New York, where he got a supporting role in "Anthony and Cleopatra" on Broadway. TV work followed in 1949 – he received rave notices for his Rochester – in 'Jane Eyre'. It lead to a contract with Hal Wallis and his film debut, in 1950, in *Dark City,* with Lizbeth Scott. His career took off when he was chosen by Cecil B. De Mille for *The Greatest Show on Earth.* Four years later, De Mille gave him another boost by casting him as Moses, in *The Ten Commandments.* It made him a star and three years after that, he won a Best Actor Oscar for *Ben-Hur.* He remained at the top for fifteen years. His box-office appeal plummeted after the mid-1970s. In 2002, Chuck was diagnosed with Alzheimer's disease and was rarely seen in public up until his death, from related symptoms, six years later, in Beverly Hills.

The Greatest Show on Earth (1952)
Ruby Gentry (1952)
The Naked Jungle (1954)
The Ten Commandments (1956)
Touch of Evil (1958)
The Big Country (1958) Ben-Hur (1959)
The Wreck of the Mary Deare (1959)
El Cid (1961) 55 Days at Peking (1963)
The Agony and the Ecstasy (1965)
Major Dundee (1966)
The War Lord (1966) Khartoum (1966)
Planet of the Apes (1968)
Will Penny (1968) Soylent Green (1973)
The Three Musketeers (1973)
Midway (1976) True Lies (1994)
In the Mouth of Madness (1995)

Dame Wendy **Hiller**
5ft 7in
(WENDY MARGARET HILLER)

Born: **August 15, 1912**
Bramhall, Cheshire, England
Died: **May 14, 2003**

With the support of her mother, Marie, Wendy convinced her father to allow her to become an actress. To get rid of her Cheshire accent, her father Frank Hiller – a wealthy cotton manufacturer – sent her south to be educated at Winceby House School, in Bexhill, in East Sussex. Wendy then went to the Manchester Repertory Theater, to learn how to act, and it was her intimate knowledge of northern accents that led to her triumph as a mill girl called Sally Hardcastle, in her first stage appearance, in "Love on the Dole". She remained in it for the London production, and in 1936, enjoyed great success in New York City. Its writer, Ronald Gow, married her in 1937, after she had returned to England to make her film debut, in *Lancashire Luck.* Shaw asked her to star in his *Pygmalion* and she, complete with an authentic cockney accent, was 'deluverly'. Wendy then turned down Hollywood offers and was given another film role from a Shaw play – *Major Barbara.* Until the late 1950s, most of her work was on the stage, but there were films like *Separate Tables,* for which she won a Best Supporting Actress Oscar. Wendy was created a Dame of the British Empire in 1975. She survived her husband by ten years and passed away peacefully at her home in Beaconsfield, Buckinghamshire. She had two children - a son and a daughter.

Pygmalion (1938)
Major Barbara (1941)
I Know Where I'm Going (1945)
Outcast of the Islands (1952)
Sailor of the King (1953)
Something of Value (1957)
Separate Tables (1958)
Sons and Lovers (1960)
Toys in the Attic (1963)
A Man for All Seasons (1966)
The Elephant Man (1980)
Miss Morison's Ghosts (1981)
The Lonely Passion of
Judith Hearne (1987)
The Countess Alice (1992)

Valerie **Hobson**
5ft 6in
(VALERIE BABETTE LOUISE HOBSON)

Born: **April 14, 1917**
Larne, County Antrim, Ireland
Died: **November 13, 1998**

Although she started her life in Ireland, both of Valerie's parents were English. Her father, a naval officer, took his wife and daughter back to England when she was fourteen, and she enrolled at the Royal Academy of Dramatic Art, in London. A successful stage debut, in "Ball at the Savoy", at London's Drury Lane Theater, was soon followed in 1933, by her film debut as the star of a B picture called *Eyes of Fate.* After only four more films, Valerie went to Hollywood, where she was a blonde in *Strange Wives.* By 1937, she had returned to Britain, where she so impressed producer Alexander Korda, he cast her in two films, *The Drum* and *Q Planes.* In 1939, she married the producer Anthony Havelock-Allen, and benefited from his film contacts until their divorce in 1952 – most notably with roles in David Lean's *Great Expectations,* the Ealing comedy, *Kind Hearts and Coronets* and a second helping of Guinness, in *The Card.* After her divorce, Valerie married the Tory politician, John Profumo. Ten years later, he would provide more drama than any of her movies. In 1954, she co-starred with the French heart-throb, Gérard Philipe, in *Knave of Hearts,* and then retired. When the scandal erupted over her husband's relationships with prostitutes and spies, she stood by him. Until she died of a heart attack at her home in London, she poured her heart and soul into charity work.

The Drum (1938)
Q Planes (1939)
A Spy in Black (1940)
Contraband (1940)
The Years Between (1946)
Great Expectations (1946)
The Small Voice (1948)
Blanche Fury (1948)
Kind Hearts and Coronets (1949)
The Interrupted Journey (1949)
The Rocking Horse Winner (1950)
The Card (1951)
Murder Will Out (1952)
Knave of Hearts (1954)

Dustin **Hoffman**
5ft 6³⁄₄in
(DUSTIN LEE HOFFMAN)

Born: **August 8, 1937**
Los Angeles, California, USA

Dustin's parents, Harry Hoffman, who worked as a prop supervisor at Columbia Pictures, and his wife, Lillian, a jazz pianist, were from a Polish Jewish background. They named him after the silent film star, Dustin Farnum. After Los Angeles High School, Dustin attended Santa Monica City College, but due to concentrating on an acting course, he dropped out. From 1956, he spent two years at the Pasadena Playhouse along with fellow actor, Gene Hackman. They both went to New York, where after struggling initially, Dustin landed a small role on Broadway, in 1961. He did TV commercials while studying at the Actors Studio. After his film debut, in a small role in *The Tiger Makes Out,* he got his big breakthrough in the same year's *The Graduate,* for which he was Oscar-nominated. From then onwards, screen credits have been in the main, a catalog of successes. Two Best Actor Oscars – for *Kramer vs. Kramer* and *Rain Man,* plus another four nominations – for *Midnight Cowboy, Lenny, Tootsie,* and *Wag the Dog* seem scant reward for his contributions – during more than forty years of movie-making. From his two marriages, to Anne Byrne, and his current wife Lisa, he has six children. Four of them are actors.

The Graduate (1967)
Midnight Cowboy (1969)
Little Big Man (1970)
Straw Dogs (1971) Papillon (1973)
Lenny (1974)
All the President's Men (1976)
Marathon Man (1976)
Kramer vs. Kramer (1979)
Tootsie (1982) Rain Man (1988)
Accidental Hero (1992)
Outbreak (1995)
American Buffalo (1996)
Sleepers (1996) Mad City (1997)
Finding Neverland (2004) Perfume:
The Story of a Murderer (2006)
Stranger Than Fiction (2006)
Mr. Magorium's Wonder
Emporium (2007)
Last Chance Harvey (2008)

Philip Seymour **Hoffman**
5ft 9¹⁄₂in
(PHILIP SEYMOUR HOFFMAN)

Born: **July 23, 1967**
Fairport, New York, USA

Phil's mother, Marilyn, was a judge in Rochester. He first became interested in acting at Fairport High School. In 1989 he graduated from New York University's Tisch School of the Arts. His film debut in 1991, was in the independent production, *Triple Bogey on a Par Five Hole.* After a number of strong supporting roles, Phil made his breakthrough in *Boogie Nights.* He soon established a reputation as one of the screen's finest actors – in indies like *Happiness* – and major features, such as *Magnolia* and *The Talented Mr. Ripley.* In 2000, Phil appeared on Broadway, in "True West", for which he was nominated for a Best Actor Tony. He has taken over as Co-Artistic Director of the LAByrinth Theater Company where he's directed a number of stage productions. He won a Best Actor Oscar for his great portrayal of Truman Capote, in *Capote.* Phil has two children with his girlfriend, Mimi O'Donnell. He can never be left out of the reckoning when it comes to awards. He was Oscar-nominated as Best Supporting Actor – for *Charlie Wilson's War* and *Doubt.*

When a Man Loves a Woman (1994)
Nobody's Fool (1994)
Sydney (1996) Twister (1996)
Boogie Nights (1997) Montana (1998)
The Big Lebowski (1998)
Happiness (1998) Magnolia (1999)
The Talented Mr. Ripley (1999)
State and Main (2000)
Almost Famous (2000)
Love Liza (2002)
Punch-Drunk Love (2002)
Red Dragon (2002) 25th Hour (2002)
Owning Mahowny (2003)
Cold Mountain (2003)
Along Came Polly (2004)
Capote (2005) Mission
Impossible III (2006)
Before the Devil Knows
You're Dead (2007)
The Savages (2007)
Charlie Wilson's War (2007)
Synecdoche, New York (2007)
Doubt (2008)

William **Holden**
5ft 11in
(WILLIAM FRANKLIN BEEDLE JR.)

Born: **April 17, 1918**
O'Fallon, Illinois, USA
Died: **November 12, 1981**

Bill's parents, William Beedle Sr., and his wife, Mary, took the family to California when he was three. He attended South Pasadena High School and Pasadena Junior College. While at the latter, he acted in plays on local radio stations. In 1937, he was playing an eighty-year-old man, in "Manya" at a private theater called the Playbox, when his performance was noted by a talent scout from Paramount. After uncredited roles in *Prison Farm,* and *Million Dollar Legs,* Bill was given the star treatment in 1939, as violin-playing boxer, Joe Bonaparte, in *Golden Boy.* It didn't make him a star. Neither did ten more unremarkable movies, up until 1942. In 1941, he married Brenda Marshall and then joined the U.S. Army. He didn't begin to rebuild his film career until 1947, when he appeared in *Blaze of Noon.* A loan out to RKO, for a Loretta Young vehicle, *Rachel and the Stranger,* got the fan mail pouring in. He was in almost every scene in the classic, *Sunset Boulevard* and acted as Judy Holliday's tutor that same year, in *Born Yesterday.* A Best Actor Oscar for *Stalag 17,* was followed by a number of top productions including *The Bridge on the River Kwai* and *The Wild Bunch.* In 1966, Bill was convicted of manslaughter in Italy and started drinking heavily. A bad fall in his Santa Monica apartment, while intoxicated, killed him.

Golden Boy (1939) Our Town (1940)
Arizona (1940) Texas (1941)
The Remarkable Andrew (1942)
Dear Ruth (1947)
Rachel and the Stranger (1948)
Streets of Laredo (1949)
Sunset Boulevard (1950) Born
Yesterday (1950) Stalag 17 (1953)
Escape from Fort Bravo (1953)
Sabrina (1954) The Country Girl (1954)
The Bridges at Toko-Ri (1954)
Picnic (1955) The Bridge on
the River Kwai (1957)
The Wild Bunch (1969)
Network (1976)

Judy **Holliday**
5ft 8in
(JUDITH TUVIM)

Born: **June 21, 1921**
New York City, New York, USA
Died: **June 7, 1965**

The only child of Abe and Helen Tuvim – who were Jewish immigrants from Russia – Judy's stage name came easily. "Tuvim" is Yiddish for "Holiday". Her entry into show business was almost as easy. From the age of four, while Judy was at PS 150, an elementary school in Queens, she started attending ballet classes. At sixteen she was working on the switchboard at Orson Welles's Mercury Theater. At the end of 1938, she formed a nightclub act called "The Revuers" with four others, including Adolph Green and Betty Comden. One of their accompanists was the composer Leonard Bernstein. It survived on the New York circuit until 1944 when the group was signed by 20th Century Fox, but all their scenes in *Greenwich Village,* were cut out. Judy had a small role (on her film debut) in *Something for the Boys.* The following year, she made her Broadway debut in "Kiss Them for Me". In 1946, she replaced Jean Arthur, in Garson Kanin's "Born Yesterday". She had enjoyed four years in the role by the time she appeared in the film version and won an Oscar for Best Actress. 1950 was also the year she was investigated for her alleged involvement in the Communist Party. Nothing was proven, but she was blacklisted from performing on television or radio for three years, and certainly her film career lost its momentum. By the time of her final movie, *Bells Are Ringing,* she was beginning to suffer from the breast cancer which took around four years to kill her. Judy had a son, Jon, from her ten-year marriage to song-writer Dave Oppenheim. He is now working as a film editor.

Winged Victory (1944) **Adam's Rib** (1949)
Born Yesterday (1950)
The Marrying Kind (1952)
It Should Happen to You (1954)
Phffft! (1954)
The Solid Gold Cadillac (1956)
Full of Life (1956)
Bells Are Ringing (1960)

Stanley **Holloway**
5ft 7in
(STANLEY AUGUSTUS HOLLOWAY)

Born: **October 1, 1890**
East Ham, Essex, England
Died: **January 30, 1982**

Born in what became the East End of London, Stanley grew up in a working class family environment. He was educated at The Worshipful School of Carpenters in nearby Stratford, and at fifteen years of age, he started his first job as a clerk in Billingsgate Fish Market. When he was seventeen, he started performing at seaside resorts such as Clacton-on-Sea, and from 1911, he was resident comedian at the West Cliff Theater. Stanley had a good singing voice and spent a few months studying in Milan, Italy. At the beginning of World War I, he joined the Connaught Rangers and in 1920, was with the "Black and Tans" in Ireland. From 1921, he was back in show business in the hit show, "The Co-Optimists". That year, he made his film debut in *The Rotters.* His film work during the 1930s was generally in cheaply made comedies, but his second marriage to Violet Lane, in 1939, spurred him into a change to his approach. His reputation as a character actor grew after the comedy classics, *Passport to Pimlico* and *The Lavender Hill Mob.* His career reached its peak in the stage hit "My Fair Lady" and he was nominated for a Best Supporting Actor Oscar for the film version. Stanley died in a Littlehampton nursing home.

This Happy Breed (1944) **The Way Ahead** (1944) **Champagne Charlie** (1944)
The Way to the Stars (1945) **Brief Encounter** (1945) **Wanted for Murder** (1946) **Carnival** (1946) **Nicholas Nickleby** (1947) **One Night with You** (1948) **Hamlet** (1948) **The Winslow Boy** (1948) **Passport to Pimlico** (1949)
The Lavender Hill Mob (1951)
The Titfield Thunderbolt (1953)
A Day to Remember (1953)
Meet Mr. Lucifer (1953) **Fast and Loose** (1954) **No Love for Johnnie** (1961) **My Fair Lady** (1964)
In Harm's Way (1965)
Ten Little Indians (1965)
The Private Life of Sherlock Holmes (1970)

Celeste **Holm**
5ft 6in
(CELESTE HOLM)

Born: **April 29, 1917**
New York City, New York, USA

Celeste was the only child of a father from a Norwegian background, Theodor Holm. Her mother, Jean, was an author and portrait painter. After studying acting at the University of Chicago, Celeste made her stage debut with a stock company in Pennsylvania. Her second husband converted her to Catholicism in 1940, but neither the marriage nor the faith, lasted very long. She appeared with Leslie Howard, in a production of "Hamlet" and by the time she played Ado Annie, in "Oklahoma" in 1943, she was a Broadway star. She made her film debut for 20th Century Fox, in *Three Little Girls in Blue* and in 1947, she won a Best Supporting Actress Oscar for Elia Kazan's powerful *Gentleman's Agreement.* In the *early* 1950s, following her role in the stage-themed *All About Eve,* Celeste decided that she preferred working in the theater, and asked to be released from her movie contract. Her main body of good film work is very small. A mention should be made of two good later showings – in *The Tender Trap* and *High Society* – before, for fifty years, gracing television. In 1968, she received the Sarah Siddons Award for her distinguished achievement in Chicago Theater. Celeste is a spokesperson for UNICEF. On her birthday in 2004, she married for the fifth time – opera singer – Frank Basile. She has occasionally made appearances in films over the past twenty years. Celeste's most recent movie role, was in *Alchemy,* in 2005.

Three Little Girls in Blue (1946)
Gentleman's Agreement (1947)
Road House (1948)
The Snake Pit (1948)
Chicken Every Sunday (1949)
Come to the Stable (1949)
Everybody Does It (1949)
Champagne for Caesar (1950)
All About Eve (1950)
The Tender Trap (1955)
High Society (1956)
Tom Sawyer (1973)
Still Breathing (1997)

Sir Ian **Holm**
5ft 6in
(IAN HOLM CUTHBERT)

Born: **September 12, 1931**
Goodmayes, Essex, England

Ian was the son of Dr. James Cuthbert, a psychiatrist in a mental hospital, and his wife, Jean Holm, who worked as a nurse. Ian was educated at Chigwell School, in Essex. After the war, he went to RADA. He established himself with the Royal Shakespeare Company in the 1950s and was strictly a stage actor for about fifteen years. In 1958, he made an uncredited appearance in a comedy called *Girls at Sea,* but his film debut proper was in *The Bofors Gun,* ten years later. To begin with, Ian earned a reputation with a series of small but significant roles in major films such as *Young Winston.* In terms of the weight of his own contribution, his first important part was as the evil android, in Ridley Scott's *Aliens.* Soon after that, he was nominated for an Oscar, as Best Supporting Actor, for *Chariots of Fire.* Throughout the following two decades, he was a familiar supporting figure in some high profile movies. Ian's third wife, whom he divorced in 2001, was the popular actress, Penelope Wilton. Of five children from earlier marriages – three of them are in show business. Ian's next movie project is called *This Side of the Looking Glass.*

Alien (1979)
Chariots of Fire (1981)
Time Bandits (1981)
Dance with a Stranger (1985)
Dreamchild (1985)
Another Woman (1988)
Henry V (1989) Hamlet (1990)
Kafka (1991)
Naked Lunch (1991)
The Madness of King George (1994)
Night Falls on Manhattan (1997)
The Fifth Element (1997)
The Sweet Hereafter (1997)
eXistenZ (1999)
The Fellowship of the Rings (2001)
Garden State (2004)
The Day After Tomorrow (2004)
The Aviator (2004)
Lord of War (2005)
The Treatment (2006)
O Jerusalem (2006)

Tim **Holt**
5ft 10in
(CHARLES JOHN HOLT III)

Born: **February 5, 1918**
Beverly Hills, California, USA
Died: **February 15, 1973**

Tim and his younger sister, Jennifer, were the children of the popular movie cowboy, Jack Holt, and his wife, Margaret. Tim was eight years old when he made his first film appearance, in the comedy short, *Young Hollywood.* A year later, he had a small role in his father's western, *The Vanishing Pioneer.* After his junior schooling, Tim attended the Culver Military Academy, in Culver, Indiana. After his graduation, he followed his dad into movies with an uncredited appearance in the 1937 Jean Arthur, Charles Boyer, drama, *History Is Made at Night.* Tim's official debut as an adult actor, was in the Barbara Stanwyck movie, *Stella Dallas.* It was natural that he drifted towards westerns – mainly B's, but two of them – *Stagecoach* and *My Darling Clementine* are all-time greats. In addition, he had roles in two other highly-regarded films – *The Magnificent Ambersons* and *The Treasure of the Sierra Madre.* The latter features Tim's best performance as a film actor. He ended his career as a cowboy star and played his father Jack's son, in *The Arizona Ranger.* In 1972, Tim was diagnosed with bone cancer and died the following year, in Shawnee, Oklahoma.

Stella Dallas (1937)
I Met My Love Again (1938)
The Law West of Tombstone (1938)
Stagecoach (1939)
5th Ave Girl (1939)
Swiss Family Robinson (1940)
Wagon Train (1940)
Back Street (1941)
Land of the Open Range (1942)
The Magnificent Ambersons (1942)
Hitler's Children (1943)
The Avenging Rider (1943)
My Darling Clementine (1946)
Thunder Mountain (1947)
The Treasure of the
Sierra Madre (1948)
The Arizona Ranger (1948)
Gun Smugglers (1949)
His Kind of Woman (1951)
Road Agent (1952)

Oscar **Homolka**
6ft
(OSCAR HOMOLKA)

Born: **August 12, 1898**
Vienna, Austro-Hungary
Died: **January 27, 1978**

In 1915, Oscar began training at the Academy of Music and Performing Arts, in Vienna. He made his stage debut at the Komödienhaus, in 1918. By 1924, he was appearing on the Berlin stage. He made his film debut in Germany in 1926, in *Adventures of a Ten Mark Note.* Oscar remained a big name there, both in the cinema and in the theater until, because he was Jewish, Adolf Hitler's jackbooted bullies forced him to leave. In 1935 he emigrated to London, where he co-starred with Walter Huston, in *Rhodes of Africa.* During his second year there, he made an impact in Alfred Hitchcock's *Sabotage.* He left for Hollywood in 1937 – making the movie *Ebb Tide* – shortly after arriving there and getting good roles in many top quality productions – sometimes supporting – sometimes starring. For one such film, *I Remember Mama,* he was nominated for a Best Supporting Actor Oscar. His bushy brows and thick accent were perfect for cold-war thrillers. He'd been an actor for more than fifty years, when he retired in 1976. Married four times, Oscar was badly affected a year later, by the death of his fourth wife, the actress Joan Tetzel. He died sad and alone in Sussex, England, of pneumonia.

Sabotage (1936)
Ebb Tide (1937)
Seven Sinners (1940)
Comrade X (1940)
The Invisible Woman (1940)
Ball of Fire (1941)
Mission to Moscow (1943)
The Shop at Sly Corner (1947)
I Remember Mama (1948)
Anna Lucasta (1949)
The White Tower (1950)
Top Secret (1952)
The Seven Year Itch (1955)
War and Peace (1956)
Mr. Sardonicus (1961)
Funeral in Berlin 1966)
Assignment to Kill (1968)
The Tamarind Seed (1974)

Bob **Hope**
5ft 10in
(LESLIE TOWNES HOPE)

Born: **May 29, 1903**
Eltham, London, England
Died: **July 27, 2003**

Bob was the fifth of seven boys born to a stonemason and his wife. In 1908, the family caught a boat to New York and settled in Cleveland, Ohio, where Bob grew up like any other American boy. The only difference being that he had the talent, from the age of twelve, to entertain with his singing, dancing, and impersonation of Charlie Chaplin. He was seen by Fatty Arbuckle, who in 1925, got him a job with "Hurley's Jolly Follies" and small parts in short silent movies. He played a vaudeville performer in his first Broadway show, "Ballyhoo" in 1933, and the following year, married the singer, Dolores Reade. He was signed by Paramount, who gave him his first featured film role in *The Big Broadcast of 1938,* in which he first sang "Thanks for the Memory". In 1939, in *The Cat and the Canary* – he introduced his cowardly hero personality. He became popular through his association with Bing Crosby in the series of 'Road' movies, and remained in the top-ten moneymakers up to 1953. From 1960, he was mainly seen in TV specials and concert dates. Bob donated land he owned at Rancho Mirage in California, to house the Eisenhower Medical Center. He kept himself fit by playing golf and, unlike his grandfather, who died aged ninety-nine years, eleven months and twenty-five days, Bob was successful in reaching his century! He died at Toluca Lake, California, of pneumonia.

The Cat and the Canary (1939)
The Ghost Breakers (1940)
Caught in the Draft (1941)
Nothing But the Truth (1941)
My Favorite Blonde (1942)
Road to Morocco (1942)
The Princess and the Pirate (1944)
Road to Utopia (1944)
My Favorite Brunette (1947)
Road to Rio (1947) The Paleface (1948)
Fancy Pants (1950) Road to Bali (1952)
That Certain Feeling (1956)
Alias Jesse James (1959)
The Facts of Life (1960)

Sir Anthony **Hopkins**
5ft 8½in
(PHILIP ANTHONY HOPKINS)

Born: **December 31, 1937**
Port Talbot, West Glamorgan, Wales

Tony was the son of a baker, named Richard Hopkins, and Muriel Yeats, who was related to the poet, W.B. Yeats. He had a sad life at Cowbridge Grammar School, where he suffered from dyslexia. Later, with encouragement from Richard Burton, whom he met briefly, he enrolled at the Cardiff College of Music and Drama. In 1959, after completing two years' National Service, he studied at RADA. He gained experience with repertory companies before, in 1965, he was asked by Laurence Olivier to join the National Theater. When Olivier was sidelined with appendicitis, Tony substituted successfully in Strindberg's "The Dance of Death". He made his film debut in 1967, in Lindsay Anderson's *The White Bus,* and was soon getting roles in important films – he worked with Richard Attenborough five times. He won a Best Actor Oscar for his chilling portrayal of Hannibal Lecter, in *The Silence of the Lambs,* and was nominated for *The Remains of the Day, Nixon,* and *Amistad.* Tony was knighted in 1993 but became a United States citizen, in 2000. He's been married three times. His third wife is the Columbian-born actress, Stella Arroyave. In 2010, Tony will star in the title role of Shakespeare's *King Lear.*

The Lion in Winter (1968)
Juggernaut (1974)
The Elephant Man (1980)
The Bounty (1984)
The Good Father (1985)
84 Charing Cross Road (1987)
The Dawning (1988)
The Silence of the Lambs (1991)
Howard's End (1992)
The Remains of the Day (1993)
Shadowlands (1993)
Legends of the Fall (1994)
Nixon (1995)
Surviving Picasso (1996)
The Edge (1997) Amistad (1997)
Meet Joe Black (1998)
Red Dragon (2002) Proof (2005)
Bobby (2006) Slipstream (2007)
Beowulf (2007)

Miriam **Hopkins**
5ft 2in
(ELLEN MIRIAM HOPKINS)

Born: **October 18, 1902**
Savannah, Georgia, USA
Died: **October 9, 1972**

After her father left, Miriam was brought up by her mother in Barre, Vermont. She attended the Goddard Seminary, in nearby Plainfield. At eighteen, she was a chorus girl in Irving Berlin's "Music Box Revue". She rose to prominence as a Broadway actress, before being offered a contract by Paramount. Miriam was the star of her debut film *Fast and Loose,* in 1930. She appeared in a series of memorable movie roles – opposite the top leading men of the day – which included Frederic March, Gary Cooper and Maurice Chevalier. Miriam was nominated for a Best Actress Oscar in *Becky Sharp* – the first feature film to benefit from 3-color Technicolor. She was unpopular with other actors. One reason was her tendency (and ability) to upstage them at every opportunity. Edward G. Robinson reprimanded her in front of the crew when they made *Barbary Coast.* After joining Warners in the late 1930s, she played second leads – only meeting her match in the great Bette Davis. She returned to Broadway in 1944, and later worked on TV. From the early 1960s, the four-times married star was often alone and drinking heavily. She died in New York City, of a heart attack.

The Smiling Lieutenant (1931)
24 Hours (1931)
Dr. Jekyll and Mr. Hyde (1931)
Trouble in Paradise (1932)
The Stranger's Return (1933)
She Loves Me Not (1934)
The Richest Girl in the World (1934)
Becky Sharp (1935)
Barbary Coast (1935)
Splendor (1935)
These Three (1936)
Wise Girl (1937)
The Old Maid (1939)
Virginia City (1940)
Old Acquaintance (1943)
The Heiress (1949) The Mating
Season (1951) Carrie (1952)
The Children's Hour (1961)
The Chase (1966)

Dennis **Hopper**
5ft 9in
(DENNIS LEE HOPPER)

Born: **May 17, 1936**
Dodge City, Kansas, USA

The son of Jay Millard Hopper, a post office manager, and his wife, Marjorie – who was a lifeguard instructor – Dennis started out on a farm. He was educated at Wooster School, in Connecticut, but his family moved to San Diego when he was a teenager. At Helix High School, in La Mesa, where Dennis first took an interest in acting, he was voted 'most likely to succeed'. He studied at the Old Globe Theater in San Diego before he spent five years under the tutorage of Lee Strasberg, in New York.Dennis made his acting debut in 1955, in an episode of the TV series, 'Medic'. It was followed soon after with featured roles in James Dean's last two movies. His reaction to Dean's death resulted in a bad frame of mind – leading to a serious confrontation with the director Henry Hathaway, on the set of *From Hell to Texas* – and virtual blacklisting. His cocaine habit added to his problems until it became an asset in the landmark film, *Easy Rider,* which he co-wrote, directed and acted in. His health was affected by his excesses to the point where he underwent a rehab program in 1983. He was Oscar nominated for a supporting role in *Hoosiers,* and in 1988, he was praised as director of a movie about L.A. gangs, titled *Colors.* Dennis is still acting with great energy. His five wives (the current one is Victoria Duffy) were all actresses.

Rebel Without a Cause (1955)
Gunfight at the O.K. Corral (1957)
Easy Rider (1969)
Apocalypse Now (1979)
Rumble Fish (1983)
Blue Velvet (1986)
River's Edge (1986)
Hoosiers (1986) Paris Trout (1991)
The Indian Runner (1991)
Red Rock West (1992)
True Romance (1993)
Speed (1994) Basquiat (1996)
Jesus' Son (1999)
Leo (2002) Americano (2005)
10th & Wolf (2006) Elegy (2008)
Swing Votes (2008)

Lena **Horne**
5ft 4¹/₂in
(LENA MARY CALHOUN HORNE)

Born: **June 30, 1917**
Brooklyn, New York City, New York, USA

Lena's father, Teddie Horne, was a New York bookmaker, and her mother, Edna Scottron – the daughter of an inventor – was an actress. After her father decided to abandon his family when Lena was three years old, she was raised in a comfortable black middle-class home, in Brooklyn, by her grandparents. While in her teens, she sang in clubs, backed by jazz musicians. She had a great voice, but more than that, she was extremely beautiful. Yet in those days, the prospects for a black girl of a movie career were limited – unless you accepted the kind of roles which Hattie McDaniel played. Lena did try to keep her integrity. She made her film debut, as the star of *The Duke is Tops,* in 1938. But it was another four years before she was offered a contract by MGM. During the 1940s, there were a couple of featured roles with all-black casts, including her best early film, *Cabin in the Sky* – directed by Vincente Minnelli. In 1947, she married MGM arranger, Lennie Hayton. Usually, her roles were no more than guest spots. When she acted in a 'white' film, her scenes were deleted for showing in southern states. Because of that, she is rarely an integral part of the story. In 1951, she was lined up for *Showboat* – having sung in a sequence from the show – in *Till the Clouds Roll By.* Sadly, the production code at that time didn't allow racial mixing. In the 1950s, she was blacklisted for her political views and her loyal support for the 'Communist', Paul Robeson. A recording career and a long spell as a popular nightclub singer culminated in a show entitled "Lena Horne: The Lady and Her Music". She sang on Sinatra's "Duets II" album and her own "Being Myself".

Panama Hattie (1942)
Cabin in the Sky (1943)
Stormy Weather (1943)
Swing Fever (1943)
Ziegfeld Follies (1946)
Till the Clouds Roll By (1946)
Words and Music (1948)
Death of a Gunfighter (1969)

Edward Everett **Horton**
6ft
(EDWARD EVERETT HORTON JR.)

Born: **March 18, 1886**
Brooklyn, New York City, New York, USA
Died: **September 29, 1970**

Edward's dad, Edward Everett Horton Sr., was a proof-reader at The New York Times. His mother, Isabella was born in Cuba to Scottish immigrants. Edward was educated at Baltimore City College High School. After that, he attended Brooklyn Polytechnic and Columbia University. He made his stage debut with the drama club and after that, toured with various stock companies. In 1922, Edward made his film debut in the silent film, *A Front Page Story.* His stage experience gave him an easy entry into 'talkies'. Edward's output during the first years of sound was prolific – in 1929, he made ten films comprising two-reelers and features. His rather effete style (he was gay) made it difficult to cast him as a romantic lead. By the early 1930s, he was a popular supporting actor in comedies with Cary Grant and musicals starring Astaire and Rogers. By the end of World War II, he saw the writing on the wall – his future in films was limited. For a quarter of a century, he kept his career going by acting on television. In 1966, he was asked about retirement. "Dear Lord!" he cried, "I would go right out of my mind". Edward died of cancer at his home in Encino, California, shortly after finishing his final film, *Cold Turkey.*

Trouble in Paradise (1932)
Easy to Love (1934)
The Merry Widow (1934)
The Gay Divorcee (1934)
The Night is Young (1935)
The Devil is a Woman (1935)
Top Hat (1935)
Lost Horizon (1937)
Shall We Dance (1937)
The Great Garrick (1937)
Bluebeard's Eighth Wife (1938)
Holiday (1938)
Ziegfeld Girl (1941)
Here Comes Mr. Jordan (1941)
The Magnificent Dope (1942)
The Gang's All Here (1943)
Lady on a Train (1945)
Sex and the Single Girl (1964)

Bob **Hoskins**
5ft 6in
(ROBERT WILLIAM HOSKINS)

Born: **October 26, 1942**
Bury St. Edmunds, Suffolk, England

Bob's father, Robert William Hoskins Sr., was a bookkeeper. To escape the London bombing, Bob's mother, Elsie, moved to Suffolk weeks before he was born. Despite a fairly limited education he had a passion for reading. At fifteen, he began earning money by working in a variety of jobs, including fire eater. Bob used most of his income to pay for seats in the 'Gods' in West End theaters. On one of those trips, he auditioned for a part in a play – by sheer accident – and got the job. He also got married and his new responsibilities (two children) pushed him to get TV work – in series such as 'Villains' and 'Thick as Thieves'. In 1974, he made his film debut in *Inserts.* Four years later, there was true international recognition, after he played Arthur Parker, in the hit TV mini-series, 'Pennies from Heaven' by Dennis Potter. Bob's first major movie role was in *The Long Good Friday.* In 1982, he married his current wife, Linda Barnwell. After that, there were few years when he didn't make a worthwhile appearance on the big screen. He was nominated for an Oscar for *Mona Lisa,* and aside from a number of Hollywood films, he is a big supporter of independent movies as well as interesting projects, like the BBC-funded, black and white film – *TwentyFourSeven.*

The Long Good Friday (1980)
Pink Floyd The Wall (1982)
Brazil (1985) **Mona Lisa** (1986)
Short Circuit (1986)
A Prayer for the Dying (1987)
Who Framed Roger Rabbit (1988)
Shattered (1991) Nixon (1995)
Felicia's Journey (1999)
Enemy at the Gates (2001)
Last Orders (2001)
The Sleeping Dictionary (2003)
Vanity Fair (2004)
Beyond the Sea (2004)
Danny the Dog (2005)
Mrs. Henderson Presents (2005)
Stay (2005) Hollywoodland (2006)
Sparkle (2007)
Doomsday (2008)

Robert **Hossein**
5ft 10in
(ROBERT HOSSEINOFF)

Born: **December 30, 1927**
Paris, France

Son of the Russian-Iranian composer, André Hossein, and a concert pianist mother, Robert took drama lessons from René Simon. He made his stage debut in "Les Voyous" in 1946. Shortly after that, he directed several plays, including "Dr. Jekyll & Mr. Hyde". Two years later he made his movie debut (a walk-on part) in *Les Souvenirs ne sont pas à vendre.* His first credited role was in *Maya,* in 1949. His movie acting career was launched in 1955, in Jules Dassin's masterpiece, *Rififi.* Following that, Robert portrayed gangsters in several French films. In 1956, he directed for the first time, and also acted in, *The Wicked Go to Hell,* with his first wife, Marina Vlady. They continued to appear together until they split up in the early 1960s. In 1962, he co-starred with both Brigitte Bardot and Sophia Loren, but neither film was anything to be proud of. In 1964, he appeared opposite Michèle Mercier, in the romantic movie, *Angélique, marquise des anges* – the first of four on that subject. In 1965, he appeared with an international cast including Henry Fonda, and Robert Ryan, in *The Dirty Game.* In 1970, at the height of his success, he left Paris to become director of the Théatre Populaire, in Reims. Robert has continued working on the stage, television, and in films right up to 2009. He is an energetic man – still active in his eighties.

Rififi (1955)
Crime and Punishment (1956)
No Sun in Venice (1956)
Toi, le venin (1958)
La Sentence (1959)
Le Jeu de la Vérité (1962)
Le Monte-Charge (1962)
Chair de poule (1963)
Nell'anno del Signore (1969)
Forbidden Priests (1973)
Bolero (1981)
The Professional (1981)
Les Enfants du désordre (1989)
The Wax Mask (1997)
Venus Beauty Institute (1999)
Un homme et son chien (2008)

Leslie **Howard**
5ft 10½in
(LESLIE HOWARD STEINER)

Born: **April 3, 1893**
Forest Hill, London, England
Died: **June 1, 1943**

The son of Ferdinand Steiner, a Hungarian Jewish immigrant, and an English-born, Jewish mother, Lillian Blumberg, Leslie grew up to be the archetypal Englishman, who American movie audiences adored. He turned out that way through his exclusive schooling at Dulwich College. In 1917 he was serving in the British Army during World War I, and suffered shell-shock on the Western Front. His mother helped his recovery by getting him work with a touring company. His first film was that year, in *The Happy Warrior.* By 1928, he had acted in several films and also appeared on the Broadway stage. Warner Brothers put him under contract in 1930 – starring him in a film version of his stage success – *Outward Bound.* A year later he was with MGM – opposite Norma Shearer – in *A Free Soul.* Leslie was too sensitive to enjoy Hollywood – believing that he and other stars were not worth their salaries. He worked in Britain for Alexander Korda but acted in plays as frequently as possible. Signing for Warners suited him better – they even helped him to set up his own production company in England. In 1939, he acted in *Gone with the Wind,* but when the war started, Leslie became a leading figure in the British film industry. He was especially good in the movie about the Spitfire designer – *The First of the Few.* In 1943, he went to Portugal to lecture on the theater. He was flying back to London from Lisbon, when his plane was shot down – the Germans wrongly believing that Winston Churchill was on board.

The Animal Kingdom (1932)
Berkeley Square (1933)
The Scarlet Pimpernel (1934)
The Petrified Forest (1936)
Romeo and Juliet (1936)
Pygmalion (1938)
Intermezzo (1939)
Gone with the Wind (1939)
'Pimpernel' Smith (1941)
49th Parallel (1941)
The First of the Few (1942)

Trevor **Howard**
5ft 11in
(TREVOR WALLACE HOWARD-SMITH)

Born: **September 29, 1913**
Cliftonville, Kent, England
Died: **January 7, 1988**

Trevor was the only son of a Lloyd's insurance broker, Arthur Howard-Smith, and his Canadian wife, Mabel. After Clifton College in Bristol, he studied acting at the Royal Academy of Dramatic Art, London. He acted on the West End stage – his debut was in 1934. That was how he made his living before serving in the Royal Artillery during World War II. He was injured and honorably discharged in 1943. The following year, he married the actress, Helen Cherry, who remained with him until his death. Trevor made his film debut with an uncredited appearance in *The Way Ahead,* which was followed by a featured role, in *The Way to the Stars.* Then came the film he is best remembered for – David Lean's *Brief Encounter.* His standing as an actor was assured after an important but supporting role in *The Third Man.* For over twenty-five years, Trevor regularly acted in big-budget movies. In 1960, he was nominated for a Best Actor Oscar, for playing Dean Stockwell's father, Walter Morel, in the superb, *Sons and Lovers.* Trevor kept on working until the end. Not long after he died of influenza and bronchitis, at his home in Bushey, Hertfordshire, one of his regular haunts – the Orange Tree Theater in Richmond, Surrey, honored him by naming their bar the "Trevor Howard Bar".

The Way to the Stars (1945)
Brief Encounter (1945) **Green for Danger** (1946) **They Made Me a Fugitive** (1947) **The Third Man** (1949)
Odette (1950)
The Clouded Yellow (1951)
Outcast of the Islands (1952)
The Heart of the Matter (1953)
Sons and Lovers (1960)
Mutiny on the Bounty (1962)
Von Ryan's Express (1965)
The Charge of the Light Brigade (1968)
Ryan's Daughter (1970)
Mary Queen of Scots (1971)
Gandhi (1982) **Time After Time** (1986) **Shaka Zulu** (1987)
White Mischief (1988)

Kate **Hudson**
5ft 6in
(KATE GARRY HUDSON)

Born: **April 19, 1979**
Los Angeles, California, USA

Katie's father is the heavy metal guitarist, Bill Hudson of the Hudson Brothers Band. Her mother is movie star, Goldie Hawn. Being her daughter meant that Katie was in the limelight from day one. As she got a bit older she sang and danced at every opportunity. Her parents divorced when she was 18 months old and she considers Goldie's long-time partner, Kurt Russell, to be her dad. Katie and her brother Oliver were raised by the couple in Colorado and educated in the Jewish faith. She was later a graduate of Crossroads School, in Santa Monica – which focussed on the performing arts. She rejected an offer to attend New York University, in order to pursue her acting career. In 1996, she made her television debut in an episode of 'Party of Five'. Her film debut was in *Ricochet River* and her breakthrough role was as Penny Lane, in *Almost Famous* – for which she was nominated for a Best Supporting Actress Oscar. Katie, who is popular with fellow actors and directors, is the celebrity model for 'Kamiseta' – a line of fashions from the Philippines. She has her own production company, Cosmic Entertainment, and recently directed the short film *Cutlass,* which features Kurt Russell and Virginia Madsen. In her leisure time she writes music, plays guitar and piano to entertain her friends. From New Year's Eve, 2000, Katie was married for seven years to the "Black Crowes" lead singer, Chris Robinson. They have a son named Ryder.

Ricochet River (1998)
Desert Blue (1998)
200 Cigarettes (1999)
About Adam (2000)
Almost Famous (2000)
The Four Feathers (2002)
How to Lose a Guy in 10 Days (2003)
Raising Helen (2004)
The Skeleton Key (2005)
Fool's Gold (2008)
My Best Friend's Girl (2008)
Bride Wars (2009) **Nine** (2009)

Rock **Hudson**
6ft 5in
(ROY HAROLD SCHERER JR.)

Born: **November 17, 1925**
Winnetka, Illinois, USA
Died: **October 2, 1985**

Rock was the son of auto mechanic, Roy Harold Scherer Sr., and Katherine Wood, who worked as a telephone operator, after her husband abandoned his family. She later married Wally Fitzgerald, who adopted her son. Rock did little acting at New Trier High School, but he did sing in the glee club. In 1943, he joined the navy as an aviation mechanic. After the war, he worked as a truck driver. A Hollywood agent saw him and got him a small part in the 1948 film, *Fighter Squadron.* A year later, he was signed by Universal, who renamed him Rock Hudson. Nothing of any note happened until 1952, when he was fourth-billed in *Bend of the River.* in 1954, Douglas Sirk's *Magnificent Obsession* and the follow-up, with its co-star, Jane Wyman, brought him stardom. Rock oozed masculinity – which made him as popular with men as with girls. His studio knew differently. In November 1955, to hide the career-destroying reality that he was homosexual, a sham marriage was arranged with Phyllis Gates, who was a lesbian. It stopped the rumors for a few years, and in 1957, Rock was voted the 'number one star' by American Exhibitors. Two years later, Rock made the first of a series of comedies with Doris Day. They helped keep him in the top three at the box-office until 1966 – the year he made what was arguably his best film, *Seconds.* His career stalled and by 1979, he was in the TV-series, 'The Martian Chronicles'. In 1981 he had open-heart surgery. Four years later he died of AIDS in Beverly Hills.

Bend of the River (1952) **The Lawless Breed** (1953) **Magnificent Obsession** (1954) **Giant** (1956)
Something of Value (1957) **The Tarnished Angels** (1958) **Pillow Talk** (1959)
Lover Come Back (1961) **Man's Favorite Sport?** (1964) **Send Me No Flowers** (1964) **Blindfold** (1965)
Seconds (1966) **Ice Station Zebra** (1968)
The Undefeated (1969)
Darling Lili (1970)

Tom **Hulse**
5ft 8in
(THOMAS EDWARD HULCE)

Born: **December 6, 1953**
Whitewater, Wisconsin, USA

When he was a small boy, Tom and his brother and two sisters were taken by their parents to live in Michigan. While at school, he planned a singing career, but after his voice broke he turned to acting. He studied at the North Carolina School of the Arts in Winston-Salem, before heading for New York via London, England. His first stage role on Broadway was in Peter Schaffer's "Equus". After his first film in 1975, a short, called *Song of Myself,* he made his feature film debut, in 1977, in *September 30, 1955* – a story about the effect of James Dean's death on a young boy. Tom worked tirelessly during those early years – in movies; on TV; and in many stage productions such as "The Seagull", "Romeo and Juliet", and "Julius Caesar". In 1984, Tom fought off a lot of intense competition to play Mozart, in the movie version of Peter Schaffer's play, *Amadeus.* It was a triumph for all concerned and awards were up for grabs. What he hadn't considered was the competition from his co-star, F. Murray Abraham, who beat him to the Best Actor Oscar. In 1988, he did win a Best Actor Award – at the Seattle Film Festival – for his outstanding acting as a mentally handicapped young man, in *Dominick and Eugene.* In 1995, he won an Emmy for his excellent work in 'The Heidi Chronicles'. In 1998, he directed the marathon two-day stage production of "The Cider House Rules" in his adopted city, Seattle, where he lives with his wife Cecilia Ermini, and their daughter, Anya.

Animal House (1978)
Those Lips, Those Eyes (1980)
Amadeus (1984) Echo Park (1986)
Dominick and Eugene (1988)
Parenthood (1989)
Black Rainbow (1989)
The Inner Circle (1991)
Fearless (1993)
Frankenstein (1994)
Wings of Courage (1995)
Stranger than Fiction (2006)
Jumper (2008)

Helen **Hunt**
5ft 8in
(HELEN ELIZABETH HUNT)

Born: **June 15, 1963**
Los Angeles, California, USA

The daughter of film director and drama coach, Gordon Hunt, and mother, Jane Novis, who is a successful photographer, Helen's background is Jewish and Methodist. She had plenty of exposure to the visual arts. By the early 1970s, with her dad's help, she was registered as a child actress – making her first appearance on television, in 1973, in 'Pioneer Woman' – which was followed by the role of Jill Prentiss, in 'Amy Prentiss'. Helen made her movie debut at the age of fourteen, in the thriller, *Rollercoaster.* She graduated from Providence High School in Burbank before spending one month at UCLA. She then concentrated on acting. Her first film as an adult was in the independent, *Waiting to Act.* She was generally lucky with her choice of film roles after that – getting starring roles in low budget films and small but strong parts in A-List movies. In 1997 she won a Best Actress Oscar for *As Good as it Gets,* and has continued acting in highly-rated films ever since. Helen made her movie-directing debut in 2007, with *Then She Found Me.* She was married to actor, Hank Azaria, for eighteen months, from 1999 until 2000.

Waiting to Act (1985)
Trancers (1985)
The Frog Prince (1986)
Peggy Sue Got Married (1986)
Project X (1987)
Stealing Home (1988)
Next of Kin (1989)
The Waterdance (1992)
Bob Roberts (1992)
Mr. Saturday Night (1992)
Sexual Healing (1993)
Kiss of Death (1995)
Twister (1996)
As Good as it Gets (1997)
Pay It Forward (2000)
Cast Away (2000)
What Women Want (2000)
The Curse of the Jade Scorpion (2001)
A Good Woman (2004)
Bobby (2006)
Then She Found Me (2007)

Holly **Hunter**
5ft 2in
(HOLLY HUNTER)

Born: **March 20, 1958**
Conyers, Georgia, USA

The youngest of seven children, Holly grew up on a farm which her father, Charles ran in tandem with a job selling sporting goods. Her homemaker mother, Opal encouraged her to learn to play the piano and to act. When she was in the fifth-grade, she played Helen Keller, in the "Miracle Worker". In 1976, she attended a drama course, at Carnegie Mellon University. After graduating, she was in New York in a stalled elevator, with the playwright Beth Henley. They got talking and the contact led to roles in Henley's plays, including "Crimes of the Heart". Following a one line film debut in *The Burning,* a year earlier, Holly went to live in Los Angeles in 1982. Later that year she had her first featured film role, in *Crimes of the Heart.* She built up to her stardom rather slowly, with low-profile film and TV roles, until 1987, when she co-starred with Nick Cage, in *Raising Arizona.* There were more decent roles before her keyboard prowess paid off, with a Best Actress Oscar, for *The Pianist.* Holly was also nominated for a Best Supporting Actress Oscar for *The Firm,* and has featured in key movies such as *Crash* and *O Brother, Where Art Thou?* In her private life, Holly married the Oscar-winning cinematographer, Janusz Kaminski, in 1995, but it ended in divorce six years later. For the past two years, Holly has played Grace Handarko, in the popular television series, 'Saving Grace'.

Swing Shift (1984)
Raising Arizona (1987)
Broadcast News (1987)
Miss Firecracker (1989)
Always (1989)
Once Around (1991)
The Piano (1993) The Firm (1993)
Copycat (1995) Crash (1996)
A Life Less Ordinary (1997)
Living Out Loud (1998)
O Brother, Where
Art Thou? (2000)
Levity (2003) Thirteen (2003)
The Big White (2005)

Jeffrey **Hunter**
6ft
(HENRY HERMAN MCKINNIES JR.)

Born: **November 25, 1926**
New Orleans, Louisiana, USA
Died: **May 27, 1969**

Jeff was raised in Milwaukee, Wisconsin and was a graduate of Whitefish Bay High School. He started his acting career on local radio and amateur theater during his high school years, and then served in the United States Navy during World War II. He completed his education by studying Drama at Northwestern University, near Chicago. In 1950, Jeff was a graduate student in Radio, at UCLA, when he was seen by 20th Century Fox talent scouts as he performed in a college play. it resulted in a two-year contract and his film debut – with an uncredited role in *Julius Caesar.* Jeff was first noticed by movie audiences in *Fourteen Hours,* and received third billing the following year, in the adventure film, *Red Skies of Montana.* He co-starred with Jean Peters in *Lure of the Wilderness.* His career went from strength to strength and in John Ford's western *The Searchers* he acted with John Wayne, and in *The Last Hurrah,* with Spencer Tracy. The peak was reached when he was cast as Jesus, in Nicholas Ray's *King of Kings.* After that, apart from the interesting *Brainstorm,* his last few years in films were uninspired. He married three times and fathered four children. In 1969, Jeff suffered a stroke and died in Los Angeles.

Fourteen Hours (1951)
Belles on Their Toes (1952)
Lure of the Wilderness (1952)
Dreamboat (1952) Single-handed (1953)
White Feather (1955)
Seven Angry Men (1955)
Seven Cities of Gold (1955)
The Searchers (1956)
The Proud Ones (1956)
The Great Locomotive Chase (1956)
A Kiss Before Dying (1956)
The True Story of Jess James (1957)
No Down Payment (1957) The Last
Hurrah (1958) In Love and War (1958)
Sergeant Rutledge (1960) Hell to
Eternity (1960) Man-Trap (1961)
King of Kings (1961) The Longest
Day (1962) Brainstorm (1965)

Kim **Hunter**
5ft 3½in
(JANET COLE)

Born: **November 12, 1922**
Detroit, Michigan, USA
Died: **September 11, 2002**

Kim was the daughter of Donald and Grace Cole. Her parents took her to live in Florida when she was twelve-years-old. After graduating from Miami Beach High School, she studied at the Actors Studio. In 1939, she made her first professional stage appearance in Miami – playing Penny – in "Penny Wise". A David O. Selznick talent scout saw Kim performing at the Pasadena Playhouse. Shortly after that, she signed a seven-year contract and changed her name to Kim Hunter. She made her movie debut in *The Seventh Victim,* a superior horror film produced in 1943, at RKO. In England, during World War II, a small but impressive part in the Powell/Pressburger film, *A Canterbury Tale,* led to a role that took her to the peak of her popularity. She then starred with David Niven, in their fantasy classic, *A Matter of Life and Death,* which was also shot in England. She was not so popular with certain politicians in the United States. Although she had never been a Communist, Kim was a firm advocate of civil rights – sponsoring the 1949 World Peace Conference, in New York. She was blacklisted from making films or working on television for some time. Her personal triumph was a Supporting Oscar winning performance as Stella Kowalski, in the film, *A Streetcar Named Desire.* Kim's final movie appearance was in *Here's to Life!* in 2000. She died from a heart attack in New York City. She was married twice.

The Seventh Victim (1943)
When Strangers Marry (1944)
A Matter of Life and Death (1946)
A Streetcar Named Desire (1951)
Deadline – USA (1952)
Storm Center (1956)
The Young Stranger (1957)
Lilith (1964) Planet of the Apes (1968)
The Swimmer (1968)
Midnight in the Farden of
Good and Evil (1997)
A Price Above Rubies (1998)
The Hiding Place (2000)

Tab **Hunter**
6ft
(ARTHUR ANDREW KELM)

Born: **July 11, 1931**
New York City, New York, USA

The son of immigrants from Germany – Tab's father, Charles Kelm, was Jewish, and his mother, Gertrude Gelien, was a Roman Catholic, who later converted to Judaism. When his folks split up, he and his older brother, Walter, went with their mother to California and changed their names to her maiden name of Gelien. When he left school at fifteen – Arthur as he was then known – lied about his age in order to enlist as a coastguard. He was found out and returned home to get a job at a riding academy, which he loved. His good looks soon brought him to the notice of Hollywood talent scouts. With no acting experience or training, he signed a contract with Warner Bros. and was renamed Tab Hunter. In 1950, he made his film debut, with a small role in *The Lawless* – a drama directed by Joseph Losey, and for five years, he was groomed for stardom. That started to become a reality after *Track of the Cat* and *Battle Cry.* The emerging teenage market in Europe and America reacted favorably – following his every move in the film magazines. In 1957, he had a hit record with "Young Love". In the 1960s, Tab's appeal evaporated. He worked on television and made his last film appearance in 1992, in a story he had written, *Dark Horse.* He finally 'came out' as gay in his 2005 memoir – 'Tab Hunter Confidential'. He lives with his partner, Allan Glaser, in Montecito, California.

Track of the Cat (1954)
Battle Cry (1955)
The Sea Chase (1955)
Lafayette Escadrille (1958)
Gunman's Walk (1958)
Damn Yankees (1958)
That Kind of Woman (1959)
They Came to Cordura (1959)
The Pleasure
of His Company (1961)
The Loved One (1965)
The Life and Times of
Judge Roy Bean (1972)
Polyester (1981)
Dark Horse (1992)

Isabelle **Huppert**
5ft 3in
(ISABELLE ANN HUPPERT)

Born: **March 16, 1953**
Paris, France

The youngest of four children, Isabelle grew up in a comfortable middle-class home in the suburb of Ville d'Avray. Her mother, who taught English, gave her and her older sister, Elisabeth, encouragement to act in school plays. By the time she was in her early teens, Isabelle was well known in the French theater world. She won an acting prize while at the Versailles Conservatory and went on to study at the Conservatoire d'Art Dramatique' in Paris. After acting in television dramas, she made her film debut in 1972, in *Faustine et le bel été*. Later that year, she got good reviews for playing Romy Schneider's sister in *César et Rosalie*. By the time she shared a Best Actress Award at Cannes (with Jill Clayburgh) for *Violette Nozière* in 1978, she was one step away from stardom. She won a BAFTA Most Promising Newcomer Award, for *La Dentellière* and for the next quarter of a century, Isabelle was in a class of her own. In 2001, she was voted Best Actress at the Cannes Film Festival, for *La Pianiste*. Whilst she was never considered the most beautiful of French actresses, she has undeniable sex-appeal. Since 1982, Isabelle has been married to the director, Ronald Chammah. They have two children.

César et Rosalie (1972)
Les Valseuses (1974)
Le Juge et l'assassin (1976)
La Dentellière (1977)
Violette Nozière (1978)
Loulou (1980) Heaven's Gate (1980)
Coup de torchon (1981)
Passion (1982)
Coup de foudre (1983)
The Bedroom Window (1987)
Une affaire de femmes (1988)
Malina (1991) Amateur (1994)
La Séparation (1994)
La Cérémonie (1995)
La Pianiste (2001)
8 femmes (2002) Gabrielle (2005)
Private Property (2006)
Home (2008)
The Sea Wall (2008)

John **Hurt**
5ft 9in
(JOHN VINCENT HURT)

Born: **January 22, 1940**
Shirebrook, Derbyshire, England

John was the son of a mathematician turned vicar, Arnould Herbert Hurt, and his wife Phillis, who was an amateur actress. His mother was a great influence and John knew he wanted to become an actor at the age of nine. He was at St. Michael's prep school in Sevenoaks, when he was featured in the play – "The Bluebird". At seventeen, he went to Grimsby Art School and in 1959, to St. Martin's School of Art, in London. There, he was in the middle of theaterland and within a year, he had won a scholarship to RADA. In 1962, he made his stage debut, as well as his film debut, in *The Wild and the Willing*. That same year, he married the actress, Annette Robertson – it lasted eighteen months and Annette would be the first of four wives. During the mid-1960s, John performed with the Royal Shakespeare Company, but a serious drink problem hampered his progress. His portrayal of Quentin Crisp, in the 1975 television play, 'The Naked Civil Servant', made John's reputation. He was nominated for a Best Supporting Actor Oscar in *Midnight Express,* and the good movie roles came thick and fast. John is already the winner of three BAFTA's and when something extraordinary is required, his is the first name to go on to the film-maker's cast-list.

Midnight Express (1978)
Alien (1979)
The Elephant Man (1980)
Heaven's Gate (1980)
Night Crossing (1981)
Champions (1984) The Hit (1984)
Nineteen Eighty-Four (1984)
La Nuit Bengali (1988)
Scandal (1989) The Field (1990)
Rob Roy (1995)
The Climb (1998)
Crime and Punishment (2002)
Shooting Dogs (2005)
The Skeleton Key (2005)
The Oxford Murders (2008)
Indiana Jones and the Kingdom of
the Crystal Skull (2008)
Hellboy II: The Golden Army (2008)

Mary Beth **Hurt**
5ft 4in
(MARY SUPINGER)

Born: **September 26, 1948**
Marshalltown, Iowa, USA

She was the daughter of Forrest Clayton and Delores Supinger. Mary Beth had an early link with the movie world. When she was a little girl, her babysitter was the future film actress, Jean Seberg. Following high school, she studied drama at the University of Iowa, and then at Tisch School of the Arts, at New York University. In 1971, she began a ten year marriage to the actor, William Hurt, so as Mary Beth Hurt, she made her New York stage debut as well as her television debut, in 1974. After their divorce, she kept his name. She was nominated for Tony awards, for her Broadway performances in "Trelawney of the Wells", "Crimes of the Heart" and "Benefactors". Mary Beth made her film debut, as Joey, in Woody Allen's *Interiors,* for which she was nominated for a Most Promising Newcomer Award. For her work on the stage, she was nominated for three Tony Awards. In 1983, she married the director/writer, Paul Schrader. They have a daughter and a son. After her role as Helen Holm Garp, in *The World According to Garp,* she's appeared in a dozen or so good movies. Mary Beth has been able to combine raising a family with acting in films directed by such talents as Martin Scorsese, Gregory Hoblit, and not forgetting her husband, Paul.

Interiors (1978)
Head Over Heels (1979)
The World According to
Garp (1982) Compromising
Positions (1985)
Parents (1989)
Light Sleeper (1992)
Shimmer (1993)
The Age of Innocence (1993)
Six Degrees of Separation (1993)
Affliction (1997)
Bringing Out the Dead (1999)
The Family Man (2000)
The Exorcism of Emily Rose (2005)
Lady in the Water (2006)
The Dead Girl (2006)
The Walker (2007)
Untraceable (2008)

William **Hurt**
6ft 2in
(WILLIAM M. HURT)

Born: March 20, 1950
Washington, D.C., USA

William's father, Alfred McCord Hurt, worked for the U.S. State Department in Washington. His mother, Claire, worked at Time, Inc. When his parents divorced, his mother actually married the founder of Time Magazine. He attended Middlesex School, in Concord, Massachusetts and studied theology at Tufts University. He later went to the Juilliard Drama School at the same time as Christopher Reeve. After stage experience and a few episodes of 'Kojak' on TV, he made his film debut in *Altered States*. Five years later, he won a Best Actor Oscar, for *Kiss of the Spider Woman*. Almost twenty years after that he received his third nomination, for *A History of Violence*. He hasn't ignored the theater either – recently starring on stage in Portland Oregon – in a production of Chekhov's "Uncle Vanya". William, who is fluent in French, has a daughter with the actress, Sandrine Bonnaire. He has appeared in so many good movies, it is impossible to compile a shortlist of his best work – and it's still growing. So here's a long list.

Altered States (1980)
Eyewitness (1981)
Body Heat (1981) The Big Chill (1983)
Gorky Park (1983)
Kiss of the Spider Woman (1985)
Children of a Lesser God (1986)
Broadcast News (1987)
The Accidental Tourist (1988)
I Love You to Death (1990)
Alice (1990) The Doctor (1991)
Second Best (1994)
Smoke (1995) Dark City (1998)
Artificial Intelligence: AI (2001)
Rare Birds (2001)
Truck Everlasting (2002)
The Village (2004)
A History of Violence (2005)
Syriana (2005)
The Good Shepherd (2006)
Into the Wild (2007) Noises (2007)
Yellow Handkerchief (2008)
Vantage Point (2008)
The Incredible Hulk (2008)

Olivia **Hussey**
5ft 5in
(OLIVIA OSUNA)

Born: April 17, 1951
Buenos Aires, Argentina

Olivia's father, Andreas Osuna, was an Argentine opera singer. Her mother, Joy Alma Hussey, was a legal secretary from England. They divorced when Olivia was two-years old. She spent her first seven years in Buenos Aires, where she was raised as a Catholic. Olivia's mother then took her and her younger brother to live in England. They settled in London, where, following junior school, Olivia spent five years at the Italia Conti Academy. In 1964, she made her first appearance on TV in an episode of 'Drama 60-67' and a year later, she made her film debut, in *The Battle of the Villa Fiorita* – which starred Maureen O'Hara and Rossano Brazzi. After a brief role in the 1965 soccer film, *Cup Fever,* she made her stage debut in the London production of "The Prime of Miss Jean Brodie". Olivia's performance was noted by the great Italian director, Franco Zeffirelli who had little hesitation in casting her as Juliet, in his superb movie version of *Romeo and Juliet*. Olivia was ideally cast, but co-starring with Robert Mitchum's son, Chris – in *Summertime Killer,* wasn't going to make her a star. The year before, she married the son of another star – Dean Paul Martin. She was in the successful horror movie, *Black Christmas* and played the Virgin Mary in Zeffirelli's 1977 TV mini-series, 'Jesus of Nazareth'. Since 2000, she's made some welcome appearances. In 2003, she was superb as 'Mother Teresa' on television. Olivia lives near Los Angeles with her third husband, David Glen Eisley.

The Battle of the
River Fiorita (1965)
Romeo and Juliet (1968)
Summertime Killer (1972)
Black Christmas (1974)
Death on the Nile (1978)
The Cat and the Canary (1979)
Day of Resurrection (1980)
The Man with Bogart's Face (1980)
Turkey Shoot (1982)
The Jeweller's Shop (1989)
El Grito (2000) Three Priests (2008)

Ruth **Hussey**
5ft 5in
(RUTH CAROL HUSSEY)

Born: October 30, 1911
Providence, Rhode Island, USA
Died: **April 19, 2005**

Ruth was only seven years old when her father was the victim of a flu epidemic. Her mother, who remarried – to a man named William O'Rourke, raised her well – she went to Pembroke College, but strangely, considering her good looks and confident manner, she was never accepted for parts in school plays. It was at the University of Michigan School of Drama, where she came into her own – working in summer stock for two seasons. She briefly became a fashion reporter on the local radio in Providence, but was unsuccessful when she auditioned to act at the Providence Playhouse. She had better luck in New York, where she landed small stage roles and also worked as a Powers model. After she toured in a stage production of "Dead End" in 1937, Ruth was spotted by an MGM talent scout and made her film debut that year, in *Big City*. In 1940, for her first big role, in *The Philadelphia Story,* she was nominated for a Best Supporting Actress Oscar. Her career ticked over nicely after that, although her marriage in 1942, to talent agent, Bob Longenecker resulted in three children and the need to spend more time at home. She was third-billed below Bob Hope and Lucille Ball in *The Facts of Life*. Ruth continued acting – mainly on television, until 1973. She and her husband celebrated their sixtieth wedding anniversary before his death in 2002. She died in Newbury Park, California, of complications of appendectomy.

Rich Man, Poor Girl (1938)
Fast and Furious (1939)
Northwest Passage (1940)
Susan and God (1940)
The Philadelphia Story (1940)
Free and Easy (1941)
H.M. Pulham, Esq. (1941)
The Uninvited (1944)
The Great Gatsby (1949) Louisa (1950)
That's My Boy (1951)
Stars and Stripes Forever (1952)
The Lady Wants Mink (1953)
The Facts of Life (1960)

Anjelica **Huston**
5ft 10in
(ANJELICA HUSTON)

Born: **July 8, 1951**
Santa Monica, California, USA

Anjelica is the daughter of the great film director, John Huston, and his fourth wife, the ballerina, Enrica Soma. One of four children, she grew up in Ireland, where she attended Kylemore Abbey – an all-girls boarding school in Connemara. She had an uncredited role in *Casino Royale,* in 1967, and two years later she starred in her father's, *A Walk With Love and Death.* She was harshly treated by the critics and for the next few years, worked as a model in the United States. She came back in small supporting roles, and in 1985, her confidence was boosted when she was awarded a Best Supporting Actress Oscar for *Prizzi's Honor.* It was also directed by her dad, but on that occasion, she received only the praise she deserved. There were two more Oscar nominations and several high profile roles including Morticia Addams, in *The Addams Family* and its sequel. In 2004, following eight 'near things' she finally won a Golden Globe Award as Best Supporting Actress, in the TV program 'Iron Jawed Angels'. Following in her dad's footsteps, she has directed three movies. After living with Jack Nicholson for sixteen years, Anjelica married sculptor, Robert Graham Jr. in 1992. They live in Venice, California.

Prizzi's Honor (1985)
The Dead (1987)
A Handful of Dust (1988)
Crimes and Misdemeanors (1989)
The Witches (1990)
Enemies: A Love Story (1990)
The Grifters (1990)
The Addams Family (1991)
Addams Family Values (1993)
Buffalo '66 (1998)
Phoenix (1998)
Ever After (1998)
The Royal Tenenbaums (2001)
Blood Work (2002)
These Foolish Things (2006)
Art School Confidential (2006)
Seraphim Falls (2006)
The Darjeeling Limited (2007)
Choke (2008)

Walter **Huston**
6ft
(WALTER HOUGHSTON)

Born: **April 6, 1884**
Toronto, Ontario, Canada
Died: **April 7, 1950**

Walter's parents were from Scottish backgrounds. On leaving school, Walter took acting classes while attending a course in electrical engineering. In 1902, he chose his path after acting with a local stock company. He went to New York, where he worked in vaudeville. Marriage and a son, the future director, John Huston, made him think about his career. He moved to Missouri, where he worked in a water and electricity plant. After two years, he formed a dance act with Bayonne Whipple – who became his second wife. Following the title role in "Mr. Pitt", he became the toast of Broadway. In 1928, talkies beckoned. He signed for Paramount and made his film debut in 1929, in *Gentlemen of the Press.* His film and stage work was then of equal importance – standing comparison with the best actors of both genres. Walter was superb in *Dodsworth,* for which he was Oscar nominated, but as he grew older, he turned into a great character actor – sometimes in walk-on roles in his son's movies. His last play on Broadway was "The Apple of His Eye". In 1948, he won a Best Supporting Actor Oscar for *Treasure of the Sierra Madre* directed by the 'apple of his eye'. Walter went out with a bang in *The Furies* – dying in Hollywood, from aneurysm, the year of its release. His third wife, Ninetta, was by his side.

Abraham Lincoln (1930)
A House Divided (1931)
The Beast of the City (1932)
American Madness (1932)
Rain (1932) Dodsworth (1936)
The Light That Failed (1939)
The Devil and Daniel Webster (1941)
Swamp Water (1941)
The Shanghai Gesture (1941)
Yankee Doodle Dandy (1942)
And Then There Were None (1945)
Dragonwyck (1946)
Duel in the Sun (1946)
The Treasure of the
Sierra Madre (1948)
The Furies (1950)

Betty **Hutton**
5ft 4in
(ELIZABETH JUNE THORNBURG)

Born: **February 26, 1921**
Battle Creek, Michigan, USA
Died: **March 11, 2007**

When Betty's father, Percy Thornburg, left his wife for another woman in 1923, her mother, Mabel, was left to bring up Betty and her older sister, Marion. She opened a speakeasy, where the two girls sang to entertain customers. They ended up in Detroit, totally destitute. To earn money, thirteen-year-old Betty sang in bars. She was hired as a band singer – as Betty Darling, by Vincent Lopez, but just like her sister – who sang with Glenn Miller, she adopted the name Hutton. In 1939, she exploded on the screen, in the short, *Public Jitterbug No.1.* Her work in the Broadway show, "Panama Hattie" won her a Paramount contract. They put her in *The Fleet's In,* and she sang two good songs. In 1942, she was one of the first singers to sign for Capitol Records. Her third teaming with Eddie Bracken, in *The Miracle of Morgan's Creek,* made her a star. She proved good in a dramatic role, in *Incendiary Blonde,* but her forte was musical comedy. Her best work was in *Annie Get Your Gun* – a part she only got because of the illness of Judy Garland. She married dance director, Charles O'Curran, but her insistence that he direct future projects, met with no offers. Four divorces, a serious drink problem, and a nervous breakdown, turned her to God. A priest helped her earn a bachelors degree and she lived until she was eighty-six.

Happy Go Lucky (1943)
Let's Face It (1943)
The Miracle of Morgan's Creek (1944)
And the Angels Sing (1944)
Here Come the Waves (1944)
Incendiary Blonde (1945)
Cross My Heart (1946)
The Perils of Pauline (1947)
Dream Girl (1948)
Red, Hot and Blue (1949)
Annie Get Your Gun (1950)
Let's Dance (1950)
The Greatest Show on Earth (1952)
Somebody Loves Me (1952)
Spring Reunion (1957)

Timothy **Hutton**
5ft 11³/₄in
(TIMOTHY HUTTON)

Born: **August 16, 1960**
Malibu, California, USA

Tim's father was the actor Jim Hutton. His mother, Maryline, was a teacher who ran a small publishing house. Tim made his film debut at five, in *Never Too Late,* which starred his father. After attending Fairfax High School and Berkeley High School, in Los Angeles – which he left at eighteen – he made a string of television drama appearances during the late 1970s – most notably in the award-winning 'Friendly Fire'. In 1980, he became the youngest-ever recipient (aged twenty) of a Best Supporting Actor Oscar, for his fine and moving portrayal of Conrad Jarrett, in *Ordinary People.* Sadly, his father died the year before his triumph. In 1986, Tim married the actress Debora Winger, with whom he had a son. They divorced in 1990. Since his Oscar, Tim's built a very successful career which is continuing long after he lost his boyish looks. He's won one Golden Globe and has been nominated twice. In 1996, he was highly praised for his acting opposite a precocious teenager, played by Natalie Portman, in *Beautiful Girls.* He is currently co-owner of P.J.Clarke's Bar and Restaurant, in New York City. His second wife Aurore, is the niece of the former President of France, Valéry Giscard d'Estaing. They have a son named Milo, who was born in Paris.

Ordinary People (1980)
Taps (1981)
Iceman (1984)
Made in Heaven (1987)
Everybody's All-American (1988)
French Kiss (1995)
Beautiful Girls (1996)
Deterrence (1999)
Sunshine State (2002)
Kinsey (2004)
Last Holiday (2006)
The Kovak Box (2006)
Heaven's Fall (2006)
The Good Shepherd (2006)
The Last Mimzy (2007)
The Alphabet Killer (2008)
Lymelife (2008)
The Killing Room (2009)

Wilfred **Hyde-White**
6ft 0¹/₂in
(WILFRED HYDE-WHITE)

Born: **May 12, 1903**
Bourton-on-the-Water, Gloucester, England
Died: **May 6, 1991**

Wilfred was the son of the Canon of Gloucester Cathedral, William White, and his wife Ethel. His uncle, was an actor, and while attending Marlborough College, Wilfred decided to follow his path rather than that of his father's. He went to London where he studied at the Royal Academy of Dramatic Art. In 1922, he made his stage debut, at Ryde, on the Isle of Wight, in the comedy, "Tons of Money" and his London debut, three years later, in "Beggar on Horseback". In 1927, Wilfred married the actress, Blanche Aitken, and they toured together in South Africa. Wilfred made his film debut in 1934, in *Josser on the Farm,* but he was hardly noticed until he had a role in the George Formby comedy, *Turned Out Nice Again,* in 1941. His film roles were rather like his character – laid-back and unassuming. 1949 was the year he broke through as a character actor, but he was hardly on the radar until he was featured in the Marilyn Monroe film, *Let's Make Love,* and Danny Kaye's last good movie, *On the Double.* Wilfred later played the role he will always be remembered for – Colonel Pickering in *My Fair Lady.* He retired in 1983 after he had acted in a series of films – in which he was merely going through the motions. Wilfred died in Woodland Hills, California, of congestive heart failure. His son is the actor, Alex Hyde-White.

Britannia Mews (1949)
Adam and Evelyne (1949)
The Third Man (1949)
Mr. Denning Drives North (1952)
Top Secret (1952)
The Million Pound Note (1953)
The Vicious Circle (1957)
North West Frontier (1959)
Libel (1959)
Let's Make Love (1960)
Two Way Stretch (1960)
On the Double (1961)
My Fair Lady (1964)
Fragment of Fear (1970)
The Cat and the Canary (1979)

Martha **Hyer**
5ft 6in
(MARTHA HYER)

Born: **August 10, 1924**
Fort Worth, Texas, USA

Following high school, Martha majored in drama and speech at Northwestern University, in Chicago – where classmates included Charlton Heston and Patricia Neal. She then gained experience at the Pasadena Playhouse, before being signed by RKO, in 1946. She got the first of three uncredited roles, in *The Locket,* in 1946, before co-starring with Tim Holt, in the western, *Thunder Mountain.* That pairing was so successful, they appeared twice more together. Martha stepped up a division in 1949, but was a B-film star by the time she met her first husband, the Writer/Director, Ray Stahl, in 1950, on the set of his poor quality, *Oriental Evil.* Ray did little to help her career and by 1954, he was history. Martha proceeded to do a lot better alone. She landed some good roles in big movies – the high point being her Best Supporting Actress Oscar-nominated role – as Gwen French, in *Some Came Running* where she was in the hot company of Frank Sinatra, Dean Martin and Shirley MacLaine. In 1966, after her marriage to the producer, Hal Wallis, she took it easy. Martha made her last film, *Day of the Wolves,* in 1973. In 1990, she published her autobiography, "Finding My Way: A Hollywood Memoir".

Roughshod (1949)
The Judge Steps Out (1949)
So Big (1953)
Riders to the Stars (1954)
Down Three Dark Streets (1954)
Sabrina (1954)
Cry Vengeance (1954)
Showdown at Abilene (1956)
Battle Hymn (1957)
Houseboat (1958)
Some Came Running (1958)
The Best of Everything (1959)
The Man from the Diner's Club (1963) Fuego (1964)
The Carpetbaggers (1964)
First Men in the Moon (1964)
The Sons of Katie Elder (1965)
The Chase (1966)
Day of the Wolves (1973)

I

Ice Cube
5ft 8in
(O'SHEA JACKSON)

Born: **June 15, 1969**
Los Angeles, California, USA

Ice Cube was born in the South Central area of Los Angeles. His father, Andrew Jackson, worked as a groundskeeper at California State University. His mother, Doris, was a hospital clerk. During his early years, Ice Cube was known by his birth name, O'Shea Jackson. When he was sixteen, at Taft High School, in Woodland Hills, he became interested in hip hop music and began writing raps in his music class. In 1987 he went to the Phoenix Institute of Technology to study Architectural Drafting. He didn't give up his music – forming a group with his friend Sir Jinx, which they called the "C.I.A." They released an EP, titled "My Posse" and started performing their songs at parties. In 1988, Ice Cube, as he was then known, appeared on a debut album "N.W.A. and the Posse". In 1990, his solo album, "AmeriKKa's Most Wanted" was released. The following year, he made his movie debut in *Boyz n the Hood* and won the Chicago Film Critics' Most Promising Actor Award. In 1992, Ice Cube married his present wife Kimberly, with whom he has four children. Ice Cube's acting skills have been used in two dozen more movies since then – not all successful. He has been praised for the one's that were, and was nominated for an Outstanding Supporting Image Award, for *Higher Learning*. His most high-profile film so far was the war story, *Three Kings* – in which he co-starred with George Clooney and Mark Wahlberg. Ice Cube has provided soundtracks for several movies. It's been a while since he had a hit movie. Maybe the upcoming *Janky Promoters* will be one.

Boyz n the Hood (1991)
Trespass (1992)
The Glass Shield (1994)
Higher Learning (1995)
Friday (1995)
Three Kings (1999)
Next Friday (2000)
All About the Benjamins (2002)
Barbershop 2: Back in Business (2002)

Rhys Ifans
6ft 2in
(RHYS EVANS)

Born: **July 22, 1968**
Haverfordwest, Pembroke, Wales

Rhys was the son of Eurwyn, a primary school teacher, and Beti-Wyn Evans, who taught in nursery school. He was brought up in Ruthin, in North Wales – where he learned the Welsh language. He received his secondary school education at Ysgol Maes Garmon, in Mold, Flintshire. He then attended youth acting school, at Theatr Clwyd, in the same town. Rhys made his TV debut in the Thames Television series 'Spatz', in 1990. He appeared in several Welsh-language TV programs before he performed in stage productions – at the Royal National Theater, in London and the Royal Exchange, Manchester. In 1993, he was briefly lead vocalist for the Welsh rock band, "Super Furry Animals". Rhys made his film debut, two years later, in the gritty drama, *Streetlife* – which was shot in Wales. He graduated from the Guildhall School of Music and Drama, in 1997. His first major movie role was in *Notting Hill,* where he played the Welsh flatmate of Hugh Grant. He was nominated for a Best Supporting Actor BAFTA and kept up the good work – both in films and on TV. In 2005, Rhys won a BAFTA Best Actor TV Award, for his portrayal of Peter Cook, in 'Not Only But Also'. In the summer of 2008, he became a bachelor again, after the break-up of his relationship with the English actress, Sienna Miller. That September, Rhys co-starred with Tom Wilkinson in a TV play, 'The Number'.

Streetlife (1995)
Twin Town (1997)
Dancing at Lughnasa (1998)
Heart (1999)
Notting Hill (1999)
You're Dead (1999)
Love, Honour and Obey (2000)
The Replacements (2000)
Human Nature (2001)
The Shipping News (2001)
Chromophobia (2005)
Four Last Songs (2007)
Hannibal Rising (2007)
Elizabeth: The Golden Age (2007)
The Informers (2009)

Jill Ireland
5ft 6in
(JILL DOROTHY IRELAND)

Born: **April 24, 1936**
London, England
Died: **May 18, 1990**

Jill's great love of dancing and acting was encouraged by her parents. She attended ballet classes from the age of seven, and made her stage debut, when she was twelve, at London's Chiswick Empire, in a production of "Sleeping Beauty". Jill was a talented child, and it wasn't long before she was touring all over Europe as a ballet dancer. It was probably her mistake that she never undertook any kind of formal training as an actress. She did appear in a decorative manner in some early British TV commercials, and made her film debut in 1955, as a dancer, in *Oh, Rosalinda!* In 1957 Jill married the young Scottish actor, David McCallum, who would later find fame as a Russian – Illya Kuryakin, in the very popular 1960s television series, 'The Man from U.N.C.L.E.' Jill appeared with him in three episodes. It didn't enhance her reputation as an actress, but it got her some work in a number of American TV shows such as 'Shane' and 'Star Trek'. On the set of a 1968 movie, *Villa Rides,* Jill met and fell in love with Charles Bronson, who was introduced to her by her first husband, David McCallum. They were married and he helped her to a new level of popularity by casting her in most of his films. Unhappily for the couple, Jill was diagnosed with breast cancer in 1984, and died in Malibu, California, after a brave but losing six-year battle.

Three Men in a Boat (1956)
Hell Drivers (1957)
Carry on Nurse (1959)
Twice Round the Daffodils (1962)
Le Passager de la pluie (1969)
Violent City (1970)
The Valachi Papers (1972)
The Mechanic (1972)
Breakout (1975)
Hard Times (1975)
Breakheart Pass (1975)
From Noon Till Three (1976)
Love and Bullets (1979)
Death Wish II (1982)

John **Ireland**
6ft 1in
(JOHN BENJAMIN IRELAND)

Born: **January 30, 1914**
Vancouver, British Columbia, Canada
Died: **March 21, 1992**

The son of a racehorse breeder, as a small boy, John was taken to live in New York. At school, he proved more of an athlete than an academic. His first job was as a swimmer in a water carnival. John started getting small roles in stage productions and in 1937, he joined a Shakespeare company. He was in several Broadway shows before getting married, in 1940. Following war service, he got his first film role, in the Lewis Milestone war movie, *A Walk in the Sun*. John went on to appear in two of the greatest westerns of all time – *My Darling Clementine* and *Red River*. On the set of the latter, he met and later married, his second wife, Joanne Dru. In 1949, with a series of good parts under his belt, he became the first Vancouver-born actor to be nominated for an Oscar, as Best Supporting Actor, in *All the King's Men*. During the 1950s, he starred in some B-pictures, but much of his later work was on TV. After his marriage had ended, in 1959, he raised a few eyebrows when he had an affair with sixteen-year-old Tuesday Weld. During the 1980s, John ran a restaurant called "Ireland's" in Santa Barbara. His last role was as King Arthur, in a 1992 film, *Waxwork II: Lost in Time*. He was married to his third wife, Daphne, for thirty years at the time of his death from leukemia, in Santa Barbara, California.

A Walk in the Sun (1945)
My Darling Clementine (1946)
Railroaded (1947)
Open Secret (1948)
Raw Deal (1948)
Red River (1948)
All the King's Men (1949)
The Scarf (1951)
Little Big Horn (1951)
Hannah Lee:
An American Primitive (1953)
Queen Bee (1955)
Gunfight at the O.K. Corral (1957)
Party Girl (1958)
Spartacus (1960)
55 Days at Peking (1963)

Jeremy **Irons**
6ft 1½in
(JEREMY JOHN IRONS)

Born: **September 19, 1948**
Cowes, Isle of Wight, England

The son of Paul and Barbara Irons, Jeremy became a seasoned entertainer at Sherborne School, in Dorset, where he was the drummer and harmonica player in the "The Four Pillars of Wisdom". He then went to Bristol to study acting, at the Old Vic Theater School – supporting himself by busking in the streets. He then gained good acting experience with Bristol Old Vic Repertory Company. His first big stage role, was in 1972, as John the Baptist, in the London production of the rock musical "Godspell". He'd already been in a TV episode of Sherlock Holmes, and it was in that medium where for a few years he got most of his employment. In 1978, Jeremy married Irish actress, Sinéad Cusack. She brought him luck: he made his film debut in *Nijinsky* in 1980, and a year later found fame in a popular TV series, 'Brideshead Revisited'. On Broadway, in 1984, Jeremy triumphed in "The Real Thing", opposite Glenn Close. His fine work earned him a Tony Award. He won further praise as Professor Higgins, in a 1987 London revival of "My Fair Lady". His good luck continued with major parts leading up to a Best Actor Oscar, for *Reversal of Fortune*. Jeremy needs to keep earning money, after purchasing Kilcoe Castle, in County Cork, Ireland. He has just completed work on a forthcoming western, *Appaloosa*.

Moonlighting (1982)
Betrayal (1983)
The Mission (1986)
Dead Ringers (1988)
Reversal of Fortune (1990)
Kafka (1991) **Damage** (1992)
M. Butterfly (1993)
The House of the Spirits 1993)
Die Hard: With a Vengeance (1995)
Stealing Beauty (1996)
Chinese Box (1997) **Lolita** (1997)
The Man in the Iron Mask (1998)
Callas Forever (2002)
The Merchant of Venice (2004)
Being Julia (2004)
Inland Empire (2006)
Appaloosa (2008)

Amy **Irving**
5ft 4in
(AMY DAVIS IRVING)

Born: **September 10, 1953**
Palo Alto, California, USA

Amy had show business in her blood. Her father was Jules Irving, a film and stage director, and her mother was the actress Priscilla Pointer. She first appeared on stage when she was only two – in a play directed by her dad. At twelve years of age, she then had a walk-on role in the Broadway show, "The Country Wife". It was directed by Robert Symonds, who in the 1980s, would become her stepfather after her dad's death. Although she is of Jewish ancestry from his branch of the family, Amy was raised as a Christian Scientist. In the early 1970s, she studied acting at the London Academy of Music and Dramatic Art. After returning to Los Angeles she made her television debut, in a 1975 episode of 'The Rookies'. Half a dozen TV roles led to her movie debut, in the key role of Sue Snell, in Brian De Palma's gripping horror/drama, *Carrie*. Amy picked her films fairly carefully and they were often on target. Even so, her only Oscar nomination so far was as Best Supporting actress, in Barbra Streisand's *Yentl*. She was Mrs. Steven Spielberg from 1985 until 1989. All three husbands were directors – she married number three, Ken Bowser, in 2007. She has two sons.

Carrie (1976)
The Fury (1978)
Voices (1979)
Honeysuckle Rose (1980)
The Competition (1980)
Yentl (1983)
Micki + Maude (1984)
Rumplestiltskin (1987)
Crossing Delancey (1988)
A Show of Force (1990)
Carried Away (1996)
I'm Not Rappaport (1996)
Deconstructing Harry (1997)
The Confession (1999)
Bossa Nova (2000)
Traffic (2000)
13 Conversations (2001)
Truck Everlasting (2002)
Hide and Seek (2005)
Adam (2009)

Burl **Ives**
6ft 1in
(BURL ICLE IVANHOE IVES)

Born: June 14, 1909
Hunt, Illinois, USA
Died: April 14, 1995

Burl was the son of Levi and Cordelia Ives. His first ambition upon leaving school was to become a teacher. He changed his mind two years into a course at the Illinois State Teachers College. During the early 1930s, there was little chance of employment, but Burl went on the road with his banjo and managed to eke out a living. He eventually settled in New York, where his positive attitude and his friendly smile, resulted in a stage debut, in "Pocahontas Preferred". After that he was in a number of Broadway shows, including "Heavenly Express" and "The Boys from Syracuse". In 1940 Burl started his own radio show, 'The Wayfaring Stranger'. It helped sell some of the phonograph records he made – his first hit being "Lavender Blue". From the start of 1942, he spent eighteen months in the Army Air Force, and was in the cast of Irving Berlin's "This Is The Army". Burl was discharged for medical reasons and went to work for CBS Radio in New York. He made his movie debut, as a singing cowboy, in *Smokey.* It was going pretty well until he was hauled before the HUAC in 1950, and grilled about his communist ties. After he cooperated, he was back with a bang. The high point of his film career was a Best Supporting Actor Oscar, for *The Big Country.* After he retired in 1988, he lived quietly with his second wife, Dorothy. Burl died of mouth cancer, in Anacortes, Washington.

Smokey (1946)
Station West (1948)
So Dear to My Heart (1948)
East of Eden (1955)
Cat on a Hot Tin Roof (1958)
The Big Country (1958)
Day of the Outlaw (1959)
Let No Man Write
My Epitaph (1960)
Summer Magic (1963)
The McMasters (1970)
Baker's Hawk (1976)
Just You and Me, Kid (1979)
White Dog (1982)

Eddie **Izzard**
5ft 7in
(EDWARD JOHN IZZARD)

Born: February 7, 1962
Aden, Yemen

Eddie was the youngest son of a couple of English expatriates living in Yemen. Harold Izzard, an accountant at British Petroleum, and his wife Dorothy, who was a midwife and nurse. Sadly she died of cancer when Eddie was six years old. It had a deep effect on him. The remaining family moved back to live in England, where Eddie attended St. Bede's Preparatory School and Eastbourne College – where he first developed a love of comedy – especially Monty Python and stand-ups like Richard Pryor. When he went to the University of Sheffield to study Accountancy, he began to experiment with some stand-up of his own. He was kicked off his course and began to work as a street performer, in Europe and the United States. In 1987, Eddie made his first appearance at The Comedy Store, in London. He worked hard on refining his act, and in 1993, he won a British Comedy Award, for "Live at the Ambassadors" in London's West End. Six years later, he was well received in America, after his live show, "Dressed to Kill" – in San Francisco – which won him Emmys (for performance and writing) was screened on HBO. He had first appeared in a film in 1996, when he acted in Damien Hirst's short, *Hanging Around.* His first feature-length movie, was *The Secret Agent,* and by the beginning of the present century, Eddie had proved himself an important character actor in several movies – the most high-profile of which are *Ocean's Thirteen* and *Valkyrie.*

The Secret Agent (1996)
Velvet Goldmine (1998)
Mystery Men (1999)
Circus (2000)
Shadow of the Vampire (2000)
The Cat's Meow (2001)
Revengers Tragedy (2002)
Ocean's Twelve (2004)
Romance and Cigarettes (2005)
My Super Ex-Girlfriend (2006)
Ocean's Thirteen (2007)
Across the Universe (2007)
Valkyrie (2008)

Hugh **Jackman**
6ft 2¹/₂in
(HUGH MICHAEL JACKMAN)

Born: **October 12, 1968**
Sydney, New South Wales, Australia

Both of Hugh's parents, Chris and Grace Jackman, were English immigrants, who divorced when he was eight. It was then left to his father to raise the family. Hugh was the youngest of five children, which made him intensely competitive as a boy at Pymble School and especially as a young actor, at Knox Grammar School. In 1987, he spent a gap year working at Uppingham School in England. Eventually, he graduated from the University of Technology in Sydney, with a degree in Communications. And communicate he did. After Hugh had studied drama at the Western Australian Academy of Performing Arts, in Perth, he landed a starring role in the TV prison drama, 'Correlli'. His co-star in that, Deborra-Lee Furness, became his wife a year later, in 1996. They have two adopted children. After a couple more years of television work, Hugh made his movie debut in the Australia-shot comedy/drama *Paperback Hero*. By 2000, he had 'star in the making' written all over him and he was helped on his way with key roles of Logan/Wolverine, in his first American film, the Sci-Fi thriller, *X-Men*. There have been two more in the series – which were equally successful. He won a Saturn Award for *X-Men* and has since been nominated for *The Fountain*. In 2004, he won a Best Actor Tony for his work in the Broadway musical, "The Boy From Oz". Apart from his tuneful singing, Hugh plays piano and guitar.

Paperback Hero (1999)
Erskinville Kings (1999)
X-Men (2000)
Someone Like You... (2001)
Swordfish (2001)
Kate and Leopold (2001)
X-2 (2003)
Standing Room Only (2004)
X-Men: The Last Stand (2006)
Scoop (2006)
The Fountain (2006)
The Prestige (2006) **Deception** (2008)
Australia (2008)
X-Men Origins: Wolverine (2009)

Glenda **Jackson**
5ft 6¹/₂in
(GLENDA MAY JACKSON)

Born: **May 9, 1936**
Birkenhead, Cheshire, England

A bricklayer's daughter, Glenda grew up in a working-class household and left school at sixteen. For two years, she worked in a pharmacy, but acting in local amateur productions gave her the urge to better herself. She then got a scholarship to RADA in London, in 1954, and made her professional debut in Worthing. In 1956, Glenda first appeared in a film (appropriately as an extra) in *The Extra Day*. Two years later, while she was acting in the play "Separate Tables" in Crewe, she met her husband Roy Hodges. Glenda had an uncredited role as a singer in *This Sporting Life* in 1963, after which, she joined the Royal Shakespeare Company, the following year. An early role was Ophelia – to David Warner's Prince – in "Hamlet". The post included work with Peter Brook's experimental group. Glenda made her New York debut in "Marat Sade" in 1966, and she was in the film version as well. Her big success was also Ken Russell's best film, *Women in Love.* She won a Best Actress Oscar and went on to earn two more nominations – for *Sunday Bloody Sunday* and *Hedda.* Glenda won a second Best Actress Oscar for *A Touch of Class.* She kept going in films and on television until 1992 - when making her final appearance, in Ken Russell's 'The Secret Life of Arnold Bax'. Shortly after that Glenda went into politics as a British Labor Party Member of Parliament. In case any of her fans want her to make a comeback as an actress, Glenda believes that there is more than enough drama in her present job!

Marat/Sade (1967)
Women in Love (1969)
The Music Lovers (1970)
Sunday Bloody Sunday (1971)
The Triple Echo (1972)
Mary, Queen of Scots (1972)
A Touch of Class (1973)
Hedda (1975)
House Calls (1978)
Stevie (1978)
Hopscotch (1980)
Turtle Diary (1985)

Gordon **Jackson**
5ft 8in
(GORDON CAMERON JACKSON)

Born: **December 19, 1923**
Glasgow, Scotland
Died: **January 15, 1990**

The youngest of five children born to a printer and his wife, young Gordon was educated at Glasgow's Hillhead High School. His interest in acting was spurred by a class visit to the BBC drama department in Glasgow. He later worked on radio – in programs such as 'Children's Hour'. He left school at fifteen to train as a draughtsman with Rolls-Royce, and was able to get stage work in Glasgow. His BBC connection paid off in 1941, when they were contacted by Ealing Studios and asked to recommend a Scot for a role in a an forthcoming film. The result was Gordon's debut, in *The Foreman Went to France*. His work for Rolls-Royce made him exempt from army service, but he appeared in uniform many times on the screen. One of his early star vehicles, *Floodtide,* brought him contact with his future wife, Rona Anderson. They married in 1951, and had two sons. That same year, Gordon made his London stage debut in "Seagulls Over Sorrento". He worked regularly in films – largely as a supporting actor. Gordon became famous with TV viewers for two shows – 'Upstairs, Downstairs' and 'The Professionals'. He died in London from cancer of the spine.

Millions Like Us (1943)
Pink String and Sealing Wax (1946)
The Captive Heart (1946)
Floodtide (1949)
Whisky Galore! (1949)
Bitter Springs (1950)
Happy Go Lovely (1951)
The Quatermass Xperiment (1955)
Sailor Beware (1956)
Seven Waves Away (1957)
Hell Drivers (1957) **Blind Spot** (1958)
The Navy Lark (1959) **Yesterday's Enemy** (1959) **Blind Date** (1959)
Tunes of Glory (1960) **Mutiny on the Bounty** (1962) **The Great Escape** (1963)
The Ipcress File (1965)
The Prime of Miss Jean Brodie (1969)
Hamlet (1969) **Scrooge** (1970)
Shaka Zulu (1987)

Joshua **Jackson**
6ft 2in
(JOSHUA CARTER JACKSON)

Born: June 11, 1978
Vancouver, British Columbia, Canada

Josh's parents were John Carter, who hailed from Texas, and Fiona Jackson, an Irish-born lady who worked as a casting director. He was the grandson of opera singers. Josh spent the first eight years of his life living in California. When his parents got divorced, his name was changed to Joshua Jackson. He was a few months old when he made a brief appearance in the George C. Scott horror movie, *The Changeling*. The family moved to Seattle – where he attended Eistein Middle School, in Shoreline. After returning to Canada, he attended the Ideal Mini School, before going to Kitsilano Secondary School, in Vancouver. Josh then became seriously interested in acting and by the age of eleven, he had decided that it was where his future lay. His mother took him to an audition, which although unsuccessful, got him a part in a television commercial for Keebler's Potato Chips. In 1991, Josh made his film debut in *Crooked Hearts,* which was cast by his mother and shot in Canada. He later appeared as Charlie, in Walt Disney's *The Mighty Ducks* series. Television provided early fame when he played Pacey Witter, in Warner Brother's teen drama, 'Dawson's Creek' – from 1998 until 2003. That exposure coincided with his work in a number of interesting adult movies such as *Apt Pupil* and *Cruel Intentions*. Since 2005, and his positive revues for *Aurora Borealis,* that aspect of his career has taken over. His sister, Aisleagh Jackson, is an actress. In his leisure hours, Josh is a keen harmonica player. He is unmarried.

The Mighty Ducks (1992)
Apt Pupil (1998)
Cruel Intentions (1999)
The Safety of Objects (2001)
The Laramie Project (2002)
Lone Star State of Mind (2002)
Americano (2005)
Aurora Borealis (2005)
The Shadow Dancer (2005)
Bobby (2006) **Battle in Seattle** (2007)
One Week (2008)

Samuel L. **Jackson**
6ft 2¹⁄₂in
(SAMUEL LEROY JACKSON)

Born: December 21, 1948
Washington, D.C., USA

An only child, Sam was raised by his mother, Elizabeth Jackson, together with her parents, in Chattanooga, Tennessee. He attended Riverside High School, where in the school orchestra, he played trumpet and French horn. Sam was an usher at the funeral of Martin Luther King Jr. in 1968, and was actively involved in the Black Power movement. He gave it up when he went to Morehouse College in Atlanta – initially to major in Architecture and then changing to Drama. He acted in plays and TV films before making his feature film debut in 1972, in *Together for Days*. Moving to New York brought more opportunities to appear on stage with the Negro Ensemble as well as the New York Shakespeare Company. It also exposed him to temptation – he got addicted to heroin and alcohol. Luckily, he was helped by Morgan Freeman, who became his mentor, and Spike Lee, who gave him small film roles. Rehabilitation was hard, but he turned the corner after he made a film on the subject in 1991 – *Jungle Fever.* The door opened to stardom. Since 1980 Sam has been married to actress LaTanya Richardson. They have a daughter named Zoè, who attended Vassar College.

True Romance (1993) **Fresh** (1994)
Pulp Fiction (1994)
Die Hard: With a Vengeance (1995)
A Time to Kill (1996)
The Long Kiss Goodnight (1996)
Eve's Bayou (1997)
Jackie Brown (1997)
The Negotiator (1998)
Rules of Engagement (2000)
Unbreakable (2000)
Changing Lanes (2002)
Basic (2003)
Kill Bill: Vol. 2 (2004)
Coach Carter (2005)
Snakes on a Plane (2006)
Black Snake Moan (2006)
Resurrecting the Champ (2007)
1408 (2007) **Cleaner** (2007)
Lakeview Terrace (2008)
Soul Men (2008)

Ulla **Jacobsson**
5ft 4in
(ULLA JACOBSSON)

Born: May 23, 1929
Gothenburg, Västra Götalands län, Sweden
Died: August 20, 1982

Following her secondary schooling, Ulla attended the Gothenburg City Theater training program in 1947. Helped by her charming personality and good looks, she quickly developed into a successful stage actress. Then, in 1951, she was lured by the prospect of a few days in the sun, to make her film debut in *Bärande hav,* which was shot in the Canary Islands. It was Ulla's second film, Arne Mattsson's *One Summer of Happiness,* which brought her instant fame, in the Art House theaters of the United States and Europe. The brief love scene next to a lake where Ulla bared her breasts provoked a huge reaction outside modern, free-thinking Scandinavia, A title role in *Karin Månsdotter* provided her with more serious material but she acted in only one Ingmar Bergman film – *Smiles of a Summer Night.* In the 1960s, Ulla was seen in English language films: *Love Is a Ball,* with Glenn Ford, *Zulu,* with Michael Caine, and *The Heroes of Telemark,* which starred Kirk Douglas and Richard Harris. After that, her career declined as she entered her forties, and she retired from acting in 1978. Ulla was twice married. She died in Vienna, of bone cancer.

One Summer of
Happiness (1951)
Karin Månsdotter (1954)
Sir Arne's Treasure (1954)
Smiles of a Summer Night (1955)
Crime et châtiment (1956
The Song of the
Scarlet Flower (1956)
Körkarlen (1958)
The Restless Night (1958)
Und das am
Montagmorgen (1959)
Love Is a Ball (1963)
Zulu (1964)
The Heroes of Telemark (1965)
Next Year Same Time (1967)
The Tender Age (1968)
La Servante (1970)
One or the Other (1974)
Faustrecht der Freiheit (1975)

Irène **Jacob**
5ft 4in
(IRÈNE MARIA JACOB)

Born: **July 15, 1966**
Suresnes, France

Irène was the youngest of three children. Her father Maurice Jacob, was a physicist and her mother was a psychologist. She was raised in a cultured and highly-educated family environment which produced a musician and two scientists. When she was three, the family moved to Geneva in Switzerland. It was there that she began to show an interest in acting – making her stage debut in 1977. The films of Charlie Chaplin inspired her. She was a student at the Geneva Conservatory of Music and earned a degree in Languages. In 1984 she studied acting at the French National Drama Academy in Paris. With her fluency in English, Irène went to London, where she attended the Dramatic Studio. Back in Paris, she made her film debut in 1984, in *Au revoir, les enfants* – as a piano teacher. She was cast by the Polish film director, Krzysztof Kieslowski, to play the dual roles in *The Double Life of Véronique*. Her performance won her the Best actress Award at Cannes. Irène then furthered her international standing in the same director's *Three Colors: Red*. She was soon working for the great Italian maestro, Michelangelo Antonioni, in his *Beyond the Clouds,* and was building an international fan-base with movies like *U.S. Marshalls, Cuisine américaine* and *Automne,* which spread the word. Frustratingly, for the past several years the material she's been given has rarely been worthy of her talents.

Au revoir les enfants (1987)
The Gang of Four (1988)
Double vie de Véronique (1991)
Claude (1993)
The Secret Garden (1993)
The Prediction (1993)
Three Colors: Red (1994)
Victory (1995) Fugueuses (1995)
Beyond the Clouds (1995)
Othello (1995) Incognito (1997)
U.S. Marshalls (1998)
Cuisine américaine (1998)
Automne (2004)
Fallen Heroes (2007)
The Dust of Time (2008)

Sir Derek **Jacobi**
5ft 10in
(DEREK GEORGE JACOBI)

Born: **October 22, 1938**
Leytonstone, London, England

Derek was the only child of a working class couple – Alfred and Daisy Jacobi. Despite Hitler's bombers battering London, he had a happy childhood. He was a very bright boy – attending Leyton County High School – where he was an enthusiastic part of the drama club – "The Players of Leyton" and from there he went on to win a scholarship to Cambridge. He honed his acting skills in that environment – stimulated by contemporaries including Ian McKellen and Trevor Nunn. When he graduated in 1960, he was invited to join Birmingham Repertory Company. A few years later, Derek became one of the eight founding members of Laurence Olivier's National Theater, in London. During eight years there, he played many great roles including Laertes in "Hamlet" with Peter O'Toole. In 1965, Derek made his film debut as Cassio, in Olivier's *Othello,* and five years later was in his *Three Sisters.* He appeared in more commercial films up until his artistic breakthrough, in 1976, when he was highly praised for his title role in the BBC TV series 'I, Claudius'. Derek made his Broadway debut in 1980, in "The Suicide" then spent four years with the Royal Shakespeare Company. Apart from his stage work, he played several classic roles on film. In March 2006, Derek officialy registered his civil partnership with Richard Clifford after twenty-seven years of living together.

Othello (1965)
The Day of the Jackal (1973)
The Odessa File (1974)
Little Dorrit (1988) Henry V (1989)
Dead Again (1991) Hamlet (1996)
Love is the Devil: Study for a
portrait of Francis Bacon (1998)
Gladiator (2000)
Gosford Park (2001)
Revengers Tragedy (2002)
The Riddle (2007)
Anastezsi (2007)
Adam Resurrected (2008)
A Bunch of Amateurs (2008)
Endgame (2009)

Richard **Jaeckel**
5ft 7in
(RICHARD HANLEY JAECKEL)

Born: **October 10, 1926**
Long Beach, Long Island, New York, USA
Died: **June 14, 1997**

By the time he was in his early teens, Jake, as he was known and his family moved to Los Angeles. He graduated from Hollywood High School and was lucky that his mother was very friendly with Louella Parsons, the Hollywood columnist. She got him a job in the mailroom at 20th Century Fox, where he was discovered by a casting director. Without any previous acting experience, Jake was given a strong debut role in *Guadalcanal Diary*. It was the first film in a career lasting 50 years. Much of his work would be in westerns and war movies, and although he was rarely the star, he made an impact in every role he played. He was one of *The Dirty Dozen,* but the high point in terms of recognition was when he was nominated for a Best Actor Oscar after Paul Newman recommended him for a role in *Sometimes a Great Notion.* In 1995 he was forced to file for bankruptcy and he lost his home in Brentwood. He remained a surprisingly youthful-looking man until after he and his wife, Antoinette Marches, moved to the Woodland Hills Retirement Center. In a short time, his wife was diagnosed with Alzheimer's disease and Jake with a malignant melanoma – which killed him at the age of seventy.

Sands of Iwo Jima (1949)
The Gunfighter (1950)
Come Back Little Sheba (1952)
Attack! (1956)
3.10 to Yuma (1957)
Cowboy (1958)
The Lineup (1958)
Town Without Pity (1961)
The Dirty Dozen (1967)
Chisum (1970)
Sometimes a Great Notion (1971)
Ulzana's Raid (1972)
Pat Garrett and Billy the Kid (1973)
The Outfit (1973)
The Drowning Pool (1975)
Twilight's Last Gleaming (1977)
Cold River (1982)
Starman (1984)

Sam Jaffe
5ft 7½in
(SHALOM JAFFE)

Born: **March 10, 1891**
New York City, New York, USA
Died: **March 24, 1984**

Sam's parents were New York Jews, As a young boy he appeared with his actress mother in Yiddish theater productions. He was academically bright throughout his childhood, and after graduating from the City College, he studied engineering at Columbia University. He then taught mathematics at a school in the Bronx, but in 1916, he joined the Washington Square Players and decided that an actor's life was for him. After making his Broadway debut in "Youth", Sam Jaffe became a regular name in many stage productions and before long, Hollywood beckoned. He refused all offers to appear in silent movies. In 1934, he made his film debut – third-billed below Marlene Dietrich – in von Sternberg's, *The Scarlet Empress.* Sam picked his parts carefully – only accepting roles which were a challenge. As soon as filming finished he was back on his beloved Broadway. He was absent from the screen throughout the war years, but made just as much impact when he returned, for Elia Kazan's *Gentleman's Agreement.* In 1951 he was a victim of the HUAC's communist witch hunt. It cost him his livelihood for seven years. In 1957, he reappeared in Henri-Georges Clouzot's entertaining French drama, *The Spies,* and after that he kept fairly busy – mostly on television. His final screen appearance was in the 1984 film, *On the Line.* Sam died of cancer, in Beverly Hills, California.

The Scarlet Empress (1934)
We Live Again (1934)
Lost Horizon (1937)
Gunga Din (1939)
13 Rue Madeleine (1948)
Gentleman's Agreement (1947)
The Accused (1949)
The Asphalt Jungle (1950)
Under the Gun (1951)
I Can Get It for You Wholesale (1951)
The Day the Earth Stood Still (1951)
The Spies (1957) Ben Hur (1959)
Guns for San Sebastian (1968)
Bedknobs and Broomsticks (1971)

Saeed Jaffrey
5ft 5in
(SAEED JAFFREY)

Born: **January 8, 1929**
Maler Kotla, Punjab, India

Saeed was educated at St. George's College, in Mussoorie, and has an MA in History from the University of Allahabad. He founded Unity Theater, in New Delhi and acted in many plays. From 1951 until 1956, he was Director of All India Radio. He studied at RADA in London before going to the U.S.A. and earning an MA in Drama from the Catholic University of America, in Washington, D.C. From 1958, he was head of publicity at the Indian Tourist Office in the U.S.A. He went to England, where he made his first TV appearance for the BBC, in 1965, in a 'Play of the Month'. After acting with Jack Hawkins in a short film, Saeed made his feature film debut in James Ivory's rather unsuccessful *The Guru.* Six years later, he secured his future as a leading character actor with a role in *The Man Who Would Be King.* He has three children from his marriage to Madhur Jaffrey – a cookbook writer and actress. He has been with his second wife, Jennifer, since 1980.

The Wilby Conspiracy (1975)
The Man Who Would Be King (1975)
The Chess Players (1977) Chasme
Buddoor (1981) Gandhi (1982)
Kissi Se Na Kehna (1983) Mandi (1983)
Masoom (1983) Mashal (1984)
A Passage to India (1984)
My Beautiful Launderette (1985)
Beyond the Next Mountain (1987)
Khudgarz (1987)
Just Ask for Diamond (1988)
Hero Hiralal (1988)
The Deceivers (1988)
Ram Lakhan (1989)
Chaal Baaz (1989)
Dil (1990) Masala (1991)
Henna (1991) Aaina (1993)
The Journey (1997)
Judaai (1997)
Deewana Mastana (1997)
Guru in Seven (1998)
Being Considered (2000)
On Wings of Fire (2001)
Snapshots (2002)
Chicken Tikka Masala (2005)

Dean Jagger
6ft 2in
(IRA DEAN JAGGER)

Born: **November 7, 1903**
Columbus Grove, Ohio, USA
Died: **February 5, 1991**

Dean grew up on an Ohio farm. To begin with, he wasn't a good scholar and twice dropped out of high school. He finally graduated from Wabash College, in Crawfordsville, Indiana, where he was a member of Lambda Chi Alpha. He was a schoolteacher for a short while, but after becoming interested in an acting career, Dean soon enrolled at the Lyceum Art Conservatory in Chicago. In 1929, following a few stage roles, he was spotted by Fox, who cast him in one of their last silents – *The Woman From Hell.* He was prematurely bald and it was really only after the studios stopped forcing him to wear wigs, that he made it in movies. In 1935, Dean celebrated his recent first marriage to Antoinette Lawrence, with a supporting role in the Myrna Loy/Cary Grant film *Wings in the Dark.* Although he starred in several films, he was at his best as a character actor. His most famous role, as Major Harvey Stovall, in *Twelve O'Clock High,* won him an Oscar as Best Supporting Actor. He continued to work in some good movies including *Bad Day at Black Rock* and *Elmer Gantry,* for a further fifteen years. After that he was most often seen on television. His final film was the mediocre, *Evil Town,* in 1987. Dean was married three times – lastly to Etta Jagger, who was by his side when he died of heart disease, in Santa Monica, California.

Brigham Young (1940)
Western Union (1941)
Sister Kenny (1946)
Pursued (1947)
Driftwood (1947)
Twelve O'Clock High (1949)
Sierra (1950) Dark City (1950)
Rawhide (1951) Warpath (1951)
The Robe (1953) Executive Suite (1954)
Private Hell 36 (1954)
White Christmas (1954)
Bad Day at Black Rock (1955)
Red Sundown (1956)
The Nun's Story (1959)
Elmer Gantry (1960)

Thomas **Jane**
5ft 10¾in
(THOMAS ELLIOTT III)

Born: **February 22, 1969**
Baltimore, Maryland, USA

Tom is the son of Michael Elliott, who was then a biogenetic engineer, and his wife Cynthia, who ran an antiques business. After attending local junior school he was educated at Thomas Sprigg Wooton High School, in Montgomery County. While there Tom developed a taste for acting, and on a visit to India in 1986, he made his film debut in *Padamati Sandhya Raagam* – the story of a young Indian girl falling in love with an American boy. The film was sensitively directed by Hasya Brahma Jandhyala. After he graduated in 1987 Tom decided on an acting his career – so a year later, he headed for Los Angeles. His priority was to improve his acting skills – at the famous Lee Strasberg Theater Institute, in Hollywood. Tom married Rutger Hauer's daughter, Aysha, in 1989. He made his American film debut, in *I'll Love You Forever...Tonight* – an Indie drama shot in black and white. In 1992, he followed up with a small role in *Buffy the Vampire Slayer*, and co-starred with his wife in a good comedy, *At Ground Zero.* His big break came with *The Last Time I Committed Suicide,* when he was billed above Keanu Reeves and Adrien Brody. 1997 was a very good year for Tom – he added *Face Off* and *Boogie Nights* to his list of credits and the good roles continued. In 2000, he made his directorial debut, with *Jonni Nitro.* He reached his peak in *The Punisher* and *The Mist.* Tom and his second wife, Patricia Arquette, have a daughter who was born in 2003.

At Ground Zero (1994)
The Last Time I Committed
Suicide (1997) **Face Off** (1997)
Boogie Nights (1997)
Thursday (1998)
The Thin Red Line (1998)
Deep Blue Sea (1999)
Molly (1999) **Magnolia** (1999)
Under Suspicion (2000)
Original Sin (2001) **Stander** (2003)
The Punisher (2004) **The Mist** (2007)
The Mutant Chronicles (2008)
Killshot (2009)

Emil **Jannings**
6ft
(THEODOR FRIEDRICH EMIL JANENZ)

Born: **July 23, 1884**
Rorschach, Switzerland
Died: **January 3, 1950**

Emil was born to German parents who were residing in Switzerland. They took him to live in New York during his childhood and after returning to Germany, they sent him to Zürich for his secondary education. Following that, Emil studied in one of the most beautiful towns in Germany, Görlitz. Its cultural life was a big attraction and after he'd watched a play at the Görlitz Theater, Emil took acting lessons and made his stage debut there, around 1906. He became a member of a roving stock company which toured the country in wagons until through a friend, he was invited to join the Darmstadt Royal Theater in Berlin – studying under Max Reinhardt. He acted in several stage productions but after he worked with fellow actor, Ernst Lubitsch (later one of the great Hollywood directors) in 1914, Emil was persuaded to appear in the film, *Passionels Tagebuch.* He divided his time between stage and screen but by the mid-1920s, after making his breakthrough film, *Jealousy,* he abandoned theater for the screen. He went to Hollywood at the tail-end of the silent era and became the first male recipient of an Oscar for two films – *The Way of All Flesh* and *The Last Command.* Emil's career suffered with the coming of sound – his German accent did not appeal to audiences, but after returning to Germany he had a major hit with *The Blue Angel.* He became a great supporter of the Nazi regime and starred in a number of their propaganda films. Married four times, Emil died of cancer at Strobl, in Austria.

The The Way of All Flesh (1927)
The Last Command (1928)
The Patriot (1928)
Sins of the Fathers (1928)
The Blue Angel (1930)
The Making of a King (1935)
The Dreamer (1936)
The Broken Jug (1937)
Robert Koch (1939)
Uncle Krüger (1941)
The Dismissal (1942)

Claude **Jarman Jr.**
6ft 3in
(CLAUDE JARMAN JR.)

Born: **September 27, 1934**
Nashville, Tennessee, USA

Claude was the son of a railroad accountant and his wife. He was at his elementary school in Nashville when he learned that MGM were conducting a nationwide search for a good-looking young boy to play the role of Jody Baxter, in their forthcoming film, *The Yearling* – based on Marjorie Kinnan Rawling's novel. Claude was chosen from several hundred candidates and under the skilful direction of Clarence Brown, the youngster delivered the most memorable performance of an enchanting film. His reward was a special Oscar, as "most promising child performer". That promise was fulfilled to some degree, in *Roughshod,* and even more so, in *Intruder in the Dust* – also directed by Clarence Brown. But the major step from child star to adult star, didn't happen. Nonetheless, he was was a lucky charm in that all eleven pictures he acted in were at the very least, worthwhile and some, like *Rio Grande,* in which he played John Wayne's son, were excellent. After 1953, the parts dried up and following his final film, *The Great Locomotive Chase,* at the age of twenty-two, Claude returned to Nashville – completing his high school education and studying pre-law at Vanderbilt University. He married the first of three wives in 1959, and served three years in the United States Navy. Moving to San Francisco, he was Director of Cultural Affairs – involved with the San Francisco Opera House and the film festival. He had two sons and five daughters – two of them with his current wife, Katherine.

The Yearling (1946)
High Barbaree (1947)
The Sun Comes Up (1949)
Roughshod (1949)
Intruder in the Dust (1949)
The Outriders (1950)
Rio Grande (1950)
Inside Straight (1951)
Hangman's Knot (1952)
Fair Wind to Java (1953)
The Great Locomotive
Chase (1956)

Lionel **Jeffries**
5ft 10in
(LIONEL JEFFRIES)

Born: **June 10, 1926**
Forest Hill, London, England

The son of Bernard and Elsie Jeffries, Lionel was raised as a Roman Catholic and educated at the Queen Elizabeth Grammar School, in Wimborne, Dorset. After active service during World War II, for which he was awarded the Burma Star, he trained for the stage at the Royal Academy of Dramatic Art in London, and joined the Garrick Theater, in Lichfield, where, being prematurely bald, he was able to take on older roles from the start. A year after marrying Eileen Walsh, with whom he had three children, he made his film debut with a small role in the comedy, *Will Any Gentleman?* From the mid-1950s onwards, Lionel was seen regularly in all kinds of British films. He was especially good in *Two Way Stretch* and *The Wrong Arm of the Law*. His mature appearance enabled him to play Dick Van Dyke's father in *Chitty Chitty Bang Bang,* even though he was six months younger than the American actor. In 1970, Lionel turned his hand to directing – most notably with the charming family films – *The Railway Children* and *The Amazing Mr. Blunden*. He was last seen on the television screen in 2001, in an episode of 'Lexx'.

The Colditz Story (1955)
The Quatermass Xperiment (1955)
Bhowani Junction (1956) **Lust for Life** (1956) **The Vicious Circle** (1957)
Decision Against Time (1957) **Barnacle Bill** (1957) **Blue Murder at St. Trinian's** (1957) **Girls at Sea** (1958)
Up the Creek (1958) **The Revenge of Frankenstein** (1958) **Law and Disorder** (1958) **Orders to Kill** (1958)
Idle on Parade (1959)
The Nun's Story (1959) **The Trials of Oscar Wilde** (1960)
Two Way Stretch (1960) **Fanny** (1961)
The Wrong Arm of the Law (1963)
First Men in the Moon (1964)
Camelot (1967)
Chitty Chitty Bang Bang (1968)
Eyewitness (1970)
Royal Flash (1975)
A Chorus of Disapproval (1988)

Richard **Jenkins**
6ft 1in
(RICHARD JENKINS)

Born: **May 4, 1947**
DeKalb, Illinois, USA

The son of dentist – Dale Jenkins, and his wife Elizabeth – Richard grew up in the small Illinois farming town of DeKalb. His parents took him to the movies every week regardless of what was showing. By his mid-teens, he'd seen a lot of films, but didn't ever dream that he would one day be acting in them. When he left high school and told his parents that he was going to be an actor, the response was positive. At eighteen, Richard took his first steps down that starry road by studying theater at Illinois Wesleyan University in Bloomington. After graduation, it didn't look so starry. He spent nine fruitless months in Hollywood. He joined the Trinity Repertory Company in Rhode Island and stayed there for fifteen years – during which he had a few TV roles – starting with 1974's 'Feasting with Panthers' and made his movie debut with a small part in the western, *Silverado*. Subsequent roles were of a similar size, but they included *Hannah and Her Sisters*. Richard's first featured role was in *The Witches of Eastwick*. After around 70 films, Richard got top billing, in *The Visitor,* for which he was nominated for an Oscar. He is married to Sharon Frederick and has two children.

The Witches of Eastwick (1987)
How I Got Into College (1989) **Sea of Love** (1989) **Blaze** (1989) **Undercover Blues** (1993) **Wolf** (1994) **It Could Happen to You** (1994) **Trapped in Paradise** (1994)
The Indian in the Cupboard (1995) **Flirting with Disaster** (1996) **Absolute Power** (1997) **Eye of God** (1997) **The Confession** (1999) **Outside Providence** (1999) **Snow Falling on Cedars** (1999) **Me, Myself & Irene** (2000)
One Night at McCool's (2001)
The Man Who Wasn't There (2001)
Changing Lanes (2002)
The Mudge Boy (2003) **Intolerable Cruelty** (2003) **Shall We Dance** (2004)
Fun with Dick and Jane (2005)
The Kingdom (2007) **The Visitor** (2007)
The Brøken (2008) **Step Brothers** (2008)
Burn After Reading (2008)

Julia **Jentsch**
5ft 5in
(JULIA JENTSCH)

Born: **February 20, 1978**
Berlin, Germany

Both of Julia's parents were successful lawyers. She was an expressive child who not only applied herself to her schoolwork, she showed a natural aptitude for music and became proficient on the piano when she was quite young. After graduating from high school – the Waldoberschule, she decided on an acting career. In 1997 she began a four-year drama course at the Hochschule für Schauspielkunst Ernst Busch, in Berlin, during a period which also produced that fine young actor, August Diehl. In 1999, she made her film debut in the religious-themed, *Zornige Küsse,* which was filmed in Switzerland. Julia began her career in the theater with a performance in Aischylos' "The Persians," at the Fledermaus Studio Theater in Berlin. It won her the Max Reinhardt Prize. She became a member of the ensemble of the Munich Kammerspiele, where her many performances included Desdemona, in Shakespeare's "Othello" and Elektra, in a production of "Orestie" – by Euripides. In the same period, she built up her portolio of supporting roles in films and also acted in television movies. Julia's first starring role was in the critically acclaimed *The Edukators,* for which she won a Bavarian Film Award as Best Young Actress. Her subsequent movie appearances have confirmed the early promise and she won a Best Actress Silver Bear, at the Berlin Film Festival, for the title-role in the Oscar-nominated *Sophie Scoll – The Final Days*. She also picked up European and German Film Awards for the same movie. Julia has made her home in Munich, where she keeps her private life very private.

Julietta (2001)
Mein Bruder, der Vampir (2001)
The Edukators (2004)
Der Untergang (2004)
Snowland (2005)
Sophie Scholl – The Final Days (2005)
I Served the King of England (2006)
33 Scenes from Life (2008)
Effi Briest (2009)

Marlène **Jobert**
5ft 4½in
(MARLÈNE JOBERT)

Born: November 4, 1940
Algiers, Algeria

After moving to France when she was eight years old, Marlène finished her high school education before going to Dijon, where she studied drama at the Conservatoire. Following that, she spent two years at the Conservatoire de Paris – adding fine art to her skills and working as a photographic model. She made her stage debut in 1963. After experience in the theater, she made her film debut opposite Jean-Pierre Léaud, in Jean-Luc Godard's *Masculin, féminin*. A year later, she was in the company of Jean-Paul Belmondo, in Louis Malle's *Le Voleur*. She then did a fair amount of television work before she shining brightly in the comedy *Alexandre le bienheureux*. An international film with Kirk Douglas wasn't a hit and acting with Anthony Perkins didn't jell either. She was a lot better with a European cast, especially in films like *Nous ne Viellirons pas ensemble*. Marlène's movies during the 1970s and early 1980s were generally of a very high standard. In 1983, she became an author. She continued to appear in French TV productions up to 1998, when after acting in 'Maintenant et pour toujours', she retired to devote her time to writing books for children. Marlène's very beautiful daughter, the actress, Eva Green was born in 1980. Her father was a Swedish dentist, Walter Green. Eva is beginning to make a name for herself in high profile movies – she was featured in *Kingdom of Heaven* – and became a Bond Girl – in *Casino Royale*.

Masculin, féminin (1966)
Le Voleur (1967)
Alexandre le bienheureux (1968)
L'Astragale (1969)
Le Passager de la pluie (1969)
Dernier domocile connu (1970)
The Scarlet Buccaneer (1971)
Nous ne viellirons pas
ensemble (1972)
Pas si méchant que ça (1974)
Le Secret (1974)
Le Bon et les méchants (1976)
L'Amour nu (1981)

Scarlett **Johansson**
5ft 3in
(SCARLETT JOHANSSON)

Born: November 22, 1984
New York City, New York, USA

The third youngest of four children – and with a twin brother, Scarlett has Danish blood from her father, Karsten Johansson. There was Polish Jewish blood, from her mother, Melanie Sloan, who was a "movie buff". Scarlett first revealed a passion for acting when she was three. At junior school she appeared in plays at every opportunity. Her first film appearance was in 1994, as Laura, in *North*. In 1996, in *Manny & Lo,* her older sister, Vanessa, made a brief appearance. Two years later, Scarlett was noted as a major star of the future when she received world-wide acclaim for her fine portrayal of Grace MacLean, in *The Horse Whisperer*. Since then her movie career has gone according to the script. In 2002, she graduated from the Professional Children's School in New York City. She won a BAFTA, a year after that, for *Lost in Translation*. Four Golden Globe nominations have kept up the pressure and her recent efforts confirm that she is improving as an actress with each passing year. *Match Point* gave her an opportunity to work with her hero, Woody Allen. Along with super-model Kate Moss, Scarlett is involved in helping the Breast Cancer Charity, by designing charm bracelets. In January 2008, Scarlett, who is a Democrat supporter, campaigned on behalf of Barack Obama, in Iowa.

Just Cause (1995)
Manny & Lo (1996)
The Horse Whisperer (1998)
The Man Who Wasn't There (2001)
Ghost World (2001)
An American Rhapsody (2001)
Lost in Translation (2003)
Girl with a Pearl Earring (2003)
A Love Song for Bobby Long (2004)
A Good Woman (2004)
In Good Company (2004)
Match Point (2005)
The Prestige (2006)
The Nanny Diaries (2007)
The Other Boleyn Girl (2008)
Vicky Cristina Barcelona (2008)
He's Just Not That Into You (2009)

Glynis **Johns**
5ft 4in
(GLYNIS JOHNS)

Born: October 5, 1923
Pretoria, South Africa

The daughter of the Welsh-born Mervyn Johns - who was a character actor in British films, and an Australian mother, Glynis returned to England with her parents in 1929. When she was twelve, she danced in "Buckie's Bears" at London's Garrick Theater and made her film debut three years later, in *South Riding*. She had her first leading role in 1941, in Michael Powell's *49th Parallel*. After a huge success the previous winter as a stage "Peter Pan", Glynis and her dad acted as father and daughter in the 1944 ghost story, *The Halfway House*. She became a star in Britain over the next four years, especially after playing a sexy mermaid in *Miranda*. It was followed by high profile movies with Douglas Fairbanks Jr., James Stewart, Robert Donat and Alec Guinness. It was their exalted company which aroused some interest in America. Glynis gained a foothold in that market in 1952, with her Broadway triumph, in "Gertie". She also met her second husband there. A brilliant showing opposite Danny Kaye, in *The Court Jester,* seemed to auger well. She settled in America and once again scored on Broadway – in "Major Barbara". She was nominated for a Best Supporting Actress Oscar for *The Sundowners*. Glynis made her last film appearance in 1999, in the rather weak comedy, *Superstar.*

49th Parallel (1941)
The Halfway House (1943)
Perfect Strangers (1945)
Frieda (1947)
An Ideal Husband (1947)
Miranda (1948)
State Secret (1950)
No Highway (1951)
The Magic Box (1951)
The Card (1952)
The Court Jester (1955)
The Sundowners (1960)
Mary Poppins (1964)
Under Milk Wood (1972)
The Vault of Horror (1973)
The Ref (1994)
While You Were Sleeping (1995)

Ben **Johnson**
6ft 2in
(BEN JOHNSON)

Born: **June 13, 1918**
Foraker, Shidler, Oklahoma, USA
Died: **April 8, 1996**

Like his Rodeo-competing father, Ben Johnson Sr., Ben was a real-life cowboy. Like him, he became a champion steer roper. Ben grew up on his dad's ranch, working with cattle and horses for $1 a day. In 1939, he was hired by producer Howard Hughes, to take a large number of horses to California. While there, he made an uncredited appearance in the B-western, *The Fighting Gringo*. Ben married Carol Jones, in 1941, and made a living as a stunt man and working as a double – often (because of his size) for John Wayne. He had an uncredited role in *The Outlaw*, in 1943, and when John Ford starred him in *Wagonmaster,* Ben had made nine movies without a mention of his name. He co-starred with Terry Moore in *Mighty Joe Young,* but fell out with Ford during the making of *Rio Grande*. Ben was persona non grata, until a small role in *Cheyenne Autumn,* in 1964. He won a Best Supporting Actor Oscar for *The Last Picture Show*. His final film appearance was in 1996, in *The Evening Star*. Ben died of a heart attack, in Mesa, Arizona.

3 Godfathers (1948)
Mighty Joe Young (1948)
She Wore a Yellow Ribbon (1948)
Shane (1953)
Rebel in Town (1956)
One-Eyed Jacks (1961)
Major Dundee (1965)
Will Penny (1966)
Hang 'Em High (1968)
The Wild Bunch (1969)
Chisum (1970)
The Last Picture Show (1971)
Junior Bonner (1972)
The Getaway (1972)
The Train Robbers (1973)
Dillinger (1973)
Sugarland Express (1974)
Bite the Bullet (1975)
Breakheart Pass (1975)
**My Heroes Have Always
Been Cowboys** (1991)
Radio Flyer (1992)

Dame Celia **Johnson**
5ft 6in
(CELIA ELIZABETH JOHNSON)

Born: **December 18, 1908**
Richmond, Surrey, England
Died: **April 26, 1982**

The daughter of Robert Johnson and his wife Ethel, Celia was educated at St. Paul's Girls School in London. She studied at RADA and made her stage debut in "Major Barbara" in Huddersfield when she was twenty. The following year, she made her London West End stage debut, in "A Hundred Years Old". She appeared on Broadway for the one and only time in 1931 – playing Ophelia – to Raymond Massey's Prince – in "Hamlet". In 1936, Celia married the travel writer, Peter Fleming (the elder brother of Ian) and remained with him until his death in 1971. She had success on the London stage, playing the leading role in "Rebecca" just before the war. Celia made her first film in 1941, in a short directed by Carol Reed called *A Letter from Home,* which was aimed at the American market and especially the anti-war lobby. She appeared in a trio of patriotic flag-wavers before her Oscar-nominated role as Laura Jesson, in David Lean's *Brief Encounter*. It is the quintessentially English tear-jerker, written by Noel Coward. Celia herself epitomized old-fashioned Englishness, who was very unlikely to appeal to American audiences. She was first and foremost a stage actress – more interested in her happy home life with her husband, Celia had a number of successful seasons on the West End stage, before returning to films one last time, in *The Prime of Miss Jean Brodie*. Celia retired to her home in Nettlebed, Oxfordshire, after playing Mrs. Gladstone, in an episode of the television series 'Number 10'. She died of a stroke.

In Which We Serve (1942)
Dear Octopus (1943)
This Happy Breed (1944)
Brief Encounter (1945)
The Astonished Heart (1950)
The Holly and the Ivy (1952)
The Captain's Paradise (1953)
A Kid for Two Farthings (1955)
**The Prime of
Miss Jean Brodie** (1969)

Don **Johnson**
5ft 11in
(DONNIE WAYNE JOHNSON)

Born: **December 15, 1949**
Flat Creek, Missouri

The son of a farmer, and a mother who was a beautician, Don was six when he was taken to live in Wichita Kansas. In 1967, he graduated from South High School in Wichita, and then attended the University of Kansas, in Lawrence. After graduating, Don had an ambition to become a professional bowler, but he turned instead to music. He had a good voice and used it as a member of the psychedelic rock band called "Horses". He first tasted the excitement of acting when he got small roles in theatrical plays. After appearing on a TV show 'The Dating Game, he decided to become an actor. He studied drama at the American Conservatory Theater in San Francisco and made his pro stage debut in the rock musical, "Your Own Thing". Don's movie debut was in 1970, in *The Magic Garden of Stanley Sweetheart*. In 1971, he met the fourteen year old Melanie Griffith, and they moved in together. They married twice – in 1976, for six months, and again in 1989 – when they stayed together for six years and had a child. His career was slow moving for a time but in 1984 he had a change of luck when he was cast as Sonny Crockett, in the TV series ' Miami Vice' and won a Golden Globe Award. His movies have been a mixed bag, but two more good TV roles – in 'Nash Bridges' and 'Just Legal', kept his name alive and he has recently acted in some good films. He has been married to Kelley Phleger, since 1999. They have a daughter.

Return to Macon County (1975)
A Boy and His Dog (1975)
Melanie (1982) **Cease Fire** (1985)
Sweethearts Dance (1988)
Dead Bang (1989)
The Hot Spot (1990)
Paradise (1991)
Guilty as Sin (1993)
Tin Cup (1996)
Goodbye Lover (1998)
Moondance Alexander (2008)
Long Flat Balls II (2008)
Torno a vivere da solo (2008)

Rita **Johnson**
5ft 4¹/₄in
(RITA MCSEAN)

Born: August 13, 1913
Worcester, Massachusetts, USA
Died: October 31, 1965

After showing great promise as a pianist, Rita graduated from high school and went to study at New England Conservatory of Music, in Boston. Apart from her talents as a musician, she was a good swimmer. She was only prevented by lack of finance from competing for the USA at the Los Angeles Olympics, in 1932. Finishing her studies during the Great Depression, her chances of making a living from music weren't good. She appeared in summer stock, but her drama teacher told her she'd never become an actress. Rita's determination proved him wrong. In 1937, MGM co-starred her with George Murphy in *London by Night*. By the outbreak of World War II, Rita had appeared in a dozen movies – sometimes in supporting roles, alongside Walter Pidgeon. In 1939 she was top-billed in Jacques Tourneur's first American film-noir *They All Came Out*. In 1940, Rita was pushing towards movie stardom – first playing opposite Spencer Tracy in *Edison the Man* and following up with *Here Comes Mr. Jordan* and a strong supporting role in the good Ginger Rogers comedy, *The Major and the Minor*. She was married and divorced twice during a six-year spell, but her career was fine until 1948, when she required brain surgery after a hair dryer fell on her. Rumors that she had been beaten up by her gangster boyfriend were supported by evidence of bruising all over her body. She made a few films and was often on TV until 1957. She had earlier succumbed to alcoholism and was fifty-two when she died in Hollywood, of a brain hemorrhage.

They All Came Out (1939)
Edison the Man (1940)
Here Comes Mr. Jordan (1941)
The Major and the Minor (1942)
My Friend Flicka (1943)
The Affairs of Susan (1945)
They Won't Believe Me (1947)
The Big Clock (1948)
Susan Slept Here (1954)
All Mine to Give (1957)

Van **Johnson**
6ft 1in
(CHARLES VAN DELL JOHNSON)

Born: August 25, 1916
Newport, Rhode Island, USA
Died: December 12, 2008

The product of a broken home, young Van used to sing and dance to escape the reality of his early life. After high school he was in the chorus of the Broadway show "New Faces". He then sang in vaudeville before touring in the Rogers and Hart musicals "Too Many Girls" and "Pal Joey". In the latter, he was understudying Gene Kelly when he was seen by a Warner Brothers talent scout. He made his film debut for them in 1942, in *Murder in the Big House,* but it was MGM who gave him a contract. A major road accident rendered him ineligible to serve his country during World War II, but in his early films, he was usually in uniform. One of them *A Guy Named Joe* was with Spencer Tracy. After appearing with June Allyson and Esther Williams in musicals he was at the peak of his popularity. In 1947 he married the wife of his good friend Keenan Wynn. Van's biggest hit was *In the Good Old Summertime,* with Judy Garland. As he entered the 1950s, Van found himself in supporting roles much of the time. He went freelance – appearing in stage shows such as "The Music Man", "Bye Bye Birdie" and "La Cage aux Folles" - his last hit. But there were few quality film parts – other than a small role in Woody Allen's *The Purple Rose of Cairo*. He was last seen in 1992, in *Clowning Around*. Van lived quietly in retirement until he died of natural causes, in Nyack, New York.

A Guy Named Joe (1944)
Thirty Seconds over Tokyo (1944)
Thrill of a Romance (1945)
Weekend at the Waldorf (1945)
Easy to Wed (1946)
Command Decision (1948)
In the Good Old Summertime (1949)
Battleground (1949)
Easy to Love (1953) The Caine
Mutiny (1954) Brigadoon (1954)
Miracle in the Rain (1956)
Slander (1956) 23 Paces to
Baker Street (1956)
Divorce American Style (1967)

Angelina **Jolie**
5ft 8in
(ANGELINA JOLIE VOIGHT)

Born: June 4, 1975
Los Angeles, California, USA

The daughter of the Hollywood actor, Jon Voight, Angie dreamed of following in his footsteps. She was seven when she appeared with him, in *Lookin' to Get Out*. After her parents separated in 1976, she and her brother, James, were raised by their mother, actress Marcheline Bertrand, who first got her interested in movies. They eventually moved to Los Angeles, where she attended Beverly Hills High School. It's very hard to believe, but Angie was an unattractive kid during those years. At fourteen, she dropped out of the acting classes her mother had encouraged her to join and spent two years floundering in a kind of mental wilderness. By the time she was sixteen, she'd sorted out her life and become a model, which was great for her confidence. After that, Angie graduated from high school and returned to Lee Strasberg's acting classes. She began her career in 1993, playing a robot, in *Cyborg 2*. She met her first husband, Jonny Lee Miller, when making her first good movie, *Hackers*. She won a Golden Globe for her work in the television movie 'George Wallace'. In 1999, Angie put the icing on the cake, by winning a Best Supporting Actress Oscar, for *Girl, Interrupted*. In May 2000, Angie married Billy Bob Thornton, but they got divorced exactly three years later. Since 2005, she has been in a relationship with Brad Pitt. In May 2006 she gave birth to their child – a daughter named Shiloh. Angie's ambition to be a great actress shows in her role in *A Mighty Heart*. She was in the running for a Best Actress Oscar, for *Changeling*.

Hackers (1995)
Playing by Heart (1998)
The Bone Collector (1999)
Girl, Interrupted (1999)
Lara Croft: Tomb Raider (2001)
Beyond Borders (2003)
Mr. & Mrs. Smith (2005)
The Good Shepherd (2006)
A Mighty Heart (2007)
Beowulf (2007) Changeling (2008)
Wanted (2008)

Al **Jolson**
5ft 8in
(ASA YOELSON)

Born: May 26, 1886
Srednik, Lithuania, Russian Empire
Died: October 23, 1950

Al was the fourth of the five children of Moses Yoelson and his wife Naomi. The Jews were persecuted in Czarist Russia and the Yoelsons emigrated to the United States in 1891. When, after three years, he had established himself as a rabbi and cantor in a synagogue, in Washington D.C., he sent for his family. Al's mother died shortly after they arrived. He and his brother sang at the synagogue and were introduced to show business in 1895, by singing for coins in the street, as "Al and Harry". When he was fourteen Al ran away from home but lived in poverty for two years until he was taken on by Walter L. Maim's Circus. That folded after one year and Al was hired for a Burlesque show, "Dainty Duchess". Over the next twenty years, he worked in vaudeville and plays and became popular singing old Stephen Foster songs in blackface, which was accepted by his black friends, who knew that he was fighting discrimination and promoting them whenever possible. Al's movie debut was in the uncompleted *Mammy's Boy,* in 1923. His breakthrough was in his second film – the part-talkie *The Jazz Singer.* He remained popular until Bing Crosby took over as the nation's number one. Al said (and sang) his farewell to movie audiences in *Swanee River.* His recordings are still very popular in the 21st century. Against his doctor's orders, Al went to Korea to entertain the troops. Shortly after his return, he died of a heart attack while playing cards in his San Francisco hotel suite. His four wives included the movie dancer, Ruby Keeler.

The Jazz Singer (1927)
The Singing Fool (1928)
Say It with Songs (1929)
Mammy (1930) Big Boy (1930)
Hallelujah I'm a Bum (1933)
Wonder Bar (1934)
Go Into Your Dance (1935)
The Singing Kid (1936)
Rose of Washington Square (1939)
Swanee River (1939)

Dean **Jones**
5ft 11in
(DEAN JONES)

Born: January 25, 1931
Decatur, Alabama, USA

Dean was the son of a construction worker, Andrew Jones and his wife, Nolia. After he'd dropped out of Asbury College, in Wilmore, Kentucky, Dean served during the Korean War, in the United States Air Corps. In the early 1950s, he was a blues singer on the nightclub circuit. He then turned to acting at the Bird Cage Theater, Knott's Berry Farm, California and met his first wife, Mae Entwhistle, with whom he had two children. In 1956, he was signed by MGM and made his film debut that year with a small role in *Somebody Up There Likes Me.* He was kept busy by the studio in tiny supporting roles until a good part in Elvis Presley's *Jailhouse Rock,* made him slightly more visible. Breaking away from MGM was the answer but for three years it meant specializing as a TV actor. A featured role in *Under the Yum Yum Tree,* with Jack Lemmon, gave Dean a chance to play comedy, but it still took two more years before he got a Disney contract and became a star – after *That Darn Cat.* The peak of his popularity was probably *The Love Bug* series, which included both films and TV versions. In 1973, Dean became a devout born-again Christian. He has made a few religious movies - the best of which was the 1986 film, *St. John in Exile* – which was originally a one-man show. Even though he is now semi-retired, Dean can't resist the temptation to work in front of the cameras. In 2007, he appeared in a short comedy entitled *Lavinia's Heist,* and recently completed work on *Mandie and the Secret Tunnel.* Dean lives in California.

Jailhouse Rock (1957)
Imitation General (1958)
Torpedo Run (1958)
Under the Yum Yum Tree (1963)
That Darn Cat! (1965)
The Ugly Dachshund (1966)
Blackbeard's Ghost (1968)
The Love Bug (1968)
St. John in Exile (1986)
Beethoven (1992)
Clear and Present Danger (1994)

Carolyn **Jones**
5ft 5in
(CAROLYN SUE JONES)

Born: **April 28, 1930**
Amarillo, Texas, USA
Died: **August 3, 1983**

Carolyn's parents, Julius Alfred Jones and his wife, Cloe, separated before she was born. Her father returned, but finding it difficult to get work in the Great Depression, he abandoned his family. Carolyn was a sickly child who suffered from asthma, but she dreamed that she would make it on the silver screen. She studied hard and won awards at school for her poetry and her appearances in plays. After graduating from high school she went to California to be nearer Hollywood. Carolyn joined the Pasadena Playhouse and gained good experience in stage presentations in the Los Angeles area. She eventually acted on television in 1952, in an episode of 'Gruen Guild Playhouse'. She made her film debut that same year, in *The Turning Point.* She was first noticed in *House of Wax,* and things were fine until she was forced by illness to miss out on *From Here to Eternity.* Despite that set-back she kept working and even had a walk-on part in *East of Eden.* Supporting roles in *The Seven Year Itch* and *The Tender Trap* led to the original sci-fi classic – *Invasion of the Body Snatchers.* Carolyn was nominated for a Best Supporting Actress Oscar for *The Bachelor Party,* and starred opposite Elvis in *King Creole.* Good film roles dried up in the 1960s but she reached the peak of her popularity as Morticia Addams, in the TV series 'The Addams Family'. In 1982, she was diagnosed with colon cancer. She died at her Hollywood home – a month after marrying her third husband, Peter.

House of Wax (1953) The Big
Heat (1953) The Saracen Blade (1954)
Three Hours to Kill (1954) The Seven
Year Itch (1955) The Tender Trap (1955)
Invasion of the Body Snatchers (1956)
The Man Who Knew to Much (1956)
Johnny Trouble (1957) Baby Face
Nelson (1957) Marjorie
Morningstar (1958) King Creole (1958)
A Hole in the Head (1959)
Last Train from Gun Hill (1959)
How the West Was Won (1962)

Griffith **Jones**
6ft 2in
(GRIFFITH HAROLD JONES)

Born: **November 19, 1909**
London, England
Died: **January 30, 2007**

The youngest of five children, Griffith was a brilliant scholar, despite parents who were not academic. His father was a Welsh-speaking former lead miner and his mother was a Londoner. After secondary school, Griffith began studying law at the University of London. He had already appeared in amateur theatrical productions and school plays, when with a year's legal studies under his belt, he dropped out to go to the Royal Academy of Dramatic Art. While he was there, he made his London stage debut under the name Harold Jones, in "Carpet Slippers". In 1932, he had reverted to his real name Griffith Jones when he made his film debut in *Money Talks* and established himself on the London West End stage. His first role as a star was in 1937, in *The Wife of General Ling,* but it was the British-filmed Hollywood production, *A Yank at Oxford* – starring Robert Taylor and Vivien Leigh, which got him known to moviegoers. In World War II Griffith served in the British Army, but spent much of his five years in uniform with a touring concert party and was able to continue acting in films such as Olivier's *Henry V.* In 1945, he starred in "Lady Windermere's Fan" in the West End and after his screen career faded, he was a stalwart of the Royal Shakespeare Company. He was married to Robin Isaac from 1932 until her death, in 1985. Their children are actors Gemma and Nicholas Jones. Griffith was ninety when he retired. He died at his home in London.

Catherine the Great (1934)
A Yank at Oxford (1938)
The Four Just Men (1939)
Atlantic Ferry (1941)
The Day Will Dawn (1942)
Henry V (1944)
The Wicked Lady (1945)
The Rake's Progress (1945)
They Made Me a Fugitive (1947)
Miranda (1948)
Good-Time Girl (1948)
The Sea Shall Not Have Them (1954)

James Earl **Jones**
6ft 1½in
(JAMES EARL JONES)

Born: **January 17, 1931**
Arkabutla, Mississippi, USA

Jim's dad, Robert Earl Jones, who was among other things an actor, butler and boxer, left his wife before Jim was born. From the age of five, he was raised by his mother's parents on their farm in Jackson, Michigan. The upheaval and trauma of his early life caused him to develop a severe stutter. He was functionally mute for eight years until a teacher at his high school saw that he wrote poetry, and forced him to recite them to the class every day. Jim went on to graduate from the University of Michigan and became an officer in the Army during the late 1950s. His growing passion for acting led to a small role in *Dr. Strangelove.* Six years later, in his first big role, he was nominated for a Best Actor Oscar, when he portrayed Jack Jefferson, in the film version of *The Great White Hope.* in 1969, he was involved in making test films for the television series, 'Sesame Street'. Jim became known for his non-appearances in the *Star Wars* films when he only provided the sinister voice for the character 'Darth Vader'. He has also been heard as 'Mufusa', in Disney's animated films of *The Lion King.* In 1979, he played the great singer in the television film, 'Paul Robeson'. Jim has been married to Cecilia Hart since 1982. Much of Jim's recent film work has been as a voice-over.

The Comedians (1967)
The Great White Hope (1970)
The Man (1972)
Conan the Barbarian (1982)
Gardens of Stone (1987)
Matewan (1987)
Coming to America (1988)
Field of Dreams (1989)
The Hunt for Red October (1990)
Convicts (1991)
Patriot Games (1992)
Sneakers (1992)
The Sandlot (1993)
Cry, the Beloved Country (1995)
On the Q.T. (1999)
Undercover Angel (1999)
The Annihilation of Fish (1999)
Finder's Fee (2001)

Jennifer **Jones**
5ft 7in
(PHYLIS ISLEY)

Born: **March 2, 1919**
Tulsa, Oklahoma, USA

Being the daughter of actors, Phillip and Flora Mae Isley – who ran a traveling tent show, Jennifer began appearing in plays performed by their stock company when she was very young. She studied at the American Academy of Dramatic Arts in New York, where she met and married Robert Walker. She was briefly registered with the Powers Model Agency. She and her husband worked together at a Tulsa radio station before testing unsuccessfully for Paramount. She did get film work in 1939, with John Wayne, in a B-western called *New Frontier.* After an audition at David O. Selznick's New York office, she was re-named Jennifer Jones. Selznick built her up to stardom over three years. The right role came along and she won a Best Actress Oscar in *Song of Bernadette.* In 1944, while filming *Since You Went Away* with her husband, Jennifer filed for divorce. Jennifer appeared in big movies like *Duel in the Sun* and *Portrait of Jenny.* In 1949, she married Selznick who would continue to master-mind her movie career – sometimes interfering to a point which handicapped her. Her hypnotic quality began to fade in the mid-1950s, but he kept plugging away on her behalf until his death in 1965. She was to suffer badly for a few years, but in 1971, she married the millionaire Norton Simon, and returned just once to the screen, in *The Towering Inferno.* Simon died in 1993. Jennifer is chairman of the Norton Simon Museum.

Song of Bernadette (1943)
Since You Went Away (1944)
Love Letters (1945) **Cluny Brown** (1946)
Duel in the Sun (1946)
Portrait of Jenny (1948)
We Were Strangers (1949)
Madame Bovary (1949)
Carrie (1952) **Ruby Gentry** (1952)
Beat the Devil (1953)
Love Is a Many-Splendored Thing (1953) **The Man in the Gray Flannel Suit** (1956)
The Barretts of Wimpole Street (1957)
A Farewell to Arms (1957)

Shirley **Jones**
5ft 5¹/₂in
(SHIRLEY MAE JONES)

Born: March 31, 1934
Charleroi, Pennsylvania, USA

The daughter of Paul and Marjorie Jones – owners of the Jones Brewing Company, Shirley was named after the popular child star, Shirley Temple. She didn't disappoint her movie-mad mother – Shirley began to show signs of real singing talent when she was six-years old - as the youngest member of her church choir. Shirley grew into a lovely young woman – winning a beauty pageant as a teenager and after graduating from South Huntingdon High School she was crowned "Miss Pittsburgh". She took acting lessons at the Pittsburgh Playhouse and then headed for New York City. She auditioned with 85 other hopefuls for a part in "South Pacific" and made her stage debut as one of the nurses. In the early 1950s, she had a couple of roles in TV dramas before being given her movie debut in *Oklahoma*. She and her co-star Gordon MacRae were so good together, the following year they were in another Rogers and Hammerstein hit, *Carousel.* It was the year she married Jack Cassidy. Shirley acted with Pat Boone and James Cagney before winning a Best Supporting Actress Oscar, for *Elmer Gantry*. From 1970 to 1973, Shirley starred with her step-son David Cassidy, in the successful TV-series, 'The Partridge Family'. Her marriage had turned sour and two years before Jack (who suffered from manic depression) died, Shirley got a divorce. Since 1977, she's been married to Marty Ingels. She was recently seen as Colleen Brady, in the TV show, 'Days of our Lives'.

Oklahoma (1955)
Carousel (1956)
April Love (1957)
Never Steal Anything Small (1959)
Elmer Gantry (1960)
Two Rode Together (1961)
The Music Man (1962)
The Courtship of
Eddie's Father (1963)
Bedtime Story (1964) **Fluffy** (1965)
The Happy Ending (1969)
The Cheyenne Social Club (1970)
Grandma's Boy (2006)

Tommy Lee **Jones**
6ft
(TOMMY LEE JONES)

Born: September 15, 1946
San Saba, Texas, USA

Tommy's father, Clyde C. Jones, worked on a Texas oil field, and his mother, Lucille, was at different times, a police officer, school teacher, and beauty shop owner. After St. Mark's School of Texas, Tommy won a scholarship to Harvard from where he graduated with a BA in English literature. He also played for the varsity football team which was undefeated during 1968. Although he had never taken an acting class, he moved to New York and got a role on Broadway, in "A Patriot for Me" before making his film debut in *Love Story*. His first big role was opposite Laurence Olivier in *The Betsy*. In 1983, Tommy won an Emmy for his portrayal of Gary Gilmore in a television special, 'The Executioner's Song'. Tommy has since appeared in a number of high-profile movies – including *The Fugitive,* for which he won a Best Supporting Actor Oscar. He directed *The Three Burials of Melquiades Estrada,* which won him the Best Actor award at Cannes. More recently, he was nominated for a Best Actor Oscar, for *In the Valley of Elah.* Tommy lives with his third wife, Dawn Laurel, in San Antonio, Texas, where he is a part-time cattle rancher.

Rolling Thunder (1977)
Coal Miner's Daughter (1980)
Stormy Monday (1988)
JFK (1991)
Under Siege (1992)
The Fugitive (1993)
The Client (1994)
Natural Born Killers (1994)
Blue Sky (1994) **Cobb** (1994)
Batman Forever (1995)
Men in Black (1997)
U.S. Marshalls (1998)
Rules of Engagement (2000)
Space Cowboys (2000)
The Missing (2003)
The Three Burials of Melquiades
Estrada (2005)
A Prairie Home Companion (2006)
No Country for Old Men (2007)
In the Valley of Elah (2007)
In the Electric Mist (2009)

Vinnie **Jones**
6ft 2in
(VINCENT PETER JONES)

Born: January 5, 1965
Watford, Hertfordshire, England

Vinnie's dad, Peter, was a gamekeeper, so by the time he was seven years old, Vinnie knew how to fire a shotgun. He was soon playing the far less aggressive game of soccer, and by his early teens he was strongly-built and his natural enthusiasm left bruises on anyone he tackled. After he left school, he was an amateur before becoming a semi-pro at Wealdstone, in West London. To supplement his income and bulk up his physique, Vinnie worked on building sites. He made progress to the point that after helping the Swedish club IFK Holmsund, to win the second division title, he was signed by the then English first division side, Wimbledon. As part of their so-called "crazy gang" he got an FA Cup winner's medal in 1988. When he retired from the game in 1998, he'd played for Chelsea, represented his mother's nation - Wales and been player/coach at Queens Park Rangers. His hard man image, which during his career had been the target for a lot of criticism, suddenly became a source of new employment as a wrestler and an actor. He made his film debut in Guy Ritchie's *Lock, Stock and Two Smoking Barrels* and appeared in a music video for Westlife's "Bop Bop Baby" and TV commercials for Bacardi and Red Devil. His propensity for violence helped his career as a screen gangster. In 2003, he was convicted of air rage offenses on a flight to Tokyo. Banned by Virgin Atlantic, he marched on and improved his acting technique. Vinnie lives in Los Angeles with his wife, Tanya, and their two children.

Lock, Stock and Two Smoking
Barrels(1998) **Snatch** (2000)
Swordfish (2001) **Mean Machine** (2001)
EuroTrip (2004)
Survive Style 5+ (2004)
The Other Half (2006)
Johnny Was (2006)
She's the Man (2006)
X-Men: The Last Stand (2006)
The Condemned (2007) **7-10 Split** (2007)
Strength and Honour (2007)
The Midnight Meat Train (2008)

Richard **Jordan**
6ft 1in
(ROBERT ANSON JORDAN)

Born: **July 19, 1938**
New York City, New York, USA
Died: **August 30, 1993**

Richard was born into a family of lawyers - he was the grandson of Judge Learned Hand. His mother, Constance Jordan, married Newbold Morris, a member of the New York City Council. While attending Hotchkiss High School, in Lakeville, Connecticut, Richard received such good notices for his acting in a production of "Mister Roberts", he was invited to join the Sharon summer stock company. He went to England as an exchange student at the famous old Sherbourne School. On his return to the United States he went to Harvard University, where he continued to appear on stage while earning his BA. He made his New York stage debut at the Shakespeare Festival and he performed there for nearly eight years, in several highly-praised productions. He made his television debut in 1961, in an episode of 'Naked City'. In 1964, Richard married his "Juliet", Kathleen Widdoes, and their eight year marriage produced a daughter, Nina. By the time he made his film debut, in *Lawman,* Richard had acted in dozens of on and off-Broadway plays. His first movie starring role was in the Canadian-made, *Kamouraska* – opposite Geneviève Bujold. He reached his peak in a hit sci-fi movie, *Logan's Run,* and Woody Allen's *Interiors* and enjoyed further successes on stage and had one final big screen triumph, in *Gettysburg,* before his early death from a brain tumor, in Los Angeles.

Lawman (1971) Valdez Is
Coming (1971) Chato's Land (1972)
Kamouraska (1973)
The Friends of Eddie Coyle (1973)
The Yakuza (1974)
Rooster Cogburn (1975)
Logan's Run (1976) Interiors (1978)
A Nightingale Sang in
Berkeley Square (1979)
A Flash of Green (1984) Dune (1984)
The Secret of My Succe$s (1987)
Romero (1989) The Hunt for
Red October (1990)
Gettysburg (1993)

Victor **Jory**
6ft 1½in
(VICTOR JORY)

Born: **November 23, 1902**
Dawson City, Yukon Territory, Canada
Died: **February 12, 1982**

Victor grew up in the area which became known as Alaska. His family moved to the United States when he reached his teens and he attended high school in California. He was determined to become an actor and to that end, he joined the Pasadena Playhouse. A year or so later, Victor signed on as a United States Coast Guard and during his two years service, he was both boxing and wrestling champion. After that, he married his sweetheart, the actress Jean Inness, and concentrated on getting his stage career started. Victor made his New York City debut in 1929, and his Broadway debut in 1930, in "Berkeley Square" – where his superb voice and his burly physique attracted the attention of Hollywood studios. His first film role was an uncredited one, in *Renegades,* made that same year. Two years later, he starred in *Pride of the Legion.* Victor was soon co-starring with such talents as Jean Arthur, supporting stars like Flynn and Cagney, and acting in *Gone With the Wind,* but by the 1940s he played villains in 'Hopalong Cassidy' films. Victor worked on TV a lot during the 1950s, but reappeared in a handful of good movies – including *The Fugitive Kind*, *The Miracle Worker* and *Papillon.* He worked in films for fifty years before his death in Santa Monica.

State Fair (1933) Sailor's Luck (1933)
Madame DuBarry (1934) Party
Wire (1935) A Midsummer Night's
Dream (1935) Meet Nero Wolfe (1936)
First Lady (1937) The Adventures of Tom
Sawyer (1938) Dodge City (1939)
Man of Conquest (1939)
Susannah of the Mounties (1939)
Each Dawn I Die (1939) Gone With the
Wind (1939) The Shadow (1940) The Green
Archer (1940) Lady with Red Hair (1940)
Bad Men of Missouri (1941)
Charlie Chan in Rio (1941)
Fighting Man of the Plains (1949)
The Fugitive Kind (1959) The Miracle
Worker (1962) Cheyenne Autumn (1964)
A Time for Dying (1969) Papillon (1973)

Erland **Josephson**
5ft 10¾in
(ERLAND JOSEPHSON)

Born: **June 15, 1923**
Stockholm, Stockholms län, Sweden

The son of a cultured Jewish couple, it was natural that he pursued an academic career at Stockholm University, but his passion was acting. From 1945 he was with the Municipal Theater in Helsingborg. He became a close friend of Ingmar Bergman and although his focus was very much on a stage career, in 1946 he took a small role in the director's second feature film *It Rains on Our Love.* Four years later, he played another anonymous role, in Bergman's *To Joy.* Until 1956, he preferred his work with the Gothenburg Theater. He then played two substantial film parts, in the great director's – *Brink of Life* and *The Magician.* But transferring to the Royal Dramatic Theater in Stockholm, he had no thoughts of being a film actor. Bergman lured him back ten years later for a role in his horror film *The Hour of the Wolf,* and as a change of mood, Erland acted in Mai Zetterling's 1968 movie, *The Girls.* He has acted in fourteen Bergman movies – *The Passion of Anna, Cries and Whispers* and *Scenes from a Marriage* are just three. He made his first non-Swedish film – playing Friedrich Nietzsche, in *Beyond Good and Evil,* and his talents were used in many more. He played his old friend Bergman in *Faithless* – directed by Liv Ullman, but now suffers from Parkinson's disease.

Brink of Life (1958)
The Magician (1958)
The Hour of the Wolf (1968)
The Girls (1968) The Passion of
Anna (1969) Cries and Whispers (1972)
Scenes from a Marriage (1973) Face to
Face (1976) Beyond Good and
Evil (1977) I Am Afraid (1977)
Autumn Sonata (1978)
To Forget Venice (1979)
The Memory Haunts My Memory (1981)
Fanny and Alexander (1982)
Nostalgia (1983) Saving Grace (1985)
The Sacrifice (1986) The Unbearable
Lightness of Being (1988)
Hanussen (1988) Oxen (1991)
Sofie (1992) Ulysses' Gaze (1995)
Faithless (2000)

Louis **Jourdan**
6ft 1in
(LOUIS GENDRE)

Born: **June 19, 1919**
Marseille, Bouches-du-Rhône, France

Louis was the son of Henri Gendre, who managed and sometimes owned hotels. His mother, Yvonne Jourdan, would provide his stage name. As a youngster, Louis moved around Europe with his parents – receiving his early education in France, England and Turkey. In 1937, he began training for an acting career under René Simon, at L'Ecole Dramatique in Paris. He made his movie debut in *Le Corsaire* – directed by Marc Allégret and featuring Charles Boyer. Louis continued working in films during the Nazi occupation, but he drew the line when he was asked to appear in German propaganda films. After his father was arrested by the Gestapo, Louis and his two brothers joined the French resistance. Following the liberation of his country in 1944 he married Berthe Frederique and had a son named Louis Henry – who in 1981, committed suicide by drug overdose. In 1947, he attempted what has always been difficult for French actors, a successful career in Hollywood. Louis had a featured role in Alfred Hitchcock's *The Paradine Case* and followed that with starring roles in a number of big budget movies on both sides of the Atlantic. The most fondly remembered was as the suavely handsome Gaston Lachaille, in the hit movie *Gigi*. He kept working in TV and films into his 70s. After the romantic comedy *Year of the Comet* in 1992, Louis retired to enjoy a relaxing life at his home in the South of France.

The Paradine Case (1947)
**Letter from an Unknown
Woman** (1948)
Madame Bovary (1949)
Anne of the Indies (1951)
Three Coins in the Fountain (1954)
The Swan (1951) **Julie** (1956)
Gigi (1958) **The Best of
Everything** (1959) **Can-Can** (1960)
A Flea in Her Ear (1968)
Silver Bears (1978)
Swamp Thing (1982)
Octopussy (1983)
Grand Larceny (1987)

Ashley **Judd**
5ft 7in
(ASHLEY TYLER CIMINELLA)

Born: **April 19, 1968**
Granada Hills, California, USA

Ashley's father, Michael Ciminella Jr., worked in the United States Horse-Racing industry. Her mother, Naomi Judd, worked as a nurse and was a future country music singer, who only took up singing after her divorce – when teaming up with her other daughter, Wynonna. The two sisters were raised by their mother in Kentucky, and both adopted her surname in their professional lives. Ashley grew up as a Baptist. She attended a dozen schools including Paul G. Blazer High School, before she majored in French (spending a semester in France) at the University of Kentucky, where she was also involved in theatrical studies. Ashley went to Hollywood, where she was coached by Robert Carnegie, at Playhouse West. Her first professional assignment was in two 1991 episodes of 'Star Trek: The Next Generation'. She made her movie debut in *Kuffs,* in 1992 and has enjoyed more than a dozen years at the top. In December 2001, Ashley married the Scottish racing driver, Dario Franchitti (who was the winner of the 2007 Indianapolis 500). Drawing on modeling experience from her early years, Ashley has recently worked for Estée Lauder, and also features in a fashion campaign – boasting her name – for Goody's. Ashley will soon be seen in the new film drama, *Crossing Over,* in which she co-stars with Harrison Ford and Ray Liotta.

Ruby in Paradise (1993)
The Passion of Darkly Noon (1995)
Smoke (1995) **Heat** (1995)
A Time to Kill (1996)
Normal Life (1996)
The Locusts (1997)
Kiss the Girls (1997)
Simon Birch (1998)
Double Jeopardy (1999)
Where the Heart Is (2000)
Someone Like You (2001)
High Crimes (2002)
Frida (2004)
De-Lovely (2004)
Come Early Morning (2006)
Bug (2006) **Helen** (2008)

Raul **Juliá**
6ft 2in
(RAUL RAFAEL CARLOS JULIA Y ARCELAY)

Born: **March 9, 1940**
San Juan, Puerto Rico
Died: **October 24, 1994**

The son of Raúl Juliá Sr. and his wife, Olga – who gave up a promising career as a mezzo-soprano to get married and raise a family. Young Raúl grew up in the Floral Park area of San Juan, where his father ran a successful restaurant called "La Cueva del Chicken Inn". It ensured Raúl and his brothers and sisters a good education and a strict Jesuit upbringing. After completing his studies at the local Colegio San Ignacio de Loyola, he spent a year at New York's Jesuit University, Fordham, then attended the University of Puerto Rico. His parents wanted him to become a lawyer, but early on in his life, Raúl had caught the acting bug. He went to New York City to study with Wynn Handman, and got work in off-Broadway productions and open air plays in Central Park. He made his film debut in 1969, in *Stiletto,* but his heart was in the theater – and Shakespeare. He later acted in several movies, including *The Panic in Needle Park,* but he didn't make much impression until *One from the Heart* and *The Escape Artist.* Raúl returned to Puerto Rico to appear in *La Gran fiesta,* and then performed his star-making role, as Valentin Arregui, in *Kiss of the Spider Woman.* In 1993, Raúl was diagnosed with cancer. He died of a stroke the following year. An Emmy and a Golden Globe were awarded posthumously, for 'The Burning Season'.

One from the Heart (1982)
The Escape Artist (1982)
Tempest (1982)
La Gran fiesta (1985)
Kiss of the Spider Woman (1985)
The Morning After (1986)
Trading Hearts (1988)
The Penitent (1988)
Moon Over Parador (1988)
Tango Bar (1988)
Tequila Sunrise (1988)
Romero (1989) **Presumed
Innocent** (1990) **The Addams
Family** (1991) **La Peste** (1992)
Addams Family Values (1993)

Curt **Jurgens**
6ft 4in
(CURD GUSTAV ANDREAS GOTTLIEB FRANZ JÜRGENS)

Born: **December 13, 1915**
Solin, Bavaria, Germany
Died: **June 18, 1982**

Curt's father was a trader who hailed from Hamburg. His mother taught French. Shortly after leaving school, Curt began a career as a journalist with a Munich newspaper. He met and fell in love with an actress called Louise Basler. Soon after their marriage, she persuaded him to go with her to Vienna, where he was able to work with her on the stage. The German Cinema was at its peak when Curt made his film debut, in 1935, for UFA, as Kaiser Franz Josef of Austria, in *Königwalzer*. He appeared in fifteen more German films up until 1944, when his outspoken criticism of the Nazi regime, landed him in a concentration camp for 'political unreliables'. On his release at the end of the war, Curt went back to Vienna where he became an Austrian citizen. It was in a musical drama titled *Das Haus Singende,* that he re-started his film career in 1948. He continued making German language films in Vienna and also returned to the country of his birth to help the film industry back on its feet. In 1955, one film, *The Devil's General,* did just that. A year later, after acting opposite Brigitte Bardot, Hollywood beckoned. Curt starred in dozens of movies – several were English language productions. His last screen role was in 'Smiley's People' – a television drama starring Alec Guinness. Curt loved acting on the stage more than anything – dying of a heart attack while appearing in a play in Vienna.

Der Engel mit der Posaune (1948)
The Devil's General (1955)
Bitter Victory (1957)
The Enemy Below (1957)
The Inn of the
Sixth Happiness (1958)
The Longest Day (1962)
Lord Jim (1964)
Battle of Britain (1969)
The Mephisto Waltz (1970)
The Vault of Horror (1973)
Cagliostro (1974)
The Spy who Loved Me (1977)
Tegeran – 43 (1981)

John **Justin**
6ft
(JOHN JUSTINIAN DE LEDESMA)

Born: **November 24, 1917**
London, England
Died: **November 29, 2002**

John was a few months old when he was taken from his Knightsbridge home to Argentina, where his Argentinian father owned a ranch. When he was eleven, John was sent back to England where he attended Bryanston School, in Dorset. When he was sixteen he made his father very angry by leaving school to join the Plymouth Repertory Company. After a few months, he was forced to go to a farming college in Norfolk. Eventually, when he was eighteen, he got a job with the Liverpool Repertory Company. His father was almost proved right when, after a frustrating period in London, John went home to Buenos Aires. Life there was even worse but his grandmother came to his rescue in 1935, by paying his living expenses to attend the Royal Academy of Dramatic Art. He found work on the West End stage with John Gielgud's company – making his debut in 1938 – in "Dear Octopus" and a year later, was in "The Importance of Being Earnest". He made his film debut in *The Thief of Bagdad,* and a short time later, served in the RAF. He went back to the stage in 1945, and the theater made up the bulk of his work. His last public appearance was in 1983, in a BBC TV drama called 'Good at Art'. John was married three times. He and his second wife, the actress Barbara Murray, had three daughters. His third wife, Alison, was with him when he died of natural causes, at their home in London.

The Thief of Bagdad (1940)
The Gentle Sex (1943)
The Angel with the Trumpet (1950)
The Sound Barrier (1952)
King of the Khyber Rifles (1953)
The Man Who Loved
Redheads (1954)
Untamed (1955)
Safari (1956)
Island in the Sun (1956)
Savage Messiah (1972)
The Big Sleep (1978)
Trenchcoat (1983)

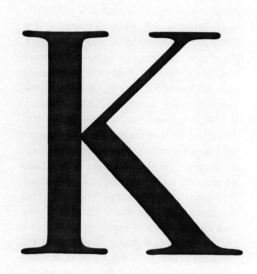

Anil **Kapoor**
5ft 11in
(ANIL KAPOOR)

Born: **December 24, 1959**
Chembur, Maharashtra, India

Anil, who is known by the nickname, "Lakkhan" is the son of the film producer, Surinder Kapoor, and his wife, Nirmal. It is a Hindu family. Anil's two brothers would also go into the movie business. He was educated at Our Lady of Perpetual Succor School, in Chembur, and during that time he became a big fan of Bollywood movies – especially those starring Raj Kapoor. When he was a child, Anil was cast in an unreleased movie called *Tu Payal Main Geet* – featuring Raj's son, Shashi. He had intended to complete his schooling in Mumbai, at St. Xaviers College, but was expelled during his second year there. He failed the written exam to join the Pune Film Institute and things looked bleak until he was accepted at Roshan Taneja's Acting School. He made his Bollywood film debut in 1979, with a supporting role in *Hamare Tumhare*. Anil's first leading role came four years later, in the Hindi film, *Woh 7 Din*. In 1984, he married Sunita Bhambhani, and his career took off. Anil won a Film Fare Best Supporting Actor Warad for *Mashaal,* and again for *Taal*. He has been Film Fare Best Actor three times – for *Tezaab in Acid, Beta,* and *Viraset*. Anil's daughter, Sonam, made her film debut, in *Saawariya*, in 2007. His recent work includes *Slumdog Millionaire,* which has taken the whole world by storm.

Mashaal (1984) **Saaheb** (1985)
Yudh (1985) **Meri Jung** (1985)
Chameli's Marriage (1986)
Janbaaz (1986) **Mr. India** (1987)
Thikana (1987) **Tezaab Is Acid** (1988)
Ram Lakhan (1989) **Essshwar** (1989)
Awaargi (1990) **Khel** (1991)
Lamhe (1991) **Beta** (1992)
1942: A Love Story (1993) **Virasat** (1997)
Judaai (1997) **Taal** (1999)
Pukar (2000) **Nayak: The Real
Hero** (2001) **Lajja** (2001)
Om Jai Jagadish (2002)
Calcutta Mail (2003)
My Wife's Murder (2005)
No Entry (2005) **Black & White** (2008)
Slumdog Millionaire (2008)

Raj **Kapoor**
5ft 8in
(RANBIR RAJ KAPOOR)

Born: **December 14, 1924**
Peshawar, North West Frontier, British India
Died: **June 2, 1988**

Raj was the eldest of four children. He was the son of a stage and movie actor named Prithviraj Kapoor, and his wife Rama. His brothers – Shammi and Shashi would also become actors. Raj grew up in the Punjab province of what is now Pakistan. He got his first small film role at the age of eleven – in *Inquilab.* By the time he was sixteen, he was working as a clapper boy for Kidar Nath Sharma. His next role was in the 1943 film, *Hamari Baat.* Four years later, Raj made his breakthrough, in Sharma's film, *Neel Kamal* – with Madhubala. He married Krishna Malhotra in a traditional Hindu wedding and they had five children. In 1948, Raj opened his own studio and had a first experience as producer/director with *Aag* (fire) which he also acted in, with his frequent co-star, Nargis. He was busy as both an actor and director, with major films such as *Awaara* and *Shree 420,* and his production company flourished. Raj had twenty years of success as an actor before taking six years to complete his personal brainchild – *My Name Is Joker.* It was a financial disaster on release but has since been acknowledged as a classic. He the acted with his son Randhir – who was making his directorial debut with *Kal Aaj Aur Kal.* Raj then concentrated mainly on producing and directing and made his final screen appearance in 1982, in *Vakil Babu.* He suffered increasingly from asthma and died in New Delhi, of complications from that condition and heart failure.

Neel Kamal (1947) **Aag** (1948)
Andaz (1949) **Barsaat** (1949)
Awaara (1951) **Shree 420** (1955)
Jagte Raho (1956) **Chori Chori** (1956)
Sharada (1957) **Main Nashe Men
Hoon** (1959) **This Country Where
the Ganges Flows** (1960)
Dil Hi To Hai (1963)
Sangam (1964) **Dulha Dulhan** (1964)
The Third Oath (1966)
Sapnon Ka Saudagar (1968)
My Name Is Joker (1970)
Kal Aaj Aur Kal (1971)

Anna **Karina**
5ft 7in
(HANNE KAREN BLARKE BAYER)

Born: **September 22, 1940**
Copenhagen, Denmark

Anna's father, who was a captain on a merchant ship, abandoned Anna and her mother, when she was a baby. She spent much of her childhood in foster homes where she was so terribly miserable, she attempted to run away several times. By the time she left school at fourteen, she was singing in cabarets and modeling for painters, in Copenhagen. In 1958, she acted in an eleven minute film called *Pigen og skoene.* The following year, Anna packed her suitcase and went to Paris. She found a room through the priest at a Danish church and sold her sketches of Paris to tourists just to stay alive. She got to know Pierre Cardin and Coco Chanel when she began working as a fashion model and they persuaded her to change her name. After a Jacques Brel musical short film, she was spotted by Jean-Luc Godard, who starred her in *A Woman Is a Woman* and married her. They remained a team until their divorce in 1967. That was a period which produced some of their best work as a team – she won a Silver Bear as Best Actress, at the 1961 Berlin Film Festival, for *A Woman Is a Woman* and Jean-Luc was given a special prize. They had more successes – with *Le Petit Soldat, Bande à part, Alphaville,* and *Pierrot le fou.* Anna made a few films outside France – the best was the German *Chinese Roulette* – for Rainer Fassbinder. Anna's four husbands were all film actors or directors. There were no children.

Une femme est une femme (1961)
Ce soir ou jamais (1961)
Vivre sa vie (1962) **Le Petit
soldat** (1963) **Bande à part** (1964)
De l'amour (1964) **Alphaville** (1965)
Le Soldatesse (1965) **Pierrot le
fou** (1965) **La Religieuse** (1966)
Made in the U.S.A. (1966)
Lo Straniero (1967) **Laughter in
the Dark** (1969) **Carlos** (1971)
Pane e cioccolata (1973)
L'Assassin musicien (1976)
Chinese Roulette (1976)
L'Oeuvre au noir (1988)

Boris **Karloff**
5ft 11in
(WILLIAM HENRY PRATT)

Born: **November 23, 1887**
Camberwell, London, England
Died: **February 2, 1969**

Boris, who was known as Billy, during his acting career, was the youngest of nine children. He was educated at Merchant Taylor's School and London University. He avoided following his father's career in the diplomatic service, by emigrating to Canada and went to work on a farm in Ontario. Influenced by a brother who was an actor, he answered an ad by a touring company, in a newspaper, got the job, and changed his name to Boris Karloff. For ten years or so, he appeared in a huge variety of roles, and doubled as a stage manager. In 1919, down, and out of work in Los Angeles, he began working as a film extra. Throughout the rest of the silent era, he kept appearing in films, but did little of note. He made his first sound picture, *The Unholy Night,* in 1929. Two years later, he became a big star after being cast as the monster, in *Frankenstein.* During seven years at Universal, he did occasionally play conventional roles, but it was his horror films – often teamed with Bela Lugosi – which had the audiences gasping. Billy was a remarkable ladies man in his early days, but he was married to his sixth wife, Evelyn, from 1946, until his death at his Midhurst, Sussex, home, from emphysema. His last three films were released after he died. They were all very bad. He shared a birthday with his only child, Sara.

Frankenstein (1931)
The Mummy (1932)
The Ghoul (1933)
Bride of Frankenstein (1935)
Charlie Chan at the Opera (1936)
Devil's Island (1939)
The Body Snatcher (1945)
Isle of the Dead (1945)
Bedlam (1946)
The Secret Life of Walter Mitty (1947)
Abbott and Costello Meet
the Killer (1949)
The Black Castle (1952)
Corridors of Blood (1958)
The Raven (1963)
The Comedy of Terrors (1964)

Danny **Kaye**
5ft 11in
(DAVID DANIEL KAMINSKI)

Born: **January 18, 1913**
Brooklyn, New York City, New York, USA
Died: **March 3, 1987**

Starting at junior school, Danny, who was the son of Jewish immigrants, Jacob and Clara Kaminski, from the Ukraine, was happy to sing and dance in front of an audience. When he left Thomas Jefferson High School at thirteen, his first job was touring the Orient with the A.B. Marcus Show. In 1935, he appeared in a short film called *Moon Over Manhattan.* He had a negative response for his cabaret act in London, at the Dorchester Hotel, in 1938, but was successful on Broadway, in the "Straw Hat Revue", the following year. In 1940, he married Sylvia Fine, who would be his wife for forty-seven years. A year later, Danny was shooting to prominence in New York with his comic rendition of the song, 'Tchaikovsky' – in "Lady in the Dark". Danny appeared in several comedy shorts before Goldwyn offered him a contract and made him a big movie star, in *Up in Arms.* He retained his popularity in such films as *The Secret Life of Walter Mitty –* right through to *The Five Pennies.* For two years Danny hosted 'The Danny Kaye Show' on CBS radio. There were further successes for him in both 1948 and 1949, at the London Palladium, and he worked throughout the 1950s, with his star shining brightly. In 1954, Danny was awarded a special Oscar. Although he was official Ambassador for UNICEF, it was reported that he wasn't always kind to children who pursued him for his autograph. Danny died of a heart attack, in Los Angeles.

Up in Arms (1943)
Wonder Man (1945)
The Kid from Brooklyn (1946)
The Secret Life of Walter Mitty (1947)
A Song is Born (1948)
The Inspector General (1949)
On the Riviera (1951)
Hans Christian Anderson (1952)
Knock on Wood (1954)
White Christmas (1954)
The Court Jester (1955)
The Five Pennies (1959)
On the Double (1961)

Stacy **Keach**
5ft 11½in
(WALTER STACY KEACH JR.)

Born: **June 2, 1941**
Savannah, Georgia, USA

Stacy was born with a cleft lip and a partial cleft of the hard palate. He underwent several operations as a child, and it made him determined to succeed – starting with his education. The son of an actor, Stacy Keach Sr., who was teaching drama at Armstrong Junior College, and his wife Mary. Keach Sr., was hired as actor and director by the Pasadena Playhouse when Stacy was a year old. The family settled in California, where he graduated from Van Nuys High School, in 1959, getting BAs in English and Dramatic Art from the University of California at Berkeley. Not content with those qualifications, he received an M.F.A, from Yale School of Drama and was a Fulbright Scholar at the London Academy of Music and Dramatic Art. In 1965, Stacy won a Tony on his Broadway debut – as Buffalo Bill – in "Indians". Stacy made his film debut in *The Heart is a Lonely Hunter* in 1969 ,and was a successful stage actor throughout the 1970s. His portrayal of 'Mike Hammer' in the cult 1980s TV drama, brought him fame and also his fourth wife, Malgosia, a Polish girl who had a small role in the show. They have a son and a daughter. In 1984, Stacy spent six months in England's Reading Prison for smuggling cocaine into the United Kingdom. It taught him a hard lesson because although he cleaned up his act, it effected his chances of stardom. He's kept going in supporting roles and television work. On stage, he recently acted with Julian Sands, in the American Premiere of Brecht's "The Life of Galileo".

The Heart is a Lonely
Hunter (1968)
Brewster McCloud (1970)
Fat City (1972)
Luther (1973)
The Killer Inside Me (1976)
The Long Riders (1980)
The Ninth Configuration (1980)
American History X (1998)
Unshackled (2000)
Come Early Morning (2006)
Jesus, Mary and Joey (2006)

Diane **Keaton**
5ft 6½in
(DIANE HALL)

Born: **January 5, 1946**
Los Angeles, California, USA

Diane was the eldest of five children born to Jack Hall and Dorothy Keaton. She was raised as a Methodist. In 1964, she graduated from Santa Ana High School and attended Santa Ana college. For one year, she was ar Orange Coast College, as an acting student. Diane then studied Drama at Manhattan's Neighborhood Playhouse. In 1968, she understudied for the rock musical, "Hair". While on Broadway, Diane met Woody Allen. He cast her in his 1969 stage hit, "Play It Again, Sam" and later in the film. Diane made her film debut in *The Godfather*. Its sequel and more movies for Allen, who she had become involved with, increased her profile. *Looking for Mr. Goodbar*, earned her a Golden Globe nomination and secured her star status. There were three more films for Woody during the decade – one of them, *Annie Hall*, brought her a Best Actress Oscar. She became involved with Warren Beatty and appeared in his film *Reds*. In the 1980s, Diane's film roles were rare, but she turned director – beginning with *Heaven*, in 1987. She played more mature roles, had a hit with *Father of the Bride* and was back with Woody, in *Manhattan Murder Mystery*. She proved her sex appeal was intact when playing a nude scene in *Something's Gotta Give*. Diane has loved but never married. She has two adopted children – Dexter and Duke – who were named after jazz greats.

The Godfather (1972)
Play It Again, Sam (1972)
Sleeper (1973) The Godfather:
Part II (1974) Love and Death (1975)
Annie Hall (1977) Looking for Mr.
Goodbar (1977) Interiors (1978)
Manhattan (1979) Reds (1981) Shoot
the Moon (1982) The Godfather:
Part III (1990) Father of the Bride (1991)
Manhattan Murder Mystery (1993)
Marvin's Room (1996)
Something's Gotta Give (2003)
The Family Stone (2005)
Mama's Boy (2007)
Mad Money (2008)

Michael **Keaton**
5ft 9in
(MICHAEL JOHN DOUGLAS)

Born: **September 5, 1951**
Coraopolis, Pennsylvania, USA

Michael attended Montour High School, before starting to study speech at Kent State University, in Ohio. He dropped out halfway through the course and moved to Pittsburgh, where his attempt to launch a career as a stand up comic, was unsuccessful. Working as a TV cameraman helped him make up his mind to become an actor. Because there was already a Michael Douglas, he changed his surname to Keaton, after reading an article about Diane. In 1977, he found work in Los Angeles, in the television series 'Maude'. After five years of TV experience, he made his film debut in the comedy, *Night Shift*. That year, 1982, he married a television actress from Seattle – called Caroline McWilliams. There were a number of okay comedies before Michael worked with Tim Burton, in the hit, *Beetlejuice*. Tim made him a star the following year, when he cast him in the title role, in his bug budget movie, *Batman*. Michael matched Jack Nicholson ("The Joker") in every scene. There was a sequel, but before that he had roles of a different kind – in *Pacific Heights* and *One Good Cop*. His work during the 1990s was pretty successful, but since the new millennium, a hit film role has proved hard to find. Now, his first effort as a director and actor – *The Merry Gentleman*, has been warmly received.

Night Shift (1982)
Mr. Mom (1983)
Beetle Juice (1988)
Clean and Sober (1988)
The Dream Team (1989)
Batman (1989)
Pacific Heights (1990)
One Good Cop (1991)
Batman Returns (1992)
My Life (1993) The Paper (1994)
Jackie Brown (1997)
Desperate Measures (1998)
A Shot at Glory (2000)
Quicksand (2003)
Game 6 (2005)
White Noise (2005)
The Merry Gentleman (2008)

Lila **Kedrova**
5ft 3in
(LILA KEDROVA)

Born: **October 9, 1918**
Petrograd, Russia
Died: **February 16, 2000**

Lila's parents escaped from Russia after the communist regime took over, and her birth certificate was lost. The family settled in France, where as a natural linguist, Lila grew up to be fluent in Russian (through her parents), French and English – having spent two years in London before World War II. In 1938, after studying drama in Paris and acting on stage, Lila made her film debut, in *Ultimatum*. The movie was interesting for two reasons unrelated to its modest quality: it starred the legendary Erich von Stroheim, and halfway through filming its director, Robert Wiene, died of a heart attack and was replaced by Robert Siodmak, who would find fame in 1940s Hollywood. Lila didn't make another film for over fifteen years, but continued to act on stage. She returned to the screen in 1953, in a West German film titled *No Way Back*. She was soon appearing regularly in European films, but it was the pulsating *Zorba the Greek* which brought her fame all around the world and won her the Best Supporting Actress Oscar. In 1968, Lila married Richard Howard. She won a Tony for the musical version of "Zorba the Greek" and worked until retiring, in 1994, to live in Paris and Canada. Lila suffered from Alzheimer's disease and died in Sault Ste. Marie, Ontario, of pneumonia.

Razzia sur la Chnouf (1955)
People of No Importance (1956)
Modigliani of Montparnasse (1958)
La Femme et le pantin (1959)
Jons und Erdme (1959)
Zorba the Greek (1964)
A High Wind in Jamaica (1965)
Torn Curtain (1966) Penelope (1966)
Maigret à Pigalle (1967)
The Kremlin Letter (1970)
The Night Child (1975)
The Tenant (1976)
Le Cavaleur (1979)
Les Égouts du paradis (1979)
Clair de femme (1979)
Tell Me a Riddle (1980)
Some Girls (1988)

Howard **Keel**
6ft 4in
(HAROLD CLIFFORD KEEL)

Born: April 13, 1919
Gillespie, Illinois, USA
Died: November 7, 2004

After Howard's father, Homer, who was a coal miner, died when he was a young boy, his mother, Grace, took him to live in California. After graduating from Fallbrook High School, when he was seventeen, he started work as a trainee mechanic at Douglas Aircraft Company in Los Angeles – for whom he became a traveling rep. He used to sing when he was working and his employers were so impressed, they sent him on a concert tour. After winning first prize at a music festival, he acquired an agent who introduced him to the lyricist, Oscar Hammerstein II. With his new name Howard Keel, he played 'Curly' in the 1947 London production of "Oklahoma". While in England, he made his film debut in the very inappropriately titled, *The Small Voice* – in a non-singing role. When he returned to America, Howard was tested by MGM for the starring role of Frank Butler, in Irving Berlin's, *Annie Get Your Gun*. The decision to cast him was instant and unanimous. The movie was a great success, but it was a difficult act to follow. Even so, *Calamity Jane, Kiss Me Kate* and *Seven Brides for Seven Brothers,* have long been regarded as classics. Howard was a musical star when they were going out of fashion. After 1955, he acted in a few films and was often seen on television. Howard toured in a nightclub act with his old co-star, Kathryn Grayson – remaining popular wherever he appeared. He later won a new set of fans during eight seasons of 'Dallas'. Howard died of colon cancer at home in Palm Desert, California. His third wife, Judy, was by his side.

Annie Get Your Gun (1950)
Pagan Love Song (1950)
Show Boat (1951)
Callaway Went Thataway (1951)
Desperate Search (1952)
Lovely to Look at (1952)
Calamity Jane (1953)
Kiss Me Kate (1953)
Seven Brides for Seven Brothers (1954)
Jupiter's Darling (1955)

Ruby **Keeler**
5ft 4in
(ETHEL HILDA KEELER)

Born: August 25, 1909
Halifax, Nova Scotia, Canada
Died: February 28, 1993

Ruby was one of six children born to Irish Catholic, immigrant parents. Her father was a truck driver, who delivered ice to local homes. Ruby was three years old when her dad moved the family to New York, where he could earn more money. She attended St. Catherine of Siena, a Catholic school on New York's East Side. Although they had very little money, her mother recognized Ruby's potential as a performer. So when she was twelve, she persuaded her husband to pay for dance classes at the Jack Blue School of Rhythm and Taps. Ruby was so good, she was was soon performing in theaters – carefully chaperoned by her mother. A woman called Texas Guinan, hired her to dance in the chorus at her nightclub. She added two years to her age when, in 1923, she made her Broadway debut, in "The Rise of Rosie O'Reilly". In 1928, in Chicago with Bob Hope, in "Sidewalks of New York", Al Jolson and Florenz Ziegfeld saw her. Al married her and Ziggy starred her, in "Show Girl". Jolson was a big name, but didn't encourage Ruby's movie career. She finally got her break – signing a contract in 1933, and making her film debut in the classic Busby Berkeley choreographed, *42nd Street*. Four films later, she was a bigger star than Jolson. Ruby and the crooner Dick Powell were dynamite together in *42nd Street, Gold Diggers* and *Dames*. No great singer, Ruby was very likeable, but by 1936 she'd lost her appetite for movies. She divorced Jolson and married a wealthy land developer, John Homer Lowe, with whom she had four children. After his death, she starred on Broadway, in 1971, in "No No Nanette" – doing 861 performances. Ruby died of cancer, at Rancho Mirage, in California.

42nd Street (1933)
Gold Diggers of 1933 (1933)
Footlight Parade (1933)
Dames (1934)
Flirtation Walk (1934)
Go Into Your Dance (1935)

Harvey **Keitel**
5ft 7½in
(HARVEY KEITEL)

Born: May 13, 1939
Brooklyn, New York City, New York, USA

The son of Harry and Miriam Keitel – Jewish immigrants from Poland and Rumania – Harvey grew up in the Brighton Beach district. After attending Abraham Lincoln High School, he joined the U.S. Marines at the age of sixteen. When he returned to civilian life, he worked as a freelance reporter. Harvey's interest in film acting took him to New York, where he studied with Stella Adler, and later with Lee Strasberg. Harvey landed small off-Broadway roles and met the young filmmaker, Martin Scorsese. Harvey then starred in the director's first film, *Who's That Knocking at My Door.* It led to work in Scorsese classics – *Mean Streets, Alice Doesn't Live Here Any More* and *Taxi Driver.* Inexplicably, Harvey seemed to lose some of his star quality during the mid-1980s. He appeared in good productions, but it took a trio of movies – *Thelma & Louise, Bugsy,* and *Reservoir Dogs,* to get his name back on the A-Track. *Bugsy* earned him a Best Supporting Actor Oscar nomination. He now runs his own production company, "The Goatsingers", with Peggy Gormley. Since 2001, Harvey's been married to his second wife, actress Daphna Kastner.

Mean Streets (1973)
Alice Doesn't Live Here
Anymore (1974)
Taxi Driver (1976)
The Duellists (1977)
Blue Collar (1978) Bad Timing (1980)
The Border (1982)
Falling in Love (1984)
The Last Temptation of Christ (1988)
Thelma & Louise (1991) Bugsy (1991)
Reservoir Dogs (1992)
The Piano (1993) Rising Sun (1993)
Pulp Fiction (1994) Smoke (1995)
Taking Sides (2001)
Red Dragon (2002) Crime
Spree (2003) Dreaming of Julia (2003)
The Shadow Dancer (2005)
A Crime (2006)
My Sexiest Year (2007) National
Treasure Book of Secrets (2007)

Brian **Keith**
6ft 1in
(ROBERT KEITH RICHEY JR.)

Born: **November 14, 1921**
Bayonne, New Jersey, USA
Died: **June 24, 1997**

With stage actors, Robert Keith and Helena Shipman as his parents, Brian was given plenty of private coaching. He was able to make his film debut at three years of age, in *Pied Piper Malone*. By the time he was twenty, he was acting on the stage and in radio shows. He had a walk-on role – in *Knute Rockne All American,* before World War II meant serving with the U.S. Marines as an aerial gunner. He returned to the stage in 1946 and he was an extra in three movies before starting a long TV career, in 1952. He made an impact with his first featured film role in the western, *Arrowhead*. Brian married Judy Landon in 1955, and his film career began to keep pace with his TV work – he made three good movies during that period – *The Violent Men, Tight Spot* and *Storm Center.* It was also the year that he acted in an endorsement advertising campaign for Camel Cigarettes – which he would one day regret. He was well liked and got work right up to the year of his death – when he acted in *Follow Your Heart.* But tragedy was about to invade his world. In April that year, his daughter Daisy, took her own life. Two months later, Brian, who had been diagnosed with emphysema and lung cancer, shot himself at his home in Malibu. Brian had been married to his third wife, Victoria, for twenty seven years.

Arrowhead (1953)
The Violent Men (1955)
Tight Spot (1955)
Storm Center (1956)
Nightfall (1956)
Run of the Arrow (1957)
The Young Philadelphians (1959)
The Deadly Companions (1961)
The Parent Trap (1961)
The Hallelujah Trail (1965)
The Rare Breed (1966)
The Russians Are Coming the
Russians Are Coming (1966)
Nevada Smith (1966)
The Yazuka (1974)
Welcome Home (1989)

Gene **Kelly**
5ft 7in
(EUGENE CURRAN KELLY)

Born: **August 23, 1912**
Pittsburgh, Pennsylvania, USA
Died: **February 2, 1996**

Gene's father was road manager for Al Jolson, but didn't do anything to help his son's career. Gene decided to do things for himself. A bright, ambitious kid, he worked his way through college – paying tuition fees by bricklaying and performing as a dancer with his brother, Fred. After majoring in economics at Pittsburgh University, he went to New York. In 1938, he got a job on Broadway, in the chorus of "Leave it to Me" – starring Mary Martin. When he danced in the show "The Time of Your Life", he impressed Richard Rogers so much he was given the title role, in "Pal Joey". In 1940, Gene married the actress, Betsy Blair. That, and the birth of their daughter, pushed him to greater effort. Under contract to David O. Selznick, he was loaned to MGM for his film debut, in *For Me and My Gal.* Gene and Judy Garland worked well together, but it was six years before they did so again – in *The Pirate*. His contract was bought from Selznick, but his next big picture was a loan-out to Columbia, for their innovative *Cover Girl,* where he worked on his on choreography. Quite different from Astaire, his was a more physical style. He enjoyed success until musicals were no longer fashionable. He was nominated for a Best Actor Oscar for *Anchors Aweigh* and made three classics – *On the Town, An American in Paris* and *Singin' in the Rain.* Gene died at his home in Beverly Hills, after a series of strokes.

For Me and My Gal (1942)
Cover Girl (1944)
Anchors Aweigh (1945)
The Pirate (1948)
The Three Musketeers (1948)
Take me out to the Ball Game (1949)
On the Town (1949)
Summer Stock (1950)
An American in Paris (1951)
Singin' in the Rain (1952)
Brigadoon (1954)
It's Always Fair Weather (1955)
Les Girls (1957)

Grace **Kelly**
5ft 7in
(GRACE PATRICIA KELLY)

Born: **November 12, 1929**
Philadelphia, Pennsylvania, USA
Died: **September 14, 1982**

Born into a wealthy Philadelphia family of Irish American Catholics, Grace, who was the third of four children, attended Ravenhill Academy, before transferring to Stevens High School, where she modeled clothes at social events. She graduated in 1947, and enrolled at the American Academy of Dramatic Arts, in New York. There was plenty of stage work available, but she first needed voice training, which she got from Sanford Meisner, at the Neighborhood Playhouse. After summer stock, Grace acted in television plays for a year or so, before making her film debut in *Fourteen Hours.* Her low-key portrayal of the sheriff's wife in that marvellous western, *High Noon,* wasn't universally appreciated, but she was able to show more passion opposite Clark Gable, in *Mogambo,* and was Oscar nominated. She then worked three times with Alfred Hitchcock, who was totally obsessed with her. He directed her in *Dial M for Murder, Rear Window* and *To Catch a Thief,* but it is unlikely that he ever enjoyed her favors like some of her male co-stars did. By the time she appeared in *To Catch a Thief,* she was a big star – who had won the Best Actress Oscar, for *The Country Girl.* It was a sad day for her male fans when Grace met and fell in love with Prince Rainier. After starring with Frank Sinatra and Bing Crosby, in *High Society,* she retired from the screen to have three royal children and to reign as the popular Princess Grace of Monaco for over a quarter of a century. She died when, after suffering a stroke, she lost control of the car she was driving on the road to Monaco.

High Noon (1952)
Mogambo (1953)
Dial M for Murder (1954)
Rear Window (1954)
The Country Girl (1954)
The Bridges as Toko-Ri (1954)
To Catch a Thief (1955)
The Swan (1956)
High Society (1956)

Kay **Kendall**
5ft 9in
(JUSTINE KAY KENDALL-MCCARTHY)

Born: May 21, 1926
Withernsea, Yorkshire, England
Died: **September 6, 1959**

Kay's parents were dancers, and her grandmother, Marie Kendall, had been a music hall star. Long-legged Kay was also a good dancer. She was barely twelve years old when she was considered tall enough to join the chorus line, at the London Palladium. She and her sister then formed a music hall act, but split up when Kay began to get movie bit parts in British musical comedies – the first of which was *Fiddlers Three,* in 1944. Two years later, she played a featured role in what was a disastrous attempt at a Hollywood-style musical, namely *London Town.* The whole experience shattered her confidence. She escaped by going to work in Germany and Italy. She then joined provincial repertory companies in England, got small roles in films, and was featured in a television play entitled 'Sweethearts and Wives'. It so impressed Rank, she was given a bigger role, in *Lady Godiva Rides Again.* In 1953, Kay was given a seven-year Rank contract following her good work in the enchanting very English comedy, *Genevieve.* She was loaned out for *The Constant Husband* – playing one of Rex Harrison's six wives – which, two years later, she became. But tragically, by the time the couple starred together in *The Reluctant Debutante,* she was already seriously ill with Leukemia. Although her final film, *Once More, with Feeling,* which co-starred Yul Brynner, was not reviewed very kindly by the critics, Kay's performance in it is pretty special. She died in London before its release.

Lady Godiva Rides Again (1951)
Curtain Up (1952)
Street of Shadows (1953)
Genevieve (1953)
Fast and Loose (1954)
Doctor in the House (1954)
The Constant Husband (1955)
Simon and Laura (1955)
Quentin Durward (1955)
Les Girls (1957)
The Reluctant Débutante (1958)
Once More, with Feeling! (1960)

Arthur **Kennedy**
5ft 10in
(JOHN ARTHUR KENNEDY)

Born: February 17, 1914
Worcester, Massachusetts, USA
Died: **January 5, 1990**

The son of a dentist, Arthur was known as "Johnny' during his early years. He was a graduate of Worcester Academy, and then studied acting at the Carnegie Mellon School of Drama before working with a number of groups – including the Globe Theater Company, in which he performed shortened versions of Shakespeare's plays. In 1937, Arthur was appearing in "Richard II" when he was seen by the prominent stage actor, Maurice Evans, and engaged to make his Broadway debut in "Everywhere I Roam". That same year, he married his only wife, Mary Cheffrey. They moved to Los Angeles, where Arthur was spotted by James Cagney, when he was acting in a play. He was cast as Cagney's brother in *City for Conquest,* and was given a Warner Bros. contract. After supporting roles in some big films, he served in the U.S. Army. Returning to the stage after the war, he specialized in Arthur Miller's plays before getting his movie career back on track. He was nominated for Best Supporting Actor Oscars, for *Champion, Trial, Peyton Place* and *Some Came Running* and for a Best Actor Oscar, in *Bright Victory.* Arthur died of a brain tumor in Branford, Connecticut, weeks after making his final film, *Grandpa.*

High Sierra (1941)
They Died with Their
Boots On (1941)
Boomerang (1947)
Cheyenne (1947)
Champion (1949)
The Window (1949)
The Glass Menagerie (1950)
Bright Victory (1951)
Bend of the River (1952)
Rancho Notorious (1952)
The Man from Laramie (1955)
The Desperate Hours (1955)
Trial (1955)
Some Came Running (1958)
Peyton Place (1957)
Elmer Gantry (1960)
Lawrence of Arabia (1962)

George **Kennedy**
6ft 3in
(GEORGE KENNEDY)

Born: February 18, 1925
New York City, New York, USA

George's father was a band leader and his mother was a ballet dancer. After making his stage debut at the age of two, little George was raised in a one-parent family after his father died in 1929. He started a career as a radio performer, during World War II, and that experience to broadcast on the Armed Forces radio. He enjoyed the life so much, he remained a soldier for sixteen years. When George came out, it proved useful when he became a technical adviser for the television series, 'Sergeant Bilko'. Appearing in a few episodes gave him the taste for the actor's life. Following his film debut, in *The Little Shepherd of Kingdom Come,* in 1961, George came to prominence in *The Sons of Katie Elder,* opposite John Wayne, and won a Best Supporting Actor Oscar, in *Cool Hand Luke.* On television in 1984, he starred in the series, 'The Love Boat'. He was already well-known to audiences of the small screen for his portrayal of Carter McKay, in the even more successful, 'Dallas'. For the past twenty years, his movie output has included too few quality productions. George used his voice to good effect for the animated, *Cat's Don't Dance,* in 1997, and the children's action film, *Small Soldiers,* the following year. He lives in Eagle, Idaho, with his third wife, Joan. George will be soon be seen again on the big screen, in the comedy western spoof, *Mad Mad Wagon Party.*

Lonely are the Brave (1962)
Charade (1964) Hush...Hush,
Sweet Charlotte (1964)
Flight of the Phoenix (1965)
The Dirty Dozen (1967)
Cool Hand Luke (1967)
The Boston Strangler (1968)
Airport (1970) Earthquake (1974)
The Double McGuffin (1979)
Just Before Dawn (1981)
The Naked Gun: From the Files
of Police Squad! (1988)
The Naked Gun 2½: The Smell
of Fear (1991)
Don't Come Knocking (2005)

Deborah **Kerr**
5ft 6in
(DEBORAH JANE KERR-TRIMMER)

Born: **September 30, 1921**
Helensburgh, Scotland
Died: **October 16, 2007**

There was no theatrical tradition in Deborah's family – her father was a civil engineer, but somehow she revealed a keen interest in dramatics. She entered the Hicks-Smale Drama School, run by her Aunt Phyllis, in Bristol, where she took lessons in acting, singing and ballet. It was as a dancer that she made her first appearance – in the corps de ballet, at Sadler's Wells, in 1938. After appearing in Shakespeare plays in the Regents Park Open Air Theater, she was offered a film contract. Her debut should have been in *Contraband,* in 1940, but her scenes were cut out. She was in *Major Barbara,* a year later and became a star in Britain after her lovely performance in *The Life and Death of Colonel Blimp.* Co-starring with the Oscar winner, Robert Donat, in *Perfect Strangers,* won the hearts of Hollywood moguls and MGM gave her a contract. Her ladylike demeanor limited her until she fought for the role in *From Here to Eternity.* Deborah was nominated for Best Actress Oscars for that performance, as well as for *Edward, My Son, The King and I, Heaven Knows Mr. Allison* and *Separate Tables.* In 1994, Deborah received an Honorary Oscar. She died in Suffolk, England – of complications from Parkinson's disease.

**The Life and Death of
Colonel Blimp** (1943)
Perfect Strangers (1945)
I See a Dark Stranger (1946)
Black Narcissus (1947)
The Hucksters (1947)
Edward My Son (1949)
King Solomon's Mines (1950)
Quo Vadis (1951)
From Here to Eternity (1953)
The King and I (1956)
Heaven Knows, Mr. Allison (1957)
An Affair to Remember (1957)
Separate Tables (1958)
The Sundowners (1960)
The Innocents (1961)
The Night of the Iguana (1964)
The Assam Garden (1985)

Evelyn **Keyes**
5ft 4in
(EVELYN LOUISE KEYES)

Born: **November 20, 1916**
Port Arthur, Texas, USA
Died: **July 4, 2008**

After her father died when Evelyn was a toddler, her mother moved the family to Atlanta, Georgia. Although very poor, Evelyn revealed a number of talents at school. She was good at Art, and showed a natural feel for music so she started piano and dancing lessons. The latter got her a job when she was eighteen – in a nightclub chorus, as "Goldie Keyes", but she had more ambition than that. In 1937, she signed with Cecil B. DeMille who gave her a small role in his 1938 swashbuckler, *The Bucanneer.* She got married, but her husband committed suicide two years later after she sued for a divorce. By that time, she'd become famous after playing Suellen O'Hara, in *Gone With the Wind.* In the 1940s, there were a steady stream of hits and romances. Evelyn was briefly married to director Charles Vidor. He was replaced by director John Huston – who was introduced to her by his father, Walter. Evelyn's love of animals and an unwanted son John brought home for adoption, after he'd been filming in Mexico, didn't help their relationship. Her marriage to Artie Shaw lasted from 1957 until 1985. Some of her amorous adventures are related in her autobiography, "Scarlett O'Hara's Younger Sister: My Lively Life in and Out of Hollywood" – published in 1977. Evelyn died of uterine cancer and Alzheimer's disease at her home in Montecito, California.

Gone with the Wind (1939)
Before I Hang (1940)
The Face Behind the Mask (1941)
Here Comes Mr. Jordan (1941)
Ladies in Retirement(1941)
The Adventures of Martin Eden (1942)
The Desperadoes (1943)
Nine Girls (1944)
**A Thousand and
One Nights** (1945)
The Jolson Story (1946)
Johnny O'Clock (1947)
Enchantment (1948)
The Prowler (1951)
99 River Street (1953)

Shahrukh **Khan**
5ft 8in
(SHAHRUKH KHAN)

Born: **November 2, 1965**
New Delhi, India

Both Shahrukh's parents were Muslims. Taj Mohammed, his father, was a freedom fighter from Peshwar, who came to New Delhi before the partition of India. Lateef Fatima, his mother, was the adopted daughter of Major General Shah Nawaz Khan. He was educated at St. Columba's School – excelling as an academic and in sports and drama. At Hausraj College he obtained an Honors in Economics. He began studying for his Masters in Mass Communications, but dropped out when the lure of Bollywood became too strong. Shahrukh studied at the Theater Action Group under director, Barry John, and made his TV debut in 1988, in 'Fauji'. He moved to Mumbai following the death of his parents and in 1991, married Gauri Khan, in a Hindu wedding ceremony. They had a son and a daughter. He made his film debut in *Deewana,* which earned him a Filmfare Best Male Debut Award. His second movie, *Maya Memsaab,* sparked controversy because of an unusually explicit sex scene. Shahrukh scored high marks in *Darr* and *Baazigar* – the second of which won him his first Filmfare Best Actor Award. He won another for Aditya Chopra's directorial debut film, *The Brave Heart Will Take the Bride.* It was a critical and commercial success and secured his place as India's top male star – endorsed in 2007 by Madame Tussaud's Museum in London – with his life-sized statue.

Kabhi Haan Kabhi Naa (1993)
Maya (1993) **Baazigar** (1993) **Darr** (1993)
Ram Jaane (1995) **The Brave Heart
Will Take the Bride** (1995)
Koyla (1997) **Yes Boss** (1997)
The Heart Is Crazy (1997)
From the Heart (1998)
Kuch Kuch Hota Hai (1998)
Hey Ram (2000)
Mohabbatein (2000) **Asoka** (2001)
Happiness & Tears (2001) **Devdas** (2002)
Shakti: The Power (2002) **Kal Ho Naa
Ho** (2003) **Veer-Zaara** (2004)
Swades: We, the People (2004)
Bhoothnath (2008)

Margot **Kidder**
5ft 6½in
(MARGARET RUTH KIDDER)

Born: October 17, 1948
Yellowknife, Northwest Territories, Canada

Because Margot's father was a mining engineer, she and her siblings spent much of their early lives in remote parts of Canada. She went to eleven different schools in twelve years, but during that time she was developing a great love of acting. She studied at the University of British Columbia before joining the Canadian Broadcasting Corporation, in Vancouver. Margot began her acting career in Toronto – her film debut was in 1968, in *The Best Damn Fiddler from Calabogie to Kaladar.* A year later, she made her first U.S. movie – in her fellow Canadian, Norman Jewison's, *Gaily, Gaily.* She left for New York to study acting for a while. Settling in Hollywood, she roomed with Jennifer Salt and met some young filmmakers. She became involved with Brian De Palma, who cast her in his thriller, *Sisters.* It set her career moving, but she became a wife and mother. After divorce, her portrayal of Lois Lane, in the huge hit, *Superman* and its sequel, made her a star. The first Gulf War caused her to speak out against U.S. military action, and she was heavily criticized. In 1990, a car crash rendered her unable to work for two years. There had been some problems in her life before, but in 1996, she cracked. After taking part in a mental wellness program she came back. In 2005, she took out United States Citizenship. In the past six years or so, Margot has responded well to therapy and involved herself in several film and television projects. Her performances were especially good in the short, *Solace,* in 2006, and in the recent, *Universal Signs* and *On the Other hand, Death.*

Sisters (1973)
A Quiet Day in Belfast (1974)
The Gravy Train (1974)
Black Christmas (1974)
The Great Waldo Pepper (1975)
Superman (1978) **Superman II** (1980)
White Room (1990)
Crime and Punishment (2002)
Universal Signs (2008)
On the Other Hand, Death (2008)

Nicole **Kidman**
5ft 10½in
(NICOLE MARY KIDMAN)

Born: June 20, 1967
Honolulu, Hawaii, USA

As she was born to Australian parents, in Honolulu, Nicole holds duel citizenship. Her father, Dr. Anthony Kidman, took his family back to Sydney in 1971. She and her younger sister were raised as Catholics and Nicole started ballet lessons when she was five. After North Sydney High School, she studied voice production and theater history, at the Australian Theater for Young People. In 1983, she had a small role in the television film, "Chase Through The Night' and made her movie debut, later that year, in *BMX Bandits.* In 1985, she was a regular in the Australian TV-series, "Five Mile Creek". After appearing in an Australian/American drama, *Dead Calm,* Nicole was ready for Hollywood. *Days of Thunder* wasn't the right vehicle, but it introduced her to future husband, Tom Cruise. *Far and Away,* did the trick for her – giving her a run of six hits in a row. Good things don't last forever and Nicole lost her magic for a while in the late 1990s. She came bouncing back to stardom in *Moulin Rouge,* and won her first Best Actress Oscar, for *The Hours.* The six years since then have been a mixed bag, with *Dogville, Cold Mountain, The Interpreter* and *Australia,* the high points. Nicole is now married to country musician, Keith Urban. The couple have a baby daughter, named Sunday.

Dead Calm (1989) **Flirting** (1991)
Far and Away (1992) **Malice** (1993)
My Life (1993) **To Die For** (1995)
The Portrait of a Lady (1997)
Moulin Rouge (2001)
The Others (2001) **Birthday Girl** (2001)
The Hours (2002) **Dogville** (2003)
The Human Stain (2003)
Cold Mountain (2003)
The Stepford Wives (2004) **Birth** (2004)
The Interpreter (2005)
**Fur: An Imaginary Portrait of
Diane Arbus** (2006)
The Invasion (2007)
Margot at the Wedding (2007)
The Golden Compass (2007)
Australia (2008)

Val **Kilmer**
6ft
(VAL EDWARD KILMER)

Born: December 31, 1959
Los Angeles, California, USA

One of three boys born to an aerospace equipment distributor and real estate developer, Eugene Kilmer, and his wife Gladys, Val grew up in the San Fernando Valley. Raised as a Christian Scientist, he was educated at the faith's, Berkeley Hall School, and Chatsworth High School, at the same time as Kevin Spacey. At the age of seventeen, Val was the youngest student to be accepted into Juilliard's drama program. In 1981, he starred in a play he had co-authored, called "How It All Began". Two years later, he was in a short film with Michelle Pfeiffer, about the dangers of drink-driving. He made his feature film debut in 1984, in *Top Secret* – playing a rock and roll star and singing all the songs. Val's star-making role was "Iceman" in the action movie, *Top Gun.* He met his future wife, Joanne Whalley, when he co-starred with her in *Willow,* and a year later, the appeared for a second time together, in *Kill Me Again.* Val reached star-status when he played Jim Morrison, in *The Doors.* From that point on he's been in some interesting and worthwhile movies. He and Joanne Whalley divorced in 1996, but they both continue to take a keen interest in the progress of their two children. Val owns a ranch in New Mexico which is a wildlife haven.

Real Genius (1985) **Top Gun** (1986)
Willow (1988) **Kill Me Again** (1989)
The Doors (1991) **Thunderheart** (1992)
Tombstone (1993)
True Romance (1993)
Batman Forever (1995) **Heat** (1995)
**The Ghost and the
Darkness** (1996) **Pollock** (2000)
The Salton Sea (2002)
Wonderland (2003)
The Missing (2003)
Spartan (2004)
Mindhunters (2004)
Kiss Kiss Bang Bang (2005)
Deja Vu (2006) **The Ten
Commandments: The Musical** (2006)
Have Dreams, Will Travel (2007)
Felon (2008)

Sir Ben **Kingsley**
5ft 8in
(KRISHNA BHANJI)

Born: **December 31, 1943**
Scarborough, Yorkshire, England

Ben's father, Rahimtulla Harji Bhanji, was an Ismaili doctor of Indian origin, who went over to England from Kenya, when he was fourteen. Ben's mother, Anna Goodman, was an English actress and model. Ben grew up in Pendlebury, Lancashire, and attended Manchester Grammar School at the same time as Robert Powell. It was there that he first became interested in acting. After the University of Salford, he studied drama at Pendleton College. Ben married actress Angela Morant, in 1966. They had two children. After work on television, including 'Coronation Street', Ben made his film debut in 1972, in *Fear is the Key*. He was virtually unknown until his career-defining performance, in the title role of Richard Attenborough's *Gandhi*. It was a once-in-a-lifetime part for which he deservedly won an Oscar. Maybe its uniqueness was the reason he avoided being type-cast in subsequent films. Ben shone in a variety of roles. For three of them – *Bugsy, Sexy Beast,* and *House of Sand and Fog,* he received further Oscar nominations. In September 2007, Ben married Daniela Barbosa de Carneiro – an actress from Brazil. She's his fourth wife.

Gandhi (1982) Betrayal (1983)
Turtle Dairy (1985) Maurice (1987)
Pascali's Island (1988)
Without a Clue (1988) Testimony (1988)
Una Vita scellerata (1990)
Bugsy (1991) Dave (1993)
Searching for Bobby Fischer (1993)
Schindler's List (1993)
Death and the Maiden (1994)
Twelfth Night: Or What You Will (1996)
The Assignment (1997)
Photographing Fairies (1997)
Rules of Engagement (2000)
Sexy Beast (2000) Tuck
Everlasting (2002) House of Sand and
Fog (2003) Lucky Number
Slevin (2006) You Kill Me (2007)
The Wackness (2008)
Transsiberian (2008) Elegy (2008)
Fifty Dead Men Walking (2008)

Greg **Kinnear**
5ft 10in
(GREG KINNEAR)

Born: **June 17, 1963**
Logansport, Indiana, USA

Greg's parents were Edward Kinnear, a career diplomat, who worked for the U.S. State Department, and his wife Suzanne. He has two brothers – James and Steve. Because of his dad's job, he was moved around quite a bit during his early years – living in Lebanon and then Greece, where at the American Community School, in Athens, he began his show business career as a talk show host with his own radio show, "School Daze With Greg Kinnear". He then returned to the United States and in 1985, graduated from the University of Arizona with a degree in broadcast journalism. He landed a job in L.A. as a marketing assistant with Empire Entertainment and got bit parts in TV shows like 'L.A. Law'. In 1994, for NBC, he hosted 'Later with Greg Kinnear'. That year, he made his film debut in *Blankman*. Since then, he's worked steadily in movies. One of the early highlights was a Best Supporting Actor Oscar nomination for *As Good As It Gets.* He's added to his list of credits since then with such entertaining fare as *Auto Focus, Little Miss Sunshine, Invincible,* and *Feast of Love.* Greg and his English wife, Helen Labdon, have two young daughters.

Sabrina (1995)
As Good as It Gets (1997)
You've Got Mail (1998)
Mystery Men (1999)
What Planet Are You From? (2000)
Nurse Betty (2000)
The Gift (2000)
Someone Like You (2001)
We Were Soldiers (2002)
Auto Focus (2002)
Stuck on You (2003)
The Matador (2005)
Fast Food Nation (2006)
Little Miss Sunshine (2006)
Invincible (2006)
Unknown (2006)
Feast of Love (2007)
Baby Mama (2008)
Ghost Town (2008)
Flash of Genius (2008)

Klaus **Kinski**
5ft 8in
(NIKOLAUS GÜNTHER NAKSZYNSK)

Born: **October 18, 1926**
Zoppot, Danzig, Poland
Died: **November 23, 1991**

The son of a pharmacist and a pastor's daughter – Klaus certainly didn't follow in his parents' footsteps. In 1930, the family moved to Berlin. He attended the Prinz-Heinrich-Gymnasium, and when he was eighteen, he joined the German Army. Klaus went AWOL while serving in the Netherlands and surrendered to British troops. In an English POW camp outside Colchester, he discovered his acting talent and performed in front of fellow prisoners. When he returned home, he changed his name to Klaus Kinski, and established himself as a legend of the German stage. He made his film debut in 1948, in a war movie called *Morituri,* but didn't pursue a movie career until the mid-1950s. In Germany he made more than a dozen films based on Edgar Wallace mysteries, and in 1958, had a small role in Douglas Sirk's, *A Time to Love and a Time to Die.* His second marriage produced Nastassja. Two other children are actors. Klaus's fame came from his work with Werner Herzog. Many of his other 170 films are best forgotten, but his final movie, *Kinski Paganini,* although self-indulgent, is worth seeing. His autobiography alienated many people including his family. After he died of a heart attack at Laguitas, California, only his son, Nikolai, attended his funeral. As has been the popular last request with a number of actors, Klaus's ashes were scattered into the Pacific Ocean.

The Counterfeit Traitor (1962)
For a Few Dollars More (1965)
Doctor Zhivago (1965)
Il Grande Silenzio (1968)
Aguirre, Wrath of God (1972)
Footprints (1975)
Nosferatu: Phantom of
the Night (1979)
Woyzeck (1979)
La Femme enfant (1980)
Fitzcarraldo (1982)
The Little Drummer Girl (1984)
Cobra Verde (1987)
Kinski Paganini (1989)

Nastassja Kinski
5ft 6½in
(NASTASSJA AGLAIA NAKSZYNSKI)

Born: **January 24, 1959**
Berlin, West Germany

The daughter of Klaus Kinski, and the actress, Brigitte Tocki, Nastassja lived with her mother in a Munich commune from her early teens. She was beautiful, so she soon began working as a photo model. Through a friendship with the actress, Lisa Kreuzer, she made her film debut at sixteen, in the Wim Wenders drama, *The Wrong Move.* Two years later, she featured nude, in the Hammer Horror film, *To the Devil a Daughter.* She started a relationship with director Roman Polanski, who recommended that she should take acting lessons from Lee Strasberg. In 1979, he cast her in the title role in his film, *Tess,* and she won a New Star Golden Globe. Her face became known all around the world. She then worked with Francis Ford Coppola, in his, *One from the Heart;* was superb as the pianist, Clara Schumann, in *Frühlingssinfonie;* then appeared with Gérard Depardieu and Dudley Moore, in *Unfaithfully Yours* – before Wenders used her again in his fascinating, *Paris Texas.* Nastassja had much of her father's fire and spirit, but with a Bergman-like grace. She was unlucky to be miscast in the flop, *Revolution,* because it took her four years to recover – mainly in Italian movies. But recover she did. Her eight year marriage to the producer, Ibrahim Moussa, resulted in two children. She also had a daughter with the jazz giant, Quincy Jones.

Tess (1979) **One from the Heart** (1982) **Cat People** (1982)
Frühlingssinfonie (1983)
Unfaithfully Yours (1984)
Paris Texas (1984)
Maria's Lovers (1984)
In una notte di chiaro di luna (1989)
Il Sole anche di notte (1990)
Faraway, So Close! (1993)
Little Boy Blue (1997) **Savior** (1998)
Your Friends & Neighbors (1998)
The Lost Son (1999)
The Magic of Marciano (2000)
The Claim (2000)
An American Rhapsody (2001)
Paradise Found (2003)

Kyôko Kishida
5ft 1½in
(KYÔKO KISHIDA)

Born: **April 29, 1930**
Suginami, Tokyo, Japan
Died: **December 17, 2006**

Kyôko's father was Kunio Kishida – one of the leading playwrights in pre-World War II Japan. Her older sister, Eriko, became a poet and a best-selling author of children's books. Their mother took care of their creature comforts. Young Kyôko thrived on the creative environment provided by that talented family and she was a good scholar. She was involved in a number of theatrical productions during her schooldays and when she finished, her first idea was to become an actress. She joined the Bungaki-za – a theater company based in Tokyo. She was naturally competitive and worked extremely hard in both modern and classical productions. In 1954, she married the actor, Noburu Nayaka. Kyôko was working exclusively in the theater until 1957, when she was given her film debut by Daiei Studios, in their crime drama, *Futeki na otoko.* She acted in three more fairly nondescript movies before her big breakthrough – in the title role of the Japanese stage version of Oscar Wilde's "Salome". Its success got her praise and better film roles – starting with the gripping drama *Her Brother* and an anti-war movie – *The Human Condition III.* Kyôko then became internationally famous for two leading roles – in the erotic, *Woman in the Dunes,* and in *Manji* – one of the first Japanese films to have a lesbian theme. In the sensational *School for Sex,* she was a middle-aged woman seeking the comfort of a young male prostitute. She died in Tokyo of a brain tumor, after completing her final film.

Bokuto kidan (1960) **Her Brother** (1960)
Get 'em All (1960)
The Human Condition III (1961)
Ten Dark Women (1961)
The Outcast (1962)
An Autumn Afternoon (1962)
Bushido (1963) **Woman in the Dunes** (1964) **Manji** (1964)
School for Sex (1965)
The Face of Another (1966)
Spring Snow (2005) **Wool 100%** (2006)

Kevin Kline
6ft 2in
(KEVIN DELANEY KLINE)

Born: **October 24, 1947**
St. Louis, Missouri, USA

Kevin was the second of four children. His father, Robert, owned the "Record Bar", the biggest toy and record store in St. Louis. Both Robert and Kevin's mother, Margaret – who was a Catholic, encouraged his creative side with piano lessons. From Saint Louis Priory School, he went to study music at Indiana University, in Bloomington, in 1965, but switched to drama. Awarded a scholarship to Juilliard, he performed Shakespeare with the City Center Acting Company. In 1976, Kevin settled in New York – and won his first Tony, in "On The Twentieth Century". Another Tony followed for "The Pirates of Penzance" – which was later filmed. Kevin's film debut was opposite Meryl Streep, in *Sophie's Choice* – which earned a Golden Globe nomination. He then had a remarkable run, which included a Best Supporting Actor Oscar, for *A Fish Called Wanda* and Golden Globe nominations for *Soapdish, Dave, In & Out* and *De-Lovely.* Kevin has remained very choosy about his film roles. He was also selective in his private life – remaining a bachelor until he was forty-two. In 1989, he married the actress, Phoebe Cates. They have two children, one of whom – their son Owen, suffered from juvenile diabetes. Kevin is active in a diabetes research foundation.

Sophie's Choice (1982)
The Big Chill (1983)
The Pirates of Penzance (1983)
Silverado (1985)
Violets are Blue (1986)
Cry Freedom (1987)
A Fish Called Wanda (1988)
Grand Canyon (1991)
Soapdish (1991) **Dave** (1993)
French Kiss (1995)
The Ice Storm (1997)
In & Out (1997)
The Anniversary Party (2001)
Life as a House (2001)
The Emperor's Club (2002)
De-Lovely (2004)
As You Like It (2006) **Trade** (2007)
Definitely, Maybe (2008)

Shirley **Knight**
5ft 3in
(SHIRLEY ENOLA KNIGHT)

Born: **July 5, 1936**
Goessel, Kansas, USA

Shirley spent her first few years living in Mitchell, Kansas. She was certainly a child prodigy. When she was only eight years of age, she entered a radio contest with her younger sister, who narrowly beat Shirley. It only made her more determined to succeed. When she was eleven, she began studying to be an opera singer, The family moved to Lyons, Kansas, where Shirley graduated from high school. She loved literature and had a story published in a magazine when she was fourteen. She then attended Phillips University, in Enid, Oklahoma, Wichita State University – and also obtained a Fine Arts Degree from Lake Forrest College. Before starting her career as an actress, Shirley studied drama at the Pasadena Theater School. Later, she took coaching classes from Jeff Corey and Lee Strasberg, and became a member of the Actor's Studio. Her film debut with an uncredited role in *Picnic,* and she was listed in the cast of *Five Gates to Hell,* in 1959. Her first big film role was *The Dark at the Top of the Stairs* – for which she was nominated for a Best Supporting Actress Oscar. Two years later she was nominated for a second Oscar, in the same category – for *Sweet Bird of Youth.* She was married to the writer John Hopkins, until his death in 1998. Shirley currently lives in New York City.

The Dark at the Top of the Stairs (1960)
Sweet Bird of Youth (1962)
The Group (1966) Dutchman (1967)
Petulia (1968) The Rain People (1969)
Secrets (1971) Juggernaut (1974)
The Sender (1982)
Somebody Is Waiting (1996)
Little Boy Blue (1997)
As Good as It Gets (1997)
Angel Eyes (2001)
P.S. Your Cat Is Dead! (2002)
Divine Secrets of
the Ya-Ya Sisterhood (2002)
A House on a Hill (2003)
Grandma's Boy (2006)
Thanks to Gravity (2006)
The Other Side of the Tracks (2008)

Keira **Knightley**
5ft 7in
(KEIRA CHRISTINA KNIGHTLEY)

Born: **March 26, 1985**
Teddington, Middlesex, England

The daughter of actor, Will Knightley, and the award-winning playwright, Sharman MacDonald, Keira attended Teddington School. She had no formal training, but started her career when she was seven, in 'Ballykissangel', on TV. Two years after that, she made her first film appearance, in *A Village affair.* She was a regular face in TV dramas like 'The Bill' before her first high profile role, in 1999, in *Star Wars. Episode 1: The Phantom Menace.* She went to Esher College where, in 2001, she sat her exams – receiving six A-levels. Keira's breakthrough film was *Bend It Like Beckham,* where she played the role of Jules Paxton, a girl footballer. Its success led to her appearance in the big budget movie, *Pirates of the Caribbean: The Curse of the Black Pearl,* starring Johnny Depp and Orlando Bloom. After such huge successes, the only way should have been up. But her next three movies got negative reviews, and she had to rely on a lady called Jane Austen to rescue her. Keira's fine portrayal of Elizabeth Bennet, in *Pride and Prejudice,* earned a Best Actress Oscar nomination. Another couple of *Pirates* and good performances in two films, *Atonement* and *The Edge of Love* – with screenplay by Keira's mom, signal a bright future for the beautiful face of Chanel's "Coco mademoiselle".

Bend It Like Beckham (2002)
Pure (2002) Pirates of the Caribbean:
The Curse of the Black Pearl (2003)
Love Actually (2003)
King Arthur (2004)
The Jacket (2005)
Pride and Prejudice (2005)
Domino (2005)
Stories of Lost Souls (2006)
Pirates of the Caribbean:
Dead Man's Chest (2006)
Pirates of the Caribbean:
At World's End (2007)
Atonement (2007)
Silk (2007)
The Edge of Love (2008)
The Duchess (2008)

Patric **Knowles**
6ft 2in
(REGINALD LAWRENCE KNOWLES)

Born: **November 11, 1911**
Horsforth, Yorkshire, England
Died: **December 23, 1995**

When he left school at fourteen, Patric was expected to join his father's book binding business in Leeds. He then ran away from home, hoping to become an actor, but an empty stomach soon saw him return. He had his way – eventually working in regional theaters and made his film debut, in 1932, in Zoltan Korda's *Men of Tomorrow.* He made a dozen or so films in Britain before his Hollywood debut, in *Give Me Your Heart,* in 1936, when he was fourth-billed behind Kay Francis. His future looked bright after he played Errol Flynn's younger brother, in *The Charge of the Light Brigade,* and even more so when he was Will Scarlet in the classic Errol Flynn vehicle, *The Adventures of Robin Hood.* Throughout the 1940s, Patric freelanced for different studios, which gave him a dozen years of employment in Hollywood. In 1950, he was happy to move into television dramas, which kept him working, with the occasional movie role, right up to the 1970s. After his retirement he wrote a novel titled "Even Steven" and spent a several years lecturing at colleges. When he grew too old to do that, he was one of the volunteers who helped organize functions for elderly show business folk at the nearby Woodlands Hills retirement home. He was happily married to Enid Percival, for sixty years, and she was with him when he died of a brain hemorrhage at their home in Woodland Hills. The couple had two children.

The Charge of the
Light Brigade (1936)
It's Love I'm After (1937)
The Adventures of Robin Hood (1938)
A Bill of Divorcement (1940)
The Wolf Man (1941) Kitty (1945)
Of Human Bondage (1946)
Monsieur Beaucaire (1946)
The Big Steal (1949)
Three Came Home (1950)
Auntie Mame (1958)
Chisum (1970)
The Man (1972)

Alexander **Knox**
5ft 10½in
(ALEXANDER KNOX)

Born: **January 16, 1907**
Strathroy, Ontario, Canada
Died: **April 25, 1995**

His father was a Presbyterian minister. Alex attended the Collegiate Institute in London, Ontario where he revealed a fine talent for writing – especially poetry. His father died when he was fourteen, but because his mother converted their home into a boarding house, he was able to go to the University of Western Ontario, in 1925. He became seriously interested in acting, and in 1928, he played "Hamlet". Before he'd had time to graduate, he accepted a job with a Boston repertory company. The stock market crashed, and the job went with it. Following a spell with a newspaper, he went to London, England. He acted on BBC radio and in a few stage roles, but the war began and he returned to Canada. In 1940, in San Francisco, he appeared with Laurence Olivier and Vivien Leigh, in "Romeo and Juliet". A role in a Broadway flop called "Jupiter Laughs" impressed Warner Bros. and they gave him his a leading role in *The Sea Wolf*. The peak of his Hollywood career was when he played Woodrow Wilson in *Wilson*. He won a Golden Globe and was nominated for a Best Actor Oscar. After that he had supporting roles in English and Canadian films and on TV in the U.K. and in the USA. Alex was married to the actress Doris Nolan from 1943 until he died at their home in Berwick-upon-Tweed, Northumberland, England, after a long battle with bone cancer.

The Sea Wolf (1941) **This Above All** (1942) **None Shall Escape** (1944)
Wilson (1944) **Sister Kenny** (1946)
The Judge Steps Out (1949)
I'd Climb the Highest Mountain (1951)
The Night My Number Came Up (1955)
Reach For the Sky (1956)
Chase a Crooked Shadow (1957)
The Vikings (1958)
Oscar Wilde (1959)
The Damned (1963)
Khartoum (1966) **Accident** (1967)
Fräulein Doktor (1969)
Gorky Park (1983)

Sebastian **Koch**
5ft 11¼in
(SEBASTIAN KOCH)

Born: **May 31, 1962**
Karlsruhe, Germany

Sebastian was raised in Stuttgart. When he left school, his intention was to become a musician, but witnessing a theater production by the director, Claus Peymann, steered him towards an acting career. In order to achieve this, he enrolled at the Otto Falckenberg School of Acting, in Munich. He graduated in 1985, and began his career on stage at Munich's Theater der Jugend, where he performed in such classics as "Die Raeber" by Schiller, and Goethe's "Iphigenie" as well as the contemporary repertoire. He worked in Ulm and Berlin, before, in 1986, appearing in his first TV role, as Commissioner Helmut Fischer, in the crime series, 'Tatort – Die Macht des Schicksals'. Sebastian's film debut was as the star of the French drama, *Transit*. It had limited distribution and it was 1997, before he made a real impact, in the German TV 'Movie of the Week' two-parter, 'Todesspiel'. Five years later, he won the Grimme Prize for his work in two television films and a three part drama. 2002 was also the year of his big breakthrough – in the mini-series, 'Napoleon', where he was acting in the illustrious company of Isabella Rossellini, Gérard Depardieu, and John Malkovich. Sebastian went up another level and won a lot of fans internationally with his performance in the award-winning movie, *Black Book*. His co-star in that film, the beautiful and talented Dutch actress, Carice van Houten, is his current flame. Sebastian has a couple of major films in post-production, including *Effi Briest*.

Transit (1991)
Flirt (1995)
An Almost Perfect Affair (1996)
Gloomy Sunday (1999)
The Tunnel (2001)
Eyewitness (2002)
The Flying Classroom (2003)
The Lives of Others (2006)
Black Book (2006)
The Return of the Racing Pig (2007)
At Any Second (2008)
Effi Briest (2009)

Sylva **Koscina**
5ft 10½in
(SYLVA KOSCINA)

Born: **August 22, 1933**
Zagreb, Yugoslavia
Died: **December 26, 1994**

Sylva's family decided to make a new life after peace returned following World War II. They moved to Naples, where she soon acquired a good knowledge of the Italian language. When she was eighteen, Sylva studied physics at the University of Naples. Her unusual height coupled with her beauty were exceptional attributes, and in 1952, while still a student, she was voted "Miss Da Tapa" in a beauty contest. The prize was a visit to the Lux Film Studios in Rome, where she was given a screen test. Nothing happened immediately, but two years later, after acting classes, she was given her movie debut, with a small role in *Siamo uomini o caporali*, which starred the Italian comedian, Totò. Sylva was third-billed in her next film – the Pietro Germi-directed movie drama, *Il Ferroviere,* but showed her inexperience. As it was a Dino De Laurentis production, she received star-grooming and got work in European films – appearing alongside such 'names' as Marcello Mastroianni and Michèle Morgan. Sylva's first English language film, was *Hot Enough for June* – which was shot in Italy. She acted for Fellini, and with Paul Newman and Rock Hudson, before seeing out her career in Italy. She made her last movie in 1994 and died in Rome, from heart problems.

La Nonna Sabella (1957)
Totò a Paragi (1958)
Racconti d'estate (1958)
Ladro lui, ladra lei (1958)
La Gerusalemme liberata (1958)
La Cambiale (1959)
Crimen (1961)
Il Fornaretto di Venezia (1963)
Judex (1963)
Hot Enough for June (1964)
Let's Talk About Women (1964)
L'Arme à gauche (1965)
Giulietta degli spiriti (1965)
Made in Italy (1965)
Deadlier Than the Male (1967)
The Secret War of Harry Frigg (1968)
The Italian Connection (1972)

Kris **Kristofferson**
5ft 11½in
(KRISTOFFER KRISTOFFERSON)

Born: **June 22, 1936**
Brownsville, Texas, USA

Because Kris's father, Lars Kristofferson, (who was from a Swedish background) was a major general in the U.S. Air Force, the family moved home a lot. Eventually with his wife, Mary, they settled in San Mateo, California, where Kris graduated from the local high school. Although, good at various sports, it was his writing skills that earned him a Rhodes Scholarship to Merton College, Oxford. While in England, he began writing songs – recording an album as 'Kris Carson'. He graduated with a masters in English Literature and then married his girlfriend, Fran. He pleased his dad by joining the Army, but resigned his commission and moved to Nashville. After hard times, including a divorce, he put aside his music to work as a helicopter pilot. Then, in 1966, his single "Viet Nam Blues" was successful and he was introduced by Johnny Cash at the Newport Folk Festival. Kris was in a relationship with Janis Joplin when she died – the year he made his film debut, in *The Last Movie.* In 1970, he won the Country Music Song of the Year Award with "Sunday Morning Coming Down". He married Rita Coolidge in 1973, and along with a successful record career, he has appeared in more than fifty films and also written an Oscar nominated score, for *Songwriter.* In 2004, Kris was inducted into the Country Music Hall of Fame and he's still acting.

Cisco Pike (1971) Blume in Love (1973)
Pat Garrett and Billy the Kid (1973)
Alice Doesn't Live Here Any More (1974)
Bring me the Head of Alfredo
Garcia (1974) Semi-Tough (1977)
Heaven's Gate (1980)
Rollover (1981) Songwriter (1984)
Trouble in Mind (1985)
No Place to Hide (1992)
Paper Hearts (1993) Lone Star (1995)
Blue Rodeo (1996) Blade (1998)
Payback (1999) Blade II (2002)
The Jacket (2005) Dreamer (2005)
Fast Food Nation (2006)
Powder Blue (2009) He's Just Not
That Into You (2009)

Diane **Kruger**
5ft 7in
(DIANE HEIDKRÜGER)

Born: **July 15, 1976**
Algermissen, Lower Saxony, Germany

Diane, who has a younger brother called Stefan, is the daughter of Hans-Heinrich Heidkrüger, a computer specialist. Her mother, Maria-Theresa, worked in a bank. When she was a little girl, Diane displayed great potential as a classical dancer, so her proud and enthusiastic parents sent her to London, to be trained at the Royal Ballet Company. Unfortunately, when well into the course, she seriously injured herself, and that dream evaporated. Being a positive sort of girl, she picked herself up and went to Paris, where she worked as a model with the world-famous Elite agency. In 1992, Diane was a finalist in their "Look of the Year" competition. She went back to Germany to complete her education and by the mid-1990s, was a successful model in both Germany and France. In Paris she took acting lessons at Cours Florent and dated French actor/director Guillaume Canet, whom she married in 2001. Diane acted in a short film, *Point le lendermain* and she made her feature film debut, as Erika, in *The Piano Player.* She then starred in her husband's directorial debut, *Mon Idole.* In 2004, she co-starred with Sean Bean, in *Troy.* Apart from her French and German, Diane speaks perfect English, For *National Treasure,* she was nominated for a Best Supporting actress Award by the Academy of Science Fiction, Fantasy & Horror Films. Since then, Diane has been a star name.

The Piano Player (2002)
Not for or Against (2002)
Mon Idole (2002) Troy (2004)
Wicker Park (2004)
National Treasure (2004)
Joyeux Noël (2005)
Frankie (2005)
Tiger Brigades (2006)
Copying Beethoven (2006)
Goodbye Bafana (2007)
Days of Darkness (2007)
The Hunting Party (2007)
National Treasure: Book of
Secrets (2007)
Anything for Her (2008)

Hardy **Krüger**
5ft 8in
(FRANZ EBERHARD AUGUST KRÜGER)

Born: **April 12, 1928**
Berlin-Wedding, Germany

Growing up in pre-war Nazi Germany, as a thirteen-year-old boy, like Hardy did, there was only one choice – you joined the Hitler Youth. He even made his film debut on the subject – in 1944, in *The Young Eagles.* A year later, Hardy was drafted into the German Army, but he was taken prisoner by the American forces. He managed to escape, but only returned to acting well after the war was over. From 1949, he was in German films for seven years before he was signed by J.Arthur Rank. He made his first English-speaking film, *The One That Got Away,* in 1957 and soon became a minor star in Europe and eventually, on the international screens. After appearing with John Wayne, in *Hatari!,* he bought a home in Tanzania – living there until political unrest forced him out in 1979. Hardy was always uncomfortable about his Nazi past. During the shooting of *A Bridge Too Far,* he would cover up his uniform immediately the cameras stopped rolling. Among Hardy's films, was the final one starring Montgomery Clift, in 1966 – *The Defector.* Hardy had three children from his three marriages – two of them, Hardy Jr. and Christiane, are professional actors. Hardy and his third wife, Anita have been together since 1978. His last major role was in 1988, as Rommel, in the TV mini-series, 'War and Remembrance'. Hardy finally retired in 1997.

The Girl on the Roof (1953)
Alibi (1955)
The One That Got Away (1957)
Bachelor of Hearts (1958)
Blind Date (1959)
Hatari! (1962)
Sundays and Cybele (1962)
The Flight of the Phoenix (1966)
The Secret of Santa Vittoria (1969)
Le Solitaire (1973)
Paper Tiger (1975)
Barry Lyndon (1975)
A Bridge Too Far (1977)
The Wild Geese (1978)
Blue Fin (1978)
Wrong Is Right (1982)

Otto **Kruger**
5ft 9in
(OTTO KRUGER)

Born: **September 6, 1885**
Toledo, Ohio, USA
Died: **September 6, 1974**

Otto was born into a family with strong Prussian ancestry. He was the grand-nephew of Paul Kruger, a true pioneer in 19th century South Africa, and eventually its State President. As a boy, Otto was keenly interested in music and after high school, he studied the subject - firstly at the University of Michigan and then Columbia University. Due to involvement with the college drama group, Otto began to focus on an acting career. He learned his trade with stock companies and in 1915, he made his stage debut, in "The Natural". That same year he made his film debut in a drama titled *Runaway Wife.* His stage roles on Broadway during that silent film era assumed more importance with notable roles in "Adam and Eve", "Alias Jimmy Valentine" and "The Royal Family". Otto's first feature-length talkie – *The Prizefighter and the Lady,* was significant because the cast included boxers, Primo Carnera, Max Baer and Jack Dempsey. The 'Lady' was Myna Loy. Apart from that, 1933 was a good year for him. Otto was extremely lucky – there were few bad films on his huge list of credits. In 1960, he had the first of several strokes which killed him. He died celebrating his 89th birthday.

Turn Back the Clock (1933)
Beauty for Sale (1933)
Ever in My Heart (1933)
Gallant Lady (1933) **The Women in His Life** (1933) **Treasure Island** (1934)
Dracula's Daughter (1936) **They Won't Forget** (1937) **Counsel for Crime** (1937)
Housemaster (1938) **Another Thin Man** (1939) **Dr. Ehrlich's Magic Bullet** (1940) **The Man I Married** (1940)
A Dispatch from Reuter's (1940)
The Men in Her Life (1941)
Saboteur (1942) **Friendly Enemies** (1942) **Cover Girl** (1944)
Murder My Sweet (1944)
Wonder Man (1945)
Duel in the Sun (1946)
High Noon (1952)
Magnificent Obsession (1954)

Jarl **Kulle**
6ft 1in
(JARL KULLE)

Born: **February 28, 1927**
Ekeby, Malmöhus län, Sweden
Died: **October 3, 1997**

Jarl, like a lot of Swedes born at the beginning of the Great Depression, was from a poor family. At junior school, he revealed a precocious talent for acting. His parents couldn't afford to send him on to higher education, but at secondary school, a teacher raised the money for him to train as an actor. He applied three times to the Royal Dramatic Theater in Stockholm and was finally accepted when he was nineteen. In 1946, a year after his sister, Gerthi was born, Jarl made his film debut – with a bit part in *Det är min modell.* Jarl made his professional stage debut in 1952, for Ingmar Bergman, in "The Day Ends Early". That was followed, the same year by the first of his six screen roles for the great director, in *Waiting Women.* In 1956, he was in the Stockholm cast of the world premier of Eugene O'Neill's, "Long Day's Journey Into Night". In the 1960s he tried his hand at directing and continued on the stage. Jarl's final film appearance was in the 1995 biography of the father of the Nobel Peace Prize – *Alfred.* He also pro-vided one of the voices for the 1998 ani-mated film, titled *H.C. Andersen og den skæve skygge.* His daughter Maria Kulle, who is from his first marriage to Louise Hermelin, is an actress. Jarl's second wife, Anne Nord, was with him until his death in Gregersboda, from bone cancer.

Waiting Women (1952)
Karin Månsdotter (1954)
Smiles of a Summer Night (1955)
Song of the Scarlet Flower (1956)
Fröken April (1958)
The Devil's Eye (1960)
Do you Believe in Angels? (1961)
All These Women (1964)
Dear John (1964)
My Sister, My Love (1966)
Ministern (1970)
Rasmus and the Vagabond (1981)
Fanny and Alexander (1982)
Babette's Feast (1987)
Herman (1990)
The Telegraphist (1990)

Meena **Kumari**
5ft 3in
(BEGUM MAHJABEEN BUX)

Born: **August 1, 1932**
Bombay, India
Died: **March 31, 1972**

Meena's parents were unable to pay the fees to the doctor who delivered her. Her father Ali – a poet, actor, and musician, even considered giving her to an orphan-age. Meena's mother, Iqbal, had been a stage actress. She converted from Hinduism to Islam and raised Meena in that faith. She began acting at the age of seven, when billed as 'Baby Meena', she made her film debut, in *Leatherface.* During the 1940s she was the income source for her family. After a series of fan-tasy movies, she gained fame when she played the heroine in *Baiju Bawra.* For that role, she became the first Filmfare Best Actress winner. In 1952, Meena married director Kamal Amrohi, who was older and already married. Although specializing in suffering women, she proved adept at playing in lighter fare, like *Miss Mary.* She was unhappy at home and her best known role – as an alcoholic wife – in *Sahib Bibi Aur Ghulam,* reflected her own problems. Drink and young male lovers drained her physically and financially but she still performed well – winning another Filmfare Best Actress Award for *Aarti,* in a year she was nominated for four roles. Meena lost her looks by the late 1960s and made her final film, *Gomti Ke Kinare,* in 1971. She died of cirrhosis of the liver. Ironically, like when she was born, there was no money to pay her hospital bills.

Baiju Bawra (1952) **Parineeta** (1953)
Daera (1953) **Azaad** (1955)
Miss Mary (1957) **Yahudi** (1958)
Satta Bazaar (1959)
Chirag Kahan Roshi Kahan (1959)
Dil Apna Aur Preet Parai (1960)
Zindagi Aur Khwab (1961)
Sahib Bibi Aur Ghulam (1962)
Main Chup Rahungi (1962)
Aarti (1962) **Kinari Kinare** (1963)
Dil Ek Mandir (1963)
Sanjh Aur Savera (1963)
Chitralekha (1964) **Phool Aur Patthar** (1966) **Majhli Didi** (1967) **Mere Apne** (1971) **Pakeezah** (1972)

Olga **Kurylenko**
5ft 10in
(OLGA KONSTANTINOVNA KURYLENKO)

Born: **November 14, 1979**
Berdyansk, Ukraine, USSR

Olga's parents, Konstantin and Marina Kurylenko, got divorced shortly after she was born. Like most people during the days of the Soviet Union, they struggled to do much more than survive in the harsh world of Communism. Marina, a single mother and her daughter moved in with Olga's grandmother, Raisa. Luckily for the pair of them, Marina was able to earn a reasonable income as an art teacher and having big ambitions for her only child, she paid for Olga's piano lessons as well as five years of ballet classes. In 1992, the two women went to Moscow. The tall and beautiful Olga was spotted by a talent scout and offered the chance to become a model. She finished her schooling, and at the age of sixteen, she received some basic training and went to live in Paris. Within two years she had established herself on the French fashion scene and appeared on several magazine covers. In addition to that, her lovely face was used to endorse the products of Clarins and Helena Rubinstein, Lejaby lingerie and Bebe fashions. Olga married the French photographer, Cedric Van Mol, but after they divorced three years later, she decided to become an actress. She took drama classes and made her film debut in Diane Bertrand's *L'Annaire*. She was then one of a whole host of starry faces in the feel-good portmanteau film, *Paris, je t'aime.* Being fluent in both French and English soon paid off with roles in *Hitman* and *Max Rayne*. A second failed marriage, to Damian Gabrielle, did nothing to halt her progress. On Christmas Eve, 2007, she was informed that she would play Bond girl, Camille, in *Quantum of Solace*. She appeared in the TV series, 'Tyranny' and featured in the French film, *À l'est de moi.*

L'Annulaire (2005)
Paris, je t'aime (2006)
Le Serpent (2006)
Hitman (2007)
Max Payne (2008)
Quantum of Solace (2008)
À l'est de moi (2008)

Nancy **Kwan**
5ft 3in
(KA SHIN KWAN)

Born: **May 19, 1939**
Hong Kong

Nancy was the daughter of a mixed-race couple. Her Chinese father, Kwan Wing Hong, was an architect. Her mother, was a Scottish-born former model, Marquita Scott. They divorced when Nancy was two-years old, and in 1941, she and her brother, Ka Keung, were taken away by their father, who was forced to flee Hong Kong during the Japanese invasion. They stayed in western China until the end of the war. In the mid-1950s, Nancy went to England, where she studied ballet at the Royal Ballet School, in London. She performed in a number of productions at Covent Garden, including "Sleeping Beauty" and "Swan Lake". When she was eighteen, she was discovered by the film producer, Ray Stark, who was looking for a genuine Asian beauty to star in the movie version of the smash-hit stage show, "The World of Suzie Wong". That film and the following year's *The Flower Drum Song,* made her a star. In her private world, Nancy married the first of her three husbands – Austrian ski-instructor, Peter Pock. Sadly, their son Bernie, would die of AIDS in 1996. Nancy returned to Hong Kong in 1972, After she remarried – to producer, Norbert Meisel, she became a United States resident, and is now politically active – as a spokesperson for the Asian American Voters Coalition.

The World of Suzie Wong (1960)
Flower Drum Song (1961)
Tamahine (1963)
The Wild Affair (1963)
Honeymoon Hotel (1964)
Fate Is the Hunter (1964)
Lt. Robinson Crusoe (1966)
The Corrupt Ones (1967)
Nobody's Perfect (1968)
The Wrecking Crew (1969)
The McMasters (1970)
Walking the Edge (1983)
Night Children (1990)
Dragon: The Bruce Lee Story (1993)
Rebellious (1995)
The Golden Girls (1995)
Mr. P's Dancing Sushi Bar (1998)

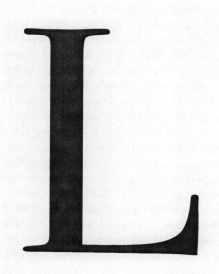

Alan **Ladd**
5ft 5in
(ALAN WALBRIDGE LADD)

Born: **September 3, 1913**
Hot Springs, Arkansas, USA
Died: **January 29, 1964**

Alan's parents were Alan Ladd Sr., and his wife, Ina Raleigh – who had emigrated from England when she was nineteen. When Alan was four, his father died. His mother took him to live in Oklahoma City, where she found a new husband, who was unemployed for long spells. They went to California, but were so poor, Alan had to work from the age of eight. He was not very academic, but at high school, he excelled at track and swimming – training for the 1932 Olympic Games. Injury prevented his participation, so he opened a hamburger stand. He got walk-on parts in two movies at Universal – the first in 1932, was *Tom Brown of Culver*. It led to more uncredited film roles and for seven years, that was as good as it got – apart from a job as a grip at Warner's. In 1936, he got married and had a son to support. He concentrated on radio work and was heard by a talent scout, Sue Carol. She worked hard to get him started. By the time that happened he had left his wife and married Sue. From his first featured role, in *This Gun for Hire,* Alan was a major star for over twelve years. As his career slumped he began to get more and more depressed and was drinking heavily. Alan died in Palm Springs, California, from an overdose of sedatives and alcohol, shortly after he'd finished work on his last movie.

This Gun for Hire (1942)
Salty O'Rourke (1945)
The Blue Dahlia (1946)
Two Years Before
the Mast (1946)
Calcutta (1947)
Whispering Smith (1948)
Appointment with Danger (1950)
Branded (1950)
The Red Beret (1953)
Shane (1953)
Drum Beat (1954)
Hell Below Zero (1954)
The Badlanders (1958)
The Proud Rebel (1958)
The Carpetbaggers (1964)

Diane **Ladd**
5ft 7in
(ROSE DIANE LANIER)

Born: **November 29, 1942**
Meridian, Mississippi, USA

Diane was the daughter of Preston and Mary Ladner. There was certainly plenty of drama in Diane's family background – her father, who ran a small poultry farm, was related to the great American playwright, Tennessee Williams. Her mother had been an actress. Diane, who was raised in the Catholic religion, went from high school to a New Orleans finishing school. She studied fencing, sang in a church choir, and was spotted by a touring company, who cast her in "Tobacco Road" – with John Carradine. She was seventeen when she went to New York (as a chorus girl at the 'Copacabana') before making her stage debut, in "Orpheus Descending". Diane made her first film appearance in 1961 – with an uncredited part in *Something Wild*. Her first featured role was five years later, in Roger Corman's, *The Wild Angels*. She was raising Laura – her daughter from her marriage to Bruce Dern, and television remained her screen medium, for most of the 1960s. It was 1974 before her film career began to register. After that, her good movie roles were more frequent. Remarkably, Diane's three nominations for Best Supporting Actress Oscars were for *Alice Doesn't Live Here Anymore, Wild at Heart* and *Rambling Rose* – all films in which her daughter Laura appears.

Chinatown (1974)
Alice Doesn't Live Here Anymore (1974)
All Night Long (1981)
Something Wicked This
Way Comes (1983)
Black Widow (1987) Plain Clothes (1988)
Wild at Heart (1990)
Rambling Rose (1991)
Hold Me, Thrill Me,
Kiss Me (1992)
The Cemetery Club (1993)
Citizen Ruth (1996)
Primary Colors (1998)
Charlie's War (2003)
The World's Fastest Indian (2005)
Come Early Morning (2006)
Inland Empire (2006)
Jake's Corner (2008)

Veronica **Lake**
4ft 11½in
(CONSTANCE FRANCES MARIE OCKELMAN)

Born: **November 14, 1919**
Brooklyn, New York City, New York, USA
Died: **July 7, 1973**

Veronica's father, Harry E. Ockelman, who worked for an oil company, was killed in an industrial explosion when she was nine. Her mother, Constance, remarried – to a newspaper staff artist, and the little girl was known as Connie Keane, when she was sent to a Catholic Girls boarding school, in Montreal, Canada. After she'd graduated from high school in Miami, her family moved to Beverly Hills, in 1938. Her mother enrolled her beautiful daughter in the Bliss-Hayden School of Acting and she progressed so quickly, she made her film debut the following year, in *Sorority House,* for RKO. Paramount producer, Arthur Hornblow Jr., changed her name to Veronica Lake, and in her private life, she changed it again when she became Mrs. John Detlie, in 1940. Her breakthrough film role was in *I Wanted Wings,* in 1941, but her star-making vehicle was in the Preston Sturges classic, *Sullivan's Travels,* later that year. Veronica had first come to prominence at the same time as Alan Ladd, and they were great together in such hits as *This Gun for Hire* and *The Blue Dahlia*. She may have looked like an angel, but she was apparently very difficult to work with. Veronica married director André de Toth, in 1944, but it didn't lead to happiness. She began drinking heavily, and around 1948, her Paramount contract was terminated. She did TV and stage work until 1959, when she fell and broke her ankle. Two more bad marriages and mental trouble led to her early death in Burlington, Vermont, from hepatitis. Her final film was in 1970, in a cheap horror picture called *Flesh Feast.*

Sullivan's Travels (1941)
This Gun for Hire (1942) The Glass
Key (1942) I Married a Witch (1942)
So Proudly We Hail! (1943)
Miss Susie Slagle's (1945)
Out of this World (1945)
The Blue Dahlia (1946)
Ramrod (1947)
Slattery's Hurricane (1949)

Hedy **Lamarr**
5ft 7in
(HEDWIG EVA MARIA KIESLER)

Born: **November 9, 1913**
Vienna, Austro-Hungary
Died: **January 7, 2000**

Hedy was the daughter of a rich Jewish couple – a Viennese banker, Emil Kiesler, and his wife, Gertrud. The 'most beautiful woman in films' as she would be known, was also a very beautiful child. A pianist, her mother sent her to piano classes and also to learn ballet. Hedy was a student at Art school, studying design, when she made her film debut, in *Geld auf der Strasse,* in 1930. Her fifth film, *Ekstase,* which was made in Germany, catapulted her to fame and notoriety. She appeared nude in some scenes – which caused the US government to ban it. Her first husband, Fritz Mandl was so upset he tried to buy up all the prints. He stopped her from making any more films, but she divorced him after *Ekstase* was shown in America in 1937, and she was offered a contract by Louis B. Mayer. A loan out to Walter Wanger first introduced her to American audiences, as Hedy Lamarr. *Algiers* was a big hit for her and co-star Charles Boyer. In the 1940s she acted with most of the big stars of the day and was certainly on the A-List for a time. She had children with her husbands Gene Markey, and the actor, John Loder. Her biggest success was *Samson and Delilah,* and her final movie was *The Female Animal,* in 1958. On two occasions, after retiring, Hedy was caught shoplifting. Her autobiography was titled "Ecstasy and Me". She died from natural causes, in Orlando, Florida.

Ecstasy (1933) **Algiers** (1938)
I Take This Woman (1940)
Boom Town (1940) **Comrade X** (1940)
Come Live with Me (1941)
HM Pelham Esq (1941)
Ziegfeld Girl (1941) **Tortilla Flat** (1942)
The Heavenly Body (1944)
The Conspirators (1944)
Experiment Perilous (1944)
The Strange Woman (1946)
Samson and Delilah (1949)
A Lady Without Passport (1950)
Copper Canyon (1950)
My Favorite Spy (1951)

Dorothy **Lamour**
5ft 5in
(MARY LETA DOROTHY SLATON)

Born: **December 10, 1914**
New Orleans, Louisiana, USA
Died: **September 22, 1996**

By the time Dorothy was in her teens, her mother, Carmen, had divorced her father, John Watson Slaton, as well as Clarence Lamour, her second husband, who had given the girl her new name. The family finances were so bad that she dropped out of school when she was fifteen. In 1931, Dorothy was crowned "Miss New Orleans". She got a job as female vocalist with a band led by Herbie Kay – whom she married. In 1934, she was hired for the 'Dreamer of Songs' radio program. When she was singing in a nightclub, she met MGM boss, Louis B. Mayer. A screen test was arranged but mislaid, and Paramount stepped in with a contract. After three uncredited roles she got star billing in 1936 (wearing a sarong) in *The Jungle Princess.* It was bound to type cast her - and it did, in a series of films set in exotic places, with Jon Hall or Ray Milland as her romantic interests. In 1940, she made the first of six 'Road' pictures, as the lovely lady fought over by Hope and Crosby. By 1949, her box-office appeal had worn as thin as her old sarongs. In the early 1950s, she sang in Las Vegas. She retired to raise her two sons with her second husband, William Ross Howard. Later, she did television work and a few more movies – the last was *Creepshow 2,* in 1987. Dorothy died of a heart attack, in Los Angeles.

High, Wide and Handsome (1937)
The Hurricane (1937)
The Last Train from Madrid (1937)
Swing High, Swing Low (1937)
Spawn of the North (1938)
Johnny Apollo (1940)
They Got Me Covered (1943)
Road to Utopia (1945)
My Favorite Brunette (1947)
Road to Rio (1947)
Lulu Belle (1948)
Manhandled (1949)
The Greatest Show on Earth (1952)
Road to Bali (1952)
Donovan's Reef (1963)

Burt **Lancaster**
6ft 1in
(BURTON STEPHEN LANCASTER)

Born: **November 2, 1913**
New York City, New York, USA
Died: **October 20, 1994**

Burt, one of five children, was the son of Jim Lancaster, a mail man, and his wife, Elizabeth. He showed great ability as an athlete and gymnast, at DeWitt Clinton High School. At seventeen Burt joined a circus – eventually forming an acrobatic duo with a little guy called Nick Cravat. He was just twenty-two when he married the first of his three wives, June Ernst. By 1940, after suffering an injury, he'd quit the circus and ended up at Marshall Fields Store, in Chicago, as a floorwalker in the lingerie department. Luckily for Burt he was drafted into the U.S. Army, where he entertained the troops in USO shows. After the war, he decided to try his luck as an actor – making a big impression in a small role in a Broadway show. In 1946, he made his film debut, in *The Killers.* He went on to star in several 'noir' thrillers and used his athletic ability in action films. Later, Burt's partnership with producer Harold Hecht, helped him to escape the studio system. Four-times nominated, he won a Best Actor Oscar for *Elmer Gantry.* He died of a heart attack in Century City, California, but his winning smile will continue to light up the screen.

The Killers (1946)
Brute Force (1947)
Sorry, Wrong Number (1948)
Criss Cross (1949)
The Flame and the Arrow (1950)
Come Back Little Sheba (1952)
The Crimson Pirate (1952)
From Here to Eternity (1953)
Vera Cruz (1954)
Gunfight at the OK Corral (1957)
Sweet Smell of Success (1957)
Elmer Gantry (1960)
Birdman of Alcatraz (1962)
The Leopard (1962)
The Swimmer (1968)
Ulzana's Raid (1972)
Atlantic City USA (1980)
Local Hero (1983)
Tough Guys (1986)
Field of Dreams (1989)

Elsa **Lanchester**
5ft 4½in
(ELSA SULLIVAN LANCHESTER)

Born: **October 28, 1902**
Lewisham, London, England
Died: **December 26, 1986**

Elsa's rather unconventional parents, Jim Sullivan and Edith Lanchester, did not believe in marriage. When she was ten, Elsa went to Paris to study dance under Isadora Duncan. At the outbreak of the war, she came back to England. In exchange for teaching Dance, she attended boarding school, in King's Langley. In 1920, she founded the Children's Theater in Soho, in London and a nightclub – the 'Cave of Harmony' where she performed short plays and sang cabaret songs. She made her stage debut in 1922, in "Thirty Minutes in a Street". Elsa's screen debut was in 1925, in the comedy/short, *The Scarlet Woman: An Ecclesiastical melodrama*. She was no oil-painting, so it was natural for her to concentrate on comedy – even when acting serious roles. Charles Laughton found her appealing enough to marry her in 1929. It was her portrayal of Anne of Cleves, in his Oscar-winning, *The Private Life of Henry VIII,* which first aroused interest in Hollywood. Her quite astonishing *Bride of Frankenstein* make-up and weird appearance, secured Elsa a place in film history. In the second of her two autobiographies – which was written after he died, Elsa claimed that Laughton was homosexual. She should have known – they were married for thirty-three years! Elsa died of bronchial pneumonia.

**The Private Life of
Henry VIII** (1933)
Bride of Frankenstein (1935)
David Copperfield (1935)
The Ghost Goes West (1935)
Lassie Come Home (1943)
The Razor's Edge (1946)
The Spiral Staircase (1946)
The Big Clock (1948)
The Inspector General (1949)
Come to the Stable (1949)
Mystery Street (1950)
Witness for the Prosecution (1957)
That Darn Cat! (1965)
Blackbeard's Ghost (1968)
Murder by Death (1976)

Martin **Landau**
6ft 3in
(MARTIN LANDAU)

Born: **June 20, 1931**
Brooklyn, New York City, New York, USA

Martin was the son of a Jewish couple – Maurice and Selma Landau. His father was born in Austria. As a young boy, Martin was a naturally gifted artist. After leaving school when he was seventeen, he worked for the New York Daily News, as a cartoonist. He always loved the cinema, and in the early 1950s, he decided to pursue an acting career. To set things in motion, he enrolled at the Actors Studio, where he was in the same class as Steve McQueen. After marrying another of the students, the actress Barbara Bain, Martin made his Broadway debut, in 1957, in "Middle of the Night". For a time, Martin worked as an acting coach to future stars like Jack Nicholson and Anjelica Huston. In 1959, he made his film debut in the war movie, *Pork Chop Hill,* and later that year, impressed audiences in Alfred Hitchcock's *North by Northwest.* From then on, Martin found steady work in a big variety of films and television dramas – being well known from 1966-69, for his role as Rollin Hand, in the popular series, 'Mission Impossible'. After two Oscar nominations in the same category – for *Tucker: The Man and His Dream,* and *Crimes and Misdemeanors,* Martin won a Best Supporting Actor Oscar, for *Ed Wood.*

Pork Chop Hill (1959)
North By North West (1959)
The Gazebo (1959)
The Hallelujah Trail (1965)
Nevada Smith (1966)
Tucker: The Man and His Dream (1988)
Crimes and Misdemeanors (1989)
Paint it Black (1989) **Fatal Love** (1992)
Legacy of Lies (1992)
No Place to Hide (1992)
Ed Wood (1994) **City Hall** (1996)
Rounders (1998)
Very Mean Men (2000)
The Majestic (2001)
The Commission (2003)
The Aryan Couple (2004)
Love Made Easy (2006)
Lovely, Still (2008)
City of Ember (2008)

Carole **Landis**
5ft 5in
(FRANCES LILLIAN MARY RIDSTE)

Born: **January 1, 1919**
Fairchild, Wisconsin, USA
Died: **July 5, 1948**

The youngest of five children born to a Norwegian father, Alfred Ridste, and a Polish mother, Clara Stentek, Carole – as she would become known, grew into a stunningly beautiful, but unhappy young woman. Her father abandoned his family before she was born and Carole had to endure poverty and sexual abuse from her stepfather when she was a child. By contrast, there was some justice when she regularly won beauty contests while she was at high school. She dropped out at fifteen to get married to a neighbor named Irving Wheeler, but it was a rocky relationship which didn't last. Carole got a job as a nightclub singer in San Francisco, and made her first appearance on celluloid (as an extra) in the 1937 film, *A Star is Born.* After that, she dyed her hair blonde, got divorced from Irving, changed her name to Carole Landis, and was given a Warner Brothers contract. Following a few bit parts, she was able to reveal some of her curvy figure, as a cave girl, in *One Million B.C.* After a relationship with Darryl F. Zanuck, she moved to 20th Century Fox, becoming a star – mostly in musical comedies, where she used her own sweet singing voice. She twice co-starred with Betty Grable. After four disastrous marriages, Carole had an affair with Rex Harrison, who was married to Lili Palmer. When he ended it, she committed suicide at home, in Pacific Palisades, California.

Turnabout (1940)
Topper Returns (1941)
Moon Over Miami (1941)
Dance Hall (1941)
I Wake Up Screaming (1941)
A Gentleman at Heart (1942)
Orchestra Wives (1942)
The Powers Girl (1943)
Wintertime (1943) **Having
Wonderful Crime** (1945)
Thieves' Holiday (1946)
Out of the Blue (1947)
Noose (1948)
Brass Monkey (1948)

Diane Lane
5ft 7in
(DIANE LANE)

Born: **January 22, 1965**
New York City, New York, USA

Diane was only a small baby when her parents divorced. Her mother, Colleen Farrington, was a singer who had been the Playboy magazine's 'Playmate of the Month' in October 1957. Her father, the acting coach, Burt Lane, raised Diane, and encouraged her to act. She made her stage debut at the age of six, at La MaMa Experimental Theater, off Broadway. She later appeared in such serious highbrow dramas as "Medea" and "The Cherry Orchard". Her reputation spread to Hollywood and when she was given her movie debut opposite Sir Laurence Olivier, in *A Little Romance,* she was only thirteen years of age. The following year, she was featured on the cover of "Time". A member of the 'Brat Pack', Diane made the transition from child to teenager in films like *Rumble Fish*. At the age of nineteen, smarting from criticism her efforts had received, she retired from films. In 1988, she married Christopher Lambert, and returned to work, in a TV mini-series called 'Lonesome Dove'. Oscar-nominated for *Unfaithful,* her recent efforts have been good. Diane has been married to the actor, Josh Brolin, since 2004.

A Little Romance (1979)
Touched By Love (1979)
Cattle Annie and
Little Britches (1981)
The Outsiders (1983)
Rumble Fish (1983)
Chaplin (1992)
Knight Moves (1992)
Judge Dredd (1995)
Wild Bill (1995)
Jack (1996)
Gunshy (1998)
A Walk on the Moon (1999)
My Dog Skip (2000)
The Perfect Storm (2000)
Unfaithful (2002)
Under the Tuscan Sun (2003)
Fierce People (2005)
Must Love Dogs (2005)
Hollywoodland (2006)
Jumper (2008) Killshot (2008)

Priscilla Lane
5ft 2½in
(PRISCILLA MULLICAN)

Born: **June 12, 1915**
Indianola, Iowa, USA
Died: **April 4, 1995**

Priscilla was the youngest of the five daughters of a dentist – Dr. Lorenzo Mullican, and his wife, Cora. She was the one who encouraged her children to sing and learn to play musical instruments. The eldest daughter, Leota, played piano for a silent screen movie house when she was twelve and was the first to leave home – followed by Dorothy, who, after they both got parts in "Greenwich Village Follies" changed her name to Lola Lane. The younger sisters all became Lanes – Rosemary and Priscilla getting their first professional engagement in 1930, singing at the premier of sister Lola's movie *Good News*. They both studied dancing, while at high school. Priscilla attended Eagin School of Dramatics and at sixteen, she got a screen test for MGM. She failed it, but so did Kate Hepburn. Cora left her husband, to help get her girls into show business. Rosemary and Priscilla sang with Fred Waring and his Pennsylvanians and in 1937, the band and the girls were featured in Dick Powell's musical, *Varsity Show*. The next big break for Priscilla, was in *Four Daughters,* which co-starred her two sisters and John Garfield. She shone in *The Roaring Twenties* and Alfred Hitchcock's *Saboteur*. Priscilla retired from movies in 1948 – rearing four children with her second husband, Colonel Joseph Howard, USAF. She died of lung cancer nineteen years after he did.

Four Daughters (1938)
Brother Rat (1938)
Daughters Courageous (1939)
Dust Be My Destiny (1939)
The Roaring Twenties (1939)
Three Cheers for the Irish (1940)
Blues in the Night (1941)
Saboteur (1942)
Silver Queen (1942)
The Meanest Man in
the World (1943)
Arsenic and Old Lace (1944)
Fun on a Weekend (1947)
Bodyguard (1948)

Hope Lange
5ft 1¾in
(HOPE ELISE ROSS LANGE)

Born: **November 28, 1933**
Redding Ridge, Connecticut, USA
Died: **December 19, 2003**

Hope's father, John George Lange, was musical arranger for Florenz Ziegfeld. Her mother, Minnette, had been an actress before she opened a swish restaurant in Greenwich Village. One day, twelve-year-old Hope's photograph was taken while she was out walking Eleanor Roosevelt's dog. The picture appeared in a paper and it landed her a role on Broadway, in "The Patriots". In 1954, following a blind date, she got engaged to the actor, Don Murray. Hope made her film debut with him (and Marilyn Monroe) in *Bus Stop*. It resulted in a 20th Century Fox contract and a Best Supporting Actress Oscar nomination for *Peyton Place*. She and Murray divorced in 1961, and after she had married Alan J. Pakula, she was in semi-retirement until becoming well known again for the television series, 'The Ghost and Mrs. Muir' – which earned her two Emmys. After an absence of thirty years, Hope returned to the Broadway stage in 1977, in "Same Time Next Year" – co-starring with former husband, Don Murray. On the movie front, Hope received very good notices for her acting in *Death Wish*. In 1986, she married her third husband, Charles Hollerith Jr. Hope was seen in small supporting roles in movies during the 1990s. In 1998, she made her final screen appearance, in the television drama, 'Before He Wakes'. Hope died of an ischemic colitis infection, in Santa Monica, California.

Bus Stop (1956)
Peyton Place (1957)
The Young Lions (1958)
In Love and War (1958)
The Best of Everything (1959)
Wild in the Country (1959)
Pocketful of Miracles (1961)
Love Is a Ball (1963)
Death Wish (1974)
I Am the Cheese (1983)
Blue Velvet (1986)
Tune in Tomorrow (1990)
Clear and Present Danger (1994)
Just Cause (1995)

Jessica **Lange**
5ft 8in
(JESSICA PHYLLIS LANGE)

Born: April 20, 1949
Cloquet, Minnesota, USA

Jessica was the third of four children – with two older sisters and a younger brother. Their father Albert Lange, was a teacher and salesman who changed jobs a lot, so the family lived a nomadic lifestyle. Their mother, Dorothy, who was of Finnish descent, took care of the children. As soon as Jessica finished high school, she went to the University of Minnesota to study Art. She fell for a visiting photography professor named Paco Grande, and for two years, they traveled extensively together. They married in 1970, and went to live in Soho, but after seeing Jean-Louis Barrault in *Les Enfants du Paradis,* she left for Paris, where she spent two years studying mime. It was very bad for her marriage, but good for her ambition. She took over the apartment when Paco left – working as a fashion model with the Wilhelmina Agency. Dino DeLaurentis went there looking for a new face to star in *King Kong.* It launched her film career, but the movie took a pasting from the critics. Jessica then began a relationship with the Russian dancer, Mikhail Baryshnikov. In 1981, they had a daughter, Alexandra. Since 1982, Jessica has been in a relationship with actor, Sam Shepherd. They have two children – a daughter, Hannah, and a son named Walker. They live in New York City. Sam's influence may have helped her to a Best Actress Oscar nomination – for *Frances.* Jessica won two Supporting Actress Oscars – for *Tootsie,* and *Blue Sky.*

All That Jazz (1979)
How to Beat the High Cost of
Living (1980) Frances (1982)
Tootsie (1982) Country (1984)
Sweet Dreams (1985)
Crimes of the Heart (1986)
Music Box (1989)
Men Don't Leave (1990)
Cape Fear (1991) Blue Sky (1994)
Rob Roy (1995) Big Fish (2003)
Broken Flowers (2005)
Don't Come Knocking (2005)
Neverwas (2005) Bonneville (2006)

Frank **Langella**
6ft 3in
(FRANK A LANGELLA JR.)

Born: January 1, 1938
Bayonne, New Jersey, USA

The son of Italian-American parents – young Frank first appeared in a school play at the age of eleven – portraying the 83-year-old Abe Lincoln. When he was in his teens, he virtually lost his American accent by listening to the recordings of John Gielgud reading Shakespeare. He studied acting at Syracuse University before making his professional stage debut in 1960, in "The Pajama Game" in New York. Frank made his Broadway debut five years later, in "Yerma". In 1977, he achieved stardom when he portrayed "Dracula" in the play which ran for 925 performances, at the Martin Beck Theater in New York. Frank resisted working in films until a small role in *Diary of a Mad Housewife,* in 1970, was quickly followed by a starring one, in *The Twelve Chairs,* which was directed by Mel Brooks. In 1979, he played Count Dracula to Laurence Olivier's Van Helsing, in a film version of *Dracula.* He proved a versatile actor after that – mostly on the stage, where he's performed in everything from Strindberg to Coward to Shakespeare – winning a Best Featured Actor Tony, for "Fortune's Fool" in 2002. In 1996, he and Ruth Weil were divorced. Frank then lived with Whoopi Goldberg until 2001. He is scheduled to star on Broadway, as Sir Thomas More, in a revival of "A Man for All Seasons". He was nominated for several awards, including an Oscar, for his playing of Richard Nixon, in *Frost/Nixon.*

Diary of a Mad Housewife (1970)
The Twelve Chairs (1970)
Dracula (1979) Those Lips, Those
Eyes (1980) True Identity (1991)
Dave (1993) Brainscan (1994)
Lolita (1997) The Ninth Gate (1999)
Sweet November (2001)
House of D (2004) Breaking the
Fifth (2004) How You Look to Me (2005)
Good Night, and Good Luck (2005)
Superman Returns (2006)
The Novice (2006)
Starting Out in the Evening (2007)
Frost/Nixon (2008)

Angela **Lansbury**
5ft 8in
(ANGELA BRIGID LANSBURY)

Born: October 16, 1925
London, England

Angela was the daughter of Edgar Lansbury, a London businessman. Her mother was the actress, Moyna McGill. Her grandfather was former British Labour Party leader, George Lansbury. After South Hampstead High School she studied dancing, singing and dramatic art. In 1940, she was evacuated from the London Blitz and moved to New York City with her mother. They later settled in Hollywood. Angela was working in a Los Angeles store when spotted by a movie scout and cast in the role of the cockney maid, in *Gaslight.* She was nominated for a Best Supporting Actress Oscar, and a year later, she was nominated for *Dorian Gray* – which also featured her mother. It was a terrific start to her Hollywood, career. Her marriage to actor, Richard Cromwell, lasted one year. She married Peter Shaw in 1949, and was playing substantial supporting roles. He managed her after her MGM contract ended, but her film work during the 1950s was limited. In 1960, she had a Broadway hit in "A Taste of Honey". Angela was nominated for a Best Supporting Actress Oscar, for *The Manchurian Candidate,* and in 1966, she enjoyed her biggest success, in "Mame" on Broadway. TV appearances in 'Murder She Wrote' have kept her name famous.

Gaslight (1944)
National Velvet (1944)
The Picture of Dorian Gray (1945)
The Private Affairs of Bel Ami (1947)
State of the Union (1948)
The Three Musketeers (1948)
Samson and Delilah (1958)
The Court Jester (1955)
The Reluctant Debutante (1958)
The Dark at the Top of the Stairs (1960)
All Fall Down (1962)
The Manchurian Candidate (1962)
Dear Heart (1964)
Bedknobs and Broomsticks (1971)
Death on the Nile (1978)
The Pirates of Penzance (1983)
The Company of Wolves (1984)
Nanny McPhee (2005)

Mario **Lanza**
5ft 7¾in
(ALFRED ARNOLD COCOZZA)

Born: **January 31, 1921**
Philadelphia, Pennsylvania, USA
Died: **October 7, 1959**

Mario's parents were Italian immigrants. His father, Antonio Cocozza, was from Filignano, and his mother, Maria Lanza, arrived in America at the age of six months. They were married in 1919. He was given a piano and lessons by his parents, but even as a boy, Mario appeared to lack the self-discipline which would later damage his career. But he had a golden voice. After Southern High School, Mario was discovered – moving pianos and singing, rather than whistling – while he worked. He was heard by the concert manager of the Philadelphia Academy of Music. Serge Koussevitsky invited him to Tanglewood. In 1942, he sang in "The Merry Wives of Windsor", but U.S. Army service delayed his career. That began in 1946 with an RCA contract and an appearance at the Hollywood Bowl. Following his operatic debut, in "Madame Butterfly", Mario was signed by MGM. He made his film debut in *That Midnight Kiss,* but that and *The Toast of New Orleans,* were slow burners until the song "Be My Love" became a hit all over the world. He later starred in the incredibly successful, *The Great Caruso.* Food, drink, women and finally, drugs would cause his early demise, but even though he reportedly behaved badly towards his co-star, Doretta Morrow, *Because You're Mine* became another massive hit. Sadly, Mario had become too fat to appear on screen. in *The Student Prince* – actor Edmond Purdom mimed to his singing. Mario was an inspiration to many, before he died of a heart attack in Rome, after making his last film there – ironically titled *For the First Time.* He was only thirty-eight. He had four children with his wife, Betty, who died five months later, from a drug overdose.

That Midnight Kiss (1949)
The Toast of New Orleans (1950)
The Great Caruso (1951)
Because You're Mine (1952)
Serenade (1956)
For the First Time (1959)

Anthony **LaPaglia**
5ft 11in
(ANTHONY LAPAGLIA)

Born: **January 31, 1959**
Adelaide, South Australia, Australia

Tony was the son of Eddie LaPaglia, an auto mechanic and car dealer, and his wife, Maria, who was a secretary. Tony and his brothers had two big passions when they were growing up – movies and soccer. Although not especially tall by Australian standards, Tony excelled as a goalkeeper at Rostrevor College – a Catholic boys school which is beautifully situated in the foothills of the Mount Lofty Ranges – outside Adelaide. In the 1980s, he played for two of the city's teams in the National Soccer League. He left Australia in 1985, intending to pursue a teaching career in the United States. Somehow, he drifted into part-time acting after completely losing his Aussie accent. Small roles on television began auspiciously in the Steven Spielberg series, "Amazing Stories". His first film role was in 1987, in the poorly received detective drama, *Cold Steel* – starring Sharon Stone. By 1989, he had become a full-time actor. The following year, he was praised for his work as a mobster, in *Betsy's Wedding.* Tony kept his name in the public eye through regular television appearances in high profile shows like 'Murder One' and 'Frasier' and currently is in his seventh season as Jack Malone, in 'Without a Trace'. In 1998 he married the Australian actress, Gia Carides. The couple have a six-year-old daughter named Bridget. Tony's voice is heard on the animated film, *$9.99.*

Betsy's Wedding (1990)
One Good Cop (1991)
Innocent Blood (1992)
Whispers in the Dark (1992)
The Custodian (1993)
The Client (1994)
Empire Records (1995)
Trees Lounge (1996)
Phoenix (1998)
Sweet and Lowdown (1999)
Lantana (2001) **The Bank** (2001)
The Salton Sea (2002)
The Guys (2002) **Happy Hour** (2003)
Winter Solstice (2004)
The Architect (2006)

Queen **Latifah**
5ft 10in
(DANA ELAINE OWENS)

Born: **March 18, 1970**
Newark, New Jersey, USA

Dana was raised in the Baptist religion by her policeman father, Lance Owens, and her schoolteacher mother, Rita. When she was a little girl, her eventual stage-name Latifah, meaning "Nice' in Arabic, was given to her by a cousin. By the time her parents divorced when she was ten, Dana had already showed promise as a singer. At high school, she appeared in "The Wiz" and was also a key member – as a power forward – of the basketball team. In 1988, Dana's demo version of "Princess of the Posse" led to a contract with Tommy Boy Records, who released her first album, "All Hail the Queen", when she was nineteen. The 'Royal' title has been with her ever since. The album received critical acclaim and its commercial success resulted in more albums and hit singles. She went on to sing at LA's Hollywood bowl, backed by a 10-piece orchestra, and released a jazz album which included a guest spot by Stevie Wonder. Queen made her movie debut in 1991, with a small role in Spike Lee's star-studded, *Jungle Fever.* From 1993 until 1998, Queen furthered her reputation with a five-year stint, as Khadijah James in the Fox television-sitcom, 'Living Single'. By the end of the decade she was as well known for her acting as for her music. Her performance as Matron Mama Morton, in *Chicago,* was nominated for a Best Supporting Actress Oscar.

Juice (1992) **My Life** (1993)
Set It Off (1996)
Hoodlum (1997)
Living Out Loud (1998)
The Bone Collector (1999)
Chicago (2002)
Bringing Down the House (2003)
Scary Movie 3 (2003)
Barbershop 2: Back in Business (2004)
Beauty Shop (2005)
Last Holiday (2006)
Stranger Than Fiction (2006)
Life Support (2007)
Hairspray (2007)
What Happened in Vegas (2008)

Charles **Laughton**
5ft 8in
(CHARLES LAUGHTON)

Born: **July 1, 1899**
Scarborough, Yorkshire, England
Died: **December 15, 1962**

Charles, the son of Robert and Elizabeth Laughton, was originally destined for a career in the family hotel business. He was probably quite lucky that after Stonyhurst College, he had to serve in the army – towards the end of World War I. On his release, he defied his father by going to London to study at RADA. He made his stage debut in 1925, and went on to appear with great success in the West End. In one play, "Mr.Prohak" he met Elsa Lanchester and appeared in one of her comic two-reelers. He married her, but it would take her thirty-three years to decide that he was gay. In 1929, Charles made his feature film debut, in *Piccadilly*. He and Elsa went to New York to star in "Payment Deferred" and stayed on so that he could make his first American film, *Devil and the Deep*. He returned to London for his Oscar-winning role in *The Private Life of Henry VIII*. During the 1930s, his movies were usually very successful. A 'mixed bag' best describes his work in the 1940s – due to a paucity of good roles rather than any fault of his. Every once in a while Charles would produce the goods – even his one-off directing effort resulted in the classic film fantasy, *The Night of the Hunter,* and he was perfectly cast in his final film, *Advise & Consent*. Charles died in Hollywood, of gall bladder cancer.

Island of Lost Souls (1932)
The Sign of the Cross (1932)
The Private Life of Henry VIII (1933)
The Barretts of Wimpole Street (1934)
Les Misérables (1935)
Mutiny on the Bounty (1935)
Ruggles of Red Gap (1935)
Rembrandt (1936)
St. Martin's Lane (1938)
The Hunchback of Notre Dame (1939)
The Big Clock (1948) Young Bess (1953)
Hobson's Choice (1954)
Witness for the Prosecution (1957)
Under Ten Flags (1960)
Spartacus (1960)
Advise and Consent (1962)

Stan **Laurel**
5ft 8in
(ARTHUR STANLEY JEFFERSON)

Born: **June 16, 1890**
Ulverston, Cumbria, England
Died: **February 23, 1965**

Stan's father, A.J. Jefferson, was a Victorian actor and theater manager. At a local grammar school in his early teens, Stan starred in Christmas pantomimes. He first worked in music halls, but his big break was when he toured America with Fred Karno's Circus in 1910. On a subsequent trip there, he understudied Charles Chaplin. Stan then left Karno to try his luck in vaudeville and got his first film role in 1918, in *Nuts in May*. He worked for Hal Roach on a casual basis before signing a contract, which resulted in some fifty shorts. Nearly all of them featured Oliver Hardy, who he teamed up with in 1927. It brought them fame and fortune – which neither were able to hang on to. They were funny in Silents, but Talkies were to give them a whole new dimension. An Oscar for *The Music Box,* in 1932, enabled them to extend the fun to feature length films. Stan was always the one with brains and his domination almost caused a split in 1935. By 1940, they were both getting old and following a tour called "The Laurel and Hardy Revue", there were worrying signs that they'd lost their appeal. The final eight features all failed at the box-office and only *The Bullfighters* is worth watching. Stan married five times – firstly to the silent screen actress, Lois Nelson (with whom he had two children) and twice to Virginia Ruth Rogers. His last wife, Ida Kitaeva, was with him when he died of a heart attack, in Santa Monica, California.

Pack Up Your Troubles (1932)
The Devil's Brother (1933)
Sons of the Desert (1933)
Babes in Toyland (1934)
Bonnie Scotland (1935)
Bohemian Girl (1936)
Our Relations (1936)
Way Out West (1937)
Blockheads (1938)
Swiss Miss (1938)
A Chump at Oxford (1940)
Saps at Sea (1940)
The Bullfighters (1945)

Hugh **Laurie**
6ft 2½in
(JAMES HUGH CALUM LAURIE)

Born: **June 11, 1959**
Oxford, Oxfordshire, England

Hugh's father, Doctor William Laurie, won a gold medal in the coxless pairs, at the 1948 Olympic Games in London. Hugh attended the Dragon preparatory school before going to Eton College. At Selwyn College, Cambridge, he got a Third-class Honors degree in Archaeology and Anthropology. Hugh was also an accomplished oarsman – rowing for the beaten light blues, in the 1980 Oxford and Cambridge Boat Race. Hugh joined the Cambridge Footlights where he met Emma Thompson, who introduced him to Stephen Fry. They took their review "The Cellar Tapes" to the Edinburgh Festival Fringe, and they won the Perrier Comedy Award. After a West End run and a TV version, they worked in a series called 'Alfresco' for Granada. Hugh's network of contacts led to key roles in 'Blackadder' and 'A Bit of Fry and Laurie' for the BBC. They teamed up again in the delightful 'Jeeves and Wooster'. Hugh's first film appearance was a small role in 1985's *Plenty*. Although he's appeared in movies with Hollywood connections, he has yet to land a part which will make him a star. The American accent he uses in the role of Dr. Gregory House, in the television series, 'House M.D.' is as good as I've ever heard from an English actor. Since 1989, Hugh has been married to Jo Green. They live in London with their three children. He was seen recently in a rare 'serious' movie role, in the crime drama, *Street Kings*.

Strapless (1989)
Peter's Friends (1992)
Sense and Sensibility (1995)
101 Dalmatians (1996)
The Borrowers (1997)
The Man in the
Iron Mask (1998)
Cousin Bette (1998)
Stuart Little (1999)
Maybe Baby (2000)
Stuart Little 2 (2002)
Flight of the Phoenix (2004)
The Big Empty (2005)
Street Kings (2008)

Piper **Laurie**
5ft 4¹/₂in
(ROSETTA JACOBS)

Born: **January 22, 1932**
Detroit, Michigan, USA

The daughter of a Jewish furniture dealer, Alfred Jacobs, and Charlotte, who was from a Russian background, Piper moved to Los Angeles with her family when she was six years old. She was a shy kid, so in addition to her Hebrew schooling, her parents sent her to elocution lessons. After high school, she studied acting and landed a contract with Universal when she was barely seventeen. During her film debut in *Louisa,* in 1950, she became good friends with Ronald Reagan. The studio gave her what she felt were unsatisfying roles in B-westerns and Ali Baba fantasies, and by 1955, Piper had had enough. She went to New York to study acting and began to get some interesting parts in serious television dramas. In 1961, her efforts were recognized when she was nominated for a Best Actress Oscar for her role as Sarah, in *The Hustler.* In 1962, she married writer/reporter, Joe Morgenstern. She had a daughter before returning to mainstream films in 1976, with the key role of Carrie's mother, Margaret, in Brian De Palma's classic, *Carrie.* Piper's regular stream of TV roles has kept her in the public eye and recent movies – including the controversial *Hounddog,* confirm that she is alive and kicking.

Louisa (1950)
Has Anybody Seen
My Girl? (1952)
The Mississippi Gambler (1953)
Ain't Misbehavin' (1955)
Until They Sail (1957)
The Hustler (1961)
Carrie (1976) Tim (1979)
Children of a
Lesser God (1986)
Distortions (1987)
Other People's Money (1991)
Wrestling Ernest
Hemingway (1993)
The Crossing Guard (1995)
The Grass Harp (1995)
Eulogy (2004)
The Dead Girl (2006)
Hounddog (2007)

Jude **Law**
5ft 11³/₄in
(DAVID JUDE LAW)

Born: **December 29, 1972**
Lewisham, London, England

Jude was the son of teachers, Peter and Maggie Law, who went on to open their own drama school in France. Following his junior education, Jude attended the independent Alleyn's School in Dulwich, South-East London. In 1987, he began his acting career with the National Youth Music Theater in London – appearing on stage that year, in "Bodywork" at the Edinburgh Fringe. In 1989, he acted on television as a stableboy, in 'The Tailor of Gloucester'. Jude's first major stage role was in 1997, as 'Foxtrot Darling', in "The Fastest Clock in The Universe", at the Hampstead Theater. Following a featured role in *Bent,* he got his big screen break that year, when he portrayed Lord Alfred Douglas, opposite Steven Fry, in the film *Wilde.* It was followed by an important role in his first Hollywood movie, as a wheelchair-bound Olympic athlete, in *Gattaca.* At the 2000 Academy Awards, Jude was nominated for a Best Supporting Actor Oscar, in *The Talented Mr. Ripley,* and four years later, he was nominated as Best Actor, for *Cold Mountain.* For six years – until 2003, Jude was married to the actress, Sadie Frost. The couple had three children. Jude was later engaged for two years, to Sienna Miller.

Bent (1997) Gattaca (1997)
Midnight in the Garden of
Good and Evil (1997) Wilde (1997)
The Wisdom of Crocodiles (1998)
Final Cut (1998) eXistenZ (1999)
The Talented Mr Ripley (1999)
Love, Honour and Obey (2000)
Enemy at the Gates (2001)
Road to Perdition (2002)
Cold Mountain (2003)
I Heart Huckerbees (2004)
Alfie (2004) Closer (2004)
The Aviator (2004)
All the King's Men (2006)
Breaking and Entering (2006)
The Holiday (2006)
My Blueberry Nights (2007)
Sleuth (2007)
Rage (2009)

Peter **Lawford**
6ft
(PETER SYDNEY LAWFORD)

Born: **September 7, 1923**
London, England
Died: **December 24, 1984**

Peter was the son of Sir Sydney Turing Barlow Lawford, a World War I hero, and his wife, Lady May Lawford. They were not married when Peter was conceived and along with his lack of education, it was to remain a source of great embarrassment to him. One of the reasons for his limited education was his family's travelling and spending his early years in France. He was spoilt by his mother who dressed him in girl's clothes until he was eleven. He made his film debut in Britain, in 1931, in *Poor Old Bill.* Peter may have had little formal education, but he was almost fluent in four languages. A collision with a glass door severely injured his arm. It kept him from serving in World War II, but enabled him to work in movies without interruption. He moved to Hollywood, where he had his first starring role, in 1942, in *A Yank at Eton.* He gave Elizabeth Taylor her first screen kiss, had a controversial affair with actress Dorothy Dandridge, and he first introduced Marilyn Monroe to John F. Kennedy, whose sister, Patricia, was the first of his four wives. An original member of the "Rat Pack" and a bisexual, Peter lived a full life in every sense. He died in Los Angeles of liver and kidney disease.

The White Cliffs of Dover (1944)
Mrs. Parkington (1944)
The Picture of Dorian Gray (1945)
Son of Lassie (1945)
Two Sisters from Boston (1946)
Cluny Brown (1946)
It Happened in Brooklyn (1947)
Good News (1947)
On an Island with You (1948)
Easter Parade (1948)
Julia Misbehaves (1948)
Little Women (1949)
Royal Wedding (1951)
Just This Once (1952)
Rogue's March (1953)
It Should Happen To You (1954)
Ocean's Eleven (1960)
Sylvia (1965) Buona Sera,
Mrs. Campbell (1968)

Jean-Pierre **Léaud**
5ft 8in
(JEAN-PIERRE LÉAUD)

Born: **May 28, 1944**
Paris, France

Jean-Pierre was the son of screenwriter Pierre Léaud, and the actress Jacqueline Pierreux. After a small role in a Jean Marais 1958 swashbuckler, he was only fourteen when he made his official film debut, as the star of François Truffaut's, French New Wave classic, *The 400 Blows.* He followed that with an uncredited role in Jean Cocteau's, *Testament d'Orphée,* in 1960. He was the young Jojo, in the Julien Duvivier film, *Boulevard,* then played a young guy who wasn't yet very confident with the mademoiselles, in *L'Amour à vingt ans* – J-P was only eighteen when he made it! He had uncredited walk-ons in a couple of Jean-Luc Godard hit movies – becoming an adult star in the great man's *Masculin féminin,* and winning the Best Actor Award at the Berlin Film Festival. He was top man for top directors including Truffaut, for a dozen years. From the mid-1980s, things slowed down due to inferior material, but Jean-Pierre bounced back with the help of the younger French film-makers and is still performing in front of the cameras. He has recently completed *Visages,* a film shot in Paris with finance from Taiwan, Belgium and France, which is directed by Malaysian, Ming-liang Tsai.

The 400 Blows (1959)
Le Testament d'Orphee (1960)
Love at Twenty (1962)
Masculine Feminine (1966)
Made in USA (1966) Weekend (1967)
La Chinoise (1967) Stolen Kisses (1968)
Bed and Board (1970)
Last Tango in Paris (1972)
Day for Night (1973)
La Maman et la putain (1973)
Out 1: Spectre (1974) L'Amour en
Fuite (1979) Détective (1985)
Jane B. par Agnès V. (1988)
I Hired a Contract Killer (1990)
Paris s'éveille (1991)
The Birth of Love (1993)
Pour rire! (1996)
L'Affaire Marcorelle (2000)
Ni na bian ji dian (2001)
J'ai vu tuer Ben Barka (2005)

Cloris **Leachman**
5ft 6in
(CLORIS LEACHMAN)

Born: **April 30, 1926**
Des Moines, Iowa, USA

The eldest of three sisters, Cloris was the daughter of Buck and Cloris Leachman. Her father owned a lumber company. A clever outgoing kid, Cloris started getting her voice heard outside her family when she was eleven – appearing on a local radio show and six years on, in amateur plays. She went on to major in Drama at Northwestern University. When she was twenty, she represented Chicago in the "Miss America" contest. She then went to New York, where she studied at the Actor's Studio, under Elia Kazan. In 1947, she was an extra in the classical music film, *Carnegie Hall,* and a year later, made her television debut in an episode of 'The Ford Hour', titled 'Night Must Fall'. In 1949, Cloris played in five of the Actor's Studio TV productions and understudied Mary Martin, in the original run of "South Pacific". For five years, Cloris, who married the actor/producer George Englund, in 1953, was mostly in television dramas. The couple had five children, but divorced in 1979. Cloris made her film debut, as Christina Bailey, in Robert Aldrich's classic *Kiss Me Deadly.* She then won a Best Supporting Actress Oscar, as the 'lonely older woman', Ruth, in *The Last Picture Show,* and has continued acting with her usual passion right up to 2008, when she acted in two star-studded movies – *The Women* and *New York, I Love You.*

Kiss Me Deadly (1955)
The Rack (1956)
Butch Cassidy and the
Sundance Kid (1969)
Lovers and Other Strangers (1970)
The People Next Door (1970)
The Last Picture Show (1971)
Dillinger (1973)
Young Frankenstein (1974)
High Anxiety (1977)
History of the World: Part 1 (1981)
Never Too Late (1997)
Sky High (2005)
Beerfest (2006)
The Women (2008)
New York, I Love You (2008)

Heath **Ledger**
6ft 1in
(HEATH ANDREW LEDGER)

Born: **April 4, 1979**
Perth, Western Australia, Australia
Died: **January 22, 2008**

Heath's father, Kim, was a mining engineer who loved fast cars, and his mother, Sally, was a teacher of French. After his early years at Mary's Mount Primary School, Heath attended Guildford Grammar School in Perth. He left school at sixteen to pursue an acting career in Sydney, in the company of his girlfriend, Jenna Sorrell. Following a couple of uncredited appearances, Heath made his TV debut – as Snowy Bowles, in the Australian series 'Sweat' in 1996, and the following year, he made his film debut, in the thriller *Black Rock.* He was too far down the cast list to make much of an impact, but he did just that when he starred in his first American film – *10 Things I Hate About You.* That promise was confirmed when he returned to Australia later that year, to make *Two Hands.* For three seasons, he starred as Conor, in the TV-series 'Roar' and he resumed his film career with a role alongside Mel Gibson, in *The Patriot.* He returned home to play Australian outlaw, *Ned Kelly.* He was nominated for a Best Actor Oscar for his role as gay cowboy, Ennis Del Mar, in the award winning, *Brokeback Mountain.* He was reported to have been very depressed when actress Michelle Williams – mother of his daughter, broke off their engagement in September, 2007. Heath died four months later, in his Manhattan apartment, from an accidental overdose of pills. His maniacal acting as 'The Joker', in *The Dark Knight,* resulted in posthumous awards – a Best Supporting Actor BAFTA and an Oscar.

10 Things I Hate About You (1999)
Two Hands (1999)
The Patriot (2000)
A Knight's Tale (2001)
Monster's Ball (2001)
Ned Kelly (2003)
Lords of Dogtown (2005)
Brokeback Mountain (2005)
Casanova (2005) Candy (2006)
I'm Not There (2007)
The Dark Knight (2008)

Virginie **Ledoyen**
5ft 5¼in
(VIRGINIE FERNANDEZ)

Born: November 15, 1976
Paris, France

Of Spanish descent on her father's side, Virginie took her paternal grandmother's name, Ledoyen, when she began her career. Her grandmother had been an actress on the Paris stage. Virginie was truly an infant prodigy. She acted in television commercials when she was only two years old and at nine she was attending the École des Enfants du Spectacle. She was eleven years old when she made her movie debut, in *Les Exploits d'un jeune Don Juan*. Virginie appeared in a French TV mini-series titled 'La Vie en panne' the following year, but finished her studies before starring in her second film – *Mima*. She was in the good company of Marcello Mastroianni and Michel Piccoli in *Le Voleur d'enfants* and was nominated for a César as the Most Promising Actress, for *Les Marmottes*. She played in any kind of movie with equal skill and even acted in a Taiwanese film, *Ma Jiang*. She worked internationally and was in the James Ivory drama, *A Soldier's Daughter Never Cries*. Her breakthrough role was as Françoise, in *The Beach,* when she co-starred with Leonardo DiCaprio. In September 2007, Virginie married film director, Iain Rogers. She has a daughter named Lilas.

Mima (1991)
Le Voleur d'enfants (1991)
Les Marmottes (1993)
Cold Water (1995)
A Single Girl (1995)
La Cérémonie (1995)
Ma Jiang (1996)
Ma 6-T va cracker-er (1997)
Héroïnes (1997) Marianne (1997)
Jeanne et le garçon
formidable (1998) A Soldier's
Daughter Never Cries (1998)
Late August, Early September (1998)
En plein coeur (1998)
The Beach (2000)
All About Love (2001) 8 femmes (2002)
Bon Voyage (2003)
The Valet (2006) BackWoods (2006)
Holly (2006) Shall We Kiss (2007)
Mes amis, mes amours (2008)

Sir Christopher **Lee**
6ft 5in
(CHRISTOPHER FRANK CARANDINI LEE)

Born: May 27, 1922
Belgravia, London, England

The son of Lieutenant-Colonel Geoffrey Trollope Lee, of the 60th King's Royal Rifle Corps, Christopher certainly was blessed with a military bearing. From his mother, Estelle, an Italian Contessa, he got his dark good looks. His parents split up when he was young and his mother took him to Switzerland. Back in England, he attended Wellington College. During the war, he served in the RAF. He was only prevented from flying due to eyesight problems discovered in training. As his great grandmother, Marie Carandini, had been an opera singer, Christopher was assured of a dramatic future. He was taken on by the Rank "Charm School", where he was taught to act. He made his film debut, in *Corridor of Mirrors,* in 1948. Nine years later *The Curse of Frankenstein* made him a star. The answer to Hammer Films' prayers, Christopher strode with menace along dimly-lit corridors, biting soft throats and terrifying audiences for thirty years. He has been married to Gitte Lee since 1961 and he celebrated sixty years of filmmaking with a knighthood.

The Curse of Frankenstein (1957)
Dracula (1958) The Hound of the
Baskervilles (1959)
The Treasure of San Teresa (1959)
Scream of Fear (1961)
Corridors of Blood (1962)
Dracula – Prince of Darkness (1965)
The Face of Fu Manchu (1965)
Theater of Death (1966)
The Private Life of Sherlock
Holmes (1970) The Three
Musketeers (1973) The Man with
the Golden Gun (1974)
Return from Witch Mountain (1978)
House of the Long Shadows (1983)
Shaka Zulu (1987) The Rainbow
Thief (1990) Jinnah (1998)
Sleepy Hollow (1999)
The Two Towers (2002) The Return of
the King (2003) Revenge of the
Sith (2005) Charlie and the
Chocolate Factory (2005)
The Golden Compass (2007)

Janet **Leigh**
5ft 5½in
(JEANETTE HELEN MORRISON)

Born: July 6, 1927
Merced, California, USA
Died: October 3, 2004

She was the only child of a poor couple, Frederick and Helen Morrison, who during the Great Depression, moved around the country looking for work. Janet dropped out of high school when she was fifteen and after a stupid first marriage which was annulled due to her age, she had a couple of years dreaming of stardom every time she sat in a movie house. Eventually, her parents found jobs at a ski resort, and when Janet was visiting them one afternoon, she was discovered by the former MGM star, Norma Shearer. After Janet impressed in her screen test, she signed a contract with the studio in 1946, and then made her second big mistake by entering another short-lived marriage. Janet's film debut came a year later, in *The Romance of Rosy Ridge*. Within three years, she was a bigger star than Tony Curtis, whom she married in 1951. Daughters, Jamie Lee and Kelly became actresses. Janet was a delightful personality who rarely got the chance to display her ability as an actress. When she did, as in *Touch of Evil* and especially Alfred Hitchcock's *Psycho,* she created unforgettable characters. In the latter, the shower scene image is among the best known in the whole of cinema history. Janet finished work on her final film, *Bad Girls from Valley High,* the year she died in Beverly Hills, of vasculitis.

The Romance of Rosy Ridge (1947)
Act of Violence (1948)
Little Women (1949)
Two Tickets to Broadway (1951)
Scaramouche (1952)
Houdini (1953) The Naked Spur (1953)
The Black Shield of Falworth (1954)
Rogue Cop (1954)
My Sister Eileen (1955)
Pete Kelly's Blues (1955)
Safari (1956) Touch of Evil (1958)
The Vikings (1958) Who Was That
Lady? (1960) Psycho (1960)
The Manchurian Candidate (1962)
Bye Bye Birdie (1963)
The Moving Target (1966)

Jennifer Jason Leigh
5ft 3in
(JENNIFER LEE MORROW)

Born: **February 5, 1962**
Hollywood, California, USA

Jennifer's father was Vic Morrow, who had burst on to the movie scene in 1955, in *Blackboard Jungle* – the film which first introduced Rock 'n' Roll to the world's postwar teenagers. Her mother was the screenwriter, Barbara Turner. Jennifer was fourteen when she began attending Lee Strasberg acting workshops. She got her first work two years later, in an episode of the TV-series 'Baretta'. She adopted the middle name Jason as a mark of respect for a family friend, Jason Robards Jr. In 1980, Jennifer made her film debut, as a seriously handicapped rape victim, in *Eyes of a Stranger.* In 1982, her father was killed when the helicopter being used on the set of *Twilight Zone: The Movie,* spun out of control. He'd lived just long enough to see his little girl making it as an actress. From the mid-1980s, Jennifer started her move towards stardom in interesting and challenging roles. In 1990, she got awards as well – from Boston and New York film critics, for *Last Exit to Brooklyn* and *Miami Blues.* In 2005, she married director Noah Baumbach. Recent character roles such as Pauline, in *Margot at the Wedding* have not diminished her appeal.

The Hitcher (1986)
Last Exit to Brooklyn (1989)
Buried Alive (1990)
Miami Blues (1990)
Backdraft (1991)
Single White Female (1992)
Short Cuts (1993)
The Hudsucker Proxy (1994)
Mrs. Parker and the Vicious Circle (1994)
Dolores Claiborne (1995)
Georgia (1995)
eXistenZ (1999)
Skipped Paris (2000)
The Anniversary Party (2001)
Road to Perdition (2002)
Palindromes (2004)
Childstar (2004)
The Jacket (2005)
Margot at the Wedding (2007)
Synecdoche, New York (2008)

Vivien Leigh
5ft 3½in
(VIVIEN MARY HARTLEY)

Born: **November 5, 1913**
Darjeeling, West Bengal, British India
Died: **July 7, 1967**

Vivien's parents were resident in India. Her father, Richard Hartley, was a British officer in the Indian Army Cavalry. He married her mother, Gertrude, in Kensington, London, in 1912, and took her out to India. Vivien's mother wanted her to grow up as a Catholic, so she was sent to to a convent school in Roehampton, to get an English education. While there, Vivien befriended the future movie star, Maureen O'Sullivan. In 1932, she married a barrister, Herbert Leigh, and they had a daughter they named Suzanne. Vivien spent a year at RADA before making her film debut, in 1934, in *Things Are Looking Up.* In 1935, her West End stage debut, in "The Mask of Virtue" brought her overnight fame. She was signed by Alexander Korda, who co-starred her with Olivier in *Fire Over England.* MGM borrowed her for *A Yank at Oxford.* Vivien was already involved with Laurence Olivier when she played Ophelia to his stage "Hamlet". She joined him in the States, and she tested successfully for *Gone with the Wind* – winning the Best Actress Oscar. Vivien married Larry in 1940. They starred in *That Hamilton Woman* but Selznick wouldn't allow her to play a small role in *Henry V.* She retaliated by refusing to leave Britain for several years. She won a second Oscar for playing the neurotic Blanche, in *A Streetcar Named Desire,* but Vivien's real-life mental problems proved too much for Laurence Olivier. Seven years after their divorce, Vivien died at her home in London, of chronic tuberculosis.

Fire Over England (1937)
Sidewalks of London (1938)
A Yank at Oxford (1938)
Gone with the Wind (1939)
Waterloo Bridge (1940)
That Hamilton Woman (1941)
Anna Karenina (1948) **A Streetcar Named Desire** (1951) **The Deep Blue Sea** (1955) **The Roman Spring of Mrs. Stone** (1961)
Ship of Fools (1965)

Margaret Leighton
5ft 10½in
(MARGARET LEIGHTON)

Born: **February 26, 1922**
Barnt Green, Worcestershire, England
Died: **January 13, 1976**

The daughter of a local businessman and his wife, Margaret joined the Birmingham Repertory company straight from school. She made her stage debut for them in 1938, as Dorothy, in the comedy "Laugh With Me", which was filmed that year and screened on BBC television. Margaret went on to study at Sir Barry Jackson's theater school, in Birmingham, before working her way to theatrical stardom with the Old Vic. She made her Broadway debut on the company's United States tour of 1946, in "Henry IV", which also starred Laurence Olivier and Ralph Richardson. On returning to England, she married the first of her three husbands, publisher, Max Reinhardt. She made her film debut, in the highly-rated British drama, *The Winslow Boy,* and worked with Hitchcock, in *Under Capricorn.* A scene stealer – Margaret's height would often dominate her leading men. She was nominated for a Best Supporting Actress Oscar, for *The Go-Between.* Margaret made her final screen appearance in 1976, in *Trial by Combat.* Her second and third husbands were actors Laurence Harvey, and Michael Wilding. Mike was with her when she died in Chichester, West Sussex, of multiple sclerosis.

The Winslow Boy (1948)
The Astonished Heart (1949)
Under Capricorn (1949)
Calling Bulldog Drummond (1951)
Home at Seven (1952)
The Good Die Young (1954)
Carrington V.C. (1955)
The Constant Husband (1955)
A Passionate Stranger (1957)
The Sound and the Fury (1959)
The Best Man (1964)
The Loved One (1965)
7 Women (1966)
The Go-Between (1970)
Lady Caroline Lamb (1972)
Zee and Co. (1972)
Galileo (1975)
Trial by Combat (1976)

Jack **Lemmon**
5ft 9in
(JOHN UHLER LEMMON III)

Born: **February 8, 1925**
Newton, Massachussets, USA
Died: **June 27, 2001**

Jack's mother, Mildred gave birth to him in a hospital elevator. His father, John, was president of a doughnut company. It sounds like a comedy sketch and it may explain Jack's future career. After Phillips Academy, Jack earned a degree in War Service Sciences from Harvard, where he was active in the University drama club. He joined the U.S. Navy as an ensign before working in radio and TV – appearing in dozens of programs, from 1948 onwards. He was spotted by Columbia, and made his film debut, opposite Judy Holliday, in *It Should Happen To You*. An Oscar, as Best Supporting Actor, in *Mister Roberts,* was followed by four years as an 'emerging star'. That all changed when he co-starred with Tony Curtis and Marilyn Monroe, in *Some Like It Hot.* The 1960s were good for him – by the end of that decade he was one of the top-ten box office stars. In 1962, he married second wife, Felicity Farr. He made his directorial debut in 1971, with *Kotch,* and two years later, won a Best Actor Oscar, for *Save The Tiger*. In 1998, he appeared with his pal, Walter Mattheu, in *The Odd Couple II.* Walter died two years later. Jack was to succumb to bladder cancer, less than a year after his final screen appearance – on television – in 'Tuesdays with Morrie'.

It Should Happen to You (1954)
Phffft! (1954) Mister Roberts (1955)
My Sister Eileen (1955)
Fire Down Below (1957)
Some Like it Hot (1959)
The Apartment (1960)
Days of Wine and Roses (1962)
Irma La Douce (1963)
The Great Race (1965)
How to Murder your Wife (1965)
The Odd Couple (1968)
Save the Tiger (1973)
The China Syndrome (1979)
Tribute (1980)
Missing (1982)
Glengarry Glen Ross (1992)
Hamlet (1996)

Téa **Leoni**
5ft 8in
(ELIZABETH TÉA PANTALEONI)

Born: **February 25, 1966**
New York City, New York, USA

Téa's father, Anthony Pantaleoni, was a corporate lawyer. Her mother, Emily, was a dietician and nutritionist, who hailed from Texas. Téa's background is Italian, Polish and English. Her paternal grandmother, "Helenka" Tradusa Adamoska, was a silent film actress who served as president of the U.S. fund for UNICEF for 25 years. That helped to inspire Téa to become a Goodwill Ambassador in 2001. She was educated at the all-girls' Brearley School in New York City, and The Putney school, in Vermont. She dropped out of the Sarah Lawrence College in 1988, after attending an audition for a planned television remake of 'Charlie's Angels'. Due to a screenwriter's strike in Hollywood, it was never made, but it fired her enthusiasm for a career. In 1989, Téa made her first small screen appearance, in an episode of 'Santa Barbara'. Two years later, she made her movie debut, with a small role in the Blake Edwards comedy, *Switch*. She married her first husband, Neil Tardio, but her acting career didn't take off until after their divorce in 1995. Up until 1998, Téa acted in the TV series, 'The Naked Truth'. *Deep Impact, The Family Man* – for which she won a Saturn Best Actress Award, and *Jurassic Park III,* are significant movie career landmarks. The recent film, *You Kill Me,* was her second venture as executive producer. Téa married the actor, David Duchovny, in 1997. They have a daughter and a son, and live in Malibu, California.

Wyatt Earp (1994)
Bad Boys (1995)
Flirting with Disaster (1996)
Deep Impact (1998)
The Family Man (2000)
Jurassic Park III (2001)
Hollywood Ending (2002)
People I Know (2002)
House of D (2004)
Spanglish (2004)
Fun with Dick and Jane (2005)
You Kill Me (2007)
Ghost Town (2008)
Manure (2009)

Joan **Leslie**
5ft 4in
(JOAN AGNES THERESA SADIE BRODEL)

Born: **January 26, 1925**
Detroit, Michigan, USA

Joan's father worked in a bank until he lost his job during the Great Depression. From the age of three, Joan was encouraged by her parents to perform with her two older sisters. She acted on stage and was so pretty, by the age of ten she was getting work through the Powers agency, as an advertising model for childrens' clothes. She was also musical. She and her sisters formed a novelty trio – Joan played the accordion, Mary the Banjo and Betty was on Saxophone. Joan was spotted by a talent scout and was taken to Hollywood, where she made her screen debut, (uncredited) in Greta Garbo's *Camille.* In 1939, she was billed as Joan Brodel, in *Winter Carnival.* She took acting lessons as well as mathematics and French in the studio school. In 1940, when she starred in *Alice in Movieland,* a short about a girl who wins a screen test, she'd changed her name to Leslie to avoid confusion with Joan Blondell. Her star-making film was playing opposite Gary Cooper, in *Sergeant York.* She made a brave effort to keep up with Astaire in *The Sky's the Limit,* but she was no Ginger Rogers. She married Dr. William Caldwell, in 1950, and a few years later she quit her acting career to raise her identical twin daughters – Patrice and Ellen. Most of Joan's later work was on television, and her last role before retiring was in the 1991 drama, 'Fire in the Dark'.

High Sierra (1941)
The Wagons Roll at Night (1941)
Thieves Fall Out (1941)
Sergeant York (1941)
The Male Animal (1942)
Yankee Doodle Dandy (1942)
The Sky's the Limit (1943)
Rhapsody in Blue (1945)
Janie Gets Married (1946)
Two Guys from Milwaukee (1946)
Repeat Performance (1947)
Born to Be Bad (1950)
Man in the Saddle (1951)
Jubilee Trail (1954)
Hell's Outpost (1954)
The Revolt of Mamie Stover (1956)

Tony **Leung**
5ft 7½in
(TONY LEUNG)

Born: June 27, 1962
Hong Kong

Tony's parents came to settle in Hong Kong from Taishan, Guandong, China. He and his younger sister were left with their mother when his father, a gambling addict, abandoned the family. Tony was only seven at the time. For a while, it affected his confidence. His mother worked hard to send him to a private school, but at fifteen, he was forced to leave because of financial pressures. He did a variety of jobs before heeding the advice of the actor comedian, Stephen Chow, and he entered show business. In 1982, Tony hosted a children's TV show called '430 Space Shuttle' and that same year, he made his movie debut, in *Forced Vengeance*. He was first noticed internationally when he was featured in the 1990 Venice Golden Lion winner, *City of Sadness*. Tony's major breakthrough came three years later, in John Woo's action movie, *Hard-Boiled*. After a four-year relationship with the actress, Margie Tsang, he began an affair with another actress, Carina Lau. After twenty years together, they got married in 2008. In addition to his prolific film career, Tony has released seven albums of Mandarin and Cantonese songs. Tony adds "Chiu Wai" to his name to avoid confusion with his namesake. He speaks good English and now has an agent in the United States.

People's Hero (1988)
The City of Sadness (1989)
My Heart Is That Eternal Rose (1989)
Bullet in the Head (1990)
Hard-Boiled (1992) Chunking
Express (1994) Cyclo (1995)
Doctor Mack (1995)
Happy Together (1997)
Timeless Romance (1998)
Your Place or Mine (1998)
In the Mood for Love (2000)
Heroes (2002)
Infernal Affairs (2002) 2046 (2004)
New Police Story (2004)
Confessions of Pain (2006)
Lust, Caution (2007)
Red Cliff (2008) Red Cliff II (2009)

Geoffrey **Lewis**
5ft 9in
(GEOFFREY LEWIS)

Born: July 31, 1935
San Diego, California, USA

Geoffrey grew up on farmland which had belonged to the Lewis family since the 17th century. He used to entertain himself by dressing up in his parents' clothes. By the age of six, he had made up his mind to become an actor. When he was ten, he moved to a remote area of California, where among other things, he learned to ski. At high school, he staged one-man shows. His drama teacher recommended him to the Plymouth Summer Theater Festival. After that, he studied at New York's Neighborhood Playhouse, and appeared in Off-Broadway shows. His film debut in 1963 – a bit part in *The Fat Black Pussycat,* didn't lead to a flood of offers from Hollywood, so he continued on stage until 1970, when he acted in a variety of TV series. His first good movie role was in *The Culpepper Cattle Co.* Since then, he has been a popular character actor. Twice married, he fathered ten children – five of whom are in show business. Juliette Lewis has made quite a name for herself as a movie actress. Geoffrey, along with Geoff Levin, is in a musical/storytelling group known as "Celestial Navigations".

The Culpepper Cattle Co. (1972)
Bad Company (1972)
High Plains Drifter (1973)
Dillinger (1973)
My Name Is Nobody (1973)
Thunderbolt and Lightfoot (1974)
Macon County Line (1974)
The Great Waldo Pepper (1975)
The Wind and the Lion (1975)
Tom Horn (1980)
Bronco Billy (1980)
Heaven's Gate (1980)
The Man Without a Face (1993)
Maverick (1994)
Midnight in the Garden of
Good and Evil (1997)
The Way of the Gun (2000)
Formosa (2005)
The Devil's Rejects (2005)
Down in the Valley (2005)
Fingerprints (2006)
Chinaman's Chance (2008)

Jerry **Lewis**
6ft
(JOSEPH LEVITCH)

Born: March 16, 1926
Newark, New Jersey, USA

Jerry's parents, Danny and Rae Levitch, made their living as entertainers on the Borscht Circuit – resorts in upstate New York – frequented by Jews. Jerry was only five when he made his debut in their show, singing "Brother, Can You Spare A Dime?" He was soon earning more than that with an act – miming to phonograph records. But the break he needed took some time. So meanwhile, he worked in burlesque. It was the summer of 1946 when he began his partnership with the singer, Dean Martin. When Hal Wallis saw them at the Copacabana, in New York, he gave them a Paramount contract. Their debut movie, *My Friend Irma,* was the first of sixteen they made together and they were hugely popular for half-a-dozen years. But not everyone loved them: In 1952, when they headlined at the London Palladium, in England, they were booed by the opening night audience. They split in 1957, and Jerry erased the memory of Dean Martin, with his first solo film, *The Delicate Delinquent*. He then had a run of hits, but the 1960s saw a decline in his popularity – other than in France, where he is regarded as "DIEU". In the 1990s, Jerry made a number of movie appearances including *Arizona Dream,* in which he co-starred with Johnny Depp. Jerry has five sons, a daughter, and seven grandchildren from his two marriages.

The Stooge (1951)
Scared Stiff (1953)
Artists and Models (1955)
Hollywood or Bust (1956)
The Geisha Boy (1958)
Li'l Abner (1959)
The Bellboy (1960)
The Ladies' Man (1961)
The Nutty Professor (1963)
The Disorderly Orderly (1964)
The Patsy (1964)
Three on a Couch (1966)
Silent Treatment (1968)
The King of Comedy (1982)
Arizona Dream (1993)
Funny Bones (1995)

Juliette **Lewis**
5ft 6in
(JULIETTE LEWIS)

Born: **June 21, 1973**
Los Angeles, California, USA

The daughter of actor Geoffrey Lewis and his wife Glenis, who is a graphic designer. Juliette was only two when they divorced, but she grew up with show business ambitions. She was fourteen, when she played the part of Maty, in the TV film, 'Home Fires'. A year later, she made her movie debut, with a small role in *My Stepmother Is an Alien*. She was third-billed after Chevy Chase and Beverly D'Angelo, in the best of the National Lampoon series – *Christmas Vacation*, but it was *Cape Fear* that turned her into a future star. She was Oscar nominated as Best Supporting Actress – the result of which was that throughout the 1990s she was seen regularly in good and interesting films. In 1999, she married professional skateboarder, Stephen Berra, but they were divorced five years later. In 2001, Juliette was nominated for an Emmy for her starring role in the television drama, 'My Louisiana Sky'. She is the lead singer in the rock band called "Juliette and the Licks" which has released several recordings. In June 2006, she appeared at the Apollo Theater in London, in "Fool for Love" – taking time off to sing with her band at the Hyde Park Festival. Juliette's new film, *Whip It!* co-stars Ellen Page and is directed by Drew Barrymore.

Christmas Vacation (1989)
Cape Fear (1991)
Husbands and Wives (1992)
Kalifornia (1993)
What's Eating Gilbert Grape (1993)
Natural Born Killers (1994)
From Dusk till Dawn (1995)
Strange Days (1995)
The Evening Star (1996)
Some Girls (1998)
Gaudi Afternoon (2001)
Old School (2003)
Starsky and Hutch (2004)
Aurora Borealis (2005)
The Darwin Awards (2006)
Grilled (2006)
Catch and Release (2006)
Whip It! (2009)

Gong **Li**
5ft 7in
(GONG LI)

Born: **December 31, 1965**
Shenyang, China

Gong was the fifth child of an economics professor and his wife – who worked as a teacher. She was raised and went to school, in Jinan – the capital of Shandong Province. After leaving school at eighteen, she decided to become an actress. She was accepted at Beijing Central College of Drama, from where she graduated after four years of study. Gong was still finishing her studies when Yimou Zhang cast her in the leading role, in the war drama, *Red Sorghum*, which marked his directorial debut. The two combined their talents in further films including *Ju Dou*, and his Oscar-nominated, *Raise the Red Lantern*. After that, Gong was named Best Actress at the Venice Film Festival, for the comedy drama, *The Story of Qui Ju*. She was then recognized in North America, with a Best Supporting Actress Award from NTFCC, for *Farewell My Concubine*, and shared a Best Actress Award, from the Montréal World Film Festival, for *Breaking the Silence*. Following *Memoirs of a Geisha*, she worked stateside, in *Miami Vice*. Gong was married to a tobacco company executive, but they are now separated.

Red Sorghum (1987)
The Empress Dowager (1989)
A Terra-Cotta Warrior (1990)
Ju Dou (1990) Back to Shanghai (1991)
Raise the Red Lantern (1991)
The Story of Qui Ju (1992)
Awakening (1992) Farewell My
Concubine (1993) Flirting Scholar (1993)
Soul of a Painter (1994)
To Live (1994) The Great
Conqueror's Concubine (1994)
Shanghai Triad (1995)
Temptress Moon (1996)
Chinese Box (1997) The Assassin (1998)
Breaking the Silence (2000)
Zhou Yu's Train (2002)
2046 (2004) Eros (2004)
Memoirs of a Geisha (2005)
Miami Vice (2006)
Curse of the Golden Flower (2006)
Hannibal Rising (2007)
Shanghai (2008)

Viveca **Lindfors**
5ft 4in
(ELSA VIVECA TORSTENSDOTTER LINDFORS)

Born: **December 29, 1920**
Uppsala, Sweden
Died: **November 25, 1995**

Viveca was brought up in a comfortable home by her father, Torsten, and mother, Karin. Viveca completed her secondary education at sixteen, and left home in 1937, to study acting at the Royal Dramatic Theater in Stockholm. Following a short period of stage work she made her film debut in 1940, in *Snurriga Familjen*. For six years, throughout World War II, she appeared on the Swedish stage and occasionally in films. The best of them was in 1945, when she starred in *Maria På Kvarngåden*, for her home town-born director, Arne Mattsson. In 1946, she moved to Hollywood, when Warner Bros offered her a contract in the hope that she would be another Garbo or Bergman. She wasn't. She then divorced her second husband, Folke Rogard, and after her Hollywood film debut, in *To the Victor*, in 1948, and co-starring with Errol Flynn, in *Don Juan*, she married the young director, Don Siegel. He directed her in *Night Unto Night* – which co-starred Ronald Reagan. Viveca kept busy both on TV and in films and turned her hand to directing in 1987, with *Unfinished Business*. Viveca went on working until the year she died – at her home in Uppsala – from complications linked to rheumatoid arthritis.

Adventures of Don Juan (1948)
Backfire (1950)
No Sad Songs for Me (1950)
Dark City (1950)
Die Vier im Jeep (1951)
Moonfleet (1955)
Run for Cover (1956)
I Accuse! (1958)
King of Kings (1961)
The Damned (1963)
Sylvia (1965) Brainstorm (1965)
Coming Apart (1969)
The Way We Were (1973)
Welcome to LA (1976)
A Wedding (1978)
The Linguini Incident (1991)
Stargate (1994)
Last Summer in the Hamptons (1995)

Margaret **Lindsay**
5ft 5in
(MARGARET KIES)

Born: **September 19, 1910**
Dubuque, Iowa, USA
Died: **May 9, 1981**

Margaret was the daughter of Catholic parents. She was the eldest of five children – one of whom was a boy. Their father was a pharmacist. While attending Visitation Convent, near Saint Paul, Minnesota, Margaret was regarded as a tomboy – climbing trees and throwing stones. To turn her into a lady, her parents sent her to the Catholic girls' finishing school, National Park Seminary, in Washington, D.C. When she left there, Margaret decided on a stage career. She persuaded her parents that it was her dream, so they financed her acting studies at the American Academy of Dramatic Arts. In the early 1930s, after her movie debut in a 1932 drama, *Okay, America!* and then acting in a Tom Mix western, she went to England to gain stage experience. She got a role in the Oscar-winning film, *Cavalcade,* because she was able to pass as English. Warners signed her, and her Hollywood career took off. Margaret was admired by men but she never married. She died in Los Angeles, of emphysema.

Cavalcade (1933)
Private Detective 62 (1933)
Baby Face (1933) Voltaire (1933)
Captured! (1933)
The World Changes (1933)
The House on 56th Street (1933)
Lady Killer (1933)
Merry Wives of Reno (1934)
Fog Over Frisco (1934)
The Dragon Murder Case (1934)
Bordertown (1935)
Devil Dogs of the Air (1935)
The Case of the Curious Bride (1935)
'G' Men (1935) Personal Maid's
Secret (1935) Frisco Kid (1935)
Dangerous (1935) Green Light (1937)
Back in Circulation (1937)
Jezebel (1938)
When Were You Born (1938)
Garden of the Moon (1938)
The House of the Seven
Gables (1940) The Spoilers (1942)
Scarlet Street (1945)

Laura **Linney**
5ft 7in
(LAURA LEGGETT LINNEY)

Born: **February 5, 1964**
New York City, New York, USA

Laura's mother, Ann Leggett, was a nurse at the Memorial Sloan-Kettering Cancer Center in New York City. Laura was born into a well-known theatrical family – her father being the prolific playwright and novelist, Romulus Linney. Her parents divorced when she young but Laura kept up the contact with her dad. She was a graduate of Northfield Mount Hermon School, in Massachusetts, in 1982. She then attended Northwestern University before earning a Bachelor of Arts degree from Brown University, four years later. After deciding on an acting career, she went to Juilliard, and the Arts Theater School, in Moscow. In New York, she appeared on Broadway with positive reviews for her work in "Hedda Gabler" and "Six Degrees of Separation". Laura made her film debut in 1992, with a small role in *Lorenzo's Oil.* Her movie career advanced swiftly. She was nominated for Best Actress Oscars for *You Can Count on Me, Kinsey,* and *The Savages,* and as Best Supporting Actress, for *Kinsey.* Laura divorced David Adkins, in 2002, and in August 2007, she became engaged to a real estate agent, Marc Schauer.

Dave (1993)
A Simple Twist of Fate (1994)
Primal Fear (1996)
Absolute Power (1997)
The Truman Show (1998)
You Can Count on Me (2000)
The House of Mirth (2000) Maze (2000)
The Laramie Project (2002)
The Life of David Gale (2003)
Mystic River (2003) Love Actually (2003)
P.S. (2004) Kinsey (2004)
The Squid and the Whale (2005)
The Exorcism of Emily Rose (2005)
Driving Lessons (2006)
Jindabyne (2006)
Man of the Year (2006)
The Savages (2007) Breach (2007)
The Nanny Diaries (2007)
The City of Your Final
Destination (2007)
The Other Man (2008)

Ray **Liotta**
6ft
(RAYMOND LIOTTA)

Born: **December 18, 1954**
Newark, New Jersey, USA

Ray was adopted by Alfred and Mary Liotta, from a Newark, New Jersey, orphanage, when he was six months old. The couple were the owners of a chain of automotive-supply stores – so Ray and another adoptee, a sister, Linda Ontario, lived their early years in a comfortable home. Ray was a bright boy, who after graduating from Union High School, went on to the University of Miami, where he studied acting. While he was there, he befriended Steven Bauer, and they both benefited from some healthy on-stage competition. Ray's first few years as a professional actor were spent in a number of television-series such as 'Another World' and 'St. Elsewhere. In 1983, he made his movie debut, in *The Lonely Lady* – which didn't get nominated for an Oscar. In 1986, he was able to take some pride in having acted in *Something Wild.* Since then, he has had a pretty good ratio of worthwhile movies. *Goodfellas* being the kind of film any actor would be happy to have on his cv. In 2004, Ray's seven year marriage to the producer/actress, Michelle Grace came to an end. They first met while appearing in the made-for-television movie, 'The Rat Pack' and have a young daughter named Karsen

Something Wild (1986)
Dominick and Eugene (1988)
Field of Dreams (1989)
Goodfellas (1990)
Unlawful Entry (1992)
Operation Dumbo Drop (1995)
Cop Land (1997)
Turbulence (1997)
Phoenix (1998)
A Rumor of Angels (2000)
Hannibal (2001)
Heartbreakers (2001)
Blow (2001) Identity (2003)
Control (2004) Revolver (2005)
Local Color (2006)
Smokin' Aces (2006)
Battle in Seattle (2007)
Hero Wanted (2008)
Chasing 3000 (2008)

Virna **Lisi**
5ft 5in
(VIRNA LISA PIERALISI)

Born: **September 8, 1937**
Ancona, Marche, Italy

After leaving school, Virna studied at a technical and business college. She was discovered by the film director, Francesco Maselli, and gave up any thoughts of a secretarial career. Virna made her screen debut in 1953, in *La Corda d'aciaio*. Following a number of small parts, her first starring role came three years later, in *La Donna del Giorno*. She built up a big fan base in Europe during the late 1950s, and in 1960, she married the industrialist, Franco Pesci. Virna starred regularly in Italian films, but had to wait until 1965 before she was given her first Hollywood role, in the comedy, *How to Murder Your Wife*, starring Jack Lemmon and Terry-Thomas. She won a César and a Cannes Film Festival Award, for her portrayal of Catherine de Medici, in *La Reine Margot*. Virna has limited her film appearances in subsequent years, but she has been very active on Italian television since the start of the millennium, and was in an episode of 'Fidati de me', as recently as 2008.

La Donna del giorno (1956)
Totò, Peppino e le fanatiche (1958)
Sua Eccellenza si fermò
a mangiare (1961)
Eva (1962)
Les Bonnes causes (1963)
La Tulipe noire (1964)
Signore & signori (1965)
La Donna del largo (1965)
How to Murder Your Wife (1965)
Le Bambole (1965)
Casanova '70 (1965)
Made in Italy (1965)
Una Vergine per il principe (1966)
Not with My Wife,
You Don't! (1966)
La Vingt-cinquième heure (1967)
The Secret of
Santa Vittoria (1969)
Un beau monstre (1971)
The Serpent (1973)
Beyond Good and Evil (1977)
Ernesto (1979)
La Reine Margot (1994)
The Best Day of My Life (2002)

John **Lithgow**
6ft 4in
(JOHN ARTHUR LITHGOW)

Born: **October 19, 1945**
Rochester, New York, USA

The Lithgows were a somewhat nomadic family until John's father, Arthur, was hired to run the McCarter Theater, in Princeton, New Jersey. John attended Princeton High School. Although growing up with acting in his blood – his mother, Sarah Jane, had been an actress – it wasn't until Harvard University, when he appeared in a performance of Gilbert and Sullivan's, "Utopia Limited" that he gave the idea of a thespian career any serious thought. John then won a Fulbright Scholarship to study at the London Academy of Music and Dramatic Art. In 1972, he made his film debut, in *Dealing: Or the Berkeley-to-Boston Forty-Brick Lost-Bag Blues*. A year after that, he was on Broadway, in "The Changing Room" – winning a Tony Award and a Drama Desk Award as 'Best Featured Actor in a Play'. John's stage successes continued, and in the 1980s, he made a big impression in movies – with Best Supporting Actor Oscar nominations – for *The World According to Garp* and *Terms of Endearment*. From 1996, he was a famous face on television, in '3rd Rock from the Sun'. John's most recent movie role was a small supporting one, in *Dreamgirls*. He has three children from his two marriages. His second wife is Mary Yeager. They have a son and a daughter.

Obsession (1976)
The Big Fix (1978)
Rich Kids (1979)
All That Jazz (1979)
Blow Out (1981)
The World According to Garp (1982)
Terms of Endearment (1983)
2010 (1984)
Memphis Belle (1990)
Ricochet (1991)
At Play in the Fields of the
Lord (1991) Cliffhanger (1993)
The Pelican Brief (1993)
A Civil Action (1998)
Orange County (2002)
The Life and Death of Peter
Sellers (2004) Kinsey (2004)
Dreamgirls (2006)

Roger **Livesey**
5ft 11½in
(ROGER LIVESEY)

Born: **June 25, 1906**
Barry, Wales
Died: **February 4, 1976**

Roger's parents were Sam and Mary Livesey. Sam was very well known on the West End stage and in the British cinema – where he appeared in films until 1937. He also ran a travelling theater booth. Roger attended the Italia Conti School and made his stage debut when he was twelve, in "Loyalty" at St. James's Theater, in London. He completed his education at Westminster City School, and had his first credited film role when he was fifteen, in an early version of *The Four Feathers*. In 1931, after more stage experience, Roger made his talkie debut in *East Lynne on the Western Front*. During the 1930s, he became an important stage actor in London – often appearing with his wife, Ursula Jeans. His first major film role was in the fine Alexander Korda production of *Rembrandt*. That same year he made his Broadway debut, in "The Country Wife". At the outbreak of World War II, he was too old to join the R.A.F., so he worked in an Aircraft factory. His movie fame was established when he played the lead in Michael Powell's *The Life and Death of Colonel Blimp*, and made absolute with three more excellent roles in the 1940s. Roger continued his stage work and made his final movie appearance, in the Ronnie Barker comedy, *Futtock's End*. In 1975, he was featured in the television series, 'The Pallisers'. Ursula died in 1973. Three years later, Roger died of bowel cancer, at his home in Watford, Hertfordshire.

Rembrandt (1936)
The Drum (1938)
The Girl in the News (1940)
The Life and Death of
Colonel Blimp (1943)
I Know Where I'm Going (1945)
A Matter of Life and Death (1946)
Vice Verse (1947)
That Dangerous Age (1949)
The Master of Ballantrae (1953)
The League of Gentlemen (1960)
The Entertainer (1960)
Hamlet (1969)

Harold **Lloyd**
5ft 10in
(HAROLD CLAYTON LLOYD)

Born: **April 20, 1893**
Burchard, Nebraska, USA
Died: **March 8, 1971**

Harold's parents were James and Elizabeth Lloyd. His paternal grandparents were Welsh. Harold made his stage debut at the age of twelve, in "Tess of the D'Urbervilles" – with the Burwood Stock company of Omaha. The Lloyds lived for a while in Denver, Colorado, where Harold attended high school. When his father was awarded substantial damages of $6000, in a personal injury case, they re-located to California. Harold completed his education, at San Diego High School. In 1913, he began his movie career with an uncredited role in that year's, *The Old Monk's Tale,* for the locally-based Edison Company. He joined Hal Roach, and by 1915, starred in the popular "Lonesome Luke" series – comprising over fifty, two-reelers. After a very passionate affair with his co-star, Bebe Daniels, ended, Harold fell for another film actress, Mildred Davis. She was his wife until her death forty-six years later. Harold's silent film career went from strength to strength and from around the mid-1920s, he made a number of comedy classics, which I've included in the list below. Harold's first talkie, in 1929 – *Welcome Danger,* was poor by compar-ison, but he soon found his *Feet First.* Harold retired in 1938, produced a couple of loss-making films, then made a come-back, for Preston Sturges, in *The Sin of Harold Diddlebock.* In 1962, he produced a compilation of his films, titled *Harold Lloyd's World of Comedy.* He died of prostate cancer, in Beverly Hills.

Girl Shy (1924)
Hot Water (1924)
The Freshman (1925)
For Heaven's Sake (1926)
The Kid Brother (1927)
Speedy (1928) **Feet First** (1930)
Movie Crazy (1932)
The Cat's-Paw (1934)
The Milky Way (1936)
Professor Beware (1938)
**The Sin of Harold
Diddlebock** (1947)

Sondra **Locke**
5ft 4in
(SONDRA LOCKE)

Born: **May 28, 1947**
Shelbyville, Tennessee, USA

Sondra grew up in a small town, with no idea of what was waiting for her in the world outside. She was very pretty, but her acting experience, when she graduated from Shelbyville Central High School, was limited. Sondra spent one year at Middle Tennessee State University – dropping out to concentrate on an acting career. The first surprise of her life was when, after a nationwide talent search, she was chosen by Warner Bros to appear in the film, *The Heart is a Lonely Hunter.* She married her sweetheart, Gordon Anderson, before shooting began, and there was further joy when she was nominated for a Best Supporting Actress Oscar. TV and more movies followed, including the very good horror film, *Willard.* But there was a tricky domestic problem for Sondra to solve when Gordon suddenly discovered that he was gay. Sondra then began a twelve-year relationship with Clint Eastwood and co-starred in six of his films – most notably *The Outlaw Josey Wales.* The end of the affair was ugly. His lawyer told her that the locks to the house they were living in had been changed. Her possessions were awaiting collection outside. It wasn't all bad: Clint's Malpaso company put up the money for her directorial debut – *Ratboy,* in 1986. After seeking compensation from both Eastwood and Warners – who had reneged on a directing deal, she settled out of court. Sondra's last film was *The Prophet's Game,* in 1999. Nowadays, she lives in the Hollywood Hills, with Scott Cunneen, a director of surgery at Cedars Sinai Hospital.

**The Heart is a
Lonely Hunter** (1968)
Willard (1971)
A Reflection of Fear (1973)
Death Game (1976)
The Outlaw Josey Wales (1976)
The Gauntlet (1977)
**Every Which Way
But Loose** (1978)
Bronco Billy (1980)
Sudden Impact (1983)

Gene **Lockhart**
5ft 6½in
(EUGENE LOCKHART)

Born: **July 18, 1891**
London, Ontario, Canada
Died: **March 31, 1957**

Gene was six when he made his stage debut. When he was fifteen, he acted in sketches with the famous Beatrice Lillie. He played professional football for the Toronto Argonauts, before he made his Broadway debut, in 1916, in a musical called "The Riviera Girl". In 1919, Gene wrote the lyrics to the song, 'The World Is Waiting for the Sunrise' – music by Ernest Seitz, a composer from Toronto. Gene was a good enough singer to appear in "Die Fledermaus' with the San Francisco Opera Association. Gene made his film debut, in 1922, in *Smilin' Through,* but spent the next twelve years appearing in plays. In 1924, he married the English actress, Kathleen Arthur, whom he acted with in films as well as on the stage. He began to concentrate on film work from 1934 onwards – he and his wife played Mr and Mrs Bob Cratchit, in *A Christmas Carol.* Gene was extremely versatile – playing contrasting characters in films before becoming a regular on TV, from 1950. His final film, *Jeanne Eagels,* was released after he died of coronary throm-bosis, in Santa Monica, California.

Of Human Hearts (1938)
Algiers (1938) **A Christmas
Carol** (1938) **His Girl Friday** (1939)
A Dispatch from Reuters (1940)
Daniel and the Devil (1941)
They Died with Their Boots On (1941)
Mission to Moscow (1943)
Northern Pursuit (1943)
Going My Way (1944)
The House on 92nd Street (1945)
Leave Her to Heaven (1945)
Miracle on 34th Street (1947)
Apartment for Peggy (1948)
Down to the Sea in Ships (1949)
The Inspector General (1949)
Madame Bovary (1949)
**I'd Climb the
Highest Mountain** (1951)
Androcles and the Lion (1952)
Carousel (1956) **The Man in the Gray
Flannel Suit** (1956)

Margaret **Lockwood**
5ft 5in
(MARGARET MARY LOCKWOOD DAY)

Born: **September 15, 1916**
Karachi, British India
Died: **July 15, 1990**

Margaret's father was a chief operating engineer, on the Indian North Eastern Railway. When she was two, she went back to England with her mother, who was Scottish. At Sydenham Girls' High School, Margaret appeared in plays and discarded an early ambition to become a missionary, by going to London and making her stage debut, aged twelve, in "A Midsummer Night's Dream". She studied drama at the Italia Conti School and the Royal Academy of Dramatic Art. Her first film appearance was in 1934, in *Lorna Doone*. A British Lion contract followed and in 1935, she co-starred with Maurice Chevalier, in *The Beloved Vagabond*. After a loan out for *Dr. Syn*, Gainsborough bought her contract. In 1937, she married Rupert de Leon and had a daughter. A Hitchcock film, *The Lady Vanishes*, propelled her towards Hollywood. It wasn't a happy stay – she made one movie with Shirley Temple and another with Douglas Fairbanks Jr., before going home. She was elevated to stardom in Britain at least, by way of *The Man in Grey*, and by 1946, was the U.K.'s top female star at the box-office. In the space of about six years, that stardust disappeared. She was seen on the stage and television, and made her final film appearance, in *The Slipper and the Rose*. Margaret was a virtual recluse when she died in Kensington, West London, of cirrhosis of the liver.

Bank Holiday (1938)
The Lady Vanishes (1938)
Susannah of the Mounties (1939)
The Stars Look Down (1940)
Girl in the News (1940)
Night Train to Munich (1940)
The Man in Grey (1943)
Love Story (1944)
A Place of One's Own (1945)
The Wicked Lady (1945)
Jassy (1947)
Trent's Last Case (1952)
Cast a Dark Shadow (1955)
The Slipper and the Rose (1976)

John **Loder**
6ft 3in
(JOHN MUIR LOWE)

Born: **January 3, 1898**
London, England
Died: **December 26, 1988**

John's father, General Lowe, was the British officer whom Patrick Pearse (leader of the Easter rising in Dublin) surrendered to in 1916. Like most young men from his background, John was expected to follow his father with an army career. Leaving Eton College, he went to the Royal Military College, and then served with the 15th Hussars. John was captured by the Germans in Galipoli, and upon his release, remained in Germany – running a pickle factory and appearing in small roles in German films. A short visit to England convinced him that Hollywood – at the birth of the talkies – was the place to be. He was in Paramount's first talking picture, *The Doctor's Secret,* but he was too English for American audiences. He returned home and found regular work in movies, including Alfred Hitchcock's *Sabotage.* At the outbreak of World War II, John had another crack at Hollywood where, apart from enjoying a long career as a supporting player, he became a United States citizen, in 1947, after he'd had two children with Hedy Lamarr. John made his last movie, *The Firechasers,* in 1971, and then retired to a ranch owned by his fifth wife, Alba Julia Lagomarsino, an Argentinian heiress. John wrote an autobiography called "Hollywood Hussar". He died from natural causes, at his home in Selbourne, England.

Lorna Doone (1934)
Java Head (1935)
The Man Who Changed
His Mind (1936)
Sabotage (1936)
Dr.Syn (1937)
Owd Bob (1938)
Confirm or Deny (1941)
How Green Was My Valley (1941)
Gentleman Jim (1942)
Old Acquaintance (1943)
The Brighton Strangler (1945)
Dishonored Lady (1947)
The Story of Esther Costello (1957)
Gideon's Day (1958)

Robert **Loggia**
5ft 10in
(SALVATORE LOGGIA)

Born: **January 3, 1930**
New York City, New York, USA

Robert was the son of Benjamin Loggia, an Italian shoemaker, and his wife, Elena. Surprisingly, Robert grew up to be a very serious scholar and loved reading. Just to balance things nicely, he also developed a liking for physical exercise while at high school. He studied Journalism at the University of Missouri, but before he left, he'd caught the acting bug. After serving in the U.S. Army for two years, he studied at the Actors' Studio, in New York. He appeared in numerous stage productions up until 1956, when he decided to give Hollywood a try. Robert made a brief appearance in *Somebody Up There Likes Me,* which was followed by a featured role in *The Garment Jungle.* In 1958, Robert starred in the Walt Disney TV-series, 'The Nine Lives of Elfego Baca'. In fact, most of his work in the 1960s was on television – and the bulk of it was aimed at younger audiences, such as in 1966 – when he played the cool, acrobatic, Thomas Hewitt Edward Cat – 'T.H.E. Cat' for short. Unfortunately it only ran for one season and Robert was back to playing character roles on TV and in films without his name being known. In 1985, Robert's career was given a boost by an Oscar-nominated performance – in *Jagged Edge.* It led to more appearances in films of the caliber of *Prizzi's Honor* and *Independence Day.* In his private life, Robert is the father of four children from his two marriages.

The Garment Jungle (1957)
The Ninth Configuration (1980)
S.O.B. (1981)
An Officer and a Gentleman (1982)
Scarface (1983) Jagged Edge (1985)
Prizzi's Honor (1985) Big (1988)
Triumph of the Spirit (1989)
Coldblooded (1995)
Independence Day (1996)
The Proposition (1998)
Wide Awake (1998)
Return to Me (2000)
All Over Again (2001)
The Deal (2005)
Her Morbid Desires (2008)

Lindsay **Lohan**
5ft 5in
(LINDSAY DEE LOHAN)

Born: July 2, 1986
New York City, New York, USA

Lindsay's folks, Michael and Dina Lohan, were both financial experts in the days when the profession carried respect. Her father was a Wall Street trader, and her mother had been a Wall Street analyst, before becoming Lindsay's manager. Lindsay is the oldest of four children. She always got on well with her two brothers, Michael Jr. and Dakota, and her sister, Ali. When she was three years old, she became a Ford model. In a few years, she appeared in more than sixty television commercials, including spots for Pizza Hut, The Gap, Wendy's, and Jell-O – in a spot which featured Bill Cosby. In 1992, at Halloween, she dressed up as "garbage" for a sketch on 'Late Night with David Letterman'. Lindsay's professional acting debut was in 1996, as Ali Fowler, in the TV drama, 'Another World'. Her first feature film was for Walt Disney Pictures (in the Hayley Mills role) in a remake of their 1961 hit, *The Parent Trap.* The new version was successful – Lindsay receiving critical acclaim and an award for Best Leading Young Actress. She attended Cold Spring Harbor School on Long Island until, after her family moved to Merrick, she transferred to Sanford H. Calhoun High School. In 2002, she began a recording career with help from Emilio Estefan Jr. and made two rock albums for Casablanca/Universal – the first of which was called "Speak". Her first single release was "Rumors". Films such as *Mean Girls, Bobby,* and *Chapter 27,* have helped to keep her name in the spotlight. But there's been a price to pay: Lindsay's 100% effort in everything she does has resulted in burn out and two spells in hospital.

The Parent Trap (1998)
Freaky Friday (2003)
Mean Girls (2004)
Herbie Fully Loaded (2005)
A Prairie Home
Companion (2006)
Bobby (2006)
Chapter 27 (2007)
Georgia Rule (2007)

Alison **Lohman**
5ft 2in
(ALISON MARION LOHMAN)

Born: September 18, 1979
Palm Springs, California, USA

Alison's father, Gary Lohman, was an architect. Her mother Diane, owned and ran a bakery. She has a younger brother named Robert. Although there were no show business connections, because of where she grew up, she was breathing the same air as some of the celebrities in the industry. When she was nine, she had her first taste of performing in front of an audience when she played Gretl, on stage, in "The Sound of Music", at Palm Desert's McCallum Theater. In 1990, Alison was voted the Desert Theater League's 'Most Outstanding Actress in a Musical', for her performance in "Annie". By the time she was seventeen, she'd worked as a backing singer for Sinatra. After graduating from high school in 1997, she headed for Los Angeles. Her movie debut was in *Kraa! The Sea Monster,* in 1998, but with her heart set on something artistically more demanding, she went to London to study at RADA. She continued to work in other rather forgettable projects until *The Thirteenth Floor.* Alison's big break came with *White Oleander,* but her important year was 2003, when she appeared in two high-profile films – *Matchstick Men* with Nicolas Cage, and the massive hit, *Big Fish.* She was voted 'Supporting Actress of the Year' at the Hollywood Film Festival and 'Superstar of Tomorrow' at the Young Hollywood Awards. Two recent releases – *Things We Lost in the Fire* and *Beowulf* will help turn that promise into reality. Alison can be seen in the Sci-Fi thriller, *Game.*

The Thirteenth Floor (1999)
Delivering Milo (2001)
Alex in Wonder (2001)
White Oleander (2002)
Matchstick Men (2003)
Big Fish (2003)
Where the Truth Lies (2005)
The Big White (2005)
Delirious (2006)
Flicka (2006)
Things We Lost in the Fire (2007)
Beowulf (2007)
Game (2009)

Gina **Lollobrigida**
5ft 5in
(LUIGINA LOLLOBRIGIDA)

Born: July 4, 1927
Subiaco, Lazio, Rome, Italy

One of six children born to a carpenter and his wife, Gina and her family lived in a cramped, one-bedroom apartment in the hillside town of Subiaco. At school she was bright enough to win a scholarship to a college, where she studied commercial art. One day, she was spotted by a talent scout as she was walking along the street. A test at Cinecittà studios, just outside Rome, and an uncredited appearance in *Lucia di Lammermoor,* resulted in her film debut, in 1946, in a big screen version of the opera, *Elisir d'Amore* – starring the great Italian baritone, Tito Gobbi. After finishing third in the 1947 "Miss Italy" contest, Gina (her voice dubbed) starred with Gobbi in two more opera films, before she showed what was to follow, in *The Bride Can't Wait,* in 1949. At that time, her films weren't seen outside her own country. She married a Yugoslav refugee, Dr. Milko Skofic, who took some glamour shots of her for magazines. They interested RKO, who brought her to Hollywood, but it was Howard Hughes who signed Gina, on a seven-year contract. He had nothing to offer her, but wouldn't let her make any films in the USA. She made one in France – *Fanfan la Tulipe,* and appeared with Bogart in *Beat the Devil,* but it was the Italian, *Bread, Love and Dreams, which* brought her fame. Her marriage ended in 1966. In the 1970s, she gave up making films to concentrate on photography.

Fanfan la Tulipe (1951)
Les Belles de Nuit (1952)
Beat the Devil (1953)
Bread, Love and
Dreams (1953)
Trapeze (1956)
La Legge (1959)
Come September (1961)
Woman of Straw (1964)
Le Bambole (1965)
Le Piacevoli notti (1966)
Hotel Paradiso (1966)
Buona Sera, Mrs Campbell (1968)
Un Bellissimo Novembre (1969)
King, Queen, Knave (1972)

Herbert **Lom**
5ft 9¼in
(HERBERT CHARLES ANGELO K. SCHLUDERPACHERU)

Born: September 11, 1917
Prague, Czech Republic

Herbert was from a privileged background – receiving the very best in education and earning a degree from Prague University. In 1937, he made his film debut for the Slavia Film Studio, in *Zena pod krízem,* but with war clouds threatening he moved to London, where he improved his English and completed his stage education at the Old Vic and London Embassy. In 1942, Herbert made his English-language film debut, as Napoleon, in *The Young Mr. Pitt.* His accent and 'foreign' appearance got him a lot of work – usually in supporting roles, where he was often sinister. Herbert first came to international prominence in the classic Ealing comedy, *The Ladykillers,* which starred Alec Guinness. One of his co-stars in that film – Peter Sellers, was instrumental in taking him to lasting fame, starting in 1961, with a good role in a film Peter directed, called *Mr. Topaze.* He then secured it, in the *Pink Panther* series, from *A Shot in the Dark* onwards, where Herbert played Inspector Dreyfus. Herbert was married to Dina Schea, from 1948 until their divorce in 1971. His recent films were failures. His last appearance was on British television in 2004, in 'The Murder at the Vicarage'.

Hotel Reserve (1944)
The Seventh Veil (1945)
Dual Alibi (1946)
Good-Time Girl (1948)
Night and the City (1950)
State Secret (1950)
The Ladykillers (1955)
War and Peace (1956)
Hell Drivers (1957)
Chase a Crooked
Shadow (1958)
I Accuse! (1958)
North West Frontier (1959)
Spartacus (1960)
A Shot in the Dark (1964)
The Return of the
Pink Panther (1975)
The Pink Panther
Strikes Again (1976)
Hopscotch (1980)

Carole **Lombard**
5ft 2in
(JANE ALICE PETERS)

Born: October 6, 1908
Fort Wayne, Indiana, USA
Died: January 16, 1942

Carole's parents were Frederick Peters, who was of German stock, and his wife, Elizabeth, whose ancestors emigrated from England in 1634. After they divorced, her mother took Carole and her two older brothers to live in Los Angeles. Carole was twelve when she was spotted by the director, Allan Dwan and given her first film role, in *A Perfect Crime.* She went from high school to acting classes – landing a contract with Fox – and changing her name. An automobile accident put her out of action for more than a year and the contract was torn up. She returned, in Mack Sennett two-reelers. Her first all-talkie – in 1929, was *High Voltage,* which co-starred the future 'Hopalong Cassidy' – William Boyd. In 1931, after securing a Paramount contract, Carole co-starred in *Man of the World,* with William Powell – and married him a year later. She wasn't satisfied with her work and kept on at the studio to give her better parts. It was a combination of the popularity of 'screwball comedies' – from the mid-1930s onwards, and competition from Colbert, Arthur, and Dunne, which forced Carole to grab the opportunities she needed. They were to be found at other studios: Three of the genre – *Twentieth Century, My Man Godfrey* and *Nothing Sacred,* are all-time classics. She married her second husband, Clark Gable in 1939. He was heartbroken and never really recovered, after Carole was killed in a plane crash, on Table Rock Mountain, Nevada, when she was traveling back home to see him after taking part in a War bond rally.

We're Not Dressing (1934)
Twentieth Century (1934)
Hands Across the Table (1935)
My Man Godfrey (1936)
Nothing Sacred (1937)
True Confession (1937)
In Name Only (1939)
Vigil in the Night (1940)
Mr. and Mrs. Smith (1941)
To Be or Not to Be (1942)

Julie **London**
5ft 5in
(GAYLE PECK)

Born: September 26, 1926
Santa Rosa, California, USA
Died: October 18, 2000

Julie was the daughter of a successful vaudeville song-and-dance team – Jack and Josephine Peck. She completed her junior schooling in Santa Rosa, but when she was fourteen, she moved with her parents, to Los Angeles. Julie finished her education at the Hollywood Professional School and when she was eighteen, while working part-time as an elevator operator, she was discovered by the talent agent, Sue Carol. In 1944, Julie made her movie debut – as Buster Crabbe's co-star, in a jungle adventure called *Nabonga.* Julie looked great, but the film was not. It was followed by minor parts in four films. Then, in 1947, she not only appeared in a good movie, *The Red House,* she married the actor, Jack Webb. They both shared a love of jazz and she often got up to sing a number when they visited night-clubs. Their six years together produced two daughters. Following her divorce, Julie disappeared from the movie scene for a while, but from the mid-1950s, she was seen in several movies, including the excellent *Man of the West* – opposite Gary Cooper. Apart from acting, Julie began to develop as a very appealing singer. With encouragement from second husband, composer/musician, Bobby Troup, she recorded a number of smooth jazz albums and a hit single, "Cry Me a River". They remained together until his death in 1999. Julie herself had suffered a stroke four years earlier and was in quite poor health until her death at her home in Encino, California, after a fatal stroke.

The Red House (1947)
Tap Roots (1948) Task Force (1949)
The Great Man (1956)
Drango (1957)
Saddle the Wind (1958)
A Question of Adultery (1958)
Voice in the Mirror (1958)
Man of the West (1958)
The Wonderful Country (1959)
The 3rd Voice (1960)
The George Raft Story (1961)

Jennifer **Lopez**
5ft 6in
(JENNIFER LYNN LÓPEZ)

Born: July 24, 1969
The Bronx, New York City, New York, USA

Jennifer was the second of three daughters born to David Lopez, a computer specialist, and his wife, Guadalupe, who was a kindergarten teacher. Both were from Puerto Rico. Jennifer grew up in the Castle Hill section of the Bronx. It was a very musical family and she took singing lessons from the age of five. Jennifer was educated at Catholic schools and at high school she excelled at softball, tennis and gymnastics. She left home when she was eighteen to pursue a show business career – making her film debut in 1987, in *My Little Girl*. In 1990, Jennifer appeared in the first of 16 episodes of the TV-series, 'In Living Color' and went to live in Los Angeles. She danced in Janet Jackson's shows and videos, including "That's The way Love Goes". She also worked on rap artists' videos and was a backup dancer for "New Kids on the Block". There was plenty of TV work, so she didn't attempt to act in another movie until 1995. In her first major film, *Blood and Wine* – Jennifer was third-billed below Jack Nicholson. It was quickly followed by *Selena,* which brought her good reviews and an ALMA Award, as Outstanding Actress. Jennifer – known as J-Lo to her friends and admirers, hasn't given up her music. In 2002, she released her third album "This is Me...Then" and she has already sold over 50 million records worldwide. Jennifer's third husband is the actor, Marc Anthony – one of the stars of her recent movie, the salsa celebration, *El Cantante.*

My Family (1995)
Jack (1996)
Blood and Wine (1996)
Selena (1997)
U Turn (1997)
Out of Sight (1998)
The Cell (2000)
Jersey Girl (2004)
Shall We Dance (2004)
Monster-in-Law (2005)
An Unfinished Life (2005)
Bordertown (2006)
El Cantante (2006)

Sergi **López**
5ft 7in
(SERGI LÓPEZ)

Born: December 22, 1965
Vilanova i la Geltrú, Barcelona, Spain

After growing up as a Catalan, in a Spain ruled by a strict dictator, Sergi welcomed the new freedom that came after Franco's death in 1975. By the time he had finished his education, he gravitated towards an acting career. Having been an admirer of French movie-making, he went to Paris to study drama and, by 1991, he was fluent enough in French to look for work. He auditioned for the Peruvian-born director, Manuel Poirier, in Normandy and made his movie debut, in *La Petite amie d'Antonio.* His success in that led to Sergi becoming a big favorite with the director and films like *Marion* and *Western* were good for both men. He was finally appreciated in his own country when he was cast in a Catalan-speaking role, in the drama, *Carícies,* which was directed by another man from Barcelona, Ventura Pons. Sergi began dividing his time between France and Spain and won the 2001 Best Actor César Award for his role as the villain, in the title role, in *Harry Is Here to Help.* An even more important role in terms of international recognition was his pro-Franco Captain Vidal, in *Pan's Labyrinth.* Sergi and his girlfriend have two children.

La Petite amie d'Antonio (1992)
...à la campagne (1995)
Marion (1997) **Western** (1997)
Carícies (1998) **Entre las piernas** (1999)
The New Eve (1999) **Lisboa** (1999)
Une liason pornographique (1999)
Empty Days (1999)
Ataque verbal (1999)
Morir (o no) (2000)
Harry Is Here to Help (2000)
Ten Days Without Love (2001)
Reines d'un jour (2001)
Les Femmes...ou les enfants d'abord... (2002)
Dirty Pretty Things (2002)
Jet Lag (2002)
Janis et John (2003)
Les Mots bleus (2005)
To Paint or Make Love (2005)
Pan's Labyrinth (2006)
La Maison (2007)

Sophia **Loren**
5ft 8½in
(SOFIA VILLANI SCICOLENE)

Born: September 20, 1934
Rome, Lazio, Italy

Sophia was the illegitimate daughter of Riccardo Scicolone and Romilda Villani, in the days when the term carried a great social stigma. Sophia grew up in a poor suburb of Naples, but she had one big advantage over most other girls – she was beautiful. After Sophia had won her first beauty contest, at fourteen, her mother took her to Rome to get her into movies. She became a model for 'photoromanzi' magazines, and starting with *Cuori sul Mare,* in 1950, got dozens of small film roles. She met Carlo Ponti at the "Miss Rome" contest. He changed her name to Loren, but it was Vittorio De Sica, who guided her to international recognition. *The River Girl* in 1955, was dubbed into English and widely shown in the USA and Britain. It got her roles in American films, but they were not as good as Vittorio De Sica's powerful, *Two Women,* which won Sophia a deserved Best Actress Oscar. In 1962, her five-year marriage to Ponti was annulled due to bigamy charges. With his first wife's help, they re-married in 1966, had two children, and were together until his death in 2007. Their son, Edoardo Ponti, who had acted with her in *Aurora,* eighteen years earlier, directed Sophia in *Between Strangers,* which was filmed in Canada in 2002. Sophia plays 'Mamma' in the star studded 2009 release, *Nine.*

Gold of Naples (1954)
Lucky to Be a Woman (1955)
Houseboat (1958)
Heller in Pink Tights (1960)
The Millionairess (1960)
Two Women (1960)
El Cid (1961) **Yesterday, Today and Tomorrow** (1963)
Matrimonio all'Italiana (1964)
Lady L (1965) **Arabesque** (1966)
More than a Miracle (1967)
Ghosts – Italian Style (1967)
Man of La Mancha (1972)
Blood Feud (1978)
Aurora (1984)
Grumpier Old Men (1995)
Between Strangers (2002)

Peter **Lorre**
5ft 5in
(LÁSZLÓ LÖWENSTEIN)

Born: **June 26, 1904**
Rózsahegy, Austro-Hungary
Died: **March 23, 1964**

After an unhappy childhood, Peter ran away from home when he was fifteen to work as a bank clerk. From his wages, he paid for acting lessons in Vienna, and made his stage debut in Zurich. From the age of twenty, he acted in Switzerland, Austria and Germany, but was unknown when Fritz Lang chose him to play the psychotic child killer in M. Being Jewish, Peter fled Germany when the Nazis came to power. First going to London, where he acted in Alfred Hitchcock's The Man Who Knew Too Much. In 1935, he went to Hollywood, where he performed as a character actor as well as the star of the Mr. Moto movies. In 1941, he began a successful screen partnership with the larger than life, Sydney Greenstreet, in The Maltese Falcon. They appeared together in seven other movies. After divorcing his second wife, Kaaren, Peter returned to Germany in 1951, as writer, director and star of Der Verlorene. He put on a lot of weight and was a comical figure in his last years as an actor. Appropriately, his final film was a Jerry Lewis comedy, The Patsy. Peter died of a stroke in Los Angeles.

M (1931) **The Man Who Knew Too Much** (1934)
Crime and Punishment (1935)
Mad Love (1935)
Secret Agent (1936)
Strange Cargo (1940)
Stranger on the Third Floor (1940)
The Maltese Falcon (1941)
All through the Night (1942)
Casablanca (1942)
Background to Danger (1943)
Arsenic and Old Lace (1944)
The Mask of Dimitrious (1944)
The Beast with Five Fingers (1946)
The Chase (1946) **The Verdict** (1946)
Casbah (1948) **Beat the Devil** (1953)
Silk Stockings (1957)
Voyage to the Bottom of the Sea (1961)
The Raven (1963)
The Comedy of Terrors (1964)

Anita **Louise**
5ft 6in
(ANITA LOUISE FREMAULT)

Born: **January 9, 1915**
New York City, New York, USA
Died: **April 25, 1970**

Anita was a child prodigy – making her Broadway debut at the age of six in "Peter Ibbetson". She was a brilliant young pianist – winning five trophies during her course at the Professional Children's School, in New York. She made her film debut in 1924, in The Six Commandments – still using the name Fremault. She became Anita Louise, in 1929, in The Marriage Playground. The transition from child actress, to teenager, to adult, was painless – she was part of the Warner Brothers family. One of Anita's best early adult roles was with the legendary Will Rogers in Judge Priest. She often complained that her beauty prevented her from getting the serious roles she was capable of playing. Even so, her looks kept her employed in quality films throughout the 1930s. In 1940, as her career began to fade, she married producer, Buddy Adler. From 1953 she worked exclusively on TV. Anita devoted her final years to various philanthropic causes before dying in Los Angeles, from a stroke.

The Phantom of Crestwood (1932)
Our Betters (1933)
The Most Precious Thing in Life (1934) **Judge Priest** (1934)
Madame DuBarry (1934)
Personal Maid's Secret (1935)
A Midsummer Night's Dream (1935)
The Story of Louis Pasteur (1935)
Anthony Adverse (1936)
Green Light (1937)
Call It a Day (1937)
The Go Getter (1937)
That Certain Woman (1937)
First Lady (1937)
Tovarich (1937)
My Bill (1938)
Marie Antoinette (1938)
The Sisters (1938)
The Little Princess (1939)
Casanova Brown (1944)
Love Letters (1945)
The Devil's Mask (1946)
Retreat, Hell! (1952)

Frank **Lovejoy**
5ft 10in
(FRANK LOVEJOY)

Born: **March 28, 1912**
The Bronx, New York City, New York, USA
Died: **October 2, 1962**

Frank's father was a salesman for the Pathé Film Studio. After high school, Frank started a career as a "runner" on Wall Street, but lost his job when the Stock Market crashed in 1929. He went into acting to keep the wolf from the door – starting as an apprentice at the Theater Mart in Philadelphia. He then toured with stock theater companies before his debut on Broadway in 1935 – in "Judgement Day". He found that he had the right kind of voice for radio – acting in dramas, like 'Gangbusters' and in the 'Damon Runyon Theater'. In 1940, Frank married actress, Joan Banks, and they had two children. He continued as a radio and stage actor to spend time with his young family and he didn't make his film debut until 1948 when he played Mark Lorimer in Black Bart – a western starring Dan Duryea and Yvonne De Carlo. His next two films, Home of the Brave and In a Lonely Place, got him as close to movie stardom as he was ever going to be. He was a reliable character actor and occasionally, first or second lead in big war films such as Strategic Air Command and crime dramas like Finger Man. Frank starred in two very popular television dramas in the late 1950s – 'Man Against Crime' and 'Meet McGraw'. His last film appearance was in 1958, in the title role of Cole Younger, Gunfighter. After that, he worked exclusively on TV. Before he died in New York of a heart attack, he appeared in an episode of 'Bus Stop' – directed for television, by Robert Altman.

Home of the Brave (1949)
In a Lonely Place (1950)
Three Secrets (1950)
The Sound of Fury (1950)
Force of Arms (1951)
I'll See You in My Dreams (1951)
House of Wax (1953)
The Hitch-Hiker (1953)
Strategic Air Command (1955)
Finger Man (1955)
Three Brave Men (1956)
Cole Younger, Gunfighter (1958)

Rob **Lowe**
5ft 11in
(ROBERT HEPLER LOWE)

Born: **March 17, 1964**
Charlottesville, Virginia, USA

Rob's parents were Charles Lowe, who was a lawyer, and his wife Barbara, who worked as a teacher. Young Rob did some modeling as a child in Dayton, Ohio, and began acting after moving to Los Angeles, where he attended Santa Monica High School at the same time as Emilio Estevez. Rob's first television appearance was in 1979, as Tony Flanagan, in the series 'A New Kind of Family'. His movie debut was in the crime film about gangs, titled *The Outsiders*. It also featured his fellow "Brat Packer" Estevez. In 1988, Rob served twenty hours community service after a scandal involving a sexually explicit video tape. He then overcame drugs and alcohol problems and emerged a better and healthier man. In 1991, he married the make-up artist, Sheryl Berkoff, and she and their two sons have helped him stay on the straight and narrow. When making *Wayne's World,* he became a close friend of Mike Myers – who's also been a good influence. In 2001, Rob was nominated for an Emmy in the TV-drama series, 'The West Wing'. Rob hasn't appeared in a film since *Thank You for Smoking.* He has had four Golden Globe nominations including one for his work in the movie, *Square Dance.* In recent times he has been seen in the role of Senator Robert McAllister, in the TV series, 'Brothers and Sisters'.

The Outsiders (1983)
The Hotel New Hampshire (1984)
St. Elmo's Fire (1985)
About Last Night (1986)
Square Dance (1987)
Bad Influence (1990)
Wayne's World (1992)
Frank & Jesse (1994)
Tommy Boy (1995)
Contact (1997)
Austin Powers: The Spy
Who Shagged Me (1999)
The Specials (2000)
Austin Powers in
Goldmember (2002)
Thank You for Smoking (2005)
Intention of Lying (2009)

Myrna **Loy**
5ft 6in
(MYRNA ADELE WILLIAMS)

Born: **August 2, 1905**
Radersburg, Montana, USA
Died: **December 14, 1993**

Myrna's mother was widowed in 1914. Four years later, she took her daughter to live in Los Angeles. Myrna attended Westlake School for Girls, then Venice High School. She danced in the chorus at Grauman's Chinese Theater. A small role in *What Price Beauty,* in 1925, was the first of sixty movies she made, up until her talent was recognized by Irving Thalberg, who signed her. It took her fine work on loan to RKO in *The Animal Kingdom,* to stir the MGM lion. They teamed her with Clark Gable, which worked well, but it was the classic *Thin Man* series – with William Powell which made her a bona fide star. Apart from two broken marriages, Myrna rarely put a foot wrong during the 1930s. She spent most of the war years working for the Red Cross. A third husband and a top film – *The Best Years of Our Lives,* made 1946 a very good year. The 1950s arrived and good film roles dried up. She made her last movie in 1978 – aptly titled *The End.* Her autobiography – "Myrna Loy: Being and Becoming", was published in 1987. In 1991, Myrna was presented with an Honorary Oscar. She died in New York, of complications following surgery – having undergone two mastectomies.

Arrowsmith (1931)
The Animal Kingdom (1932)
Love Me Tonight (1932)
The Prizefighter and the Lady (1933)
When Ladies Meet (1933)
Topaze (1933)
The Thin Man (1934)
The Great Ziegfeld (1936)
Libeled Lady (1936)
Wife vs. Secretary (1936)
Test Pilot (1938)
Too Hot to Handle (1938)
I Love You Again (1939)
Love Crazy (1941)
The Best Years of Our Lives (1946)
The Bachelor and the
Bobby-Soxer (1947)
Mr. Blandings Builds
His Dream House (1948)

Bela **Lugosi**
6ft 1in
(BÉLA FERENC DEZSO BLASKÓ)

Born: **October 20, 1882**
Lugos, Austro-Hungary
Died: **August 16, 1956**

Raised as a Roman Catholic, Bela was the youngest of four children born to a banker, István Blasko and his wife, Paula. After leaving school, Bela began learning to act by appearing in very small roles in Shakespearean plays – using the stage name, Arisztid Olt. Towards the end of World War I, after being wounded three times – while serving in the Austro-Hungarian army, he made his silent film debut, in *Nászdal* – billed as Bela Lugosi. That year, 1917, he married the first of his five wives, Ilona Szmik. Following thirteen films made in Germany, he left her to go to the United States in 1920, where he settled in New York City. He made a reasonable living as a character actor in fifteen American films, before striking gold in *Dracula.* The worldwide fame that came with it and the pride he felt in becoming a United States citizen, evaporated quickly as his divorces and alimony payments forced him to take any part he was offered. He slipped into drug addiction which he concealed on the set by sipping burgundy from a crystal glass. By the time Bela died at his home in Los Angeles from a heart attack, his final film *The Black Sleep,* had been released. Frank Sinatra paid for his funeral.

Dracula (1931)
Murders in the
Rue Morgue (1932)
Island of Lost Souls (1932)
International House (1933)
The Black Cat (1934)
Mark of the Vampire (1935)
The Raven (1935)
The Invisible Ray (1936)
Son of Frankenstein (1939)
Ninotchka (1939)
Black Friday (1940)
The Wolf Man (1941)
Night Monster (1942)
The Body Snatcher (1945)
Abbott and Costello Meet
Frankenstein (1948)
The Black Sleep (1956)

Paul **Lukas**
6ft 1½in
(PÁL LUKÁCS)

Born: **May 26, 1887**
Budapest, Austro-Hungary
Died: **August 15, 1971**

Paul was born in a railway carriage on a train bound for Budapest. His father ran a publicity company and was able to afford Paul's private education. At the outbreak of World War I, he joined the army, but was invalided out with shell-shock. He left home to join a theatrical company in Kosice and became famous after a leading role in "Liliom" at the beautiful old Comedy Theater, in Budapest. He made his film debut in 1918, in a silent film called *A Sphynx*. He was a star of the Hungarian cinema by the time he represented his country at the 1924 Olympic Games in Paris – as a wrestler. He worked in Austrian films before he sailed for America with his young bride, Gizella, and settled in Hollywood in 1927. His first American film was *Two Lovers,* in 1928. He improved his English and in 1930, played in eight talkies. With his distinctive accent, he was used as a 'foreign' character throughout the decade – *The Lady Vanishes* being a good example. His talent won him the Best Actor Oscar, for *Watch on the Rhine.* Paul did TV and stage work and a few films until the year before his death. He died from heart failure in Morocco.

Little Women (1933)
Affairs of a Gentleman (1934)
Dodsworth (1936)
Ladies in Love (1936)
Espionage (1937)
The Lady Vanishes (1938)
Confessions of a Nazi Spy (1939)
Strange Cargo (1940)
The Ghost Breakers (1940)
They Dare Not Love (1941)
Watch on the Rhine (1943)
Address Unknown (1944)
Experiment Perilous (1944)
Deadline at Dawn (1946)
Berlin Express (1948) **Kim** (1950)
20,000 Leagues
Under the Sea (1954)
Tender Is the Night (1962)
55 Days at Peking (1963)
Lord Jim (1965)

John **Lund**
6ft 0½in
(JOHN LUND)

Born: **February 6, 1911**
Rochester, New York, USA
Died: **May 10, 1992**

Both John's parents were of Norwegian origin – his father was a glassblower. They encouraged their boy to develop his fine writing talent, and were very proud when he got a job in a New York advertising agency. He was making his living as an ad man until 1939, when he was invited to work as a presenter for an industrial show at the World's Fair, in New York. The opportunity to address a large audience fired John's imagination and he made up his mind to pursue an acting career. After two years of drama lessons and summer stock, he was ready for the bigger stage. In 1941, John made his Broadway debut in William Shakespeare's, "As You Like It". A year later, he married his sweetheart, Marie, and they were together until her death in 1982. John wrote the book and lyrics for the Broadway show, "New Faces of 1943". For his acting in "The Hasty Heart", he received the Theater World Award in 1945. Paramount put him under contract and they gave him his film debut, in *To Each His Own.* Perhaps he was lacking the charisma needed to become a top star, but at least he rubbed shoulders with the best, in *High Society.* He was vice-president of the Screen Actor's Guild during the period when he was making B-westerns. John never acted on television. In 1952 he was 'Johnny', on a CBS Radio show, 'Yours Truly, Johnny Dollar'. He retired to San Diego in 1963, after making his last film – *If a Man Answers.* Twenty-nine years later, he died of natural causes, in Los Angeles.

To Each His Own (1946)
The Perils of Pauline (1947)
A Foreign Affair (1948)
Miss Tatlock's Millions (1948)
No Man of Her Own (1950)
Duchess of Idaho (1950)
The Battle at Apache Pass (1952)
Bronco Buster (1952)
High Society (1956)
Dakota Incident (1956)
If a Man Answers (1962)

Dolph **Lundgren**
6ft 5in
(HANS DOLPH LUNDGREN)

Born: **November 3, 1957**
Stockholm, Stockholms län, Sweden

Dolph was one of four children born to an engineer and his wife – he has two sisters and a brother. At high school, he was interested in music and the Arts, but after graduating, he decided to follow in his father's footsteps. Dolph first did his compulsory military service, before enrolling at the Royal Institute of Technology, in Stockholm. Always a superb athlete, he took up Kyokushin Karate and captained the Swedish team at the Tokyo Open Tournament in 1979. Dolph then attended Sydney University – and gained a master's degree in chemical engineering. While he was in Australia, he won a heavyweight Karate competition. He was awarded a Fulbright Scholarship to the United States, but aged twenty-five, Dolph decided to pursue an acting career. He went to New York City, where he studied at the Warren Robertson Theater Workshop and worked as a bodyguard for Grace Jones, whom he lived with for four years. She helped him get his start in motion pictures in a film she featured strongly in – the Roger Moore Bond film, *A View to Kill.* Later that year, he beat off competition from 5000 rivals for the role of Ivan Drago, in *Rocky IV.* Like most action-stars, he isn't always favored by the critics, but sometimes he's received their grudging praises. Since 1994, Dolph has been married to a Swedish girl, Anette Qviberg - who works as an interior decorator. The couple have two young daughters – Ida and Greta, and currently live in London, England.

A View to Kill (1985)
Rocky IV (1985)
Dark Angel (1990)
Showdown in Little Tokyo (1991)
Universal Soldier (1992)
Men of War (1994)
Silent Trigger (1996)
Direct Action (2004)
The Defender (2004)
The Mechanik (2005)
L'Inchiesta (2006)
Missionary Man (2007)
Direct Contact (2009)

William **Lundigan**
6ft 2in
(WILLIAM LUNDIGAN)

Born: **June 12, 1914**
Syracuse, New York, USA
Died: **December 20, 1975**

Bill's father owned a large building, which housed the WFBL radio station. From an early age, he would listen to the broadcasts and while still at high school, he did a few hours a week as an announcer. Bill went to Syracuse University to study Law, but spent most of his time playing basketball, football and tennis. He dropped out when he was offered full time employment at WFBL – working as an announcer and news reader and reading out commercial messages. One of them was heard by Charles R. Rogers, head of production at Universal Studios in Hollywood, who was impressed by Bill's mellifluous voice. The athletic twenty-three year old went for a screen test and made his film debut, in 1937, in *Armored Car*. Most of his early movies were B's, but he began branching out with supporting roles in Errol Flynn's *Dodge City* and *The Old Maid,* starring Bette Davis. From 1942, he served in the United States Marines. His return to films proved difficult until 1947, when he had a five-year run in movies of varying quality. He worked on Chrysler Motors sponsored TV programs. In 1959, he featured in the series, 'Men in Space'. From 1945 until his death from lung and heart congestion, Bill was married to Rena Morgan.

Wives Under Suspicion (1938)
The Missing Guest (1938)
Three Smart Girls Grow Up (1939)
Dodge City (1939) **The Old Maid** (1939)
Three Cheers for the Irish (1940)
The Man Who Talked Too Much (1940)
The Sea Hawk (1940)
Santa Fe Trail (1940) **A Shot in the Dark** (1941) **Highway West** (1941)
Apache Trail (1942)
The Fabulous Dorseys (1947)
Dishonored Lady (1947)
The Inside Story (1948)
Follow Me Quietly (1949) **Pinky** (1949)
I'll Get By (1950)
I'd Climb the Highest Mountain (1951)
The House on Telegraph Hill (1951)
Inferno (1953)

Ida **Lupino**
5ft 4in
(IDA LUPINO)

Born: **February 4, 1914**
Camberwell, London, England
Died: **August 3, 1995**

The daughter of the popular comedian, Stanley Lupino, and his wife, Connie Emerald, Ida was coached for the stage from the age of seven. She and her kid sister, Rita, performed adult roles. By the time she was ten, Ida knew all of the Shakespeare heroines' roles by heart. When she was sixteen, she began training at RADA. In 1931, she made her film debut, in *The Love Race,* and a year later, starred as a girl who tempts an older man in *Her First Affaire.* Ida was ambitious, so in 1934, she traveled to Hollywood and signed for Paramount. She had supporting roles, but worked with top names like Cooper, Crosby and George Raft. In *Artists and Models,* with Jack Benny, she outshone everyone. She married Louis Hayward, who brought her luck, left Paramount, and got a seven-year contract at Warners. Her first three for them were all hits, starting with *They Drive by Night.* But she wasn't the Bette Davis they hoped for. She married Columbia executive Collier Young, and directed inexpensive films with a message. With third husband, Howard Duff, she starred in TV's 'Mr. Adams and Eve'. Her last film role was in 1978, in *My Boys Are Good Boys.* While battling with colon cancer, in Los Angeles, Ida suffered a stroke and died.

Peter Ibbetson (1935)
Anything Goes (1936) **Artists and Models** (1937) **The Adventures of Sherlock Holmes** (1939)
The Light That Failed (1939)
They Drive by Night (1940)
High Sierra (1941) **The Sea Wolf** (1941)
Out of the Fog (1941) **Ladies in Retirement** (1941) **Moontide** (1942)
The Hard Way (1943) **The Man I Love** (1947) **Road House** (1948)
On Dangerous Ground (1952)
Beware My Lovely (1952)
Jennifer (1953) **The Bigamist** (1953)
Private Hell 36 (1954) **The Big Knife** (1955) **While the City Sleeps** (1956)
Junior Bonner (1972)

Carol **Lynley**
5ft 5in
(CAROLE ANN JONES)

Born: **February 13, 1942**
New York City, New York, USA

Carole began a career as a child model – posing for kids' nightwear catalogs, and later appearing in commercials on TV, for early teens' sportswear – using the name 'Carolyn Lee'. When Carole was fifteen, her picture appeared on the cover of Life magazine. Later that year, without any formal training, and having become Lynley, to avoid confusion with Caroline Jones, she made her film debut, in Disney's *Light in the Forest*. In 1960, Carol married her teenage sweetheart, Michael Selsman, with whom she had a daughter named Jill. They were divorced four years later. The image Carol projected in her films is pretty much exactly as she was – wholesome and clean. She did appear in both the Broadway and the film versions of *Blue Denim,* which dealt with the controversial subject of an unwanted pregnancy. She was nominated for a Golden Globe as Most Promising Female Newcomer, and by the early 1960s, was the dream-girl for many American teenage boys. Of all the films Carol acted in, her favorite is *Bunny Lake is Missing.* Throughout that decade, she was most frequently seen on TV, but had a good part in the film, *The Poseidon Adventure,* where she lip-synched to a recording of the Oscar-winning theme song. Nowadays, she is enjoying life as a painter, in Malibu. In 2006, Carol acted in a short movie called *Vic* – directed by Sly Stallone's son, Sage.

The Light in the Forest (1958)
Holiday for Lovers (1959)
Blue Denim (1959)
The Last Sunset (1961)
The Stripper (1963)
Under the Yum Yum Tree (1963)
The Cardinal (1963)
Shock Treatment (1964)
The Pleasure Seekers (1964)
Bunny Lake is Missing (1965)
The Shuttered Room (1967)
Once You Kiss a Stranger (1969)
The Poseidon Adventure (1972)
Blackout (1988)
Neon Signs (1996)

M

James **MacArthur**
5ft 8in
(JAMES GORDON MACARTHUR)

Born: December 8, 1937
Los Angeles, California, USA

Jim was adopted as a baby by a famous show business couple – the playwright Charles MacArthur, and legendary stage and screen actress, Helen Hayes. His early life was spent growing up in Nyack, New York. Jim was educated at the Allen Stevenson School, in New York City. In 1948, he appeared with his mother on the radio in a "Theater Guild of the Air" presentation, in front of a live audience. He then attended Solebury School, in New Hope, Pennsylvania. Jim blossomed into a star sportsman – at basketball, football and baseball. He was class president and also edited his school paper, "The Scribe". He was president of the Drama Club, and while at Solebury, he played the role of Scrooge, in "A Christmas Carol". Jim made his stage debut when he was twelve, in "The Corn is Green", in Olney. Maryland. He gained good experience in summer stock and was a backroom boy at the Helen Hayes Festival, in Falmouth – working as a set painter and electrician's assistant, among other tasks. Jim made his TV debut in 1955, in 'Deal a Blow' – for which he was praised. It led to his movie debut in *The Young Stranger*, directed by John Frankenheimer. Jim went to Harvard to study History, but his movie career took over, and for seven years he appeared in a string of successes. A brief appearance in *Hang 'Em High*, resulted in a long run in TV's 'Hawaii Five-O.' Now semi-retired, Jim lives with his third wife, H.B. Duntz. He has four children and six grandchildren.

The Young Stranger (1957)
The Light in the Forest (1958)
Third Man on the Mountain (1959)
Kidnapped (1960)
Swiss Family Robinson (1960)
The Interns (1962)
Spencer's Mountain (1963)
Cry of Battle (1963)
The Truth About Spring (1964)
The Bedford Incident (1965)
Battle of the Bulge (1965)
Ride Beyond Vengeance (1966)
Hang 'Em High (1968)

Jeanette **MacDonald**
5ft 4in
(JEANETTE ANNA MACDONALD)

Born: June 18, 1903
Philadelphia, Pennsylvania, USA
Died: January 14, 1965

Jeanette was the youngest of three daughters born to Daniel and Anne MacDonald. She and her sister, Blossom, were schooled in singing and dancing. By the age of thirteen, Jeanette was winning singing competitions and performing at school and church functions. Jeanette was sixteen when she made her New York debut, in the chorus of "The Demi-Tasse Revue" – a free entertainment, performed between double-bill film shows at the Capital Theater, on Broadway. During the 1920s, she worked her way up until "Boom Boom" in 1929 (which introduced a young Cary Grant) led to the famous film director, Ernst Lubitsch, who cast her in his first sound film, *The Love Parade.* Jeanette and co-star, Maurice Chevalier, were huge hits with audiences all over the world. It started a recording and film career for Jeanette, which continued with Chevalier, but reached its peak when she was teamed with the baritone, Nelson Eddy, in Victor Herbert's *Naughty Marietta,* in 1935. The couple were known as "America's Singing Sweethearts" and they appeared in eight films. In 1937, Jeanette married her own sweetheart – Gene Raymond. Still with ambitions to perform serious music, she made her operatic debut, in Canada, in 1944. Her last film, *The Sun Comes Up,* was in 1949, but she continued on TV and stage – sometimes with Nelson Eddy. She remained happily married to Gene until her death from a heart attack, in Houston, Texas.

The Love Parade (1929)
Love Me Tonight (1932)
One Hour with You (1932)
The Cat and the Fiddle (1934)
The Merry Widow (1934)
Naughty Marietta (1935)
San Francisco (1936) **Maytime** (1937)
The Girl of the Golden West (1938)
Sweethearts (1938) **Bitter Sweet** (1940)
New Moon (1940)
Smilin' Through (1941) **Cairo** (1942)
Three Daring Daughters (1948)

Kelly **MacDonald**
5ft 3in
(KELLY MACDONALD)

Born: February 23, 1976
Glasgow, Scotland

After her parents split up when she was nine, Kelly and her younger brother were raised by their mother on a council estate in Newton Means, on the outskirts of Glasgow. Poverty was always a factor during her early years and the upheavals affected Kelly's attitude and destroyed her confidence. She did manage to go to Eastwood High School, which helped her to believe in herself, but following her departure from home at seventeen, she dropped out of a college course and was working as a barmaid. One evening she was given a printed flyer, asking for young girls to audition for a film role. The result was the role of Diane, in *Trainspotting* – the movie which launched her career. She has now appeared in more than twenty films and begun to enjoy success in the USA. In 2005, she acted in the TV-movie, 'The Girl in the Café' – which won her an Emmy as the Outstanding Supporting Actress. Kelly's role in *No Country for Old Men*, received a Best Supporting Actress BAFTA nomination. She's married to the Glasgow-born musician, Dougie Payne, who has his own success, as the bass player in the rock band, "Travis". Their son Freddie, was born in March, 2008.

Trainspotting (1996)
Stella Does Tricks (1996)
Cousin Bette (1998)
Elizabeth (1998) **Entropy** (1999)
My Life So Far (1999)
Two Family House (2000)
Some Voices (2000)
Gosford Park (2001)
Intermission (2003)
Finding Neverland (2004)
The Hitchhiker's Guide to
the Galaxy (2005)
A Cock and Bull Story (2005)
All the Invisible Children (2005)
Nanny McPhee (2005)
Lassie (2005) **No Country**
for Old Men (2007)
The Merry Gentleman (2008)
Choke (2008) **In the**
Electric Mist (2009)

Andie MacDowell
5ft 8in
(ROSALIE ANDERSON MACDOWELL)

Born: **April 21, 1958**
Gaffney, South Carolina, USA

Andie was the daughter of a successful lumber executive, Marion St. Pierre Macdowell, and his wife Paula, who was a music teacher. As a teenager, Andie earned money to buy the latest fashions by working at Pizza Hut and McDonalds. She dropped out of Winthrop College, in Rock Hill to join her sister Babs as a waitress in a Disco Night Club called "Stage Door". She was discovered there and became an Elite model in New York City. Andie's international exposure in cosmetics advertising for L'Oreal, and a series of commercials for Calvin Klein led, in 1984, to her film debut, as Jane Porter, in *Greystoke: The Legend of Tarzan, Lord of the Apes*. Because of her strong Carolina accent, her lines in the film were dubbed by Glenn Close. Andie soon acquired the necessary polish to use her own voice – starting with the 'Brat Pack' film *St. Elmo's Fire*. in 1986, she married fellow model, Paul Qualley, after they had featured together in GAP ads. They had a son and two daughters before divorcing in 1999. She made it to another level when director Steven Soderbergh cast her in *Sex, Lies and Videotape*, and her pairing with the French icon, Gerard Depardieu, resulted in the popular comedy, *Green Card*. Three years later, Andie won a Best Actress Saturn Award for *Groundhog Day*, but her biggest success so far is *Four Weddings and a Funeral*. For some time her roles have been inconsistent in quality.

Sex, Lies, and Videotape (1989)
Green Card (1990)
The Object of Beauty (1991)
Groundhog Day (1993)
Short Cuts (1993)
**Four Weddings
and a Funeral** (1994)
Unstrung Heroes (1995)
Multiplicity (1996)
The Muse (1999)
Harrison's Flowers (2000)
Crush (2001)
Beauty Shop (2005)
Intervention (2007)

Ali MacGraw
5ft 8in
(ALICE MACGRAW)

Born: **April 1, 1938**
Pound Ridge, New York, USA

Ali was the daughter of commercial artists. Her maternal grandfather was a Jewish immigrant from Hungary. Although they were far from perfect parents, they did give her an interest in the visual arts from an early age – when she was a pupil at Choate Rosemary Hall, in Wallingford, Connecticut. After that, Ali attended Wellesley College, a women's liberal arts college, in Massachusetts. Her first job, in 1960, was as a photographic assistant at Harper's Bazaar. She became assistant to Diana Vreeland at Vogue, and was later a fashion model in New York City. During those years she appeared in TV commercials and started to think seriously about an acting career. She made her film debut in 1968, with a small role in *A Lovely Way to Die*. She next co-starred with Richard Benjamin, in the hit romantic comedy, *Goodbye Columbus*. Ali married the actor-turned-producer, Robert Evans, and the following year, she played the role she is most famous for – the leukemia-victim Jennifer Cavalleri, in the classic tear-jerker, *Love Story*. Ali was nominated for a Best Actress Oscar, but narrowly missed out to Glenda Jackson. She was a big star, with a one-year-old son, when she appeared with Steve McQueen in *The Getaway*. She had an affair with him and after divorcing Evans, she married him. The five years with McQueen was an unproductive time for Ali – she missed out on several projects Evans had lined up for her, including *The Great Gatsby* and *Chinatown*. To say that McQueen was difficult to live with would be a gross understatement. By the time they divorced in 1978, Ali had an alcohol problem. After Betty Ford sorted her out, she was in her forties. She made her Broadway debut, in 2006 – in "Festen".

Goodbye Columbus (1969)
Love Story (1970)
The Getaway (1972)
Convoy (1978)
**Just Tell Me What
You Want** (1980)
Natural Causes (1994)

Kyle MacLachlan
6ft 0½in
(KYLE MERRITT MACLACHLAN)

Born: **February 22, 1959**
Yakima, Washington, USA

When he was a kid, Kyle used to amuse his family by acting out the parts in the "Hardy Boys" adventure books. After early years at Eisenhower High School, in Yakima, Kyle graduated from Seattle's University of Washington, in 1982, with a BA in Fine Arts. After some stage experience, he made his film debut, in David Lynch's *Dune*. It was his second outing for the director – in *Blue Velvet*, that brought him to the threshhold of movie stardom. It was consolidated after an international success as Special Agent Dale Cooper, in the director's absorbing series for ABC TV, 'Twin Peaks', in 1990. That portrayal earned Kyle a Golden Globe Award. For a complete change of pace and image, he played Ray Manzarek, in *The Doors*, and just to heighten the contrast, he was back as the neatly-groomed, Cooper, in David Lynch's mind-blowing *Twin Peaks* movie. He then endured a six year spell when his movie roles were decidedly off-target. It was William Shakespeare who got his career back on track, in a modern version of *Hamlet*, but the last few years have been lower profile. He lives in Manhattan with his wife Desiree Gruber and their two dogs, Mookie and Sam. Since 2006, Kyle has appeared in more than forty episodes of the TV series, 'Desperate Housewives'.

Dune (1984)
Blue Velvet (1986)
The Hidden (1987)
The Doors (1991)
**Twin Peaks: Fire Walk
With Me** (1992)
Where the Day Takes You (1992)
Rich in Love (1993)
Roswell (1994) **One Night
Stand** (1997)
Xchange (2000)
Hamlet (2000)
Timecode (2000)
Me Without You (2001)
Miranda (2002)
Northfork (2003)
Touch of Pink (2004) **Manure** (2009)
Mao's Last Dancer (2009)

Shirley **Maclaine**
5ft 7in
(SHIRLEY MACLEAN BEATY)

Born: **April 24, 1934**
Richmond, Virginia, USA

Shirley's parents were devout Baptists, and teachers. Her mother, Kathlyn, taught drama, but her father, Ira, had a deeper interest in the world of philosophy and psychology. Shirley was named after child star, Shirley Temple, whose birthday was a day earlier. Encouraged by her mother to learn ballet, she fractured her ankle, and gave up her ambition to be a dancer. By the time she left Washington Lee High School, where she starred in several plays, she had the confidence to go to New York. She understudied Carol Haney, in "The Pajama Game". Carol broke her ankle. Hal Wallis saw Shirley perform, and gave her a Paramount contract. In 1955, she appeared in two episodes of the TV series 'Shower of Stars' before her film debut in Hitchcock's black comedy, *The Trouble with Harry*. Shirley has enjoyed a long career and after being nominated six times, she won a Best Actress Oscar for *Terms of Endearment*. She was married to Steve Parker from 1954-1982. The best of Shirley's recent work is in Director Richard Attenborough's, *Closing the Ring*.

Artists and Models (1955)
The Sheepman (1958) Hot Spell (1958)
The Matchmaker (1958)
Some Came Running (1958)
Can-Can (1960) The Apartment (1960)
All in a Night's Work (1961)
Two for the Seesaw (1962)
Irma la Douce (1963)
The Bliss of Mrs. Blossom (1968)
Sweet Charity (1969)
Two Mules for Sister Sara (1970)
The Turning Point (1977)
Being There (1979)
Terms of Endearment (1983)
Steel Magnolias (1989)
Postcards from the Edge (1990)
Wrestling Ernest Hemingway (1993)
Guarding Tess (1994)
The Evening Star (1996)
Bruno (2000) Carolina (2003)
In Her Shoes (2005)
Rumor Has It... (2005)
Closing the Ring (2007)

Aline **MacMahon**
5ft 8in
(ALINE LAVEEN MACMAHON)

Born: **May 3, 1899**
McKeeport, Pennsylvania, USA
Died: **October 12, 1991**

Despite her Irish-sounding name, Aline was Jewish. She grew up in New York City and was educated at the Erasmus High School, in Brooklyn, and Barnard College. Following some private acting lessons, in her late teens, Aline began to work in the theater. By the early 1920s, she was getting starring roles in Broadway plays – after her debut there in 1921, in "The Madras House". She first came to the screen following her success in "Winter Bound". Her film debut was in 1931, with a supporting role in the Oscar-nominated *Five Star Final*. Aline didn't neglect her stage work, but a Warners contract led to a series of good films, in which she was third or fourth billed. One of them was the classic Busby Berkeley musical, *Gold Diggers of 1933*. Although not beautiful, Aline had a lovely, sympathetic face, and the camera liked her. Her first starring role was opposite Richard Barthelmess, in *Heroes for Sale*. Aline's period of stardom was brief, but she lent quality to whatever she did. She was nominated for a Best Supporting Actress Oscar, for *Dragon Seed,* but her favorite role was in *The Search*. She retired in 1975, following the death of her husband, the architect Clarence S. Stein, and she died in New York, of pneumonia sixteen years later.

Five Star Final (1931) Life Begins (1932)
One Way Passage (1932)
Once in a Lifetime (1932)
Gold Diggers of 1933 (1933)
The Life of Jimmy Dolan (1933)
Heroes for Sale (1933)
The World Changes (1933)
Heat Lightning (1934)
While the Patient Slept (1935)
Ah, Wilderness! (1935)
Back Door to Heaven (1939)
Out of the Fog (1941) Dragon
Seed (1944) The Search (1948)
The Flame and the Arrow (1950)
The Man from Laramie (1955)
Cimarron (1960)
All the Way Home (1963)

Fred **MacMurray**
6ft 2½in
(FREDERICK MARTIN MACMURRAY)

Born: **August 30, 1908**
Kantakee, Illinois, USA
Died: **November 5, 1991**

Fred was the son of Frederick MacMurray, a violinist, and his wife, Maleta. When Fred was five, his father moved the family to Beaver Dam, Wisconsin. After graduating from high school, he got a scholarship to the liberal arts, Carroll College, in Waukesa, where he was a contemporary of future film actor, Dennis Morgan. While there, Fred used to gig on tenor sax with local bands. He also possessed a fine singing voice and was featured as vocalist on a Gus Arnheim Orchestra recording, "All I Want Is Just One Girl". In 1929, he made his first appearance on film, as an extra, in *Girls Gone Wild*. After college, Fred appeared on Broadway, in "Three's a Crowd" and, with Bob Hope and Sydney Greenstreet, in the original cast of Kern and Harbach's "Roberta". His debut in a featured film role came in 1935, in *Grand Old Girl* and that year, he co-starred with Katherine Hepburn in *Alice Adams*. Fred was popular with his female co-stars, but in 1936, he married Lillian Lamont. His standout film is *Double Indemnity,* but he was rarely anything other than excellent. When Lillian died in 1953, June Haver gave up the prospect of a convent life to be with him until his death from Leukemia.

Alice Adams (1935) Hands across
the Table (1935) The Texas
Rangers (1936) True Confession (1937)
Remember the Night (1940)
Dive Bomber (1941) Above
Suspicion (1943) No Time for
Love (1943) Double Indemnity (1944)
Murder He Says (1945)
Pardon My Past (1945) Smoky (1946)
The Egg and I (1947)
Singapore (1947)
An Innocent Affair (1948)
A Millionaire for Christy (1951)
The Caine Mutiny (1954)
Pushover (1954)
Woman's World (1954)
The Apartment (1960)
The Absent Minded Professor (1961)
Follow Me, Boys! (1966)

Gordon MacRae
5ft 8in
(ALBERT GORDON MACRAE)

Born: **March 12, 1921**
East Orange, New Jersey, USA
Died: **January 24, 1986**

As a boy, Gordon lived in Syracuse, New York. While at Deerfield Academy, in Massachusetts, he joined the Drama Club and demonstrated his singing ability. He played piano, clarinet and saxophone, and by the age of eighteen, was the complete entertainer. In 1939, he won a singing contest and a two-week gig at the World's Fair in New York, backed by the bands of Harry James and Les Brown. He was hired by Horace Heidt's Band and stayed for two years. In 1942, Gordon joined the U.S. Airforce, serving as a navigator until the end of the war. In late 1945, he made his Broadway debut in "Junior Miss". His next job was a high-profile one, in Ray Bolger's 1946 revue, "Three To Make Ready". He was spotted by Capitol Records, who gave him a contract. In 1948, he starred on ABC Radio, in 'The Railroad Hour', which gave him an opportunity to test himself with various female singers, in operetta and lighter forms of music. In 1948, he made his film debut in *The Big Punch,* before starring with June Haver, in *Look for the Silver Lining.* Two other co-stars, Doris Day and Shirley Jones, helped him become a big star. Considering his career, the cause of his death – cancer of the mouth and jaw, was particularly tragic. He had four children with first wife, Sheila, and one child with his second wife, Elizabeth. His daughters, Meredith and Heather are both actresses.

Look for the Silver Lining (1949)
The Daughter of Rosie
O'Grady (1950)
Tea for Two (1950)
The West Point Story (1950)
On Moonlight Bay (1951)
By the Light of the
Silvery Moon (1953)
The Desert Song (1953)
Three Sailors and a Girl (1953)
Oklahoma! (1955)
The Best Things in Life are
Free (1956) Carousel (1956)
The Pilot (1980)

George MacReady
6ft 1in
(GEORGE PEABODY MACREADY JR.)

Born: **August 29, 1899**
Providence, Rhode Island, USA
Died: **July 2, 1973**

After graduating from Brown University, George worked as a journalist with a New York newspaper for several years. He claimed to be descended from the 19th century Shakespearean actor, William Macready. In 1925, a close friend of his, Richard Boleslawski, a Polish-born stage director (who was later a Hollywood film director) recommended that the young man indeed had the potential to be a good actor. On that advice, George took a few lessons and made his Broadway debut in 1926, in "The Scarlet Letter". He was an immediate success and for fifteen years, worked in most of Shakespeare's plays – opposite such great names as Helen Hayes and Katherine Cornell. During the 1930s, George had a car accident which left him with a scar on his right cheek. It added something sinister to his film roles, which began in 1942, with *Commandos Strike at Dawn.* It was the year he married his wife, Elizabeth. He later owned an art gallery in Los Angeles with Vincent Price. George's last film was *The Return of Count Yorga,* in 1971. He retired and died from emphysema, two years later, at his home in Los Angeles.

The Seventh Cross (1944)
I Love a Mystery (1945)
Counter-Attack (1945)
Gilda (1946)
The Man Who Dared (1946)
Down to Earth (1947)
The Swordsman (1948)
The Big Clock (1948)
Coroner Creek (1948)
Beyond Glory (1948)
Knock on Any Door (1949)
Alias Nick Beal (1949)
Johnny Allegro (1949)
The Desert Fox (1951)
Detective Story (1951)
Julius Caesar (1953)
Vera Cruz (1954)
Paths of Glory (1957)
Seven Days in May (1964)
Tora! Tora! Tora! (1971)

Amy Madigan
5ft 5½in
(AMY MADIGAN)

Born: **September 11, 1950**
Chicago, Illinois, USA

Amy's father, John Madigan, was a local celebrity: he was a broadcaster, a media personality, and a lawyer. Her mother, Dolores, was a union worker. Early on, Amy showed potential as a musician as well as acting, which she did regularly at the local St. Philip Neri grammar school and Aquinas High School. She then studied philosophy at Marquette University, in Milwaukee, and after that, she perfected her piano playing skills at the Chicago Conservatory. It wasn't enough for Amy – she went to New York to study at Lee Strasberg's Theater and Film Institute. In 1970, she moved to Los Angeles, where she won a Drama-Logue Award for her work in the Los Angeles Theater Center production of "Stevie Wants to Play the Blues". In between acting assignments, she used her keyboard ability to play in local rock bands including 'Jelly'. In 1981, she made her TV debut in an episode of 'Hart to Hart'. Amy's first film appearance was in the drama, *Love Child.* In 1983, she married Ed Harris, after they worked together in *Places in the Heart,* and the couple have appeared in a total of seven movies. In 1984, Amy was named Best Actress at the Catalonian International Film Festival, for *Streets of Fire.* Amy's one Oscar nomination so far, was for Best Supporting Actress, in *Twice in a Lifetime.* She and Ed have a daughter named Lily.

Love Letters (1983)
Places in the Heart (1984)
Streets of Fire (1984)
Alamo Bay (1985)
Twice in a Lifetime (1985)
Field of Dreams (1989)
Uncle Buck (1989)
The Dark Half (1991)
Pollock (2000)
The Sleepy Time Gal (2001)
Just a Dream (2002)
In the Land of Milk and
Money (2004)
Winter Passing (2005)
Gone Baby Gone (2007)
Gary's Walk (2009)

Guy **Madison**
6ft
(ROBERT OZELL MOSELY)

Born: **January 19, 1922**
Bakersfield, California, USA
Died: **February 6, 1996**

Guy's father was employed on a ranch, and when his son was still a small boy, he taught him to ride horses – later a useful tool in Guy's film career. Before that began, he left Bakersfield Junior College in 1940, and worked as a telephone lineman. From 1942, Guy served for three years in the United States Coast Guard. While enjoying liberty in Hollywood, one weekend, his boyish good looks caught the eye of David O. Selznick's head of talent, Henry Willson, when Guy sat in the audience at a Lux Radio Theater broadcast. A glowing report was followed by a change of name and a small role in Selznick's weepie, *Since You Went Away*. Thousands of fan letters poured in following its release, but by then, the debutant was away completing his war service. In 1946, Guy was given a contract by RKO and co-starred with Dorothy Maguire, in *Till The End of Time*. He was admired but didn't get a chance to play against type. He improved his acting ability by studying and working in the theater. In 1949, he married the beautiful but troubled actress, Gail Russell. From 1951, Guy starred for seven years in the TV series 'Adventures of Wild Bill Hickock'. After that his work was in minor European movies and B-westerns. Guy married the Irish actress, Sheila Connolly. They had three daughters and a son. He died of emphysema at his home in Palm Springs, California.

Till The End of Time (1946)
Honeymoon (1947)
Texas, Brooklyn and
Heaven (1948) Drums in
the Deep South (1951)
The Charge at Feather River (1951)
5 Against the House (1955)
The Last Frontier (1955)
On the Threshold of
Space (1956)
Hilda Crane (1956)
Reprisal! (1956)
Renegade Riders (1967)
Where's Willie? (1978)

Michael **Madsen**
6ft 2in
(MICHAEL SOREN MADSEN)

Born: **September 25, 1958**
Chicago, Illinois, USA

Mike's father, Cal, was a fireman from a Danish background. His mother, Elaine, is an Emmy Award winning poet, who became a successful playwright. They were traveling down different roads and when Mike was nine, they separated. It was a traumatic time for the boy and his sister Virginia, who also became a famous movie star. Mike in particular suffered from the frequent changes of schools and began to steal. In a way, he was growing up like his hero, Robert Mitchum. By his late teens he'd sorted himself out to the extent that he made an honest living as a motor mechanic, a hospital orderly, and a gas pump attendant. He broke away from that life by going to Chicago, and being taught acting by John Malkovich, at the Steppenwolf Theater. In 1982, Mike made his film debut, as an alcoholic in *Against All Hope*. Two years later, he had a supporting role in a big movie, *The Natural*, and got his first really good notices for playing the deranged Vince Miller, in *Kill Me Again*. His breakthrough came as 'Mr. Blonde', in Tarantino's powerful hit film, *Reservoir Dogs*. Apart from blockbuster movies, Mike is a supporter of independent film making. He has five children from his three marriages. He's enjoyed a flurry of activity during the past year or so, with roles in around two dozen movies.

Kill Me Again (1989)
The Doors (1991)
Thelma & Louise (1991)
Reservoir Dogs (1992)
Season of Change (1994)
Wyatt Earp (1994)
Donnie Brasco (1997)
Welcome to America (2002)
Kill Bill (2003)
Kill Bill: Vol. 2 (2004)
Sin City (2005)
Strength and Honor (2007)
Tooth & Nail (2007)
House (2008) Hell Ride (2008)
45 R.P.M. (2008)
Serbian Scars (2008)
Break (2009)

Virginia **Madsen**
5ft 5in
(VIRGINIA MADSEN)

Born: **September 11, 1961**
Chicago, Illinois, USA

Gina, as she is known, is the daughter of Calvin Madsen, a Chicago fireman, and his wife, Elaine, a poet and playwright. Gina inherited most of her talent from her mother. She has Irish and native American blood from her mother, and has Danish ancestry from her father. A big influence on her future career was her older brother, Michael, who performed magic shows for the family, with little Gina acting as his assistant. At New Trier High School in Winnetka, she was a regular in their drama productions. During the early 1980s she attended Ted Liss's Acting Studio. Before she launched her career, she spent some time at Harand Camp Adult Theater Seminar, at Elkhart Lake, Wisconsin. In 1983, Gina made her movie debut in the comedy/drama, *Class*. That bit part was quickly followed by a more substantial role, as Princess Irulan, in David Lynch's *Dune*. Film work has been plentiful and Gina will soon be completing twenty-five years in films. She was nominated for a Best Supporting Actress Oscar, for *Sideways*. She was briefly married to Danny Huston, and has a son, Jack, with Antonio Sabato Jr.

Dune (1984)
Slam Dance (1987)
The Dead Can't Lie (1988)
Mr. North (1988)
The Hot Spot (1990)
Victim of Love (1991)
Candyman (1992)
Someone's Watching (1993)
The Prophecy (1994)
Ghosts of Mississippi (1996)
The Rainmaker (1997)
Almost Salinas (2001)
American Gun (2002)
Sideways (2004)
A Prairie Home
Companion (2006)
The Astronaut Farmer (2006)
The Number 23 (2007)
Cutlass (2007)
Diminishing Capacity (2008)
Amelia (2009)

Anna **Magnani**
5ft 3in
(ANNA MAGNANI)

Born: **March 7, 1908**
Rome, Lazio, Italy
Died: **September 26, 1973**

Anna was an illegitimate child who never knew the identity of her father. She grew up in abject poverty, in a slum district of Rome. She was quickly abandoned by her mother and raised by her maternal grandmother, who made sure that she got a minimal education at a convent school in Rome. When she was sixteen, Anna sang in cabarets and nightclubs in order to support herself while she was studying at the Academy of Dramatic Art. She then toured the country with small repertory companies, but in 1927, after impressing in a production of "La Nemica e Scampolo", she made her first screen appearance in a film version of it – *Scampolo*. It didn't lead to offers of more movie work, so she concentrated on the theater until the mid-1930s. She made what is considered her official film debut, in 1934, in *The Blind Woman of Sorrento*. In 1935, she married – for the only time – film director, Goffredo Alessandrini. Anna remained a stage actress apart from appearances in low budget Italian movies, including one of her husband's. She needed a genius to bring out her own special qualities and this she got in 1941, from Vittorio De Sica, in his film, *Do You Like Women*, and even more so, under Roberto Rossellini's direction, in *Roma, città aperta*. It elevated her into another league and eventually, Hollywood. She won a deserved Oscar, for *The Rose Tattoo*, and gave superb performances in two more English language movies. Anna retired in the early 1970s, and died of pancreatic cancer, at her home in Rome.

Rome, Open City (1945)
L'Amore (1948)
Belissima (1951)
The Golden Coach (1953)
The Rose Tattoo (1955)
Wild is the Wind (1957)
The Fugitive Kind (1960)
Risate di gioia (1960)
Mamma Roma (1962)
Made in Italy (1965)
The Secret of Santa Vittoria (1969)

Tobey **Maguire**
5ft 8½in
(TOBIAS VINCENT MAGUIRE)

Born: **June 27, 1975**
Santa Monica, California, USA

Tobey's parents, Vincent Maguire, who was a construction worker, and Wendy Brown, who worked as a secretary, were both unmarried teenagers when he was conceived. Although they soon married, they split up two years after he was born. His mother moved home regularly and Tobey spent his early years living in California, Oregon, and Washington State. When he was at high school his ambition was to be a chef, but his mother, who was a screenwriter, gave him $100 dollars to encourage him to study drama. During his freshman year, Tobey dropped out of school and didn't take his GED test until 2000. When he was fifteen, after appearing on a Rodney Dangerfield TV show, he made his movie debut as a video games competitor in *The Wizard*. He had no lines in the film and he stuck to television work for three years. At many movie auditions during 1990, he found himself competing with the young Leonardo DiCaprio. They became and have remained, firm friends after they both worked on *This Boy's Life*. To begin with, Tobey wasn't as lucky as his pal in terms of getting suitable roles. He was still being cast as a teenager, but things began to get better after *Wonder Boys*. His role as *Spider-Man* made him a star – *The Good German* enhanced his reputation. Tobey is married to Jennifer Meyer, with whom he has a baby daughter named Ruby.

This Boy's Life (1993)
The Ice Storm (1997)
Deconstructing Harry (1997)
**Fear and Loathing in
Las Vegas** (1998)
Pleasantville (1998)
The Cider House Rules (1999)
Ride with the Devil (1999)
Wonder Boys (2000)
Spider-Man (2002)
Seabiscuit (2003)
Spider-Man 2 (2004)
The Good German (2006)
Spider-Man 3 (2007)
Brothers (2009)

Marjorie **Main**
5ft 7in
(MARY TOMLINSON)

Born: **February 24, 1890**
Acton, Indiana, USA
Died: **April 10, 1975**

Marjorie's father, the Reverend Samuel Tomlinson, was a minister in the Church of Christ. She was educated at nearby Franklin College, but at seventeen years of age, Marjorie went to Lexington, Kentucky to attend the Hamilton School of Dramatic Expression. Her parents wouldn't have approved, so she claimed to be training as a teacher. In fact, she taught drama for one year after graduating. To save them embarrassment, she changed her name and joined a stock company which toured throughout the State of Indiana. She then began a career in vaudeville which led to her debut on Broadway, in 1916. In 1921, Marjorie married Dr. Stanley Krebs, who was a doctor of psychology. She gave up the stage to tour with him when he lectured. Marjorie returned to Broadway in W.C.Fields shows, and made her film debut, in 1931, in an uncredited role, in *A House Divided*. By the late 1930s, following her husband's death, Marjorie was an in-demand character actress in many good movies, including *Meet Me in St. Louis*. She was nominated for a Best Supporting Actress Oscar, for *The Egg and I*. A series of *Ma and Pa Kettle* comedies kept her busy until retiring, after an episode of TV's 'Wagon Train' in 1958. She died of lung cancer, in Los Angeles.

Music in the Air (1934)
Stella Dallas (1937) **Dead End** (1937)
Test Pilot (1938) **The Women** (1939)
Dark Command (1940)
A Woman's Face (1941)
The Shepherd of the Hills (1941)
Honky Tonk (1941) **Heaven Can
Wait** (1943) **Meet Me in
St. Louis** (1944) **Murder, He
Says** (1945) **The Harvey Girls** (1946)
Bad Bascomb (1946)
Undercurrent (1946)
The Egg and I (1947) **The Wistful
Widow of Wagon Gap** (1947)
Ma and Pa Kettle (1949) **Big Jack** (1949)
Summer Stock (1950)
The Belle of New York (1952)

Karl **Malden**
6ft 0½in
(MLADEN SEKULOVICH)

Born: **March 22, 1912**
Chicago, Illinois, USA
Died: **July 1, 2009**

Karl was the eldest of three boys born to a Serb father, Petar Sekulovich, and a Czech mother, named Minnie. He spoke Serbian until he started to go to kindergarten. When he was five years old, the family moved to Gary, Indiana. His dad was active in the local church and Karl was given his first opportunity to act in plays. At his high school, Karl twice broke his nose when he played for the basketball team. He enrolled at Emerson School for Visual and Performing Arts and after he'd graduated, bang in the middle of the Great Depression, he had to work in the steel industry for three years. At that point, he changed his name and made up his mind to become an actor. He trained at the Goodman School and the Chicago Art Institute. In 1937, Karl went to New York, where he appeared on stage and married Mona Greenberg, with whom he had two children. His film debut in 1940, in *They Knew What They Wanted* was followed by U.S. Army Air Force service. He resumed his stage career with the help of Elia Kazan, and became one of the great film characters – with a Best Supporting Actor Oscar, for *A Streetcar Named Desire,* and a nomination, for *On the Waterfront.* Karl's last film appearance was in *Nuts,* with Barbra Streisand, in 1997. On TV he acted in an episode of 'West Wing' in 2000. In December, 2008, his marriage to Mona had lasted seventy years! Karl died of natural causes – in Brentwood, California.

The Gunfighter (1950)
Halls of Montezuma (1950)
A Streetcar Named Desire (1951)
I Confess (1953) On the
Waterfront (1954) Baby Doll (1956)
Fear Strikes Out (1957)
One-Eyed Jacks (1961) Gypsy (1962)
Cheyenne Autumn (1964)
The Cincinnati Kid (1965)
Nevada Smith (1966) Blue (1968)
Patton (1970) Wild Rovers (1971)
Summertime Killer (1972)
Billy Galvin (1986) Nuts (1987)

John **Malkovich**
6ft 1in
(JOHN GAVIN MALKOVICH)

Born: **December 9, 1953**
Christopher, Illinois, USA

John's father, Daniel, a state conservation director and publisher of "Outdoor Illinois", was from a Croatian background. His mother, Joanne, who owned the "Benton Evening News", was a mixture of Scottish and German. In his early years, John was a big overweight kid, but by the time he attended high school, he had slimmed down and began to excel as an athlete. At Illinois State University, he spent one semester studying Ecology before switching to a Drama major. In 1976, John joined the Steppenwolf Theater in Chicago, then newly founded by his friend, Gary Sinise. He stayed until 1983, when he went to New York. He won an Obie, in the play, "True West". In 1984, he won an Emmy for his performance with Dustin Hoffman, in the revival of "Death of a Salesman". Since making his Best Supporting Actor Oscar nominated screen debut, in *Places in the Heart,* John has gone from strength to strength. He received a second Best Supporting Actor nomination, for *In the Line of Fire* and has continued to impress. John has a son and a daughter with his second wife, Nicoletta Peyran.

The Killing Fields (1984)
Places in the Heart (1984)
Death of a Salesman (1985)
Empire of the Sun (1987)
The Glass Menagerie (1987)
Dangerous Liaisons (1988)
Miles from Home (1988)
The Object of Beauty (1991)
Queen's Logic (1992)
In the Line of Fire (1993)
Mary Reilly (1995)
Mulholland Falls (1996)
The Portrait of a Lady (1996)
Con Air (1997)
Being John Malkovich (1999)
Shadow of the Vampire (2000)
Ripley's Game (2002)
The Libertine (2004)
Art School Confidential (2006)
In Tranzit (2007)
Burn After Reading (2008)
Afterwards (2008)

Dorothy **Malone**
5ft 6in
(DOROTHY ELOISE MALONEY)

Born: **January 30, 1925**
Chicago, Illinois, USA

Dorothy was one of five children – two of whom died very young. She worked as a child model and was spotted by an RKO Studios talent scout, when she was in a supporting role in a high school play. At seventeen, Dorothy was given a screen test and made her film debut, in a B-picture, *The Man Who Wouldn't Die.* She began her studies at Southern Methodist University, in Dallas, but dropped out in 1943, to pursue a film career. She wasn't really noticed in twelve subsequent films until, in *The Big Sleep,* in 1946, when she played the rather intellectual-looking girl Humphrey Bogart encounters in the Acme bookstore. From that stage on, she slowly built up to stardom by going freelance and acting in a variety of supporting roles. By the mid-1950s, Dorothy reached her peak, after turning blonde. She won a Best Supporting Actress Oscar, for *Written on the Wind.* Dorothy was married three times – the first of them to French actor, Jacques Bergerac, with whom she had two daughters. After her film career tailed off, she did lots of TV work, including the popular series 'Dr. Kildare', 'Peyton Place' and 'Rich Man Poor Man'. Her last movie appearance was in *Basic Instinct.*

To the Victor (1948)
To Guys from Texas (1949)
Colorado Territory (1949)
Scared Stiff (1953)
Pushover (1954)
Private Hell 36 (1954)
Young at Heart (1955)
Battle Cry (1955)
Artists and Models (1955)
Tension at Table Rock (1956)
Written on the Wind (1956)
The Tarnished Angels (1957)
Tip on a Dead Jockey (1957)
Too Much, Too Soon (1958)
Warlock (1959)
The Last Sunset (1961)
Fate Is the Hunter (1964)
Golden Rendezvous (1977)
Winter Kills (1979)
Basic Instinct (1992)

Silvana **Mangano**
5ft 6in
(SILVANA MANGANO)

Born: **April 21, 1930**
Rome, Lazio, Italy
Died: **December 16, 1989**

Silvana's father was a Sicilian, who worked as a conductor on the railroad. Her mother was an Englishwoman. It was a hard period for her family, what with the Great Depression – followed by World War II, but somehow they raised the money for Silvana to go to dancing classes when she was a seven-year-old girl. By the age of sixteen, she was paying her own way, by working as a photo model. She made her first screen appearance in a French resistance film called *Le Jugement dernier,* at the end of the war, and in 1946, she won the "Signorina Roma" beauty pageant, The prize was a movie contract at the city's Cinnecittà Studios, and an appearance in the movie of the Opera, *L'Elisir d'amore.* The following year she competed in the "Miss Italia" contest – won by a future Italian star, Lucia Bosé. In 1949, she signed for Lux Films and was selected to appear in *Bitter Rice* – a great success in Art Houses around the world. Silvana married its producer, Dino De Laurentis, with whom she had four children. Silvana never became as internationally famous as Loren and Lollobrigida, but she was popular in Italy for thirty years. She died of lung cancer, in Madrid, Spain.

Bitter Rice (1949)
Il Brigante Musolino (1950)
Anna (1951)
Mambo (1954)
Ulysses (1954)
The Gold of Naples (1954)
This Angry Age (1957)
The Great War (1959)
5 Branded Women (1960)
Barabbas (1961)
My Wife (1964)
Il Disco volante (1964)
Le Streghe (1967)
Oedipus Rex (1967)
Teorema (1968)
Death in Venice (1971)
Ludwig (1972)
**Gruppo di famiglia
in un interno** (1974)

Jayne **Mansfield**
5ft 5in
(VERA JAYNE PALMER)

Born: **April 19, 1933**
Bryn Mawr, Pennsylvania, USA
Died: **June 29, 1967**

Jayne was the daughter of a successful lawyer, Herbert Palmer, and his wife, Vera. Jayne was of English ancestry on her father's side and German on her mother's. Soon after Jayne was born, the family moved to Phillipsburg, New Jersey, where her father established a law practice. When she was barely three-years old, young Jayne had a most traumatic experience. She was in the family car driven by her dad, when he died of a heart attack. Her mother worked as a teacher after that – later remarrying and moving to Dallas. Jayne also got married – at the early age of sixteen. She was studying drama at Southern Methodist University and had to give that up after she became Mrs. Mansfield and had a baby daughter. Her husband Paul was in the US. Army, so she completed her education in fits and starts. Between winning beauty contests, she was credited with an I.Q. of 163. In 1953, after some acting classes with Sidney Lumet's father, Baruch, she made her stage debut, in "Death of a Salesman". Jayne moved to Los Angeles with her family and studied drama at UCLA. Her stage work at the Pasadena Playhouse led to a Warner Brothers contract and her film debut, in 1954, in *Female Jungle.* The following year, she was a hit on Broadway in "Will Success Spoil Rock Hunter", and two years later, starred in the film version. She had three children with her second husband, Mickey Hargitay. After 1961, her films were unbelievably poor. Jayne had just divorced her third husband, Matt Cimber, when she was killed in an horrific automobile crash, on U.S. Highway 90, in Slidell, Louisiana, in a head-on collision with a tractor-trailer.

Illegal (1955) **The Burglar** (1956)
The Girl Can't Help It (1956)
The Wayward Bus (1957)
Will Success Spoil Rock Hunter (1957)
The Sheriff of Fractured Jaw (1958)
Too Hot to Handle (1960)
The George Raft Story (1961)

Joe **Mantegna**
5ft 11³/₄in
(JOSEPH ANTHONY MANTEGNA JR.)

Born: **November 13, 1947**
Chicago, Illinois, USA

Joe's parents, Joseph Sr., who worked as an insurance salesman, and Mary Ann, who was a shipping clerk, were both from Italian backgrounds. Joe was educated at Morton East High School, in Cicero – a town where the infamous mobster, Al Capone once took refuge, to escape the attentions of the Chicago police force. When Joe was growing up it had a largely Italian population – providing a lot of material for his future characterizations. Joe graduated with an acting degree from the Goodman School of Drama, in Chicago, but he was also a keen musician – playing bass guitar in a band called "The Apocryphals". The year he left drama school was the year he made his stage acting debut, in the musical "Hair". Joe continued gaining stage experience, and in 1975, he married Arlene Vrhel, with whom he has two children. In 1977, he made his film debut, in a short called *Medusa Challenger.* One year later, Joe made his Broadway debut, in "Working". Among the seventy films Joe's made, there are several which are close to being genuine modern-day classics.

The Money Pit (1986)
House of Games (1987)
Things Change (1988)
The Godfather: Part III (1990)
Alice (1990) **Queen's Logic** (1991)
Bugsy (1991) **Homicide** (1991)
**Searching for
Bobby Fischer** (1993)
Forget Paris (1995)
Above Suspicion (1995)
Eye for an Eye (1996)
Up Close & Personal (1996)
Jerry and Tom (1998)
**The Wonderful Ice Cream
Suit** (1998) **Celebrity** (1998)
Liberty Heights (1999)
Laguna (2001) **Uncle Nino** (2003)
Pontormo (2004)
Nine Lives (2005) **Edmond** (2005)
Club Soda (2006)
Elvis and Annabelle (2007)
My Suicide (2008)

Jean **Marais**
5ft 10in
(JEAN-ALFRED VILLAIN-MARAIS)

Born: **December 11, 1913**
Cherbourg, Manche, France
Died: **November 8, 1998**

Jean was the son of a veterinarian, who left to fight in World War I, but was abandoned by his wife and family when he returned home. Jean was taken to Paris by his mother, Rosalie, when he was four, to live with his grandmother. He attended the prestigious private school – the Lycee Condorcet. Among its alumni were Louis de Funes and Jean Cocteau – both of whom would feature strongly in Jean's life. He left there when he was thirteen years old and after several other establishments he was then sent to a Catholic boarding school. At sixteen, he worked as a photographer's assistant and model, and became involved in acting on the amateur stage. In 1933, Jean made his film debut with a bit part in *L'Épervier*. His career was changed forever after meeting Jean Cocteau (who called him "Jeannot") four years later – Jean would appear in most of his films, including the classic, *La Belle et La Bête*. He saw the war out in occupied Paris and, although he was Cocteau's lover, in 1942, he was briefly married to the actress, Mila Parély. Jean made his final film appearance, in Bertolucci's *Stealing Beauty*. Jean died in Cannes, of cardio-vascular disease.

L'Éternel retour (1943) **Voyage Without Hope** (1943) **La Belle et la Bête** (1946)
Eagle with Two Heads (1948)
Les Parents Terribles (1948)
Orphée (1950) **Royal affairs in Versailles** (1953) **Napoléon** (1955)
Elena et les Hommes (1956)
White Nights (1957)
Un amour de poche (1957)
Chaque jour a son secret (1958)
Life as a Couple (1958)
Le Bossu (1960) Le Capitan (1960)
Le Capitaine Fracasse (1961)
Fantômas (1964)
Fantômas se déchaîne (1965)
Fantômas Against Scotland Yard (1967) **Donkey Skin** (1970)
Les Misérables (1995)
Stealing Beauty (1996)

Sophie **Marceau**
5ft 8in
(SOPHIE DANIÈLE SYLVIE MAUPU)

Born: **November 17, 1966**
Paris, France

Sophie was the second child born to Benoît and Simone Maupu, who ran a small brasserie in Paris, called 'Le Pharaon'. Much of her childhood was spent in the suburbs of Paris – first in Chelles, and later, when her parents got divorced, in a council flat in Gentilly. Although she enjoyed her school she was impatient to leave her boring existence. When Sophie was twelve, and already very pretty, her mother suggested that she register with a children's modeling agency. It was an attractive possibility, but after they took her photo she didn't really expect anything to happen. A month later, the agency contacted her and told her to attend an audition for a movie, requiring a good-looking teenager. She was seen by Gaumont's casting director. After further visits, the fourteen-year-old was offered the lead in *La Boum,* which made her a star under her new name, Marceau. In 1981, she recorded with François Valéry and appeared in a commercial for Lux Beauty soap. Adult roles exposed her to a wider audience – acting with Mel Gibson, in *Braveheart,* performing in Shakespeare, and being a Bond Girl. In her private life, Sophie has children from relationships with two film producers – a son with Andrzej Zulawski and a daughter with Jim Lemley. She has also directed three films.

La Boum (1980)
Fort Saganne (1984)
Police (1985)
Chouans! (1988)
Fanfan (1993)
D'Artagnan's Daughter (1994)
Braveheart (1995)
Beyond the Clouds (1995)
Anna Karenina (1997)
Marquise (1997)
Firelight (1997)
A Midsummer Night's Dream (1999)
The World Is Not Enough (1999)
La Fidélité (2000)
Anthony Zimmer (2005)
Female Agents (2008)

Frederic **March**
5ft 10in
(ERNEST FREDERICK MCINTYRE BICKEL)

Born: **August 30, 1897**
Racine, Wisconsin, USA
Died: **April 14, 1975**

Frederic was the son of John and Cora Bickel. Following his attendance at local schools – Winslow Elementary and Racine High School, Frederic went to Wisconsin University, in Madison, where he studied Economics. Frederic began a career as a banker, but following an emergency appendectomy, in 1920, he changed his mind and became an actor. He got work as an extra in films made in New York City, starting with *The Great Adventure,* which starred Lionel Barrymore. He shortened his mother's maiden name, Marcher, and made his stage debut, in "Deburau" and appeared on Broadway, in 1926. Three years later, Frederic had a contract with Paramount and starred with Ann Harding in her first film, *Paris Bound*. Nominated for a Best Actor Oscar, for *The Royal Family of Broadway,* he won for *Dr.Jeckyll and Mr. Hyde* and had his pick of the best scripts. He was Oscar-nominated four more times. Fifteen years later he won a second Oscar, for *The Best Years of Our Lives*. He left films on a high when he co-starred with Lee Marvin, in *The Iceman Cometh*. His second wife, the actress Florence Eldridge, was with him from 1927 – right up until his death, in Los Angeles, from prostate cancer.

Laughter (1930) **The Royal Family of Broadway** (1930) **Dr. Jekyll and Mr. Hyde** (1931) **Strangers in Love** (1932) **The Sign of the Cross** (1932)
The Eagle and the Hawk (1933)
Design for Living (1933) **Death Takes a Holiday** (1934) **The Barretts of Wimpole Street** (1934) **Anna Karenina** (1935)
A Star Is Born (1937) **Nothing Sacred** (1937) **So Ends Our Night** (1941)
I Married a Witch (1942) **The Best Years of Our Lives** (1946)
Another Part of the Forest (1948)
Death of a Salesman (1951)
The Desperate Hours (1956)
Inherit the Wind (1960) **Seven Days in May** (1964) **Hombre** (1967)
The Iceman Cometh (1973)

Janet Margolin

5ft 4in

(JANET MARGOLIN)

Born: **July 25, 1943**
New York City, New York, USA
Died: **December 17, 1993**

Janet was the daughter of a Russian-born accountant, Benjamin Margolin – who was founder and president of the Nephrosis Society. At Walden School, near Central Park, it was clear that Janet was destined to be an actress. She attended the New York High School of Performing Arts and began her career working as a prop girl, at the Central Park Shakespeare Festival. Soon she was on the Broadway stage. The film director, Frank Perry, saw her act in the role of an emotionally disturbed teenage girl, in the play "Daughter of Silence". It earned her a Tony nomination and a starring role on her film debut (as a schizophrenic girl) in Perry's *David and Lisa,* opposite Keir Dullea. It was a huge artistic success and the critics were unanimous in their praise for the young actress. Looking back on Janet's 1960s film work it isn't possible to say why she didn't make the big time. A bad first marriage, to Jerry Brandt, which lasted barely two years, may have contributed, and by the time they divorced, in 1970, Janet's movie career had slowed down and she was doing a lot of television work. A second marriage in 1979, to the actor, Ted Wass, was a happier one and it produced two children. Janet played her last film role in 1989, in *Ghostbusters II.* Sadly, in the early 1990s, she was diagnosed with ovarian cancer, Janet was only fifty years old when she died, in Los Angeles.

David and Lisa (1962)
**Bus Riley's Back
in Town** (1965)
**The Saboteur, Code
Name Moriati** (1965)
**The Greatest Story
Ever Told** (1965)
Nevada Smith (1966)
Enter Laughing (1967)
Buona Sera, Mrs.Campbell (1968)
Take the Money and Run (1969)
Annie Hall (1977)
Last Embrace (1979)
Distant Thunder (1988)

Hugh Marlowe

5ft 11in

(HUGH HERBERT HIPPLE)

Born: **January 30, 1911**
Philadelphia, Pennsylvania, USA
Died: **May 2, 1982**

In the early 1930s, following radio work, and after changing his name to John Marlowe, he began his stage career at the Pasadena Playhouse, in California. In 1936, he began getting work in small supporting roles in films – the first of which was *Brilliant Marriage.* His first important film was in 1944, for MGM, when he acted in a romantic drama, *Mrs.Parkington,* in another of those small roles, but this time in the company of Greer Garson and Walter Pidgeon. It was a case of taking what he could get and being in a movie with Judy Garland wasn't hurting his image. It won him a 20th Century Fox contract and good roles in five of the studio's best films of the period – including what is still one of the greatest Sci-Fi movies ever made – *The Day the Earth Stood Still.* The 1950s was Hugh's most fruitful period in terms of film work. In later years, he was mainly seen in television productions. Hugh had three children from his marriages to actresses K.T.Stevens, and Rosemary Torri. His final film was a weak thriller, *The Last Shot You Hear,* in 1969. He died of a heart attack, in New York, at the age of seventy-one.

Meet Me in St. Louis (1944)
Come to the Stable (1949)
Twelve O'Clock High (1949)
Night and the City (1950)
All About Eve (1950)
Rawhide (1951) **The Day the
Earth Stood Still** (1951)
**Mr. Belvedere Rings
the Bell** (1951)
**Wait 'Til the Sun
Shines, Nellie** (1952)
Monkey Business (1952)
Way of a Gaucho (1952)
Casanova's Big Night (1954)
Garden of Evil (1954)
Illegal (1955)
**Earth vs. the
Flying Saucers** (1956)
Elmer Gantry (1960)
Seven Days in May (1964)

Alan Marshall

6ft 1½in

(ALAN MARSHALL)

Born: **January 29, 1909**
Sydney, Australia
Died: **July 13, 1961**

Alan was born to English actor, Leonard Willey, and his wife, the stage actress Irby Marshall, when they were on a tour of Australia, in 1908. Irby was related to the Australian cricketer, Alan Marshall, who played for Surrey, in England. The family settled in Hopewell Junction, New York, and Alan attended school there before being sent to boarding school in upper New York State. After beginning his acting career, Alan took his mother's maiden name, when he acted on stage with his father. He was seen by a Hollywood scout, and went for a screen test. He was given a seven-year contract by David O. Selznick at Selznick International Pictures and made his film debut, in *The Garden of Allah,* which starred Marlene Dietrich and Charles Boyer. MGM borrowed him for *After the Thin Man,* and he was in Greta Garbo's film, *Conquest.* Alan acted with great stars like Luise Rainer. His stock was so high by the late 1930s, he became the original choice for the role of Rhett Butler. In 1938, he married socialite, Mary Boule. A chronic nervous condition virtually ended his film career, in 1944. He made two films in 1959, the last was *Day of the Outlaw.* Alan died of a heart attack on the Chicago stage – when appearing with Mae West, in "Sextette".

The Garden of Allah (1936)
After the Thin Man (1936)
Night Must Fall (1937)
Conquest (1937)
Dramatic School (1938)
For Girls in White (1939)
**The Adventures of Sherlock
Holmes** (1939) **The Hunchback of
Notre Dame** (1939)
Married and in Love (1940)
Irene (1940)
Tom Dick and Harry (1941)
Lydia (1941) **The White Cliffs of
Dover** (1944)
Bride by Mistake (1944)
House on Haunted Hill (1959)
Day of the Outlaw (1959)

Brenda **Marshall**
5ft 3in
(ARDIS ANKERSON GAINES)

Born: **September 29, 1915**
Island of Negros, Philippines
Died: **July 30, 1992**

Brenda would keep her birth name, Ardis Anderson Gaines, long after she became a movie star and would even insist that her co-stars addressed her as that. Brenda first saw the light of day in the beautiful tropical paradise known as the Island of Negro, where her Danish father owned a sugar plantation. She spent her early years in the Philippines before being taken back to the United States by her American mother. After completing her high school education, Brenda attended the famous School of Dramatic Art, run by Russian acting coach, Maria Ouspenskaya, in New York City. Maria was a strict disciplinarian, who was a scary sight – both in films and in person. But she got the best out of her pupils and Brenda made an impressive debut on Broadway, in 1938, in "On the Rocks". Pursued by three studios – she signed for Warner Brothers and made her film debut, in *Espionage Agent,* with Joel McCrea. She divorced her first husband, Richard Gaines, and played opposite Errol Flynn, in *The Sea Hawk.* Her movie career was going along nicely, but her maternal instincts got the better of her. In 1941, she married the actor William Holden, with whom she would have two sons and an increasingly distant relationship, before they divorced in 1971. She retired in 1950, after *The Iroquois Trail.* Brenda died in Palm Springs, California, of throat cancer.

Espionage Agent (1939)
The Man Who Talked
Too Much (1940)
The Sea Hawk (1940)
Money and the Woman (1940)
East of the River (1940)
Footsteps in the Dark (1941)
Singapore Woman (1941)
The Smiling Ghost (1941)
Captain of the Clouds (1942)
You Can't Escape Forever (1942)
The Constant Nymph (1943)
Background to Danger (1943)
Strange Impersonation (1946)
Whispering Smith (1948)

E.G. **Marshall**
5ft 8in
(EVERETT EUGENE GRUNZ)

Born: **June 18, 1914**
Owatonna, Minnesota, USA
Died: **August 24, 1998**

The son of Charles and Irene Grunz, E.G. Marshall was of Norwegian ancestry. He was educated at Mechanic Arts High School, in St. Paul, Minnesota. From 1933, during the Great Depression, he worked in the theater and on radio, in St. Paul, Minneapolis, and Chicago. In 1933, he joined the Oxford Players, a touring company specializing in the works of Shakespeare. In 1935, E.G. settled in Chicago and was able to take advantage of the Federal Theater Project – a national program with the aim of employing as many struggling artists as possible. In the late 1930s, he moved to New York, where he established himself on the Broadway stage in such plays as "The Skin of Our Teeth". He was first married in 1939, to Helen Wolf, with whom he had two daughters. His entry into films was hardly dramatic. A bit part in the 1945 movie, *The House on 92nd Street,* was his debut. Two years later he got his first credit, in *Untamed Fury*. For the next fifty years, he was a popular figure in films and several television series including 'The Defenders' – his last screen appearance was in a 1998 episode, called 'Choice of Evils'. Married three times, E.G. Marshall had seven children. He died of lung cancer, in Bedford, New York.

Call Northside 777 (1948)
The Caine Mutiny (1954)
Pushover (1954)
The Mountain (1956)
The Bachelor Party (1957)
12 Angry Men (1957)
The Buccaneer (1958)
The Journey (1959)
Compulsion (1959)
Town Without Pity (1961)
The Chase (1966)
Tora! Tora! Tora! (1970)
Interiors (1978)
Superman (1980)
Power (1986) Christmas
Vacation (1989) Nixon (1995)
Absolute Power (1997)

Herbert **Marshall**
6ft
(HERBERT BROUGH FALCON MARSHALL)

Born: **May 23, 1890**
London, England
Died: **January 22, 1966**

Bart was educated at St.Mary's College in Harrow, England. He started out as an accountant in the City of London, but after showing natural ability as an actor in some amateur stage productions he turned professional. In 1911, he made his debut in London's West End, then, just as he was establishing himself, World War I broke out. Bart joined the London Scottish Regiment and saw action in Belgium, where, towards the end of the conflict, he was seriously injured and lost a leg. Rehabilitation took time and he only resumed his acting career in 1922, having adjusted his movements to draw as little attention as possible to his wooden leg. Theater work in England and New York and a single silent, *Mumsie* – made in Britain in 1927 – showed it was no handicap. He married the actress, Edna Best, and set off for Hollywood in 1929, where he made his debut in the early version of *The Letter.* His kind face and mellow voice made him a popular film actor during the 1930s and 1940s in films like *The Letter, Duel in the Sun,* and *The Razor's Edge.* Bart was seventy-five when he retired after completing his last film, *The Third Day.* He was living in Beverly Hills, Los Angeles, with his fifth wife, Dee, when he died of a heart attack.

Murder (1930)
Trouble in Paradise (1932)
The Painted Veil (1934)
Dark Angel (1935)
If You Could Only Cook (1935)
Accent On Youth (1935)
Foreign Correspondent (1940)
The Letter (1940)
The Enchanted Cottage (1945)
The Unseen (1945)
Duel in the Sun (1946)
The Razor's Edge (1946)
The Underworld Story (1950)
Anne of the Indies (1951)
Angel Face (1953) The Fly (1958)
Midnight Lace (1960) The List of
Adrian Messenger (1963)

Dean **Martin**
5ft 11in
(DINO PAUL CROCETTI)

Born: **June 7, 1917**
Steubenville, Ohio, USA
Died: **December 25, 1995**

Dino's parents were Italian Americans. He claimed to have spoken only Italian until he was five. Whatever the truth of that story, he was certainly fluent enough in English by the time he dropped out of school in tenth grade. For the next few years, he sold bootleg liquor (which he also drank), boxed at welterweight, with little success and a broken nose, and worked as a croupier. While he was working in illegal casinos, Dino established contacts with local bands, and was eventually hired by the Ernie McKay Orchestra. In the early 1940s, he got married and changed his name to Dean Martin at the suggestion of his second employer, Sammy Watkins. During the war, Dino was drafted, and served in the U.S. Army from 1944-45. In 1946, he was singing at the Glass Hat Club, in New York, when he met and befriended Jerry Lewis. Their comedy-music team was unique and their movie debut, in *My Friend Irma,* in 1949, began a seven-year partnership. One of his movie hit songs was "That's Amore". A solo career was equally successful, but with more dramatic movies, such as *The Young Lions* and *Toys in the Attic.* In 1987, his son's death in a plane crash, sent him into a state of depression he never recovered from. He lived out his life in isolation – dying from lung cancer and emphysema in Beverly Hills – on Christmas Day.

Living It Up (1954)
Artists and Models (1955)
Hollywood or Bust (1956)
The Young Lions (1958)
Some Came Running (1958)
Rio Bravo (1959)
Who Was That Lady? (1960)
Bells Are Ringing (1960)
Ocean's Eleven (1960) All in a Night's
Work (1961) Toys in the Attic (1963)
What a Way to Go! (1964)
Robin and the 7 Hoods (1964)
Kiss Me Stupid (1964)
The Sons of Katie Elder (1965)
Texas Across the River (1966)

Mary **Martin**
5ft 3in
(MARY VIRGINIA MARTIN)

Born: **December 1, 1913**
Weatherford, Texas, USA
Died: **November 3, 1990**

Mary was the youngest daughter of Preston Martin – an attorney, and his wife Juanita – who was a violin teacher. While she was still a child, Mary acted in local theater productions, and when she was twelve, she began taking voice tuition. At seventeen, she quit school in Nashville, in order to marry Benjamin J. Hagman. Their son would become the 'Dallas' star, Larry, but the marriage was already over in 1935. Mary had opened a dance school in Weatherford, but as soon as she was free, she decided to pursue a career in show business by singing on a Dallas radio program and working in clubs. After starring in Cole Porter's "Leave It To Me" in New York, she became a Broadway favorite and achieved national recognition with her recording of "My Heart Belongs to Daddy". She was signed by Paramount and made her film debut, in *The Great Victor Herbert* – the first of ten movies for the studio. She made two with Bing Crosby, but although pleasant enough to look at, she was no glamour girl. After remarrying in 1940, Mary took the wise decision to concentrate more and more on the stage. Her interpretations of many of the female leads in classic musicals, were regarded as definitive by many critics and fans. In 1949, Mary scored one of her biggest stage successes, in Rogers and Hammerstein's "South Pacific". After that came Irving Berlin's "Annie Get Your Gun". She won Tony Awards for "Peter Pan" and "The Sound of Music". Her last television appearance was a role in an episode of 'Hardcastle and McCormick' in 1985. Mary died of cancer at her home in Rancho Mirage, California.

The Great Victor Herbert (1939)
Rhythm on the River (1940)
Love Thy Neighbor (1940)
Kiss the Boys
Goodbye (1941)
Birth of the Blues (1941)
Happy Go Lucky (1943)
True to Life (1943)

Steve **Martin**
6ft
(STEPHEN GLENN MARTIN)

Born: **August 14, 1945**
Waco, Texas, USA

Steve's parents, Glenn and Mary Lee Martin, moved to Southern California in the early years of his life. His father worked in real estate, but had a yearning to be an actor. Steve was always keen on show business, and when he was a teenager, he worked in the Magic Shop, in Disneyland. While there, he learned a lot of the tricks he would later use in his act. Together with classmate, Kathy Westmoreland, he used to perform a musical act at the Bird Cage, in Knott's Berry Farm. At Long Beach College, he majored in Philosophy, but in 1967, he transferred to UCLA where he switched to acting. Steve wrote material for 'The Smothers Brothers Comedy Hour' on TV – which won him an Emmy. In 1971, he made his TV debut, on 'The Ray Stevens Show'. His 'Saturday Night Live' debut was quickly followed by comedy albums, with Dan Aykroyd. In 1977, he wrote and acted in a short, *The Absent Minded Waiter,* which was nominated for an Oscar. His third feature *The Jerk,* showed off his talents admirably and for more than twenty-five years he delivered some great comedy. He was married to the English actress, Victoria Tennant, from 1986 until 1994, and recently wed Anne Stringfield. He has no children.

The Jerk (1979)
Pennies from Heaven (1981)
Dead Men Don't Wear Plaid (1982)
The Man with Two Brains (1983)
Little Shop of Horrors (1986)
Roxanne (1987)
Planes, Trains & Automobiles (1987)
Parenthood (1989)
Father of the Bride (1991)
Grand Canyon (1991)
A Simple Twist of Fate (1994)
The Spanish Prisoner (1997)
Bowfinger (1999)
Novocaine (2001)
Bringing Down the House (2003)
Looney Tunes: Back in Action (2003)
Cheaper by the Dozen (2003)
Shopgirl (2005)
Baby Mama (2008)

Tony **Martin**
5ft 11in
(ALVIN MORRIS)

Born: **December 25, 1912**
San Francisco, California, USA

Tony was the son of Jewish immigrants from Poland. It was a very musical family and he was encouraged to learn to play an instrument. After receiving a saxophone from his grandmother on his tenth birthday, Tony became the star of his school glee club band. At high school, he formed his own outfit, "The Red Peppers" and added his beautiful singing voice to the mix. He then joined the Tom Gerun Orchestra – sitting in the reed section with future top bandleader, Woody Herman. He was with the band when they performed at the Chicago World's Fair in 1933. In the mid-1930s, he went to Hollywood, where he made his first screen appearance (as a sailor) in the Astaire/Rogers musical, *Follow the Fleet*. In 1936, he had a small featured role in Shirley Temple's *Poor Little Rich Girl*. He adopted the stage name Tony Martin and began to get bigger parts – usually in musicals starring his first wife, Alice Faye. They were married in 1937, but got divorced in 1940. By that time Tony's career looked like overtaking hers. He starred with the Marx Brothers, in *The Big Store*. Then came World War II. He served in the Navy and the Army. During that time, Tony sang with the Glenn Miller Army/Airforce band. On his return to civilian life, he worked on Walter Winchell's "Lucky Strike Hour". In 1948, the year he made one of his best films, *Casbah,* he married Cyd Charisse – his wife for sixty years, until she passed away in 2008.

Banjo on My Knee (1936)
You Can't Have
Everything (1937)
Ali Baba Goes to Town (1937)
Sally, Irene and Mary (1938)
Music in My Heart (1940)
Ziegfeld Girl (1941)
The Big Store (1941)
Till the Clouds Roll By (1946)
Casbah (1948)
Two Tickets to Broadway (1951)
Here Come the Girls (1953)
Easy to Love (1953)
Hit the Deck (1955)

Elsa **Martinelli**
5ft 6in
(ELSA TIA)

Born: **January 13, 1935**
Grosseto, Tuscany, Italy

During her mid-teens, Elsa's family moved to Rome. When she was eighteen, she took a job working in a bar. One day in 1953, she was discovered by the fashion designer, Roberto Capucci, and began a successful career as a model. She was not only chic, she was very photogenic. Her beautiful face was seen on the cover of a magazine by an Italian film producer and, that same year, she was given her debut with a small role in a portmanteau picture – *Se vincessi cento millioni*. The following year she had an even smaller role in the Gérard Philipe drama, *Le Rouge et le noir*. No matter, she had already been noticed on the cover of "Vogue" by Kirk Douglas's wife, Anne Buydens. Kirk cast her as his Sioux lover, in his own Bryna Productions western, *The Indian Fighter*. Americans and Europeans liked the look of her, and so did the judges at the Berlin International Film Festival – who awarded her a Silver Berlin Bear as Best Actress, in *Donatella*. Elsa followed it with Hollywood and British films, including *Manuela* – in which she co-starred with Trevor Howard. In the year of its release she married Count Franco di San Vito, with whom she had a daughter, Cristiana, who became an actress. Elsa continued in movies until 1999. Her second husband was the "Paris Match" photographer, Willy Rizzo.

The Indian Fighter (1955)
Donatella (1956) Four Girls in
Town (1957) Manuela (1957)
Costa Azzurra (1959)
The Big Night (1959)
Blood and Roses (1960)
Le Capitan (1960)
Love in Rome (1960)
Hatari! (1962) The Pigeon
That Took Rome (1962)
The Trial (1962)
The V.I.P.s (1963) Rampage (1963)
De l'amour (1964) Hail, Mafia (1965)
The Tenth Victim (1965)
Women Times Seven (1967)
Manon 70 (1968) Una sull'altra (1969)
La Part des lions (1971)

Fele **Martínez**
5ft 10in
(RAFAEL MARTÍNEZ)

Born: **February 22, 1975**
Alicante, Spain

Fele showed early talent as an actor. After completing his normal schooling, when he was eighteen, he went to Madrid, where he studied at the Escuela Superior de Arte Dramático. During that same period, Fele began directing plays as well as acting in them. Along with some friends, he formed an experimental theater group called "Sexpeare". He was twenty-one when he got his first big break in the film feature debut of the writer/director, Alejandro Amenábar, titled *Tesis*. The role won Fele the Goya Award as Best New Actor and helped launch his film career. Within a couple of years, he was one of the most popular movie actors in Spain, with titles like *Open Your Eyes, The Lovers from the North Pole,* and the *Art of Dying,* making people sit up and take notice. He is a big supporter of independent films and he is regularly appearing in interesting short subjects. In 2004, Fele was nominated for a European Film Award, for *Bad Education* – which won him the Jury Award at The Fort Lauderdale International Film Festival. Despite his successes, Fele remains a shy thoughtful character, who only changes his personality when he is acting.

Tesis (1996)
El Tiempo de la felicidad (1997)
Open Your Eyes (1997)
Sleepless in Madrid (1998)
The Lovers from
the North Pole (1998)
Black Tears (1998)
The Art of Dying (2000)
Captains of April (2000)
Red Ink (2000)
Hemingway, the Hunter
of Death (2001)
Just Run! (2001)
Talk to Her (2002)
Darkness (2002)
Utopía (2003)
Two Tough Guys (2003)
Bad Education (2004)
Butterfly (2007)
14, Fabian Road (2008)
The Big Old House (2008)

Lee **Marvin**
6ft 2in
(LEE MARVIN)

Born: **February 19, 1924**
New York City, New York, USA
Died: **August 29, 1987**

Lee's thuggish appearance belied the fact that he was from a sophisticated background. His father, Lamont, was a well-to-do New York advertising executive, and his mother, Courtenay, worked as a fashion writer. Lee was a rebel from the start: after being expelled from several schools, he was sent to Florida, where he attended St. Leo Preparatory College. In 1942, he left to join the U.S. 4th Marine Division. While operating as a sniper, he was wounded, in the battle of Saipan. He received a Purple Heart for his bravery and was given a medical discharge. When the war was over, Lee took a job as a plumber. It proved fortuitous. Repairing pipes at a community theater, he was asked to fill in for an actor who'd fallen ill. He was such a success, he went from amateur theater to understudy jobs off-Broadway. He moved to the West Coast in 1950, and made his film debut, in *You're in the Navy Now,* a year later. He celebrated by marrying Betty Ebeling, with whom he would have four children, but they divorced in 1967. Lee won a Best Actor Oscar for *Cat Ballou* and made significant films, including *The Dirty Dozen, Point Blank,* and *Hell in the Pacific.* When Lee died of a heart attack, in Tuscon, Arizona, he was living with his second wife, Pamela.

The Big Heat (1953) **The Caine Mutiny** (1954) **Bad Day at Black Rock** (1955) **Violent Saturday** (1955) **Attack!** (1956) **Raintree County** (1957) **The Man Who Shot Liberty Vallance** (1962) **Donovan's Reef** (1963) **The Killers** (1964) **Cat Ballou** (1965) **The Professionals** (1966) **The Dirty Dozen** (1967) **Point Blank** (1967) **Hell in the Pacific** (1968) **Paint Your Wagon** (1969) **Prime Cut** (1972) **Emperor of the North** (1973) **The Big Red One** (1980) **Gorky Park** (1983)

Chico **Marx**
5ft 6in
(LEONARD MARX)

Born: **March 22, 1887**
New York City, New York, USA
Died: **October 11, 1961**

The oldest of five sons born to Sam and Minnie Marx – an older brother, Manfred had died in infancy. Leonard grew up with an addictive personality – for women and gambling, but not necessarily in that order. His stage name and Italian persona was the result of having to be streetwise in order to survive when he was a kid. Perfecting a series of accents, including Irish and German, to keep him safe in a tough environment. Chico, as he became known, was a hustler with an exceptional memory for figures and a natural talent as a poker player. When the boys began to perform, Minnie Marx was the group's manager for a time. But when he got older, Chico took over the handling of all the business deals and contracts for the Marx Brothers act. He was a talented pianist who early on, had used those skills to earn money for his family. In 1917, he married Betty Carp, who gave him a daughter and put up with his philandering until 1940. During their years together, Chico got the Marx Brothers a booking on Broadway, a Paramount film contract, and after *Duck Soup,* an even better one with MGM. In the 1940s, he led a dance band and was the first to employ the singer, Mel Tormé. Because of his gambling and his relentless pursuit of women, which cost him a lot of money, Chico was the only Marx brother to go on working right up until a year before he died in Hollywood, from cardiovascular disease. His second wife, Mary De Vithas, was with him from 1958 until his death.

The Cocoanuts (1929)
Animal Crackers (1930)
Monkey Business (1931)
Horse Feathers (1932)
Duck Soup (1933)
A Night at the Opera (1935)
A Day at the Races (1937)
At the Circus (1939)
Go West (1940)
The Big Store (1941)
A Night in Casablanca (1946)

Groucho **Marx**
5ft 7½in
(JULIUS HENRY MARX)

Born: **October 2, 1890**
New York City, New York, USA
Died: **August 19, 1977**

As hard as it is to imagine, Julius, as he was known during his childhood, left school at twelve, and was described as a shy, introverted boy, who was never given the attention received by his four brothers. He made up for it later – after he became Groucho! It took several years in vaudeville shows (with their fifth brother, Gummo), before the Marx Brothers finally got their act together. They made a silent film in 1920, called *Humor Risk* – which was never released because, apart from Harpo, they weren't very good without dialogue. In 1924, they began a series of Broadway plays, with "I'll Say she Is". It was followed by "The Cocoanuts", which ran for nearly three years, and "Animal Crackers". The last two were brought to the screen. After hiding his talent as a singer, he 'came out' in the film *At the Circus,* when he sang the definitive version of "Lydia the Tattooed Lady". After the Marx Brothers quit filming, Groucho's solo career in films was only modest, and one of them, *A Girl in Every Port,* was a total disaster on every level. In the 1950s, he was a big success on the radio and with a television game show, 'You Bet Your Life'. Groucho's three marriages – all of them to actresses - Ruth Johnson, Kay Marvis and Eden Hartford, ended in divorce, but they did produce three lovely children – Arthur, Miriam, and Melinda. Groucho died of pneumonia, in Los Angeles.

The Cocoanuts (1929)
Animal Crackers (1930)
Monkey Business (1931)
Horse Feathers (1932)
Duck Soup (1933)
A Night at the Opera (1935)
A Day at the Races (1937)
Room Service (1938)
At the Circus (1939)
Go West (1940)
The Big Store (1941)
A Night in Casablanca (1946)
Will Success Spoil Rock Hunter? (1957)

Harpo **Marx**
5ft 5½in
(ADOLPH MARX)

Born: **November 23, 1888**
New York City, New York, USA
Died: **September 28, 1964**

Somebody suggested that being raised in a small Jewish neighborhood somehow resulted in Adolph being the smallest of the three great Marx Brothers. When he was a boy at school, he was bullied unmercifully. He quit school at the age of eight, which may explain why he never got to speak any lines. After working with his various brothers in "The Nightingales" singing group, he was given a harp by his mother and acquired the name "Harpo". He quickly learned to compensate for his lack of inches by developing a character with an unrelenting nuisance value. This would reach its peak in his subsequent film appearances. He had an easy going disposition which made people quickly forgive him. Minnie Marx died in 1929, following a stroke and Harpo was at her bedside. A string of hit movies kept the audiences smiling during the Great Depression. In 1934, Harpo was the first entertainer from the West to perform in the U.S.S.R. Although Harpo always chased girls during his movies, he was the only one of the Marx Brothers to lead a normal family life. In 1936, he married actress, Susan Fleming. They couldn't have kids so they adopted four children and were together until his death. During four years of World War II, Harpo worked as a solo act – entertaining American troops around the world. In 1961 he published his autobiography, "Harpo Speaks". He made his final appearance, in 1961, on television, in 'The Red Skelton Show'. He died in Los Angeles following open heart surgery.

The Cocoanuts (1929)
Animal Crackers (1930)
Monkey Business (1931)
Horse Feathers (1932)
Duck Soup (1933)
A Night at the Opera (1935)
A Day at the Races (1937)
At the Circus (1939)
Go West (1940)
The Big Store (1941)
A Night in Casablanca (1946)

Giulietta **Masina**
5ft 3in
(GIULIA ANNA MASINA)

Born: **February 22, 1921**
San Giorgio di Piano, Bologna, Italy
Died: **March 23, 1994**

Giulietta's father was a violinist, and her mother was a schoolteacher. She was the youngest of four children – and the cleverest. Academically, she did well. Giulietta was studying literature, but added something extra, when at Rome University, she joined a drama group. After graduating she became an actress with the Ateneo Theater Group. Her first job was on the radio, where she played Pallina, in a serial called 'Cico e Pallina' which was written by Federico Fellini. She married him in October 1943, but suffered a miscarriage when she fell down a flight of stairs in their apartment block. The couple had a son two years later only to see him die at one month old. They remained together until Fellini's death. In 1946, Giulietta made an uncredited appearance in Rossellini's film *Paisà*. She was featured for the first time in 1948, when her husband wrote the screenplay for *Without Pity*. She was one of the stars when he directed *Variety Lights* and the pair created some great cinema together – including *La Strada,* and *Nights of Cabiria*. One of her last films, *Ginger and Fred,* was a loving tribute to Fred Astaire and Ginger Rogers, by two of Italy's great stars – Giulietta, and Marcello Mastroianni. In 1991, she starred in the French movie, *A Day to Remember*. Giulietta died of cancer within five months of Fellini's death, in 1993.

Variety Lights (1950)
Housemaid (1951)
Europa '51 (1952)
The White Sheik (1952)
Via Padova 46 (1954)
La Strada (1954)
The Swindle (1955)
Nights of Cabiria (1957)
Fortunella (1958)
Wild Wild Women (1959)
Jons und Erdme (1959)
Juliet of the Spirits (1965)
The Feather Fairy (1985)
Ginger and Fred (1986)
A Day to Remember (1991)

James **Mason**
5ft 11in
(JAMES NEVILLE MASON)

Born: **May 15, 1909**
Huddersfield, Yorkshire, England
Died: **July 27, 1984**

James was the son of John and Mabel Mason. His father was a wealthy merchant and young James enjoyed a privileged upbringing – he attended Marlborough College, before gaining a B.A. degree in Architecture, at Peterhouse College, Cambridge. Without any training as an actor, he began to get work in stock companies . He made his professional debut in "Rasputin the Rascal Monk', in 1931, and in 1933, just after a first London appearance in "Gallows Glorious" he joined the Old Vic. His film debut was in *Late Extra,* in 1935. He married Pamela Kellino in 1938 and they starred together, in *I Met a Murderer,* just before the outbreak of World War II. He was a conscientious objector, which upset his parents, but did wonders for his film career. James was a big star in Britain before *Odd Man Out* led to him making it in America. He was nominated for a Best Actor Oscar in *A Star is Born* and for Best Supporting Actor in *Georgy Girl* and *The Verdict*. He died at his home in Switzerland, after a heart attack.

Hatter's Castle (1942)
The Seventh Veil (1945)
Odd Man Out (1947)
The Reckless Moment (1949)
**Pandora and the
Flying Dutchman** (1951)
The Desert Fox (1951) **5 Fingers** (1952)
The Prisoner of Zenda (1952)
The Desert Rats (1953)
Julius Caesar (1953)
The Man Between (1953)
A Star Is Born (1954)
Bigger than Life (1956)
North By North West (1959)
**Journey to the Center of
the Earth** (1959)
A Touch of Larceny (1959)
Lolita (1962)
The Pumpkin Eater (1964)
Georgy Girl (1966)
The Last of Sheila (1973)
The Verdict (1982)
The Shooting Party (1985)

Marsha **Mason**
5ft 3in
(MARSHA MASON)

Born: **April 3, 1942**
St. Louis, Missouri, USA

The daughter of Edward and Catharine Mason, Marsha was born one year before her sister Linda. She was educated at the exclusive girls-only, Nerinx High School, in Webster Groves, Missouri. And after that, Webster College, in the same town. She went to New York City to study drama and in 1965, she married the first of her two husbands, the actor, Gary Campbell. Marsha made her film debut in 1966, in the oddly named *Hot Rod Hullabaloo.* It took six years to recover! During those years, she was impressive on stage in Noel Coward's "Private Lives" directed by Francis Ford Coppola, at San Francisco's American Conservatory Theater. In 1973, she met Neil Simon, while rehearsing for his play, "The Good Doctor". They were married three weeks later. She starred in five movies adapted from his plays and her stage work clinched her first important film role – in *Cinderella Liberty,* for which she was Best Actress Oscar-nominated. She was nominated for a Best Actress Oscar on three other occasions – for *The Goodbye Girl, Only When I Laugh* and *Chapter Two* – the last-named was based on her early relationship with Neil Simon. The couple divorced in 1984. Marsha has continued with her acting career, but the bulk of her work since 1990 has been on television – most recently in episodes of 'Nightmares and Dreamscapes: From the Stories of Stephen King', 'Lipstick Jungle' and 'Army Wives'.

Blume in Love (1973)
Cinderella Liberty (1973)
Audrey Rose (1977)
The Goodbye Girl (1977)
The Cheap Detective (1978)
Promises in the Dark (1979)
Chapter Two (1979)
Only When I Laugh (1981)
Max Dugan Returns (1983)
Heartbreak Ridge (1986)
Stella (1990)
Nick of Time (1995)
Two Days in the Valley (1996)
Bride & Prejudice (2004)

Raymond **Massey**
6ft 1in
(RAYMOND HART MASSEY)

Born: **August 30, 1896**
Toronto, Ontario, Canada
Died: **July 29, 1983**

The son of the head of the Massey-Ferguson Tractor Company, Raymond was educated at Appleby College, an international private boarding school, in Oakville, Ontario. Raymond finished his academic career at the University of Toronto and Balliol College, Oxford. He graduated shortly before the outbreak of World War I. With little hesitation, he joined the Canadian Army and served on the Western Front in Belgium and France. He returned home suffering from shell-shock and worked at Yale as an army instructor. He then used his love of theater to entertain American troops in Siberia. In 1922, he was on the stage in London in "In the Zone". Seven years later, he made a part-talkie film, *High Treason.* In his first sound film, *The Speckled Band,* in 1931, he played Sherlock Holmes. He married his second wife, Adrianne Allen, in 1929, and fathered Anna and Daniel Massey. Raymond's most famous role was as Abe Lincoln, who he portrayed four times – most memorably in *Abe Lincoln in Illinois.* He became an American Citizen in 1944. Raymond's third wife, Dorothy Whitney, was with him when he died of pneumonia in Los Angeles.

The Scarlet Pimpernel (1935)
Things to Come (1936)
Fire Over England (1937)
The Prisoner of Zenda (1937)
The Drum (1938)
Abe Lincoln in Illinois (1940)
49th Parallel (1941)
Desperate Journey (1942)
Action in the North Atlantic (1943)
Arsenic and Old Lace (1944)
The Woman in the Window (1945)
A Matter of Life and Death (1946)
Possessed (1947)
The Fountainhead (1949)
Come Fill the Cup (1951)
Battle Cry (1955)
East of Eden (1955)
How the West Was Won (1962)
Mackenna's Gold (1969)

Mary Stuart **Masterson**
5ft 4in
(MARY STUART MASTERSON)

Born: **June 28, 1966**
New York City, New York, USA

Mary was one of the three children born to struggling New York actors, who decided to give the West Coast a try. Her father, Peter Masterson, was a director, writer and actor, and her mother was Carlin Gynn, an actress. They moved back to the Big Apple in 1968, and their careers took off. When she was eight years old, Mary had her first movie role, in *The Stepford Wives,* which featured her father. She attended The Nightingale-Bamford School in Manhattan, and when she was fourteen, she went to a performing arts camp in the Catskills, known as Stagedoor Manor – taking drama lessons from Estelle Parsons. When she was sixteen, she made her Broadway debut, in "Alice in Wonderland". After two summers at Robert Redford's Sundance Institute, she was given her first teenage movie role, in *Heaven Help Us.* For eight months after that, Mary attended New York University to study Anthropology. In the 1980s and 1990s her work included big-budget films, independents, and television movies. In 2007, Mary directed her first feature film, *The Cake Eaters,* which won her awards at two Independent Film Festivals. Mary was recently seen on TV in episodes of 'Law & Order: Special Victims Unit'. Her third husband is actor, Jeremy Davidson.

Heaven Help Us (1985)
At Close Range (1986)
Some Kind of Wonderful (1987)
Gardens of Stone (1987)
Mr. North (1988)
Chances Are (1989)
Immediate Family (1989)
Married to It (1991)
Fried Green Tomatoes (1991)
Benny & Joon (1993)
Bed of Roses (1996)
Heaven's Prisoners (1996)
Dogtown (1997)
Digging to China (1998)
The Book of Stars (1999)
The Florentine (1999)
Leo (2002)
The Sisters (2005)

Mary Elizabeth **Mastrantonio**
5ft 4in
(MARY ELIZABETH MASTRANTONIO)

Born: **November 17, 1958**
Lombard, Illinois, USA

The daughter of Italian immigrants – Frank and Mary Mastrantonio, Mary grew up in Oak Park, Illinois. Her prettiness got her roles in plays at Oak Park River Forest High School, but it was her natural acting ability that made people look up and admire her. In her teens, she trained as an opera singer, but although nothing came of it, she has been able to use her singing ability during her acting life. At the University of Illinois, she became heavily involved in drama productions and is fondly remembered for her role as Sarah Brown, in "Guys and Dolls". In 1981, she went to live in New York and was first seen there in another musical, "West Side Story". After appearing in a bit part in the 1983 movie, *The King of Comedy,* she starred as Gina Montana, opposite Al Pacino and Michelle Pfeiffer, in *Scarface.* For her next big film, *The Color of Money,* she was nominated for a Best Supporting Actress Oscar. In 1990, she married the director, Pat O'Connor. They have two children and since 2001, the family has lived in London. There have been fewer film opportunities of late, but from 2005 until 2006, she was in several episodes of the television drama, 'Without a Trace' and in 2008, she acted in the quality TV drama, 'The Russell Girl'.

Scarface (1983)
The Color of Money (1986)
Slam Dance (1987)
The January Man (1989)
The Abyss (1989)
Fools of Fortune (1990)
Class Action (1991)
Robin Hood:
Prince of Thieves (1991)
White Sands (1992)
Consenting Adults (1992)
Three Wishes (1995)
Two Bits (1995)
Limbo (1999)
My Life So Far (1999)
The Perfect Storm (2000)
Tabloid (2001)
Stories of Lost Souls (2004)

Chiara **Mastroianni**
5ft 5in
(CHIARA MASTROIANNI)

Born: **May 28, 1972**
Paris, France

Chiara had not one, but two extremely hard acts to follow, when she was born to European movie superstars – Marcello Mastroianni, from Italy, and Catherine Deneuve, from France. She took it all in her stride, when at the age of seven, she was given her first taste of film-making while her mother was on location – acting in the film *À nous deux,* in Canada. That brief debut was followed by her education, and she was twenty-one by the time she had a supporting role in *Ma Saison préfer-ée,* which also starred her mother and Daniel Auteuil. Chiara was praised for her effort in the movie and nominated for a César Award, as Most Promising Actress. A role in the poorly received *Prêt-à-Porter* did her no harm and actually gave her some exposure internationally. For the time being she used her fluency in French and Italian to get work in both countries. She had her first starring role in *Le Journal d'un Séducteur,* and supported her father in one of his final films, *Three Lives and Only One Death.* In 1997, she gave birth to her son Milo, and in 2002, she married the singer, Benjamin Biolay. A daughter Anna, was born to them a year later and they recorded an album called "Home". Trouble was, their home life wasn't happy and they were divorced in 2005. Chiara and her mother can be seen acting together again, in *A Christmas Tale.*

Don't Forget You're
Going to Die (1995)
Le Journal du Séducteur (1996)
Three Lives & Only
One Death (1996)
For Sale (1998)
Le Temps retrouvé (1999)
La Lettre (1999)
Libero Burro (1999)
Drugs (2000)
The Words of
My Father (2002)
Carnages (2002)
L'Heure zéro (2007)
Les Chansons d'amour (2007)
A Christmas Tale (2008)

Marcello **Mastroianni**
5ft 9¼in
(MARCELLO VINCENZO DOMENICO MASTROIANNI)

Born: **September 28, 1924**
Fontana Liri, Lazio, Italy
Died: **December 19, 1996**

Marcello's family moved to Rome by the time he was old enough to go to school. He began working as a draftsman, but in 1943, he was interned by the Nazis and escaped to Venice. The intrigue may have sparked the prospect of an acting career because in 1945, he began studying at Centro Universitario Teatrale. He went to work for a film company as an accountant and made his screen debut in 1947, with a small role in *I Miserabili.* Visconti took a liking to him after seeing him on stage, in "Angelica", and cast him in his production of "A Streetcar Named Desire". In 1957, he went from supporting roles to stardom in Fellini's *La Dolce Vita,* and was three-times Oscar-nominated, for *Divorce Italian Style, A Special Day,* and *Dark Eyes.* His daughter, Chiara – from his relationship with Catherine Deneuve, acted with him in his penultimate film, *Three Lives and Only One Death.* Marcello was married to Flora Carabella, from 1948 until his death in Paris, from pancreatic cancer.

Le Notte Bianche (1957)
Big Deal (1958) La Dolce vita (1960)
Il Bell'Antonio (1960) Love a la
Carte (1960) Fantasmi a Roma (1961)
La Notte (1961) Divorce Italian
Style (1961) 8½ (1963)
Yesterday, Today and Tomorrow (1963)
Marriage Italian Style (1964)
The 10th Victim (1965)
The Stranger (1967)
Jealousy Italian Style (1970)
Sunflower (1970) Allonsanfan (1973)
La Grande Bouffe (1973)
Mogliamante (1977)
Todo modo (1977)
A Special Day (1977)
Traffic Jam (1979)
La Nuit de Varennes (1982)
O Melissokomos (1986)
Ginger and Fred (1986)
Dark Eyes (1987)
Che ora è (1989)
Three Lives and Only
One Death (1996)

Richard **Masur**
6ft 1in
(RICHARD MASUR)

Born: **November 20, 1948**
New York City, New York, USA

From a Jewish family, Richard's father was a pharmacist and his mother was a school teacher. Richard was educated at P.S. 28, Walt Whitman Junior High School, and Roosevelt High School, in Yonkers. While a freshman at State University NY-Stony Brook, he joined a friend to audition for a school play and after trying out, he got the part. He studied acting at Yale School of Drama and began his career on the stage. In 1971, he was an actor and technical director with the Hartford Stage Company. In 1973, Richard made his Broadway debut in "The Changing Room". He was seen by a TV producer and invited to make his debut in an episode of 'All in the Family'. In 1974, Richard moved to Los Angeles. He made his name in a TV sit-com, 'Hot L Baltimore' and the following year he made his film debut, in *Whiffs*. He made his directing debut in 1986, with an Oscar-nominated live-action short, called *Love Struck,* which was produced by his then wife, Fredda Weiss. Richard has been active ever since as an in-demand supporting actor in movies and on TV. From 1995, he served two terms as the president of the Screen Actors Guild. His second wife, Eileen Henry, is currently SAG branch president.

Semi-Tough (1977)
Who'll Stop the Rain? (1978)
Heaven's Gate (1980)
The Thing (1982)
Risky Business (1983)
The Mean Season (1985)
Deadly Pursuit (1988)
Flashback (1990)
My Girl (1991)
The Man Without A Face (1993)
Six Degrees of
Separation (1993)
Patriots (1994)
Forget Paris (1995)
Multiplicity (1996)
Palindromes (2004)
Lovely by Surprise (2007)
Vote and Die: Liszt for
President (2008)

Samantha **Mathis**
5ft 5in
(SAMANTHA MATHIS)

Born: **May 12, 1970**
Manhattan, New York City, New York, USA

After her parents divorced when she was three, Sammy was raised by her mother, an aspiring actress called Bibi Besch. Theater was in the family. Her maternal grandmother Gusti Huber, an Austrian actress, was famous in German films and the Viennese theater, before World War II. Initially, her mother tried to discourage her daughter from an acting career. They went to Los Angeles together where, because of her mother's work, the youngster was soon immersed in the atmosphere of show business. On top of her school work, Sammy took acting classes, and in 1988, made her television debut, as Roseanne Miller, in the first of several episodes of 'Aaron's Way'. The following year she made her first film appearance in the independent production, *Forbidden Sun.* That was no great shakes, and for a while, she carried on with TV work. Her luck changed with a supporting role in *Pump Up the Volume,* and her name began to creep up the cast list. She co-starred with tragic young talent, River Phoenix, in *The Thing Called Love* and they were close – she was with him at The Viper Room on the night he died. Sammy has a couple of new movies in production – including *Order of Chaos* and *The New Daughter,* but until their release, she can frequently be seen on television. At the time of writing, this lovely lady is still single.

Pump Up the Volume (1990)
This Is My Life (1992)
The Music of Chance (1993)
The Thing Called Love (1993)
Little Women (1994)
Jack & Sarah (1995)
How to Make
an American Quilt (1995)
The American President (1995)
Broken Arrow (1996)
Sweet Jane (1998)
The Simian Line (2000)
American Psycho (2000)
The Punisher (2004)
Believe in Me (2006)
Local Color (2006)

Walter **Matthau**
6ft 3in
(WALTER JOHN MATTHOW)

Born: **October 1, 1920**
New York City, New York, USA
Died: **July 1, 2000**

The son of Russian-Jewish immigrants, Walter and his brother Henry, were raised on the Lower East Side of New York City. Their mother brought them up alone, after their father deserted them. They were so poor, there was no such thing as pocket money. Walter sold soft drinks on the street until at the age of eleven, he made a bit of extra cash by playing small roles in a Yiddish theater. He graduated from Seeward Park High School, and worked when he could in the Great Depression. He served in the U.S. Army Corps during World War II. After acting classes with Raiken Ben-Ari and Irwin Piscator, he became an actor. In 1950, he made his first TV appearance, in an episode of 'Lux Theater' called "Shadow on the Heart". In 1955, he made his film debut, in *The Kentuckian.* There wasn't much fun in his early films, but he teamed up with Jack Lemmon and won a Best Supporting Actor Oscar, for *The Fortune Cookie* – which was very funny. Walter was later nominated for Best Actor Oscars, for *Kotch* and *The Sunshine Boys.* Walter died of a heart attack in Santa Monica. He was married twice and had three children.

Lonely Are the Brave (1962)
Charade (1963)
Fail-Safe (1964)
The Fortune Cookie (1966)
A Guide for the
Married Man (1967)
The Odd Couple (1968)
Hello, Dolly! (1969)
Cactus Flower (1969)
Kotch (1971)
Charley Varrick (1973)
The Taking of Pelham One
Two Three (1974)
The Front Page (1974)
The Sunshine Boys (1975)
House Calls (1978)
Hopscotch (1980)
Grumpy Old Men (1993)
Grumpier Old Men (1995)
I'm Not Rappaport (1996)

Victor **Mature**
6ft 2½in
(VICTOR JOHN JOSEPH MATURE)

Born: **January 29, 1913**
Louisville, Kentucky, USA
Died: **August 4, 1999**

Vic's father, Marcellino Mature, was a South Tyrolean, from Italy, and his mother Clara was of Swiss ancestry. Vic was a disruptive influence at his schools, and was expelled several times. He loved his parents and when he was a teenager, he developed his splendid physique by helping his dad deliver butcher's supplies. When he attended Kentucky Military Academy, one of his classmates was the future actor, Jim Backus. Vic was such a hit with the opposite sex it went to his head so he decided to become an actor. In his early twenties, Vic moved to California, where he studied and practiced his acting techniques, at the Pasadena Playhouse. In 1939, his film career started with his debut, in *The Housekeeper's Daughter.* A couple of years later it was interrupted by World War II. To start with, Vic served in the Coast Guard, and was able to make nine more movies. When he left for service overseas, his fan-mail was pouring in. He saw action in Europe and was on Okinawa, when the A-bomb was dropped on Japan. Fox took him back with open arms on his return and they cast him in probably the finest of John Ford's westerns – *My Darling Clementine,* quickly followed by the classic film-noir, *Kiss of Death.* Vic had twenty good years in the movies and five beautiful wives. His only child, Victoria, was born in 1975, to his fifth wife, Loretta. He died of leukemia at Rancho Santa Fe, in California.

I Wake Up Screaming (1941) **Song of the Islands** (1942) **My Gal Sal** (1942)
Footlight Serenade (1942)
My Darling Clementine (1946)
Kiss of Death (1947)
Cry of the City (1948)
Samson and Delilah (1949)
Wabash Avenue (1950)
Million Dollar Mermaid (1952)
Affair With a Stranger (1953)
The Glory Brigade (1953)
Violent Saturday (1955) **The Last Frontier** (1955) **Interpol** (1957)

Virginia **Mayo**
5ft 5in
(VIRGINIA CLARA JONES)

Born: **November 30, 1920**
St. Louis, Missouri, USA
Died: **January 17, 2005**

The daughter of a newspaper man and his wife, one of Ginny's ancestors had served in the American Revolution, and later founded East St. Louis, Illinois, just across the Mississippi. On a more modern footing was a show business connection – her aunt operated a dance studio, where Ginny took lessons from the age of six. She also had a good singing voice – when she graduated from high school in 1937, she joined the chorus of the St. Louis Municipal Opera. She went to New York still using the name Virginia Jones and got work as a dancer on Broadway. In 1939, she made her first screen appearance in a short, called *Gals and Gallons.* Its significance was that after working with Andy and Florence Mayo (who played Pansy the Horse) she changed her name. In 1943, she signed with Samuel Goldwyn, who gave her small roles, until *The Princess and the Pirate,* co-starring Bob Hope, made her a star. Four successful films with Danny Kaye ensured Ginny's lasting popularity. In 1947 she married her only husband, actor Michael O'Shea. Ginny's later films are of little value. She made her last appearance in 1997, in *The Man Next Door.* She died of pneumonia and heart failure, at Thousand Oaks, California.

The Princess and the Pirate (1944)
Wonder Man (1945)
The Kid from Brooklyn (1946)
The Best Years of Our Lives (1946)
Out of the Blue (1947)
The Secret Life of Walter Mitty (1947
A Song Is Born (1948)
Flaxy Martin (1949)
Colorado Territory (1949)
The Girl from Jones Beach (1949)
White Heat (1949) **Backfire** (1950)
The Flame and the Arrow (1950)
Captain Horatio Hornblower R.N. (1951)
Great Day in the Morning (1956)
The Proud Ones (1956)
The Tall Stranger (1957)

Rachel **McAdams**
5ft 5in
(RACHEL ANNIE MCADAMS)

Born: **November 17, 1978**
London, Ontario, Canada

The daughter of a truck driver, Lance McAdams, and his wife, Sandra, who was a nurse, Rachel grew up in the small town of St.Thomas, with younger siblings, Daniel and Kayleen. When she was four years old, Rachel began figure skating at a competitive level. At thirteen, she attended a summer theater camp called 'Original Kids', where she gained her first acting experience. After her secondary school – Central Elgin Collegiate Institute – she starred in the award-winning play, "I Live in a Little Town", at Sears Drama Festival. Rachel then graduated with Honors and a Bachelor of Fine Arts degree in Theater, from York University, in Toronto. She then participated in David Rotenberg's on-camera acting classes, in Toronto, before getting work – starting with a pilot in 2001, for a Canadian television series called 'Shotgun Love Dolls'. Rachel's film debut came a year later, in a Canadian/Italian co-production, *My Name Is Tanino,* and that same year, she made her first appearance in an American movie, in a comedy titled, *The Hot Chick.* She was one of MTV Movie Award Team's winners for *Mean Girls,* and confirmed her promise in the romantic film, *The Notebook* – she shared a Best Kiss Award with Canadian co-star Ryan Gosling. They were an item after that, but split up during 2007. Rachel's recent movie – the Neil Burger-directed comedy, *The Lucky Ones,* co-starring Tim Robbins, received good reviews and it registered her seventh hit in a row. Her upcoming – *The Time Traveler's Wife,* with Eric Bana, is eagerly awaited by her fans – *State of Play* is already a winner.

My Name Is Tanino (2002)
Perfect Pie (2002) **The Hot Chick** (2002)
Mean Girls (2004)
The Notebook (2004)
Wedding Crashers (2005)
Red Eye (2005)
The Family Stone (2005)
Married Life (2007)
The Lucky Ones (2008)
State of Play (2009)

James McAvoy
5ft 7in
(JAMES ANDREW MCAVOY)

Born: April 21, 1979
Glasgow, Scotland

When Jimmy was seven, his parents got divorced. He and his sister Joy, went to live with their maternal grandmother. For a while, Jimmy went with his dad to support the Glasgow Celtic soccer team, but now hasn't spoken to him for twenty-one years. Young Joy became a singer with the Scottish girl group "Streetside". Jimmy was attending the St. Thomas Aquinas Secondary School, when director, David Heyman paid a visit. Jimmy asked him if he could give him some work experience on his next film project and ended up with a small role in *The Near Room*. Jimmy then won a place at the Royal Scottish Academy of Music and Drama. That was followed by television work. When he was twenty, he moved down to London where he was a roommate of the young Australian actor, Jesse Spencer. They both appeared in the 2000 television movie, 'Lorna Doone'. The following year, Jimmy acted in a German made horror film, *Swimming Pool*. His breakthrough came when the multi-talented Stephen Fry put on his director's hat, and chose the young Scot for a leading role in *Bright Young Things*. Jimmy secured his status with a trio of good movies including the children's fantasy, *Narnia*. He has since given fine performances in *The Last King of Scotland* and *Atonement* – both of which got him BAFTA nominations. For Jimmy McAvoy, the only way is up. In 2006, he married English actress, Anne-Marie Duff. They live in London. His next film, *The Last Station*, looks promising.

Bright Young Things (2003)
Wimbledon (2004)
Inside I'm Dancing (2004)
The Chronicles of Narnia:
The Lion, the Witch and
the Wardrobe (2005)
The Last King of Scotland (2006)
Penelope (2006)
Starter for 10 (2006)
Becoming Jane (2007)
Atonement (2007)
Wanted (2008)

Andrew McCarthy
5ft 9in
(ANDREW MCCARTHY)

Born: November 29, 1962
New York City, New York, USA

Andrew spent his early years in Westfield, New Jersey. When he was fifteen, he attended Pingry Preparatory School, in Bernardsville. It was while there that he developed a passion for acting and skills as a basketball player. His next stop was New York University, where he was a theater major. After graduating, he made his film debut in the 1983 teen-flick, *Class*. He was one of the nine original members of the "Brat Pack". During the making of *St. Elmo's Fire*, Andrew took up smoking and after a long struggle, kicked the habit ten years later. To get away from Hollywood, he attended drama studies at the Circle in Square Theater School in New York and made his Broadway debut, in "The Boys in Winter", in 1985. Apart from overcoming his smoking habit, Andrew has dealt in the same determined way with an alcohol problem, which began when he was twelve. He entered detox in 1992, and has been sober ever since then. His television work includes the 2005 series, 'E-Ring'. In 1999, he married his college sweetheart, Carol Schneider – twenty years after they first met. They have a son named Sam, but due to Andrew's personal problems, got divorced in 2005. Andrew has continued with his career since then and has been seen in several episodes of the TV comedy drama series, 'Lipstick Jungle'. On the big screen he was in the popular family fantasy movie – *The Spiderwick Chronicles*. His next film will be the horror thriller, *Camp Hope*.

Class (1983)
The Beniker Gang (1985)
Heaven Help Us (1985)
St. Elmo's Fire (1985)
Pretty in Pink (1986)
Waiting for the Moon (1987)
Less than Zero (1987)
Weekend at Bernie's (1989)
Mrs. Parker and the
Vicious Circle (1994)
New Waterford Girl (1999)
The Orphan King (2005)
The Spiderwick Chronicles (2008)

Kevin McCarthy
5ft 10in
(KEVIN MCCARTHY)

Born: February 15, 1914
Seattle, Washington, USA

Kevin was the son of Roy and Martha McCarthy. His father was from a wealthy Irish family. Kevin and his older sister, the future author, Mary McCarthy, were orphaned when both their parents died in the great flu epidemic of 1918. The two children were initially taken in by their father's Catholic parents, in Minneapolis, Minnesota. They were then raised by their maternal grandparents in Seattle. Kevin graduated from Campion High School, in Prairie du Chien, Wisconsin, in 1932. After the University of Minnesota, he studied at the Actor's Studio. Kevin worked in stock productions before his Broadway debut in "Abe Lincoln in Illinois" in 1938. World War II came along and he served in the U.S. Air Force. In 1941, he married the actress, Augusta Dabney, with whom he had three children. They divorced in 1961. He toured in the play "Winged Victory" – making his film debut in a bit part in the 1944 screen version. He did stage and television work after the war and seemed on the brink of a major movie career when he was nominated for a Best Supporting Actor Oscar for *Death of a Salesman*. His most famous role was as Miles Bennell in the classic film *Invasion of the Body Snatchers*. He was in the 1978 version as well. Kevin lives with his second wife, Kate, whom he married in 1979, and was still making films in 2008.

Death of a Salesman (1951)
Drive a Crooked Road (1954)
Stranger on Horseback (1955)
An Annapolis Story (1955)
Invasion of the Body Snatchers (1956)
Nightmare (1956) **The Misfits** (1961)
The Prize (1963) **A Gathering of**
Eagles (1963) **The Best Man** (1964)
Mirage (1965)
Big Deal at Dodge City (1966)
Kansas City Bomber (1972)
Invasion of the Body
Snatchers (1978)
The Howling (1981)
Looney Tunes:
Back in Action (2003)
Her Morbid Desires (2008)

Matthew **McConaughey**
6ft
(MATTHEW DAVID MCCONAUGHEY)

Born: **November 4, 1969**
Uvalde, Texas, USA

Of Irish heritage, Matthew was the youngest of three brothers born to the former Green Bay Packers footballer, J.D.McConaughey, who owned a gas station. His mother, Mary, was a school teacher. When Matthew was eleven, the family moved to Longview, Texas, where he graduated from Longview High school after being voted "Most Handsome". It suggested a dramatic future, but before that, Matthew spent a year as an exchange student in New South Wales, Australia. On his return to the USA, he went back to Austin, where he took film direction studies at the University of Texas. He'd appeared in a few student films and some television commercials by the time he made his professional TV acting debut in a 1992 episode of 'Unsolved Mysteries'. He also directed a short called *Chicano Chariots*. A year later, he had a small role in his first movie, *My Boyfriend's Back,* but it was that year's, *Dazed and Confused* which got him noticed. The year when he became real star material was 1996, when he played a sheriff in *Lone Star* and a young lawyer in John Grisham's *A Time to Kill* – for which he won an MTV Movie Award. In 1998, he wrote, directed, and starred in a short, *The Rebel*. Success is now his and in 2007, he purchased a dream home in Malibu.

Dazed and Confused (1993)
Judgement (1995)
Boys on the Side (1995)
Lone Star (1996)
A Time to Kill (1996)
Contact (1997) Amistad (1997)
Edtv (1999) U-571 (2000)
Thirteen Conversations
About One Thing (2001)
Frailty (2001)
How to Lose a Guy
in 10 Days (2003)
Two For the Money (2005)
We Are Marshall (2006)
Fool's Gold (2008)
Tropic Thunder (2008)
Surfer, Dude (2008)

Joel **McCrea**
6ft 3in
(JOEL ALBERT MCCREA)

Born: **November 5, 1905**
South Pasadena, California, USA
Died: **October 20, 1990**

Joel grew up in Los Angeles. His father worked for the L.A. Gas and Electric Co. and his mother was a professional Christian Scientist. He was educated at Hollywood High School and Pomona College in Claremont. Joel graduated in 1929 from the University of Southern California. He got stage experience at Pasadena Playhouse before venturing into the movies. His grandfather, who'd been a stagecoach driver, taught young Joel to ride so well that he was able to get extra work from 1927 onwards. He was considered one of the best horsemen in westerns. His first important film role, in 1929, was in *The Jazz Age*. From MGM, he moved to RKO, where his friendship with Will Rogers (a fellow rancher) helped his career. Initially, he was a romantic lead and in comedies, and it wasn't until he appeared in B-movies that he was given the cowboy roles he most enjoyed. In 1933, he married the young actress, Frances Dee. They were together for fifty-seven years. Joel worked for Sturges – *Sullivan's Travels, The Palm Beach Story,* and Hitchcock – *Foreign Correspondent*. His last western was in 1976, in *Mustang Country*. Joel died in Woodlands Hills, California, of pulmonary complications.

The Hounds of Zaroff (1932)
The Lost Squadron (1932)
The Silver Chord (1933)
Gambling Lady (1934)
Barbary Coast (1935)
Banjo on My Knee (1936)
Dead End (1937)
Union Pacific (1939)
Foreign Correspondent (1940)
Sullivan's Travels (1940)
The Palm Beach Story (1942)
The More the Merrier (1943)
The Unseen (1945)
Ramrod (1947) Saddle
Tramp (1950) Rough Shoot (1952)
Wichita (1955)
The Tall Stranger (1957)
Ride the High Country (1963)

Hattie **McDaniel**
5ft 2in
(HATTIE MCDANIEL)

Born: **June 10, 1895**
Wichita, Kansas, USA
Died: **October 26, 1952**

The youngest of thirteen children, Hattie's parents were former slaves. Her father, Henry, had fought in the Civil War, and her mother, Susan, was a fine singer of religious music. In 1900, the family moved to Colorado, where Hattie attended East Denver High School. At fifteen, she was the only black person to compete in the Women's Christian Temperance Union event, and won a gold medal for reciting a poem titled "Convict Joe". Flushed with success, she saw her future as a performer. She then dropped out of school during her sophomore year to join two of her brothers in their father's traveling minstrel show - for which she wrote songs. In 1926, she began singing on a radio show in Denver and two years later, she was making records. In 1931, she joined other members of her family in Los Angeles, and made her film debut in *The Golden West,* in 1932. To say she was type-cast by her color is an understatement. She made her living impersonating maids. In 1939, she won a Best Supporting Actress Oscar, for playing one in *Gone With the Wind*. She was married four times. Hattie's first husband died, but she divorced the other three. She made her final appearance on TV, in 'Beula' in 1952 – the same year that she died at Woodlands Hills, from breast cancer – after a two-year illness.

Show Boat (1936)
Saratoga (1937)
The Shining Hour (1938)
Zenobia (1939)
Gone With the Wind (1939)
Maryland (1940)
The Great Lie (1941)
The Male Animal (1942)
In This Our Life (1942)
George Washington
Slept Here (1942)
Johnny Come Lately (1943)
Thank Your Lucky Stars (1943)
Since You went Away (1944)
Margie (1946)
Song of the South (1946)

Christopher McDonald
6ft 3in
(CHRISTOPHER MCDONALD)

Born: **February 15, 1955**
New York City, New York, USA

Chris was one of seven children born to James McDonald, a high school principal and his wife, Patricia, a nursing professor. Chris grew up close to his school, at Romulus, in upstate New York. He attended Hobart College, in Geneva, N.Y. and after graduating, he went to London, where he studied at the Royal Academy of Dramatic Art and the London Academy of Music and Dramatic Art. He returned to New York, where he took more coaching from the Stella Adler Acting Conservatory. Chris was first seen on the small screen in the television comedy, 'Getting Married' in 1978. He made his film debut two years later in a dreary horror movie, called *The Hearse*. Then came TV work including an episode of 'Cheers' and some below par movies. In 1985, things brightened up when he worked on *The Boys Next Door*, with Charlie Sheen. Of his fifty movies since then, there have been enough good ones – *Thelma & Louise, Quiz Show, Requiem for a Dream, My Sexiest Year* – to mention a few – to keep his name in the minds of casting directors. Since 1992 Chris has been married to Lupe Gidley. The couple have four children and live in Southern California.

The Boys Next Door (1985)
Chances Are (1989)
Thelma & Louise (1991)
Dutch (1991)
Grumpy Old Men (1993)
Terminal Velocity (1994)
Quiz Show (1994)
Happy Gilmore (1996)
Unforgettable (1996)
Lawn Dogs (1997)
Dirty Work (1998) SLC Punk! (1998)
The Faculty (1998)
Gideon (1999) Takedown (2000)
Requiem for a Dream (2000)
The Perfect Storm (2000)
The Man Who Wasn't There (2001)
Broken Flowers (2005)
My Sexiest Year (2007)
Awake (2007)
Player 5150 (2008)

Mary McDonnell
5ft 8in
(MARY MCDONNELL)

Born: **April 28, 1952**
Wilkes-Barre, Pennsylvania, USA

Mary's family relocated shortly after she was born and she was raised in Ithaca, New York. After high school, she was a Liberal Arts Major at Fredonia State University, in New York. From drama school she joined the Long Wharf Theater Company in New Haven, Connecticut, with whom she was active for more than twenty years. In 1980, Mary won an Obie for her role in "Still Life" and went on to perform in several Broadway productions including "The Heidi Chronicles". Mary made her first TV appearance in 1980, in the soap opera, 'As the World Turns'. In 1984, she made her film debut, with a small role in Sidney Lumet's *Garbo Talks,* which starred Anne Bancroft. Her first major film role was as Elma Radnor, in the highly-rated *Matewan,* but it was her performance as 'Stands With A Fist' a white American girl raised by Sioux Indians, in Kevin Costner's epic *Dances with Wolves,* which brought her to the brink of stardom. It also earned her a first Oscar nomination as Best Supporting Actress. Two years later, she was nominated for a Best Actress Oscar, for *Passion Fish*. Mary is married to the drama teacher, Randle Mell, and teaches acting classes with him. The couple have two children, Olivia and Michael. Being a star can sometimes create problems. In September, 2007, Mary was forced to get a court order against an obsessive female fan, who was stalking her. Mary has appeared as President Laura Roslin, in over seventy episodes of the TV series, 'Battlestar Galactica'.

Matewan (1987)
Dances with Wolves (1990)
Grand Canyon (1991)
Passion Fish (1992)
Sneakers (1992)
Blue Chips (1994)
Independence Day (1996)
You Can Thank Me Later (1998)
Mumford (1999)
Donnie Darko (2001)
Nola (2003)
Crazy Like a Fox (2004)

Frances McDormand
5ft 6in
(FRANCES LOUISE MCDORMAND)

Born: **June 23, 1957**
Chicago, Illinois, USA

Fran was the third adopted child of a Canadian Disciples of Christ minister, Vernan McDormand and his wife, Noreen. She was raised in Monessen, near Pittsburgh, Pennsylvania. She attended Bethany College in West Virginia, where she earned a B.A. in Theater, before her MFA from Yale Drama School. Fran then traveled all over the country and gained experience in a variety of stage theater productions. In 1984, she made her film debut as Abby – in the Coen Brothers' first movie, *Blood Simple.* She married Joel Coen that same year. A year later, she had a supporting role (as a nun) in their crime comedy, *Crimewave.* It was followed by TV work, and a Tony nomination for her acting on Broadway, in "A Streetcar Named Desire". The Coen's *Raising Arizona,* helped to raise her profile and she got juicier roles. One of which, *Mississippi Burning,* earned her the first of four Oscar nominations. Success at the Academy Awards came her way when her portrayal of Marge Gunderson, in *Fargo,* won Fran a Best Actress Oscar. She was subsequently nominated as Best Supporting Actress – for *Almost Famous* and *North Country.* The recent Coen brothers film, *Burn After Reading,* provided her with another great role.

Blood Simple (1983)
Raising Arizona (1987)
Mississippi Burning (1988)
Darkman (1990)
Hidden Agenda (1990)
Short Cuts (1993)
Beyond Rangoon (1995)
Fargo (1995) Palookaville (1995)
Primal Fear (1996) Paradise Road (1997)
Almost Famous (2000)
The Man Who Wasn't There (2001)
Laurel Canyon (2002)
City by the Sea (2002)
Something's Gotta Give (2003)
North Country (2005)
Miss Pettigrew Lives
for a Day (2008)
Burn After Reading (2008)

Roddy **McDowall**
5ft 10in
(RODERICK ANDREW ANTHONY JUDE MCDOWALL)

Born: **September 17, 1928**
Herne Hill, London, England
Died: **October 3, 1998**

Roddy's father, Thomas McDowall, was in the Merchant Navy. His mother, Irish-born Winsfriede, was an aspiring actress. Both Roddy's parents were theater enthusiasts. They paid for his elocution lessons from the age of five. With their encouragement, he made his film debut when he was ten in *Murder in the Family,* which starred Jessica Tandy. By the time he left war torn London for America, he was a veteran of seventeen British films. In Hollywood, he began his career in the patriotic film, *Man Hunt,* set in England and starring Walter Pidgeon and Joan Bennett. A whole host of roles came his way, including a starring one in the film which introduced Elizabeth Taylor to American audiences – *Lassie Come Home.* When he was eighteen, Roddy went to New York to act on Broadway. In 1960, he won a Tony Award as Best Supporting Actor in the Broadway play, "The Fighting Cock". His stage work didn't affect his movie work – although there was a ten-year break when he grew out of young roles – and worked on TV. By the time he acted in his last film, in 1998's *Something to Believe In,* he'd made over 150 movies. After his death from cancer, this popular actor's ashes were scattered into the Pacific Ocean.

How Green Was
My Valley (1941)
My Friend Flicka (1943)
Lassie Come Home (1943)
The White Cliffs of Dover (1944)
The Keys of the Kingdom (1944)
Macbeth (1948)
Kidnapped (1948)
The Longest Day (1962)
That Darn Cat (1965)
Lord Love a Duck (1966)
Planet of the Apes (1968)
Bedknobs and Broomsticks (1971)
Conquest of the Planet of
the Apes (1972)
The Life and Times
of Judge Roy Bean (1972)
The Poseidon Adventure (1977)

Malcolm **McDowell**
5ft 8½in
(MALCOLM JOHN TAYLOR)

Born: **June 13, 1943**
Leeds, Yorkshire, England

The son of a pub owner who became an alcoholic, Malcolm's parents weren't rich, but they raised the money to send him to boarding school when he was eleven. At Cannock House School, in Eltham, Kent, he got involved in plays – making his debut in 1956, as Feste, in Shakespeare's "Twelfth Night". Malcolm's first job was working at the family pub as a barman until his father was made bankrupt. Malcolm worked as a coffee salesman to pay for acting classes at the London Academy of Music and Art. Eventually, he was able to start working as an extra with the Royal Shakespeare Company. He first appeared on television in the series, 'Crossroads' in 1964, and three years later, was in demand for roles in 'Z Cars' and 'Dixon of Dock Green'. After a small role in the film *Poor Cow,* from which his scenes were deleted, he made an impressive starring debut, as Mick Travis, in Lindsay Anderson's *If....* Stanley Kubrick's *A Clockwork Orange* made him a star. He is divorced from actresses Margot Bennett and Mary Steenburgen, and now lives in a suburb of Los Angeles with his third wife, Kelley Kuhr, and their young sons, Beckett and Finnian. Busier than ever, he was recently on TV, in several episodes of 'Metalocalypse' and 'Heroes'.

If.... (1968) Figures in
a Landscape (1970)
A Clockwork Orange (1971)
O Lucky Man! (1973)
Time after Time (1979)
Cat People (1982)
Blue Thunder (1983)
Out of Darkness (1990)
Assassin of the Tsar (1991)
Bopha! (1993)
Cyborg 3: The Recycler (1994)
Gangster No.1 (2000)
The Company (2003)
Bobby Jones:
Stroke of Genius (2004)
The List (2007)
Halloween (2007)
Doomsday (2008)

Darren **McGavin**
5ft 10in
(WILLIAM LYLE RICHARDSON)

Born: **May 7, 1922**
San Joaquin, California, USA
Died: **February 25, 2006**

Darren's parents, Grace and Reid Delano Richardson, got divorced when he was a small boy. His father, who was literally left holding the baby, was at his wit's end, and placed Darren in an orphanage. It was the first of three, and apart from the third, which he quite liked, he regularly tried to run away. Darren's first job was as a painter at Columbia Pictures. Although he'd had no formal training as an actor, Darren made his movie debut, in 1945, with an uncredited appearance in *A Song to Remember.* After three equally invisible film roles, Darren moved to New York, where he trained as an actor – firstly at the Neighborhood Playhouse and then at the Actors Studio. He married Melanie York, who gave up her own acting career to have a family. Although they got divorced twenty-five years later, they brought four children into the world. Television work dominated the next few years, but in 1951, Darren had his first featured role in a modest comedy called *Queen for a Day.* In 1955, he was fourth billed below Katherine Hepburn, Rossano Brazzi and Isa Miranda in *Summertime,* and he had a pretty good run for the next forty-five years – on stage, television and in films. Darren was eighty-three when he passed away peacefully at home in Los Angeles – from natural causes. His second wife, Kathie, had died in 2003.

Summertime (1955)
The Court Martial of Billy
Mitchell (1955)
The Man with the
Golden Arm (1955)
Beau James (1957)
The Delicate Delinquent (1957)
Bullet for a Badman (1964)
The Night Stalker (1971)
Airport '77 (1977)
A Christmas Story (1983)
From the Hip (1987)
Dead Heat (1988)
Billy Madison (1995)
Small Time (1996)

Bruce McGill
5ft 9¼in
(BRUCE TRAVIS MCGILL)

Born: **July 11, 1950**
San Antonio, Texas, USA

Bruce's father, Woodrow Wilson McGill, was a real estate agent who later worked for an insurance company. His mother Adriel, was an artist and homemaker. Bruce was educated at the Douglas MacArthur High School and graduated from the University of Texas at Austin, with a Drama degree. His film debut, at the age of twenty-seven, was a strong role in the comedy/drama, *Handle with Care.* His follow-up, as "D-Day Day", in *Animal House,* was another success. He then spent one season in the television-series, 'Delta House' and following a couple of disappointing movies, he was back on track in the exceptional *Silkwood.* After playing Ernest Hemingway, in *Waiting for the Moon,* the good film roles dried up for a while, but *The Last Boy Scout* and *My Cousin Vinny,* gave him a platform to launch from. Since then, it's mostly been a smooth ride. Bruce is one of Hollywood's great supporting actors. When he has time, he works in the theater. He has been married to Gloria Lee since 1994.

Handle with Care (1977)
Animal House (1978)
Silkwood (1983) Wildcats (1986)
Waiting for the Moon (1987)
The Last Boy Scout (1991)
My Cousin Vinny (1992)
Cliffhanger (1993) Timecop (1994)
Perfect Alibi (1995)
Black Sheep (1996)
Courage Under Fire (1996)
Rosewood (1997) Lawn Dogs (1997)
The Insider (1999)
The Legend of Bagger Vance (2000)
Shallow Hal (2001) Ali (2001)
The Sum of All Fears (2002)
Matchstick Men (2003)
Runaway Jury (2003)
Collateral (2004)
Cinderella Man (2005)
Elizabeth Town (2005) American
Fork (2007) The Good Life (2007)
The Lookout (2007)
King of the Evening (2008)
Vantage Point (2008)

Kelly McGillis
5ft 10in
(KELLY ANN MCGILLIS)

Born: **July 9, 1957**
Newport Beach, California, USA

A doctor's daughter, with no theatrical links in her family background, Kelly grew up with a natural acting ability. When she was at high school, she won an award and went on to study at the Juilliard School's Drama Division. Her career was interrupted by a bad first marriage in 1979, but within two years she was free again. In 1982, Kelly endured a most horrific experience when two men broke into her apartment and sexually assaulted her. The following year, she made her film debut, with Tom Conti in *Reuben, Reuben.* It was praised by the critics, but audiences didn't rush to see it. Even so, her performance impressed Australian director, Peter Weir, who cast her as an Amish widow in his powerful film, *Witness.* Having co-starred with Harrison Ford, she was regarded as a bankable star – ideal for the blockbuster, *Top Gun.* Despite her beauty and obvious acting talent, Kelly never quite made it to the top. In *The Accused,* her performance alongside Jodie Foster was a career highlight. She is believed to have drawn on her earlier experience in this harrowing tale of rape. In 1989, she settled down to a second marriage, with Fred Tillman, with whom she founded the restaurant "Kelly's" in Key West, Florida. The couple have two daughters, Kelsey and Sonora, but were divorced in 2002. In 2004, Kelly toured as Mrs. Robinson, in a stage production of "The Graduate". Kelly has been recently on television in a couple of episodes of 'The L Word'.

Witness (1985)
Top Gun (1986)
Made in Heaven (1987)
The House on
Carroll Street (1987)
The Accused (1988)
Winter People (1989)
The Babe (1992)
Ground Control (1998)
The Settlement (1999)
At First Sight (1999)
Morgan's Ferry (1999)
The Monkey's Mask (2000)

John C. McGinley
6ft 2in
(JOHN CHRISTOPHER MCGINLEY)

Born: **August 3, 1959**
New York City, New York, USA

John's father, Gerald McGinley, was a stockbroker, and his mother, Patricia, was a schoolteacher. Although he was born in Greenwich Village, one of five children, John's parents moved when he was very young and raised him in Milburn, New Jersey. He attended Milburn High School before studying acting at Syracuse University. He then earned his Master of Fine Arts degree at New York University. In New York he began getting small roles in off-Broadway and Broadway productions. In 1985, John made his television debut in the series 'Another World'. When he was understudying at the Circle-In-The-Square he was spotted by Oliver Stone. The following year, after making his film debut, in Alan Alda's *Sweet Liberty,* John was given a featured role in Stone's highly-rated Vietnam-themed, *Platoon.* He has been married twice in the past ten years, first to Lauren Lambert, and since 2007, to Nichole Kessler, with whom he lives in Malibu, California. Since 1999, he hasn't really acted in a hit movie, but for seven years, he's been starring as Dr. Perry Cox in the popular TV series, 'Scrubs'.

Platoon (1986)
Wall Street (1987)
Talk Radio (1988)
Prisoners of Inertia (1989)
Fat Man and Little Boy (1989)
Born on the Fourth of July (1989)
Point Break (1991)
Article 99 (1992)
A Midnight Clear (1992)
Watch It (1993)
Surviving the Game (1994)
The Rock (1996) Mother (1996)
Set It Off (1996)
Colin Fitz (1997)
Truth or Consequences, N.M. (1997)
Nothing to Lose (1997)
Office Space (1999)
Any Given Sunday (1999)
Identity (2003)
Two Tickets to Paradise (2006)
Puff, Puff, Pass (2006)
Wild Hogs (2007)

Patrick McGoohan
6ft 2in
(PATRICK JOSEPH MCGOOHAN)

Born: **March 19, 1928**
Astoria, New York City, New York, USA
Died: **January 13, 2009**

Patrick was the son of a United States based Irish couple, Thomas McGoohan and his wife Rose. He moved to Ireland with his family when he was seven. A few years later, they went across to England, where they settled in Sheffield, Yorkshire. After leaving Ratcliffe School, he worked for the British Rope Company, in Sheffield and was then the manager of the small branch of a bank. It wasn't terribly stimulating, nor for that matter, was his next job, as a chicken farmer. Almost in desperation, Patrick applied to Sheffield Repertory. He was taken on as a stage manager and when he left, four years later, had become their leading man. In 1951, he married the actress, Joan Drummond. They had three daughters, and were still happy together fifty-seven years later! Patrick did stage work until 1954, when he began getting TV work. He next signed with the Rank Organization and made his film debut in 1955, in *Passage Home*. Although he continued with stage, film and TV roles, it wasn't until 1964, that he finally achieved international fame, with the role of John Drake, in the series, 'Danger Man'. When that was over, after four seasons, he was in the mini-series, 'The Prisoner'. A few good film roles came his way after that, most notably, his warden, in *Escape from Alcatraz,* his Dr. Paul Ruth, in *Scanners* and King Edward I, in *Braveheart.* After a short illness, Patrick passed away at St. John's Health Center, in Santa Monica.

Hell Drivers (1957)
Two Living, One Dead (1961)
All Night Long (1962)
Life for Ruth (1962)
The Quare Fellow (1962)
The Three Lives of Thomasina (1964)
Ice Station Zebra (1968)
Mary Queen of Scots (1972)
Silver Streak (1976)
Escape from Alcatraz (1979)
Scanners (1981)
Braveheart (1995)
A Time to Kill (1996)

Elizabeth McGovern
5ft 9in
(ELIZABETH MCGOVERN)

Born: **July 18, 1961**
Evanston, Illinois, USA

Elizabeth was the daughter of William Montgomery McGovern, a law professor at Northwestern University, in Evanston, and his wife, Katharine, who was a high school teacher. Elizabeth's sister, Cammie, became a prominent novelist. Elizabeth moved with her family when her father accepted a position at UCLA. By the time she was at North Hollywood High School, Elizabeth had starred in several plays. After she'd graduated from The Oakwood School, an agent, Joan Scott, saw her perform in Thornton Wilder's, "The Skin of Our Teeth" and recommended that she took acting lessons. She joined the American Conservatory Theater, in San Francisco and later, Juilliard, in New York. While at Juilliard, Elizabeth acted in a short film made at UCLA, *Last Year's Model.* In 1980, she dropped out to make her first feature film, Robert Redford's *Ordinary People.* After a Best Supporting Actress Oscar nomination for *Ragtime,* she completed studying and acted off-Broadway. In 1984, Elizabeth was engaged to Sean Penn, after falling in love with him during the filming of *Racing with the Moon.* An accomplished guitarist, she sings and plays with her own band, "Sadie And The Hotheads". Since 1992, Elizabeth has been married to English-born producer, Simon Curtis.

Ordinary People (1980)
Ragtime (1981)
Once upon a Time in
America (1984)
Racing with the Moon (1984)
Native Son (1986)
The Bedroom Window (1987)
Aunt Julia and the
Scriptwriter (1990)
Women and Men: Stories of
Seduction (1990)
King of the Hill (1993)
The Wings of the Dove (1997)
The House of Mirth (2000)
Buffalo Soldiers (2001)
The Truth (2006)
Inconceivable (2008)

Ewan McGregor
5ft 9½in
(EWAN GORDON MCGREGOR)

Born: **March 31, 1971**
Crieff, Perthshire, Scotland

The son of teachers, James McGregor, and his wife, Carol, Ewan was born in the Perth Royal Infirmary, and grew up in the small town of Crieff, where he attended the independent fee-paying school, Morrisons Academy. He was encouraged to go into show business by his uncle, the actor Denis Lawson. So, at sixteen years of age, with his parents' blessing, he left school to join the Perth Repertory Theater. In 1988, he went to London to study drama at the Guildhall School of Music and Drama, where his contemporaries were future stars Daniel Craig and Alistair McGowan. Before graduating, Ewan made his first appearances on television – in 'Family Style' and Dennis Potter's mini-series, 'Lipstick on Your Collar', which were both aired in 1993. The following year, Ewan made his film debut in the Black Comedy, *Shallow Grave.* He put himself on the international map with a dynamic performance in the brilliant *Trainspotting.* Since then, he has been a top star in several important movies. Ewan is married to the French production designer, Eve Mavrakis, whom he met in 1995, while working on the television drama, 'Kavanagh QC'. They have three daughters and live in North London.

Shallow Grave (1994)
Trainspotting (1995)
Emma (1996)
Little Voice (1998)
Moulin Rouge (2001)
Black Hawk Down (2001)
Down with Love (2003)
Young Adam (2003)
Big Fish (2003)
Revenge of the Sith (2005)
The Island (2005)
Stay (2005)
Scenes of a
Sexual Nature (2006)
Miss Potter (2006)
Cassandra's Dream (2007)
Incendiary (2008)
Deception (2008)
I Love You Phillip Morris (2009)

Dorothy McGuire
5ft 6in
(DOROTHY HACKETT MCGUIRE)

Born: **June 14, 1916**
Omaha, Nebraska, USA
Died: **September 13, 2001**

Showing early talent, Dottie made her stage debut when she was thirteen, at the Omaha Community Playhouse – opposite Henry Fonda, in "A Kiss for Cinderella". She continued her education at Omaha Junior School, the Ladywood Convent in Indianapolis and finally, Pine Manor Junior College in Wellesley, Massachusetts. Her early experience was gained in summer stock and in 1938, she appeared in shows like "Bachelor Born". After understudying Martha Scott, for the role of Emily Gibb, Dottie made her Broadway debut – in Thornton Wilder's, "Our Town". She was seen by David O. Selznick who signed her to a personal contract and loaned her to 20th Century Fox for her movie debut – recreating her Broadway role, in *Claudia*. Her honest, sympathetic face graced many good films for twenty more years, but she was unfairly overlooked when it came to awards. Her only nomination was for a Best Actress Oscar, in *Gentleman's Agreement*. In 1947, together with her co-stars in that film – Gregory Peck and Mel Ferrer, she founded La Jolla Playhouse. She was the star of successful films during the 1950s – most importantly, *Three Coins in the Fountain* and *Friendly Persuasion*. Dottie's marriage to photographer, John Swope, lasted thirty-six years – until his death in 1979. Her last appearance on a screen was in 1990, in a television drama, 'The Last best Year'. Dottie suffered a short illness before she died of cardiac arrest, in Santa Monica, California.

Claudia (1943)
The Enchanted Cottage (1945)
A Tree Grows in Brooklyn (1945)
The Spiral Staircase (1946)
Claudia and David (1946)
Gentleman's Agreement (1947)
Mister 880 (1950) I Want You (1951)
Three Coins in the Fountain (1954)
Friendly Persuasion (1956)
The Dark at the Top of the Stairs (1960)
Swiss Family Robinson (1960)
The Greatest Story Ever Told (1965)

Sir Ian McKellen
5ft 11in
(IAN MURRAY MCKELLEN)

Born: **May 25, 1939**
Burnley, Lancashire, England

At the outbreak of World War II, Ian's parents, Denis and Margery McKellen, took him and his sister Jean to live in the coal mining town of Wigan. Through visits to the local cinema and encouragement from his parents, Ian soon developed a passion for acting and the theater. They took him to see Shakespeare plays, and at Bolton School, he acted his first role, as Malvolio, in a production of "Twelfth Night". In 1961, armed with a Bachelor of Arts degree, he began his career on the London stage. Because of the laws at that time, he was forced to hide the fact that he was a homosexual. He made his first TV appearance in an episode of 'The Indian Tales of Rudyard Kipling', in 1964, and five years later, after stage and television work, he made his film debut, in *A Touch of Love*. His many fine screen portrayals since included two Oscar nominations – Best Actor in *Gods and Monsters,* and Best Supporting Actor in *The Fellowship of the Ring*. Ian came out in 1988, when the British Prime Minister, Margaret Thatcher, tried once again to make being gay a crime. Ian has since more than proved that he is one of the greatest British male actors in movie history. In 2008, Ian played the title role of Trevor Nunn's video version of Shakespeare's *King Lear*.

The Keep (1983) Scandal (1988)
Last Action Hero (1993)
Six Degrees of Separation (1993)
I'll Do Anything (1994)
The Shadow (1994)
Cold Comfort Farm (1995)
Jack & Sarah (1995)
Restoration (1995)
Richard III (1995)
Rasputin (1996)
Apt Pupil (1997)
Gods and Monsters (1998)
The Fellowship of the Ring (2001)
Emile (2003)
Asylum (2005)
Neverwas (2005)
The Da Vinci Code (2006)
X-Men: The Last Stand (2006)

Virginia McKenna
5ft 7½in
(VIRGINIA MCKENNA)

Born: **June 7, 1931**
London, England

Virginia was part of a sophisticated family. Her father was a member of Christies, the London auctioneers, and her mother was a pianist who wrote a song for Eartha Kitt, entitled "An Englishman Needs Time." Virginia was educated at Heron's Ghyll School in Uckfield, Sussex, and in Cape Town. She trained as an actress at the Central School of Speech and Drama, in London, before joining Dundee Repertory Company in Scotland. She made a name for herself in London's West End, when she appeared in "The River Line" and "A Penny for a Song" and was given her film debut, with a small role in the 1952 comedy, *Father's Doing Fine*. In 1954, she spent nine unhappy months as the wife of actor, Denholm Elliott. Throughout the 1950s she was an extremely popular actress in Britain. In 1966, she had a spell as an international star, after playing the role of Joy Adamson, in *Born Free*. Her co-star in that film was Bill Travers, who had become her second husband in 1957, and remained so until his death in 1994. Together, they had set up the Born Free Foundation in 1984. After Bill's death, she opened the Violet Szabo Museum, in Hereford. Violet was an heroic true-life character she played in one of her best movies – *Carve Her Name with Pride*. Virginia has kept on working – mainly on television, but she's had plenty to occupy her mind, with her six grandchildren, from her three sons and one daughter. Virginia was awarded an OBE in 2004.

The Cruel Sea (1953)
The Ship That Died of Shame (1955)
A Town Like Alice (1956)
The Smallest Show on Earth (1957)
Carve Her Name with Pride (1958)
The Wreck of the Mary
Deare (1959) Born Free (1966)
Ring of Bright Water (1969)
Swallows and Amazons (1974)
The Disappearance (1977)
Blood Link (1982)
Staggered (1994)
Sliding Doors (1998)

Leo **McKern**
5ft 6in
(REGINALD MCKERN)

Born: **March 16, 1920**
Sydney, New South Wales, Australia
Died: **July 23, 2002**

Leo was the third son of Norman McKern, who was a refrigerator engineer, and his wife, Vera. Nothing of consequence had happened in Leo's life when he attended Sydney Technical School. After leaving school at fifteen, he became apprenticed to an engineering firm. An accident at work, cost him his left eye. He had a glass eye fitted, and studied commercial art for a few years – getting involved in amateur theater productions at the same time. After serving in the Australian Army, at the beginning of World War II, he made his stage debut, in Sydney, in 1944, in "Uncle Harry". He met his future wife, Jane Holland, who had decided to emigrate to England. Leo followed her to London where they were married. By 1947, he made his Old Vic debut in "Love's Labor's Lost". Theater work helped him lose his Aussie accent but his film debut in *Murder in the Cathedral,* in 1952, didn't require him to talk. He featured in TV's, 'The Adventures of Robin Hood' and was a fully-fledged Brit by the time he portrayed a Greek, in *All For Mary,* in 1955. He became a top character actor, and won an Australian Film Institute Best Actor Award for *Travelling North.* He co-starred with Alec Guinness, in *A Foreign Field,* and played his final movie role, in *Molokai: The Story of Father Damien.* Leo died in Bath, England, following a long illness.

Yesterday's Enemy (1959)
The Day the Earth Caught Fire (1961)
Lisa (1962) King & Country (1964)
Help! (1965)
A Man for All Seasons (1966)
Ryan's Daughter (1970)
The Adventure of Sherlock Holmes'
Smarter Brother (1975)
Candleshoe (1977) The French
Lieutenant's Woman (1981)
Ladyhawke (1985)
Travelling North (1987)
A Foreign Field (1993)
Molokai: The Story of
Father Damien (1999)

Victor **McLaglen**
6ft 3in
(VICTOR ANDREW DE BIER EVERLEIGH MCLAGLEN)

Born: **December 10, 1886**
Tunbridge Wells, Kent, England
Died: **November 7, 1959**

Victor was a small boy when his father, a bishop, took the family to Claremont, just outside Cape Town, in South Africa. Victor returned to England when he was fourteen to join the British Army. His plan to fight in the Boer War was thwarted when, stationed at Windsor with the Life Guards, his true age was discovered. In 1904, he moved to Canada and used his massive physique to earn a living as a wrestler and boxer – once taking on the great World Heavyweight Champion, Jack Johnson, in an exhibition bout. During World War I, he served with the Middlesex Regiment and was Heavyweight Champion of the British Army, in 1918. He tried his luck in Hollywood, in 1920, and made his debut in the film, *The Call of the Road.* He was a star when talkies arrived – with thirty-five movies under his belt. Sound didn't diminish his popularity, and in 1935, he won an Oscar for *The Informer.* Victor appeared in three of John Ford's greatest westerns – starting with *Fort Apache.* He was married three times. His son, Andrew, who is 6' 7" tall, became a director. Victor died of a heart attack at Newport Beach, California, shortly after completing an episode of 'Rawhide' for TV – directed by his son.

Guilty as Hell (1932)
The Captain Hates
the Sea (1934)
The Informer (1935)
Professional Soldier (1935)
Klondike Annie (1936)
Magnificent Brute (1936)
Nancy Steele Is Missing (1937)
Wee Willie Winkie (1937)
The Devil's Party (1938)
Gunga Din (1939)
Tampico (1944)
The Princess and
the Pirate (1944)
Fort Apache (1948)
She Wore a Yellow Ribbon (1949)
Rio Grande (1950)
The Quiet Man (1952)
Many Rivers to Cross (1955)

Stephen **McNally**
5ft 11in
(HORACE VINCENT MCNALLY)

Born: **July 29, 1913**
New York City, New York, USA
Died: **June 4, 1994**

Stephen was a qualified lawyer before, because of the bad economic situation at the time, he decided to become an actor. He took a few drama classes and then launched himself on stage – still using his original name, Horace McNally. When World War II started, he realized that the shortage of leading men in Hollywood could mean work for him. He married Rita Wintrich, in 1941. Together they produced eight children. In 1942, Stephen made a seventeen-minute propaganda film for MGM with the young star, Esther Williams, titled *Inflation.* It was quickly followed by his first feature film *Grand Central Murder,* which starred Van Heflin. There were more shorts for the studio and then, in the illustrious company of Judy Garland and Gene Kelly, he had a good role in the musical *For Me and My Gal.* He changed his name to Stephen in 1946, and that, combined with breaking away from MGM, appeared to set his career on a higher level. Stephen's menacing portrayal of Locky McCormick, in *Johnny Belinda,* started a run of featured roles in good films, which included his memorable, Dutch Henry Brown, in one of the classic westerns, *Winchester '73.* Stephen retired in 1980 and died of heart failure, fourteen years later, at his home in Beverly Hills.

Grand Central Murder (1942)
Eyes in the Night (1942)
For Me and My Gal (1942)
Keeper of the Flame (1942)
An American Romance (1944)
Thirty Seconds Over Tokyo (1944)
Johnny Belinda (1948)
City Across the River (1949)
Criss Cross (1949)
Winchester '73 (1950)
Apache Drums (1951)
Diplomatic Courier (1952)
Split Second (1953)
Violent Saturday (1955)
Tribute to a Bad Man (1956)
Panic in the City (1968)
Black Gunn (1972)

Kristy **McNichol**
5ft 3in
(CHRISTINA ANN MCNICHOL)

Born: **September 11, 1962**
Los Angeles, California, USA

Her father was Scottish and her mother was from a Palestinian background. Kristy's all too short career began when she was six years old – acting in television commercials alongside her older brother, Jimmy, who was already well established as a child actor. In 1973, she appeared on television in an episode of 'Love American Style' and followed that with a two-year tenure as Virginia Apple, in 'Apple's Way'. In 1976, Kristy won the first of two Best Supporting Actress Emmys for her role as Buddy Lawrence, in the TV series 'Family'. Kristy's movie debut was in 1978, when she joined a starry line-up in the comedy, *The End.* That same year, she and Jimmy released an album which spawned the hit single, "He's So Fine". It was two years later in *Little Darlings,* that she came into her own. She was nominated for a Young Artist Award, and built up a massive teenage fan base. *Only When I Laugh* was equally successful and it earned Kristy a Golden Globe nomination. Then things began to go wrong. A hugely expensive production, *The Pirate Movie,* failed at the box office and a trip to Europe to film *Just the Way You Are,* was nearly a disaster when she left the set with seventeen days to go. She completed it a year later, but by 1984, she'd taken on a new career – as a hairdresser! In 1986, she came back to star in the TV film, 'Love Mary' and the feature, *Dream Lover.* A television sitcom, 'Empty Nest', kept her going, but severe manic depression was eating away at her and she retired at thirty-three. An episode of the TV series, 'Invasion America', in 1998, is probably the last time we will see her perform on the screen. Kristy's talent had burned brightly for only a little while.

The End (1978) **Little Darlings** (1980)
**The Night the Lights Went Out
in Georgia** (1981)
Only When I Laugh (1981)
White Dog (1981)
Just the Way You Are (1984)
Dream Lover (1986)
The Forgotten One (1990)

Steve **McQueen**
5ft 9¹/₂in
(TERENCE STEVEN MCQUEEN)

Born: **March 24, 1930**
Beech Grove, Indiana, USA
Died: **November 7, 1980**

Abandoned by his father when he was six months old, Steve's mother then left him for several years with an uncle who lived on a farm. He rejoined her in Los Angeles when he was twelve. Steve began hanging out with gangs and when it got too much for his mom, she sent him to a home for young tearaways, the California Junior Boys Republic, in Chino. It straightened him out and he never forgot that. When he left there in 1946, his mother sent him money so he could go to New York. He took a job on the "SS Alpha", but when it docked in Cuba, he jumped ship. After a short time back in the United States, Steve joined the Marines. After being honorably discharged, he went to work in the Texas oilfields, and as a lumberjack, in Canada. An actress he was dating at the time persuaded him to study with Sanford Meisner, in New York. Three years later he replaced Ben Gazzara, in "A Hatful of Rain" and met his first wife Neile Adams. He moved to Los Angeles, and got an uncredited role in the 1953 film *Girl on the Run.* Steve starred in the cult movie, *The Blob,* but was catapulted to twenty-year stardom, in *The Magnificent Seven.* Steve was especially effective in *The Great Escape, Bullitt* and *The Thomas Crown Affair.* A heavy smoker all his adult life, he died of a heart attack after surgery for lung cancer, in Juárez, Mexico.

The Blob (1958)
The Magnificent Seven (1960)
Hell Is for Heroes (1962)
The Great Escape (1963)
Love with the Proper Stranger (1963)
The Cincinnati Kid (1965)
Nevada Smith (1966)
The Sand Pebbles (1966)
Bullitt (1968) **The Thomas Crown
Affair** (1968) **The Getaway** (1972)
Junior Bonner (1972)
Papillon (1973)
The Towering Inferno (1974)
Tom Horn (1980)
The Hunter (1980)

Ralph **Meeker**
6ft 1in
(RALPH RATHGEBER)

Born: **November 21, 1920**
Minneapolis, Minnesota, USA
Died: **August 5, 1988**

When he was three years old, Ralph – the son of Ralph and Magnhild Rathgeber, moved with his parents to Chicago. After Ralph junior graduated from Leelanau School for Boys, in Glen Arbor, Michigan, he went on to study musical composition and took up acting, at Northwestern University, in Evanston – from 1938 until 1942. He served in the United States Navy for a short time during World War II – he was invalided out after injuring his neck. In 1943, Ralph went back to Chicago, where he made his stage debut, in the National Company production of "The Doughgirls". He then headed for New York where, with only $35 to his name, he was forced to work as a soda jerk until he toured with a stock company production of, "Up in Mabel's Room". On V-E day, he was in Italy with the USO, entertaining the troops in "Ten Little Indians". From 1945, he was on stage. In 1949, he replaced Brando in "A Streetcar Named Desire" and aroused interest from MGM. He made his film debut in 1951 – a small role in *Teresa,* but his Mike Hammer, in *Kiss Me Deadly,* and a key role in *Paths of Glory,* mark the high points of his career. His last movie was the Sci-Fi Horror film, *Without Warning,* in 1980. Twice married, Ralph was living with his second wife, Colleen, when dying of a heart attack in Woodland Hills, California.

Somebody Loves Me (1952)
Jeopardy (1953)
The Naked Spur (1953)
Kiss Me Deadly (1955)
Big House USA (1955)
Paths of Glory (1957)
Run of the Arrow (1957)
The Dirty Dozen (1967)
**The St. Valentine's Day
Massacre** (1967)
The Detective (1968)
I Walk the Line (1970)
The Anderson Tapes (1971)
The Mind Snatchers (1972)
Brannigan (1975)
Winter Kills (1979)

Eva **Mendes**
5ft 6in
(EVA MENDES)

Born: **March 5, 1974**
Miami, Florida, USA

After her family moved from Florida, Eva, who is from a Cuban-American background, was the youngest of four children. They were all raised by their mother in the Silver Lake-Echo Park area of Los Angeles after her parents divorced. As a Roman Catholic, her original ambition was to become a nun. While at Herbert Hoover High School, in Glendale, she took acting classes with the famous drama coach, Ivana Chubbuck. She was a marketing major at California State University, Northridge, but dropped out when she received acting offers. Eva began her professional career in 1998 – appearing first in an episode of 'ER' on television, and then in a couple of horror movies. Three years later, she gained a wider audience, with a featured role in the Denzel Washington film, *Training Day*. The success of that film, coupled with Eva's impressive performance, led to another opportunity to work with Denzel – in *Out of Time* – as his co-star. Since then she has built a reputation as a serious actress, who can turn her hand to comedy. She has already had seven award nominations, but these are early days. In addition to her acting career, Eva regularly appears in print and television advertising campaigns, for Revlon Cosmetics. Although she's reported to be an outdoor type, she loves interior design, and is in the process of writing a book aimed at very young children – entitled "Crazy Leggs Beshee".

Training Day (2001)
2 Fast 2 Furious (2003)
Once Upon a Time in
Mexico (2003)
Out of Time (2003)
Stuck On You (2003)
Hitch (2005)
The Wendell Baker Story (2005)
Guilty Hearts (2005)
Ghost Rider (2007)
Live! (2007)
We Own the Night (2007)
Cleaner (2007)
The Spirit (2008)

Adolphe **Menjou**
5ft 10in
(ADOLPHE JEAN MENJOU)

Born: **February 18, 1890**
Pittsburgh, Pennsylvania, USA
Died: **October 29, 1963**

Adolphe was half French as his name will suggest – but he was also a relative – via his mother – of the famous Irish poet and novelist, James Joyce. Adolphe's father, who had come to the United States from France, moved his family to Cleveland, Ohio, where he ran a successful group of restaurants. Young Adolphe had already expressed an interest in becoming an actor, but his father sent him to Culver Military Academy, in Indiana, which he hoped would change the boy's mind. It didn't – anymore than Cornell University in New York, where he switched from Engineering to Liberal Arts. He left in his third year, and worked as an extra for several film studios. Adolphe's first credited screen appearance was in 1916, in *A Parisian Romance*. Following sixty-five 'silents', he made his talking picture debut in the 1929 comedy, *Fashions in Love.* After he was Oscar nominated for *The Front Page*, Adolphe's elegant looks and debonair personality was enjoyed by film fans and television viewers for thirty years. Married three times, he died of hepatitis at his home in Beverly Hills.

Morocco (1930)
The Front Page (1931)
A Farewell to Arms (1932)
Morning Glory (1933)
Little Miss Marker (1934)
Gold Diggers of 1935 (1935)
A Star Is Born (1937)
One Hundred Men and a Girl (1937)
Stage Door (1937)
Golden Boy (1939)
Roxie Hart (1942)
Sweet Rosie O'Grady (1943)
Heartbeat (1946)
The Hucksters (1947)
State of the Union (1948)
My Dream Is Yours (1949)
The Tall Target (1951)
The Sniper (1952)
Man on a Tightrope (1953)
Paths of Glory (1957)
Pollyanna (1960)

Melina **Mercouri**
5ft 6½in
(MARIA AMALIA MERCOURIS)

Born: **October 18, 1920**
Athens, Greece
Died: **March 6, 1994**

Melina had a political background – her grandfather was mayor of Athens, and her father was a member of Parliament. Her parents split up when she was a kid and she went to live with her mother. During World War II, her father was one of the leaders of the Greek Resistance against German occupation. Her first lover was the actor, George Papas, but in 1941, Melina married a very wealthy man by the name of Panos Harokopos, who made her life comfortable during the three years of Axis occupation. During the war, Melina studied acting at the National School of Theater, in Athens. Melina had a clever mind and a high level of basic intelligence and sensitivity, which contrasted with the fiery personality she displayed, when she appeared in Greek tragedies. After the war, she performed on the Paris stage in three plays including "Le Moulin de la Galette" – in 1951. Her debut film, *Stella,* gave her the chance to attend the Cannes Film Festival, where she met Jules Dassin - the love of her life. He later directed her most successful film *Never on Sunday,* for which she was nominated for a Best Actress Oscar. After living in exile in France from 1967 until 1974, during the military dictatorship, Melina returned to Greece and became Minister of Culture. She quit acting in the late 1970s to concentrate on politics. A heavy smoker all her life, Melina died of lung cancer, in New York.

Stella (1955)
Celui qui doit mourir (1957)
The Gypsy and the
Gentleman (1958)
Where the Hot Wind Blows (1959)
Never on a Sunday (1960)
The Last Judgement (1961)
Phaedra (1962)
The Victors (1963)
Topkapi (1964)
A Man Could Get Killed (1966)
Promise at Dawn (1970)
Nasty Habits (1977)
A Dream of Passion (1978)

Burgess **Meredith**
5ft 5½in
(OLIVER BURGESS MEREDITH)

Born: **November 16, 1907**
Cleveland, Ohio, USA
Died: **September 9, 1997**

The youngest of three children, he was the son of a Canadian doctor, William Meredith, and his American wife, Ida. In 1920, Burgess attended the Cathedral Choir School, where he was a boy soprano. Four years after that, he graduated from Hoosac Preparatory School, and completed his education at Amherst College, where he was a member of the Class of 1931. After that, he was a Wall Street runner and a clerk before deciding to become an actor. He learned his trade with the Civic Repertory Company, and Eva Le Gallienne's Theater Company. In 1936, he made his movie debut, when he repeated his Broadway success, in *Winterset*. In 1939, Burgess attracted praise for his film work, when he portrayed George, in the film adaptation of John Steinbeck's, *Of Mice and Men.* During World War II, Burgess served for three years with the U.S. Air Force. After a promising start to his post-war movie career in *The Story of G.I. Joe* and *The Diary of a Chambermaid,* his work was halted in the late 1940s by the House Un-American Activities Committee. Burgess came back in 1958, and during his later career, he was nominated for Best Supporting Actor Oscars – for *The Day of the Locust* and *Rocky.* His four wives included Paulette Goddard. He died in Malibu, California, from a combination of melanoma and Alzheimer's disease.

Winterset (1936)
Idiot's Delight (1939)
Of Mice and Men (1939)
Castle on the Hudson (1940)
That Uncertain Feeling (1941)
Tom Dick and Harry (1941)
Story of G.I. Joe (1945)
The Diary of a Chambermaid (1946)
The Man on the Eiffel Tower (1949)
Advise and Consent (1962)
The Cardinal (1963) **Batman** (1966)
MacKenna's Gold (1969)
The Day of the Locust (1975)
Rocky (1976) **Magic** (1978)

Una **Merkel**
5ft 4in
(UNA MERKEL)

Born: **December 10, 1903**
Covington, Kentucky, USA
Died: **January 2, 1986**

Una was educated in Covington and grew up locally. At sixteen she was employed as Lillian Gish's double, in *Way Down East.* There were two more silent films, but during the 1920s she lived in New York and acting on Broadway in 1927, with Helen Hayes, in "Coquette". In 1930, she returned to Hollywood, to make her first talking picture, *Abraham Lincoln,* which was directed by D.W. Griffith. For much of that decade, she was a popular female second-lead in fifty films – giving great comic support to super-stars such as Jean Harlow and Carole Lombard. She was probably at her best – complete with peroxide blonde hair, in the great musical, *42nd Street.* When Una began getting top billing in 1937, it was mainly in B-movies. The 1940s started on a high when she featured in one of W.C. Fields' very best comedies, *The Bank Dick,* but apart from a 'Road' film with Hope and Crosby, her quality roles were rare. In 1946, Una was almost killed when her mother committed suicide by turning on the gas tap. She won a Tony Award for "The Ponder Heart". In 1956, she was nominated for a Best Supporting Actress Oscar in *Summer and Smoke.* Una was married to Ronald Burla from 1932 until 1945. She died in Los Angeles from natural causes.

Wicked (1931) **Private Lives** (1931)
Men Wanted (1932)
Red-headed Woman (1932)
Blonde Bombshell (1933)
42nd Street (1933)
The Merry Widow (1934)
Broadway Melody of 1936 (1935)
Born to Dance (1936)
Don't Tell the Wife (1937)
True Confession (1937)
Some Like It Hot (1939)
Destry Rides Again (1939)
The Bank Dick (1940)
Road to Zanzibar (1941)
I Love Melvin (1953)
The Parent Trap (1961)
Summer and Smoke (1961)

Ethel **Merman**
5ft 6¼in
(ETHEL AGNES ZIMMERMANN)

Born: **January 16, 1908**
Astoria, New York City, New York, USA
Died: **February 15, 1984**

Ethel was the daughter of an accountant, Edward Zimmermann and his wife, Agnes. Growing up in Queen's, close to the Famous Players-Lasky's studios, Ethel used to see the wealthy movie stars and dreamed of being one. Her singing in the choir at the local Episcopalian Church, led to concert appearances. The daughter of an accountant and a school teacher, Ethel graduated from William Cullen Bryant High School and worked briefly as a stenographer. Her ear for a good tune soon established a useful source of extra cash by singing at private parties in the evenings. She then acquired an agent, who got her cabaret work in Manhattan. When she was twenty-two, the Gershwins asked her to audition for their new musical, "Girl Crazy". After it opened, in October 1930, Ethel was the talk of the town. Warner Brothers signed her and put her in a short *The Cave Club,* but it was Paramount who gave her a break when, in 1934, they put her in *We're Not Dressing,* with Crosby and Lombard heading the cast. Ethel sang three songs as she did in *Kid Millions,* with Eddie Cantor. She was with Crosby in *Anything Goes,* and despite being no real glamour girl, she was briefly a movie star. Her tendency to dominate movies with her belting style wore thin by 1938, and she concentrated on the stage until the 1950s, when she repeated her great Broadway success, in *Call Me Madam.* Ethel's four husbands included actor Ernest Borgnine. She made her final appearance on TV's 'The Love Boat' and died in New York City – following an operation for brain cancer.

We're Not Dressing (1934)
Kid Millions (1934)
Anything Goes (1936)
Happy Landing (1938)
Alexander's Ragtime Band (1938)
Call Me Madam (1953)
There's No Business Like Show Business (1954) **It's a Mad Mad Mad Mad World** (1963)
Airplane! (1980)

Gary **Merrill**
5ft 10in
(GARY MERRILL)

Born: **August 2, 1915**
Hartford, Connecticut, USA
Died: **March 5, 1990**

Gary's ancestors had arrived in America on the "Mayflower" and his family tree was big in New England. He was educated at Bowdoin – the liberal arts college, in Brunswick, Maine. He started out working on New York's WOR Radio and he had established himself in the 'Batman' series before America's involvement in World War II. In 1941, after marrying his first wife, Barbara Leeds, Gary joined the United States Army Air Force Special Service unit. While he was there, he began his acting career in 1944, in a fund raiser for the Army Relief, titled "Winged Victory". He went to New York after the war and took acting classes before embarking on his professional career. In February 1946, he played Paul Verrall in "Born Yesterday" at the Lyceum Theater. Paul Douglas and Judy Holliday were its stars. Gary was still with the show when it transferred two years later to the Henry Miller Theater. He started his movie career in 1948, as the narrator for *The Quiet One*. His first screen role was in *Slattery's Hurricane*. Without ever threatening the stars, Gary had a good career in films and television. His second wife was Bette Davis. When his film career ended, Gary made a living as a voice-over artist. In 1988, he published his autobiography, "Bette. Rita. And the Rest of My Life". A heavy smoker for many years, Gary died from lung cancer, at his home in Falmouth, Maine.

Slattery's Hurricane (1949)
Twelve O'Clock High (1949)
All About Eve (1950)
Where the Sidewalk Ends (1950)
Decision Before Dawn (1951)
Phone Call from a Stranger (1952)
The Wonderful Country (1959)
The Savage Eye (1960)
The Great Impostor (1961)
Mysterious Island (1961)
A Girl Named Tamiko (1962)
Ride Beyond Vengeance (1966)
The Incident (1967)
The Power (1968)

Bette **Midler**
5ft 1in
(BETTE MIDLER)

Born: **December 1, 1945**
Honolulu, Hawaii, USA

Bette started singing when she was a kid and it wasn't long before she was winning talent contests. After Radford High School, she began studying drama, at the University of Hawaii. Then, with money she earned as an extra in the 1966 movie, *Hawaii,* she headed for New York. It didn't take her long to set Broadway alight with her role as Tzeitel, in the musical, "Fiddler on the Roof" – she sang 'Matchmaker' – to rapturous applause – eight times a week! Hired by the gay men's club, 'Continental Baths', and with a little help from Barry Manilow's piano she soon became known as the "Divine Miss M". It was the title of her first album for the New York label, Atlantic Records and in 1973, she won a Grammy as Best New Artist. Hollywood was next, and her first starring role, in *The Rose,* continued her upward climb. Her dynamic performance earned Bette a Best Actress Oscar nomination – as did the 1991 release, *For the Boys.* There were other good movies and a turkey or two, but Bette is still going strong. Her albums and live performances continue to delight her many fans. In February 2008, she opened a new show at Caesar's Palace in Las Vegas. Bette's charity work includes the New York Restoration Project. Bette's been married to the actor/director/producer, Martin von Haselberg, since 1984. They have a grown daughter named Sophie, who is now twenty-four and is a student at Yale.

The Rose (1979)
Down and Out in
Beverly Hills (1986)
Ruthless People (1986)
Outrageous Fortune (1987)
Big Business (1988)
Beaches (1988)
Stella (1990) For the Boys (1991)
Hocus Pocus (1993)
The First Wives Club (1996)
That Old Feeling (1997)
Drowning Mona (2000)
Then She Found Me (2007)
The Women (2008)

Toshirô **Mifune**
5ft 9in
(SANCHUAN MINLANG)

Born: **April 1, 1920**
Tsingtao, China
Died: **December 24, 1997**

Toshirô was born in China to Japanese parents. His father was a photographer who employed his son in the darkroom after the boy left school. Even though he had spent the first nineteen years of his life in China, his links with Japan had not been severed. During World War II, Toshirô was drafted into the Imperial Japanese Air Force, where he served in the Aerial Photography unit. In 1946, he settled in Tokyo where he began to work as a cameraman in both stills and movies. A year later, after competing with 4000 applicants, he was given a screen test by Kajiro Yamamoto. It led to his first feature film, *Shin Baka Jidai*. He also met his future wife, Sachiko Yoshmine. Family opposition was overcome with the help of director Akira Kurosawa, who after casting Toshirô in *Drunken Angel,* would use him in all but one of the films he made up to 1965 – a collaboration that resulted in top roles in masterpieces of the Japanese cinema. A Best Foreign Language Oscar for the powerful *Rashômon* gave him a chance to appear in English language movies. He died in Tokyo of organ failure.

Drunken Angel (1948)
Stray Dog (1949)
Rashômon (1950)
Seven Samurai (1954)
Throne of Blood (1957)
The Rickshaw Man (1958)
The Hidden Fortress (1958)
The Age of Gods (1959)
Yojimbo (1961)
The Important Man (1962)
Red Beard (1964)
Samarai Assassin (1965)
Grand Prix (1966)
Hell in the Pacific (1968)
Band of Assassins (1969)
Red Sun (1971)
Winter Kills (1979)
Conquest (1982)
Death of a Tea Master (1989)
Picture Bride (1994)
Deep River (1995)

Nikita **Mikhalkov**
6ft 1½in

(NIKITA SERGEYEVICH MIKHALKOV-KONCHALOVSKY)

Born: October 21, 1945
Moscow, Soviet Union

Born in the Soviet Union at a positive and optimistic time in world history, Nikita was from a distinguished family of artists and poets. His father Sergei Mikhalkov wrote Children's books and was lyricist of the Soviet and Russian national anthems. His mother, Natalia, was a poetess and grand-daughter of the painter, Vasily Surikov. Nikita studied acting at the children's studio, run by the Moscow Art Theater. In 1959, he made his film debut in *The Sun Shines for All.* When he was sixteen, he studied directing at the State Film School. In 1969, before he went behind the camera, he acted in *Home of the Gentry,* directed by his older brother, Andrei Konchalovsky. Nikita's reputation as a director came with his *Slave of Love.* He resumed acting in the early 1980s and had many successes before *Burnt by the Sun* (directed by him) established him internationally – winning a Best Foreign Film Oscar. His recent film *12* – which he wrote, directed and acted in, has received great acclaim around the world. Nikita has three children with his second wife, Tatyana Mikhalkova.

The Red Tent (1969)
Friend Among Strangers,
Strangers Among Friends (1974)
Slave of Love (1976)
An Unfinished Piece for
Mechanical Piano (1977)
Siberiada (1980)
A Railway Station for Two (1982)
Flight in Dreams and
in Reality (1982)
A Cruel Romance (1984)
Aurora Borealis (1990)
The Insulted and the Injured (1991)
Burnt by the Sun (1994)
Revizor (1996)
The Barber of Siberia (1998)
Belief, Hope and Blood (2000)
The State Counselor (2005)
Blind Man's Buff (2005)
Persona non Grata (2005)
It Doesn't Hurt (2006)
12 (2007)

Alyssa **Milano**
5ft 2in

(ALYSSA JAYNE MILANO)

Born: December 19, 1972
Brooklyn, New York City, New York, USA

Lyssa is the daughter of an Italian-American couple, Tom and Lin Milano. Her father is a film music editor and boating enthusiast. Her mother had been a fashion designer who became a talent manager. Lyssa's younger brother, Cory, is now an actor, and lead singer in a band called "Chloroform Days". Lyssa, who was raised a Catholic, grew up and went to school on Staten Island. When she was seven, her babysitter, who was an aspiring dancer, took her to an open audition for a tour of "Annie". Lyssa got a role as July – one of the orphans. After that, she established a reputation as a child actress and began to get regular work in television commercials and off-Broadway shows. In 1983, she landed the role of Samantha Micelli, in the TV-sitcom, 'Who's the Boss?'. It was a good enough reason for the Milano family to move to Hollywood and Lyssa was able to continue her education at The Buckley School, in Sherman Oaks, and win a 1984 Kids' Choice Award, as 'Favorite TV Actress'. She made her film debut in *Old Enough* when she was twelve and had her first featured adult role in *Little Sister* – eight years later. Lyssa, who has dyslexia, was advised to write down her lines by Sir John Gielgud, when they worked together in the TV play, 'The Canterville Ghost'. In 1999, Lyssa and the rock singer, Cinjun Tate, were married and divorced within a ten-month spell. Her film career went through a couple of troughs, but she kept her face in front of the public with a long run as Phoebe Halliwell, in the TV-series, 'Charmed' and was impressive in the movie, *The Blue Hour.*

Little Sister (1992)
Where the Day Takes You (1992)
Fear (1996) **Glory Daze** (1996)
Hugo Pool (1997)
Buying the Cow (2002)
Kiss the Bride (2002)
Dickie Roberts: Former
Child Star (2003)
The Blue Hour (2007)
Pathology (2008)

Sarah **Miles**
5ft 5in

(SARAH MILES)

Born: December 31, 1941
Ingatestone, Essex, England

Sarah claims to be of Royal Blood and is possibly a distant cousin of Elizabeth II. She began her secondary education at Rodean, the exclusive girls school in Sussex. When she was fifteen, she had the urge to become an actress, so she enrolled at the Royal Academy of Dramatic Art, in London. She made her film debut in *Term of Trial,* which starred Laurence Olivier and Simone Signoret, but Sarah was the one who stood out. She was even more outstanding in her next film, Harold Pinter's masterpiece – *The Servant.* Four films later and her appearance in *Blowup* was the last we saw of her for four years. Sarah had given up acting to be the playwright/screenwriter, Robert Bolt's wife. When she returned, it was for David Lean's romantic drama, *Ryan's Daughter,* for which, in the title role, she was nominated for a Best Actress Oscar. In 1971, she played Mary Queen of Scots on stage, in "Vivat! Vivat! Regina! An affair with her *Man Who Loved Cat Dancing* co-star, Burt Reynolds, didn't help her marriage, and in 1975, she got divorced. Sarah continued to work in films and on television. In 1988, she did another stint as Bolt's wife, and was with him until he died. She published her autobiography, "A Right Royal Bastard", in 1993.

Term of Trial (1962)
The Servant (1963)
Those Magnificent Men in Their
Flying Machines (1965)
I Was Happy Here (1965)
Blowup (1966)
Ryan's Daughter (1970)
Lady Caroline Lamb (1972)
The Hireling (1973) **The Man Who**
Loved Cat Dancing (1973)
The Sailor Who Fell from Grace
with the Sea (1976)
Priest of Love (1981)
Steaming (1985)
Hope and Glory (1987)
White Mischief (1987)
The Silent Touch (1992)
The Accidental Detective (2003)

Vera **Miles**
5ft 3¾in
(VERA JUNE RALSTON)

Born: **August 23, 1929**
Bolse City, Oklahoma, USA

Vera was the daughter of Thomas and Burnice Ralston. After moving from Bolse City, and spending her schooldays in Pratt and Wichita, in Kansas, where she graduated from Wichita North High School, Vera started entering beauty contests. She was crowned "Miss Kansas" in 1948. Shortly after that, she married her first husband, the stuntman/actor, Bob Miles, whose name she kept throughout her career. Her first television appearance was in a commercial for Lustre Creme Soap. In 1951, as a contestant on the TV quiz program 'You Bet Your Life' she won $4! After bit parts, kicking off with that year's *When Willie Comes Marching Home,* Vera began her movie career, in 1952, with a featured role in *For Men Only.* She used her married name because the Republic Studios had a star named Vera Ralston. Until 1954, B-pictures, television roles and B-westerns were Vera's staple diet. She married Gordon Scott, the then current Tarzan, who may have been lucky for her. A Joel McCrea western and a couple of higher profile movies brought her to the attention of that lover of beautiful blondes – Alfred Hitchcock – who cast her opposite Henry Fonda in *The Wrong Man.* It put her on the A-list for a while, and participation in his classic *Psycho,* ensured that her name would never be forgotten. It was also the year she married her third husband, Keith Larsen. She had two daughters and two sons and has been retired since 1995.

Wichita (1955)
Autumn Leaves (1956)
The Searchers (1956)
The Wrong Man (1956)
Beau James (1957)
The FBI Story (1959)
Psycho (1960)
The Man Who Shot
Liberty Valance (1962)
Those Calloways (1965)
Sergeant Ryker (1968)
One Little Indian (1973)
The Castaway Cowboy (1974)
Psycho II (1983)

Ray **Milland**
6ft 2in
(ALFRED REGINALD JONES)

Born: **January 3, 1905**
Cimla, Glamorgan, Wales
Died: **March 10, 1986**

Ray was the son of Alfred and Elizabeth Jones. After spending his childhood in Neath, a coal mining community in Wales, Ray went to live in London. By 1923, he was serving as a guardsman in the Royal Household Cavalry. In those days, due to the snobbery that existed in England, and the type of people he was mixing with in London, he claimed his surname to be Truscott-Jones. Three years later, as he began taking small stage roles and working as an extra in British films, a double-barreled name didn't fit very well on the board outside the theaters. He took his stage name from a street leading to the river Neath. By 1929, he was established enough to be given his film debut, in *The Plaything.* He went to Hollywood where a stage-trained voice was welcomed. He married Muriel Webber in 1932 – and enjoyed success in films and in his private life. They had two children and remained together until he died. Receiving his Best Actor Oscar for *The Lost Weekend,* left Ray totally speechless! He recovered his power of speech to make around another sixty movies. He died of lung cancer in Torrance, California.

We're Not Dressing (1934)
The Glass Key (1935) **Three Smart Girls** (1936) **Easy Living** (1937)
Beau Geste (1939)
French Without Tears (1940)
Arise My Love (1940) **Skylark** (1941)
Reap the Wild Wind (1942)
The Major and the Minor (1942)
The Uninvited (1944)
Ministry of Fear (1944)
Kitty (1945)
The Lost Weekend (1945)
The Big Clock (1948)
It Happens Every Spring (1949)
Close to My Heart (1951)
Rhubarb (1951)
The Thief (1952)
Dial M for Murder (1954)
The Man with the X-Ray Eyes (1963)
Love Story (1970)

Ann **Miller**
5ft 7in
(JOHNNIE LUCILLE ANN COLLIER)

Born: **April 12, 1923**
Chireno, Texas, USA
Died: **January 22, 2004**

Ann's father was a criminal lawyer, who defended some big-name hoodlums. He also liked chasing women. Ann was nine when her mother had had enough, so she was taken to live in California. She took tap-dancing lessons and began dancing in Hollywood night clubs in order to feed the two of them during the Great Depression. Ann got work as an extra, starting in 1934, with *Anne of Green Gables.* When she was fourteen, Ann went with a fake birth certificate to RKO. Her birth year was given as 1919 and her name as Lucille Ann Collier. Actually she was named Johnnie, because her dad wanted a boy. In the belief that she was eighteen, RKO put her in *The Life of the Party* and *Stage Door.* From 1939, for two years, she was appearing in the Broadway show, "George White's Scandals". In the early 1940s, most of her films featured her dynamic tap-dancing. She was more a supporting act than a star, but many of those films were better for her being in them. She married the first of three husbands in 1946. Three of her films, *Easter Parade, On the Town* and *Kiss Me Kate,* stand out. Ann starred in "Mame" on Broadway and from 1979-89, she toured in "Sugar Babes", with Mickey Rooney. She retired in 2001, after completing work on her final movie, *Mulholland Drive.* She died of lung cancer, in Los Angeles.

You Can't Take It with You (1938)
Room Service (1938)
Too Many Girls (1940)
Go West, Young Lady (1941)
Reveille with Beverly (1943)
Jam Session (1944)
The Thrill of Brazil (1946)
Easter Parade (1948)
On the Town (1949)
Two Tickets to Broadway (1951)
Lovely to Look at (1952)
Small Town Girl (1953)
Kiss Me Kate (1953)
Deep in My Heart (1954)
Hit the Deck (1955)

Sienna **Miller**
5ft 5in
(SIENNA ROSE MILLER)

Born: **December 28, 1981**
New York City, New York, USA

Sienna's father Edwin, is a New York banker and a dealer in Chinese art. Her mother, Jo, is a South African, who was once David Bowie's secretary. The family moved to England when Sienna was a child. Jo ran Lee Strasberg's acting academy in London. Her parents split up when she was six, but after attending Heathfield School, in Ascot, Sienna spent a year at the Lee Strasberg Academy, in New York City, and appeared in a number of stage plays. She also studied with Michael Margotta. While planning her acting career, Sienna made contact with Select Models in New York. When she returned to London she signed with their British branch and appeared in campaigns for Prada and Coca-Cola. In 2001, she made her film debut in *South Kensington,* which received luke-warm reviews. She shook that disappointment off quickly with two successful films – *High Speed* and *The Ride.* After that, some supporting roles in big-budget productions took her to her first starring vehicle, *Casanova* – in which she appeared opposite Heath Ledger. Since then, Sienna has hit the jackpot with each subsequent movie and is considered hot property in Hollywood. She regards herself as English and is an ardent fan of the Chelsea soccer team in London. For seven months, from 2004, she was engaged to Jude Law, whom she met when they worked on *Alfie.* Her performance in *The Edge of Love,* is certainly her best so far. In her private life, Sienna is currently unattached – which gives her plenty of time to heap lots of love on her two dogs – Porgy and Bess.

High Speed (2002)
The Ride (2002)
Layer Cake (2004)
Alfie (2004)
Casanova (2005)
Factory Girl (2006)
Interview (2007)
Camille (2007)
Stardust (2007)
The Edge of Love (2008)

Hayley **Mills**
5ft 4in
(HAYLEY CATHERINE ROSE VIVIEN MILLS)

Born: **April 18, 1946**
London, England

Hayley was the second daughter of the famous English actor, John Mills, and the novelist/playwright, Mary Haley Bell – who gave the little girl her name. Her sister, Juliet was born in 1941, so young Hayley got used to being around people older than herself. When she went to Elmhurst boarding school at the age of nine, she felt shy among her contemporaries until she began acting in school plays. When she was twelve, film director, J.Lee Thompson was visiting the Mills home prior to her dad's appearance in his upcoming *Tiger Bay.* Seeing Hayley, he knew immediately that she would be ideal to play the kid who befriends the on-the-run sailor, Horst Buchholz. It was a really wonderful film debut – winning Hayley a BAFTA award as the year's most promising newcomer. It didn't take Disney very long to get on the phone. While she was still a cute kid, things worked out pretty well. For her Hollywood film debut, in the title-role of *Pollyanna,* she was given a special Oscar. But like so many great child film actors, the difficulty for audiences is to accept that they have grown up. Hayley's adult career has focussed on the stage. A five-year marriage to Roy Boulting ended in divorce. Hayley was recently seen on television in several episodes of the series, 'Wild at Heart'.

Tiger Bay (1959)
Pollyanna (1960)
The Parent Trap (1961)
Whistle Down the Wind (1961)
The Chalk Garden (1964)
The Moonspinners (1964)
Sky West and Crooked (1965)
That Darn Cat! (1965)
The Family Way (1966)
The Trouble with Angels (1966)
Twisted Nerve (1968)
Mr. Forbush and
the Penguins (1971)
Endless Night (1972)
Deadly Strangers (1974)
Appointment
with Death (1988)

Sir John **Mills**
5ft 8in
(LEWIS ERNEST WATTS MILLS)

Born: **February 22, 1908**
North Eltham, Norfolk, England
Died: **April 23, 2005**

Being born at the Watts Naval Training School, where his father was headmaster, may explain why John was so good in all those 1950s war movies. He left Norwich High School at sixteen and after three years in the family corn business, he headed for London, where he worked as a salesman. He'd dreamt of going on the stage as a boy and he took dancing lessons which paid off when he made his professional debut, in 1929, in the chorus of "The Five O'Clock Girl" at the London Hippodrome. Three years later, John made his film debut in *The Midshipmaid.* Throughout the 1930s, he appeared in many British films before *Goodbye, Mr. Chips,* an Oscar-winner, brought him international exposure. He joined the Royal Artillery in 1939, but was discharged in 1941 – on medical grounds. He married secondly, Mary Hayley Bell, with whom he had three children, including Hayley. By the end of the war, John was a star in Britain and became a popular actor all over the world. He won a Best Supporting Actor Oscar, for *Ryan's Daughter,* but his favorite film was *Tunes of Glory.* Although he was suffering from failing eyesight and deafness, John continued working until the end of his life. He died peacefully at his home in Denham, aged ninety-seven.

The Young Mr. Pitt (1942)
The Way to the Stars (1945)
Great Expectations (1946)
The October Man (1947)
Scott of the Antarctic (1948)
Morning Departure (1950)
The Rocking Horse Winner (1950)
Hobson's Choice (1954)
The Colditz Story (1955)
Above Us the Waves (1955)
Ice-Cold in Alex (1958) Tiger Bay (1959)
Tunes of Glory (1960) Swiss Family
Robinson (1960) The Truth About
Spring (1964) The Family Way (1966)
Ryan's Daughter (1970)
Young Winston (1972)
Gandhi (1982)

Yvette **Mimieux**
5ft 4in
(YVETTE CARMEN MIMIEUX)

Born: **January 8, 1942**
Hollywood, California, USA

The daughter of a French father – and a Mexican mother – Carmen Montemayor, Yvette started turning heads while at high school. One afternoon, she was out horse riding in a suburb of Los Angeles, when a helicopter with engine trouble landed nearby. The pilot was a show business press agent, who after telling her that she ought to be in pictures, gave her his calling card. She went on to win a number of beauty contest titles – including "Los Angeles Art Directors Queen" in 1958. In 1960, she made her first TV appearance, in an episode of 'One Step Beyond' and had a small role in a minor film, *Platinum High School*. Director Vincent Minnelli, was impressed when directing her screen test prior to her starring debut, in George Pal's, *The Time Machine*. It was followed by half a dozen years as a star. In 1972, Yvette married the famous film director, Stanley Donen, who was eighteen years her senior. In 1974, Yvette starred on television in a play she'd written, called 'Hit Lady' and two years after that, she starred in the cult classic movie, *Jackson County Jail*. Ten years later, she co-wrote and acted in 'Obsessive Love'. She played her last role – in a TV-movie, 'Lady Boss', before retiring in 1992. With her second husband, Howard Ruby, Yvette runs Oakwood Worldwide Housing.

The Time Machine (1960)
Where the Boys Are (1960)
The Four Horsemen of the
Apocalypse (1962)
Light in the Piazza (1962)
The Wonderful World
of the Brothers Grimm (1962)
Diamond Head (1963)
Toys in the Attic (1963)
Joy in the Morning (1965)
The Reward (1965)
Dark of the Sun (1967)
The Picasso Summer (1969)
Skyjacked (1972)
Jackson County Jail (1976)
The Black Hole (1979)
Circle of Power (1983)

Sal **Mineo**
5ft 4in
(SALVATORE MINEO JR.)

Born: **January 10, 1939**
The Bronx, New York City, New York, USA
Died: **February 12, 1976**

Sal's father, Salvatore Mineo Sr., was a casket maker, who had emigrated from Sicily and met his wife Josephine, in the Bronx. Sal grew up in that tough neighborhood with two brothers and a sister. By the age of eight, he'd joined a street gang. After his arrest for his part in a robbery when he was ten, Sal was given an ultimatum; he had a choice of going to juvenile prison or attending a school which majored in acting. He very wisely chose the latter. He made his stage debut, in "The Rose Tattoo" – which starred Eli Wallach and Maureen Stapleton. When he was thirteen, he made his television debut in two episodes of the 'Hallmark Hall of Fame' series. Soon after that he was the young prince, in "The King and I" on Broadway, with Yul Brynner. When he was sixteen, he played a much younger boy on his film debut, *Six Bridges to Cross*. His appearance in *Rebel Without a Cause* (for which he was nominated for a Best Supporting Actor Oscar) led to friendships with James Dean and Natalie Wood. In 1957, he had a couple of minor hit records including "Start Movin". Sal's second Best Supporting Actor Oscar nomination was for *Exodus*. After a slow down in his film career, in a period when he was openly gay, Sal worked on television. He was stabbed to death by a crazy drug-addict who only wanted his cash.

Six Bridges to Cross (1955)
The Private War of
Major Benson (1955)
Rebel Without a Cause (1955)
Crime in the Streets (1956)
Somebody Up There
Likes Me (1956)
Giant (1956)
The Young Don't Cry (1957)
The Gene Krupa Story (1959)
Exodus (1960)
Cheyenne Autumn (1964)
Who Killed Teddy Bear (1965)
Escape from the Planet
of the Apes (1971)

Liza **Minnelli**
5ft 4in
(LIZA MAY MINNELLI)

Born: **March 12, 1946**
Los Angeles, California, USA

The only child from the marriage of the legendary movie star and much-loved singer, Judy Garland, and Oscar-winning film musical director, Vincente Minnelli, Liza was born to be a star herself. She was only three when she appeared in the final scene of her mother's film, *In the Good Old Summertime*. Like most young kids, she then got on with her education – in her case, Scarsdale High School, in New York. She made her stage debut, with her mother, at the Palace Theater, in 1960. In the early 1960s, she attended the Sorbonne, in Paris. Back in the United States, she studied drama with Uta Hagen and Herbert Berghof and worked in New York productions of "Best Foot Forward", "Take Me Along", "The Diary of Anne Frank", and "Flora the Menace". In 1967, she married the first of her four husbands – the Australian-born singer Peter Allen, and made her movie debut in Albert Finney's, *Charlie Bubbles*. She was then nominated for a Best Actress Oscar – for *The Sterile Cuckoo,* and won the award for her dynamic portrayal of Sally Bowles, in *Cabaret*. Liza recorded several albums of songs which her fans adored and she had one of her biggest successes in 1989, when she combined with "The Pet Shop Boys" on the album entitled "Results". Several illnesses have threatened to end her career, but she keeps coming back – she was touring again in 2007, but she collapsed on stage during a Stockholm Christmas concert. In 2008, she was back again – with dates in the USA and Italy.

Charlie Bubbles (1967)
The Sterile Cuckoo (1969)
Tell Me That You Love Me,
Junie Moon (1970)
Cabaret (1972)
Lucky Lady (1975)
A Matter of Time (1976)
New York, New York (1977)
Arthur (1981)
The King of Comedy (1983)
Stepping Out (1991)
The Oh in Ohio (2006)

Miou-Miou
5ft 4in
(SYLVETTE HÉRY)

Born: **February 22, 1950**
Paris, France

After growing up in a suburb of Paris where her father was a policeman and her mother ran a fruit and vegetable stall, the beautiful Sylvette, as she was then known, looked for a way out of 'une vie ordinaire'. One lucky day, she sold strawberries to the actor-director, Romain Bouteille, who invited her to work at a Parisian theater called Café de la Gare. Gérard Depardieu was one of the theater's principal actors, but Sylvette's job was cleaning. She soon graduated to the position of dresser and was well liked, in the way one would like a nice, attractive, pussycat. One of the company, the actor, Michel Colouche, gave her the nickname "Miou-Miou". The name stuck. She made her film debut with it in 1971, in *La Vie Sentimentale de Georges Le Tueur.* Miou-Miou then became romantically involved with the actor, Patrick Dewaere, and they had a daughter they named Angele, who was born in 1974. It was a good decade for the talented young actress, but in 1980, she caused a huge controversy, when refusing to accept a César after she was voted Best Actress, for *La Dérobade.* On nine other occasions, she was nominated, but didn't win! Miou-Miou has a second daughter, Jeanne Herry, whose father is the popular singer, Julien Clerc.

Les Grandes brulées (1973)
Les Valseuses (1974)
Victory March (1976)
La Dérobade (1979)
The Woman Cop (1980)
Coup de foudre (1983)
Evening Dress (1986)
Les Portes tournantes (1988)
La lectrice (1990)
Milou en mai (1990)
Germinal (1993)
The Long Day (1996)
Dry Cleaning (1997)
Women (1997)
Everything's Fine (2000)
The Science of Sleep (2006)
Avril (2006)
Le Grand alibi (2008)

Dame Helen **Mirren**
5ft 4in
(ILLIANA LYDIA PETROVNA MIRONOVA)

Born: **July 26, 1945**
Chiswick, London, England

Helen's grandfather, a Tsarist, found himself stranded in London at the outbreak of the Russian Revolution. He sent for his wife and son Vasiliy – Helen's father, who married Kathleen Rogers – the thirteenth of fourteen children born to a West Ham butcher. Vasiliy became Basil, and played viola with the London Philharmonic. Helen was raised as a Catholic and attended St. Bernard's High School, in Southend, Essex – where she had her first acting experience. She studied at the New College of Speech and Drama in London and in 1963, was accepted by the National Youth Theater. She made her debut, at the Old Vic, in "Antony and Cleopatra" in 1965. She worked with the Royal Shakespeare Company before making her film debut, in *Herostratus.* Without ever deserting the theater, she became a screen icon. Helen was twice nominated for Oscars – for *The Madness of King George* and *Gosford Park,* and was adjudged Best Actress – portraying *The Queen.* In 1997, Helen married American writer/director, Taylor Hackford – who later won an Oscar for *Ray.*

Herostratus (1967)
Age of Consent (1969)
Savage Messiah (1972)
O Lucky Man! (1973)
Hamlet (1976)
The Long Good Friday (1980)
Excalibur (1981)
Cal (1984) 2010 (1984)
Heavenly Pursuits (1985)
White Nights (1985)
The Mosquito Coast (1986)
The Cook the Thief his
Wife & Her Lover (1989)
Where Angels
Fear to Tread (1991)
The Madness of King George (1994)
Last Orders (2001)
The Queen (2006)
National Treasure:
Book of Secrets (2007)
Inkheart (2008)
State of Play (2009)

Cameron **Mitchell**
5ft 11in
(CAMERON MCDOWELL MITZELL)

Born: **November 4, 1918**
Dallastown, Pennsylvania, USA
Died: **July 6, 1994**

Cameron lived his early life very close to poverty – growing up during the Great Depression in a Pennsylvania Dutch community. He was one of the seven children born to the Reverend Charles Mitzell and his wife, Kathryn. The family was as poor as everyone else and little Cameron wore his older sister's "hand-me-down" coats and shoes to school. It was at High School that he first dreamed of becoming an actor and one of his teachers was so convinced that he'd make it, he urged the boy to go to drama school and lent him some money to get started. Cameron did his bit by washing dishes, but his luck changed when he met Broadway legend, Lynn Fontanne – who told him to change his name to Mitchell. In 1940, he married actress, Joanna Mendel, who was the daughter of self-made Canadian business tycoon, Fred Mendel. He worked with Lynn Fontanne and her husband Alfred Lunt until 1942, when he joined the Air Corps. He made his film debut in 1945, in a short for MGM, *The Last Installment,* and made one hundred and twenty-five movies without ever becoming a star. Most of his final thirty or so were quite bad. He completed work on his last film, *Jack-O,* before dying of lung cancer. His son and daughter are both actors.

They Were Expendable (1945)
Command Decision (1948)
Man in the Saddle (1951)
Death of a Salesman (1951)
Les Miserables (1952)
Man on a Tightrope (1953)
How to Marry a Millionaire (1953)
Hell and High Water (1954)
Garden of Evil (1954) Desirée (1954)
Love Me or Leave Me (1955)
House of Bamboo (1955)
The Tall Men (1955) Carousel (1956)
Tension at Table Rock (1956)
Monkey on My Back (1957)
No Down Payment (1957) Hombre (1967)
Buck and the Preacher (1972)
My Favorite Year (1982)

Radha **Mitchell**
5ft 5¾in
(RADHA RANI AMBER INDIGO ANUNDA MITCHELL)

Born: November 12, 1973
Melbourne, Victoria, Australia

Radha's parents were influenced by the mystic Eastern religions which became popular in the 1960's, through celebrities like the Beatles. Her mother was a fashion model in Italy during that period. Three of the names she was given at birth are of Indian Hindu origin. Early on in her life she was interested in acting and appeared in school plays. When she was fourteen she made her TV debut, as Pixie Robinson, in the Australian family comedy drama series 'Sugar and Spice'. Her next appearance on the small screen would be five years later, but during her high school years she appeared on stage in "Desire". Radha made her film debut, in *Love and Other Catastrophes* and was first seen by U.S. audiences in *High Art*. Apart from acting with Denzel Washington, in *Man On Fire* and Johnny Depp, in *Finding Neverland,* Radha has given her special aura to every film she's been in. Her percentage of good movies must be the envy of many actors. Radha, who has lived in Los Angeles since 1997, is a vegetarian and keeps her calm demeanor by practicing yoga.

Love and Other
Catastrophes (1996)
High Art (1998)
Sleeping Beauties (1999)
Kick (1999)
Everything Put Together (2000)
Pitch Black (2000)
Cowboys and Angels (2000)
Ten Tiny Love Stories (2001)
When Strangers Appear (2001)
Dead Heat (2002)
Phone Booth (2002)
Man on Fire (2004)
Finding Neverland (2004)
Melinda and Melinda (2004)
Mozart and the Whale (2005)
Silent Hill (2006)
The Half Life of
Timofey Berezin (2006)
Feast of Love (2007) Rogue (2007)
Henry Poole Is Here (2008)
The Children of Huang Shi (2008)
Thick as Thieves (2009)

Thomas **Mitchell**
5ft 10in
(THOMAS MITCHELL)

Born: July 11, 1892
Elizabeth, New Jersey, USA
Died: **December 17, 1962**

The youngest son of Irish immigrants, Tommy followed his father and his brother into journalism when he left school. Through the writing experience, he began to come up with theatrical sketches of the comical variety, and when he acted in them, he realized where his future lay. He went on tour with the future screen actor, Charles Coburn's company before a career on Broadway, which started in the early 1920s. In 1923, he made his film debut, in *Six Cylinder Love*. It would be thirteen years before his next screen role, in *Craig's Wife*. In 1930, he co-wrote a play titled "Little Accident" which would be made into Hollywood films three times. Tommy became one of the great American character actors – being nominated for an Oscar for *The Hurricane,* and winning a Best Supporting Actor Oscar. in John Ford's great western, *Stagecoach.* He was in several classics including *Gone With the Wind* and *Mr. Smith Goes to Washington.* Tommy went on performing until the year before his death from cancer in Beverly Hills. He was married twice.

Craig's Wife (1936)
Theodora Goes Wild (1936)
Lost Horizon (1937)
The Hurricane (1937)
Trade Winds (1938)
Stagecoach (1939)
Only Angels Have Wings (1939)
Mr. Smith Goes to Washington (1939)
Gone With the Wind (1939)
The Hunchback of Notre Dame (1939)
The Long Voyage Home (1940)
Out of the Fog (1941) Moontide (1942)
Tales of Manhattan (1942)
The Black Swan (1942)
Flesh and Fantasy (1943)
The Fighting Sullivans (1944)
The Dark Mirror (1946)
It's a Wonderful Life (1946)
The Romance of Rosy Ridge (1947)
High Noon (1952)
While the City Sleeps (1956)
Pocketful of Miracles (1961)

Robert **Mitchum**
6ft 1in
(ROBERT CHARLES DURMAN MITCHUM)

Born: August 6, 1917
Bridgeport, Connecticut, USA
Died: **July 1, 1997**

Bob's father, a railroad worker, died in a train accident when he was two. He was raised by his mother and his stepfather – a British army major. There was little discipline and by the time he was fourteen, Bob had been sentenced to work on a chain gang – from which he escaped. While working at Lockheed, in Long Beach, California, he joined a local amateur theater. In 1940, he married his only wife, Dorothy, who bore him three children and tolerated his transgressions until his death. In 1942, he had his first bit part, in Hitchcock's *Saboteur.* An early credit was in a Hopalong Cassidy film, *Border Patrol.* He'd been in two dozen movies before his breakthrough, in *Story of G.I. Joe* – for which he was Oscar-nominated. It is said that he was underrated as an actor, and you will be hard-pressed to name many really bad Mitchum movies. Despite a lifetime of heavy drinking, smoking, brawling and womanizing, Bob managed to survive for eighty years. He died in Santa Barbara, California, from cancer and emphysema.

Story of G.I. Joe (1945)
The Locket (1946)
Pursued (1947) Crossfire (1947)
Out of the Past (1947)
Rachel and the Stranger (1948)
The Big Steal (1949)
His Kind of Woman (1951)
The Racket (1951) Angel Face (1952)
Night of the Hunter (1955)
Heaven Knows, Mr. Allison (1957)
The Enemy Below (1957)
Thunder Road (1958) Home from
the Hill (1960) The Sundowners (1960)
Cape Fear (1962) Two for the
Seesaw (1962) El Dorado (1966)
Ryan's Daughter (1970)
The Yakuza (1974) Farewell,
My Lovely (1975) Midway (1976)
The Last Tycoon (1976)
Maria's Lovers (1984)
Scrooged (1988) Cape Fear (1991)
Dead Man (1995)
Waiting for Sunset (1995)

Matthew **Modine**
6ft 4in
(MATTHEW AVERY MODINE)

Born: **March 22, 1959**
Loma Linda, New York, USA

Raised in a Mormon family, Matthew was the youngest of seven children born to Mark and Dolores Modine. The whole family worked in drive-in movie theaters operated by Mark. Inspired by some of the films he saw – especially a documentary about the making of *Oliver!* Matthew set his mind on becoming an actor and also took tap dancing lessons. He joined the Glee Club at his junior high school. He graduated from Mar Vista High School, at Imperial Beach, California and attended Brigham Young University, in Provo, Utah. He then moved to New York to study with Stella Adler. He was a chef at "Au Natural" in Manhattan before his acting career took off. In 1980, he married Cari Rivera, with whom he has a son and a daughter. After a TV appearance in an episode of ABC 'Afterschool Specials' Matthew made his film debut, in 1983, in the high school comedy, *Baby It's You.* Later that year, he made rapid progress when he was cast by Robert Altman – in his Vietmam war themed, *Streamers* – which won a collective Best Actor Prize at the Venice Film Festival. He helped collect a similar award for *Short Cuts.* In 2008, Matthew directed a short comedy called *I Think I Thought* and a serious short, *To Kill an American.*

Streamers (1983) **Birdy** (1984)
Full Metal Jacket (1987)
Married to the Mob (1988)
Memphis Belle (1990)
Pacific Heights (1990)
Wind (1992)
Short Cuts (1993)
The Browning Version (1994)
Bye Bye Love (1995) **Fluke** (1995)
The Real Blonde (1997)
Any Given Sunday (1999)
Very Mean Men (2000)
Nobody's Baby (2001)
Hollywood North (2003)
Transporter 2 (2005)
Opa! (2005) **Kettle of Fish** (2006)
Have Dreams, Will Travel (2007)
Go Go Tales (2007)
The Garden of Eden (2008)

Gretchen **Moll**
5ft 6in
(GRETCHEN MOL)

Born: **November 8, 1972**
Deep River, Connecticut, USA

Gretchen is the daughter of a couple of schoolteachers. Her mother, Janet, is also an artist. Although she wasn't aware of it at the time, Gretchen grew up a few miles away from the home of the movie great, Katherine Hepburn. Her brother, Jim went on to work as a film editor. During her high school years Gretchen appeared in plays and musicals – frequently in the company of a classmate, Peter Lockyer, who would become a well-known actor on Broadway. After graduating, Gretchen also headed for New York, where she began her studies at the American Musical and Dramatic Academy and later, at the William Esper Studios. She was not tall enough to be a fashion model, but her perfect looks brought her beauty work and her face appeared on the covers of magazines. During a quiet spell, she was working as a hat check girl at Michael's Restaurant when she was spotted by a talent scout. The result was a leading role in a Coca-Cola commercial. Gretchen also played in summer stock until 1996, when she made her movie debut, in Spike Lee's *Girl 6.* Her career flourished for three good years including a vintage one, in 1998 – Woody Allen's *Celebrity,* with Leonardo DiCaprio and Kenneth Branagh being the highpoint. She floundered for three years, but came back strongly with *The Shape of Things* and marriage to writer/director, Tod "Kip" Williams – with whom she has a son.

The Funeral (1996)
Donnie Brasco (1997)
The Last Time
I Committed Suicide (1997)
Music from Another Room (1998)
Rounders (1998)
Celebrity (1998)
Finding Graceland (1998)
Cradle Will Rock (1999)
Just Looking (1999)
The Shape of Things (2003)
The Notorious Bettie Page (2005)
Puccini for Beginners (2006)
3:10 to Yuma (2007)
An American Affair (2009)

Alfred **Molina**
6ft 2½in
(ALFRED MOLINA)

Born: **May 24, 1953**
London, England

The son of a Spanish communist from Madrid, who was working as a waiter and chauffeur, and an Italian lady who worked as a hotel cleaner, Fred could be said to have had a modest start to life. It didn't prevent him from dreaming of a better future. He made his mind up to become an actor when he was nine years old, after he'd seen the film *Spartacus,* at a movie theater near his home in Notting Hill. He graduated from the Guildhall School of Music and Drama and after working as a kind of street comedian, he began his career on the London stage. Fred made his movie debut in the Hollywood blockbuster, *Raiders of the Lost Ark,* and four years later, he had a good role in *Letter to Brezhnev.* That success gave him the confidence to marry the actress Jill Gascoine. He secured his own acting future when he played Joe Orton's lover, Kenneth Halliwell in Stephen Frears' *Prick Up Your Ears.* Apart from his many films, Fred's done plenty of theater work. In 1998, on his Broadway debut, he received a Tony nomination for "Art". His film work since then has been of a consistently high standard. Fred is now a United States Citizen.

Raiders of the Lost Ark (1981)
Letter to Brezhnev (1985)
Ladyhawke (1985)
Prick Up Your Ears (1987)
Enchanted April (1992)
Maverick (1994)
Nervous Energy (1995)
The Perez Family (1995)
Anna Karenina (1997)
Boogie Nights (1997)
The Man Who Knew
Too Little (1997) **Magnolia** (1999)
Chocolat (2000) **Frida** (2002)
Identity (2003) **Luther** (2003)
The Da Vinci Code (2006)
As You Like It (2006)
The Hoax (2006) **Silk** (2007)
The Little Traitor (2007)
Nothing Like the Holidays (2008)
The Lodger (2008)
An Education (2009)

Michelle **Monaghan**
5ft 7in
(MICHELLE LYNN MONAGHAN)

Born: **March 23, 1976**
Winthrop, Iowa, USA

Michelle certainly grew up amongst a lot of kids. In addition to living with two older brothers, her mother Sharon ran a day care center at the family's home and there were several occasions when she was fostering children. Michelle's father, Bob was a nice easy-going guy who worked in a factory. She was a bright girl who after graduating from East Buchanan High School in 1994, moved to Chicago to study journalism at Columbia College. Her height and looks enabled her to supplement her allowance by doing some modeling – including work in Italy and the Far East during breaks from her studies. She moved to New York before completing her course and after further modeling work, in 2000 she got her first television acting role in the series, 'Young Americans'. Having had experience in the business, she made her debut in a 2001 film about models – in *Perfume* – which stank! A much better film after that was *Unfaithful*. For the time being, television made her name when she appeared in eight episodes of 'Boston Public'. It led to film work in *It Runs in the* (Douglas) *Family,* a strong role in *Winter Solstice,* and an appearance in a hit movie, *The Bourne Supremacy*. In 2005, Michelle married a graphic designer, Peter White, and things have been going well ever since then – including the arrival of her first child – a baby girl named Willow, in November 2008. In terms of Michelle's recent career, special mention should be made of her performances in *Gone Baby Gone* and *Trucker.*

Unfaithful (2002)
Winter Solstice (2004)
The Bourne Supremacy (2005)
Kiss Kiss Bang Bang (2005)
Mr. & Mrs. Smith (2005)
North Country (2005)
Mission: Impossible III (2006)
Gone Baby Gone (2007)
The Heartbreak Kid (2007)
Trucker (2008)
Made of Honor (2008)
Eagle Eye (2008)

Marilyn **Monroe**
5ft 5½in
(NORMA JEAN MORTENSEN)

Born: **June 1, 1926**
Los Angeles, California, USA
Died: **August 5, 1962**

The identity of Marilyn's father is unknown. As Norma Jean, she had a traumatic early life. Her mother, Gladys Monroe, was a film-cutter at RKO, who went insane. The little girl was sent to the Los Angeles Orphans' Home – which paid her 5 cents a month for cleaning and kitchen work. She briefly attended Van Nuys High School, then at sixteen, she married a man called James Dougherty, whom she referred to as "Daddy". While he was away during World War II, she worked at the Radioplane Company, owned by the actor, Reginald Denny. She was actually discovered by an Army photographer and signed by the Blue Book Modeling Agency. She changed her image and took acting lessons from Lee Strasberg and attended singing classes. In 1946, she signed with 20th Century Fox. She became Marilyn Monroe and was given a few bit parts, starting with *The Shocking Miss Pilgrim,* in 1947. It was in *All About Eve,* that Marilyn first displayed her star potential. By 1953, she'd become the biggest sex symbol of all time. She had two more husbands – baseball star, Joe DiMaggio, and playwright, Arthur Miller, and a host of famous lovers – including Sinatra and Jack Kennedy. Despite all this excitement Marilyn was a sad and lonely girl, who believed she was being used. When the pressure became too much, she took her own life with a drug overdose – at the early age of thirty-six.

All About Eve (1950)
The Asphalt Jungle (1950)
Don't Bother to Knock (1952)
Monkey Business (1952)
Gentlemen Prefer Blondes (1953)
How to Marry a Millionaire (1953)
Niagara (1953)
There's No Business Like Show Business (1954) **The Seven Year Itch** (1955) **Bus Stop** (1956)
Some Like It Hot (1959)
Let's Make Love (1960)
The Misfits (1961)

Ricardo **Montalban**
6ft
(RICARDO GONZALO PEDRO MONTALBAN Y MERINO)

Born: **November 25, 1920**
Mexico City, Distrito Federal, Mexico
Died: **January 14, 2009**

Ricardo and his brother and sister were raised as devout Catholics by their parents, Jenaro and Ricarda. The family moved to the United States and settled in Los Angeles. Ricardo was educated at Fairfax High School and later studied drama at L.A. High School. He made his film debut in the war drama, *Five Were Chosen,* in 1941, but when his mother fell ill, he went back to Mexico with her. One stroke of luck occurred, when he met Loretta Young's sister, Georgina. They fell in love, married in 1944, had four children together and were soul-mates. Ricardo appeared in eleven Mexican films during five years there, and when he got back to Hollywood, in 1947, it was for the Latin themed *Fiesta*. Ricardo's image and accent would ensure his future employment in a large number of leading and supporting roles. It was a good thing he resisted studio efforts to change his name to Ricky Martin! He was given the MGM build-up with a featured role in *On an Island with You,* starring Esther Williams and followed that with roles in hit movies like *Two Weeks with Love* and *Sayonara*. Ricardo's career lasted sixty-five years! His wife, Georgina, died in 2007. He died in Los Angeles, of congestive heart failure.

On an Island with You (1948)
Border Incident (1949)
Battleground (1949)
Mystery Street (1950)
Right Cross (1950)
Two Weeks with Love (1950)
Across the Wide Missouri (1951)
A Life in the Balance (1955)
Sayonara (1957)
Let No Man Write My Epitaph (1960)
The Reluctant Saint (1962)
Cheyenne Autumn (1964)
Madame X (1966)
The Train Robbers (1973)
Star Trek: The Wrath of Khan (1982)
The Naked Gun: From the Files of Police Squad! (1988)

Yves **Montand**
6ft 2in
(IVO LIVI)

Born: **October 13, 1921**
Monsummano Terme, Tuscany, Italy
Died: **November 9, 1991**

His parents were desperately poor and his father, being a staunch communist, fled Mussolini's Italy in 1923, and settled in Marseilles. When he was eleven, Yves left school and worked in a series of dead-end jobs, including delivery boy, hairdresser's apprentice, truck loader, and as a waiter in a dockside cafe. He kept a positive attitude, and after singing in musical halls around the country, he went to Paris, where he caught the eye of Edith Piaf. Yves became her lover and in 1946, got a featured film role with her, in *Étoile san Lumière*. Even better was her successfully lobbying Marcel Carné to star him in the big budget *Les Portes de la Nuit*. In 1951, his marriage to Simone Signoret did wonders for his movie career and they became great favorites with French audiences. Yves' screen breakthrough was in *The Wages of Fear*. During the filming of *Let's Make Love*, he had an affair with Marilyn Monroe. Yves enjoyed a revival of his movie career, when he appeared in two French movie classics – *Jean de Florette* and *Manon des Sources*. He died of a heart attack a few months after completing his final film. He had a son with his widow, Carole Amiel.

Les Portes de la Nuit (1946)
The Wages of Fear (1953)
Marguerite de la Nuit (1955)
Napoléon (1955) Let's Make Love (1960)
Le Joli Mai (1962)
La Guerre est Finie (1966)
Grand Prix (1966) Z (1969)
The Confession (1970)
The Red Circle (1970)
La Folie des grandeurs (1971)
César and Rosalie (1972)
The Threat (1977)
I...comme Icare (1979)
Choice of Arms (1981)
Garçon! (1983)
Jean de Florette (1986)
Manon des Sources (1986)
IP5: L'île aux
pachydermes (1992)

George **Montgomery**
6ft 3in
(GEORGE MONTGOMERY LETZ)

Born: **August 29, 1916**
Brady, Montana, USA
Died: **December 12, 2000**

George was the youngest of fifteen children born to Ukrainian immigrants. Following high school, he spent a year studying Architecture at the University of Montana. His involvement in stage productions there convinced him that an actor's life was what he wanted. In 1935, he headed for Hollywood, where his impressive physique and handsome face got him work as as stuntman and extra, using his real name, George Letz, in westerns – starting that year in the Gene Autry movie, *The Singing Vagabond*. His first featured role was three years later, in the serial, *The Lone Ranger*. There were two dozen more uncredited roles until Twentieth Century Fox featured him in *The Cisco Kid and the Lady,* and other B-westerns. They gave him a good role in *Roxie Hart* and began promoting him in other hit films such as *Orchestra Wives*. He was soon acting opposite the screen goddesses, Gene Tierney – *China Girl,* and Betty Grable – *Coney Island*. George retired in 1986, following a poorly made war film shot in Yugoslavia. George was married to the singer, Dinah Shore, from 1943 until 1963. He died of heart failure at Rancho Mirage, California.

Star Dust (1940)
The Cowboy and the Blonde (1941)
Riders of the Purple Sage (1941)
Roxie Hart (1942)
Ten Gentlemen from West Point (1942)
Orchestra Wives (1942)
China Girl (1942)
Coney Island (1943)
Bomber's Moon (1943)
Three Little Girls in Blue (1946)
The Brasher Doubloon (1947)
Dakota Lil (1950)
The Texas Rangers (1951)
The Pathfinder (1952)
Robbers' Roost (1955)
Street of Sinners (1957)
Badman's Country (1958)
Battle of the Bulge (1965)
Warkill (1968)

Robert **Montgomery**
6ft 1in
(HENRY MONTGOMERY JR.)

Born: **May 21, 1904**
Beacon, New York, USA
Died: **September 27, 1981**

Robert's father was president of the New York Rubber Company. He could afford to send his son to private schools but had lost his fortune by the time he died in the early 1920s. Robert had no alternative but to curtail his studies and work for the railway and later went to sea on a merchant ship. In 1926, he went to New York, where he became assistant property-man in a theater. He auditioned as an actor, and working on stage with George Cukor, persuaded him to go to Hollywood. Before he did so, he married the first of his two wives, the Broadway actress, Elizabeth Bryan Allen. One of their two children was Elizabeth Montgomery, of 'Bewitched' fame. He signed with MGM, and was an extra in a Garbo silent film, *The Single Standard,* in 1929. A year later, Robert was fourth-billed in Norma Shearer's, *The Divorcee*. In Robert's forty films during the 1930s, he played opposite almost every big female star. Before a break for U.S. Navy service in World War II, he was twice nominated for Best Actor Oscars – for *Night Must Fall,* and *Here Comes Mr. Jordan*. He directed five movies, including *Lady in the Lake* – an experimental film which was not liked at the time. His last movie was *Your Witness,* in 1950, which he directed and acted in. Robert retired in 1960 and died of cancer in New York City.

The Big House (1930)
When Ladies Meet (1933)
Fugitive Lovers (1934)
Riptide (1934)
Trouble for Two (1936)
Night Must Fall (1937)
Ever Since Eve (1937)
Busman's Honeymoon (1940)
Mr. & Mrs. Smith (1941)
Here Comes Mr. Jordan (1941)
Unfinished Business (1941)
They Were Expendable (1945)
Lady in the Lake (1947)
Ride the Pink Horse (1947)
June Bride (1948)
Once More, My Darling (1949)

Demi **Moore**
5ft 5in
(DEMETRIA GENE GUYNES)

Born: **November 11, 1962**
Roswell, New Mexico, USA

Demi had a pretty rough start to her life. Her father had left home before she was born and her mother's second marriage was a total disaster – her stepfather was a violent drunkard who finally committed suicide. Demi left Fairfax High School when she was sixteen and at eighteen, married the rock musician, Freddie Moore – from whom she took her stage name, but divorced in 1985. Prior to that, she became one of the nine original members of the so-called "Brat-Pack". Demi made her film debut in 1981, in the independent *Choices,* and worked in the TV series, 'General Hospital'. Her first featured role (topless), was in a mediocre Michael Caine film, *Blame it on Rio.* A much better opportunity was playing a coke addict, in *St. Elmo's Fire* – which she only got after agreeing to cut her alcohol and drugs consumption. It led to some quality roles and a thirteen year marriage to Bruce Willis, with whom she had three daughters. One movie that didn't provide any quality was the really disastrous, *Striptease,* in 1996. But Demi laughed all the way to the bank – having become the highest-paid actress in Hollywood. Following a rather lengthy lull, and an appearance in the disappointing *Charlie's Angels: Full Throttle,* it looks as if her star is shining again – with three promising looking movies scheduled for release during 2009.

St. Elmo's Fire (1985)
One Crazy Summer (1986)
The Seventh Sign (1988)
Ghost (1990)
Mortal Thoughts (1991)
A Few Good Men (1992)
Disclosure (1994)
Now and Then (1995)
The Juror (1996)
G.I.Jane (1997)
Deconstructing Harry (1997)
Passion of Mind (2000)
Half Light (2006)
Bobby (2006)
Flawless (2007)
Mr. Brooks (2007)

Dudley **Moore**
5ft 2½in
(DUDLEY STUART JOHN MOORE)

Born: **April 19, 1935**
Dagenham, Essex, England
Died: **March 27, 2002**

Although succeeding beyond his working-class parents' wildest dreams, Dudley was a victim of the English class system when he was growing up. He was born with a club foot, which, despite being corrected to some extent, was an object of verbal bullying – both at school and later, at the hands of his upper-class comedy partner, Peter Cook. But it's true to say that Dudley was also born with genius. He was a child prodigy who was a choirboy at the age of six, and was playing the church organ at weddings when he was fourteen. After winning a music scholarship to Magdalen College, Oxford, he could have become a good classical pianist. But he chose jazz – which was more fun, and also exposed him to the world of show business – and girls. He went to live in London, where he appeared in a satirical review, "Beyond the Fringe" and befriended Peter Cook, who became his partner. The successful pairing won a big following on stage, in nightclubs such as Cook's 'Establishment' and on television – where they were magic. Despite Peter's tendency to put Dudley down, they loved each other. It could have gone on, but Peter envied Dudley's success in Hollywood. Films they made together were fine, but *10* and *Arthur* – for which he was Oscar-nominated, elevated Dudley to a level above Peter. Worst of all, he was quite ordinary without "Dud". Peter's death deeply saddened Dudley, and he followed seven years later after a bout of pneumonia, in Plainfield, New Jersey. His four marriages produced two children including a son with the actress, Tuesday Weld.

The Wrong Box (1966)
Bedazzled (1967)
Monte Carlo or Bust (1969)
The Bed Sitting Room (1969)
Foul Play (1978) **10** (1979)
Derek and Clive
Get the Horn (1979)
Arthur (1981)
Unfaithfully Yours (1984)

Julianne **Moore**
5ft 4in
(JULIE ANN SMITH)

Born: **December 3, 1960**
Fayetteville, North Carolina, USA

Julianne's father, Peter Moore Smith, was a military judge – who had been an army colonel, lawyer, and helicopter pilot. Her Scottish mother, Anne, was a psychiatric social worker. She and her sister and brother grew up as "army brats' in the United States and in Frankfurt, Germany, where she went to Frankfurt American High School. Back in the USA, she earned a Bachelor's Degree from the College of Fine Arts, at Boston University. In 1983, she moved to New York, where she worked as a waitress before getting her first break in the TV soap, 'As the World Turns' for which she won a Daytime Emmy Award. Her movie debut was in the Canadian horror film, *sLaughterhouse II,* in 1988. There was some average fare up until, *The Hand that Rocks the Cradle,* which really got her film career moving. The quality of her subsequent work has resulted in four Best Actress Oscar nominations - for *Boogie Nights, The End of the Affair, The Hours,* and *Far From Heaven.* In 2005, she married her third husband, Bart Freundlich, a director, writer and actor. Julianne's acting in the recent, *Blindness,* is something else – as is most of her work.

The Hand That Rocks
the Cradle (1992)
Benny & Joon (1993)
The Fugitive (1993) **Short Cuts** (1993)
Vanya on 42nd Street (1994)
Safe (1995) **Assassins** (1995)
Boogie Nights (1997)
The Big Lebowski (1998)
Cookie's Fortune (1999)
An Ideal Husband (1999)
The End of the Affair (1999)
Magnolia (1999) **Hannibal** (2001)
The Shipping News (2001)
Far from Heaven (2002)
The Hours (2002) **The Forgotten** (2004)
The Prize Winner of Defiance,
Ohio (2005)
Children of Men (2006)
Savage Grace (2007)
I'm Not There (2007)
Blindness (2008)

Mary Tyler **Moore**
5ft 7in
(MARY TYLER MOORE)

Born: **December 29, 1936**
Brooklyn, New York City, New York, USA

Mary was the eldest of three children – two girls and a boy – born to George Tyler Moore and his wife, Marjorie. In Brooklyn, Mary attended the Saint Rose of Lima Roman Catholic School before, when she was eight, her parents took her and the other children to live in California. There, she finished her education at St. Ambrose School in Los Angeles and at the exclusive Immaculate Heart High School, on Los Feliz Boulevard in Hollywood. Mary was a pretty teenager who took dancing lessons and was soon signed by a talent agency. She was given her first assignment in a TV commercial for Hotpoint, which was aired during the popular show, 'The Adventures of Ozzie & Harriet'. Mary married her sweetheart, Dick Meeker, in 1955, and was soon pregnant with her only child, a son named Richie. Mary's first screen appearance was an uncredited one in a 1958 Rowan and Martin comedy, *Once Upon a Horse*. She had short-lived roles in more than twenty TV shows before her next movie, *X-15*. It was the same year that she made her breakthrough, as Laura Petrie, in 'The Dick Van Dyke Show'. Her good run of movies included *Thoroughly Modern Millie* and co-starring with Elvis Presley in *Change of Habit*. In 1970, she became more popular than ever (on TV at least) when she began a seven-year tenure in her own 'The Mary Tyler Moore Show'. Her next film role, as Beth Jarrett, in *Ordinary People*, was a good one and she was nominated for a Best Actress Oscar. Mary's film appearances since then have been too infrequent. She has been married to Dr. Robert Levine, since 1983.

X-15 (1961)
Thoroughly Modern
Millie (1967) What's So Bad
About Feeling Good? (1968)
Don't Just Stand There! (1968)
Change of Habit (1969)
Ordinary People (1980)
Just Between Friends (1986)
Flirting with Disaster (1996)
Cheats (2002)

Kieron **Moore**
6ft 1in
(KIERON O'HANRAHAN)

Born: **October 5, 1924**
Skibbereen, County Cork, Ireland
Died: **July 15, 2007**

Kieron's father, Peter, was a poet, who was one of the founders of the Gaelic League. Throughout his life, he did his best to keep the Irish language alive and was twice imprisoned by the British for his outspoken views. It was a very creative family, with Kieron's brother and sister working in broadcasting and music. They moved to Dublin where, after attending the Irish language school, Coáiste Mhuire, Kieron studied Medicine at University College. He dropped out when he was invited to join the famous Abbey Players. His dark good looks were soon in demand as the world returned to peace. In 1945, he made his film debut in *The Voice Within*, and fell in love with his co-star, Barbara White. They married two years later and had four children. By 1947, Kieron was being groomed for stardom by the British Film Industry and that year, he registered strongly as a post traumatic stress victim, in *Mine Own Executioner*. Starring with Vivien Leigh and Ralph Richardson in *Anna Karenina*, was as good as it would get, and enduring fame proved elusive. He kept working in films and on TV until his retirement in 1974, when, after appearing in an episode of 'The Zoo Gang' he became involved with Third World development. Kieron was in France when he died of natural causes.

Mine Own Executioner (1947)
Anna Karenina (1948)
Saints and Sinners (1949)
Ten Tall Men (1951)
The Green Scarf (1954)
The Key (1958)
Darby O'Gill and
the Little People (1959)
The League of Gentlemen (1960)
The Day They Robbed the
Bank of England (1960)
The Siege of
Sidney Street (1960)
The 300 Spartans (1962)
The Thin Red Line (1964)
Arabesque (1966)

Sir Roger **Moore**
6ft 1in
(ROGER GEORGE MOORE)

Born: **October 14, 1927**
Stockwell, London, England

Roger was the son of a London 'bobby' or police constable. He attended Battersea Grammar School and Dr. Challoner's School – in Amersham, Buckinghamshire. It was due to his artistic talent, that his first job was in Soho, as a tracer/filler, with a cartoon film company. As he was good looking, he was given work as an extra in the 1944 film, *Caesar and Cleopatra*. He was encouraged enough to spend three terms at RADA. While there, he met his first wife, Doorn van Steyn. He then spent seven years gaining acting experience with a repertory company in Cambridge. It was a slow process, with only a few bit parts to show for it. Then, in 1954, Roger was put under contract by MGM and was featured as a tennis pro, in *The Last Time I Saw Paris*. One year later he received third billing below Glenn Ford and Eleanor Parker, in the musical drama, *Interrupted Melody*. It was popular, but hardly a star-maker for Roger, whose best early exposure was as Beau Maverick, in a TV series starring James Garner. 'The Saint' and 'The Persuaders' made him a television super-star and becoming the second James Bond sealed his future. Roger has had four wives – since 2002, he's been married to 'Kiki' Tholstrup. He had three children with his third wife, the Italian actress, Luisa Mattioli.

Interrupted Melody (1955)
Diane (1956)
The Miracle (1959)
The Man Who
Haunted Himself (1970)
Live and Let Die (1973)
The Man With the
Golden Gun (1974)
Shout at the Devil (1976)
The Spy Who Loved Me (1977)
The Wild Geese (1978)
North Sea Hijack (1979)
Moonraker (1979)
The Sea Wolves (1980)
For Your Eyes Only (1981)
Octopussy (1983)
A View to Kill (1995)

Terry **Moore**
5ft 2in

(HELEN LUELLA KOFORD)

Born: **January 7, 1929**
Glendale, California, USA

Terry was raised in a strict Mormon family but during the Great Depression, her poor parents had no objections when she started bringing in extra cash as a child model. When she was eleven she made her first film appearance – a bit part in *Maryland.* While she was still at school, there were several uncredited movie roles and her name was changed from Judy Ford, to Helen Koford, to Jan Ford – which she used when appearing in the popular radio show, 'Smiths of Hollywood'. She settled on Terry Moore when she starred in her first grown-up movie, *The Return of October.* Terry became a star when she played opposite a gorilla, in *Mighty Joe Young* and she was nominated for a Best Supporting Actress Oscar, for *Come Back Little Sheba.* The 1950s were good for her career – with hit films such as *Man on a Tightrope, King of the Khyber Rifles, Daddy Long Legs, Bernadine,* and *Peyton Place* – keeping her face in the movie magazines. After that, she kept her looks and was photographed nude for 'Playboy' at the age of fifty-five. She claimed that one of her six husbands was Howard Hughes, but three of them – including LA Rams halfback, Glenn Davis, were around during that same period. Could that have been bigamy? The last one, Jerry Rivers, died in 2001. Terry didn't marry again, and after a five-year retirement, she has gone back to acting in movies.

Son of Lassie (1945) **The Return of October** (1948) **Mighty Joe Young** (1949) **The Great Rupert** (1950)
Gambling House (1951)
The Barefoot Mailman (1951)
Come Back, Little Sheba (1952)
Man on a Tightrope (1953)
Beneath the 12-Mile Reef (1953)
King of the Khyber Rifles (1953)
Portrait of Alison (1955)
Daddy Long Legs (1955)
Shack Out on 101 (1955)
Bernadine (1957) **Peyton Place** (1957)
Second Chances (1998)
The Still Life (2007)

Agnes **Moorehead**
5ft 6in

(AGNES ROBERTSON MOOREHEAD)

Born: **December 6, 1900**
Clinton, Massachusetts, USA
Died: **April 30, 1974**

Of exclusively British descent, Agnes was the daughter of a Presbyterian minister and his wife. When she was three, Agnes gave her first public performance - reciting "The Lord's Prayer" in her father's church. After the family moved to St. Louis, she began to show a keen interest in acting – encouraged every step of the way by her mother. Agnes graduated from Central High School in 1918, and at Muskingum College, Ohio, she was active on stage. While earning a Master's Degree in English at the University of Wisconsin, she taught school. In 1929, she graduated from the American Academy of Dramatic Arts. It proved hard to get work until 1937, when she joined the Mercury Theater, appearing in Orson Welles' 'The War of the Worlds' radio play. In 1941, she made her movie debut, in *Citizen Kane.* She was nominated four times for Best Supporting Actress Oscars - for *The Magnificent Ambersons, Mrs. Parkington, Johnny Belinda* and *Hush...Hush, Sweet Charlotte.* Agnes married two actors – Robert Gist, and Jack Lee, with whom she adopted a son. In the 1960s she became more popular than ever – as Endora, in the television series, 'Bewitched'. She died of cancer at her home in Rochester, Minnesota.

Citizen Kane (1941)
The Magnificent Ambersons (1942)
Mrs. Parkington (1944)
Johnny Belinda (1948)
Caged (1950)
Showboat (1951)
Magnificent Obsession (1954)
All That Heaven Allows (1955)
The Revolt of
Mamie Stover (1956)
The True Story of
Jesse James (1957)
Raintree County (1957)
Pollyanna (1960)
Jessica (1962)
How the West Was Won (1962)
Hush...Hush,
Sweet Charlotte (1964)

Nonna **Mordyukova**
5ft 4in

(NOYABRINA VIKTOROVNA)

Born: **November 25, 1925**
Konstantinovskaya, Ukraine
Died: **July 6, 2008**

Nonna was the daughter of Viktor Mordyukov and Petrovna Mordyukova. She was one of a large family raised in a Cossack village – where her mother worked as chairwoman of a collective farm. When she was twenty, and having survived the Nazi occupation, Nonna felt a strong desire to become an actress and began studying at the Soviet State Institute of Cinema, under Boris Bibikov and Olga Ryzhova. In 1948, Nonna made her film debut, in *The Young Guard.* It also featured Vyacheslav Tikhonov, who would become her husband later that year. In 1950, she joined the Theater School of Film Acting in Moscow and by the end of the decade she had become a star of the Soviet Cinema, with a choice of the best roles available. Nonna had huge success in top movies such as *Balzaminov's Marriage, The Komissar,* and *Russian Field.* The playwright, Viktor Merezhko, expanded her range with *Tyrasina,* and after her appearance in *Rodnya,* Nonna gained an international audience. In 1999, she refused to play any more old women, so she retired to write her memoirs. She died in Moscow, nine years later, of lung disease and heart failure.

Other People's Relatives (1955)
Ekaterina Voronina (1957)
A Home for Tanya (1959)
A Simple Story (1960)
The Chairman (1964)
Balzaminov's Marriage (1965)
War and Peace (1967)
The Komissar (1967)
Little Crane (1968)
The Diamond Arm (1968)
Burn, Burn, My Star (1969)
Russian Field (1971)
They Fought for the
Motherland (1975) **Tyrasina** (1978)
Rodnya (1981)
Incognito from St. Petersburg (1981)
A Railway Station for Two (1982)
Luna Park (1992)
Mama (1999)

Kenneth More
5ft 10in
(KENNETH GILBERT MORE)

Born: **September 20, 1914**
Gerrards Cross, Buckinghamshire, England
Died: **July 12, 1982**

Kenneth was educated at Worthing, in Sussex, and on the island of Jersey, where his father was manager of the Jersey Eastern Railways. Upon leaving school, Kenneth became apprenticed to an engineering firm in Shrewsbury. He didn't like it, so he set sail for Canada. They didn't like Ken, so they deported him. Back in England, he decided to give show business a try. He worked backstage at the Windmill Theater in London, where he began appearing in sketches. After two years, he started his stage career with repertory companies in Wolverhampton and Newcastle – touring in a play called "To Have and to Hold". In 1935, he had the first of three pre-war film bit parts, in *Look Up and Laugh*. In 1940, he married Beryl Johnstone. He served in the Royal Navy before going back to the stage in 1946 when he also had his first featured film role, in *School for Secrets*, as well as his first divorce. Ken became a star in 1953, following his role in the hit film *Genevieve*. He was excellent in films such as *Reach for the Sky*, in which he portrayed the legless fighter pilot, Douglas Bader, and in *A Night to Remember* – an early version of *Titanic*. He continued until 1980, when he made his final appearance – in a TV version of a 'A Tale of Two Cities'. The onset of Parkinson's disease forced his retirement and he died two years later at his home in London.

Scott of the Antarctic (1948)
The Clouded Yellow (1951)
Genevieve (1953)
Doctor in the House (1954)
The Deep Blue Sea (1955)
Reach for the Sky (1956)
The Admirable Crichton (1957)
The Sheriff of Fractured Jaw (1958)
A Night to Remember (1958)
North West Frontier (1959)
The 39 Steps (1959)
Sink the Bismark! (1960)
The Greengage Summer (1961)
Battle of Britain (1969)

Jeanne Moreau
5ft 3in
(JEANNE MOREAU)

Born: **January 23, 1928**
Paris, France

Jeanne's father, Anatole, was a restaurateur. Her mother, Katherine, was an English girl who danced at the Folies Bergere. After leaving school, Jeanne studied acting at the Paris Conservatoire with Denis d'Ines. From the age of twenty, she had four years of important experience with La Comedie Française, before joining the Theatre National Populaire and having her first major stage success, in "L'Heure Eblouissante". In 1949, she married the actor, Jean-Louis Richard. That same year, she made her film debut, in *Dernier amour*. More movie roles came quickly, and her first starring role, in *La Reine Margot*, is superior to the version made forty years later. *Les Amants, Jules et Jim* and *Diary of a Chambermaid* established Jeanne as an international star. Her contributions to the French Cinema are priceless – with the directors, Louis Malle and François Truffaut owing her as huge a debt as she owes them. In 2009, this remarkable actress is still making movies.

La Reine Margot (1954)
The Wages of Sin (1956)
Ascenseur pour l'échafaud (1958)
Les Amants (1958)
Les Liaisons dangereuses (1959)
Moderato cantabile (1960)
La Notte (1961) Jules et Jim (1962)
Eva (1962) The Trial (1962)
La Baie des anges (1963)
The Victors (1963)
Diary of a Chambermaid (1964)
The Train (1964)
Mata-Hari (1964) Viva Maria! (1965)
Mademoiselle (1966)
The Immortal Story (1968)
Monte Walsh (1970)
Les Valseuses (1974)
Monsieur Klein (1976)
The Last Tycoon (1976)
Querelle (1982) La Truite (1982)
Anna Karazamoff (1991)
A Foreign Field (1993)
Cet amour-là (2001)
Désengagement (2007)
Plus tard (2008)

Rita Moreno
5ft 2½in
(ROSITA DOLORES ALVERIO)

Born: **December 11, 1931**
Humacao, Puerto Rico

In 1937, Rita went to live in New York City with her mother. When she was five years old, she actually danced at a night club in Greenwich Village! While still at school, she began her professional career as a freelancer – dubbing Spanish-language versions of American films. She was only thirteen when she made her Broadway debut, in "Skydrift", which starred the young Eli Wallach. In 1950, as Rosita Moreno, she made her film debut, in *So Young So Bad,* which was filmed in New York City. An MGM contract followed and supporting roles in Mario Lanza's *The Toast of New Orleans* and the landmark musical, *Singin' in the Rain,* gave the young actress good cause for optimism. Unfortunately she suffered from being regarded as the Hispanic stereotype, which severely limited her range of opportunities. It did work in her favor on one occasion, when she was cast as the Puerto Rican girl, Anita, in *West Side Story* which won her a Best Supporting Actress Oscar. During the 1970s, she won a Grammy for "The Electric Company" – a soundtrack album from the TV show. She has also won a Tony and two Emmys. Since 1965, Rita has been married to a cardiologist, Lenny Gordon. They have a daughter, Fernanda, who designs jewelry. During 2007, Rita appeared on television in 'Ugly Betty' and in the role of Amalia, in the series, 'Cane'.

The Toast of New Orleans (1950)
Singin' in the Rain (1952)
Jivaro (1954)
The Yellow Tomahawk (1954)
Garden of Evil (1954)
Untamed (1955)
The King and I (1956)
West Side Story (1961)
Summer and Smoke (1961)
Popi (1969) Marlowe (1969)
Carnal Knowledge (1971)
The Ritz (1976)
The Boss' Son (1978)
The Four Seasons (1981)
Blue Moon (2000) Piñero (2001)

Dennis Morgan
6ft 2in
(EARL STANLEY MORNER)

Born: **December 20, 1908**
Prentice, Wisconsin, USA
Died: **September 7, 1994**

The son of a Wisconsin lumberman, Dennis was blessed with a very positive personality. He was a star performer in plays at Carroll College, which he left at the height of the Depression. Dennis appeared with local stock companies – performing everything from Steinbeck to Shakespeare. He broadened his scope even further and trained his voice by working as a radio announcer. Dennis' singing wasn't bad – he was a welcome addition to several traveling operetta productions. He married his sweetheart, Lillian Vedder, in 1933 - a marriage made in heaven! With a new baby, they headed for Hollywood. In 1935, he was signed by MGM – and made his film debut – as Stanley Morner – in *I Conquer the Sea!* Dennis got mainly bit parts, and changing his name to Richard Stanley didn't improve matters. In 1939, his move to Warner Brothers, starring in *Waterfront,* and finally becoming Dennis Morgan, did. He then became best friends with Jack Carson, who co-starred with him several times during his 1940s heydays - one of their best being *Two Guys from Milwaukee.* Dennis retired in 1980 after appearing in an episode of 'The Love Boat'. He was terrifically successful as a businessman in later life. When Dennis passed away, of natural causes, in Fresno, California, he and his wife, Lillian had been married for sixty-one years.

Three Cheers for the Irish (1940)
Kitty Foyle (1940) Bad Men of
Missouri (1941) Captains of the
Clouds (1942) In This Our Life (1942)
The Hard Way (1943)
Thank Your Lucky Stars (1943)
Shine on Harvest Moon (1944)
The Very Thought of You (1944)
God Is My Co-pilot (1945)
Christmas in Connecticut (1945)
Two Guys from Milwaukee (1946)
Pretty Baby (1946)
My Wild Irish Rose (1947)
Perfect Strangers (1950)
This Woman Is Dangerous (1952)

Frank Morgan
5ft 10in
(FRANCIS PHILIP WUPPERMANN)

Born: **June 1, 1890**
New York City, New York, USA
Died: **September 18, 1949**

Frank was the youngest of eleven children born to wealthy parents, who were the distributors of Angostura Bitters. He was a boy soprano at school. He later attended Cornell University, prior to following his brother Ralph, into show business. Frank began his career on the Broadway stage. In 1914, Frank married Alma Muller, who would be his wife for thirty-five years. Frank used the name Wupperman, for his film debut, in the 1916 silent drama, *The Suspect,* based on a play. Stage actors like him were in demand at film studios. It suited Frank, who got on with his stage career and had also appeared in twenty movies, before he made his first talkie in 1930, a comedy short, called *Belle of the Night.* He was even more prolific during the next decade, and was Best Actor Oscar-nominated for *The Affairs of Cellini.* He was nominated for a Best Supporting Actor Oscar, for his role as 'The Pirate', in *Tortilla Flat.* His most memorable role was as the title character of the classic fantasy, *The Wizard of Oz.* Frank died of a heart attack in Beverly Hills, after finishing work on his final film, *Key to the City.*

Hallelujah I'm a Bum (1933)
Bombshell (1933)
The Affairs of Cellini (1934)
The Good Fairy (1935)
Naughty Marietta (1935)
The Great Ziegfeld (1936) Dimples (1936)
Paradise for Three (1938)
The Crowd Roars (1938)
The Wizard of Oz (1939)
The Shop Around the Corner (1940)
The Mortal Storm (1940)
Boom Town (1940)
The Vanishing Virginian (1942)
Tortilla Flat (1942)
The Human Comedy (1943)
A Stranger in Town (1943)
The White Cliffs of Dover (1944)
Casanova Brown (1944)
The Three Musketeers (1948)
The Stratton Story (1949)
Key to the City (1950)

Harry Morgan
5ft 4in
(HARRY BRATSBURG)

Born: **April 10, 1915**
Detroit, Michigan, USA

The son of Norwegian immigrants, Harry graduated from Muskegon High School before studying Law at the University of Chicago. The Great Depression forced him to withdraw because of lack of funds, and while he was working as a salesman, he got roles in amateur stage productions. Harry set his sights on an acting career. Early on, he joined the Group Theater, in New York. It had been set up to teach the methods of Russian-born actor/director Constantin Stanislavski. Harry was taught an early version of "Method Acting". His first professional role was in 1937, when he co-starred with Frances Farmer, in "At Mrs. Beam's". In 1940, he married Eileen Detchon, with whom he had four children. Using the name Henry Morgan, he made his film debut, in 1942, in *To the Shores of Tripoli.* Henry would remain a supporting actor in several movies and on television – including 'December Bride', 'Dragnet', and 'M*A*S*H' – for which he won an Emmy, in 1980. In 1986, after the death of Eileen, he married Barbara Bushman – the granddaughter of Francis X. Bushman, a major star of the silent screen.

Crash Dive (1943)
The Ox-Bow Incident (1943)
Wing and a Prayer (1944)
A Bell for Adano (1945)
State Fair (1945)
Dragonwyck (1946)
All My Sons (1948)
The Big Clock (1948)
Moonrise(1948)
Yellow Sky (1948)
Down to the Sea in Ships (1949)
Red Light (1949)
High Noon (1952)
The Glenn Miller Story (1953)
The Teahouse of the
August Moon (1956)
Inherit the Wind (1960)
Support Your Local Sheriff! (1969)
Support Your Local
Gunfighter (1971)
The Shootist (1976)
Dragnet (1987)

Michèle **Morgan**
5ft 6in
(SIMONE RENÉE ROUSSEL)

Born: **February 29, 1920**
Neuilly-sur-Seine, France

Born in a "Leap Year", Michèle's early life was spent in Dieppe. She left home when she was fifteen – preferring to live with her grandmother in Neuilly – who was more sympathetic to her dream of becoming a film star. She went to Paris, where she studied acting with René Simon and began getting extra work – starting with *Une fille à papa,* in 1935. A fellow student, a niece of Jean Gabin's, got her a small role in *Le Mioche,* in 1936. A year later, she co-starred with Raimu, in Marc Allégret's *Gribouille,* under her new name, Michèle Morgan. She was a big success in French films, and was in the classic *Le Quai des Brumes,* directed by Marcel Carné. In 1942, she married the American actor, William Marshall, and broadened her appeal – starring in the Sinatra vehicle, *Higher and Higher,* and with Bogart, in *Passage to Marseille.* Michèle returned to France following the war – to star in *La Symphonie pastorale,* which won her the Best Actress Award, at Cannes. Following her divorce from Marshall, she starred with Henri Vidal in *Fabiola,* and they married in 1950. After his death she married a third actor, Gérard Oury – who died in 2006. Michèle published her autobiography, "Avec ces yeux-là" ("With Those Eyes") in 1977. Around that time, she marketed her own range of ties, known as "Cravates Michèle Morgan". She spends much of her leisure time nowadays painting and writing poems.

Gribouille (1937)
Le Quai des brumes (1938)
L'Entraîneuse (1940)
Les Musiciens du ciel (1940)
Remorques (1941)
Passage to Marseille (1944)
La Symphonie pastorale (1946)
The Chase (1946)
The Fallen Idol (1948) Fabiola (1949)
The Seven Deadly Sins (1952)
The Moment of Truth (1952)
Les Grandes Manoeuvres (1955)
Fortunat (1960) Benjamin (1968)
Cat and Mouse (1975)

Cathy **Moriarty**
5ft 9in
(CATHY MORIARTY)

Born: **November 29, 1960**
The Bronx, New York City, New York, USA

Her parents John and Catherine Moriarty, were both Irish Catholic immigrants. Cathy grew up in Westchester, where she graduated from high school at sixteen to pursue an acting career. She appeared in plays at local dinner theaters and her big step to stardom certainly began early enough. She was seventeen when she successfully auditioned for the role of Vicki La Motta, following a screen test for Martin Scorsese, and made her film debut – opposite Robert De Niro, in *Raging Bull,* for which she was nominated for a Best Supporting Actress Oscar. It was always going to be a hard one to follow, but her next film got negative reviews, and even worse was a serious automobile accident in 1981 – resulting in major back surgery and her absence from the screen for six years. In 1989, she made her television debut, in an episode of the CBS series, 'Wiseguy'. After that her roles were often supporting ones, but she revealed a talent as a comedienne, in *Soapdish.* In 1999, Cathy married Joseph Gentile, with whom she has three children including twins. Since she gave birth to their third child, in 2001 – a daughter, Annabella, Cathy has done very little in the way of acting, apart from appearing in one 2005 episode of the TV series, 'Law & Order: Special Victims Unit'. She and Joe own the "Mulberry Street Pizzeria" restaurant, in Los Angeles – specializing in New York style pizzas.

Raging Bull (1980)
White of the Eye (1987)
Kindergarten Cop (1990)
Soapdish (1991)
The Mambo Kings (1992)
Forget Paris (1995)
Casper (1995)
A Brother's Kiss (1997)
Dream with the Fishes (1997)
Cop Land (1997)
Digging to China (1998)
Crazy in Alabama (1999)
But I'm a Cheerleader (1999)
New Waterford Girl (1999)
Analyze That (2002)

Robert **Morley**
6ft 0½in
(ROBERT ADOLPH WILTON MORLEY)

Born: **May 26, 1908**
Semley, Wiltshire, England
Died: **June 3, 1992**

From a well-to-do military family, Robert was educated at Wellington College – which he did not enjoy, and at schools in France, Germany, and Italy. Robert was ear-marked for a diplomatic career, but his love for the theater led to him studying acting at RADA. He made his stage debut in 1929, at the Strand Theater in London in a production of "Treasure Island" and following a string of well-received West End performances, made his Broadway debut, in 1938, in the title role of "Oscar Wilde". His portly figure and double-chinned face were then transferred to the screen for his first film role – as Louis XVI, in *Marie Antoinette.* – for which Robert was nominated for a Best Supporting Actor Oscar. He was first choice when anyone needed to cast a pompous ass or a member of the aristocracy. In 1942, he married Joan Buckmaster. Their three children including the well-known film critic, Sheridan Morley. One of his best roles was as the Reverend Samuel Sayer, in *The African Queen.* Robert made his last film, *Istanbul,* in 1989. It was a poor finale. He died of a stroke at his home in Wargrave.

Marie Antoinette (1938)
Major Barbara (1941)
The Foreman Went to France (1942)
The Young Mr. Pitt (1942)
The Ghosts of Berkeley Square (1947)
The African Queen (1951)
Outcast of the Islands (1952)
The Story of Gilbert and Sullivan (1953)
Beat the Devil (1953)
Beau Brummell (1954)
Law and Disorder (1958)
Libel (1959)
The Battle of the Sexes (1959)
Oscar Wilde (1960)
The Boys (1962)
Topkapi (1964) Cromwell (1970)
Who Is Killing the
Great Chefs of Europe? (1978)
The Great Muppet Caper (1981)
High Road to China (1983)
Little Dorrit (1988)

Temuera **Morrison**
5ft 7in
(TEMUERA JACK NICOLAS DAVID MORRISON)

Born: **December 26, 1960**
Rotorua, North Island, New Zealand

Temuera's parents are Maoris, descended from the Ngati Whakaue tribe. He was one of eight children. Temuera's father, Laurie Morrison, was a musician related to the famous New Zealand entertainer, Sir Howard Morrison. His mother's name is Hana. When he was ten, Temuera toured internationally with "Ngati Rangiwewehi" a performance group led by his sister Taini. He started acting in amateur productions at the age of twelve and made his first screen appearance, in *Rangi's Catch*. After junior school, Temuera was educated at Wesley College, in Auckland. In the mid-1980s he began to get regular work in local film and TV productions, starting with the low-budget *Other Halves*. He was first taken seriously as an actor when he played a young cop in *Mauri* and received good notices when he co-starred with Rena Owen in *Once Were Warriors,* which won several awards around the world. He established himself in the Australian film industry before making his American debut in in 1996, in a weak action/sci-fi film called *Barb Wire*. But Temuera had his feet firmly planted in Hollywood and after good New Zealand movies, *Broken English* and *What Becomes of the Broken Hearted?* he was in *Star Wars* territory. He divides his time between New Zealand, Australia and the USA. He was recently in the NZ-made TV series, 'Shortland Street'.

Mauri (1988)
The Grasscutter (1990)
Once Were Warriors (1994)
Whipping Boy (1996)
Broken English (1996)
Six Days Seven Nights (1998)
What Becomes of the
Broken Hearted? (1999)
Crooked Earth (2001)
Star Wars Episode II:
Attack of the Clones (2002)
The Beautiful Country (2004)
Blueberry (2004)
Star Wars Episode III:
Revenge of the Sith (2005)
River Queen (2005)

Vic **Morrow**
5ft 9in
(VICTOR MORROW)

Born: **February 14, 1929**
The Bronx, New York City, New York, USA
Died: **July 23, 1982**

Vic's parents were Jewish, from Russian backgrounds. His father was an electrical engineer. Vic quit high school when he was seventeen to enlist in the US Navy. He was able to take advantage of the G.I. Bill to study Law at Florida Southern College. Through participating in school plays he decided that acting was the life for him, so he switched to drama studies. He went to New York, where he joined the Actors Workshop. Shortly after he graduated, he got a part in a summer stock production of "A Streetcar Named Desire". Vic's movie debut, in *Blackboard Jungle,* was memorable for two reasons – its sound-track introduced "Rock around the Clock" to the world's teenagers and his perform-ance as the tough, Artie West, was one of the best things in it. In 1957, he married the actress Barbara Turner and the couple had two daughters – one of whom is Jennifer Jason Leigh. Vic was invariably type cast in mean character roles, but he proved on several occasions that he could play a man with a heart, and got good notices for his work in the comedy, *The Bad News Bears*. In 1976, the failure of his second marriage and the death of his mother hit him hard and he turned to drink. Vic kept working in B-movies and made-for-TV films. He was killed in a freak helicopter accident at Indian Dunes, California, while filming a scene for what might have been his 'comeback' movie, *Twilight Zone: The Movie.*

Blackboard Jungle (1955)
Tribute to a Bad Man (1956)
Men in War (1957)
Hell's Five Hours (1958)
King Creole (1958)
God's Little Acre (1958)
Cimarron (1960)
Portrait of a Mobster (1961)
Posse from Hell (1961)
Dirty Mary Crazy Larry (1974)
The Bad News Bears (1976)
Treasure of Matecumbe (1976)
Twilight Zone: The Movie (1983)

Viggo **Mortensen**
5ft 11in
(VIGGO PETER MORTENSEN JR.)

Born: **October 20, 1958**
Manhattan, New York City, New York, USA

He was the eldest son of a Danish farmer, Viggo Peter Mortensen, and his American wife, Grace. After Viggo was born, the family moved to South America, where his father managed ranches in Argentina and Venezuela. At seven years of age, young Viggo was sent to a boarding school in Argentina. His parents divorced when he was eleven and he and his two brothers went with their mother back to New York. Viggo graduated from Watertown High School, in 1976, and after that attended St. Lawrence University. In 1980, in search of his roots, he went to Denmark, where he worked in a variety of jobs and began writing poetry. He fell in love with a girl and followed her back to New York, where the relationship died. He started taking acting classes and in 1985, made his film debut with a small role in *Witness*. He married his co-star, Ezxene Cervenka, after they acted together in *Salvation*. The marriage lasted ten years. It was Viggo's son, Henry, who persuaded him to accept a role in *The Lord of the Rings*, when he was doubtful about it. He did, and became a star. Viggo was nominated for a Best Actor Oscar for *Eastern Promises*. His new movie, *The Road,* is eagerly awaited by his many fans all over the world.

The Reflecting Skin (1990)
The Indian Runner (1991)
Carlito's Way (1993)
Crimson Tide (1995)
The Prophecy (1995)
Albino Alligator (1996)
G.I. Jane (1997)
A Perfect Murder (1998)
A Walk on the Moon (1999)
28 Days (2000)
The Fellowship of the Ring (2001)
The Two Towers (2002)
Return of the King (2003)
Hidalgo (2004)
A History of Violence (2005)
Alatriste (2006)
Eastern Promises (2007)
Appaloosa (2008)
Good (2008)

Emily **Mortimer**

5ft 8in

(EMILY MORTIMER)

Born: **December 1, 1971**
London, England

Emily is the eldest daughter of the late Sir John Mortimer QC and his wife, Penelope. In addition to his legal reputation, Sir John was famous as a dramatist – for "Rumpole of the Bailey" and many others. Emily was educated at St. Paul's Girls' School – where she eagerly participated in most of the student stage presentations. After that, she read Russian at Lincoln College, Oxford. At University, Emily performed in a number of plays. She also refined her acting technique with a spell at Moscow Arts Theater School. She was seen at Oxford by a producer, who cast her in a 1995 television adaptation of 'The Glass Virgin', by Catherine Cookson. Emily wrote a column for the Daily Telegraph, but in 1996, she began her career in earnest when making her movie debut, in *The Ghost and the Darkness,* which starred Val Kilmer. Within four years, she had established herself as an actress with potential. Emily won an Independent Spirit and a COFCA Best Supporting Actress Award, for *Lovely & Amazing* and she was a believable 'Lady Diana' on TV. In her first vintage year – 2003, she didn't appear in a single failure. It was a good year on the romantic front too - she got married to actor Alessandro Nivola – with whom she had appeared in *Love's Labour's Lost.* They have a son named Sam.

The Ghost and the Darkness (1996)
The Saint (1997) Elizabeth (1998)
Notting Hill (1999)
Love's Labour's Lost (2000)
The Kid (2000)
Lovely & Amazing (2001)
The 51st State (2001)
A Foreign Affair (2003)
Nobody Needs to Know (2003)
The Sleeping Dictionary (2003)
Bright Young Things (2003)
Young Adam (2003)
Dear Frankie (2004)
Match Point (2005)
Chaos Theory (2007)
Lars and the Real Girl (2007)
Transsiberian (2008) Red Belt (2008)
City Island (2009)

Armin **Mueller-Stahl**

6ft

(ARMIN MUELLER-STAHL)

Born: **December 17, 1930**
Tilsit, East Prussia, Germany

The third of five children born to a bank employee, Armin studied violin at the Berlin Conservatory and qualified as a music teacher. When he first decided to become an actor, he was turned down by the drama school on the grounds that he lacked talent! He didn't give up easily and in 1952, while still working as a concert violinist, he was accepted. Armin began a long association on stage with the Volksbühne in Berlin, in 1954. He made his film debut two years later, in *Heimliche Ehen,* but it was 1960 before he had his next movie role in the superb East German production, *Five Cartridges.* In 1973, Armin married Gabriele Scholz, with whom he had a son they named Christian. He was voted his country's favorite actor five years running, but was black-listed in 1976 when he got involved in politics. He was later allowed to emigrate to West Germany with his family, in 1981, and he immediately fitted in, playing the male lead in Fassbinder's *Lola.* In 1989, *Music Box* brought him international fame. He was nominated for a Best Supporting Actor Oscar for *Shine,* and has continued to shine in the twelve years since then. In 2006, he was a jury member at the Berlin International Film Festival.

Lola (1981)
A Love in Germany (1983)
Bitter Ernte (1985)
Music Box (1989)
Night on Earth (1991)
Kafka (1991) Utz (1992)
The House of the Spirits (1993)
The Last Good Time (1994)
Shine (1996)
The Game (1997)
The Commissioner (1998)
The X Files (1998)
The Thirteenth Floor (1999)
Jacob the Liar (1999)
Local Color (2006)
Eastern Promises (2007)
Leningrad (2007)
Buddenbrooks (2008)
The International (2009)

Dermot **Mulroney**

5ft 9½in

(DERMOT MULRONEY)

Born: **October 31, 1963**
Alexandria, Virginia, USA

Dermot's father, Michael, was a lawyer. His mother, Ellen, had been a keen amateur actress. Both parents were of Irish ancestry. Dermot grew up with three brothers and a sister. He had a good ear and was a very gifted young musician at Maury Elementary School – playing cello in the City Youth Orchestra. Dermot also acted in children's community productions, but it was in "Are Teachers Human", at George Washington Middle School, in which he made his stage debut. After graduating from T.C. Williams High School in 1981, he attended the School of Speech, at Northwestern University, from where he graduated in 1985. The following year, Dermot made his TV debut in 'Sin of Innocence'. He made his movie debut, in Blake Edwards' *Sunset,* the same year as he appeared in *Young Guns.* He married actress Catherine Keener, in 1990. Seventeen years later, they divorced. Dermot's first starring role, in *Where the Day Takes You,* won him a Golden Space Needle Award at the Seattle International Film Festival. Since then, Dermot has enjoyed sixteen years of success.

Young Guns (1988)
Longtime Companion (1990)
Where the Day Takes You (1992)
Samantha (1992)
Point of No Return (1993)
The Thing Called Love (1993)
There Goes My Baby (1994)
Living in Oblivion (1995)
Copycat (1995)
Bastard Out of Carolina (1996)
Box of Moon Light (1996)
My Best Friend's Wedding (1997)
Where the Money Is (2000)
The Safety of Objects (2001)
About Schmidt (2002)
Undertow (2004)
Must Love Dogs (2005)
The Family Stone (2005)
Griffin & Phoenix (2006)
Zodiac (2007) Gracie (2007)
Georgia Rule (2007) Jolene (2008)
Flash of Genius (2008)

Paul **Muni**
5ft 10in
(MESHILEM MEIER WEISENFREUND)

Born: **September 22, 1895**
Lemberg, Austro-Hungary
Died: **August 25, 1967**

Paul was the son of Phillip and Salli Weisenfreund. He spent his first seven years in a province of what is now the Ukraine. His parents, who were both actors in the Yiddish theater, took their young family to the United States in 1902. He was known as Moony Weisenfreund when he began his own acting career in New York, at the age of twelve. He was a cousin of Edward G. Robinson, who would offer serious competition when they appeared on stage, and later, in films. In 1921, he met and married Bella Finkel, who would be with him until he died. Paul didn't make it to Broadway until he was twenty-nine – playing an elderly Jew, in "We Americans". It was the first time he acted in English, and from then on, he made up for lost time. He was Oscar nominated for his first film, *The Valiant,* and after another spell on Broadway, returned to the screen in the powerful *Scarface.* Paul won a Best Actor Oscar for *The Story of Louis Pasteur,* and had a few vintage years. His other Oscar nominations were for *I Am a Fugitive from a Chain Gang, Black Fury, The Life of Emile Zola* and *The Last Angry Man* – which was to be his final film. Paul's failing eyesight and poor health forced him to retire in 1962, after he had finished work on an episode of 'Saints and Sinners' for television. He died of heart disease, in Montecito, California.

The Valiant (1929) Scarface (1932)
I Am a Fugitive from
a Chain Gang (1932)
The World Changes (1933)
Bordertown (1935)
Black Fury (1935)
Dr. Socrates (1935)
The Story of Louis Pasteur (1935)
The Good Earth (1937) The Life of
Emil Zola (1937) Juarez (1939)
Commandos Strike at Dawn (1942)
A Song to Remember (1945)
Counter-Attack (1945)
Angel on My Shoulder (1946)
The Last Angry Man (1959)

Audie **Murphy**
5ft 5in
(AUDIE LEON MURPHY)

Born: **June 20, 1924**
Kingston, Texas, USA
Died: **May 28, 1971**

From a family of poor Texas sharecroppers, Audie went to school until the eighth grade in Celeste, Texas. He was the sixth of twelve children – only nine of whom survived. From such humble beginnings Audie would grow up to be as famous as the President of the United States. When his father deserted the family, Audie went cotton picking to support them. In 1942, he joined the United States Army. He took part in the liberation of Sicily, and saw action at Salerno and in France – receiving a host of medals, including two Silver Stars and a Medal of Honor. He suffered from "battle fatigue" and was one of the first servicemen to draw attention to PTSD. In July 1945, Audie was on the cover of "Life" and was urged by James Cagney to go to Hollywood. Roles didn't come, and Audie was disillusioned and broke. In 1948, he made his film debut in *Texas, Brooklyn and Heaven,* but it was the smallest of bit parts. A brief marriage to actress Wanda Hendrix, raised his profile and pushed him to a featured role in *Bad Boy,* in 1949. Westerns made him a star name, which enabled him to persuade his studio to let him play himself, in *To Hell and Back* – the film version of his autobiography. He had a few years at the top, when he mostly played cowboys. Audie died when his private plane crashed in thick fog near Roanoke, Virginia. He was survived by his second wife, Pamela Archer, and their two sons.

Kansas City Raiders (1950)
The Red Badge of Courage (1951)
Column South (1953) Destry (1954)
To Hell and Back (1955)
Walk the Proud Land (1956)
Night Passage (1957)
The Quiet American (1958)
Ride a Crooked Trail (1958)
No Name on the Bullet (1959)
The Unforgiven (1960)
Posse from Hell (1961)
Bullet for a Badman (1964)
A Time for Dying (1969)

Eddie **Murphy**
5ft 9¹⁄₂in
(EDWARD REGAN MURPHY)

Born: **April 3, 1961**
Brooklyn, New York City, New York, USA

His dad, Charles Edward Murphy, who worked as a transit police officer, left the family when Ed was three. In 1969, he died of stab wounds. Ed and his brother Charlie were raised, along with a step-brother, by their mother Lilian and her new husband, Vernon Lynch. A natural-born comedian, Ed was a clever kid and a good athlete when he was a student at Roosevelt High School, in New York. After that he formed a comedy duo with Mitchell Kyser, and perfected the act at youth clubs and local bars. Before starting a full-time career, he attended Nassau Community College, on Long Island. His first solo break was at "The Comic Strip" in Manhattan. Ed then moved to the West Coast, where he did stand-up comedy at the "Bay Area Comedy Club" – and had a reputation for his off-color jokes about gays and AIDS. He featured on 'Saturday Night Live' and in 1983, was in the concert film, *Delirious.* He won a Grammy for his comedy album, "Eddie Murphy". Ed made a stunning film debut, in *48 Hrs,* but although he got close on a couple of occasions, he was not able to sustain the quality of his first two movies. Even so he won a couple of awards and a first Oscar nomination (as Best Supporting Actor) for *Dreamgirls.* He had five children with his ex-wife Nicole Mitchell.

48 Hrs. (1982)
Trading Places (1983)
Beverly Hills Cop (1984)
The Golden Child (1986)
Beverly Hills Cop II (1987)
Coming to America (1988)
Harlem Nights (1989)
Boomerang (1992)
The Distinguished
Gentleman (1992)
The Nutty Professor (1996)
Doctor Dolittle (1998)
Bowfinger (1999)
Showtime (2002)
I Spy (2002)
Daddy Day Care (2003)
Dreamgirls (2006)

George **Murphy**
5ft 11in
(GEORGE LLOYD MURPHY)

Born: **July 4, 1902**
New Haven, Connecticut, USA
Died: **May 3, 1992**

Born on the perfect day for a young American, George was the son of Irish Catholics and was raised accordingly. His father was a track and field coach, but George's first inclination was not sporting – he attempted to join the United States Navy when he was fifteen. He was under age and returned home and graduated from the Peddie Institute, in Hightstown, New Jersey. He attended Yale University for a while, but quit to start his career as a dancer in a night club. In 1926, George married Juliette Henkel and partnered her – with her stage name, Julie Johnson, in a dance act which saw its way to Broadway the following year. They started a family, and in 1935, a year after George's movie debut, in *Kid Millions,* she decided to retire and raise their two children. He was given a contract by Columbia, and over the next dozen or so years, co-starred with Jean Arthur, Eleanor Powell, Shirley Temple, Judy Garland and even John Barrymore. President of the Screen Actors Guild from 1944-1946, he was awarded a special Oscar in 1950. From 1965, he served six years as Senator of California. During that term, he developed throat cancer and had his larynx removed. He died of leukemia in Palm Beach, Florida. George was survived by his second wife, Betty.

Kid Millions (1934)
The Public Menace (1935)
Broadway Melody of 1938 (1937)
You're a Sweetheart (1937)
Little Miss Broadway (1938)
Letter of Introduction (1938)
Hold That Co-ed (1938)
Broadway Melody of
1940 (1940)
Little Nelly Kelly (1940)
Tom Dick and Harry (1941)
Ringside Maisie (1941)
For Me and My Gal (1942)
Bataan (1943)
Step Lively (1944) Big City (1948)
Border Incident (1949)
Battleground (1949)

Bill **Murray**
6ft 1in
(WILLIAM JAMES MURRAY)

Born: **September 21, 1950**
Wilmette, Illinois, USA

Bill was the son of an Irish American Catholic couple who were quite poor. Along with eight sisters and brothers, Bill earned pocket money and school fees by caddying at the local golf course. He was educated at Loyola Academy, a Jesuit preparatory school, in Wilmette. It was there that he first started developing an interest in acting. He then attended Regis College in Denver to study pre-med, only to be forced to withdraw in his sophomore year following his arrest at O'Hare Airport for possession of Marijuana . At around that time he was lead singer in a rock band, "The Dutch Masters". Bill had his first break at Second City Chicago. In 1975, an Off-Broadway version of "The National Lampoon Show" earned him a TV job with 'Saturday Night Live'. In 1979, after a few TV outings, he made his film debut in *Meatballs.* Bill married Mickey Kelley that same year and they had two children. He has since had four more with second wife, Jennifer. After he was nominated for a Best Actor Oscar, for *Lost in Translation,* there has been a run of good entertaining movies under Bill's name.

Caddyshack (1980)
Stripes (1981) Tootsie (1982)
Ghostbusters (1984)
Little Shop of Horrors (1986)
Ghostbusters II (1989)
Quick Change (1990)
What About Bob? (1991)
Groundhog Day (1993)
Ed Wood (1994)
Kingpin (1996)
The Man Who Knew
Too Little (1997)
Wild Things (1998)
Rushmore (1998)
Cradle Will Rock (1999)
The Royal Tenenbaums (2001)
Lost in Translation (2003)
Coffee and Cigarettes (2003)
Broken Flowers (2005)
The Darjeeling Limited (2007)
Get Smart (2008)
City of Ember (2008)

Don **Murray**
6ft 2in
(DONALD PATRICK MURRAY)

Born: **July 31, 1929**
Hollywood, California, USA

Don's father, Dennis Murray, was a dance director, but no relation to Arthur. His mother, Ethel, was a former Ziegfeld Girl. Don was only a few months old when the family moved to New York. Because of his dad's profession, he lived and went to school in Ohio and Texas before graduating from East Rockaway High School, in New York. He then attended the city's American Academy of Dramatic Arts, before summer stock and eventually made his Broadway debut, in 1948, in "The Insect Comedy". His reputation was secured following his sterling work in "Rose Tattoo" and some television dramas including episodes of 'Kraft Theater' and 'The Philco Hour'. In 1955, he was a hit in "The Skin of Our Teeth", on Broadway, and Hollywood beckoned. Don made his film debut, in *Bus Stop,* opposite Marilyn Monroe. Apart from being nominated for a Best Supporting Actor Oscar, he also met his first wife, Hope Lange, on the set. Don had ten years as a star before doing more television, taking supporting roles in films, and also having a new career as a director – he worked on his third film, *Elvis Is Alive,* in 2001. Don is the father of the actor Christopher Murray.

Bus Stop (1956)
The Bachelor Party (1957)
A Hatful of Rain (1957)
From Hell to Texas (1958)
Shake Hands with the Devil (1959)
These Thousand Hills (1959)
One Foot in Hell (1960)
Hoodlum Priest (1961)
Advise & Consent (1962)
Escape from East Berlin (1962)
One Man's Way (1964)
Baby the Rain Must Fall (1965)
Sweet Love, Bitter (1967)
Happy Birthday, Wanda June (1971)
Justin Morgan Had a Horse (1972)
Conquest of the Planet of
the Apes (1972)
Peggy Sue Got Married (1986)
Made in Heaven (1987)
Elvis Is Alive (2001)

Ornella **Muti**
5ft 6¼in
(FRANCESCA ROMANA RIVELLI)

Born: **March 9, 1955**
Rome, Italy

Ornella's father was from Naples and her mother was Estonian. The combination produced two beautiful daughters – the first, Claudia, who was born in 1951, and Francesca, who would become Ornella Muti. After she left school, Ornella became a teenage fashion model. Living in the city which is the home of the Italian movie industry's Cinecittà Studio, soon got her noticed by talent scouts. In 1970, as a fifteen-year-old, she made her film debut, in *The Most Beautiful Wife.* Ornella then played sexy young things in a series of movies and in 1974, she was the sexy young thing who falls for a man thirty years older than her, in *Romanzo popolare.* By the late 1970s she was a star - appearing as Princess Aura, in the action/fantasy, *Flash Gordon.* She didn't do anything else on the international scene until co-starring with Jeremy Irons, in *Swann in Love.* It is always nice to see Ornella in English language movies, and every few years she makes one. In 1994, she was voted "The Most Beautiful Woman in the World" by the readers of "Class" magazine. Twice married – she's had three children – two with Franco Faccinetti. Her first daughter, the actress/model, Naike Rivelli, made Ornella a glamorous grandmother in 1996.

La Moglie più bella (1970)
Romanzo popolare (1974)
Nest of Vipers (1977)
The Twisted Detective (1977)
Primo amore (1978)
Life is Beautiful (1979)
Flash Gordon (1980)
The Girl from Trieste (1982)
Swann in Love (1984)
Me and My Sister (1987)
Mi fai un favore (1996)
Pour rire! (1996)
Tomorrow (2001) **Cavale** (2002)
Après la vie (2002)
Un couple épatant (2002)
**The Heart Is Deceitful Above
All Things** (2002)
Friday or Another Day (2005)
L'Inchiesta (2006)

Mike **Myers**
5ft 8in
(MICHAEL MYERS)

Born: **May 25, 1963**
Scarborough, Ontario, Canada

Mike's parents both hailed from Liverpool, in England. His father worked in Canada as an encyclopedia salesman. After he appeared in a television commercial when he was nine, Mike set his sights on a show business career. He graduated from Stephen Leacock Collegiate and joined the Second City Canadian Touring Company. In 1984, Mike moved back to England, where he was one of the founders of the London Comedy Store. In 1986, he starred in the children's TV program, 'Wide Awake Club'. He returned to Canada, where in Toronto, he was one of the cast in the Second City's stage show. From 1989, Mike was a regular member of the cast of NBC's 'Saturday Night Live'. From one of the show's sketches – 'Wayne's World', he and Dana Carvey developed a full length film which became his big screen debut and was popular enough to warrant a sequel. In 1997, he introduced *Austin Powers* to movie audiences with equal success. He credits his nephew, Jeff, as being 'ideas man' for the characters. As a welcome break from his filming, Mike is a member of the band, "Ming Tea". His musical skills and physical resemblance will come in useful when he portrays "The Who" drummer, Keith Moon in an upcoming biopic. He recently got a divorce from his wife, Robin Ruzan. He's also had a long period of poorly received movies. His new creation, *The Love Guru,* has stirred up a lot of controversy and offends many people. It looks unlikely to provide the hit Mike so desperately needs.

Wayne's World (1992)
**So I Married an
Axe Murderer** (1993)
Wayne's World 2 (1993)
**Austin Powers: International
Man of Mystery** (1997)
54 (1998)
**Austin Powers: The Spy
Who Shagged Me** (1999)
Mystery, Alaska (1999)
**Austin Powers in
Goldmember** (2002)

N

Anne **Nagel**
5ft 4in
(ANNE DOLAN)

Born: **September 29, 1915**
Boston, Massachusetts, USA
Died: **July 6, 1966**

The daughter of devout Catholic parents, Anne was sent to a school with the express purpose of preparing her for the Sisterhood. She was extremely unhappy there from the start, and in defiance of her parents wishes, left in her teens. Anne worked as a photographer's model before joining a local Boston theater company. Ironically, her parents split up and her mother remarried a small-time director who starred her in several Technicolor experimental shorts, produced by Tiffany Studios. Anne made her feature length debut in the 1932 film, *Hypnotized,* and had ten bit part appearances before she landed a contract at Warner Brothers. A small role in *China Clipper* introduced her to Ross Alexander, who was recovering from the recent loss of his first wife – who'd committed suicide. A short time after marrying him, Anne discovered the probable reason why – he was a closet homosexual. In 1937, their brief marriage was over when he ended his own life by shooting himself. It affected Anne deeply and she began to drink. Her best films (even though the roles were small) were *Black Friday,* with Lugosi and Karloff, and the W.C.Fields vehicle, *Never Give a Sucker an Even Break* – as "Madame Gorgeous" – which she was. By the late 1940s, Anne was mainly employed as a supporting player in B-movies and Poverty Row productions. She was last seen on screen in 1957, in an episode of the TV show, 'Circus Boy'. She retired and ended her days virtually penniless. Anne died in Hollywood, of liver cancer.

The Footloose Heiress (1937)
Escape by Night (1937)
The Adventurous Blonde (1937)
Under the Big Top (1938) **Black
Friday** (1940) **Argentine Nights** (1940)
The Invisible Woman (1940)
Man Made Monster (1940)
Sealed Lips (1941) **Never Give a
Sucker an Even Break** (1941)
An Innocent Affair (1948)

J. Carrol **Naish**
5ft 9½in
(JOSEPH PATRICK CARROL NAISH)

Born: **January 21, 1896**
New York City, New York, USA
Died: **January 24, 1973**

His parents were comfortably off Irish immigrants. Joe was educated as a Catholic, at St. Cecilia's Academy in New York City. He left when he was sixteen to join the Merchant Navy – travelling all around the world before, in the early 1920s, starting his career in vaudeville. He then went to Paris, where as an able linguist, he performed in French with the popular dancer, Gaby Deslys. In 1926, Joe made his stage debut in a touring company production of "The Shanghai Gesture" and became a respected name in the theater. Joe's wide knowledge of languages wasn't much help during the cinema's silent era, but he did make his screen debut in 1926, in *What Price Glory.* He was brought to Hollywood from New York by Fox, and in the early 1930s he was established as a supporting actor who could do any kind of accent. Joe married in 1929 – he and his wife Gladys had a daughter. Apart from his roles in hit movies such as *The Lives of a Bengal Lancer* and *Captain Blood,* Joe was twice nominated for Oscars – for *A Medal for Benny* and *Sahara.* He died of emphysema in La Jolla, California.

The Hatchet Man (1932)
Upperworld (1934)
The Lives of a Bengal Lancer (1935)
Black Fury (1935)
Front Page Woman (1935)
Captain Blood (1935)
Anthony Adverse (1936)
**The Charge of the Light
Brigade** (1936) **We Who Are
About to Die** (1937)
Beau Geste (1939)
Down Argentine Way (1940)
Blood and Sand (1941)
Sahara (1943)
A Medal for Benny (1945)
The Southerner (1945)
Humoresque (1946)
The Fugitive (1947)
Annie Get Your Gun (1950)
Rio Grande (1950)

Dame Anna **Neagle**
5ft 5in
(FLORENCE MARJORIE ROBERTSON)

Born: **October 20, 1904**
Forest Gate, Essex, England
Died: **June 3, 1986**

Anna was the daughter of a merchant navy man, Herbert Robertson, and his wife, the former Florence Neagle. She grew up in a modest English family home until she was eleven. She raised her sights considerably after being bright enough to attend St. Albans High School. She started out as a teacher of gymnastics and dancing – she was once a finalist in the World Ballroom Dancing Championships. After working as a dancer, from 1917 onwards, in 1926, she made her featured stage debut, in "Charlot's Revue". She then appeared in London's West End, with Jack Buchanan, in "Stand Up and Sing" at the Hippodrome, and in New York, in several C.B. Cochran productions. Four years later, after a couple of uncredited bit parts, she made her film debut, in *Should a Doctor Tell?* Anna met producer/director Herbert Wilcox, in 1931, and he became her Svengali, then in 1943, her husband. His guidance was the reason for her incredible reign as the "Queen of British Cinema" for ten years – and she starred in three Hollywood musicals. By the mid-1950s, she was considered a 'square', and she completed thirty years in films, in 1959, with the aptly-titled, *The Lady Is a Square.* She returned to the stage and continued to work after Herbert's death in 1977 – making her final appearance, in 'Tales of the Unexpected', on television, in 1983. Anna died of complications from Parkinson's disease at her home in West Byfleet, Surrey.

Bitter Sweet (1933)
Nell Gwyn (1934)
Victoria the Great (1937)
Sixty Glorious Years (1938)
Nurse Edith Cavell (1939)
Irene (1940) **They Flew alone** (1942)
Forever and a Day (1943)
I Live in Grosvenor Square (1945)
The Courtneys of Curzon Street (1947)
Spring in Park Lane (1948)
Odette (1950)
The Lady with the Lamp (1951)

Patricia **Neal**
5ft 8in
(PATSY LOUISE NEAL)

Born: January 20, 1926
Packard, Kentucky, USA

Patricia's family moved soon after she was born, and she was raised throughout her childhood, in Knoxville, Tennessee. When she was eleven, she showed enough interest in drama for her parents to send her to acting school. After graduating from Northwestern University, where her classmates included Charlton Heston and Cloris Leachman, she went to New York. Patricia appeared in summer stock productions and worked as a doctor's assistant, a model, and as a jewellery store clerk before becoming an understudy in the Broadway production of "The Voice of the Turtle". In 1946, she made her first Broadway appearance, in "Another Part of the Forest" – for which she won a Tony Award as Best Actress. In 1949, she made her film debut in a Ronald Reagan comedy, *John loves Mary*. Her next film, Ayn Rand's *The Fountainhead,* was to prove dramatic in more ways than one. A passionate affair with her married co-star Gary Cooper, resulted in her pregnancy, and an abortion. In 1953, she married the author, Roald Dahl, with whom she had five children. He stuck with her when she fought her way back from a debilitating stroke, but they were divorced in 1983. Patricia won a Best Actress Oscar for *Hud* and was nominated for *The Subject Was Roses*. She has a featured role in *Flying By* – due for release during 2009.

The Fountainhead (1949)
The Hasty Heart (1949)
The Breaking Point (1950)
Three Secrets (1950)
The Day the Earth
Stood Still (1951)
Diplomatic Courier (1952)
A Face in the Crowd (1957)
Breakfast at Tiffany's (1961)
Hud (1963)
In Harm's Way (1965)
The Subject Was Roses (1968)
The Night Digger (1971)
Baxter! (1973)
The Passage (1979)
Cookie's Fortune (1999)

Liam **Neeson**
6ft 4in
(WILLIAM JOHN NEESON)

Born: June 7, 1952
Ballymena, County Antrim, Northern Ireland

Liam's father, worked as a school caretaker and his mother was a cook. There was little to suggest Liam's future celebrity. He grew up with his three sisters. Liam's first venture into the spotlight was when he attended boxing lessons. When he was eleven, he began acting in school plays, but some five years later, he was the Heavyweight Youth Champion of Northern Ireland. He worked as a fork-lift operator for Guinness and spent two years at a teachers training college in Newcastle, in England. In 1970, he had his first screen role in the BBC series, 'Play for Today'. Back in Ballymena, he got three roles for a religious film company then returned to England, where his career began in the successful movie, *Excalibur*. Liam was nominated for a Best Actor Oscar, in the blockbuster, *Schindler's List*. A year after that, Liam married Natasha Richardson – who was his co-star when he made his debut on Broadway, in "Anna Christie". Liam and their two sons were devastated when Natasha died in March, 2009, following a fall during a skiing session.

Excalibur (1981) Krull (1983)
The Bounty (1984)
The Mission (1986)
Lamb (1986) Suspect (1987)
The Dead Pool (1988)
The Good Mother (1988)
Dark Man (1990)
Under Suspicion (1991)
Husbands and Wives (1992)
Ethan Frome (1993)
Schindler's List (1993)
Nell (1994) Rob Roy (1995)
Before and After (1996)
Michael Collins (1996)
Les Misérables (1998)
K-19: The Widowmaker (2002)
Gangs of New York (2002)
Love Actually (2003) Kinsey (2004)
Kingdom of Heaven (2005)
Batman Begins (2005)
Seraphim Falls (2006)
Taken (2008)
Five Minutes of Heaven (2009)

Sam **Neill**
6ft
(NIGEL JOHN DERMOT NEILL)

Born: September 14, 1947
Omagh, County Tyrone, Northern Ireland

Sam's New Zealand-born father, Dermot Neill, was stationed in Northern Ireland with the Irish Guards. His mother, Priscilla, was English. When Sam was seven, they returned to New Zealand, to run their liquor business. Sam was educated at Christ's College, a boarding school in Christchurch and went on to read English Literature at the University of Canterbury and earn a Bachelor of Arts, from Victoria University in Wellington. He got a job with the New Zealand Film Unit as a director and actor – making his film debut in 1977, in *Sleeping Dogs*. It was the Australian classic, *My Brilliant Career,* that first made Sam famous. He began to make movies all over the world and was even on the short list to take over the James Bond role from Roger Moore. It was perhaps just as well that he wasn't selected – the quality of his films since then have been generally of a far higher level, with his work in *The Piano,* being outstanding. In 1983, Sam had a son with New Zealand actress, Lisa Harrow, but he didn't marry her. Five years later, on the set of *A Cry in the Dark*, in Australia, Sam met the girl who was to become his wife in 1989 – the Japanese make-up artist, Noriko Watanabe. The couple have a daughter named Elena.

My Brilliant career (1979)
Possession (1981)
Enigma (1983)
Plenty (1985)
A Cry in the Dark (1988)
Dead Calm (1989)
The Hunt for Red October (1990)
Death in Brunswick (1991)
The Piano (1993)
Jurassic Park (1993)
Country Life (1994)
In the Mouth of Madness (1995)
Children of the Revolution (1996)
The Horse Whisperer (1998)
The Dish (2000)
The Zookeeper (2001)
Yes (2004) Little Fish (2005)
Angel (2007)
Dean Spanley (2008) Skin (2008)

Kate **Nelligan**
5ft 4in
(PATRICIA COLLEEN NELLIGAN)

Born: **March 16, 1950**
London, Ontario, Canada

Kate's father, Patrick Nelligan, worked as a maintenance man at a recreational park and ice rink. Her mother, Josephine, was a schoolteacher, who later suffered from serious psychological problems. Kate, who was one of six children, was educated at the local South Secondary School, where she acted in "Hamlet". She then studied at the University of Toronto, but didn't graduate – choosing instead to go to England, where she attended the Central School of Speech and Drama in London. In 1972, Kate made her professional stage debut at Bristol's Little Theater, in "Barefoot in the Park". She made her film debut, in *The Romantic Englishwoman,* and built up an impressive portfolio of stage work in England. In 1978 she was nominated for an Olivier Award for Best Actress, in "Plenty", at London's National Theater and appeared in a BBC Shakespeare series. In 1983, she went to live in New York – and was nominated for four Best Actress Tonys between 1983 and 1989 – which was the year she married Robert Reale, with whom she had a son. Kate was nominated for a Best Supporting Actress Oscar, for *Prince of Tides.* She went on to play the role of Olive Worthington, in the outstanding film, *The Cider House Rules.* Although she has been seen on TV on a fairly regular basis, the past ten years has yielded little in the way of good movies.

The Romantic Englishwoman (1975)
Dracula (1979)
Mr. Patman (1980)
Eye of the Needle (1981)
Without a Trace (1983)
Eleni (1985) White Room (1990)
Frankie and Johnny (1991)
The Prince of Tides (1991)
Fatal Instinct (1993) Wolf (1994)
Margaret's Museum (1995)
How to Make an
American Quilt (1995)
Up Close & Personal (1996)
U.S. Marshalls (1998)
The Cider House Rules (1999)
Premonition (2007)

Craig T. **Nelson**
6ft 3¹/₂in
(CRAIG THEODORE NELSON)

Born: **April 4, 1944**
Spokane, Washington, USA

Craig's father was a professional drummer who at one time played in the band which accompanied Bing Crosby – when he was starting his career in Spokane. It didn't rub off on his son, Craig, who wasn't musical. He attended the University of Arizona before considering the unlikely profession of a hydroplane racer. His dad argued against it, so Craig began his working life as a comedy writer and performer. To begin with, he appeared on the radio and later as a stand-up comic in nightclubs in the Los Angeles area. In the mid-1970s, Craig decided that he was struggling with his career and disenchanted, he took his wife, Robin, and their three children to rural California. He worked as a janitor, carpenter and lumberjack. By the time he returned to L.A. his marriage was over. He produced a documentary series and successfully auditioned for his film debut in the Al Pacino movie, *...And Justice for All.* Since 1987, Craig has been married to actress, Doria Cook – a good luck charm judging by his career since then. In 1992, he won an Emmy after three years of an eight year stint in the long-running TV series, 'Coach'. Apart from films such as *The Devil's Advocate* and *Blades of Glory,* Craig has been seen more recently in quality TV productions like 'The District', but his new movie, a comedy titled *The Proposal,* could be a good one.

...And Justice for All (1979)
Where the Buffalo Roam (1980)
Stir Crazy (1980)
Poltergeist (1982)
Man, Woman and Child (1983)
The Osterman Weekend (1983)
All the Right Moves (1983)
Silkwood (1983)
The Killing Fields (1984)
Turner & Hooch (1989)
Ghosts of Mississippi (1996)
I'm Not Rappaport (1996)
The Devil's Advocate (1997)
All Over Again (2001)
The Family Stone (2005)
Blades of Glory (2007)

Judd **Nelson**
5ft 10in
(JUDD ASHER NELSON)

Born: **November 28, 1959**
Portland, Maine, USA

Judd's father, Leonard Nelson, was an attorney who became the first Jewish president of the Portland Symphony Orchestra. Prior to her marriage to Leonard, Judd's mother, Merle, had been a member of the Maine State Legislature. In addition to their son, the couple had two daughters, Eve and Julie. Judd received his education at St. Paul's School in Concord, New Hampshire, and later at Haverford College in Pennsylvania, where he majored in Philosophy. He went to live in Manhattan, and pursued an acting career. To help achieve this, he studied with Stella Adler, in New York. He served his apprenticeship in the tough arena of summer stock before he felt ready to face the challenge of Hollywood. After becoming a member of the "Brat Pack", Judd made his film debut, in 1984, in a high school comedy, *Making the Grade.* He did make the grade, especially in the golden year of 1985, when he was in three successful films – the best of which was the John Hughes drama, *The Breakfast Club.* In subsequent years, he hasn't always been so lucky, but overall, the critics have usually liked him. In 1988, Judd was nominated for a Golden Globe Award as Best Actor, in the TV Mini-Series, 'Billionaire Boys Club'. His movie career has slowed down somewhat after 2001, but he has no less than nine movies due for release during 2009. Although he was once engaged to the actress, Shannen Doherty, Judd has never married.

Fandango (1985)
The Breakfast Club (1985)
St. Elmo's Fire (1985)
From the Hip (1987)
Relentless (1989)
Primary Motive (1992)
Airheads (1994)
Light It Up (1999)
Endsville (2000)
Jay and Silent Bob
Strike Back (2001)
Netherbeast
Incorporated (2007)

Gene **Nelson**

6ft

(LEANDER EUGENE BERG)

Born: March 24, 1920
Seattle, Washington, USA
Died: September 16, 1996

Gene was thirteen when he saw Fred Astaire and Ginger Rogers, in the movie, *Flying Down to Rio*. It convinced him that he too would be a dancer when he grew up. He took dancing classes when he was at high school, but after graduating, it was as a skater that he was first employed. Gene joined the 'Sonja Henie Ice Show' in Los Angeles, in 1938, and toured with it until 1941. Through Sonja, he was given a bit part in her 1939 movie, *Everything Happens at Night*. Still using his original name, Gene Berg, he served in the United States Army during World War II. In 1943, he was one of the male dancers in the film *This Is the Army*. When peace was restored, Gene used the G.I. Bill facility to take acting lessons. Following a couple of seasons in repertory productions, he made his Broadway debut (as Gene Nelson) in 1948, in the musical revue "Lend an Ear". He and his two co-stars Carol Channing and Bob Scheerer, won the Theater World Award. The first half of the next decade was his golden period. By 1960, he had turned to directing – both on television, and with movies like Elvis' *Kissin' Cousins* and *Harum Scarum,* and a Hank Williams biopic, *Your Cheatin' Heart*. The last movie he directed was *The Cool Ones,* in 1967. After that, most of his work was on TV. His final appearance as an actor, was in a 1987 episode of 'Murder She Wrote'. Gene was married three times. He died of cancer, in Los Angeles.

The Daughter of Rosie O'Grady (1950)
Tea for Two (1950)
The West Point Story (1950)
Lullaby of Broadway (1951)
Painting the Clouds with
Sunshine (1951)
She's Working Her Way
Through College (1952)
Three Sailors and a Girl (1953)
Crime Wave (1954)
So This Is Paris (1955)
Oklahoma (1955)
Thunder Island (1963)

Franco **Nero**

5ft 11in

(FRANCESCO SPARANERO)

Born: November 23, 1941
San Prospero, Parma, Italy

Franco was brought up in a family where the father-figure was a police sergeant. While Franco attended Milan University, he earned extra money by posing for the Italian photo-novels. Through that exposure, he was given his screen debut, in 1964, with a small role in *La Celestina*. That, and some of his early movies, were dire. An appearance in the successful spaghetti western, *Django,* made him a star in Italy, and brought him his first opportunity to appear in an English language film, *Camelot*. The film's female star, Vanessa Redgrave, became his long time partner, and they had a son, Carlo. Throughout the 1970s, Franco was a very busy man – with a starring role for Luis Buñel, in *Tristana* – starting the decade on the right note. His English language films didn't work out so well and they were few and far between. His appearance in *Die Hard 2,* was a rare treat for his fans, but most of Franco's recent roles have been supporting ones in poor films. A notable exception, is the international historical drama, *Bathory,* in which he has a good role – portraying Hungarian King Mathias. He finally married Vanessa in 2007.

Django (1966)
Third Eye (1966)
Massacre Time (1966)
Camelot (1967)
Il Giorno della civetta (1968)
Revenge of a Gunfighter (1968)
Fifth Day of Peace (1969)
Tristana (1970)
The Virgin and the Gypsy (1970)
Companeros (1970)
La Vacanza (1971)
The Assassination of
Matteotti (1973)
Mussolini: Ultimo atto (1974)
Keoma (1976)
Scandal (1976) Querelle (1982)
The Falcon (1983)
10 Days That Shook
the World (1983)
Die Hard 2 (1990)
Bathory (2008)

James **Nesbitt**

5ft 11½in

(JAMES NESBITT)

Born: January 15, 1965
Coleraine, Northern Ireland

The son of a schoolmaster, Jimmy had three older sisters. He was raised in Lisnamurrican, near Ballymena, and was educated at the local primary school where his father was teaching. In 1976, the family moved home and he attended the Coleraine Academical Institution. While he was there, one of his teachers encouraged him to look for acting opportunities at the Riverside Theater. He was thirteen when he made his stage debut, as the 'Artful Dodger' in the musical "Oliver!" Although he enjoyed it, as well as other theatrical outings, Jimmy didn't consider any other future than teaching. Almost by default, he got his equity card at seventeen, when he stepped in for an injured actor. His dad then suggested that he move to London where he enrolled at the Central School of Speech and Drama. He went on a world tour, in "Hamlet", where he met his wife, Sonia Forbes-Adam, who was understudying Ophelia. They married in 1993 and have two daughters – Peggy and Mary. He got good notices for his work in *Hear My Song,* which was filmed in County Clare, but was so pleased with his effort, he sat back, and it took him months to get motivated again. When he did, there were several career highlights including *Go Now, Welcome to Sarajevo, Waking Ned,* and *Bloody Sunday,* as well as some excellent television work recently, in 'Jeckyll', 'Murphy's Law', 'The Passion' and 'Midnight Man'.

Hear My Song (1991)
Go Now (1995)
Jude (1996)
Welcome to Sarajevo (1997)
This Is the Sea (1997)
Resurrection Man (1998)
Waking Ned (1998)
Women Talking Dirty (1999)
Wild About Harry (2000)
Lucky Break (2001)
Bloody Sunday (2002)
Millions (2004)
Match Point (2005)
Five Minutes of Heaven (2009)

Anthony **Newley**
5ft 11in
(GEORGE ANTHONY NEWLEY)

Born: **September 24, 1931**
Hackney, London, England
Died: **April 14, 1999**

Tony was the illegitimate son of George Kirby and his girlfriend, Grace Newley. He didn't stick around. As a single mother, Grace endured several tough years. Then, around the time World War II started, she became "respectable" by marrying a man called Ronald Gardner, who helped her raise her son. Tony wasn't much of a scholar, but he showed a natural talent for mimicry and a great passion for popular music. The London Blitz resulted in him being evacuated to the countryside. When he returned home, he left school at the then minimum age of fourteen and took a job as an office boy. In 1946, he was shown a newspaper advertisement asking for boy actors. Tony attended an audition and was accepted at the Italia Conti Stage School. In 1947, he made his film debut, in the title role of the children's serial, *Dusty Bates*. He had a featured role in *Vice Versa* – directed by Peter Ustinov, but it was his role as the 'Artful Dodger' in David Lean's masterly, *Oliver Twist*, which launched his movie career. Tony had two miserable years doing National Service in the army. After that, he was mainly in supporting roles. Fame came his way through his song-writing talent – most notably with his two British number ones – "Why" and "Do You Mind" and the Grammy Award-winning song, "What Kind of Fool Am I?" He also wrote the musical, "Stop the World – I Want to Get Off". Tony's three wives included Joan Collins. When Tony died of renal cancer, he was living with the designer, Gina Fratini.

Oliver Twist (1948)
Vote for Huggett (1949)
A Boy, a Girl and a Bike (1949)
The Cockleshell Heroes (1955)
The Blue Peter (1955)
X: The Unknown (1956)
Fire Down Below (1957)
How to Murder a
Rich Uncle (1957)
Idle on Parade (1959)
Doctor Doolittle (1967)

Nanette **Newman**
5ft 5in
(NANETTE NEWMAN)

Born: **May 29, 1934**
Northampton, Northants, England

Nanette's father worked in cabaret and he encouraged his daughter to follow in his footsteps. After her primary education, she was sent down to London where she attended the renowned Italia Conti Academy Stage School, and then the Royal Academy of Dramatic Art. In 1953, just before starting at RADA, she made her film debut, in *Personal Affair*. In 1955, Nanette became the second wife of the actor/director, Bryan Forbes, with Roger Moore officiating as their best man. They had two daughters and are still together more than fifty years later. Nanette has appeared in several of the films Bryan directed, most notably, *Seance on a Wet Afternoon, The Whisperers* and *The Stepford Wives*. She has kept working on television, and was a regular on the BBC panel game 'What's My Line'. She even became a familiar face in a series of British commercials for 'Fairy Liquid'. Her best film role was as the wheelchair-bound girl Jill Matthews, in *The Raging Moon* (also directed by her husband) for which she was nominated for a Best Actress BAFTA Award. Nanette is the author of over thirty children's books and six cookery books – one of them, "The Summer Cookbook" was voted 'Cookery Book of the Year'. In 2006, Nanette's voice was heard in an Italian-made animated short, entitled *Cosa raccomanda lei?*

Personal Affair (1953)
The League of Gentlemen (1960)
Faces in the Dark (1960)
House of Mystery (1961)
The Rebel (1961)
The Wrong Arm of
the Law (1963)
Seance on a
wet Afternoon (1964)
The Wrong Box (1966)
The Whisperers (1967)
Oh! What a Lovely War (1969)
The Raging Moon (1971)
The Stepford Wives (1975)
The Mystery of
Edwin Drood (1993)

Paul **Newman**
5ft 9½in
(PAUL LEONARD NEWMAN)

Born: **January 26, 1925**
Shaker Heights, Ohio, USA
Died: **September 26, 2008**

Paul's father, who ran a sporting goods store, was of German-Jewish ancestry. His mother began life as a Catholic, but converted to Christian Science when Paul was five. He showed a keen early interest in acting. At seven, he made his stage debut, as the court jester, in his school's production of "Robin Hood". He graduated from Cleveland Heights High School and attended Ohio University. At the tail-end of World War II, Paul served in the U.S. Navy. After the war, he studied acting at Yale University, before moving to New York City, where he was given his "method" training by Lee Strasberg. Paul made his debut on Broadway in the original production of "Picnic". In 1954, he made his film debut, in the mediocre, *Silver Chalice*. After that he had many quality roles. His ten Oscar nominations – starting with *Cat on a Hot Tin Roof* and ending with *Road to Perdition,* yielded one win – for *The Color of Money*. He has six children from two marriages. The second one, to Joanne Woodward, lasted more than fifty years. Paul finally retired in 2006. He died at his home near Westport, Connecticut, after a battle with cancer.

Somebody Up There Likes Me (1956)
Cat on a Hot Tin Roof (1958)
The Left Handed Gun (1958)
The Long Hot Summer (1958)
The Hustler (1961)
Sweet Bird of Youth (1962)
Hud (1963) The Prize (1963)
The Moving Target (1966)
Cool Hand Luke (1967)
Butch Cassidy and the
Sundance Kid (1969)
The Life and Times of Judge
Roy Bean (1972) The Sting (1973)
The Towering Inferno (1974)
Absence of Malice (1981)
Fort Apache, the Bronx (1981)
The Verdict (1982) The Color of
Money (1986) The Hudsucker
Proxy (1994) Twilight (1998)
Road to Perdition (2002)

Robert Newton
6ft
(ROBERT NEWTON)

Born: **June 1, 1905**
Shaftesbury, Dorset, England
Died: **March 25, 1956**

Robert's father, Algernon Newton, was a highly respected landscape painter and a member of the Royal Academy in London. His mother added a talent for writing to his pedigree. He was educated in Lamorna, in Cornwall, and then Newbury Grammar School, which he left at fifteen. Robert's first job was as assistant stage manager at Birmingham Repertory Company. In 1920 he was given his stage debut, in "Captain Brassbound's Conversation", by George Bernard Shaw. For three years he received training in every aspect of theatrical management and stage craft. He toured South Africa and on his return, made his West End debut in a revue called "London Life". By the end of the decade, he was appearing in Noël Coward's popular plays. Robert married Peta Walton, with whom he had a daughter. His film debut was a small role in *Reunion,* in 1932, and when he saw the close-up, he knew that he would be a success on the screen. He had a fine speaking voice and could imitate just about any accent. He was especially good in *Odd Man Out, Oliver Twist,* and *Waterfront,* but his liking for booze began to hamper his career. His final movie appearance was a cameo, in *Around the World in Eighty Days,* a few months before he died of a heart attack and alcohol related causes, in Beverly Hills. He was married four times.

Gaslight (1940)
Hatter's Castle (1941)
Major Barbara (1941)
Henry V (1944)
This Happy Breed (1944)
Odd Man Out (1947)
Oliver Twist (1948)
Waterfront (1950)
Treasure Island (1950)
Tom Brown's Schooldays (1951)
Les Misérables (1952)
The Desert Rats (1953)
The High and the Mighty (1954)
The Beachcomber (1954) Around the
World in Eighty Days (1956)

Thandie Newton
5ft 2in
(THANDIWE NEWTON)

Born: **November 6, 1972**
London, England

She is the daughter of Nick Newton, an English laboratory technician, and his wife, Nyasha, a health care worker from the Zimbabwean tribe, Shona. Thandie lived with them in Zambia until political unrest forced them to move to Penzance, Cornwall, in the southwest of England. When she was eleven she enrolled at the Art Educational School in London, where she learned modern dance. A future in that became impossible when she injured her back. She then attempted to break into the American market, but her English accent proved a disadvantage. She went home to study at Downing College, Cambridge University, and got her degree in Anthropology. In 1991, she traveled to New South Wales, in Australia, to make her film debut, in *Flirting* – which also featured an unknown actress called Nicole Kidman. She then appeared in a TV film, 'Pirate Prince' before a return to movies in the London-set *The Young Americans.* Her career moved rapidly after 1994 when she was able to add the star-studded *Interview with the Vampire,* to her list of credits. In 1998, she married English writer/director, Ol Parker. They have a daughter named Ripley. Thandie won a Supporting Actress BAFTA for *Crash.* She has brightened several films since then – *The Pursuit of Happyness,* and *Run Fat Boy, Run,* being the pick – along with her portrayal of Condoleezza Rice, in *W.*

Flirting (1991)
The Young Americans (1993)
Interview with the Vampire (1994)
Jefferson in Paris (1995)
The Journey of August King (1995)
The Leading Man (1996)
Gridlock'd (1997)
Besieged (1998)
Mission Impossible (2000)
Shade (2003)
Crash (2004)
The Pursuit of Happyness (2006)
Run Fat Boy, Run (2007)
RocknRolla (2008)
W. (2008)

Jack Nicholson
5ft 9¾in
(JOHN JOSEPH NICHOLSON)

Born: **April 22, 1937**
Neptune, New Jersey, USA

Jack never found out who his father was. His mother was a showgirl, June Nilson, whose real name, Nicholson, was given to Jack. She then handed him over to her parents, who raised him as as a Catholic. He was educated at Manasquan High School where he was voted "class clown" in 1954. When he first went to Hollywood, he applied at Hanna-Barbera animation studios, who offered him a job as a junior artist. He turned it down to pursue a career as an actor/writer/producer. Roger Corman gave Jack his film debut in 1958, in his crime thriller, *The Cry Baby Killer.* Over the next ten years, only two or three of his films were okay, and none of them made his name. That all changed with *Easy Rider,* for which he was nominated for a Best Supporting Actor Oscar. The floodgates opened and he was nominated for eleven more Academy Awards. He won Best Actor Oscars for One Flew Over the *Cuckoo's Nest* and *As Good as It Gets* and won a Best Supporting Actor Oscar, for *Terms of Endearment.* He has had a wealth of good roles. Married once, to the actress Sandra Knight, with whom he had a daughter, he has had a lot of girlfriends and has fathered four other children.

Easy Rider (1969)
Five Easy Pieces (1970)
Carnal Knowledge (1971)
The King of Marvin Gardens (1972)
Chinatown (1974) One Flew
Over the Cuckoo's Nest (1976)
The Missouri Breaks (1976)
The Shining (1980)
Terms of Endearment (1983)
Prizzi's Honor (1985) Ironweed (1987)
A Few Good Men (1992)
Hoffa (1992) Wolf (1994)
The Crossing Guard (1995)
Mars Attacks! (1996)
As Good as It Gets (1997)
The Pledge (2001)
About Schmidt (2002)
Something's Gotta Give (2003)
The Departed (2006)
The Bucket List (2007)

Connie **Nielsen**
5ft 10in
(CONNIE INGE-LISA NIELSEN)

Born: July 3, 1965
Elling, Frederikshavn, Denmark

Connie was raised in Copenhagen, where her father was a bus driver. Her mother, who worked as an insurance clerk, had once longed to be an actress, and she encouraged her daughter to make it her career. They formed a duo and worked together on the Copenhagen variety circuit. When she reached eighteen, Connie headed for Paris, where she did modeling and also perfected her French. In 1984, she made her film debut, in a French Jerry Lewis movie, called *Par où T'es Rentré? On T'a Pas Vu Sortir*. After that, she went to a drama school in Rome and in 1988, she made her TV debut in the mini-series, 'Colletti Bianchi'. She attended classes in Milan with teacher Lydia Styx, from Il Piccolo Teatro di Milano, and was in an Italian film titled *Vacanze di Natale '91*. That same year, her son, Sebastian, was born. After some years in Italy, Connie moved to the U.S.A. in 1996. She is fluent in six languages, which gives her plenty of options and she has appeared in French, Italian and Danish productions. Her first American movie was *The Devil's Advocate* – with Al Pacino and Keanu Reeves. Her big international break came as Lucilla, in the award-winning *Gladiator*. In 2007, Connie and the rock band "Metallica" drummer – fellow Dane, Lars Ulrich, had a son they named Bryce.

The Devil's Advocate (1997)
Permanent Midnight (1998)
Rushmore (1998)
Soldier (1998)
Mission to Mars (2000)
Gladiator (2000)
One Hour Photo (2002)
Demonlover (2002)
The Hunted (2003)
Basic (2003)
Brødre (2004)
Return to Sender (2004)
The Great Raid (2005)
The Ice Harvest (2005)
The Situation (2006)
Battle in Seattle (2007)
A Shine of Rainbows (2008)

Leslie **Nielsen**
6ft 1in
(LESLIE WILLIAM NIELSEN)

Born: February 11, 1926
Regina, Saskatchewan, Canada

Leslie's father was an officer in the Royal Canadian Mounted Police, stationed at Fort Nelson (now Tulita). When the time came for him and his brother to go to school, the family left Yukon Territories and settled in Edmonton. After he had graduated from high school, Leslie joined the Royal Canadian Air Force and served as an aerial gunner towards the latter stages of World War II. The war ended a year later, so Leslie went to work as a disc jockey on a radio station in Calgary. He moved to Toronto, where he enrolled at The Lorne Greene Academy of Radio Arts. He left for New York after receiving a scholarship to study at the Neighborhood Playhouse. Following work in summer stock, he got his first television role in 1950, in an episode of 'Actor's Studio'. For six years, he was exclusively a TV actor – which was looked down upon in those days, but he made a living. In 1956, he was offered an MGM contract and made his film debut, in *Ransom!* It was a good start, but his second film, the science fiction classic, *Forbidden Planet*, made him a star. He's continued working in movies well beyond the popular *Naked Gun* series. Leslie's been married four times and he had two daughters with his second wife, Alisande Ullman. His present spouse is Barbaree Earl Nielsen.

Ransom! (1956)
Forbidden Planet (1956)
The Opposite Sex (1956)
Hot Summer Night (1957)
Tammy and the Bachelor (1957)
The Sheepman (1958)
Dark Intruder (1965)
Rosie! (1967)
The Poseidon Adventure (1972)
Airplane! (1980)
Wrong Is Right (1982)
Creepshow (1982) Nuts (1987)
The Naked Gun 2½ (1991)
Naked Gun 33⅓: The
Final Insult (1994)
Scary Movie 3 (2003)
Music Within (2007)

Alessandro **Nivola**
5ft 9in
(ALESSANDRO ANTINE NIVOLA)

Born: June 28, 1972
Boston, Massachusetts, USA

Sandro was born into an academic and creative family. His father, Pietro Nivola, is a professor of political science and is the author of the major book, "Laws of the Landscape: How Policies Shape Cities in Europe and America". His mother is an artist. Sandro, who has a brother named Adrian, has Italian blood from his father and Jewish blood from his mother. He was educated at Phillips Exeter Academy, in New Hampshire and later earned a degree in English from Yale University. While still an undergraduate, Sandro played the leading role in a Seattle production of Athol Fugard's "Master Harold...and the Boys". In 1995, he made his Broadway debut in "A Month in the Country" - as the young lover of the Helen Mirren character. The following year, he appeared on TV, in Danielle Steele's 'The Ring' and from that solid platform, he landed his first film role, a supporting one, in *Inventing the Abbotts*. Later that year, he played Nicolas Cage's schizophrenic brother, in Face/Off and was nominated for a 'Favorite Supporting Actor Award' by Blockbuster. Sandro's career had taken off, and after an Independent Spirit Award nomination, for *Laurel Canyon,* he began getting starring roles. Since January 2003, Sandro has been married to the English actress, Emily Mortimer. They have a son named Sam.

Inventing the Abbotts (1997)
Face/Off (1997)
I Want You (1998)
Reach the Rock (1998)
Best Laid Plans (1999)
Mansfield Park (1999)
Love's Labour's Lost (2000)
Jurassic Park III (2001)
Laurel Canyon (2002)
The Clearing (2004) Junebug (2005)
The Sisters (2005) Goal! (2005)
Grace Is Gone (2007)
Goal II: Living the Dream (2007)
The Girl in the Park (2007)
The Eye (2008)
$5 a Day (2008)
Who Do You Love (2008)

David **Niven**
6ft
(JAMES DAVID GRAHAM NIVEN)

Born: **March 1, 1910**
London, England
Died: **July 29, 1983**

Born on St. David's Day – David was the son of an Englishman, William Niven, and a mother, Henrietta Degacher, who was half French. His father was killed in Gallipoli in 1915 and his mother married Sir Thomas Comyn-Platt – believed by some family members, to be David's biological father. David attended the newly-founded Stowe School before going to Sandhurst. What he learned there became very much a part of his screen persona. He served in the Army for four years and after resigning his commission he had a bit part in the 1932 comedy, *There Goes the Bride*. One more small British film convinced him that he had a future. He made it to Hollywood in 1934 and with the help of Fred and Adele Astaire, met people who could help him. He worked as an extra in the 1934 version of *Cleopatra* and within two years had a featured role in his new friend Errol Flynn's *The Charge of the Light Brigade*. He won a Best Actor Oscar for *Separate Tables*. Married twice, David had four children – two with Primula Rollo, who died in 1946, and two with Hjordis Paulina Tersmeden, who was with him when he died of Lou Gehrig's disease at his home in Château-d'Oex, Switzerland.

Dodsworth (1936)
The Charge of the
Light Brigade (1936)
The Prisoner of Zenda (1937)
The Dawn Patrol (1938)
Wuthering Heights (1939)
The First of the Few (1942)
The Way Ahead (1944)
A Matter of Life and Death (1946)
The Bishop's Wife (1947)
Enchantment (1948)
Carrington, V.C. (1954)
Around the World in
Eighty Days (1956)
Separate Tables (1958)
The Guns of Navarone (1961)
55 Days at Peking (1963)
The Pink Panther (1964)
The Sea Wolves (1980)

Philippe **Noiret**
6ft 1½in
(PHILIPPE NOIRET)

Born: **October 1, 1930**
Lille, Nord, France
Died: **November 23, 2006**

Philippe was the son of Pierre Georges Noiret, who had a passion for poetry and literature. His mother, Lucy was a brilliant cook, who ensured a comfortable home life. Although a bright child, Philippe was not good when it came to exams. He failed his baccalauréat several times before deciding to become an actor. He went to Rennes to study at the Centre Dramatique de l'Ouest. For nearly seven years he toured France as a member of the Villeurbanne-based, Théâtre National Populaire. Phillipe formed a comedy duo with Jean-Pierre Darras, and they performed in nightclubs. In 1956, he was cast by director Agnès Varda in her debut film, *La Pointe Courte*. It was successful, but Phillipe didn't receive another offer of film work until *Zazie dans le Métro,* which kickstarted his movie career. He also met his future wife, Monique Chaumette, during that time, and they were married in 1962. For over thirty years Philippe was a giant of the French Cinema. He won a Best Actor BAFTA for *Cinema Paradiso*. Philippe died of cancer a few months after completing work on his final film – *3 amis*.

Zazie dans le Métro (1960)
Thérèse Desqueyroux (1962)
Lady L (1965)
La Vie de Château (1965)
The Assassination Bureau (1969)
Topaz (1969) Murphy's War (1971)
The Old Maid (1972)
La Grande Bouffe (1973)
The Clockmaker of St. Paul (1974)
Who Is Killing the Great Chefs
of Europe? (1978)
Heads or Tails (1980)
Coup de Torchon (1981)
The North Star (1982)
Le Cop (1984)
Cinema Paradiso (1988)
Uranus (1990)
I Don't Kiss (1991)
Tango (1993) Il Postino (1994)
Le Bossu (1997)
Honest Dealer (2002)

Lloyd **Nolan**
5ft 10½in
(LLOYD BENEDICT NOLAN)

Born: **August 11, 1902**
San Francisco, California, USA
Died: **September 27, 1985**

Lloyd's parents – James and Margaret Nolan, were both of Irish stock. His father owned a shoe factory in San Francisco, but Lloyd resisted joining the family business. After Santa Clara College, he attended Stanford University. Because of his preoccupation with amateur dramatics, he flunked out and went to work on a freighter. When his father died in 1927, Lloyd was left enough money to keep him going while studying acting at the Pasadena Playhouse. Following a couple of years with stock companies he went to New York. After roles in a trio of musical revues – the first of which was "Cape Cod Follies". Lloyd then made real impact on Broadway in 1933, as Biff Grimes in "One Sunday Afternoon". Lloyd's film debut was in the James Cagney starrer, *"G" Men*. He became a reliable second lead and supporting actor. He served his country in several war dramas, but by 1950, the bulk of his work was in television. Twice married, Lloyd died of lung cancer at his home in Los Angeles, after completing work on his final film, the Woody Allen comedy drama, *Hannah and Her Sisters*.

"G" Men (1935)
The Texas Rangers (1936)
Every Day's a Holiday (1937)
Wells Fargo (1937)
Johnny Apollo (1940)
The Man Who Wouldn't Die (1942)
Guadalcanal Diary (1943)
A Tree Grows in Brooklyn (1945)
The House on
92nd Street (1945)
Lady in the Lake (1947)
The Street With No Name (1948)
Easy Living (1949)
The Lemon Drop Kid (1951)
The Last Hunt (1956)
A Hatful of Rain (1957)
Portrait in Black (1960)
Susan Slade (1961)
Sergeant Ryker (1968)
Ice Station Zebra (1968)
Hannah and Her Sisters (1986)

Nick **Nolte**
6ft 1in
(NICHOLAS KING NOLTE)

Born: **February 8, 1941**
Omaha, Nebraska, USA

Nick was the son of Franklin Nolte, a salesman, of German descent, and Helen, a buyer in a department store. Nick was educated at Omaha Benson High School, where he became the star kicker in their football team. He was expelled for drinking beer, so he then transferred to West Side High School in Omaha and Pasadena City College. He stayed with sport and went on a football scholarship to Arizona State. He left academia following poor grades, and concentrated on his acting future by studying at the Pasadena Playhouse and at Stella Adler's L.A. Academy. It led to work in regional theaters, an episode of 'Disneyland' and some uncredited film roles. He scored high marks in TV's 'Rich Man Poor Man' and in 1977, was given a leading role in *The Deep.* Since then he has been nominated for Oscars for *The Prince of Tides* and *Affliction.* Nick later overcame drink and drugs problems, as well as the negative effects of three failed marriages. In 2007, Nick fathered a baby daughter with his girlfriend, Clytie Lane.

The Deep (1977)
Who'll Stop the Rain (1978)
48 Hours (1982) **Under Fire** (1983)
Extreme Prejudice (1987)
New York Stories (1989)
Cape Fear (1991)
The Prince of Tides (1991)
Lorenzo's Oil (1992)
Jefferson in Paris (1995)
Mulholland Falls (1996)
Mother Night (1996)
Nightwatch (1997)
Afterglow (1997) **U Turn** (1997)
Affliction (1997)
The Golden Bowl (2000)
The Good Thief (2002)
Northfork (2003)
The Beautiful Country (2004)
Clean (2004)
Hotel Rwanda (2004)
Peaceful Warrior (2006)
Off the Black (2006)
The Spiderwick Chronicles (2008)
Tropic Thunder (2008)

Eduardo **Noriega**
5ft 11in
(EDUARDO NORIEGA GÓMEZ)

Born: **August 1, 1973**
Santander, Cantabria, Spain

The youngest of seven brothers born to a Mexican father and a Spanish mother. There was little interest in movies in the family even though there had been a Mexican film star with exactly the same name. Eduardo was the only one of them to become an actor. During his childhood, he was crazy about music and learned to play Spanish guitar. When he was finished with his secondary schooling, Eduardo considered a law degree, but studied musical harmony and choral singing, at Santander University. He decided against both those careers in favor of an acting one – attending Madrid's School of Dramatic Art. He was twenty when he worked with Alejandro Amenábar for the first time, in a short thriller called *Luna* – for which he was named Best Actor at Alcalá de Henares Short Film Festival. Eduardo's first feature-length movie, was in 1995, when he had a small role in *Historias del Kronen.* The following year, he starred opposite Anna Galiena, in a good thriller called *Question of Luck.* His own luck was unquestioned – he became a star when, that same year, Amenábar cast him as 'Bosco' in the hugely successful *Tesis.* In 1999, Eduardo was named as one of 'European Films' Shooting Stars'. In 2008, he branched out internationally with two movies – *Transsiberian* and *Vantage Point* – a star-studded American thriller featuring Dennis Quaid and Forest Whitaker.

Question of Luck (1996)
Tesis (1996)
Open Your Eyes (1997)
Cha-cha-chá (1998)
Nobody Knows Anybody (1999)
El Invierno de las anjanas (2000)
Burnt Money (2000)
The Devil's Backbone (2001)
Warriors (2002)
El Lobo (2004) **Souli** (2004)
Mon Ange (2004)
Che Guevara (2005)
The Method (2005)
Alatriste (2006) **Transsiberian** (2008)
Vantage Point (2008)

Sheree **North**
5ft 4in
(DAWN SHIRLEY CRANG)

Born: **January 17, 1932**
Los Angeles, California, USA
Died: **November 5, 2005**

Sheree's mother, June Bethel, remarried when she was a little girl and she was known for a time as Dawn Bethel. By the time she was ten, she was dancing at USO socials in the Los Angeles area and three years later was working at the Greek Theater. Having received little parental guidance, she married Fred Bessire, in 1948, and had a baby daughter when she was sixteen. Surprisingly, the marriage lasted six years. By the early 1950s, she was dancing under the name of Shirley Bessire. In 1951, she had a bit part in the movie, *Excuse My Dust,* starring Red Skelton. In 1953, Sheree appeared on Broadway, in the musical "Hazel Flagg" which led to a role in the Martin and Lewis film, *Living It Up,* as well as the new name, Sheree North. She signed a contract with 20th Century Fox and was given the role intended for Marilyn Monroe, in *How to Be Very, Very Popular.* Following a few more movies for the studio, she had to take a back seat to their new protegee, Jayne Mansfield. In the 1960s, Sheree got a lot of television work, and always did well when offered a movie role. She had three more husbands and another child after divorcing Fred. Sheree made her final film appearance in 1998, in *Susan's Plan.* She then retired and died in Los Angeles seven years later – following complications after cancer surgery.

Living It Up (1954)
How to Be Very, Very Popular (1955)
**The Best Things in
Life are Free** (1956)
No Down Payment (1957)
In Love and War (1958)
Madigan (1968) **Lawman** (1971)
The Organization (1971)
Charley Varrick (1973)
The Outfit (1973)
Breakout (1975)
The Shootist (1976)
Telefon (1977)
Maniac Cop (1988)
Defenseless (1991)

Edward **Norton**
6ft
(EDWARD HARRISON NORTON)

Born: **August 18, 1969**
Boston, Massachusetts, USA

Edward grew up in Columbia, Maryland. His father, Edward Norton Snr., was a lawyer who specialized in environmental matters. His mother Robin, taught English. Edward's sister Molly, and brother Jim, arrived a little later. When he was twelve years old Edward began going to summer camp in Hebron, New Hampshire. He won the Acting Cup in 1984, and still visits the camp whenever he can spare the time. In 1987, Edward graduated from Wilde Lake High School, and went on to Yale. While there, he gained experience in theater productions and acted with his fellow students, Ron Livingston and Paul Giametti. Following graduation, he went to Japan to work for his grandfather's company, Enterprise Foundation. Moving to New York, he appeared in a raft of off-Broadway productions. His film debut, in the role of the disturbed, Aaron Stampler, in *Primal Fear,* made people take notice. Edward was nominated for a Best Supporting Actor Oscar for that effort. He is able to play nice or nasty with equal facility and has been lucky with nearly all the material he has been offered. He was later Oscar nominated as Best Actor, for *American History X.* He has been engaged to Courtney Love and Salma Hayek – the star of *Frida,* but he is still single.

Primal Fear (1996)
The People vs. Larry Flynt (1996)
Everyone Says I Love You (1996)
Rounders (1998)
American History X (1998)
Fight Club (1999)
Keeping the Faith (2000)
The Score (2001)
Frida (2002)
Red Dragon (2002)
25th Hour (2002)
The Italian Job (2003)
Kingdom of Heaven (2005)
Down in the Valley (2005)
The Illusionist (2006)
The Painted Veil (2006)
The Incredible Hulk (2008)
Pride and Glory (2008)

Kim **Novak**
5ft 6in
(MARILYN PAULINE NOVAK)

Born: **February 13, 1933**
Chicago, Illinois, USA

Kim's father, Josef, was a Czech, who worked for the Chicago-Milwaukee railroad and her mother, Blanche, had been a schoolteacher. Kim was educated in Chicago, at Farragut High School and Wright Junior College, where she majored in Drama. From her early teens she modeled for a local department store. After college, she demonstrated refrigerators before moving to L.A. with her mother and registering with the Caroline Leonetti Model Agency. It soon led to other opportunities, and before her twentieth birthday, she first appeared on the screen (in an uncredited role as a model) in a 3-D picture, *The French Line.* Columbia Pictures saw her and, without any great conviction, signed her to a six-months contract. Marilyn Novak was too close to MM, so they named her Kim, and she made her debut, opposite Fred MacMurray, in the film-noir, *Pushover.* That was so well received that the studio was forced to extend her contract. Kim scored high marks in *Picnic, The Man with the Golden Arm, The Eddie Duchin Story, Pal Joey* and *Vertigo.* During the late 1950s, she rivaled both Marilyn Monroe and Jayne Mansfield in terms of glamour, and won a Golden Globe as 'World Film Favorite', in 1957. Since 1976, Kim's been married to her second husband, Robert Malley. They breed horses in Oregon and California.

Pushover (1954)
Phffft! (1954)
5 Against the House (1955)
Picnic (1955)
The Man with the Golden Arm (1955)
The Eddie Duchin Story (1956)
Pal Joey (1957)
Jeanne Eagels (1957)
Vertigo (1958)
Bell Book and Candle (1958)
Middle of the Night (1959)
Strangers When We Meet (1960)
The Notorious Landlady (1962)
Boys' Night Out (1962)
Kiss Me Stupid (1964)
The Great Bank Robbery (1969)

Ramón **Novarro**
5ft 6in
(JOSE RAMÓN GIL SAMANIEGOS)

Born: **February 6, 1899**
Durango, Mexico
Died: **October 30, 1968**

In 1911, Ramón's wealthy family (his father was a dentist) fled to the United States to escape the Mexican Revolution. They then settled in California. Following his basic schooling, Ramón headed for Hollywood. He began to get work as singing waiter, a dancer, and as an extra in silent films beginning with *Joan the Woman,* in 1917. After ten uncredited parts he had his first featured role, in 1922, in *Mr. Barnes of New York.* He was a big success in the 1922 version of *The Prisoner of Zenda* and was soon being promoted as a rival to Rudolph Valentino – in action films like *Scaramouche,* and ultimately the classic 1925 production of *Ben-Hur.* In 1926, with Valentino's death, the throne was his. His first talkie *Devil-May-Care,* did nothing to reduce his popularity. For six years he was a big star at MGM – playing opposite some of the screen goddesses of the day including Greta Garbo, Helen Hayes, and Myrna Loy. When his contract lapsed in 1934, it wasn't renewed. He began acting in supporting roles and made movies in France and Mexico. One of them was the great Mexican film – *La Virgen que forjó una patria.* His final appearances were in television westerns. Ramón was gay and his appetite for sex resulted in his brutal murder by two brothers he had hired for that purpose.

Devil-May-Care (1929)
Call of the Flesh (1930)
Daybreak (1931) Son of India (1931)
Mata Hari (1931)
The Son-Daughter (1932)
The Barbarian (1933)
The Cat and the Fiddle (1934)
The Night Is Young (1935)
The Sheik Steps Out (1937)
A Desperate Adventure (1938)
La Comédie du bonheur (1940)
La Virgen que forjó
una patria (1942)
We Were Strangers (1949)
The Big Steal (1949)
The Outriders (1950) Crisis (1950)

Bill **Nunn**
6ft 3¹/₂in
(WILLIAM NUNN)

Born: **October 20, 1953**
Pittsburgh, Pennsylvania, USA

Bill's father, William G. Nunn, was a well-known journalist and the editor of the Pittsburgh Courier. He was also an NFL scout for the Pittsburgh Steelers. As a young boy, Bill dreamed of becoming a writer, so he enrolled at Morehouse College, in Atlanta, as an English major. His natural instincts pointed to drama however, and while still at college, he appeared in local theater productions including "A Soldier's Play", "Fences", and "Macbeth". After he graduated in 1976, Bill worked in nightclubs as part of a comedy team with his old friend, Al Cooper. In 1981, he tasted movies for the first time with an uncredited role in Burt Reynolds' *Sharkey's Machine.* Bill then began doing a little television work before, in 1988, he made his official film debut, in Spike Lee's comedy, *School Daze.* His first big budget film was *Regarding Henry,* and after that, there have been few years where Bill's beaming face hasn't brightened a film or TV drama. He and his wife Donna have two daughters – Jessica and Cydney.

Do the Right Thing (1989)
Mo' Better Blues (1990)
New Jack City (1991)
Regarding Henry (1991)
Sister Act (1992)
Blood Brothers (1993)
The Last Seduction (1994)
**Things to Do in Denver When
You're Dead** (1995)
Canadian Bacon (1995)
Bulletproof (1996)
Kiss the Girls (1997)
He Got Game (1998)
Ambushed (1998)
The Legend of 1900 (1998)
The Tic Code (1999)
Lockdown (2000)
Spider-Man (2002)
Spider-Man 2 (2004)
Champions (2006)
Spider-Man 3 (2007)
Randy and the Mob (2007)
**Little Bear and
the Master** (2008)

France **Nuyen**
5ft 3in
(FRANCE NGUYEN VANNGA)

Born: **July 31, 1939**
Marseilles, Bouches-du-Rhône, France

France grew up in the country she was named after. Her father was Vietnamese and her mother was French. When she was a small girl during World War II, her mixed-race parents were persecuted by the Nazis and accused of being Gypsies. France was raised by a cousin who grew orchids and drew her attention to nature and her love of art. After she left school at fifteen she worked locally as a seamstress. She was a stunningly good looking girl and one day at the beach, she caught the eye of the internationally famous Life magazine photographer, Philippe Halsman. It wasn't long before she was doing fashion modeling. France then attracted the attention of a producer, who was planning to stage an adaptation of Richard Mason's 1957 novel, "The World of Suzie Wong". In 1958, she made her London West End theater debut, opposite William Shatner and made her film debut in *South Pacific.* It was disappointing for her when, after having been cast to repeat her "Suzie" stage success, she was replaced by Nancy Kwan, in the film version. She was married to a psychiatrist from 1963 to 1966 and had a daughter. Her second husband was movie actor, Robert Culp. Since their divorce in 1970 France hasn't remarried. What she has done since 1986 – when she earned a master's degree in Clinical Psychology, is work as a counselor for abused women and children. She was named "Woman of the Year" in 1989 for her work in this field. She was seen on the screen most recently, as Dr. Pierce, in the 2007 film, *The American Standards.*

South Pacific (1958)
In Love and War (1958)
The Last Time I Saw Archie (1961)
Satan Never Sleeps (1962)
A Girl Named Tamiko (1962)
Diamond Head (1963)
Man in the Middle (1963)
One More Train to Rob (1971)
China Cry: A True Story (1990)
The Joy Luck Club (1993)
The Battle of Shaker Heights (2003)

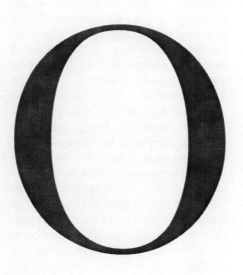

Hugh O'Brian
6ft 1in
(HUGH CHARLES KRAMPE)

Born: **April 19, 1923**
Rochester, New York, USA

Hugh's family moved to Illinois when he was a child. He received his education at the New Trier School, in Winnetka. It has an illustrious list of movie alumni, including Rock Hudson, Ann-Margret and Charlton Heston. At the Kemper Military School in Boonville, Missouri, Hugh demonstrated his prowess as an athlete in various sports including football, basketball, wrestling, and track. He spent one semester at the University of Cincinnati, but when America joined the war he enlisted in the Marine Corps. Hugh became their youngest-ever drill instructor and remained a Marine until 1946. Hugh headed for Los Angeles with the idea of studying Law at Yale University. But after being roped into joining a little theater group, by actress Ruth Roman, he had cause to change his plans. He got such good notices for his acting, in the Somerset Maugham play "Home and Beauty", he went to study drama at Los Angeles City College. In 1948 he made his film debut, with an uncredited role as a sailor, in *Kidnapped*. His first feature role in a movie was two years later, in *Rocketship X-M*. Universal offered Hugh a contract but didn't make him a star. The title role of TV's 'Wyatt Earp' did. It led to Broadway shows, plenty of TV work and a few film roles. In 1958 he founded the inspirational Hugh O'Brian Youth Leadership Program which still keeps him busy. In 2006 Hugh married for the very first time – to a lady called Virginia Barber.

The Return of Jesse James (1950
Vengeance Valley (1951)
The Cimarron Kid (1952)
The Battle of Apache Pass (1952)
Sally and Saint Anne (1952)
The Raiders (1952) Meet Me at the
Fair (1953) The Lawless Breed (1953)
Seminole (1953) The Man from
the Alamo (1953) Saskatchewan (1954)
Broken Lance (1954)
White Feather (1955)
The Fiend Who Walked the West (1958)
Ten Little Indians (1965)
The Shootist (1976) Twins (1988)

Edmund O'Brien
5ft 10in
(REDMOND O'BRIEN)

Born: **September 10, 1915**
New York City, New York, USA
Died: **May 9, 1985**

From an Irish family background, Eddy had an older brother, Liam, who grew up to become an Oscar-nominated screenwriter. The O'Briens were neighbors of the famous escapologist Harry Houdini. When he was ten, Eddy was taught conjuring tricks by the great man. While he was at high school he was nicknamed 'Tiger', because of his determination. He decided to become an actor and majored in Drama at Columbia University. In 1936, he made his Broadway debut, in "Daughters of Atrus" and performed in a modern dress version of "Julius Caesar" – with Orson Welles's Mercury Players. A bit part in 1938, was followed by a featured role, in *The Hunchback of Notre Dame,* which began a successful film career – which was interrupted by army service in World War II. He became a reliable character actor – winning a Best Supporting Actor Oscar, for *The Barefoot Contessa* and he was nominated, for *Seven Days in May.* Eddy retired in 1974 and died at his home in Inglewood, California, of Alzheimer's disease. He was married twice and had three children.

The Hunchback of Notre Dame (1939)
The Killers (1946) The Web (1947)
A Double Life (1947)
Another Part of the Forest (1948)
An Act of Murder (1948)
White Heat (1949) D.O.A. (1950)
711 Ocean Drive (1950)
The Turning Point (1952)
The Hitch-Hiker (1953)
Julius Caesar (1953)
The Bigamist (1953)
The Barefoot Contessa (1954)
Pete Kelly's Blues (1955)
The Rack (1956)
The Girl Can't Help It (1956)
The Man Who Shot
Liberty Vallance (1956)
Stopover Tokyo (1957)
Seven Days in May (1964)
The Wild Bunch (1969)
Lucly Luciano (1973)

Margaret O'Brien
4ft 9in
(ANGELA MAXINE O'BRIEN)

Born: **January 15, 1937**
San Diego, California, USA

Margaret's father, an Irishman, who was a circus performer, died before her first birthday. Her Spanish mother, Gladys Flores, performed Flamenco with her sister in theaters. When she was three, Margaret featured on the covers of family magazines and was already expressing a wish to be an actress. She had a natural talent and was given her movie debut shortly after that – a one minute scene in the Garland/Rooney musical, *Babes on Broadway*. MGM were so enchanted, they starred her in *Journey for Margaret,* which resulted in her being given the name of the role she played. She was soon the number one child star at the box office and was world famous, after she played 'Tootie' in *Meet Me in St. Louis.* She received a special Oscar as Outstanding Child Actress. She was called "America's favorite Sweetheart" and although her movie career was quite short, it was most certainly sweet. By the time she reached her mid teens, Margaret's appearances were largely confined to television. She married twice – having her only child, with her second husband, Ted Thorsen, in 1977. After a ten-year absence, Margaret made a sort of comeback, in 2002, when she had a small role in a video movie, called *Dead Season.* Seven years after that, she had leading roles in *Dead in Love* and a horror film – *Frankenstein Rising.*

Journey for Margaret (1942)
Madame Curie (1943)
Jane Eyre (1944)
The Canterville Ghost (1944)
Meet Me in St. Louis (1944)
Music for Millions (1944)
Our Vines have
Tender Grapes (1945)
Bad Bascomb (1946)
Three Wise Fools (1946)
The Unfinished Dance (1947)
Tenth Avenue Angel (1948)
Big City (1948)
Little Women (1949)
The Secret Garden (1949)
Amy (1981)

Pat O'Brien
5ft 11in
(WILLIAM JOSEPH PATRICK O'BRIEN)

Born: **November 11, 1899**
Milwaukee, Wisconsin, USA
Died: **October 15, 1983**

Pat was raised as a Catholic in an Irish American family. He served as an altar boy at Gesu Church, and attended the Marquette High School at the same time as Spencer Tracy. From there, he went on to Marquette University, but decided against joining the priesthood. He began a stage career, but like people from all walks of life he had to struggle when the Great Depression arrived. He was lucky that his stage acting reputation was important for Hollywood studios, who were having to cope with sound. Pat made an uncredited appearance, in 1930, in *Compliments of the Season,* and the following year, he married Eloise Taylor, who was his wife for fifty-two years. A most successful screen teaming was with James Cagney – they appeared in nine films together, including *Angels with Dirty Faces* and Jimmy's final movie, *Ragtime.* Pat was also featured in one of the great classic comedies, *Some Like It Hot.* His last screen appearance was in an episode of 'Happy Days'. He died of a heart attack, in Santa Monica.

The Front Page (1931)
American Madness (1932)
Bureau of Missing Persons (1933)
Bombshell (1933)
I've Got Your Number (1934)
Twenty Million Sweethearts (1934)
Here Comes the Navy (1934)
Page Miss Glory (1935)
Back in Circulation (1937)
Angels with Dirty Faces (1938)
The Fighting 69th (1940)
Castle on the Hudson (1940)
Torrid Zone (1940)
Broadway (1942)
Secret Command (1944)
Crack-Up (1946) Riffraff (1947)
The Boy with Green Hair (1948)
The Fireball (1950)
The People Against O'Hara (1951)
The Last Hurrah (1958)
Some Like It Hot (1959)
The End (1978)
Ragtime (1981)

Arthur O'Connell
5ft 11½in
(ARTHUR O'CONNELL)

Born: **March 29, 1908**
New York City, New York, USA
Died: **May 18, 1981**

Arthur started out in vaudeville and made his professional acting debut, on stage, in 1935, after accompanying a friend to an audition. His first movie was in 1938, when he had an uncredited role in *Freshman Year.* Following three more barely noticed bit parts, and a couple of short films, Arthur joined Orson Welles's Mercury Theater. He had a small role as a reporter in *Citizen Kane.* Throughout the 1940s, Arthur hardly registered in sixteen more films. He returned to Broadway, where he acted in both "Hamlet" and "Macbeth". Then, in 1953, he appeared at the Music Box Theater, in the original Broadway cast of "Picnic". It was such a huge success, Arthur was cast in the movie version two years later and he was nominated for a Best Supporting Actor Oscar. From that moment, Hollywood wanted Arthur O'Connell, and he was again Oscar-nominated, for *Anatomy of a Murder.* He was a popular guest artist on television shows in the early 1970s, but had been reduced to working on a series of toothpaste commercials for Crest, when Alzheimer's disease finally finished him off, in Woodland Hills, California.

Picnic (1955)
Bus Stop (1956)
Man of the West (1958)
Gidget (1959)
Anatomy of a Murder (1959)
The Great Imposter (1961)
Pocketful of Miracles (1961)
7 Faces of Dr. Lao (1964)
Your Cheatin' Heart (1964)
The Great Race (1965)
The Third Day (1965)
The Silencers (1966)
Fantastic Voyage (1966)
A Covenant with Death (1967)
The Power (1968)
There Was a
Crooked Man (1970)
The Last Valley (1970)
The Poseidon Adventure (1972)
The Hiding Place (1975)

Donald O'Connor
5ft 8in
(DONALD DAVID DIXON RONALD O'CONNOR)

Born: **August 28, 1925**
Chicago, Illinois, USA
Died: **September 27, 2003**

One of seven children, Donald was born into show business – his whole family worked in vaudeville. His father "Chuck" O'Connor, performed as an acrobat with Ringling Brothers-Barnum and Bailey's Circus, where Donald's mother, Effie, was a bareback rider. He was still a toddler when he witnessed his sister's death, in a road accident, and a few weeks later, had to endure the sad death of his father, who suffered a heart attack. In 1936, Donald danced on stage with the six-year-old Beverly Yissar. He made his film debut, in 1937, when he and his two brothers, Jack and Billy, performed a speciality routine in *Melody for Two.* Billy died of scarlet fever two years later. Donald got good notices for his performance in the Bing Crosby picture, *Sing You Sinners,* but it took him ten years before he could be called a star. In the meantime, he made movies which showed off his precocious talent. In 1944, he was drafted into the U.S. Army. Before leaving, he married Gwen Carter. They divorced in 1954, but a second marriage, to Gloria Noble, endured for nearly fifty years. His work in *Singin' in the Rain* – for which he won a Golden Globe, as Best Motion Picture Actor – Musical/Comedy, *Call Me Madam* and *There's No Business Like Show Business,* were Donald's career highlights. He retired in 1997. He died of heart failure, in Calabasas, California.

Sing You Sinners (1938)
Beau Geste (1939)
Chip Off the Old Block (1944)
Something in the Wind (1947)
Francis (1950)
The Milkman (1950)
Singin' in the Rain (1952)
I Love Melvin (1953)
Call Me Madam (1953)
Walking My Baby
Back Home (1953)
There's No Business Like
Show Business (1954)
Anything Goes (1956)
Ragtime (1981)

Cathy **O'Donnell**
5ft 4in
(ANN STEELY)

Born: **July 6, 1923**
Siluria, Alabama, USA
Died: **April 11, 1970**

Cathy's schoolteacher father died when she was twelve, and she moved from Alabama to Oklahoma City along with her mother and her younger brother, Joe. There she went to Harding Junior High School, before graduating from Classen High School, in 1942. She then studied stenography, until she made up her mind to become an actress. To achieve this, she enrolled at Oklahoma City University – concentrating on Dramatic Art and appearing in student plays. In 1944, she went to Hollywood and after a few weeks of knocking on doors, she was given a screen test, by producer Sam Goldwyn. He signed her to a contract, changed her name to Cathy O'Donnell and sent her to the American Academy of Dramatic Arts, in New York, to smooth out her southern accent, and improve her acting technique. Before going back to Hollywood, Cathy toured in the stage version of "Life With Father". After an uncredited appearance in Danny Kaye's *Wonder Man,* she made her official screen debut, in *The Best Years of Our Lives* and earned praise for her sensitive acting as a girl whose sailor boyfriend returns from the war, an amputee. In 1948, Cathy eloped with the director's brother, Robert Wyler, and was fired by Goldwyn. Cathy left a handful of worthwhile films – the last of which was *Ben-Hur,* in which she played the supporting role of Tirzah. Cathy died on her twenty-second Wedding Anniversary, in Los Angeles, after a long battle with cancer.

**The Best Years of
Our Lives** (1946)
Bury Me Dead (1947)
The Amazing Mr. X (1948)
They Live by Night (1948)
Side Street (1950)
The Miniver Story (1950)
Detective Story (1951)
Eight O'Clock Walk (1954)
Mad at the World (1955)
The Man from Laramie (1955)
Ben-Hur (1959)

Maureen **O'Hara**
5ft 8in
(MAUREEN FITZSIMONS)

Born: **August 17, 1920**
Ranelagh, County Dublin, Ireland

The second of six children, Maureen was from a lively and musically talented family background. Her positive-thinking father, Charles FitzSimons, was a part-owner of the Shamrock Rovers soccer club, and he gave her a love of sports. Her mother, Marguerita, possessed a beautiful contralto singing voice. Maureen was taught the Irish language at school and used that skill in a couple of her films. When she was six, she was sent to elocution classes. By the age of fourteen she had joined the famous Abbey Theater in Dublin and performed in classical plays. In 1938, she made her film debut in *Kicking the Moon Around* – filmed at Pinewood Studios. While she was there she was invited for a screen test at Elstree, where Charles Laughton – the co-owner of Mayflower Pictures was impressed enough to cast her in *Jamaica Inn.* She co-starred with him in *The Hunchback of Notre Dame,* and RKO gave her a seven-year contract. The red-haired beauty then began a very successful movie career – maintaining her star-status for over thirty years. She married three times and had a daughter named Bronwyn. Maureen's last appearance was in a television-movie, *The Last Dance,* in 2000.

**The Hunchback of
Notre Dame** (1939)
How Green Was My Valley (1941)
The Black Swan (1942)
The Immortal Sergeant (1943)
Sentimental Journey (1946)
Miracle on 34th Street (1947)
Sitting Pretty (1948)
Britannia Mews (1949)
Rio Grande (1950)
Against All Flags (1952)
The Quiet Man (1952)
**The Redhead from
Wyoming** (1953)
The Long Gray Line (1955)
The Wings of Eagles (1957)
Our Man in Havana (1959)
The Deadly Companions (1961)
The Parent Trap (1961)
McLintock! (1963)

Dan **O'Herlihy**
6ft 3in
(DANIEL O'HERLIHY)

Born: **May 1, 1919**
Wexford, Ireland
Died: **February 17, 2005**

The son of an architect, young Dan was educated at the Christian Brothers' Blackrock College, outside Dublin. He then studied architecture at the National University, in the city itself, and while he was there, began getting small stage roles at the Abbey and Gate theaters. In 1945, he married Elsie Bennett, with whom he would have five children. In 1946, he went to Belfast to make his film debut, in Carol Reed's *Odd Man Out.* Dan appeared on Broadway in "The Life of Charles Dickens" and played Macduff in the Orson Welles film of *Macbeth,* for which he designed both the costumes and the sets. He made a somewhat desperate attempt to win an Oscar, for *The Adventures of Robinson Crusoe* – hiring a small movie theater and inviting members of the Academy to a screening. He was nominated, but it was Brando's year. His career should have yielded more top performances, but in his younger days, he didn't get the breaks. Dan remained good humored despite his disappointment with his career and he worked steadily on television and in films. He played the U.S. president's father, Joe Kennedy, in the 1998 TV-film, 'The Rat Pack' and then retired. He died of natural causes in Malibu, California.

Macbeth (1948)
Soldiers Three (1951)
Actors and Sin (1952)
Operation Secret (1952)
**The Adventures of
Robinson Crusoe** (1954)
**The Black Shield of
Falworth** (1954)
The Virgin Queen (1955)
Home Before Dark (1958)
Imitation of Life (1959)
Fail-Safe (1964)
The Carey Treatment (1972)
The Tamarind Seed (1974)
MacArthur (1977)
The Last Starfighter (1984)
RoboCop (1987)
The Dead (1987)

Dennis O'Keefe
6ft 2in
(EDWARD VANCE FLANAGAN)

Born: **March 29, 1908**
Fort Madison, Iowa, USA
Died: **August 31, 1968**

Starting life as "Bud" Flanagan, Dennis was the son of a pair of Irish vaudevillians. When he was still very young, he was part of his parents' stage act and even wrote sketches for them. After finishing his high school education, Dennis got work as a film extra, starting in 1930, with *Check and Double Check*. He had appeared in over 150 uncredited roles before, in 1937, things got better for him. After changing his name to Dennis O'Keefe, he was given a featured role in a Wallace Beery western, *The Bad Man of Brimstone*. In 1940, he married his second wife, the Hungarian-born actress, Steffi Duna. Their son, James O'Keefe, became a director and film producer. Throughout the 1940s and early 1950s, Dennis carved himself a very comfortable career as a supporting actor in big-budget movies and the star of many B-pictures. After that, he was happy to work on screenplays, direct a couple of movies, and appear in television dramas while enjoying the occasional movie role. He was married to Steffi until he died of lung cancer, in Santa Monica, California.

The Chaser (1938)
That's Right – You're Wrong (1939)
Arise My Love (1940)
Topper Returns (1941)
Weekend for Three (1941)
Hangmen Also Die! (1943)
The Leopard Man (1943)
Hi Diddle Diddle (1943)
The Fighting Seabees (1944)
Up in Mabel's Room (1944)
The Story of Dr. Wassell (1944)
Getting Gertie's Garter (1945)
The Affairs of Susan (1945)
Brewster's Millions (1945)
Doll Face (1946)
Dishonored Lady (1947)
T-Men (1947) Raw Deal (1948)
Sirens of Atlantis (1949)
Cover-Up (1949) Abandoned (1949)
The Great Dan Patch (1949)
The Company She Keeps (1951)
Dragoon Wells Massacre (1957)

Patrick O'Neal
6ft
(PATRICK O'NEAL)

Born: **September 26, 1927**
Ocala, Florida, USA
Died: **September 9, 1994**

Patrick's father had the lovely name of Coke Wisdom O'Neal. His mother was simply Martha. They were both of Irish descent so they named their boy Patrick. He was a bright lad who graduated from the University of Florida in Gainesville. As soon as he'd finished there, towards the end of World War II, he was drafted for service into the U.S. Air Force. He wasn't sent overseas, so he used the time well – directing training films. At the end of the war, he finished his stint and moved to New York City. He made his mind up to become an actor, and his first stop was the Neighborhood Playhouse. In 1946, he went looking for summer work, and was used as stand-in for Gregory Peck, during the shooting of *The Yearling*. He always credited that actor for steering him in the right direction. That direction was via television's Kraft Theater in 1952. Patrick's film debut, was in *The Mad Magician*, in 1954. Film work didn't exactly come thick and fast, but he kept the wolf from the door with TV work. He needed the income: in 1956 Patrick had married his sweetheart, Cynthia. The pair produced three children and remained together until his death in New York, following a battle with tuberculosis and cancer.

The Black Shield of
Falworth (1954)
From the Terrace (1960)
In Harm's Way (1965)
King Rat (1965)
A Fine Madness (1966)
Alvarez Kelly (1966)
Where Were You When the
Lights Went Out? (1968)
Assignment to Kill (1968)
Castle Keep (1969)
The Kremlin Letter (1970)
The Way We Were (1973)
The Stepford Wives (1975)
New York Stories (1989)
Q & A (1990) Alice (1990)
For the Boys (1991)
Under Siege (1992)

Ryan O'Neal
6ft 1in
(PATRICK RYAN O'NEAL)

Born: **April 20, 1941**
Los Angeles, California, USA

The son of the writer, Charles O'Neal, and his wife Patricia, who had once been an actress, Ryan had a creative pedigree. When he was a kid, his father was in the Army, stationed in West Germany. Ryan was educated at the U.S. Army School in Munich, where he was a pretty useful amateur boxer. Before he left Germany, he became a stuntman for a TV series called 'Tales of the Vikings'. After he returned to the United States, he was at one time, a Golden Gloves contender. He later worked as a lifeguard until he got his first role on the small screen in a 1960 episode of 'The Many Loves of Dobie Gillis'. He made his film debut in 1962, with Richard Egan and Charles Bronson, in *This Rugged Land,* and later appeared in Egan's television series, 'Empire'. In 1963, Ryan married Joanna Cook Moore, and fathered a daughter, the future movie star, Tatum. There was lots of television work and a few movies before he got his big break in *Love Story,* for which he was nominated for a Best Actor Oscar. He was the star when his little girl became the youngest ever Oscar winner, when she was Best Supporting Actress, at the age of ten, in *Paper Moon.* From 1980-97, Ryan lived with Farrah Fawcett. In 2007, he was in a short, called *Waste Land.* He has since suffered from leukemia, but is now in remission following treatment. In 2008, Ryan appeared on television – as Max Keenan, in 'Bones'. Ryan remained close to Farrah and it hit him hard when she died of cancer in June 2009.

The Games (1970)
Love Story (1970) Wild Rovers (1971)
What's Up Doc? (1972)
The Thief Who Came to Dinner (1973)
Paper Moon (1973)
Barry Lyndon (1975) Nickelodeon (1976)
A Bridge Too Far (1977)
The Driver (1978)
Irreconcilable Differences (1984)
Chances Are (1989) Faithful (1996)
Zero Effect (1998)
People I Know (2002)

Tatum O'Neal
5ft 7in
(TATUM BEATRICE O'NEAL)

Born: **November 5, 1963**
Los Angeles, California, USA

Ryan's daughter was named after the jazz piano great, the legendary Art Tatum. Her mother, Joanna Cook Moore, struggled with amphetamine and alcohol addiction before her divorce in 1968. She got worse after taking her two children – Tatum and her brother, Griffin, to live on a rundown ranch outside Los Angeles. The kids lived in squalor and were beaten and abused by their drunken mother's men friends. They were eventually sent to a boarding school, but in 1971, Tatum left to go and live with her dad in Malibu. He'd become a big star and although it was heaven compared with her earlier life, she had to share him with a string of beautiful women. Her success in the movie, *Paper Moon,* destroyed their relationship. He stayed away from the Award ceremony. Life became unbearable: she slashed her wrists and overdosed on drugs. Her career stalled, and at sixteen, she lived in a rented apartment and hung out with bad people. She fell for tennis star, John McEnroe, married him and had three kids, but they clashed too often for it to work. When they divorced in 1992, he was given custody – and Tatum turned to heroin. That was yesterday. Today she's clean and enjoys pretty good relationships with her children. She published her memoirs "A Paper Life" in 2004, and is now working regularly again. Since 2005, she has been seen in the role of Maggie in the TV series, 'Rescue Me' and Blythe Hunter in 'Wicked Wicked Games'. Tatum's just completed work on the film drama, *Saving Grace B. Jones* – written and directed by the singing star/actress, Connie Stevens.

Paper Moon (1973)
The Bad News Bears (1976)
Nickelodeon (1976)
International Velvet (1978)
Circle of Two (1980)
Little Darlings (1980)
Little Noises (1992)
Basquait (1996)
The Scoundrel's Wife (2002)
My Brother (2006)

Jennifer O'Neill
5ft 8in
(JENNIFER O'NEILL)

Born: **February 20, 1948**
Rio de Janeiro, Brazil

Jennifer's father was a businessman of Irish-Spanish descent, and her mother was English. They moved to Connecticut when she was a little girl and later, to New York. She was a fifteen year old student at the Dalton School in Manhattan, when she started getting modeling jobs. She bought her first horse with the money she made, but an accident put a stop to any prospects of riding for a while. When she was seventeen, Jennifer married the first of her nine husbands, and gave birth to a daughter. After appearing on magazine covers, she was accepted at the prestigious Neighborhood Playhouse. In 1968, she made her film debut with a small role in *For Love of Ivy* – a comedy written by, and starring, Sidney Poitier. Two years after that, Jennifer was cast by Howard Hawks in the John Wayne western, *Rio Lobo.* She then secured brief stardom when she played war widow, Dorothy, in the beautiful romantic drama, *Summer of '42.* Apart from Luchino Visconti's final film *L'Innocente,* she never again had a role of anywhere near that quality. An accident with a firearm, in 1982 – when she shot herself in the abdomen could have ended her career, but she continued to act. In 1997, Jennifer married Mervyn Louque, and lives with him on a ranch in Nashville where she can ride horses to her heart's content. She also works for charitable causes and derives much comfort from being a born again Christian. She has a daughter and two sons. Jennifer had a small role in the recent biopic about Billy Graham – *Billy: The Early Years.*

Rio Lobo (1970)
Summer of '42 (1971)
Such Good friends (1971)
The Carey Treatment (1972)
The Reincarnation of Peter Proud (1975)
L'Innocente (1976)
Sette note in nero (1977)
Caravans (1978)
Scanners (1981)
The Ride (1997)

Maureen O'Sullivan
5ft 3in
(MAUREEN PAULA O'SULLIVAN)

Born: **May 17, 1911**
Boyle, County Roscommon, Ireland
Died: **June 23, 1998**

Maureen was born into a fairly wealthy Irish family. Her father, Charles Joseph O'Sullivan, served with The Connaught Rangers (an Irish regiment of the British Army) during World War I. Her mother, Mary, was a traditional homemaker. After a period at a convent school in Dublin, Maureen was sent to London where she attended the Convent of the Sacred Heart in Roehampton. While she was there, she befriended one of her classmates – the future Vivien Leigh. Maureen then went to finishing school in France. She returned to Dublin to work with poor people. The Hollywood director, Frank Borzage, was shooting location footage for the John McCormack film, *Song o' My Heart.* He saw her, gave her a screen test, and the next thing Maureen knew, she was in Hollywood. In 1930, she made her debut in *So This Is London,* starring Will Rogers. Maureen's fame arrived when she became Tarzan's Jane, in *Tarzan the Ape Man.* The 1930s was good for her, with many films she acted in considered among the best of each year. She married film director, John Farrow, and their seven children included Mia. Maureen died at home in Scottsdale, Arizona – from complications following heart surgery.

Tarzan the Ape Man (1932)
Tugboat Annie (1933)
Stage Mother (1933)
Tarzan and His Mate (1934)
The Thin Man (1934)
Hide-Out (1934)
The Barretts of Wimpole Street (1934)
David Copperfield (1935)
West Point of the Air (1935)
Anna Karenina (1935)
A Day at the Races (1937)
A Yank at Oxford (1938)
The Crowd Roars (1938)
Pride and Prejudice (1940)
Tarzan's Secret Treasure (1941)
The Big Clock (1948)
Where Danger Lives (1950)

Annette O'Toole
5ft 4in
(ANNETTE O'TOOLE)

Born: **April 1, 1952**
Houston, Texas, USA

Annette's parents, William and Dorothy O'Toole, encouraged their little girl to begin dancing lessons at the age of three. Her mother owned a dance studio in Houston. It gave her poise and confidence which resulted in opportunities to act in school plays and also develop her sweet singing voice. Around about the time of Annette's thirteenth birthday, the O'Toole's moved to Los Angeles. During her high school years, Annette re-focussed her attention on acting, and with that aim in mind she attended drama classes with Peggy Feury – at the Loft Studios, in L.A. The reward for her efforts were guest appearances on several television shows including 'My Three Sons' 'This Is the Life', 'The Virginian' and 'Gunsmoke'. When she was eighteen she was an extra in the Dustin Hoffman movie *Little Big Man* but her true movie debut was five years later, as Beauty Queen "Miss Anaheim" in *Smile*. Her first starring role was opposite Robby Benson, in *One on One*. Annette achieved stardom in *48 Hours,* a popular hit for Eddie Murphy and Nick Nolte. After appearing in the disastrous *Superman III* she wisely waited five years for her next film role – in a light and pleasant comedy, *Cross My Heart*. Her movies have been in short supply since then and it does appear that she has been much luckier with her opportunities on television. She has been heard singing from time to time. In 2007 she did backing vocals during a Live Earth concert in London, with husband, Michael McKean – an actor, composer, comedian, musician and impersonator.

Smile (1975)
One on One (1977)
King of the Gypsies (1978)
Foolin' Around (1980)
Cat People (1982)
48 Hours (1982)
Cross My Heart (1987)
Love at Large (1990)
Imaginary Crimes (1994)
Temptation (2003)
The Golden Door (2008)

Peter O'Toole
6ft 2in
(PETER SEAMUS O'TOOLE)

Born: **August 2, 1932**
Connemara, County Galway, Ireland

Peter and his parents moved to Leeds in England when he was one year old. For several years, he and his mother, Connie, used to journey to the racetracks with his father, Patrick – a traveling bookmaker. Because of that, he didn't attend school regularly until he was eleven. Then, after being terrorized by the nuns, he lasted only two years – leaving school to work as a teaboy, and eventually a reporter at the Yorkshire Evening News. He enjoyed his two years National Service in the Royal Navy, but when that ended he decided to become an actor. In 1952, after being rejected by the Abbey Theater's Drama School, because he couldn't speak Irish, he went to RADA, in London. Two of his classmates were Alan Bates and Albert Finney. In 1955, he joined the Bristol Old Vic and the following year, made his TV debut in 'The Scarlet Pimpernel'. He married actress Siân Phillips, in 1959, and a year later, made his movie debut, with a very small role in *Kidnapped*. The epic *Lawrence of Arabia* made him a huge star and he was nominated for a Best Actor Oscar. It was the first of eight – the others were *Becket, The Lion in Winter, Goodbye Mr, Chips, The Ruling Class, The Stunt Man, My Favorite Year* and *Venus*.

The Day They Robbed the
Bank of England (1960)
Lawrence of Arabia (1962)
Becket (1964) Lord Jim (1965)
What's New Pussycat (1965)
How to Steal a Million (1966)
The Night of the Generals (1967)
The Lion in Winter (1968)
Goodbye Mr. Chips (1969)
Murphy's War (1971)
The Ruling Class (1972)
The Stunt Man (1980)
My Favorite Year (1982)
The Last Emperor (1987)
The Rainbow Thief (1990)
Wings of Fame (1990)
Global Heresy (2002) Lassie (2005)
Venus (2006) Stardust (2007)
Dean Spanley (2008)

Jack Oakie
5ft 11in
(LEWIS DELANEY OFFIELD)

Born: **November 12, 1903**
Sedalia, Missouri, USA
Died: **January 23, 1978**

After Jack had graduated from De La Salle High School, in New York, his parents were hoping he would go into a respectable business when he left school, but early experience answering telephone queries for a brokerage company, convinced him otherwise. In 1919, his career was decided following his appearance in a charity show mounted by Wall Street executives on behalf of the Cardiac Society. It resulted in a teaming with Lulu McConnell, who performed with him until 1927. They made their stage debuts in the chorus of George M. Cohen's, 1922 musical, "Little Nellie Kelly". After several Broadway shows, and bit parts in movies, Jack went to Hollywood, where he made his debut, in the 1928 silent, *Finders Keepers*. He made the transition to sound without a hitch, when in 1929, he had a small role in *The Dummy*. During the 1930s, his career declined, but he came back with a bang in *The Great Dictator* – for which he was nominated for a Best Supporting Actor Oscar. Jack went on working until the early 1970s, when he made his last appearance, in an episode of the TV series, 'Night Gallery'. He was twice married. Jack died in Los Angeles, from aortic aneurysm.

If I Had a Million (1932)
The Eagle and the Hawk (1933)
Murder at the Vanities (1934)
Call of the Wild (1935)
King of Burlesque (1936)
The Texas Rangers (1936)
The Affairs of Annabel (1938)
The Great Dictator (1940)
Song of the Islands (1942)
Hello Frisco, Hello (1943)
The Merry Monahans (1944)
When My Baby
Smiles at Me (1948)
Thieves Highway (1949)
Tomahawk (1951)
The Wonderful Country (1959)
The Rat Race (1960)
Lover Come Back (1961)

Warren **Oates**
5ft 11in
(WARREN MERCER OATES)

Born: **July 5, 1928**
Depoy, Kentucky, USA
Died: **April 3, 1982**

Warren was the son of Bayless E. Oates and his wife, Sarah. Following high school in Louisville he served in the United States Marines. After that he studied at the University of Louisville, where he began acting. He went to New York and got his first television job, as the "gags" tester, on 'Beat the Clock'. In the early 1950s, he did menial jobs at night while attending auditions during the day. He made his debut in a television drama in 1956, as Private Lear in the U.S. Steel Hour comedy, 'Operation Three R's'. Warren worked steadily in small screen westerns until making his film debut in 1959 – with an uncredited role in *Up Periscope*. He had a bigger part in *Yellowstone Kelly* that year, and was in demand for character roles, for the next twenty five years. Warren's style suited westerns and his several good ones included *Ride the High Country* and *The Wild Bunch*. In 1975 he sang in the back-up chorus on the Kris Kristofferson album "Who's to Bless ...Who's to Blame". He made his last film appearance in *Tough Enough*. Warren was married three times and had two children. He died of a heart attack, in Los Angeles.

The Rise and fall of
Legs Diamond (1960) **Ride the**
High Country (1962)
Mail Order Bride (1964)
Major Dundee (1965)
The Shooting (1967)
Welcome to Hard Times (1967)
In the Heat of the Night (1967)
Crooks and Coronets (1969)
The Wild Bunch (1969)
There Was a Crooked Man (1970)
Two-Lane Blacktop (1971)
The Hired Hand (1971)
Dillinger (1973) **Badlands** (1973)
Bring Me the Head of Alfred
Garcia (1974) **Race with the**
Devil (1975) **92 in the Shade** (1975)
The Brinks Job (1978)
1941 (1979) **Stripes** (1981)
The Border (1982) **Blue Thunder** (1983)

Merle **Oberon**
5ft 2in
(ESTELLE MERLE O'BRIEN THOMPSON)

Born: **February 19, 1911**
Bombay, British India
Died: **November 23, 1979**

Even if Merle could see that she was an exceptionally pretty girl, she endured a very unhappy childhood. As the daughter of Arthur Thompson, a British-born railway engineer, and Charlotte, who was an Anglo-Sinhalese nurse, young Merle grew up with a distinct feeling of inferiority. Her situation worsened when her father died at the beginning of World War I, and for four years, she lived in poverty with her mother in Bombay. Things began to look better when, in Calcutta, she received a foundation scholarship to attend the exclusive La Martiniere College. But it was never going to work: her life was made so miserable by the other girls, Merle was forced to leave and take lessons at home. She matured into a beautiful girl, who not only performed with the Calcutta Amateur Dramatic Society, she was courted by older men. In 1928, she and her mother went to France, and after an uncredited role in *The Three Passions*, directed by Rex Ingram, she re-invented herself as Australian, Queenie O'Brien, and went to London. Korda liked her, re-named her Merle Oberon, became her lover, and turned her into a major star with a series of big roles, starting with Anne Boleyn, in *The Private Life of Henry VIII*. They married in 1939. Merle was Oscar-nominated for *The Dark Angel*. She made her last movie in 1973. Merle had three more husbands before dying of a stroke, in Malibu.

The Private Life of Henry VIII (1933)
The Scarlet Pimpernel (1934)
Folies Bergère de Paris (1935)
The Dark Angel (1935)
These Three (1936) **Beloved**
Enemy (1936) **I, Claudius** (1937)
The Divorce of Lady X (1938)
Wuthering Heights (1939)
'Til We Meet Again (1940)
That Uncertain Feeling (1941)
The Lodger (1944) **Dark Waters** (1944)
A Song to Remember (1945)
Berlin Express (1948)
Desirée (1954)

Warner **Oland**
5ft 11in
(JOHAN VERNER ÖLUND)

Born: **October 3, 1879**
Nyby, Västerbottens län, Sweden
Died: **August 6, 1938**

Warner was the son of a shopkeeper, Johan Olund, and his wife, Maria. In October 1892, the family emigrated to the United States and settled in Boston. By the time Warner finished his education, he spoke fluent English and Swedish. As a young man he decided to be a stage actor. After Dr. Curry's Drama School, he toured with Alla Nazimova's troupe. In 1907, he married the playwright, Edith Gardener Shearn, who helped him build a big reputation as a translator of the complete works of August Strindberg. Following a bright start to his Broadway career, he ventured into silent films for the first time, in the 1912 drama, *Pilgrim's Progress*. His rather sinister looks, made him ideal for the Pearl White dramas starting with *The Romance of Elaine,* in 1915. Thirty films later, in 1927, Warner had a major role in the first 'talkie' – *The Jazz Singer.* He was cast as Chinese characters for most of his career, and made his final movie, *Charlie Chan at Monte Carlo,* the year before he died in Stockholm, Sweden, of bronchial pneumonia.

The Jazz Singer (1927)
The Mighty (1929)
Dangerous Paradise (1930)
The Vagabond King (1930)
The Return of
Dr. Fu Manchu (1930)
The Drums of Jeopardy (1931)
Dishonored (1931)
Charlie Chan Carries On (1931)
The Black Camel (1931)
Shanghai Express (1932)
A Passport to Hell (1932)
The Son-Daughter (1932)
Before Dawn (1933)
Charlie Chan's Greatest Case (1933)
Mandalay (1934) **Bulldog**
Drummond Strikes Back (1934)
The Painted Veil (1934)
Werewolf of London (1935)
Shanghai (1935)
Charlie Chan's Secret (1936) **Charlie**
Chan at the Race Track (1936)

Gary **Oldman**
5ft 9in
(LEONARD GARY OLDMAN)

Born: **March 21, 1958**
New Cross, London, England

Gary's dad was a welder who had been a sailor. He turned out to be an abusive alcoholic – leaving the family when Gary was seven. Shortly after that, his mother Kathleen, encouraged him to learn the piano. He was good enough on the instrument to consider a musical career, and his singing was not far behind. At some point, he changed direction and decided to become an actor. He won a scholarship to the Rose Bruford College, near London, and in 1979 he received a B.A. in Theater Arts. Gary then appeared on stage with Greenwich Young People's Theater – and he won The British Theater Association Award for Best Actor, in 1985. Gary made his film debut, as Sid Vicious, in *Sid and Nancy.* For over twenty years he's hardly ever failed to come up with something special. He has been less successful in his private life:- three marriages (his wives included actresses, Lesley Melville, and Uma Thurman) ended in divorce. He has three sons. Gary's sister, Maureen, is an actress who uses the stage name (which was suggested by him) of 'Laila Morse'.

Sid and Nancy (1986)
Prick Up Your Ears (1987)
Track 29 (1988)
Rosenkrantz and Guildenstern
are Dead (1990)
State of Grace (1990)
JFK (1991) Dracula (1992)
True Romance (1993)
Romeo Is Bleeding (1993)
Léon (1994)
Immortal Beloved (1994)
Murder in the First (1995)
Basquiat (1996)
The Fifth Element (1997)
Air Force One (1997)
The Contender (2000)
Nobody's Baby (2001)
Hannibal (2001)
Interstate 60 (2002)
Batman Begins (2005)
The Goblet of Fire (2005)
The Order of the Phoenix (2007)
The Dark Knight (2008)

Edna May **Oliver**
5ft 7in
(EDNA MAY NUTTER)

Born: **November 9, 1883**
Malden, Massachusetts, USA
Died: **November 9, 1942**

The daughter of Charles and Ida Nutter, and a descendant of the sixth American president, John Quincy Adams, Edna was a bony, rather plain-looking girl, but she quit school at the age of fourteen with the intention of pursuing a career on the stage. She worked in a junior capacity for several companies – and toured as pianist in an all girl orchestra. Slowly but surely, she was given small roles to play. Her first real success was nearly twenty years after she'd started – in the 1917 Broadway production of Jerome Kern's musical, "Oh, Boy!". Edna's horse-like features were not ideal for playing heroines, but she was a great character in dramas and comedies. She could be harsh and warm in the same role. In 1923, she made her film debut, in *Wife in Name Only.* She was in the original "Show Boat" and in 1928, married David Pratt. It lasted five years. Her nomination for an Oscar was as Best Supporting Actress – in *Drums Along the Mohawk.* Edna May died in Los Angeles, from an intestinal disorder, while celebrating her fifty-ninth birthday.

The Conquerors (1932)
Penguin Pool Murder (1932)
Ann Vickers (1933)
Little Women (1933)
Alice in Wonderland (1933)
The Poor Rich (1934)
The Last Gentleman (1934)
We're Rich Again (1934)
David Copperfield (1935)
Murder on a Honeymoon (1935)
No More Ladies (1935)
A Tale of Two Cities (1935)
Romeo and Juliet (1936)
Rosalie (1937)
Paradise for Three (1938)
Little Miss Broadway (1938)
The Story of Vernon and
Irene Castle (1939)
Second Fiddle (1939)
Drums Along the Mohawk (1939)
Pride and Prejudice (1940)
Lydia (1941)

Sir Laurence **Olivier**
5ft 10in
(LAURENCE KERR OLIVIER)

Born: **May 22, 1907**
Dorking, Surrey, England
Died: **July 11, 1989**

Larry was brought up in a strict, religious home, with a disciplinarian father named Gerard, who was an Anglican priest. His mother gave him all the love and attention, but sadly, she died when he was twelve. In 1918, his father was transferred to Hertfordshire, and Larry and his older brother and sister lived at the Old Rectory in Letchworth. Not long after that he went as a boarder, to St. Edward's School, in Oxford. When he was fifteen, he played Katherine, in the school's production of "The Taming of the Shrew". His father then suggested that he should consider an acting career. He went to the Central School of Dramatic Art, in London, and in 1926, joined Birmingham Rep. In 1930, he made his screen debut, in a short, *Too Many Crooks,* and married Jill Esmond, with whom he had a son. His other wives were Vivien Leigh, and Joan Plowright, with whom he had three children. Nominated nine times for Best Actor Oscars – for *Wuthering Heights, Rebecca, Henry V, Hamlet, Richard III, The Entertainer, Sleuth, Marathon Man,* and lastly, *The Boys from Brazil,* Larry won just once, in the title role of *Hamlet.* He died at Steyning, West Sussex, following a hip replacement operation.

Fire Over England (1937)
The Divorce of Lady X (1938)
Q Planes (1939) Wuthering
Heights (1939) Rebecca (1940)
Pride and Prejudice (1940)
That Hamilton Woman (1941)
49th Parallel (1941) Henry V (1944)
Hamlet (1948) Carrie (1952)
Richard III (1955)
The Devil's Disciple (1959)
The Entertainer (1960)
Spartacus (1960) Othello (1965)
Bunny Lake Is Missing (1965)
Khartoum (1966)
Battle of Britain (1969) Sleuth (1972)
Marathon Man (1976)
The Boys From Brazil (1978)
The Bounty (1984)

Clive **Owen**
6ft 2in
(CLIVE OWEN)

Born: **October 3, 1962**
Keresley, Coventry, Warwickshire, England

Clive was one of five brothers abandoned by their father, a Country Western singer, when Clive was three. He was raised by his mother and later her low-earning second husband. Clive attended Binley Park Comprehensive and after joining a youth theater, had his first success, as the 'Artful Dodger' in "Oliver". Following a period of being jobless, in 1984, he was accepted at the Royal Academy of Dramatic Art, in a class which included Ralph Fiennes. He graduated in 1987, and was taken on by the Young Vic, where he acted in several Shakespeare plays – in one of which, "Romeo and Juliet", he met his future wife Sarah-Jane Fenton. Clive made his TV debut in 1987, as a cop, in 'Rockcliffe's Babies'. His first film was a year later, in *Vroom*. There were three more years of TV work before he was cast in the drama, *Close My Eyes*. It's theme of incest raised a few eyebrows and Clive's next project (as a bisexual) in a stage production of Nöel Coward's "Design For Living", raised a few more. Clive has since established himself as a top flight Hollywood movie star. For his role as Larry, in *Closer,* he was nominated for a Best Supporting Actor Oscar. He played 'The Driver' in a series of shorts directed by John Woo, Tony Scott, Kar Wai Wong, Guy Ritchie, Ang Lee, Joe Carnahan and John Frankenheimer.

Close My Eyes (1991)
Century (1993)
The Turnaround (1995)
Bent (1997) Croupier (1998)
Greenfingers (2000)
Gosford Park (2001)
The Bourne Identity (2002)
I'll Sleep When I'm Dead (2003)
Beyond Borders (2003)
King Arthur (2004) Closer (2004)
Sin City (2005)
Derailed (2005)
Inside Man (2006)
Children of Men (2006)
Shoot 'Em Up (2007)
Elizabeth: The Golden Age (2007)
The International (2009)

Reginald **Owen**
6ft
(JOHN REGINALD OWEN)

Born: **August 5, 1887**
Wheathampstead, Hertfordshire, England
Died: **November 5, 1972**

Immediately after leaving school, Reg studied at Sir Herbert Beerbohm Tree's Academy of Dramatic Art. He made his professional stage debut in 1905, and became the first winner of the Bancroft Gold Medal. In 1911, he made his debut on screen, in a short version of *Henry VIII*. He later acted in two more European silents. After fifteen years of doing everything on the stage – from Shakespeare roles to musical comedy, Reg moved to New York and became a Broadway star. He went to Hollywood in 1929, where his first film role was in a Paramount short, *Pusher-in-the-Face*. It was followed by the Oscar-nominated movie, *The Letter,* which starred Jeanne Eagels. He became one of the busiest character actors in Hollywood films and acted in two Dickens' classics, *A Tale of Two Cities,* and as Ebenezer Scrooge, in the highly-rated version of *A Christmas Carol*. Reg died from a heart attack, in Idaho, at the age of eighty-five. Married three times, he had two children.

The Letter (1929) Platinum
Blonde (1931) A Study in
Scarlet (1933) Queen Christina (1933)
Mandalay (1934)
The House of Rothschild (1934)
Of Human Bondage (1934)
Madame DuBarry (1934)
Music in the Air (1934)
The Good Fairy (1935) The Call of
the Wild (1935) Anna Karenina (1935)
The Bishop Misbehaves (1935)
A Tale of Two Cities (1935)
The Great Ziegfeld (1936)
Madame X (1937) Conquest (1937)
Kidnapped (1938) A Christmas
Carol (1938) The Real Glory (1939)
A Woman's Face (1941)
Charley's Aunt (1941)
Mrs. Miniver (1942)
Random Harvest (1942)
National Velvet (1944)
The Three Musketeers (1948)
Mary Poppins (1964)
Bedknobs and Broomsticks (1971)

P

Al **Pacino**
5ft 7in
(ALFREDO JAMES PACINO)

Born: **April 25, 1940**
New York City, New York, USA

Al's parents, Salvatore and Rose, were from Sicilian backgrounds. They got divorced when he was a young boy. He and his mother then moved in with his grandparents. As a single child, he lived in a fantasy world among adults – frequently re-enacting the scenes from his favorite movies. He enjoyed appearing in his school plays, because he showed little enthusiasm for the academic world. Al knew times would be tough financially when he enrolled at the High School of Performing Arts, but he worked as a messenger and theater usher to make ends meet. He moved on to the Actors Studio in 1966, learning the "method" from Lee Strasberg. His professional stage debut, was in "The Seagull". He won a Tony for "Does a Tiger wear a Necktie?" He made his movie debut in 1969, in *Me Natalie,* and three years later, he was nominated for a Best Supporting Actor Oscar for *The Godfather* and Best Actor for its sequel. There were five other near misses before he won the Best Actor Oscar, for *Scent of a Woman.* Al is justifiably rated as one of the greatest actors of all time. He had a daughter with acting coach, Jan Tarrant, and twins with Beverly D'Angelo.

The Godfather (1972)
Serpico (1973)
The Godfather: Part II (1974)
Dog Day Afternoon (1975)
...And Justice for All (1979)
Scarface (1983) Sea of Love (1989)
Frankie & Johnny (1991)
Glengarry Glen Ross (1992)
Scent of a Woman (1992)
Carlito's Way (1993)
Heat (1995) City Hall (1996)
Donnie Brasco (1997)
Any Given Sunday (1999)
The Insider (1999)
Insomnia (2002)
People I Know (2002)
The Recruit (2003)
The Merchant of Venice (2004)
Two for the Money (2005)
Righteous Kill (2008)

Ellen **Page**
5ft 1in
(ELLEN PHILPOTTS PAGE)

Born: **February 21, 1987**
Halifax, Nova Scotia, Canada

Ellen's father, Dennis, is a designer in the advertising industry. Her mother, Martha, is a schoolteacher. Ellen was educated at Halifax Grammar School and Shambhala School, from where she graduated in 2005. During her schooldays, she developed a love for sports – participating in soccer, track and field and swimming. She is also a good skier and snowboarder. She received her training as an actress from the Neptune Theater in Halifax, which had opened its school in 1997. Ellen's first appearance on a screen was that year, when she played Maggie McLean, in the TV movie,' Pit Pony'. It was an impressive debut - earning her a Canadian TV award nomination. She was very honest with her proud parents – when she was twelve. She felt uncomfortable with them present on the set. She told them so and they've complied. Ellen's movie debut, was in the Canadian drama, *Marion Bridge.* Her petite build got her the role of the fourteen-year old, Hayley Stark, in her first Hollywood picture, *Hard Candy.* It was quickly followed by the blockbuster, *X-Men:The Last Stand.* In 2008, Ellen was nominated for a Best Actress Oscar, for her performance in the outstanding independent movie, *Juno.* Still only twenty-two, she's already laid a solid foundation for a long and successful movie career. In the meantime, she enjoys her leisure hours – as a winter-sports enthusiast. In the summer months, she loves swimming and cycling. Ellen's upcoming movies are the thriller, *Peacock,* and the comedy drama, *Whip It!*

Marion Bridge (2002)
Love That Boy (2003)
Wilby Wonderful (2004)
Hard Candy (2005)
X-Men:
The Last Stand (2006)
An American Crime (2007)
The Tracey Fragments (2007)
Juno (2007)
The Stone Angel (2007)
Smart People (2008)

Geneviève **Page**
5ft 8in
(GENEVIÈVE BRONJEAN)

Born: **December 13, 1930**
Paris, France

Geneviève was a graduate of the Conservatoire National Supérieur d'Art Dramatique de Paris, before joining the famous Comédie Française, and acting in many stage productions of famous French plays, including "Lorenzaccio" and "Les Caprices de Marianne". She continued in classical repertoire at Theatre de l'Odeon in works such as "Le Soulier de satin", "Andromaque" and "La Nuit des Rois". Geneviève made her film debut in 1951, in *Pas de pitié pour les femmes* – a title which translates as *No Pity for Women.* it was followed by a strong supporting role in one of the most popular French swashbuckler's of all time, *Fanfan la Tulipe.* Geneviève was a young actress with the elegance and wit (and fluency in English) to transfer without problems to American films, beginning with Robert Mitchum's *Foreign Intrigue.* Later, she would add her charming presence to hit movies such as *El Cid* and *Grand Prix.* From a career perspective, one of her most important films was *Belle de Jour,* which was directed by Luis Buñuel. She married Jean-Claude Bujard, in 1959. They have two children. Geneviève retired from acting in 2003 after appearing in *Don't Worry, Be Happy.*

Fanfan la Tulipe (1952)
L'Étrange désir de
Monsieur Bard (1954)
Foreign Intrigue (1956)
Michel Strogoff (1956)
Un amour de poche (1957)
Song Without End (1960)
El Cid (1961)
Le Jour et l'heure (1963)
Youngblood Hawke (1964)
Grand Prix (1966)
Tendre voyou (1966)
Belle de jour (1967)
The Private Life of Sherlock
Holmes (1970)
Buffet Froid (1979)
Dark Woods (1989)
Stranger in the House (1992)
Lovers (1999)
Don't Worry, Be Happy (2003)

Geraldine **Page**
5ft 8in
(GERALDINE SUE PAGE)

Born: **November 22, 1924**
Kirksville, Missouri, USA
Died: **June 13, 1987**

The daughter of a physician and his wife, Gerry and her older brother, Donald, moved with them to Chicago when she was five years old. She soon showed keen interest in the arts and could have become a painter, or a pianist. They took a back seat after she joined her church drama club and she started appearing in plays. Following graduation from high school in 1942, she enrolled at the Goodman Theater Dramatic School, in Chicago, and later studied with Uta Hagen. She began her career in 1945, by appearing at the summer theater, in Lake Zurich. She then went to New York, where she found the going tough. Three years of summer stock led in 1948, to her New York debut, in "Seven Mirrors". On her film debut, Gerry was Oscar-nominated as Best Supporting Actress, for *Hondo*. Seven more Oscar nominations followed – Supporting, for *You're a Big Boy Now, Pete 'n' Tillie* and *The Pope of Greenwich Village* and Best Actress, for *Summer and Smoke, Sweet Bird of Youth, Interiors* and *The Trip to Bountiful* – which she won. When she died of a heart attack, Gerry was starring in "Blithe Spirit" on Broadway to great critical acclaim. She is widely regarded as one of the greatest American stage and film actresses of all time. From June 1963, Gerry was married to her second husband, the actor, Rip Torn. They had three children – a daughter and twin sons.

Hondo (1953)
Summer and Smoke (1961)
Sweet Bird of Youth (1962)
Toys in the Attic (1963) Dear Heart (1964)
You're a Big Boy Now (1966)
Whatever Happened to Aunt
Alice? (1969) The Beguiled (1971)
Happy as the Grass was Green (1973)
The Day of the Locust (1975)
Interiors (1978)
I'm Dancing as Fast as I Can (1982)
The Pope of Greenwich Village (1984)
White Nights (1985)
The Trip to Bountiful (1985)

Debra **Paget**
5ft 2in
(DEBRALEE GRIFFIN)

Born: **August 19, 1933**
Denver, Colorado, USA

Debra's family were fanatical about show business. Her mother was determined that her three lovely daughters and her handsome son would succeed. They all studied dance and drama, and when Debra was thirteen years old, she made her stage debut, in "The Merry Wives of Windsor". She was given a 20th Century Fox contract and a supporting role in *Cry of the City* – where she appeared to good effect in two key scenes. Debra decorated several movies in the 1950s, but wasn't considered able to carry a film on her own. She acted in major movies including the biblical epic, *The Ten Commandments* and co-starred with Elvis Presley, on his debut, in *Love Me Tender*. In 1958, she married an actor, David Street, who was sixteen years older and not at all on her wavelength. The marriage lasted three months. She did no better with number two, the director Bud Boetticher – that one survived twenty two days! In 1959, Debra starred in two of the great German film director Fritz Lang's final movies – *The Tiger of Bengal* and *The Indian Tomb*. Debra retired in 1964, after marrying a Chinese oil millionaire, Louis Kung. They were divorced in 1980.

Cry of the City (1948)
House of Strangers (1949)
Broken Arrow (1950)
Fourteen Hours (1951)
Anne of the Indies (1951)
Belles on Their Toes (1952)
Les Misérables (1952)
Stars and Stripes Forever (1952)
Prince Valiant (1954)
Demetrius and
the Gladiators (1954)
White Feather (1955)
Seven Angry Men (1955)
The Last Hunt (1956)
The Ten Commandments (1956)
Love Me Tender (1956)
The River's Edge (1957)
Tiger of Bengal (1959)
Tales of Terror (1962)
The Haunted Palace (1963)

Jack **Palance**
6ft 4in
(VOLODYMYR PALANYUK)

Born: **February 18, 1918**
Lattimer Mines, Pennsylvania, USA
Died: **November 10, 2006**

The son of a coalminer, young Jack set his mind on getting out of that environment as early as possible. He studied hard at high school and attended the University of North Carolina, where he was one of their star athletes. When he graduated in the late 1930s, there wasn't much work to be had, so he fought as a professional boxer in the heavyweight division. Using the name Jack Brazzo, he won his first fifteen fights – twelve of them by KOs. In December 1940, he was stopped by the future contender, Joe Baksi. At the point of America's involvement in World War II, Jack was drafted into the U.S. Air Force, and served as a bomber pilot. His plane was shot down in flames during combat and he needed extensive plastic surgery because of facial burns sustained. After the war, he studied drama at Stanford University. In 1947, Jack made his New York stage debut, in "The Big Two". The leading role in "A Streetcar Named Desire" aroused interest from Hollywood and after marrying Virginia Baker, he made an impressive movie debut, in *Panic in the Streets*. An Oscar nomination, as Best Supporting Actor, for *Sudden Fear,* was followed by a second, one year later, for his role as the evil Jack Wilson, in *Shane*. Thirty-eight years later, Jack won the award, for *City Slickers*. A violent man in many of his films, he lived a quiet private life and died peacefully at his home in Montecito, California.

Panic in the Streets (1950)
Halls of Montezuma (1950)
Sudden Fear (1952) Shane (1953)
The Big Knife (1955) Attack! (1956)
House of Numbers (1957)
Ten Seconds to Hell (1959)
Barabbas (1961) Once a Thief (1965)
The Professionals (1966)
Torture Garden (1967)
Monte Walsh (1970)
Oklahoma Crude (1973)
Young Guns (1988) Batman (1989)
City Slickers (1991)

Michael **Palin**
5ft 10in
(MICHAEL EDWARD PALIN)

Born: **May 5, 1943**
Ranmoor, Sheffield, Yorkshire, England

The son of a steel company engineer, Michael was educated at the Birkdale Preparatory School in Sheffield, where he had his first experience as an actor, in Charles Dickens' "A Christmas Carol". He attended the Shrewsbury School before reading modern history at Brasenose College, Oxford. Michael developed his writing and acting gifts while he was at the university – enjoying comic collaborations with his fellow students, Terry Jones and Robert Hewison. After finishing university, he married a girl called Helen Gibbins, whom he'd first met seven years earlier. Michael got together with Jones to write sketches for various BBC TV program's including 'The Frost Report', and in the early 1970's he got involved with 'Monty Python' as both writer and actor. In 1971, Michael made his movie debut, in the anthology, *And Now for Something Completely Different,* but it was after the Python bubble had finally burst that he established himself as an actor – both comic and serious – most notably for *A Fish Called Wanda,* for which he won a BAFTA as Best Supporting Actor. Another talent was first revealed in 1980, when a film about his childhood train spotting was aired by BBC television and was much admired. His last film appearance was in *Fierce Creatures.* TV programs, with some fascinating glimpses of Michael's round-the-world travels, have kept him famous.

And Now for Something
Completely Different (1971)
Monty Python and the
Holy Grail (1975)
Jabberwocky (1977)
Life of Brian (1979)
Time Bandits (1981)
The Missionary (1982)
The Meaning of Life (1983)
A Private Function (1984)
Brazil (1985)
A Fish Called Wanda (1988)
American Friends (1991)
The Wind in the Willows (1996)
Fierce Creatures (1997)

Eugene **Pallette**
5ft 9in
(EUGENE PALLETTE)

Born: **July 8, 1889**
Winfield, Kansas, USA
Died: **September 3, 1954**

Gene's theatrical parents traveled a lot, which resulted in their son seriously neglecting his education. Until his mid-teens, he often appeared with them in shows, but in an effort to make it on his own, he spent two seasons working as a jockey. When he was eighteen, he took a job as a streetcar conductor, but in 1908, he re-started his show business career by touring with a stock company. In 1913, Gene appeared in five shorts directed by Allan Dwan, the first being *When the Light Fades.* It was a prolific year for the young actor with thirteen films to his name. In 1914, he appeared in more than double that – dramas, westerns, comedies, you name it. Although not credited, he played a Union soldier in the epic, *Birth of a Nation.* His first talkie, *The Canary Murder Case,* in 1929, was his 138th picture! His sound films introduced him to a whole new generation of moviegoers, and he made a new career as a rotund, rasping-voiced character actor – never better than in *The Adventures of Robin Hood, Mr. Smith Goes to Washington, The Lady Eve,* and *Heaven Can Wait.* Gene, who was twice married, retired in 1946. He died of cancer at his home in Los Angeles.

Shanghai Express (1932)
Storm at Daybreak (1933)
I've Got Your Number (1934)
Bordertown (1935)
The Ghost Goes West (1935)
My Man Godfrey (1936)
Topper (1937) One Hundred Men
and a Girl (1937)
The Adventures of Robin Hood (1938)
There Goes My Heart (1938)
Mr. Smith Goes to
Washington (1939)
The Mark of Zorro (1940)
The Lady Eve (1941)
Tales of Manhattan (1942)
The Forest Rangers (1942)
It Ain't Hay (1943)
Heaven Can Wait (1943)
The Gang's All Here (1943)

Lilli **Palmer**
5ft 6in
(LILLI MARIE PEISER)

Born: **May 24, 1914**
Posen, Prussia, Germany
Died: **January 27, 1986**

Lilli was the daughter of a German Jewish surgeon. Her mother had been an actress in Austria, and encouraged her daughter to appear in school plays from the age of ten. Lilli was a keen linguist – spending her school holidays in Kent, England, where she learned English. She studied acting in Berlin before joining the State Theater in Darmstadt – where she played the lead in musicals. When the Nazis took power, she joined her sister Irene, in Paris, where they sang in cabaret. In 1933, Lilli was recommended to Gainsborough Studios, in England, who were looking for new talent. She made her screen debut that year, opposite John Mills, in *The First Offence.* Lilli's breakthrough was nearly two years later, in the film, *Crime Unlimited,* a Warner Brother's production shot at Teddington Studios. During the 1930s, she acted in *Secret Agent* for Hitchcock. In 1943, she married Rex Harrison and had a son the following year. One of her best films, *Body and Soul,* was made just after the end of the war, but she worked internationally until shortly before her death from cancer, in Los Angeles, thirty years later. Lilli's second husband, the movie actor, Carlos Thompson, whom she had married in 1957, returned to Buenos Aires, where he committed suicide, in 1990.

Crime Unlimited (1935)
Secret Agent (1936)
A Girl Must Live (1939)
Thunder Rock (1942)
The Gentle Sex (1943)
The Rake's Progress (1945)
Cloak and Dagger (1946)
Body and Soul (1947)
The Four Poster (1952)
The Devil in Silk (1956)
Between Time and Eternity (1956)
Montparnasse 19 (1958)
But Not for Me (1959)
Conspiracy of Hearts (1960)
The Counterfeit Traitor (1962)
Operation Crossbow (1965)
The Boys from Brazil (1978)

Gwyneth **Paltrow**
5ft 9in
(GWYNETH KATE PALTROW)

Born: **September 27, 1972**
Los Angeles, California, USA

Of Russian Jewish ancestry, Gwyneth is the daughter of the film producer, Bruce Paltrow and the Tony award-winning actress, Blythe Danner. She was raised in Santa Monica, where she attended Crossroads School, and then the private Spence School in New York. From the age of eleven, Gwyneth received her early training as an actress from her parents. She began studying Art History, at the University of California, in Santa Barbara, but dropped out to become an exchange student in Spain. When she got back, she focussed on her acting career – making her professional stage debut in 1990. The following year she made her movie debut in a musical drama, *Shout,* starring John Travolta. A small role in the big-budget *Hook,* led to television roles, more film work, and three years later, to *Se7en,* where, in the impressive company of Morgan Freeman and Brad Pitt (to whom she was engaged until 1997), she went from little known to world famous. Her Best Actress Oscar for *Shakespeare in Love* sealed her stardom. In 2003, she married the "Coldplay" singer, Chris Martin. They have a daughter named Apple and a son named Moses, and live in North London in a house they purchased from Kate Winslet. Gwyneth will soon be seen as Regan, in a new star-studded film version of *King Lear.*

Malice (1993)
Flesh and Bone (1993)
Jefferson in Paris (1995)
Moonlight and Valentino (1995)
Se7en (1995) Emma (1996)
Sliding Doors (1997)
Shakespeare in Love (1998)
The Talented Mr. Ripley (1999)
The Royal Tenenbaums (2001)
Shallow Hal (2001)
Sylvia (2003) Proof (2005)
Infamous (2006)
Running with Scissors (2006)
The Good Night (2007)
Iron Man (2008)
Two Lovers (2008)

Irene **Papas**
5ft 6in
(IRENE LELEKOU)

Born: **September 3, 1926**
Chilimodion, Corynth, Greece

Irene showed early promise as an actress while still a child. Encouraged by her parents, she started going to drama school at the age of twelve. When she was sixteen, she broadened her scope and danced and sang in Greek variety shows. Ultimately, it was as a serious actress in the traditional theater that she would build her reputation. After graduating from the Royal Drama School in Athens, Irene became famous on the stage for her work in such classics as "The Idiot", "Journey's End" and "The Merchant of Venice". During 1943, she changed her stage name after marrying the actor/writer, Alkis Papas. They divorced in 1947, and a year later, she made her movie debut, in the Greek film, *Lost Angels.* On the strength of that, and her continuing work on the stage, she was given a contract in Italy with Lux Films. After a number of continental productions, including *Attila,* with Anthony Quinn, she broke into English language movies, starting with *Tribute to a Bad Man.* She continued to make films in Italy and France, where she appeared in some high-quality television dramas, but she is best known overseas for *Guns of Navarone, Zorba the Greek, Z,* and *Anne of a Thousand Days.* Irene made her last film appearance in *A Talking Picture.*

Tribute to a Bad Man (1956)
The Guns of Navarone (1961)
Elektra (1962)
The Moonspinners (1964)
Zorba the Greek (1964)
Trap for the Assassin (1966)
We Still Kill the
Old Way (1967) Z (1969)
A Dream of Kings (1969)
Anne of a
Thousand Days (1969)
The Trojan Women (1971)
The Message (1976)
Lion of the Desert (1981)
Party (1996)
Captain Corelli's
Mandolin (2001)
A Talking Picture (2003)

Vanessa **Paradis**
5ft 3in
(VANESSA CHANTAL PARADIS)

Born: **December 22, 1972**
Saint-Maur-des-Fessés, Val de Marne, France

Vanessa's mother, Corinne, was about twenty-years of age when her beautiful baby was born. She and her husband, Andre, ran a business which supplied imitation wood to places like Disneyland, Paris. Vanessa was raised in leafy suburbs of the city. When she was five, she was enrolled in dance classes which she loved. She was fascinated by Gene Kelly and she could recite the dialogue from *Singin' in the Rain,* as well as sing the songs. When Vanessa was eight, she performed on the television show, 'L'Ecole des Fans' which launched her career. She recorded her first single "La Magie des Surprises Parties". It was not a hit but it led to her 1987 French Number 1 – "Joe le Taxi". She made her film debut, in *Noce Blanche* – for which she won a César Award, as Most Promising Newcomer. In 1991, she was used by Chanel to promote their new fragrance, "Coco". When she was nineteen, Vanessa went to live in the United States, where she recorded an album in English, "Vanessa Paradis", which was written and produced by her boyfriend at the time, Lenny Kravitz. One of the singles from it, "Be My Baby", did well in both the French and UK charts – where it reached the Top Ten. Vanessa met Johnny Depp in 1994, and four years later, they decided to live together. They now have a daughter, Lily-Rose Melody, and a son named John Christopher – who is known as "Jack". The Depp family has homes in Somerset, England, the South of France, Paris, the Bahamas, and Hollywood. A 2007 album "Dividylle" is already selling well. Vanessa's latest film project is as one of the voices for the 3-D animated, *Un monstre à Paris.*

Noce Blanche (1989)
Élisa (1995)
Un amour de sorcière (1997)
Une chance sur deux (1998)
La Fille sur le pont (1999)
Atomik Circus – Le retour de
James Bataille (2004)
Mon ange (2004)
La Clef (2007)

Anne **Parillaud**
5ft 6¼in
(ANNE PARILLAUD)

Born: **May 6, 1960**
Paris, France

Anne Parillaud is very guarded about her private life and little is known of her early years. What is known is that she studied ballet as a child, but her earliest ambition was to become a lawyer. When she was seventeen years old, Anne made her film debut, with a small role in *Un amour de sable*. It was followed by a bigger role as Estelle, in *L'Hôtel de la plage,* during the school summer holidays, in 1978. There were a number of teen movies and the exciting thriller entitled, *Pour la peau d'un flic* – directed by and starring, Alain Delon, with whom she had an affair and also appeared with, in *Le Battant*. After that, apart from a number of television dramas, including the Italian-made mini-series, 'Nessuno torna in dietro', nothing much happened until the Italian made comedy movie, *Che ora è?* – opposite Marcello Mastroianni. A year later, Anne became famous internationally when she starred in the imitated but never bettered original, *La Femme Nikita* – for which she won a Best Actress César. After that, she was able to switch from French to English language films like *The Man in the Iron Mask,* with no problem. Having been first married to Luc Besson, with whom she had a daughter, Juliette, Anne was a little wary about another serious commitment. As things turned out, the waiting was well worthwhile. She and the composer Jean-Michel Jarre, tied the knot in May 2005.

Pour la peau d'un flic (1981)
Le Battant (1983)
Che ora è? (1989)
La Femme Nikita (1990)
Innocent Blood (1992)
Map of the Human Heart (1993)
Frankie Starlight (1995)
Dead Girl (1996)
Passage à l'acte (1996)
The Man in the Iron Mask (1998)
Gangsters (2002)
Sex Is Comedy (2002)
Deadlines (2004)
Kid Power (2007)
The Last Mistress (2007)

Cecil **Parker**
6ft
(CECIL SCHWABE)

Born: **September 3, 1897**
Hastings, East Sussex, England
Died: **April 20, 1971**

Cecil spent his early years on the English south coast. Following his schooldays, he started to train as an actor, but shortly after World War I began, he joined the British Army. By the early 1920s, Cecil had focussed again on an acting career and he first appeared on stage in a provincial theater production, in 1922. He established himself on the West End stage, in London, before making his film debut, at the age of thirty-six, with a supporting role in *The Golden Cage*. His first major film three years later was *The Man Who Changed His Mind* – starring the master of Horror, Boris Karloff. He was third-billed, below Vivien Leigh and Rex Harrison in *Storm in a Teacup* and he was rarely the star. Cecil was reputed to have never given a poor performance. After struggling to arrive at this long short-list, who am I to argue? Cecil remained near his birthplace all his life and died in Brighton.

The Man Who Changed His Mind (1936)
Dark Journey (1937) Storm in a
Teacup (1937) The Lady Vanishes (1938)
The Citadel (1938) The Stars Look
Down (1939) Dangerous
Moonlight (1941) Caesar and
Cleopatra (1945) The Magic Bow (1946)
Hungry Hill (1947) Captain
Boycott (1947) Quartet (1948)
Dear Mr. Prohack (1949)
The Chiltern Hundreds (1949)
The Man in the White Suit (1951)
The Magic Box (1951)
I Believe in You (1952)
Father Brown (1954)
The Constant Husband (1955)
The Court Jester (1955)
The Lady Killers (1955)
23 Paces to Baker Street (1956)
The Admirable Crichton (1957)
A Tale of Two Cities (1958)
Indiscreet (1958)
I Was Monty's Double (1958)
Swiss Family Robinson (1960)
Heaven's Above! (1963)
Guns at Batasi (1964)

Eleanor **Parker**
5ft 6½in
(ELEANOR JEAN PARKER)

Born: **June 26, 1922**
Cedarville, Ohio, USA

Eleanor was the third of three children born to a mathematics teacher and his wife. At junior school she began appearing in plays and from the age of fifteen, she participated in the annual Rice Summer Theater, at Martha's Vineyard. She was offered a contract by 20th Century Fox, but she turned it down to graduate from high school and gain stage experience. Eventually, she went to live in California, where she studied acting at the Pasadena Playhouse. She signed a Warner brothers contract after finishing her course, and in 1941, was cast in *They Died with Their Boots On,* but was left on the cutting room floor. A year later, she made her movie debut, in a B-Picture called *Busses Roar*. Eleanor met her first husband, a Navy dentist, on the film set of the pro-Soviet, *Mission to Moscow*. The marriage lasted eighteen months. Her film career flourished from 1945. She was nominated for Best Actress Oscars – for *Caged,* for which she was voted Best Actress, at the Venice Film Festival, *Detective Story,* and *Interrupted Melody.* Her last big movie was *The Sound of Music,* but she went on acting until 1991, when she appeared in a TV drama, 'Dead on the Money'. She had four children from her four marriages.

Mission to Moscow (1943)
Between Two Worlds (1944)
The Very Thought of You (1944)
Pride of the Marines (1945)
The Voice of the Turtle (1947)
The Woman in White (1948)
Caged (1950)
A Millionaire for Christy (1951)
Detective Story (1951)
Scaramouche (1952)
Above and Beyond (1952)
Escape from Fort Bravo (1953)
The Naked Jungle (1953)
Interrupted Melody (1955)
The Man with the Golden Arm (1955)
A Hole in the Head (1959)
Home from the Hill (1960)
The Sound of Music (1965)
Warning Shot (1967)

Jean **Parker**
5ft 3in
(LOIS MAE GREEN)

Born: **August 11, 1915**
Deer Lodge, Montana, USA
Died: **November 30, 2005**

Jean grew up in poverty. Following her parents' long-term unemployment, she was adopted by a family in Pasadena, where she attended high school and showed talent for art, music and dancing. In 1932, she entered a poster competition and won it. The story and her photo appeared in a Los Angeles newspaper and before she knew it, she was called by Louis B. Mayer's office and invited for a screen test. Within a couple of days she was given an MGM contract and had her name changed to Jean Parker. The studio organized acting and speech classes and in 1932, she made her film debut, in *Divorce in the Family*. Next was a small uncredited role, in *Rasputin and the Empress* – the only film where John, Ethel, and Lionel Barrymore acted together. Once she got into her stride, Jean became a very big star in the 1930s. *Little Women* and *The Ghost Goes West* are her best movies. Her last was the B-western, *Apache Uprising,* in 1966. Jean was divorced four times by 1957, and didn't remarry. She died of a stroke at the Woodland Hills retirement home.

The Secret of
Madame Blanche (1933)
Gabriel Over the
White House (1933)
Storm at Daybreak (1933)
Lady for a Day (1933)
Little Women (1933)
A Wicked Woman (1934)
Limehouse Blues (1934)
Sequoia (1934)
Princess O'Hara (1935)
The Ghost Goes West (1935)
The Texas Rangers (1936)
The Flying Deuces (1940)
Son of the Navy (1940)
Beyond Tomorrow (1940)
Minesweeper (1943)
Bluebeard (1944)
The Gunfighter (1950)
Black Tuesday (1954)
A Lawless Street (1955)

Mary-Louise **Parker**
5ft 8in
(MARY-LOUISE PARKER)

Born: **August 2, 1964**
Fort Jackson, South Carolina, USA

Mary-Louise's father was a judge, who served in the United States Army, and her mother was from Sweden. She and her older siblings grew up as "army brats" on bases in different parts of the USA. She first became interested in drama at high school, and went on to major in Acting at North Carolina School of the Arts. She got her first TV bit part in the soap opera, 'Ryan's Hope'. After graduating, she went to New York. In 1989, she first appeared on the big screen, in *Signs of Life*. Mary-Louise made her Broadway debut in 1990 in "Prelude to a Kiss" – in the leading role of Rita, for which she won the Clarence Derwent Award. It was also the year when she made a big impression in the movie *Longtime Companion* – which dealt very sensitively with the difficult subject of AIDS. Strong supporting roles in films and regular stage work have helped build her reputation. In 1997, Mary-Louise acted in the critically praised play, "How I Learned to Drive". She has a son, William, from a seven year relationship with Billy Crudup and has recently adopted a baby girl from Africa. Mary-Louise's work in the western about Jesse James, is excellent, and her role in the very entertaining family fantasy film, *The Spiderwick Chronicles,* confirms her status as a major talent. From 2005, she appeared in fifty episodes of the TV comedy crime drama, 'Weeds'.

Longtime Companion (1990)
Grand Canyon (1991)
Fried Green Tomatoes (1991)
Naked in New York (1993)
Mr. Wonderful (1993)
The Client (1994)
Bullets Over Broadway (1994)
The Five Senses (1999)
Pipe Dream (2002)
Red Dragon (2002)
Saved! (2004)
Romance & Cigarettes (2005)
The Assassination of
Jesse James by the Coward
Robert Ford (2007)
The Spiderwick Chronicles (2008)

Sarah Jessica **Parker**
5ft 4in
(SARAH JESSICA PARKER)

Born: **March 25, 1965**
Nelsonville, Ohio, USA

Sarah was one of eight children from her mother Barbra's two marriages. Her father, Stephen Parker, was Jewish. Sarah started her career early in life when she was trained in ballet and singing. She studied at the Professional Children's School and at the American Ballet School. With four of her siblings, she appeared in a production of "The Sound of Music" and then landed the title role of "Annie", on Broadway. Her family moved to New Jersey around that time, and Sarah went to the local Dwight Morrow High School in Englewood. In 1982, she landed a role in the TV-movie 'My Body, My Child' and then in the high school sit-com, 'Square Pegs'. A year later, she made her film debut, in *Somewhere Tomorrow*. In 1985, she began a six year relationship with Robert Downey Jr. By the time that finished, her career had taken off: key roles with A-List stars like Johnny Depp put her firmly on the map. In 1997, she had doubts about committing herself to a TV-series, but accepted the role of Carrie Bradshaw, in the mega-hit "Sex and the City". It coincided with a slow-down in her career, and its success has rejuvenated her. Since 1997, Sarah's been married to Matthew Broderick. They have a son. Despite the quite justified critical slating aimed at the film, *Sex and the City,* Jessica's maintained her good run of successes – co-starring with Dennis Quaid in the smart comedy – *Smart People.*

Somewhere Tomorrow (1983)
Girls Just Want to Have Fun (1985)
Flight of the Navigator (1986)
L.A.Story (1991)
Honeymoon in Vegas (1992)
Hocus Pocus (1993)
Ed Wood (1994)
The Substance of Fire (1996)
The First Wives Club (1996)
Mars Attacks! (1996)
State and Main (2000)
The Family Stone (2005)
Spinning Into Butter (2007)
Smart People (2008)

Larry **Parks**
5ft 10in
(SAMUEL KLUSMAN LAWRENCE PARKS)

Born: **December 13, 1914**
Olathe, Kansas, USA
Died: **April 13, 1975**

Larry was of German and Irish descent. As a child - when he was growing up in Joliet, Illinois, Larry suffered from several serious illnesses, including rheumatic fever. He grew stronger through sheer will-power and determination, so that by the time he graduated from Joliet Township High School, he'd successfully participated in sports. His parents were delighted when he majored in Science at the University of Illinois. They were less pleased when, after involvement in college dramatics, he dropped the idea of becoming a doctor. He worked in touring shows before making the big move to New York City. He was a Radio City tour guide and a Carnegie Hall usher, while appearing in summer stock. His first film, in 1934, was *You Belong To Me.* In 1937, Larry made his Broadway debut, in the Group Theater's production of "Golden Boy". He acted in several of their plays, but was forced to return home when his beloved father died. For more than two years, he worked as a Pullman inspector and then in construction, until, in 1941, he landed a Columbia contract. After his film debut, in *Mystery Ship,* in 1941, he was with them for nine years. Larry was Oscar-nominated for *The Jolson Story.* He and his wife, Betty Garrett, were victims of blacklisting during the McCarthy era. Their sons are both in show business. Larry was on TV in the late 1950s. His final film, was *Freud.* He died of a heart attack – in Studio City, California.

The Boogie Man
Will Get You (1942)
Reveille with Beverly (1943)
Is Everybody Happy? (1943)
Hey Rookie (1944)
Counter-Attack (1945)
Renegades (1946)
The Jolson Story (1946)
Down to Earth (1947)
The Swordsman (1948)
Jolson Sings Again (1949)
Emergency Wedding (1950)
Freud (1962)

Michael **Parks**
6ft
(HARRY SAMUEL PARKS)

Born: **April 24, 1940**
Corona, California, USA

The son of a truckdriver, Mike dropped out of Sacramento High school after getting married at the age of fifteen. He had several jobs including upholstering caskets. He turned down an offer to play minor league baseball because he was earning more money doing that. In 1960, he was discovered by a talent scout who got him TV work starting with 'Zane Grey Theater' and continuing for four years, with other top shows including 'The Untouchables', 'Gunsmoke', 'Perry Mason', '77 Sunset Strip' and 'Ben Casey'. Mike made his film debut in 1965, opposite Ann-Margret, in *Bus Riley's Back in Town.* His second marriage, to actress Jan Moriarty, ended after only a few months, when she committed suicide with a pills overdose. Mike was steadily employed on TV and in films and made a number of country/blues albums during that period. In 1969, he starred in and sang the theme song for the series, 'Then Came Bronson'. A fine athlete, Mike narrowly missed out on qualification as a miler for the USA, in the 1972 Olympics. Apart from five episodes of 'Twin Peaks', the 1980s and early 1990s weren't vintage years, but since being cast by Quentin Tarantino, as Earl McGraw, in *Kill Bill,* his movie career has soared into another league. Actor James Parks, is his son.

Bus Riley's Back in Town (1965)
Wild Seed (1965) The Last Hard
Men (1976) The Private Files
of J.Edgar Hoover (1977)
North Sea Hijack (1979)
From Dusk Till Dawn (1996)
Deceiver (1997)
Niagara, Niagara (1997)
Julian Po (1997)
Big Bad Love (2001)
Kill Bill: Vol 1 (2003) Kill Bill: Vol 2 (2004)
The Listening (2006)
Grindhouse (2007) Death Proof (2007)
Planet Terror (2007)
The Assassination of Jesse James
by the Coward Robert Ford (2007)
Three Priests (2008)

Estelle **Parsons**
5ft 4in
(ESTELLE MARGARET PARSONS)

Born: **November 20, 1927**
Marblehead, Massachusetts, USA

Estelle was the daughter of Eben Parsons and Elinore Ingebore Mattson, who was born in Sweden. She was a childhood friend of Jack Lemmon. After attending the Oak Grove School for Girls, in Vassalboro, Maine, Estelle graduated from Connecticut College, in New London, in 1949. She then studied Law at Boston University Law School, but dropped out to pursue an acting career. Initially, she earned a living by teaching acting at Yale and Columbia Universities. In 1952, she was hired by NBC because of her legal knowledge, as a political news writer, producer and reporter on the 'Today Show'. In 1953, she married Richard Gehman and had twin daughters during their five year marriage. After her divorce Estelle re-focussed on acting and made her film debut, in *Ladybug Ladybug.* She then did four years on stage and acted in several television series before winning a Best Supporting Actress Oscar, for playing Blanche, in *Bonnie and Clyde.* She was nominated for *Rachel, Rachel,* and went on to get Tony nominations for her work in "The Seven Descents of Myrtle" and "And Miss Reardon Drinks a Little". Estelle also directed the Broadway productions of "Romeo and Juliet", "As You Like It", and "Macbeth". Following twelve years without a good film role – the last being Margaret, in *Looking for Richard* – directed by Al Pacino, Estelle will shortly be seen in *Salomaybe?* – also directed by the great man. Since 1983, she has been married to her second husband, Peter Zimroth. They adopted a son.

Ladybug Ladybug (1963)
Bonnie and Clyde (1967)
Rachel, Rachel (1968)
Watermelon Man (1970)
I Never Sang for My Father (1970)
I Walk the Line (1970)
Two People (1973)
For Pete's Sake (1974)
Dick Tracy (1990)
Boys On the Side (1995)
Looking for Richard (1996)

Gail **Patrick**
5ft 7in
(MARGARET LAVELLE FITZPATRICK)

Born: **June 20, 1911**
Birmingham, Alabama, USA
Died: **July 6, 1980**

Gail was the daughter of an Irishman and a woman from a Southern family. She was an outdoor girl during her formative years – swimming, riding and tennis being her favorite sports. Gail attended Howard College, in San Angelo, Texas, where she demonstrated her leadership qualities as dean of women. She was then a pre-law student at the University of Alabama before setting her sights on an acting career. She signed for Paramount, after a nationwide contest, and in 1932, she made her film debut, with an uncredited appearance in *If I Had a Million*. The following year, she featured in a western, *The Mysterious Rider*. Gail soon developed into a top-quality supporting actress. In the mid-1930s, she perfected a hard-as-nails character, as a rival to star leading ladies – Carole Lombard – in *My Man Godfrey*; Ginger Rogers – in *Stage Door*; and Irene Dunne – in *My Favorite Wife*. She retired in 1948, but was seen in one 1966 episode of Perry Mason. Gail had two children from her four marriages. She died of leukemia, in Los Angeles.

Murders in the Zoo (1933)
To the Last Man (1933)
Death Takes a Holiday (1934)
Murder at the Vanities (1934)
Mississippi (1935)
No More Ladies (1935)
Doubting Thomas (1935)
Two-Fisted (1935)
The Lone Wolf Returns (1935)
Two in the Dark (1936)
My Man Godfrey (1936)
Artists & Models (1937)
Stage Door (1937)
Mad About Music (1938)
Dangerous to Know (1938)
Man of Conquest (1939)
My Favorite Wife (1940)
The Doctor Takes a Wife (1940)
Love Crazy (1941)
We Were Dancing (1942)
Tales of Manhattan (1942)
Up in Mabel's Room (1944)

Nigel **Patrick**
6ft
(NIGEL DENNIS WEMYSS)

Born: **May 2, 1913**
London, England
Died: **September 21, 1981**

Nigel's mother was the actress, Dorothy Turner. Aided by her private coaching and enthusiastic encouragement, Nigel was good enough to make his stage debut in 1932. He established himself in the London West End over a period of seven years. In 1939, he made his first film – a low budget crime movie called *Mrs. Pym of Scotland Yard*. Frustratingly, that new career was interrupted by World War II. Nigel served as a lieutenant colonel in the British Army. His return to acting, in 1946, was in an early television drama, 'Morning Departure'. He worked his way back into movies with supporting roles in British films and developed into a smooth leading man. In 1952, his performance in *The Sound Barrier,* earned him a BAFTA nomination as Best Actor. For one of his few forays into the international arena, *Raintree County,* Nigel was nominated for a Golden Globe. For over twenty-eight years he was happily married to Irish-born actress, Beatrice Campbell – who died in 1979. Two years later, at his home in London, Nigel succumbed to lung cancer.

Spring in Park Lane (1948)
Silent Dust (1949)
Morning Departure (1950)
Trio (1950)
Pandora and the
Flying Dutchman (1951)
The Browning Version (1951)
Encore (1951)
The Sound Barrier (1952)
The Pickwick Papers (1952)
The Sea Shall Not Have
Them (1954)
All for Mary (1955)
How to Murder a Rich Uncle (1957)
Raintree County (1957)
Count Five and Die (1957)
Sapphire (1959)
The League of Gentlemen (1960)
The Trials of Oscar Wilde (1960)
The Informers (1963)
Battle of Britain (1969)
The MacKintosh Man (1973)

Paula **Patton**
5ft 4in
(PAULA MAXINE PATTON)

Born: **December 5, 1975**
Los Angeles, California, USA

When you hear that Paula's family home was just across the street from 20th Century Fox Studios, it's hardly surprising to learn that she has been a movie fan for as long as she can remember. Her father, who was a lawyer, was the more serious of her two parents, but her mother, who was a schoolteacher, was also fond of movies. When she was quite little, Paula would fantasize about playing different roles. By the time she attended Hamilton Magnet Arts High School of Music, in Los Angeles, she was one of the regular actresses in its plays. After she graduated from high school, Paula went to study Film at the University of California at Berkeley, in a summer program which quickly led to a three-month assignment. She was then making documentaries for the Public Broadcasting Service, as well as for the Howard Mandel talk show. She then worked as a producer with the Discovery Channel. Paula enjoyed the work, but at the back of her mind was the dream of becoming a performer. She started taking acting lessons. In 2005, she played Detective Angela Kellogg, in the Fox TV drama, 'Murder Book'. Close on its heels, was her film debut, for Columbia Pictures – *Hitch,* which starred Will Smith and Eva Mendes. A year later, Paula was Denzel Washington's leading lady, in the effective thriller, *Deja Vu*. She is married to the singer/songwriter, Robin Thicke – himself the son of actors. They first met at a teen club in Los Angeles, when she was fifteen and he was fourteen. The young couple are currently concentrating all their efforts on individual careers before they have the children they both want. Paula is working on a film drama titled *This Wednesday*.

Hitch (2005)
London (2005)
Idlewild (2006)
Deja Vu (2006)
Push: Based on the
Novel by Sapphire (2008)
Swing Vote (2008)
Mirrors (2008)

Bill **Paxton**
5ft 11in
(WILLIAM PAXTON)

Born: **May 17, 1955**
Fort Worth, Texas, USA

Bill's father, John, was a multi-faceted character, who at different times, had been a businessman, a lumber wholesaler, a museum executive – and when he had the opportunity – an actor. Bill's mother, Mary Lou, took care of the home and made sure that her son grew up to be a good Catholic. After leaving high school, Bill attended Southwest Texas State University, in San Marcos. He then went to Los Angeles, where he worked as a set designer on the films of Roger Corman. He made his debut in a Corman film, *Crazy Mama,* in 1975. Although it was a poor film, the experience was enough to make his mind up to become an actor. His first step was a move to New York City to study with Stella Adler. In 1980, Bill directed a comedy short called *Fish Heads* which was shown on 'Saturday Night Live'. His career in TV and movies kicked off and he was a member of the band, "Martini Ranch". After James Cameron directed the band's video, Bill got a small role in *The Terminator,* followed by a bigger one in *Aliens.* He has two children with his second wife, Louise Newbury. Since 2006, Bill has been 'Bill Henrickson' in the TV series, 'Big Love'.

The Terminator (1984)
Weird Science (1985)
Aliens (1986)
Near Dark (1987)
Brain Dead (1990)
Predator 2 (1990)
One False Move (1992)
Trespass (1992)
Indian Summer (1993)
Frank & Jesse (1994)
True Lies (1994)
Apollo 13 (1995)
The Last Supper (1995)
Twister (1996)
Traveller (1997)
Titanic (1997)
A Simple Plan (1998)
U-571 (2000)
Frailty (2001)
The Good Life (2007)

John **Payne**
6ft 1in
(JOHN PAYNE)

Born: **May 23, 1912**
Roanoke, Virginia, USA
Died: **December 6, 1989**

John's father was the grandly-named, George Washington Payne, who worked as a property developer. His mother, Ida, was a graduate from the local seminary. John also had a small piece of musical history in his family background: he was a direct descendant of John Howard Payne – the composer of the song "Home Sweet Home". John attended Roanoke College before studying Drama at Columbia University. Following that, he took some singing lessons at Juilliard. For a time he made a living as a wrestler, and from work as a crooner in vaudeville. In 1934, he was heard by a talent scout for the Shubert Theater Group and taken on as a stock player. Following two seasons performing with them and singing on radio shows, John was offered a 20th Century Fox contract. He made his film debut, in *Dodsworth,* and married the actress, Anne Shirley. By the 1940s he was a star – in hit films like *Sun Valley Serenade, The Razor's Edge* and *Miracle on 34th Street.* John's second wife was Gloria DeHaven. They had two children. He made his last film, *They Ran for Their Lives,* in 1968, and did TV work until retiring in 1975. John died of heart failure, in Malibu, California.

Dodsworth (1936)
Hats Off (1936)
College Swing (1938)
Garden of the Moon (1938)
Wings of the Navy (1939)
Star Dust (1940)
The Great Profile (1940)
Tin Pan Alley (1940)
Sun Valley Serenade (1941)
Week-End in Havana (1941)
Remember the Day (1941)
Footlight Serenade (1942)
Springtime in the Rockies (1942)
The Dolly Sisters (1945)
Sentimental Journey (1946)
The Razor's Edge (1946)
Miracle on 34th Street (1947)
Larceny (1948)
The Boss (1956)

Guy **Pearce**
5ft 10in
(GUY EDWARD PEARCE)

Born: **October 5, 1967**
Ely, Cambridgeshire, England

Guy's mother, Anne, was schoolteacher, his father, Stuart, was a New Zealand-born air force test pilot. When Guy was three, the family moved to Geelong, in Australia, where Anne ran a deer farm. His father died when he was nine and he was raised by his mother. He attended Geelong College, where he competed as an amateur bodybuilder. In his early twenties, he won the title "Mr. Natural Victoria". Guy's interest in being in the spotlight took a new turn when he started getting small roles in plays. It moved up a gear, when in 1985, he was cast in the role of Mike Young, in the popular Australian soap opera, 'Neighbours'. In 1990, he made his big screen debut in an independent film, *Friday on My Mind.* After more television work and minor films, he got international movie exposure in the funny, extraordinary, Australian hit, *The Adventures of Priscilla, Queen of the Desert.* After a poor decision to try to impersonate Errol Flynn, he shone in *Dating the Enemy,* and secured his future with his first Hollywood film role, as Ed Exley, in the excellent *L.A.Confidential.* 1997 was also the year he married psychologist Kate Mestitz. Her influence has certainly helped keep his career moving on an upward path.

The Adventures of Priscilla,
Queen of the Desert (1994)
Dating the Enemy (1996)
L.A.Confidential (1997)
Ravenous (1999)
Memento (2000)
The Count of Monte Cristo (2002)
The Hard Word (2002)
Till Human Voices
Wake Us (2002)
Deux frères (2004)
The Proposition (2005)
First Snow (2006)
Factory Girl (2006)
Death Defying Acts (2007)
Winged Creatures (2007)
Traitor (2008)
The Hurt Locker (2008)
Bedtime Stories (2008)

Gregory **Peck**
6ft 3in
(ELDRED GREGORY PECK)

Born: **April 5, 1916**
La Jolla, California, USA
Died: **June 12, 2003**

Greg's parents divorced when he was five, so he was raised by his grandmother, who took him to the movies once a week. After San Diego College, he studied Medicine at Berkeley, where he became interested in acting. He went to New York, worked at the 1939 World's Fair, and won a scholarship to the Neighborhood Playhouse. After graduating from there, Greg made his Broadway debut, in "The Morning Star" and in 1944, his film debut, in *Days of Glory*. A spinal injury suffered at college meant he was unfit for war service. It gave him an opportunity, which he grabbed with both hands. He was nominated for Oscars – for *The Keys of the Kingdom, The Yearling, Gentleman's Agreement,* and *Twelve O'Clock High,* before finally being voted Best Actor, for *To Kill a Mockingbird.* Greg had five children from his two marriages. His second wife, Veronique, was by his side when he died in Los Angeles – from a combination of cardiac arrest and bronchial pneumonia.

The Keys of the Kingdom (1944)
The Valley of Decision (1945)
Spellbound (1945) **The Yearling** (1946)
Duel in the Sun (1946)
The Paradine Case (1947)
Gentleman's Agreement (1947)
Yellow Sky (1948)
Twelve O'Clock High (1949)
The Gunfighter (1950)
Captain Horatio Hornblower R.N. (1952)
The Snows of Kilimanjaro (1965)
Roman Holiday (1953) **The Man in the Gray Flannel Suit** (1956)
Moby Dick (1956) **The Bravados** (1958)
The Big Country (1958)
Pork Chop Hill (1959)
On the Beach (1959)
The Guns of Navarone (1961)
Cape Fear (1962)
To Kill a Mockingbird (1962)
Captain Newman M.D. (1963)
Mirage (1965) **The Omen** (1976)
The Boys from Brazil (1978)
The Sea Wolves (1980) **Cape Fear** (1991)

Simon **Pegg**
5ft 9in
(SIMON JOHN BECKINGHAM)

Born: **February 14, 1970**
Gloucester, Gloucestershire, England

Simon is the son of jazz musician, John Pegg, and Gillian Smith, who was a civil servant. They divorced when he was seven. He was educated in Gloucester at the Brockworth Comprehensive School and after that, he focussed on literature and performance studies at Stratford College and was the drummer in a band called "God's Third Leg". Finally, he graduated from the University of Bristol with a BA in Theater, Film and Television. Simon moved to London in 1993 – working as a stand-up comic until moving into television and shows such as 'Asylum', 'Six Pairs of Pants', and 'Faith in the Future'. From 1998, he was a regular on BBC Radio 4's 'The 99p Challenge'. A year later, Simon was nominated for a British Comedy Award, for the Channel 4 TV-comedy 'Spaced', which co-starred his best friend, Nick Frost. He made his film debut, in *Guest House Paradiso,* in 1999, but it took another four years of television work before he really grasped the medium with the brilliant short film, *Danger! 50,000 Zombies!* and a starring role in *Shaun of the Dead* – for which he shared both a British Independent Film Award and a Bram Stoker Award. 2007 was a vintage year for Simon Pegg films – with *Hot Fuzz* (which he co-wrote), *Grindhouse* and *Run Fatboy Run* (also co-writer) being something special. Simon's married to Maureen McCann. He will next be seen in the role of 'Scotty' in a new *Star Trek* movie.

Guest House Paradiso (1999)
The Reckoning (2003)
Shaun of the Dead (2004)
The League of Gentlemen's Apocalypse (2005)
Land of the Dead (2005)
Mission Impossible III (2006)
Big Nothing (2006)
The Good Night (2007)
Hot Fuzz (2007) **Grindhouse** (2007)
Run Fatboy Run (2007)
How to Lose Friends and Alienate People (2008)
Srar Trek (2009)

Chris **Penn**
5ft 10in
(CHRISTOPHER SHANNON PENN)

Born: **October 10, 1965**
Los Angeles, California, USA
Died: **January 24, 2006**

From the multi-talented Penn family, Chris was the son of film director, Leo Penn, and the actress, Eileen Ryan. His two older brothers are the fine actor, Sean Penn, and Aimee Mann's husband – musician and songwriter, Michael Penn. Chris began acting when he was eleven, at the Loft Studio in Los Angeles. He received his training from Peggy Feury. He was an enthusiastic karate practitioner and had a black belt classification. Chris was fourteen when he made his first film appearance, in a mediocre children's fantasy, *Charlie and the Talking Buzzard.* Three years later, he was given much better material, in the TV series, 'Magnum P.I.' and the exciting crime drama movie, *Rumble Fish.* His career built steadily with the hit dance musical, *Footloose,* and he appeared with his mother and brother Sean in *At Close Range.* There were good parts in two Tarantino films and a Best Supporting Actor Award, at the 1996 Venice Film Festival, for *The Funeral.* Chris had been suffering weight problems for some time when died in Santa Monica, at only forty years of age, from the effects of an enlarged heart. His final film *Aftermath,* is currently in post-production and will be released soon.

Rumble Fish (1983)
Footloose (1984)
Pale Rider (1985)
At Close Range (1986)
Reservoir Dogs (1992)
The Music of Chance (1993)
Short Cuts (1993)
True Romance (1993)
Imaginary Crimes (1994)
Mulholland Falls (1996)
The Funeral (1996)
The Boys Club (1997)
Deceiver (1997)
Rush Hour (1998)
Murder by Numbers (2002)
Starsky & Hutch (2004)
After the Sunset (2004)
Holly (2006)

Sean **Penn**
5ft 9in
(SEAN JUSTIN PENN)

Born: **August 17, 1960**
Santa Monica, California, USA

Sean was the son of Jewish immigrants from Lithuania and Russia, on his father's side, and Italian/Irish Catholics, on his mother's. He was raised in a secular home and grew up to be an Agnostic. He was educated at Santa Monica College, where he studied Speech and Auto Mechanics, but didn't graduate. In 1974 he made his TV debut in 'Little House on the Prairie', in an episode directed by his dad, Leo. Sean studied acting at The Beverly Hills Playhouse at the same time as Michelle Pfeiffer, and made his movie debut, in *Taps*. His work is characterized by an intense and powerful style, which is not dissimilar to that of Al Pacino. Sean and his first wife, Madonna, were divorced in 1989. He married Robin Wright Penn in 1996. The couple have two children. On the professional front, Sean has already had five Best Actor Oscar nominations in his career – for *Dead Man Walking, Sweet and Lowdown, I Am Sam* and for *Mystic River* – which he won. In the 2009 Oscars Sean's Harvey *Milk* faced a 'close contest' against Mickey Rourke's *The Wrestler*. He emerged triumphant – holding aloft the Best Actor Academy Award.

Taps (1981) **Fast Times at Ridgemount High** (1982)
Bad Boys (1983)
Racing with the Moon (1984)
The Falcon and the Snowman (1985)
At Close Range (1986) **Colors** (1988)
Casualties of War (1989)
State of Grace (1990)
Carlito's Way (1993)
Dead Man Walking (1995)
She's So Lovely (1997)
U Turn (1997) **The Game** (1997)
The Thin Red Line (1998)
Sweet and Lowdown (1999)
I Am Sam (2001) **Mystic River** (2003)
21 Grams (2003)
**The Assassination
of Richard Nixon** (2004)
The Interpreter (2005)
All the King's Men (2006)
Milk (2008)

George **Peppard**
6ft
(GEORGE PEPPARD JR.)

Born: **October 1, 1928**
Detroit, Michigan, USA
Died: **May 8, 1994**

George was the son of George Peppard Sr., a building contractor, and his wife, Vernelle Rohrer. George was educated at Dearborn High School, in Dearborn, the tenth largest city in the state of Michigan. After he graduated from high school, he joined the United States Marine Corps, where during nineteen months service he achieved the rank of gunnery sergeant. On his return to civilian life, George continued his education when he attended Purdue University, in West Lafayette, Indiana, where he studied Civil Engineering and later went to Carnegie Mellon University, in Pittsburgh. Following a variety of short-term jobs, the handsome twenty-one-year-old joined the Pittsburgh Playhouse and worked as a part-time disc-jockey. In 1954, he married the first of his five wives – Helen Davies, with whom he had two children. After a number of on and off-Broadway productions, in 1956, George made his screen debut – on TV, in an episode of 'The United States Steel Hour'. A year later, he made his film debut, in the powerful drama, *The Strange One*. He was a Hollywood name after he co-starred with lovely Audrey Hepburn in *Breakfast at Tiffany's*. By 1970, his movie star faded but he became popular on TV through two series – 'Banacek' and 'The A-Team'. He overcame a drinking problem in 1978 and worked in films and TV until the year of his death, in Los Angeles, from pneumonia.

The Strange One (1957)
Pork Chop Hill (1959)
Home from the Hill (1960)
Breakfast at Tiffany's (1961)
How the West Was Won (1962)
The Victors (1963)
The Carpetbaggers (1964)
Operation Crossbow (1965)
The Third Day (1965)
The Blue Max (1966) **Tobruk** (1967)
**What's So Bad About
Feeling Good?** (1968)
Rough Night in Jericho (1968)
Five Days from Home (1979)

Vincent **Perez**
5ft 11½in
(VINCENT PEREZ)

Born: **June 10, 1962**
Lausanne, Vaud, Switzerland

Vincent, the second of three children, grew up speaking several languages – his father, who ran an import/export business, was Spanish and his mother was German. Added to this was the Swiss French location of his early schooling. Vincent was artistically gifted, and considered a career as a photographer or painter, but after seeing a Charlie Chaplin movie when he was seven years old, he made up his mind to become an actor. He began studying drama in Geneva, but at eighteen, with his mother's encouragement, Vincent went to France – where he first attended the Conservatoire in Paris, and then L'Ecole des Amandiers, in Nanterre. While he was still a student, he made his film debut, in *Gardien de la nuit,* and after finishing his studies, he gained experience on the stages of the French provincial theaters. He enjoyed a worldwide following after appearing in the huge success, *Cyrano de Bergerac.* From then on, Vincent wasn't only a star in France. He played in the Oscar-winning, *Indochine,* and in 1993, made his debut as a director, with the short, *L'Exchange.* He lives in France with his wife Karine Silla and their four children. Vincent's next appearance will be in the drama, *Inhale* – an American production with Diane Kruger and Dermot Mulroney.

Gardien de la nuit (1986)
The House of Jade (1988)
Cyrano de Bergerac (1990)
The Voyage of Captain Fracasse (1990)
Snow and Fire (1991)
Indochine (1992) **Fanfan** (1993)
Beyond the Clouds (1995)
Ligne de vie (1996)
Swept from the Sea (1997)
Le Bossu (1997)
**Those Who Loved Me Can
Take the Train** (1998)
Talk of Angels (1998)
Time Regained (1999)
Bride of the Wind (2001)
Happiness Costs Nothing (2003)
Fanfan la tulipe (2003)
The Knight Templar (2007)

Anthony **Perkins**
6ft 2in
(ANTHONY PERKINS)

Born: **April 4, 1932**
New York City, New York, USA
Died: **September 12, 1992**

Tony's father was the stage and film actor, James Ripley Osgood Perkins, whose wife was named Janet. Tony was educated at the Brooks School in New York City, and the private, Buckingham Browne & Nichols, in Cambridge, Massachusetts, after moving to Boston, following his father's death in 1942. He later attended Columbia University and Rollins College. During vacation, Tony went to Hollywood, took an MGM screen test, and had a small role in the 1953 drama, *The Actress*. He then returned to his studies and did summer stock before, in 1954, replacing John Kerr in the Broadway play, "Tea and Sympathy". Tony's next film role, in the drama, *Friendly Persuasion,* was good enough to be nominated for a Best Supporting Actor Oscar. He released three popular vocal albums during 1957-58 and appeared in some good movies. Tony became an icon of the cinema after his portrayal of Norman Bates, in *Psycho,* but at the time of the sequel twenty-three years later, he was a spent force. Prior to his marriage to Berry Berenson, in 1973, (they had two sons – Osgood and Elvis) Tony was said to have had affairs with several gay male film actors. He died in Hollywood, of pneumonia – which was a complication of AIDS. His widow died on Flight 11, during the 9/11 attacks.

Friendly Persuasion (1956)
Fear Strikes Out (1957)
The Tin Star (1957)
On the Beach (1959)
Psycho (1960)
Goodbye Again (1961)
Phaedra (1962)
The Trial (1962)
The Fool Killer (1965)
Is Paris Burning? (1966)
Pretty Poison (1968)
The Life and Times of Judge
Roy Bean (1972)
North Sea Hijack (1979)
Psycho II (1983)
Crimes of Passion (1984)

Elizabeth **Perkins**
5ft 8in
(ELIZABETH PERKINS)

Born: **November 18, 1960**
Queens, New York City, New York, USA

Elizabeth's father, James Perkins, a farmer and aspiring writer, was of Greek ancestry – his parents had immigrated to the United States from Salonika. Her mother, Jo, who worked as a drug treatment counselor, had at one time seriously considered a career as a classical concert pianist. Unfortunately, that interesting environment was destroyed when Elizabeth's parents divorced when she was barely three years old. Even so, she had inherited some of their positive genes. She was raised in Vermont and following her graduation from Northfield Mount Hermon School, she pursued her passion for acting at the Goodman School of Drama in Chicago. In 1984, Elizabeth made her Broadway debut, in Neil Simon's play, "Brighton Beach Memoirs". She went on to appear in some of the Bard's great plays with The New York Shakespeare Festival company and the Steppenwolf Theater. Although she is firstly a stage actress, Elizabeth has been in a number of good films – starting with *About Last Night*. She has a high ratio of successful films but hasn't been lucky with awards. She became a regular in the TV comedy series 'Weeds', and has been nominated for two Emmys and two Golden Globes. Her second husband is Argentinian cinematographer, Julio Macat.

About Last Night (1986)
From the Hip (1987) Big (1988)
Sweet Hearts Dance (1988)
Love at Large (1990)
Enid Is Sleeping (1990) Avalon (1990)
He Said, She Said (1991)
The Doctor (1991)
Indian Summer (1993)
Moonlight and Valentino (1995)
Lesser Prophets (1997)
Crazy in Alabama (1999)
28 Days (2000) Cats & Dogs (2001)
Try Seventeen (2002)
Jiminy Glick in Lalawood (2004)
Fierce People (2005)
The Thing About My Folks (2005)
Must Love Dogs (2005)
Kids in America (2005)

Ron **Perlman**
6ft 1in
(RONALD FRANCIS PERLMAN)

Born: **April 13, 1950**
New York City, New York, USA

The son of a Jewish jazz drummer and his wife, Dorothy, who worked for the municipality, he grew up in Washington Heights. Ron had a reasonably pleasant childhood until he became unhappy with the way he looked. He was educated at the local George Washington High School and he received a Bachelor of Fine Arts degree in Theater from Lehman College. After his dad saw him perform in a school production of "Guys and Dolls", he urged Ron to seriously consider a career as an actor. He then earned a degree in Theater Arts from the University of Minnesota. In 1975, Ron made his television debut in an episode of the series 'Ryan's Hope', but it was five more years before his movie debut, in *Quest for Fire*. Another five years elapsed before his second good film role, in *The Name of the Rose,* but after that he was a busy man. In 1989 he received a Golden Globe Award for one of the title roles in the TV series 'Beauty and the Beast'. Ron has been married to Opal Stone, a fashion and jewelry designer, since 1981. The couple had two children together, now grown up.

Quest for Fire (1981)
The Name of the Rose (1986)
When the Bough Breaks (1993)
The Adventures of Huck Finn (1993)
Cronos (1993) Romeo Is Bleeding (1993)
The City of Lost Children (1995)
Fluke (1995) The Last Supper (1995)
Alien: Resurrection (1997)
I Woke Up Early the Day I Died (1998)
Happy, Texas (1999)
Price of Glory (2000)
Enemy at the Gates (2001)
Boys on the Run (2001) Blade II (2002)
Star Trek: Nemesis (2002)
Hoodlum & Son (2003)
Hellboy (2004)
Missing in America (2005)
Local Color (2006)
The Last Winter (2006)
Outlander (2008)
Hellboy II: The Golden Army (2008)
The Mutant Chronicles (2008)
I Sell the Dead (2008)

Joe **Pesci**
5ft 4in
(JOSEPH FRANK PESCI)

Born: February 9, 1943
Newark, New Jersey, USA

From an Italian American background, Joe was the son of Angelo Pesci, a GM forklift driver, and his wife, Mary, who worked as a part-time barber. The boy's personality was magnetic from the start. At the age of five, he was getting work on the New York stage, and by the age of ten, he was appearing regularly on the television variety show, 'Startime Kids' – which featured Connie Francis. In the early 1960s, Joe began a back-up career as a barber. He was a talented singer, but not in a barbershop quartet, and he played guitar. Using the name Joseph Richie, he brought out an album "Little Joe Can Sing" and was on guitar in the group, "Joey Dee and the Starlighters" with whom he made his film debut, in 1961 – in *Hey, Let's Twist.* Joe formed a comedy duo with his pal Frank Vincent and apart from that, the 1960s yielded a couple of roles as a musician on TV shows. It was 1976 before he made his film acting debut, in *The Death Collector.* Robert De Niro persuaded Scorsese to cast him in *Raging Bull,* which earned him a nomination for a Best Supporting Actor Oscar. He went on to win it for *Goodfellas* and to contribute strongly to several big movies. His work in the past few years has slowed, but big things are expected of *Love Ranch,* in which he co-stars with Helen Mirren. Joe is divorced from the actress, Claudia Haro.

Raging Bull (1980)
I'm Dancing as Fast
as I Can (1982)
Once Upon a Time
in America (1984)
Lethal Weapon 2 (1989)
Goodfellas (1990)
Home Alone (1990)
JFK (1991)
My Cousin Vinny (1992)
Lethal Weapon 3 (1992)
The Public Eye (1992)
A Bronx Tale (1993)
Casino (1995)
Lethal Weapon 4 (1998)
The Good Shepherd (2006)

Jean **Peters**
5ft 5½in
(ELIZABETH JEAN PETERS)

Born: October 15, 1926
Canton, Ohio, USA
Died: October 13, 2000

Jean grew up in a farming family. Both her parents were from Welsh backgrounds. Apart from the occasional role in a school play, she had little interest in acting, but while studying for a teaching degree, at Ohio University, in 1946, a friend entered her for the "Miss Ohio State" beauty contest. Jean's prize for winning was a trip to Hollywood and a screen test with 20th Century Fox. The test was positive and she made her film debut opposite Tyrone Power, in *Captain from Castile.* Her best films were *Viva Zapata, Niagara, Pickup on South Street* and *Three Coins in the Fountain,* but not one of the nineteen films she made was bad. In 1957, following her divorce from her first husband, Jean married Howard Hughes, who persuaded her to give up her film career in 1956. Their marriage was finally dissolved in 1971 – after Hughes agreed to pay her a lifetime annual alimony of $70,000 – adjusted for inflation. She then agreed never to divulge any secrets about him and stayed married to Stanley Hough, a Fox executive, until his death in 1990. Jean died of leukemia, ten years later, in Carlsbad, California.

Captain from Castile (1947)
Deep Waters (1948)
It Happens Every Spring (1949)
Love That Brute (1950)
As Young as You Feel (1951)
Take Care of My Little Girl (1951)
Anne of the Indies (1951)
Viva Zapata (1952)
Wait 'Til the Sun Shines
Nellie (1952)
Lure of the Wilderness (1952)
O.Henry's Full House (1952)
Niagara (1953)
Pickup on South Street (1953)
Vicki (1953)
A Blueprint for Murder (1953)
Three Coins in the
Fountain (1954)
Apache (1954)
Broken Lance (1954)
A Man Called Peter (1955)

Michelle **Pfeiffer**
5ft 7½in
(MICHELLE MARIE PFEIFFER)

Born: April 29, 1958
Santa Ana, California, USA

Michelle was the second of four children born to Richard Pfeiffer and his wife Donna. They were raised in Midway City, thirty miles south east of Los Angeles. Michelle graduated from Fountain Valley High School in 1976. While there, she was 'Alice in Wonderland' at Disneyland. She studied for a short time at the Golden West Community College, with the idea of becoming a court reporter. In 1978, she dropped out after winning the "Miss Orange County" beauty pageant, and although unsuccessful in her effort to be "Miss California USA", she had made up her mind to be an actress. She did TV commercials before getting her first acting role in a 1979 episode of 'Delta House'. Michelle's film debut was in the following year's comedy, *The Hollywood Knights.* There was nothing of substance until her breakthrough, when she played Elvira Hancock, in *Scarface.* She has been nominated for three Best Actress Oscars – for *Dangerous Liaisons, The Fabulous Baker Boys,* and *Love Field.* Michelle has two children with her second husband, the former lawyer and now a writer/producer – David E. Kelley.

Scarface (1983)
Ladyhawke (1985)
The Witches of Eastwick (1987)
Tequila Sunrise (1988)
Dangerous Liaisons (1988)
The Fabulous Baker Boys (1989)
The Russia House (1990)
Batman Returns (1992)
Love Field (1992)
The Age of Innocence (1993)
Wolf (1994)
One Fine Day (1996)
A Thousand Acres (1997)
A Midsummer Night's
Dream (1999)
What Lies Beneath (2000)
White Oleander (2002)
I Could Never Be Your
Woman (2007) Hairspray (2007)
Stardust (2007) Chéri (2009)
Personal Effects (2009)

Gérard **Philipe**
5ft 11½in
(GÉRARD PHILIP)

Born: **December 4, 1922**
Cannes, Alpes-Maritimes, France
Died: **November 25, 1959**

Gérard's father, Marc Philip, worked for a law firm and later managed a hotel. Minou, Gérard's mother, was a beautiful woman of Slavic ancestry. For Gérard and his brother Jean, their early life was idyllic. During his childhood, he dreamed of becoming a locomotive driver, and as he grew older, he wanted to be a physician. Then, with his mother's encouragement, he turned his attention to an acting career. His father was then managing the Hotel du Parc, in Cannes, and hoped that he would study Law. When the Germans occupied France during World War II, there were plenty of visitors from Paris. Gérard's mother began reading cards for guests. One day, in 1942, movie director, Marc Allégret was having his fortune told, when he saw Gérard. He was impressed enough to ask him to read a scene from a play and fixed him up with a drama course in Nice. After he graduated, Allégret gave him his film debut in 1944, in *Les Petites du quai aux fleurs*. Gérard was a supporting actor until *Le Pays sans étoiles*, in 1946. After that, it was non-stop stardom. He married Nicole Fourcade and had two children. He built up a big female following throughout Europe with films such as *Le Diable au corps, La Beauté du diable, La Ronde,* and *Fanfan la Tulipe*. He made *La Fièvre monte à El Pao*, in Mexico, but fell ill months later. Gérard died of liver cancer, in Paris. He was almost thirty seven.

Le Diable au corps (1947)
La Chartreuse de Parme (1948)
La Beauté du diable (1950)
La Ronde (1950) Souvenirs
perdus (1950) Key of Dreams (1951)
Fanfan la Tulipe (1952) Seven Deadly
Sins (1952) Les Orgueilleux (1954)
Monsieur Ripois (1954)
Le Rouge et le noir (1954)
Les Grandes manoeuvres (1955)
Pot-Bouille (1957)
Le Joueur (1958) Les Amants de
Montparnasse (1958)
Les Liaisons dangereuses (1959)

Ryan **Phillippe**
5ft 9in
(MATTHEW RYAN PHILLIPPE)

Born: **September 10, 1974**
New Castle, Delaware, USA

Ryan's parents were Richard Phillippe, a chemist with DuPont, and his wife Susan, who ran a day care center at the family home. Ryan, who was educated at the New Castle Baptist Academy, had three sisters. He was particularly good at sports – excelling at basketball and soccer as well as earning a black belt at Tael Kwon Do. In his senior year, he was editor of the school yearbook. From the age of fifteen, he became interested in an acting career. Two years later, an agent saw him in a barbershop and started to send him to auditions. The first time he got a part, was for the role of a gay teenager, in the 1992 ABC soap opera, 'One Life to Live'. Following a move to Los Angeles, Ryan began to get regular small parts in television shows. He made his film debut, playing the role of a seaman in the 1995 blockbuster, *Crimson Tide*. It was followed by the nondescript sci-fi movie, *Invader,* and then a decent role, in *White Squall*. His career has picked up nicely since then, with an average of two opportunities each year and films of the calibre of *Crash, Flags of Our Fathers* and *Breach,* keeping his name up in lights. In 1999, there was great rejoicing when Ryan married actress Reese Witherspoon, but eight years – and a daughter and son later – the marriage ended in divorce.

White Squall (1996)
Little Boy Blue (1997)
I Know What You Did Last
Summer (1997)
Homegrown (1998) 54 (1998)
Cruel Intentions (1999)
The Way of the Gun (2000)
Antitrust (2001)
Gosford Park (2001)
Igby Goes Down (2002)
The I Inside (2003)
Crash (2004) Chaos (2005)
Five Fingers (2006)
Flags of Our Fathers (2006)
Breach (2007)
Stop-Loss (2008)
Franklyn (2008)

Joaquin **Phoenix**
5ft 8½in
(JOAQUIN RAFAEL BOTTOM)

Born: **October 28, 1974**
San Juan, Puerto Rico

Joaquin was the third child born to the nomadic Children of God missionaries, John Bottom Amram and Arlene Dunitz Jochebed, who was from Hungarian and Russian stock. The family moved home often – in Central and South America. A great admirer of brother, River, Joaquin followed him into an acting career. By the time Joaquin was six, the family had had enough of the Children of God, and settled in the Los Angeles area. Their mother found a good job as a secretary at NBC in Los Angeles and their father used his creative talent to became a landscape gardener. All five children got themselves an agent and soon gained experience in television commercials. Joaquin got his first TV acting role (as Leaf Phoenix) in 1982, in an episode of 'Seven Brides for Seven Brothers'. Four years later, he made his movie debut in a children's sci-fi film, *SpaceCamp*. His first major adult film was with Nicole Kidman and Matt Dillon, in *To Die For*. Joaquin's steady growth as a star accelerated after an Oscar nomination for Best Supporting Actor, in *Gladiator*. Five years later he was up for a Best Actor Oscar for his portrayal of Johnny Cash, in *Walk the Line*. His recording for the film's soundtrack album, won a Grammy Award. Joaquin is unattached at the present time. A serious three-year relationship with the young actress, Liv Tyler, ended in 1998.

Parenthood (1989)
To Die For (1995)
U Turn (1997)
Return to Paradise (1998)
Clay Pigeons (1998)
Gladiator (2000) Quills (2000)
Buffalo Soldiers (2001) Signs (2002)
It's All About Love (2003)
The Village (2004)
Hotel Rwanda (2004)
Ladder 49 (2004)
Walk the Line (2005)
We Own the Night (2007)
Reservation Road (2007)
Two Lovers (2008)

River **Phoenix**
5ft 10in
(RIVER JUDE BOTTOM)

Born: **August 23, 1970**
Madras, Oregon, USA
Died: **October 31, 1993**

The eldest of this talented family, his place in the sun was much too short. After their parents gave up their work with the Children of God, and all returned to the USA, they officially adopted the name "Phoenix" to represent their new life. After a tough few years, River started his show business career in the 1983 television series 'Seven Brides for Seven Brothers'. In December of that year, he appeared in the episode, "Christmas Song", with his sister, Liberty, and his brother Joaquin. After three more years of TV work, he made his movie debut, in the children's adventure, *Explorers.* River's second movie role, as Chris Chambers, in *Stand by Me,* made him a star. His fan following was enormous, and from an artistic point of view, he was highly rated. He was nominated for a Best Supporting Actor Oscar, for *Running on Empty,* and in 1991, he was voted Best Actor at the Venice Film Festival, for *My Own Private Idaho.* Apart from acting, River played guitar with his band "Aleka's Attic". For most of his short adult life he was a dedicated animal rights campaigner and environmentalist. His final film, *Thing Called Love,* was excellent, but *Silent Tongue,* released a year later, was not. Apparently depressed about the abuse he'd suffered in his early life, he found living difficult. He died in Hollywood from an overdose of heroin and cocaine, at the age of twenty-three.

Explorers (1985)
Stand by Me (1986)
The Mosquito Coast (1986)
A Night in the
Life of Jimmy Reardon (1988)
Running on Empty (1988)
Indiana Jones and the
Last Crusade (1989)
I Love You to Death (1990)
My Own Private Idaho (1991)
Dogfight (1991)
Sneakers (1992)
Dark Blood (1993)
The Thing Called Love (1993)

Michel **Piccoli**
6ft 0½in
(JACQUES DANIEL MICHEL PICCOLI)

Born: **December 27, 1925**
Paris, France

Michel's parents were both professional musicians – his father, Henri, who was from an Italian background, was a violinist and his mother, Marcelle, was a pianist. Michel appreciated music, but during his schooldays he was more interested in the theater. His parents had no objections when he enrolled at the Cours Simon, in Paris. The school had turned out many fine actors since it was founded in 1925, by the great Michel Simon. It proved to be the perfect launching pad for Michel, who after appearing on the Paris stage, made his film debut in *Le Point du jour* in 1945. After that, he progressed in the theater for most of the 1950s – making his movie breakthrough in *Le Mépris.* He was Best Actor at Cannes for *Salto nel vuoto,* and won Berlin's Silver Bear, for *Une étrange affaire.* Michel worked with Buñuel, Hitchcock, Resnais, Godard, and Malle. He's been married three times, including to the singer/actress, Juliette Gréco. He has been together with his third wife, Ludivine, for twenty-five years.

Le Mépris (1963)
Diary of a Chambermaid (1964)
Masquarade (1965)
The Sleeping Car Murders (1965)
The War is Over (1966)
La Voleuse (1966) **Les Créatures** (1966)
Paris brûle-t-il? (1966)
Belle de jour (1966) **Topaz** (1969)
The Discreet Charm
of the Bourgeoisie (1972)
La Grande bouffe (1973)
Todo Modo (1976)
The Last Woman (1976)
Spoiled Children (1977)
Salto nel vuoto (1980)
Atlantic City (1980)
Une étrange affaire (1982)
Milou en mai (1990)
Divertimento (1991)
Bête de scène (1994)
Travelling Companion (1996)
Belle toujours (2006)
Sous les toits de Paris (2007)
The Dust of Time (2008)

Walter **Pidgeon**
6ft 2½in
(WALTER DAVIS PIDGEON)

Born: **September 23, 1897**
Saint John, New Brunswick, Canada
Died: **September 25, 1984**

After attending public schools in New Brunswick, he studied Law and Drama, at the city's University. He interrupted his studies to enlist with the Canadian Field Artillery at the outbreak of World War I, but never saw combat after a serious training accident. After the war, he moved to Boston, where he worked as a bank runner to pay for classical voice studies at the New England Conservatory of Music. He went to New York, where he made his stage debut, in "At Home" and was soon in musicals – using his fine baritone on Broadway, to introduce such classics as "What'll I Do?" and "Alone". In 1926, Joseph Schenk bought him out of his stage contract and took him to Hollywood where he made his film debut in that year's *Mannequin.* Walter made fourteen silents before his first talkie, *Melody of Love.* It heralded a long career, with Best Actor Oscar nominations, for *Mrs. Miniver* and *Madame Curie* – both films co-starring Greer Garson. His first wife Muriel, died giving birth to their daughter in 1926. He married his secretary, Ruth Walker, who was with him until his fatal stroke, in Santa Monica, California.

The Shopworn Angel (1938)
Too Hot to Handle (1938)
Man Hunt (1941)
Blossoms in the Dust (1941)
How Green Was My Valley (1941)
Mrs. Miniver (1942)
Madame Curie (1943)
Mrs. Parkington (1944)
Julia Misbehaves (1948)
Command Decision (1948)
The Bad and the Beautiful (1952)
Executive Suite (1954)
Forbidden Planet (1956)
The Rack (1956)
Advise & Consent (1962)
Big Red (1962)
Warning Shot (1967)
Funny Girl (1968)
Harry in Your Pocket (1973)
Two-Minute Warning (1976)

Jada Pinkett Smith
5ft
(JADA KOREN PINKETT)

Born: **September 18, 1971**
Baltimore, Maryland, USA

Jada was the daughter of Robson Pinkett Jr. – head of a construction company, and Adrienne Banfield-Jones – a head nurse at an inner-city clinic in Baltimore. Her parents split up only a few months after her birth and her mother remarried twice. After her normal schooling, and being crowned "Miss Maryland" in 1988, Jada majored in Theater at the Baltimore School for the Arts. While there, she developed a very important friendship with the rap artist, Tupac Shakur, and was devastated when he was killed in a shooting in Las Vegas, in 1996. After graduating, Jada spent one year at North Carolina School of the Arts. In 1990, she got her first TV role in 'Moe's World' and the following year, began the first of thirty-six appearances as Lena James, in NBC's 'A Different World'. She made her film debut two years later, in the crime drama, *Menace II Society*. Co-starring with Eddie Murphy, in *The Nutty Professor,* set her on the road to stardom and helped her get good roles in some important movies – not least of which was *Ali* – in which she acted with her husband, Will Smith, with whom she now has two children – a son, Jaden Christopher Syre Smith and a daughter, Willow Camille Reign Smith. Jade did well in the *Matrix* movies. Another major film, *Collateral,* helped lift her up towards star status. She recently branched out when she wrote and directed the film *The Human Contact.*

Menace II Society (1994)
The Inkwell (1994)
Jason's Lyric (1994)
Tales from the Crypt:
Demon Knight (1995)
The Nutty Professor (1996)
Set It Off (1996)
Scream 2 (1997)
Return to Paradise (1998)
Bamboozled (2000)
Ali (2001)
The Matrix Reloaded (2003)
The Matrix Revolutions (2003)
Collateral (2004)
Reign Over Me (2007)

Brad Pitt
5ft 10¾in
(WILLIAM BRADLEY PITT)

Born: **December 18, 1963**
Shawnee, Oklahoma, USA

Brad's father Bill, ran a truck company. His mother Jane, was a high school counselor. Together with his brother, Doug, and sister, Julie, Brad was raised as a Baptist, in Springfield, Missouri, where the family settled just after he was born. He attended Kickapoo High School, which had opened for the first time in 1971. Brad was a good student – participating in debating and student government, as well as acting. He then studied Journalism at the University of Missouri. After deciding on an acting career, he went to California to study with Roy London. An uncredited role in the 1987 movie, *No Man's Land,* was followed by four episodes of 'Dallas'. Supporting parts led to his first starring role in 1991, in *Across the Tracks,* but more importantly, his appearance in the successful *Thelma & Louise.* He built to a crescendo in the 1990s. He was nominated for a Best Supporting Actor Oscar, for *Twelve Monkeys* and had reached A-list stardom, by the century's turn, via top performances in such movies as *Se7en, Fight Club,* and *Snatch.* The subsequent eight years have secured it. Divorced from Jennifer Aniston in 2005, Brad has formed a family unit with Angelina Jolie. He was nominated for a Best Actor Oscar, for *The Curious Case of Benjamin Button.*

Thelma & Louise (1991)
Kalifornia (1993)
True Romance (1993)
Interview with the Vampire (1994)
Legends of the Fall (1994) Se7en (1995)
Twelve Monkeys (1995)
Seven Years in Tibet (1997)
Meet Joe Black (1998)
Fight Club (1999) Snatch (2000)
Spy Game (2001) Ocean's Eleven (2001)
Mr. & Mrs. Smith (2005) Babel (2006)
Ocean's Thirteen (2007)
The Assassination of
Jesse James (2007)
Burn After Reading (2008)
The Curious Case of
Benjamin Button (2008)
Inglourious Basterds (2009)

Donald Pleasence
5ft 7in
(DONALD PLEASENCE)

Born: **October 5, 1919**
Worksop, Nottinghamshire, England
Died: **February 2, 1995**

Donald's parents were Thomas and Alice Pleasence. When his father got a job as stationmaster at Louth, on the East Lincolnshire Railway, the family moved to a village called Grimoldy, where Donald attended the local junior school. At seven years of age, he won medals for recitations. At twelve years of age, he was attending Ecclesfield Grammar School, in Sheffield, Yorkshire. Without any formal drama training, he joined the Jersey Repertory Company in 1939, and made his stage debut that year, in "Wuthering Heights". Donald's London debut was in "Twelfth Night" in 1942. During the early part of World War II, he was a conscientious objector, but changed his mind and joined the RAF. In 1944, his bomber was shot down and he was a POW for two years. He came back to the London stage in 1947, and built his reputation before making his screen debut, in 1952, in a BBC play 'Arrow to the Heart'. His film debut was in 1954, in *The Beachcomber.* Donald's manic style and hypnotic gaze, got him a lot of film work right up to the year he died of complications during heart valve replacement surgery, at Saint-Paul-de-Vence, in France.

Lisa (1962)
The Caretaker (1963)
The Great Escape (1963)
The Hallelujah Trail (1965)
Cul-de-sac (1966)
Fantastic Voyage (1966)
The Night of the Generals (1967)
You Only Live Twice (1967)
Will Penny (1968)
Soldier Blue (1970)
Henry VIII and His Six Wives (1972)
From Beyond the Grave (1973)
The Black Windmill (1974)
Escape to Witch Mountain (1975)
The Eagle Has Landed (1976)
Telefon (1977)
Halloween (1978)
Dracula (1979)
Escape from New York (1981)

Suzanne **Pleshette**
5ft 4in
(SUZANNE PLESHETTE)

Born: **January 31, 1937**
New York City, New York, USA
Died: **January 19, 2008**

Suzanne was the only child of Eugene Pleshette, who came from a French background. Her mother, Geraldine, who was Jewish, was a dancer who used the stage name Geraldine Rivers. Eugene was manager of the Paramount Theater in Brooklyn during the Big Band era in the 1930s and 1940s. At the age of twelve, she attended the New York High School for the Performing Arts and went on to Syracuse University. After setting her heart on an acting career, Suzanne studied at the Neighborhood Playhouse and Sanford Meisner's School. In 1957, she made her stage debut on Broadway, in the courtroom drama, "Compulsion". That same year, Suzanne made her first TV appearance, in an episode of 'Harbourmaster'. Her film debut was in the Jerry Lewis comedy, *The Geisha Boy.* Fame followed five years later, when she had a significant role in Alfred Hitchcock's *The Birds.* In January 1964, Suzanne enjoyed a whole eight months of marriage to actor, Troy Donahue. Second and third marriages endured until her husbands' deaths. She maintained a career as a likeable second lead in films and television for forty years. Suzanne died at her home in Los Angeles of respiratory failure, fifteen months after chemotherapy treatment for lung cancer.

The Geisha Boy (1958)
Rome Adventure (1962)
The Birds (1963)
Youngblood Hawke (1964)
The Ugly Dachshund (1966)
Nevada Smith (1966)
Mister Buddwing (1966)
The Adventures of
Bullwhip Griffin (1967)
Blackbeard's Ghost (1968)
The Power (1968)
If It's Tuesday,
This Must Be Belgium (1969)
Support Your Local
Gunfighter (1971)
The Shaggy D.A. (1976)
Hot Stuff (1979)

Dame Joan **Plowright**
5ft 4½in
(JOAN ANN PLOWRIGHT)

Born: **October 28, 1929**
Brigg, North Lincolnshire, England

The daughter of a newspaper editor, Joan attended Scunthorpe Grammar School. She'd always dreamed of a stage career and began her training at the Bristol Old Vic Theater School. She made her stage debut in Croydon, in 1951, and she first appeared in London's West End, three years later – it was the year she appeared as Adriana, in the BBC television production of 'The Comedy of Errors'. In 1956, Joan was signed by the English Stage Company, who cast her as Margery Pinchwife, in 'The Country Wife', at the Royal Court Theater. While acting in that, she made her film debut, with an uncredited role in John Huston's *Moby Dick.* She was in the 1957 London stage production of John Osborne's 'The Entertainer' and her first significant screen role was in the film version. The play had first introduced her to her future husband, Laurence Olivier. The couple married in 1961, and had three children, two of whom are actresses. Joan's priority has always been the stage, but although approaching her eighties, she continues to feature in some excellent movies.

Time Without Pity (1957)
The Entertainer (1960)
Uncle Vanya (1963)
Three Sisters (1970)
Equus (1977)
The Dressmaker (1988)
Drowning by Numbers (1988)
I Love You to Death (1990)
Avalon (1990)
Enchanted April (1992)
Widows' Peak (1994)
Hotel Sorrento (1995)
Jane Eyre (1996)
Surviving Picasso (1996)
Tea with Mussolini (1999)
Tom's Midnight Garden (1999)
Global Heresy (2002)
Callas Forever (2002)
I Am David (2003)
Mrs. Palfrey at the Claremont (2005)
Goose on the Loose (2006)
The Spiderwick Chronicles (2008)

Christopher **Plummer**
5ft 10½in
(ARTHUR CHRISTOPHER ORME PLUMMER)

Born: **December 13, 1929**
Toronto, Ontario, Canada

Chris was the grandson of a former Canadian Prime Minister, through his mother, Isabella Abbott. His father, John, worked at McGill University. After his parents divorced, Chris attended public and private schools and he and his mother moved to Senneville, near Montreal. An early ambition to become a concert pianist was replaced by his love for the theater which developed at high school. He began his training for the stage at the Canadian Repertory Company, in Ottawa, and started his career in both French and English, on stage and in radio plays, in Montreal. In 1953, he first appeared on TV, in an episode of 'Studio One'. The following year, he made his New York debut, with roles in two plays – "The Constant Wife" and "The Dark Is Light Enough". In 1956, he married the first of his three wives, Tammy Grimes – the mother of his actress daughter, Amanda Plummer. His film debut was in the 1958 drama, *Stage Struck.* He appeared in a wealth of good films en route to fame and fortune, including *The Sound of Music.* Almost fifty years later, in *Man in the Chair* and *Closing the Ring,* he proved he is as good as ever. Chris has been married to Elaine Taylor, since 1970.

The Fall of the Roman Empire (1964)
The Sound of Music (1965)
Inside Daisy Clover (1965)
Triple Cross (1966)
The Night of the Generals (1967)
Battle of Britain (1969)
The Royal Hunt of the Sun (1969)
Waterloo (1970)
The Man Who Would Be King (1975)
Aces High (1976) Murder by
Decree (1979) Eyewitness (1981)
Dreamscape (1984) Souvenir (1989)
Dolores Claiborne (1995)
A Beautiful Mind (2001)
Syriana (2005) Inside Man (2006)
The Lake House (2005)
Man in the Chair (2007)
Closing the Ring (2007)
Already Dead (2007)

Sidney **Poitier**
6ft 2½in
(SIDNEY POITIER)

Born: February 20, 1927
Miami, Florida, USA

Sidney's parents were West Indians, from Cat Island, in The Bahamas. Their son arrived in Miami, while they were visiting relatives in the USA. Sidney's father was a poor tomato-farmer, and there was little money to spare. The youngster had very little formal education, and when he was fifteen they sent him and his brother to live in Miami. Because of the poor treatment he suffered there, he went to New York, where he did menial jobs. Following Army service, Sidney was turned down by the American Negro Theater, but soon after smoothing out his accent, he was given a bit part in the all-black, "Lysistrata", on Broadway. He was highly praised for his movie debut, in *No Way Out.* Good roles were hard to get for a black actor, but Sidney was no ordinary talent. He made his breakthrough in *The Defiant Ones,* for which he was nominated for a Best Actor Oscar. Five years later, he won one for *Lilies of the Field.* His best films are *Porgy and Bess, To Sir, with Love, In the Heat of the Night* and *Guess Who's Coming to Dinner?* 1967 was certainly his vintage year. Sidney had four children with Juanita Hardy, and two with Joanna Shimkus – his second wife, since 1976.

No Way Out (1950)
Cry, the Beloved Country (1951)
Blackboard Jungle (1955)
Something of Value (1957)
The Defiant Ones (1958)
Porgy and Bess (1959)
A Raisin in the Sun (1961)
Paris Blues (1961)
Lilies of the Field (1963)
The Bedford Incident (1965)
A Patch of Blue (1965)
To Sir, with Love (1967)
In the Heat of the Night (1967)
Guess Who's Coming to Dinner (1967)
They Call Me Mister Tibbs! (1970)
The Organization (1971)
Buck and the Preacher (1972)
Uptown Saturday Night (1974)
Let's Do It Again (1975)
Sneakers (1992)

Kevin **Pollack**
5ft 5in
(KEVIN ELLIOT POLLAK)

Born: October 30, 1957
San Francisco, California, USA

Kevin started doing stand-up comedy when he was ten – performing lip-sync to Bill Cosy routines. Ignoring his college opportunities, he honed his skills on the Bay Area circuit. Kevin entered the 1982 San Francisco International Comedy Competition and finished a close second. After moving to Los Angels in 1984, he worked at comedy clubs such as "The Improv", where he won a lot of fans with his impressions of Peter Fall (moving one eye only) and William Shatter. He also appeared for the first time on TV, in the series, 'Flashes'. In 1987, Kevin made his film debut in *Million Dollar Mystery,* which was almost a million dollar flop. His second movie, *Willow,* was much more of a success, and he secured his big screen future in *Avalon.* Kevin became a regular guest on 'The Tonight Show'. With over fifty films to his credit, including *The Usual Suspects,* Kevin's is a familiar face. Since 1995, he has been married to actress, Lucy Webb, but recently filed for divorce. Since 2007, he has appeared on television as D.A. Leo Cutler, in 'Shark'.

Willow (1988)
Avalon (1990)
L.A. Story (1991)
A Few Good Men (1992)
Indian Summer (1993)
Grumpy Old Men (1993)
The Usual Suspects (1995)
Chameleon (1995)
Canadian Bacon (1995)
Casino (1995)
Truth or Consequences,
N.M. (1997)
Outside Ozona (1998)
Deterrence (1999)
The Whole Nine Yards (2000)
Steal This Movie (2000)
Stolen Summer (2002)
Mother Ghost (2002)
Blizzard (2003)
Our Time Is Up (2004)
Hostage (2005)
Niagara Motel (2006)
Numb (2007)

Sarah **Polley**
5ft 2in
(SARAH POLLEY)

Born: January 8, 1979
Toronto, Ontario, Canada

Sarah was the youngest of five children, born to Michael Polley, a British-born actor who became an insurance agent. His wife, Diane was an actress and casting director, who sadly died of cancer when Sarah was eleven years old. Sarah made her film debut at the age of four, in the Disney production, *One Magic Christmas.* At eight, years old she acted in the short-lived TV series, 'Ramona' and the following year, became well-known with a regular role in the popular 'Road to Avonlea'. It ran for seven years, and Sarah was "Canada's Sweetheart". She combined her acting career with television work, and movies like *The Adventures of Baron Munchausen* – together with her studies. It resulted in her dropping out before graduating from Earl Haig Secondary School. Sarah concentrated on her acting career and was rewarded with some satisfying parts. Early on, she had been politically active, but has been less so since marrying the Canadian film editor, David Wharnsby, in 2003. Sarah was Oscar nominated in 2008, for her screenplay (it was also her third directing effort) for *Away From Her,* starring Julie Christie. Sarah's next screen appearance will be in *Mr. Nobody.*

The Adventures of Baron
Munchausen (1988)
Exotica (1994)
Joe's So Mean to Josephine (1996)
The Sweet Hereafter (1997)
The Hanging Garden (1997)
Jerry and Tom (1998)
Last Night (1998)
Guinevere (1999)
eXistenZ (1999) Go (1999)
The Life Before This (1999)
The Weight of Water (2000)
The Law of Enclosures (2000)
The Claim (2000)
No Such Thing (2001)
The I Inside (2003)
My Life Without Me (2003)
Dawn of the Dead (2004)
Don't Come Knocking (2005)
The Secret Life of Words (2005)

Natalie **Portman**
5ft 3in
(NATALIE HERSHLAG)

Born: **June 9, 1981**
Jerusalem, Israel

Natalie is the only child of Avner Hershlag, an Israeli doctor, and an American mother named Shelley, who gave up being a homemaker to become her agent. They moved to the USA, when Natalie was three years old. She attended the Charles E. Smith Jewish School, in Washington, D.C. Natalie started dancing lessons at four and acted in plays at summer camps, but above all, she was an academic – excelling in everything she attempted at Syosset High School, in New York – and when studying for a bachelor's degree in Psychology from Harvard. Her research papers were published in professional scientific journals and in addition to being bilingual in English and Hebrew, she's studied Japanese, German and Arabic! How she found the time for acting is a wonder, but she made her film debut at thirteen, in the French movie, *Léon*. She never took it easy during school vacations – acting at every opportunity. Her ambition has pushed her to the front in films like *Cold Mountain*. She was nominated for a Best Supporting Actress Oscar in *Closer*, and there's more to come. She's currently dating the composer, Devendra Banhart.

Léon (1994) **Heat** (1995)
Beautiful Girls (1996)
Everyone Says I Love You (1999)
The Phantom Menace (1999)
Anywhere But Here (1999)
Where the Heart Is (2000)
Star Wars II (2002)
Cold Mountain (2003)
Garden State (2004)
Closer (2004)
Revenge of the Sith (2005)
Free Zone (2005)
V for Vendetta (2005)
Goya's Ghosts (2006)
My Blueberry Nights (2007)
Hotel Chevalier (2007)
The Darjeeling Limited (2007)
Mr. Magorium's
Wonder Emporium (2007)
The Other Boleyn Girl (2008)
New York, I Love You (2009)

Pete **Postlethwaite**
5ft 9in
(PETER WILLIAM POSTLETHWAITE)

Born: **February 16, 1946**
Warrington, Cheshire, England

Pete was the son of William and Mary Postlethwaite. He was bright enough at junior school to move on to West Park Catholic Grammar School, in St. Helen's, Merseyside – a school with a strong rugby history. From there, he went to St. Mary's College, in Strawberry Hill, near London. Pete was twenty-four when he decided to pursue an acting career, with the Old Vic Drama School, in Bristol.To begin with, he was a drama teacher, but it led to acting assignments and stage experience with companies such as the Manchester Royal Exchange and the Royal Shakespeare Company. In 1975, he made his first film – a short subject directed by Anthony Garner – called *The Racer*. Following a few years of television and low-profile movie roles, he married Jacqueline Morrish, and made an impact in *The Dressmaker*. With a wife and two children to support, Pete made steady progress. He was nominated for a Best Supporting Actor Oscar, for *In the Name of the Father*, and was then in the smash-hit, *The Usual Suspects*. Pete's become a casting director's favorite.

The Dressmaker (1988)
Distant Voices, Still Lives (1988)
Hamlet (1990) **The Grass Arena** (1991)
Alien 3 (1992) **Waterland** (1992)
The Last of the Mohicans (1992)
Anchoress (1993)
In the Name of the Father (1993)
The Usual Suspects (1995)
When Saturday Comes (1996)
Dragonheart (1996)
Romeo + Juliet (1996) **Brassed Off** (1996)
The Serpent's Kiss (1997)
The Lost World: Jurassic Park (1997)
Amistad (1997)
When the Sky Falls (2000)
Cowboy Up (2001) **The Shipping**
News (2001) **Triggermen** (2002)
Between Strangers (2002)
Strange Bedfellows (2004)
Dark Water (2005)
The Constant Gardener (2005)
Valley of the Heart's Delight (2006)
Closing the Ring (2007)

Franka **Potente**
5ft 8in
(FRANKA POTENTE)

Born: **July 22, 1974**
Münster, North Rhine-Westphalia, Germany

Franka grew up a few miles from her birthplace, in a town called Dülmen, where she and her younger brother, Stefan, were raised by a schoolteacher father, and a mother who worked as a medical assistant. Because her brother was a sickly child in his early years, Franka felt the need to play-act and clown around in order to get some of the attention he was getting. She grew out of that jealous phase and developed into a nice confident girl who was popular at high school, where she was the class spokesperson. When she was seventeen, Franka went to Houston, Texas, as an exchange student. It was there that she first thought about an acting career and acquired an American boyfriend. On her return to Europe, she enrolled at the Otto Falkenberg School of Performing Arts in Munich. In 1995, she made her screen debut, in a student film, called *Aufbruch*. Around that time, after being spotted by a casting agent in a nightclub, she made her feature film debut in *Nach Fünf im Urwald*, directed by her then boyfriend, Hans-Christian Schmid. It won her the Bavarian Film Prize for Young Talent. Franka then went to New York to finish her training at the Lee Strasberg Theater Institute. She returned home to appear on TV before landing the title role in the international hit, *Run, Lola, Run*. It was three more years before her first English-language movie, *Blow* – starring Johnny Depp. She then secured stardom in *The Bourne Identity*, and its sequel.

Nach Fünf im Urwald (1995)
Run, Lola, Run (1998)
Downhill City (1999) **Anatomie** (2000)
The Princess and the
Warrior (2000) **Blow** (2001)
Storytelling (2001)
The Bourne Identity (2002)
Try Seventeen (2002)
The Bourne Supremacy (2004)
Creep (2004)
Elementary Particles (2006)
Romulus, My Father (2007)
Guerrilla (2008)

Dick **Powell**

6ft

(RICHARD EWING POWELL)

Born: **November 14, 1904**
Mountain View, Arkansas, USA
Died: **January 2, 1963**

Dick started performing early – as a boy soprano in his local church choir. He was educated at Little Rock College, where he sang at the proms and also acted in school plays. His original dream was to make it as a recording artist, and in the 1920s, he joined the Midwest based, Charlie Davis Orchestra, and cut some sides for Vocalion. He married Mildred Maude, in 1925, but it didn't work out and he moved to Pittsburgh to take up a high-profile job as MC, at the Enright Theater. He was spotted by a Warners talent scout and given a contract. Dick made his film debut in 1932 – in a small part in *Blessed Event*. His boyish looks and pleasant voice set the tone for his 1930 films – beginning with *42nd Street*. He married co-star Joan Blondell in 1936, and was desperate to expand his range, but the studio resisted. After his contract expired, he become a big star of film noir, in *Murder My Sweet, Cornered,* and *Pitfall*. Dick proved to be a very capable director – with five movies and several TV shows to his credit. He married June Allyson in 1945, and they had two children. They were happy until his death in Los Angeles, from cancer.

42nd Street (1933)
Gold Diggers of 1933 (1933)
Footlight Parade (1933)
Dames (1934)
Gold Diggers of 1935 (1935)
A Midsummer Night's Dream (1935)
Gold Diggers of 1937 (1936)
On the Avenue (1937)
Hollywood Hotel (1937)
Christmas in July (1940)
Murder My Sweet (1944)
Cornered (1945)
Johnny O'Clock (1947)
To the Ends of the Earth (1948)
Pitfall (1948) Station West (1948)
Cry Danger (1951)
The Tall Target (1951)
You Never Can Tell (1951)
The Bad and the Beautiful (1952)
Susan Slept Here (1954)

Eleanor **Powell**

5ft 6½in

(ELEANOR TORREY POWELL)

Born: **November 21, 1912**
Springfield, Massachusetts, USA
Died: **February 11, 1982**

As a child, Eleanor was a dreamer, with very little interest in school work. From the age of eleven, she concentrated on her dancing skills – learning both ballet and acrobatics. She was twelve when she was discovered by the producer, Gus Edwards, and given her stage debut in "Vaudeville Kiddie Revue". She was seen by bandleader, Ben Bernie, who hired her to dance in his New York nightclubs. Eleanor could see that she needed to tap in order to get work, so she took lessons at Jack Donohue's Dance School. In 1927, she was in private shows with the great Bill Robinson. In 1929, she became a Broadway star in "Follow Thru" – tapping like a machine gun to "Button Up Your Overcoat". She was given a couple of bit parts in film musicals, starting with *Queen High,* in 1930, but had to wait five years before the movies were ready to showcase her talent. But even then, it was only a very small part, in *George White's 1935 Scandals*. She starred in Broadway shows and also appeared with Paul Whiteman's band at Carnegie Hall. Her spell of movie stardom began with *Born to Dance*. It finished shortly after she married Glenn Ford in 1943, and concentrated on raising their son, Peter, who was born two years later. After their divorce in 1959, Eleanor worked briefly as a night-club entertainer before becoming a minister in the Unity Church. Eleanor died of cancer at the age of sixty-nine, in Beverly Hills.

George White's 1935
Scandals (1935)
Broadway Melody of 1936 (1935)
Born to Dance (1936)
Broadway Melody of 1938 (1937)
Rosalie (1937)
Honolulu (1939)
Broadway Melody of
1940 (1940)
Lady Be Good (1941)
Ship Ahoy (1942)
I Dood It (1943)
Sensations of 1945 (1944)

Jane **Powell**

5ft 0½in

(SUZANNE LORRAINE BURCE)

Born: **April 1, 1929**
Portland, Oregon, USA

Jane took a few singing lessons and then sang on local radio, where she was soon given her own program. She also attended Agnes Peters Dancing school, in Portland, and performed on stage, before her parents took her to Los Angeles, to compete in a big talent show called "Hollywood Showcase". It was enough for MGM to take her on and place her in the experienced hands of the man who had masterminded Deanna Durbin's career – Joe Pasternak. In 1944, she was loaned to United Artists for her film debut, in the minor musical, *Song of the Open Road*. The one good thing about it, was that she adopted the character's name – Jane Powell. MGM began to pitch her as a kind of poor man's Durbin, which she wasn't, but she did her best with the material given to her. In 1949 she sang at President Harry S. Truman's inauguration ball, and married the first of five husbands, the ice skater, Geary Steffin. One of Jane's bridesmaids was Elizabeth Taylor. Jane was charming in several musicals, but none was as successful as *Seven Brides for Seven Brothers*. After her film career ended, Jane appeared in stage musicals including "South Pacific" and "The Sound of Music". Since 1988, she's been married to the former child star, Dickie Moore. Jane was seen on TV as recently as 2002.

Holiday in Mexico (1946)
Three Daring Daughters (1948)
A Date with Judy (1948)
Luxury Liner (1948)
Nancy Goes to Rio (1950)
Two Weeks with Love (1950)
Royal Wedding (1951)
Rich, Young and Pretty (1951)
Small Town Girl (1953)
Three Sailors and a Girl (1953)
Seven Brides for Seven
Brothers (1954)
Deep in My Heart (1954)
Athena (1954)
Hit the Deck (1955)
The Girl Most Likely (1957)
Marie (1985)

Robert **Powell**
5ft 8½in
(ROBERT POWELL)

Born: **May 5, 1943**
Salford, Lancashire, England

Robert was already keen on acting at the age of six, when still in his early years at junior school. When he was twelve years old, he went to Manchester Grammar School, where he excelled at Ancient History, Greek, and Latin. This led to a place at Manchester University, where he began reading Law, but he switched to Drama. He appeared on stage during that time, making his debut, with Stoke-on-Trent Repertory. In 1967, he made his film debut, with an uncredited role in the Peter Yates directed, *Robbery*. Two years later, Robert had a small role in *Walk a Crooked Path,* and then made a slightly bigger appearance in the original version of *The Italian Job*. But TV appeared to be a more obvious way for him to earn a living – with 'Doomwatch' providing more than a year's work. By the early 1970s, Robert was the popular star of several television dramas, but lacking a movie role which was big enough to propel him forward. From an artistic point of view, he had his moments. *The Asphyx* and *Mahler* were certainly two of them and *Tommy* was full of star names. But Robert was at his best as Richard Hannay, in another big screen remake of *The Thirty Nine Steps*. He repeated the role in 1988 on TV. In 1975, he married former "Pan's People" dancer, Barbara Lord. They had two children. For the past three years, Robert has been seen regularly as Mark Williams. in the TV hospital drama, 'Holby City'.

The Italian Job (1969)
Secrets (1971)
Asylum (1972)
The Asphyx (1973)
Mahler (1974)
Tommy (1975)
Beyond Good and Evil (1977)
The Thirty Nine Steps (1978)
Harlequin (1980)
Imperativ (1982)
Shaka Zulu (1987)
The Mystery of
Edwin Drood (1993)
Hey Mr DJ (2005)

William **Powell**
6ft
(WILLIAM HORATIO POWELL)

Born: **July 29, 1892**
Pittsburgh, Pennsylvania, USA
Died: **March 5, 1984**

Bill was the only child of Horatio Powell, a public accountant, and his wife, Nettie. When he was fourteen, the family moved to Kansas City, Missouri, where he later attended high school and showed an early aptitude for acting in several of the school stage productions. After graduating from high school, Bill went to New York, where he enrolled at the American Academy of Dramatic Arts. In 1912, he started his career with a spell in vaudeville, and he made his New York stage debut, in "The Ne'er Do Well". He then toured with stock companies until his first Broadway hit, in "Spanish Love", led to a movie offer and a film debut, in the John Barrymore 1922 version of *Sherlock Holmes*. Bill's first starring role was in Paramount's sound film, *Interference,* in 1928. A year later he played opposite Louise Brooks, in *The Canary Murder Case*. It was his Oscar-nominated role of Nick Charles, in *The Thin Man,* that made him a star. A year earlier, a two-year marriage to Carole Lombard, ended in divorce. Bill was successful throughout the 1930s and 1940s – with Oscar nominations for *My Man Godfrey,* and *Life with Father.* He retired after making *Mister Roberts*. Bill had been married to Diana Lewis for over twenty-four years when suffering cardiac arrest, at his home in Palm Springs, California.

One Way Passage (1932)
Manhattan Melodrama (1934)
The Thin Man (1934)
Evelyn Prentice (1934)
The Great Ziegfeld (1936)
My Man Godfrey (1936)
Libeled Lady (1936)
The Emperor's Candlesticks (1937)
I Love You Again (1940)
Ziegfeld Follies (1946)
Life with Father (1947)
The Senator Was Indiscreet (1947)
Dancing in the Dark (1949)
It's a Big Country (1951)
How to Marry a Millionaire (1953)
Mister Roberts (1955)

Tyrone **Power**
5ft 10in
(TYRONE EDMUND POWER JR.)

Born: **May 5, 1914**
Cincinnati, Ohio, USA
Died: **November 15, 1958**

Ty came from an established theatrical family. His father, the English-born, Tyrone Power Snr., had acted with Henry Irving and appeared in silent screen epics. In 1915, the Powers moved to California. After her divorce in 1920, Patia, Ty's mother, worked as a stage actress and at the age of seven, he appeared with her in "La Golondrina". On graduating from Purcell High School, in 1931, he left home to learn what he could from his father. The old man died in his arms that December. Ty made his movie debut in 1932 with a bit part in *Tom Brown of Culver.* It did little for him so he returned to the New York stage. Fox signed him in 1936, and following a couple of small roles, he shot to stardom in *Lloyd's of London.* For seven years, until military service, he was in hit after hit. He married French actress, Annabella, his co-star in *Suez*. Ty was even more popular on his return from the war and fought for the lead in *Nightmare Alley* – his best screen performance. In the 1950s, he also had success on stage. Ty was with his third wife, Debbie, when he died of a heart attack in Madrid, Spain.

Lloyd's of London (1936)
In Old Chicago (1937)
Thin Ice (1937)
Alexander's Ragtime Band (1938)
Suez (1938)
Jesse James (1939)
Johnny Apollo (1940)
The Mark of Zorro (1940)
Blood and Sand (1941)
The Black Swan (1942)
The Razor's Edge (1946)
Nightmare Alley (1947)
Captain from Castile (1947)
Rawhide (1951)
Diplomatic Courier (1952)
King of the Khyber Rifles (1953)
Untamed (1955)
The Eddy Duchin Story (1956)
Abandon Ship! (1957)
The Sun Also Rises (1957)
Witness for the Prosecution (1957)

Paula **Prentiss**
5ft 10in
(PAULA RAGUSA)

Born: **March 4, 1938**
San Antonio, Texas, USA

Paula was the daughter of a Sicilian-born father and an American mother. She and her younger sister, Ann, were two lively, talented girls who looked as if they would grow up to be beautiful. Paula did well at Randolph Macon Academy, in Front Royal, Virginia and then finished off her education by attending Northwestern University, in Evanston, Illinois. It was there, in 1958, that she was seen performing in a school play by a talent scout and given a contract with MGM. She was groomed for stardom by the studio and given her debut in the comedy, *Where the Boys Are* – which also featured the singer, Connie Francis. In 1961, Paula married Richard Benjamin, and they are still together forty-seven years later. Unusually tall compared with most actresses of that era, Paula appeared in four films with Jim Hutton, who was 6ft 5in. But she hit the big time opposite Rock Hudson – who was also tall – in the romantic comedy, *Man's Favorite Sport?* She then co-starred with Peter Sellers, in *The World of Henry Orient,* before landing a serious role in the war drama, *In Harm's Way.* Paula has continued acting – mainly in supporting roles – and she can be seen in the 2007 film, *Hard Four,* which stars one of her two children, Ross Benjamin.

Where the Boys Are (1960)
The Honeymoon Machine (1961)
Bachelor in Paradise (1961)
Man's Favorite Sport (1964)
The World of Henry Orient (1964)
Looking for Love (1964)
In Harm's Way (1965)
What's New Pussycat? (1965)
Catch-22 (1970)
Move (1970)
Born to Win (1971)
Last of the Red Hot Lovers (1972)
Crazy Joe (1974)
The Parralax View (1974)
The Stepford Wives (1975)
The Black Marble (1980)
Buddy Buddy (1981)
Hard Four (2007)

Micheline **Presle**
5ft 4in
(MICHELINE NICOLE JULIA ÉMILIENNE CHASSAGNE)

Born: **August 22, 1922**
Paris, France

Micheline's ambition from her early teens was to become an actress. Her convent school work was achieved with as little effort as she needed, and her visits to the cinema were the most important part of her week. When she was fourteen, she began taking acting classes, and in 1937, she auditioned successfully for her first film role in *La Fessée*. It won her the Prix Suzanne Bianchetti, as the most promising young actress in the French cinema. She combined her film work with acting classes from Raymond Rouleau. Her reputation was secured at the age of twenty, and she appeared on stage and in films during the occupation of Paris by the Nazis. She headed for Hollywood after *Le Diable au corps,* had been well received, and she made three films there. The first of which, *Under My Skin,* co-starred John Garfield. In America she married William Marshall. Their daughter, is the actress and director, Tonie Marshall. She had a long career in French films after that, but occasionally appeared in American productions such as *The Prize.* Micheline is still acting in movies, in 2009.

La Belle Aventure (1942)
Falbalas (1945) Boule de suif (1945)
Le Diable au corps (1947)
Under My Skin (1950) American
Guerilla in the Philippines (1950)
L'Amour d'une femme (1954)
Beatrice Cenci (1956) Les Louves (1957)
Christine (1958) Blind Date (1959)
L'Amants de cinq jours (1961)
The Seven Deadly Sins (1962)
The Devil and the Ten
Commandments (1962) If a Man
Answers (1962) The Prize (1963)
La Religieuse (1966)
The King of Hearts (1966)
Peau d'âne (1970)
Les Voleurs de nuit (1984)
Les Misérables (1995)
Bad Company (1999)
Tender Souls (2001)
Vertiges de l'amour (2001)
Saltimbank (2003)

Elvis **Presley**
6ft
(ELVIS AARON PRESLEY)

Born: **January 8, 1935**
Tupelo, Mississippi, USA
Died: **August 16, 1977**

Elvis' poor father, Vernon, had struggled through the years of the Great Depression as a sharecropper. His mother, Gladys, was a sewing machine operator. Elvis, who was the second of identical twins, (his brother was stillborn), had a United Nations of nationalities in his blood – including British, German and Cherokee Indian. As he grew up he became very close to his mother and developed a strong sense of religion and a love for gospel music. When he was ten, Elvis won second prize for singing "Old Shep" at a Dairy Show. His dad moved the family to Memphis, to escape from the law for bootlegging liquor and Elvis began to live for playing the guitar and singing. At L.C. Humes High School, his musical tastes weren't appreciated. He absorbed all kinds of sounds – most of all, those put out on the black labels. He made his first recordings, at Sun Records, in 1953. He appeared at the Grand Ole Opry, Nashville and in 1956, had a monster hit single with "Heartbreak Hotel". Later that same year, young girls drowned out the dialogue by screaming every time he appeared in his debut film, the western, *Love Me Tender.* Most of Elvis' movies were light musical comedies, but a couple – *Jailhouse Rock* and *King Creole* – required and delivered, a fair amount of dramatic acting from "The King" as he became known. His United States Army service kept him in the public eye, but good film vehicles became rare. When he died of cardiac arrhythmia, in Memphis, he left his fans a wealth of great music and a few very acceptable movies.

Love Me Tender (1956)
Loving You (1957)
Jailhouse Rock (1957)
King Creole (1958)
G.I.Blues (1960)
Flaming Star (1960)
Wild in the Country (1961)
Viva Las Vegas (1964)
Girl Happy (1965)
Change of Habit (1969)

Kelly **Preston**
5ft 7in
(KELLY KAMALELEHUA SMITH)

Born: **October 13, 1962**
Honolulu, Hawaii, USA

Kelly moved around a lot as a little girl. Although her father's position, as an agent for an agricultural company based in Hawaii, finished, the family spent a year in Iraq (during the good times) and then two years in Australia. Sadly, her father was drowned in an accident when she was young and Kelly took the name of her adoptive father, Peter Palzis. Back in Hawaii, Kelly became an Elite model, got work in TV commercials and developed an interest in acting. After she had graduated from Punahou High School, in Honolulu, she studied Drama and Theater, at the University of Southern California. Her first television role was appropriately in an episode of 'Hawaii Five-O', in 1980. More television work led to her film debut – still as Kelly Palzis – in a 1983 Charles Bronson action drama, titled *10 to Midnight*. In 1986, Kelly began a two-year marriage to the actor, Kevin Gage. In 1991, after her divorce, she married John Travolta, and gave up her career for a while to raise their son, Jett. She and her husband, who are Scientologists added a little daughter, Ella Bleu, in 2000. Kelly's return to the world of films in 1996, resulted in a trio of strong titles including *Citizen Ruth* and *Jerry Maguire*. Her recent film, *Death Sentence,* gained her high marks from critics and audiences. After mourning the death of their son, Kelly and John will be seen together, in *Old Dogs*.

Christine (1983)
Mischief (1985)
Secret Admirer (1985)
52 Pick-Up (1986) Twins (1988)
Citizen Ruth (1996)
From Dusk Till Dawn (1996)
Jerry Maguire (1996)
Nothing to Lose (1997)
For Love of the Game (1999)
What a Girl Wants (2003)
Eulogy (2004)
Return to Sender (2004)
Sky High (2005)
Broken Bridges (2006)
Death Sentence (2007)

Robert **Preston**
5ft 10in
(ROBERT PRESTON MESERVEY)

Born: **June 8, 1918**
Newton Highlands, Massachusetts, USA
Died: **March 21, 1987**

The son of a man who made a modest living in a garment factory, Robert's life took an upward turn when his parents moved to California. In Los Angeles he attended Abraham Lincoln High School, where he performed on several musical instruments at concerts, and also had his first taste of acting. After graduation, he studied at the Pasadena Community Playhouse. In 1938, when appearing in "Idiot's Delight', he was seen by a Paramount scout, and signed by the head of their B-picture department. He was ready to return to the stage but his bit part debut, in the 1938 drama, *King of Alcatraz,* led to his big break, in Cecil B. De Mille's *Union Pacific,* and another important film, *Beau Geste*. In 1940, he married actress, Catherine Craig – who was his wife for more than thirty-six years. From 1943, Robert served as an intelligence officer with the U.S. 9th Air Force. During the 1950s, Robert was most frequently on TV. He came back strongly in *The Music Man,* and near the end of his career, he was nominated for a Best Supporting Actor Oscar, for *Victor Victoria*. Robert died of lung cancer at his home in Montecito, California.

Union Pacific (1939)
Beau Geste (1939)
North West Mounted Police (1940)
The Lady from Cheyenne (1941)
Reap the Wild Wind (1942)
This Gun for Hire (1942)
Wake Island (1942)
The Macomber Affair (1947)
Blood on the Moon (1948)
Whispering Smith (1948)
Tulsa (1949)
The Sundowners (1950)
The Last Frontier (1955)
The Dark at the Top of
the Stairs (1962)
The Music Man (1962)
How the West Was Won (1962)
All the Way Home (1963)
Junior Bonner (1972)
Victor Victoria (1982)

Dennis **Price**
6ft 2in
(DENNISTOUN FRANKLYN JOHN ROSE-PRICE)

Born: **June 23, 1915**
Twyford, Berkshire, England
Died: **October 6, 1973**

Dennis was from a military background. He was educated at Radley College and Oxford University, where he won prizes for oratory. He studied at the Embassy Theater School of Acting, and made his stage debut, in Croydon, in 1937. He served in the Royal Artillery from 1949-42 and was introduced to filmgoers, in Powell & Pressburger's *A Canterbury Tale*. He was limited in the kind of roles he could play – often badly miscast – especially as a romantic hero. His best role – in the classic Ealing comedy, *Kind Hearts and Coronets,* was undervalued at the time because of Guinness's eight-part brilliance. Dennis divorced his wife of eleven years, Joan Schofield, in 1950, and his homosexuality became much more apparent on screen. A failed suicide attempt, in 1954, led to an increasing dependency on alcohol. He continued in supporting roles and was an admirable 'Jeeves' on TV in 'The World of Wooster'. Dennis died in Guernsey, of heart failure and cirrhosis of the liver, a few months after he'd completed work on his final film – *Son of Dracula*.

A Canterbury Tale (1944)
A Place of One's Own (1945)
Jassy (1947) Master of Bankdam (1947)
Good-Time Girl (1948)
Kind Hearts and Coronets (1949)
The Magic Box (1951) The House in
the Square (1951) The Intruder (1953)
Oh... Rosalinda! (1955)
Private's Progress (1956)
Fortune is a Woman (1957)
The Naked Truth (1957) Danger
Within (1959) I'm All Right Jack (1959)
School for Scoundrels (1960)
Oscar Wilde (1960)
Tunes of Glory (1960) Victim (1961)
Ten Little Indians (1965)
The Rise and Rise of Michael
Rimmer (1970)
Alice's Adventures in
Wonderland (1972)
Theater of Blood (1973)

Vincent **Price**
6ft 4in
(VINCENT LEONARD PRICE JR.)

Born: **May 27, 1911**
St. Louis, Missouri, USA
Died: **October 25, 1993**

Born into a wealthy family – his father was President of the National Candy Company – Vincent attended St. Louis Country Day School until he was fifteen. His parents then paid for him to go on a grand tour of Europe, before he went to Yale University, where he sang in Gilbert and Sullivan operettas. He worked briefly as a teacher before getting a History degree from London University and studying Art at the Courtauld Institute. During that period, he took acting classes and made his stage debut at Dublin's Gate Theater, in 1935, in "Chicago", then "Victoria Regina", which he went back to the USA with, and performed on the New York stage. In 1938, Vincent made his film debut, in *Service de Luxe* and married the first of three actress wives, Edith Barrett. He was in several excellent movies during the 1940s and 1950s – including *Song of Bernadette, Laura, Leave Her to Heaven,* and *While the City Sleeps.* Later on in his career, he specialized in horror films and presented cooking programs on television. Vincent died of lung cancer, in Los Angeles.

The House of
the Seven Gables (1940)
Hudson's Bay (1941)
The Song of Bernadette (1943)
Laura (1944) Leave Her to
Heaven (1945) Dragonwyck (1946)
Rogues' Regiment (1948)
The Three Musketeers (1948)
The Bribe (1949)
Champagne for Caesar (1950)
His Kind of Woman (1951)
House of Wax (1953)
While the City Sleeps (1956)
The Fly (1958)
House on Haunted Hill (1959)
Pit and the Pendulum (1961)
Tales of Terror (1962) The Raven (1963)
The Masque of the Red Death (1964)
Theater of Blood (1973)
House of the Long Shadows (1983)
The Whales of August (1987)
Edward Scissorhands (1990)

Richard **Pryor**
5ft 10in
(RICHARD FRANKLIN LENNOX THOMAS PRYOR III)

Born: **December 1, 1940**
Peoria, Illinois, USA
Died: **December 10, 2005**

Richie's mother, Gertrude, was a well-known local prostitute, and his father, Leroy Pryor, who was an ex-boxer, acted as her pimp. To add to that warm family atmosphere, the Pryors lived in his grand-mother's brothel. Richie was raised by her from the age of ten and miraculously, he retained a sharp sense of humor during an appalling childhood – which ended with his expulsion from school. At fourteen he began to make a life for himself as a drum-mer in a night club. In 1958, there was his two years of military service – much of it spent in army prison due to some violence triggered by a racial incident, when he was stationed in Germany. Richie got his act together in 1963, when he moved to New York and began doing stand-up, in clubs. He worked on television shows including 'Tonight' and 'Ed Sullivan' and made his movie debut, in 1967 in *The Busy Body*. In Las Vegas, he started to use profanity and words like "nigger" in his act and it was his unique ability to embarrass his audiences that made him popular. In the 1970's, Richie made records and acted in several very funny films. In his later years, he was confined to a wheelchair due to multiple sclerosis. He was married seven times – twice each to two of his wives – Flynn Belaine and Jennifer Lee. He died in Encino, California, of a heart attack.

Wild in the Streets (1968)
Lady Sings the Blues (1972)
The Mack (1973)
Hit! (1973)
Uptown Saturday Night (1974)
Silver Streak (1976)
Which Way Is Up? (1977)
Blue Collar (1978)
California Suite (1978)
The Muppet Movie (1979)
Stir Crazy (1980)
Bustin' Loose (1981)
The Toy (1982)
Brewster's Millions (1985)
See No Evil, Hear No Evil (1989)
Lost Highway (1997)

Jürgen **Prochnow**
6ft
(JÜRGEN PROCHNOW)

Born: **June 10, 1941**
Berlin, Germany

The son of an engineer, Jürgen, and his older brother, Dieter, were taken to live in Düsseldorf when the allied bombs began raining down on Berlin. Following his high school education, where he developed a keen interest in acting, Jürgen studied at the Folkwang Academy in Essen. After his graduation, he gained early experience on the German stage. His first screen job was in 1970, as a sexed-up teenager in a tele-vision drama called 'Unternehmer'. His film debut was two years later, when he had a supporting role in the romantic *Zoff*. Jürgen's first starring role was in a prison drama, *The Brutalization of Franz Blum*. A year later, *Katharina Blum,* made Jürgen a star in Germany, but the role which brought him to international attention was as the German submarine captain, in the TV-series *Das Boot*. Through the resulting fame, he went to Wales to act in his first English-language production, *The Keep*. His second, *Dune,* was almost a disaster. When filming a tricky stunt, where green smoke (simulating poison gas) was emerging from his cheek, a high-powered bulb exploded and he received first and second-degree burns. Jürgen recovered and the following year, at the Bavarian Film Awards, he was voted Best Actor, for *The Cop and the Girl*. It wasn't long before he was rubbing shoulders with Brando, and acting for David Lynch. He would become arguably the most successful German actor ever to work in Hollywood.

The Brutalization of Franz Blum (1974)
One or the Other (1974)
The Lost Honor of
Katharina Blum (1975)
Operation Ganymed (1977)
The Keep (1983)
Dune (1984) The Seventh Sign (1988)
A Dry White Season (1989)
Twin Peaks: Fire Walk with Me (1992)
The English Patient (1996)
Air Force One (1997)
The Replacement Killers (1998)
The Da Vinci Code (2006) Beerfest (2006)
La Conjura de El Escoril (2008)

Jonathan **Pryce**
6ft 2in
(JOHN PRICE)

Born: **June 1, 1947**
Holywell, Flintshire, Wales

Jon's father, Isaac Price, was a former coalminer, who ran a grocery store, where his mother, Margaret, worked as cashier. Jon did well enough during his early years at school to go on to Holywell Grammar School. When he was sixteen he had a short spell at art school before undergoing teacher training, at Edge Hill College, in Ormskirk. It was there that his gift for acting was first discovered in college plays. Fired by a friend's enthusiasm, he applied to RADA in London, and was awarded a scholarship. After graduating, he acted in a few plays before becoming Artistic Director, at Liverpool's Everyman Theater Company. While there, he fell in love with the Irish actress, Kate Fahey. They married in 1974 and had three children. Jon made his film debut, in 1976, in *Voyage of the Damned.* In 1980, he won the Olivier Award for "Hamlet" at the Royal Court Theater. Jon was voted Best actor at Cannes, for *Carrington,* and he has rarely failed to impress during the following twenty years of film work. He will soon be seen in *Echelon Conspiracy.*

Breaking Glass (1980)
The Ploughman's Lunch (1983)
Brazil (1985) The Adventures of
Baron Munchausen (1988)
The Rachel Papers (1989)
Glengarry Glen Ross (1992)
Deadly Advice (1993)
The Age of Innocence (1993)
Carrington (1995) Evita (1996)
Regeneration (1997)
Tomorrow Never Dies (1997)
Ronin (1998)
Stigmata (1999)
The Affair of the Necklace (2001)
Unconditional Love (2002)
Pirates of the Caribbean:
The Curse of the Black Pearl (2003)
De-Lovely (2004) The New World (2005)
Pirates 2 (2006)
The Moon and the Stars (2007)
Pirates 3 (2007) Leatherheads (2008)
Bedtime Stories (2008)
G.I. Joe: The Rise of Cobra (2009)

Bill **Pullman**
6ft 1½in
(WILLIAM PULLMAN)

Born: **December 17, 1953**
Hornell, New York, USA

Bill was one of seven children. His father James Pullman, who was a physician, came from an English background, and his mother, Johanna's family came from Holland. In 1971, Bill graduated from Hornell High School, and then attended the State Universities of New York at Delhi, and at Oneonta. After he'd received his Masters Degree in Fine Arts, from Massachusetts University, Bill taught Theater – at Delhi and Montana State University. Bill moved to New York City at the age of twenty-eight, to pursue his career as an actor. By the early 1980s, he was jetting between assignments with theater companies in New York and Los Angeles. In 1986, he made his television debut, in an episode of 'Cagney and Lacey' and his film debut, in *Ruthless People.* The following year, he married Tamara Hurwitz, with whom he has three children. Bill has built his career performing in strong supporting roles in a steady stream of good films. In 2001, he shared a Bronze Wrangler Award, for the TV-movie – 'The Virginian'.

Ruthless People (1986)
Spaceballs (1987)
The Serpent and the Rainbow(1988)
Rocket Gibraltar (1988)
The Accidental Tourist (1988)
A League of Their Own (1992)
Singles (1992) Sommersby (1993)
Sleepless in Seattle (1993)
Malice (1993)
Wyatt Earp (1994)
The Last Seduction (1994)
While You Were Sleeping (1995)
Independence Day (1996)
Lost Highway (1997)
Zero Effect (1998)
Brokedown Palace (1999)
The Guilty (2000)
Igby Goes Down (2002)
Dear Wendy (2005)
You Kill Me (2007)
Nobel Son (2007)
Surveillance (2008)
Your Name Is Here (2008)

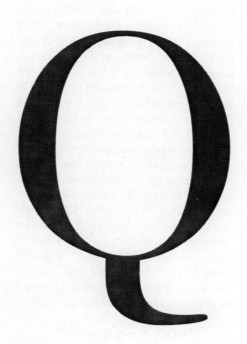

Dennis **Quaid**
6ft 1in
(DENNIS WILLIAM QUAID)

Born: **April 9, 1954**
Houston, Texas, USA

Dennis, who was raised as a Baptist, was the son of William Rudy Quaid, an electrician, and his wife, Jaunita, who worked in real estate. He was educated at Pershing Middle School in Houston, before studying at Bellaire High School, in Bellaire, Texas, where he took a keen interest in drama. At the University of Houston, he was given the opportunity to learn from the drama coach, Cecil Pickett. When his brother was Oscar nominated for *The Last Detail,* Dennis dropped out of university to pursue an acting career of his own. He moved to Los Angeles in 1975, but initially found the going hard. An uncredited role in *Crazy Mama* and a few other bit parts and TV scraps was the sum total until *Breaking Away.* In 1978, he married P.J.Soles. His rise to stardom saw him tackle all kinds of material – *The Right Stuff, The Big Easy* and *Far From Heaven* – being standouts. His second wife was Meg Ryan, with whom he had a son. Since 2004, Dennis has been married to Kim Buffington. They have twins, who were born in 2007.

Breaking Away (1979)
The Long Riders (1980) The Right
Stuff (1983) Dreamscape (1984)
Enemy Mine (1985)
The Big Easy (1987)
Innerspace (1987) D.O.A. (1988)
Everybody's All-American (1988)
Great Balls of Fire! (1989)
Come See the Paradise (1990)
Postcards from the Edge (1990)
Flesh and Bone (1993)
Wyatt Earp (1994) Dragonheart (1996)
Saviour (1998)
The Parent Trap (1998)
Any Given Sunday (1999)
Frequency (2000) Traffic (2000)
The Rookie (2002)
Far from Heaven (2002)
The Day After Tomorrow (2004)
In Good Company (2004)
American Dreamz (2006)
Smart People (2008)
Vantage Point (2008)
The Horsemen (2008)

Randy **Quaid**
6ft 4½in
(RANDALL RUDY QUAID)

Born: **October 1, 1950**
Houston, Texas, USA

Randy is the older brother of Dennis. The two had an identical early education with one difference: while Dennis was appearing in a play at university, Randy was discovered by director, Peter Bogdanovich and given his impressive film debut, in *The Last Picture Show.* He was nominated for a Best Supporting Actor Oscar, for his role as Larry Meadows, in *The Last Detail.* Randy proved his comedic talent in several of the *National Lampoon* movies - most notably, *Christmas Vacation.* In 1987, he won a Golden Globe for his TV-film portrayal of President Johnson in 'LBJ: The Early Years'. Randy's long list of more than ninety movie credits include *The Missouri Breaks, Bound for Glory, Independence Day,* and the award winning, *Brokeback Mountain.* Randy has been married twice and has a daughter, called Amanda. His second wife, Evi Motolaner, was a model for the photographer, Helmut Newton, in her early days. She directed Randy in the 1999 movie, *The Debtors.* In 2004, he appeared on stage at the Actors Drama School in New York in Sam Shepard's "God of Hell". Four years later, he was banned by Equity after problems during a Seattle production of "Lone Star Love".

The Last Picture Show (1971)
What's Up Doc? (1972) The Last
Detail (1973) The Apprenticeship
of Duddy Kravitz (1974)
Breakout (1975)
The Missouri Breaks (1976)
Bound for Glory (1976)
Midnight Express (1978)
The Long Riders (1980)
Vacation (1983) Parents (1989)
Christmas Vacation (1989)
Quick Change (1990) The Paper (1994)
Independence Day (1996)
Kingpin (1996)
Milwaukee, Minnesota (2003)
Carolina (2003) Brokeback
Mountain (2005) The Ice
Harvest (2005) Goya's Ghosts (2006)
Real Time (2008) Balls Out:
The Gary Houseman Story (2008)

John **Qualen**
5ft 7in
(JOHAN MANDT KVALEN)

Born: **December 8, 1899**
Vancouver, British Columbia, Canada
Died: **September 12, 1987**

The son of Norwegian immigrants – his father, who changed the family name to Qualen – served as a Lutheran minister in Elgin, Illinois, which is where John grew up and went to school. He won a scholarship to Northwestern University in Evanston, on the strength of his good showing in an oratory contest. After studying drama for three years, John went to live in New York. In 1924, he married Pearle Larson, a girl from a Scandinavian background. He worked in summer stock productions until getting his chance on Broadway – as a Swedish janitor in "Street Scene". In 1931 he made his screen debut, in the movie version, which was shot in New York City. By the mid-1930s he had moved up the cast list in films such as *Sing and Like It* and soon supported big stars like Cagney, Paul Muni, and Janet Gaynor. When John made his fifty-third film – the classic Cary Grant comedy – *His Girl Friday,* he was still unknown. But he acted in fine films, such as *The Grapes of Wrath, Casablanca* and *The Fugitive.* His last appearance was in a 1974 episode of TV's 'Movin' On'. John died of heart failure, in Torrance, California.

Black Fury (1935)
The Three Musketeers (1935)
The Road to Glory (1936)
Meet Nero Wolfe (1936)
Stand Up and Fight (1939)
His Girl Friday (1940)
The Grapes of Wrath (1940)
Angels Over Broadway (1940)
Knute Rockne All American (1940)
The Long Voyage Home (1940)
The Road to Glory (1940)
Out of the Fog (1941)
The Shepherd of the Hills (1941)
The Devil and Daniel Webster (1941)
Larceny, Inc. (1942) Tortilla Flat (1942)
Casablanca (1942) Dark Waters (1944)
Roughly Speaking (1945)
Captain Kidd (1945)
The Fugitive (1947) The Big Steal (1949)
Unchained (1955)
The Searchers (1956)

Sir Anthony **Quayle**
6ft 1in
(JOHN ANTHONY QUAYLE)

Born: **September 7, 1913**
Southport, Lancashire, England
Died: **October 29, 1989**

Tony was educated at the famous Rugby School. He trained for the stage at the Royal Academy of Dramatic Art in London and after appearing in music hall, made his stage debut at the Q Theater, in 1931, in a production of "Robin Hood". He joined the Old Vic Theater the following year and soon became one of the country's leading Shakespearean actors. In 1934, he married the actress, Hermione Hannen, and in 1935, made his film debut, with an uncredited role in *Moscow Nights*. It was followed by a small part in *Pygmalion*, in 1938, and television plays. During World War II, he served as an officer in the British Army and was appointed Commander of auxiliary units. He divorced his first wife in 1941, and in 1947, he married actress, Dorothy Hyson, with whom he had two children. Tony's first post-war film role was as Marcellus, in Olivier's *Hamlet*. He had a good film career with a memorable role in *Ice-Cold in Alex* and was nominated for a Best Supporting Actor Oscar, for *Anne of the Thousand Days*. He died of cancer at his home in London. Tony's daughter, Jenny Quayle, is an actress.

Hamlet (1948)
Saraband for Dead Lovers (1948)
Oh...Rosalinda! (1955)
The Battle of the River Plate (1956)
The Wrong Man (1956)
Woman in a Dressing Gown (1957)
Ice-Cold in Alex (1958)
Tarzan's Great Adventure (1959)
The Guns of Navarone (1961)
Lawrence of Arabia (1962)
The Fall of the Roman Empire (1964)
Operation Crossbow (1965)
A Study in Terror (1965)
MacKenna's Gold (1969)
Anne of the Thousand Days (1969)
The Tamarind Seed (1974)
The Eagle Has Landed (1976)
Murder by Decree (1979)
The Legend of the Holy Drinker (1988)
Buster (1988)
King of the Wind (1990)

Kathleen **Quinlan**
5ft 5in
(KATHLEEN DENISE QUINLAN)

Born: **November 19, 1954**
Pasadena, California, USA

Kathy was an only child. Her father, Robert Quinlan, was a television sports director. Her mother, Josephine, worked as a military supply supervisor. Kathy grew up near San Francisco, in Mill Valley. She attended the local Tamalplais High School, which is where she first developed her acting skills. She was a brilliant gymnast and at one time, considered teaching it as a career. In 1972, she stood in for Trish van Devere, in a highboard jumping sequence, in the film *One is a Lonely Number*. In 1973, she made her official movie debut, in *American Graffiti*. She has had two phases to her movie career – the first peaked with *I Never Promised You a Rose Garden*. The second got going in the late 1980s, after a fair amount of poor material. The one thing I would note is, Kathy got better as she matured. She was nominated for a Best Supporting Actress Oscar, for *Apollo 13*, and won a Blockbuster Entertainment Award for her supporting role, as Amy Taylor, in *Breakdown*. Since then, Kathy has produced some fine performances. In 1994, Kathy married actor, Bruce Abbott. They have two children. From 1999 until 2002, Kathy starred in the television drama series, 'Family Law'.

Lifeguard (1976)
I Never Promised You a
Rose Garden (1977)
Independence Day (1983)
Twilight Zone:
The Movie (1983)
Sunset (1988)
Clara's Heart (1988)
The Doors (1991)
Apollo 13 (1995)
Breakdown (1997)
Event Horizon (1997)
Lawn Dogs (1997)
A Civil Action (1998)
The Battle of
Shaker Heights (2003)
The Hills Have Eyes (2006)
American Fork (2007)
Breach (2007)
Made of Honor (2008)

Aidan **Quinn**
5ft 11½in
(AIDAN QUINN)

Born: **March 8, 1959**
Rockford, Illinois, USA

Retaining their historical links with Ireland, Aidan's devoutly Catholic parents raised him in Chicago and in Dublin. He has two brothers and a sister who have gone into show business. After he graduated from Rockford West High School, Aidan received his initial training as an actor, at the Piven Theater Workshop, in Evanston. He began his stage career in Chicago when he was nineteen. He then graduated from the Goodman Theater B.F.A. acting program, and is still a member of the company. Aidan's film debut was opposite Daryl Hannah, in *Reckless*. His breakthrough role was in *Desperately Seeking Susan*. In 1985, Aidan starred in a TV film 'An Early Frost' – as a young lawyer dying of AIDS. Nominated for an Emmy Award, he got plenty of exposure among casting agents. In 1987, he married actress, Elizabeth Bracco. The couple have two daughters. During the 1990s, Aidan's career moved to a higher level following *Legends of the Fall*. He was especially good in *Michael Collins*, *This Is My Father*, *Song for a Raggy Boy*, and *Nine Lives*. Recently, Aidan has been seen on TV, in several episodes of 'Canterbury's Law'.

Reckless (1984)
Desperately Seeking Susan (1985)
The Mission (1986)
Stakeout (1987)
Crusoe (1989) Avalon (1990)
At Play in the Fields of the
Lord (1991) The Playboys (1992)
Benny & Joon (1993) Blink (1994)
Frankenstein (1994)
Legends of the Fall (1994)
The Stars Fell on Henrietta (1995)
Haunted (1995)
Michael Collins (1996)
The Assignment (1997)
Music of the Heart (1999)
Songcatcher (2000)
Stolen Summer (2002)
Song for a Raggy Boy (2003)
Nine Lives (2005)
Dark Matter (2007)
Wise Child (2008)

Anthony **Quinn**
6ft 2in
(ANTONIO RUDOLFO OAXACA QUINN)

Born: **April 21, 1915**
Chihuahua, Mexico
Died: **June 3, 2001**

Tony's father, Francisco Quinn, was the son of an Irishman and his Mexican wife. His mother, Manuela, was of Aztec origin. Shortly after they moved to California, he suffered the loss of his father in an automobile accident. Tony was educated at Polytechnic High School in Los Angeles, where he trained as a draughtsman and even attended classes under Frank Lloyd Wright. But Tony's big ambition was to become an actor. A job as a janitor in a drama school led to parts in amateur productions and acting lessons from Michael Checkov. In one play, "Clean Beds", he portrayed an elderly drunk. He was seen by one, John Barrymore, and unofficially adopted. Tony made his first movie appearance in 1936, with a walk-on part in *Parole*. A series of roles as "ethnics" and pirates, were the best he could get, but in 1938, while Tony was appearing in *The Buccaneer,* he met Kathleen DeMille, the director's daughter. Their marriage did little for his career, but they had five children. Tony won Best Supporting Actor Oscars for *Viva Zapata* and *Lust for Life.* He was nominated as Best Actor, for *Wild Is the Wind* and *Zorba the Greek.* By then he was a major star and a respected painter. Tony died of throat cancer at his home in Boston, leaving his third wife, Kathy, with their two children.

Blood and Sand (1941) **The Ox-Bow Incident** (1943) Back to Bataan (1945)
Sinbad the Sailor (1947)
Viva Zapata! (1952)
La Strada (1954) Lust for Life (1956)
The Ride Back (1957)
Wild Is the Wind (1957)
Hot Spell (1958) Warlock (1959)
The Last Train from Gun Hill (1959)
The Guns of Navarone (1961)
Requiem for a Heavyweight (1962)
Lawrence of Arabia (1962)
The Visit (1964) Zorba the Greek (1964)
The Secret of Santa Vittoria (1969)
The Message (1976)
Lion of the Desert (1981)

J.C. **Quinn**
5ft 7in
(J.C. QUINN)

Born: **November 30, 1940**
Philadelphia, Pennsylvania, USA
Died: **February 10, 2004**

J.C. endured an unhappy childhood. After finishing school, he ran away from home to escape from his abusive father. He was seventeen when he began a career in the United States Airforce. He progressed well as a code-breaker and sometime spy. As a Far East field agent he watched through an oscilloscope as Gary Powers' U2 plane was shot down over the Soviet Union. In the early 1960s, J.C. left the airforce and moved to New Jersey to work as a junior executive. He began to act in plays at the Nutley Community Theater and decided it was the life for him. He landed a leading role in an off-Broadway play, in 1967, and the following year, he joined the Theater Company of Boston. In 1974 he returned to New York to study at Lee Strasberg's Actor's Studio. He made his film debut, four years later, in *On the Yard.* J.C. was kept busy as a character actor from then on, but it took a while before he was known to movie audiences. The comedy drama *Barfly,* made his name for a while but apart from the Sci-Fi thriller, called *Megaville,* he would never be the star. While working on the Goldie Hawn movie *CrissCross,* in Key West, J.C. met his dream woman, Yolande. He married for the first time, aged fifty, and had a happy life until he died in a car crash, in Mexico.

Night-Flowers (1979) **Times Square** (1980) **Eddie Macon's Run** (1983)
Silkwood (1983) **Vision Quest** (1985)
At Close Range (1986) **Barfly** (1987)
Big Business (1988) **Happy Together** (1989) Turner & Hooch (1989)
Gross Anatomy (1989) **Days of Thunder** (1990) **The Babe** (1992)
CrissCross (1992) **The Program** (1993)
The Prophecy (1995)
God's Lonely Man (1996)
Bastard Out of Carolina (1996)
Deceiver (1996)
Digging to China (1998)
Primary Colors (1998)
Across the Line (2000)
Animal Factory (2000) **Takedown** (2000)

R

Daniel **Radcliffe**
5ft 6in
(DANIEL JACOB RADCLIFFE)

Born: July 23, 1989
Fulham, London, England

Dan is the only son of literary agent, Alan Radcliffe, and Marcia Gresham, a BBC Television casting agent. He has Irish blood from his father's side of the family and Jewish from his mother. When he was ten years, old Dan made his TV debut, in the BBC two-part adaptation of Charles Dickens' 'David Copperfield. He was educated at the City of London School for Boys and appeared in several of their stage presentations. While there, in 2000, he was was seen acting with his father and invited by producer David Heyman, to audition for the role of Harry Potter, in the planned filming of J.K. Rowling's best-selling series of books. She could not imagine a "better Harry". Meanwhile, Dan made his film debut, in a supporting role, in *The Tailor of Panama,* starring Pierce Brosnan. It was quickly followed by his Potter debut in *Harry Potter and the Sorcerer's Stone,* which by 2010's, *The Deathly Hallows,* would have been the first of a seven-film run. Dan may have had enough by then – he has already branched out with more adult fare, in *December Boys,* which was shot in Australia. But the Harry Potter series – for which he has received several nominations and one National Movie Award - made him a big star all over the world and will provide him with plenty of future opportunities. In the meantime, Dan enjoys Indie rock music, supports Fulham Football Club, and he's been officially recognized as "Britain's Richest Teenager".

The Tailor of Panama (2001)
Harry Potter and the
Sorcerer's Stone (2001)
Harry Potter and the Chamber
of Secrets (2002)
Harry Potter and the Prisoner
of Azkaban (2004)
Harry Potter and the Goblet
of Fire (2005)
Harry Potter and the Order
of the Phoenix (2007)
December Boys (2007)
Harry Potter and the
Half-Blood Prince (2009)

George **Raft**
5ft 9in
(GEORGE RANFT)

Born: September 26, 1895
New York City, New York, USA
Died: November 24, 1980

George grew up in New York's "Hell's Kitchen" – a tough area which provided characters for many of his movie portrayals. His education was minimal, but he was street-wise and soon made money as a prize fighter. He later earned a living as a dance-hall gigolo and got to know members of the Mafia. He partnered Elsie Pilcer in the Broadway shows – "City Chap", "Gay Paree" and "Palm Beach Nights" – are just a few of them. He married an older woman, Grayce Mulrooney, in 1923, and took care of her, until her death in 1970. It was his mob connection that got him his first film role. He was sent (with a gun in his pocket) to protect a night club run by Texas Guinan. She liked George and got him a small role in her 1929 movie, aptly named, *Queen of the Night Clubs.* His appearance three years later, in *Scarface,* set him on the road to film stardom. From then until the late 1940s, George was a big star. His last big film role, in *Some Like It Hot,* was in character. In 1966, when running the Colony Club, in London, he was barred from re-entering the UK because of his Mafia connections. He died of leukemia, in Los Angeles, California.

Scarface (1932)
If I Had a Million (1932)
Pick-Up (1933) The Bowery (1933)
Limehouse Blues (1934)
Every Night at Eight (1935)
Yours for the Asking (1936)
Souls at Sea (1937)
Spawn of the North (1938)
Each Dawn I Die (1939)
Invisible Stripes (1939)
The House Across the Bay (1940)
They Drive By Night (1940)
Manpower (1941) Broadway (1942)
Background to Danger (1943)
Nob Hill (1945) Johnny Angel (1945)
Nocturne (1946)
Race Street (1948)
Johnny Allegro (1949) Black
Widow (1954) Rogue Cop (1954)
Some Like It Hot (1959)

Aishwarya **Rai**
5ft 7in
(AISHWARYA KRISHNARAJ RAI)

Born: November 1, 1973
Mangalore, Karnataka, India

Aishwarya's dad, Krishnaraj, was a marine biologist. Her mother, Vrinda, was a writer. Her older brother, Aditya, became an engineer in the merchant navy, and was co-producer on her 2003 film, *Dil Ka Rishta.* Aishwarya was a little girl when her father took the family to live in Mumbai. She was educated at the Arya Vidya Mandir High School, in Santa Cruz, and then attended Jai Hind College at Churchgate. After one year she switched to Ruparel College, in Matunga, where she completed her "HSC" studies. Aishwarya's ambition at the time was to become an architect, but her natural attributes resulted in modeling jobs and a crack at the "Miss India" title in 1994. She finished second, but in London, that same year, she won the "Miss World" contest. Aishwarya's victory led to further modeling work and her film debut, in the Tamil production, *Iruvar.* Her Bollywood debut film *Aur Pyaar Ho Gaya* was a flop, but two years later, *Straight from the Heart* was a huge hit and won her the first of her Filmfare Best Actress Awards. Since then, Aishwarya has become a major star and is making her name internationally through movies such as *Bride & Prejudice,* and *Mistress of Spices.* In 2007, she married the Indian actor, Abhishek Bachchan.

Iruvar (1997)
Straight from the Heart (1999)
Taal (1999)
I Have Found It (2000)
Josh (2000)
You Have My Heart (2000)
Love Stories (2000)
Devdas (2002)
Shakthi: The Power (2002)
Chokher Bali (2003)
Don't Say a Word (2003)
The Uniform (2004)
Raincoat (2004)
Bride & Prejudice (2004)
The Mistress of Spices (2005)
Provoked (2006)
Guru (2007)
Jodhaa Akbar (2008)
Sarkar Raj (2008)

Raimu
5ft 8½in
(JULES MURAIRE)

Born: **December 18, 1883**
Toulon, Var, France
Died: **September 20, 1946**

Born into humble circumstances and with very little formal schooling, he was literate enough to create the name "Raimu" by the use of a near-anagram of his birth name. With that title, he made his stage debut at the age of sixteen in the Casino de Toulon. Nine years later, the great music hall star, Félix Mayol – who was also from his town – gave him the opportunity to work as his support act on the Paris circuit. Raimu quickly graduated to the Folies Bergere. For more than twenty years he was famous as a comic and made his silent film debut, in 1912, in *Le Fumiste*. A stage production of Marcel Pagnol's play, "Marius" showcased his talent and he reprised the role in the film version. The 1930s was a golden period for Raimu with superb performances in classic movies such as *Fanny, César, L'Étrange Monsieur Victor, La Femme du Boulanger,* and *La Fille du puisatier.* Shortly after finishing his last film *L'Homme au chapeau rond,* in 1946, Raimu retired and died in hospital during a minor operation. In 1961, the French Government issued a postage stamp with his image. Perhaps even more appropriately, there is a Cinéma Raimu, in Toulon, named in his honor.

Marius (1931) **Fanny** (1932)
Ces messieurs de la santé (1933)
Le Roi (1936) **César** (1936)
Faisons ub rêve (1937)
Vous n'avez rien à déclarer? (1937)
Les Perles de la couronne (1937)
Un carnet de bal (1937)
Gribouille (1937)
L'Étrange Monsieur Victor (1938)
La Femme du boulanger (1938)
Noix de coco (1939)
La Fille du puisatier (1940)
**Les Inconnus dans
la maison** (1942)
Monsieur La Souris (1942)
Le Bienfaiteur (1942)
Untel père et fils (1943)
Le Colonel Chabert (1943)
L'Homme au chapeau rond (1946)

Luise Rainer
5ft 4in
(LUISE RAINER)

Born: **January 12, 1910**
Düsseldorf, Germany

The daughter of a Jewish couple, Heinrich Rainer and his wife Emmy, Luise was educated in Vienna. When she was eighteen, she made her stage debut, at the Dumont Theater, in Düsseldorf. In the following few years, she studied in Vienna with Max Reinhardt and appeared in a large number of plays, including "Measure for Measure", "Mademoiselle", "Saint Joan" and "Men in White". In 1932, she made her first film appearance, in *Sehnsucht 202*. She made three other German-language films before Hitler's attitude towards the Jews made remaining in Austria or Germany, highly dangerous. MGM offered her a contract and Luise arranged to emigrate to the USA. She made her Hollywood film debut in 1935, when she replaced Myrna Loy, opposite William Powell, in *Escapade.* It had a luke-warm reception, but there was a bonus during its filming – she met and fell in love with the playwright, Clifford Odets – whom she married in 1937. In the meantime, Powell had asked for her to co-star with him in *The Great Ziegfeld.* His wish was granted and she won the first of her consecutive Best Actress Oscars - the second was for *The Good Earth.* She divorced Odets in 1940 and disappeared from the screen for three years. In 1945, Luise married a New York publisher, Robert Knittel, and had a daughter, Francesca. At the age of eighty-seven, she reappeared on the big screen in a new version of Dostoyevsky's famous novel, *The Gambler.* As of the summer of 2009, Luise is still the oldest living Oscar winner.

Sehnsucht 202 (1932)
Escapade (1935)
The Great Ziegfeld (1936)
The Good Earth (1937)
**The Emperor's
Candlesticks** (1937)
Big City (1937)
The Toy Wife (1938)
The Great Waltz (1938)
Dramatic School (1938)
Hostages (1943)
The Gambler (1997)

Claude Rains
5ft 6½in
(WILLIAM CLAUDE RAINS)

Born: **November 10, 1889**
Camberwell, London, England
Died: **May 30, 1967**

Claude made his stage debut at the age of ten, when he and other boys from his school were invited to provide a crowd scene in "Nell of Old Drury", at London's Haymarket Theater. That experience convinced him to become an actor. For seven years, he worked as a call-boy at His Majesty's Theater and in 1911, began to get small parts in plays. Sir Herbert Beerbohm Tree, the founder of RADA, recognized the boy's talent and paid for elocution lessons to smooth out his south London accent. He toured Australia, and in 1913, married the first of his six wives, actress Isabel Jeans. Claude served in World War I with the London Scottish Regiment. After his film debut in 1920, in *Build Thy House,* he concentrated on the theater until *The Invisible Man.* He was at his peak in the 1930s and 40s. He was nominated for four Oscars – for *Mr. Smith Goes to Washington, Casablanca, Mr, Skeffington,* and *Notorious.* He worked up until 1965. Claude died of an intestinal hemorrhage, in Laconia, New Hampshire.

The Invisible Man (1933)
Crime Without Passion (1934)
Anthony Adverse (1936)
They Won't Forget (1937)
**The Adventures of
Robin Hood** (1938) **Juarez** (1939)
Mr. Smith Goes to Washington (1939)
The Sea Hawk (1940)
Here Comes Mr. Jordan (1941)
Kings Row (1942) **Moontide** (1942)
Now, Voyager (1942)
Casablanca (1942)
Phantom of the Opera (1943)
Passage to Marseille (1944)
Mr. Skeffington (1944)
Notorious (1946)
Angel on My Shoulder (1946)
The Unsuspected (1947)
Rope of Sand (1949)
**The Man Who Watched the
Trains Go By** (1952)
Lawrence of Arabia (1962)
The Greatest Story Ever Told (1965)

Ella **Raines**
5ft 3in
(ELLA WALLACE RAINES)

Born: **August 6, 1920**
Snoqualmie Falls, Washington, USA
Died: **May 30, 1988**

Ella's father, Ernest Raines, was a foreman at a lumber-mill near their home. In 1938 after graduating from Snoqualmie High School, she went against her mother's wishes when she switched from music and studied Drama at the University of Washington in Seattle. It was a lucky day when she was seen in a stage production by the film director, Howard Hawks, who signed her to work for the new production company he had set up with Charles Boyer. In 1942, she married the first of two husbands, Kenneth Trout. She made her film debut, for Universal in 1943, with Randolph Scott, in *Corvette K-225* – the wartime story of a ship in the Royal Canadian Navy. For seven years, Ella had a good career – appearing in some top films – including the moving *Cry Havoc,* the Preston Sturges' comedy hit, *Hail the Conquering Hero,* and the Burt Lancaster film-noir classic, *Brute Force.* Her work tapered off after she married the fighter pilot, Robin Olds, in 1947 and had two daughters. In 1954 and 1955, Ella was starring on television as 'Janet Dean, Registered Nurse.' She made her last film, *The Man in the Road,* in England, in 1957, and appeared on television in 1984, in one episode of 'Matt Houston'. Ella died of throat cancer in Sherman Oaks, California.

Corvette K-225 (1943)
Cry 'Havoc' (1943)
Phantom Lady (1944)
Hail the Conquering Hero (1944)
Tall in the Saddle (1944)
The Suspect (1944)
The Strange Affair of
Uncle Harry (1945)
The Runaround (1946)
The Web (1947)
Brute Force (1947)
The Senator Was Indiscreet (1947)
The Walking Hills (1949)
Impact (1949)
Singing Guns (1950)
The Second Face (1950)
Ride the Man Down (1952)

Charlotte **Rampling**
5ft 7in
(CHARLOTTE RAMPLING)

Born: **February 5, 1946**
Sturmer, Essex, England

Charly's father, Godfrey Rampling, had been a gold medal-winner in the 4x400 metres relay, at the 1936 Berlin Olympics. He served in the British Army and was later a NATO commander. Charly's early life was sprinkled with overseas postings. She was educated at the Jeanne d'Arc Académie pour Jeunes Filles, in Paris and St. Hilda's School in Bushey, near Windsor. In the early 1960's, she traveled round Europe before working as a model on the London fashion scene and appearing in television commercials. Just ike her dad, Charly was athletic. She made her film debut in 1965, as a water skier, in *The Knack.* A fluency in French was another useful tool for the young actress. There were controversial films such as Visconti's *The Damned,* and Cavani's *The Night Porter* – both featuring Dirk Bogarde. In 1996, she ended her twenty-year marriage to French composer, Jean-Michel Jarre. Charly's still making movies in 2008.

Georgie Girl (1966)
The Damned (1969)
Three (1969)
Henry VIII and His Six Wives (1972)
Asylum (1972)
The Night Porter (1974)
The Purple Taxi (1977)
Stardust Memories (1980)
The Verdict (1982)
Viva la vie! (1984)
Max mon amour (1986)
Angel Heart (1987)
Asphalt Tango (1996)
The Wings of the Dove (1997)
The Cherry Orchard (1999)
Aberdeen (2000)
Under the Sand (2000)
Embrassez qui
vous voudrez (2002)
Swimming Pool (2003)
The Statement (2003)
Le Chiavi di casa (2004)
Lemming (2005)
Heading South (2005)
Chaotic Anna (2005)
The Duchess (2008)

Tony **Randall**
5ft 8in
(ARTHUR LEONARD ROSENBERG)

Born: **February 26, 1920**
Tulsa, Oklahoma, USA
Died: **May 17, 2004**

From a Jewish family, Tony was the son of art dealer, Mogsa, and his wife, Julia. He was educated at Tulsa Central High School and then spent one year at Northwestern University. After deciding to become an actor, he attended New York's Neighborhood Playhouse, where he studied drama and speech under Sanford Meisner, Martha Graham, and Henry Jacobi. As Anthony Randall, he acted in radio soaps and made his New York stage debut in 1941, in "The Circle of Chalk". In 1942, he married Florence Mitchell, and soon after, served in the United States Army Signal Corps. After the war, he worked for two years at the Olney Theatre, in Maryland. In 1947, he made his Broadway debut as Scarus in "Antony and Cleopatra". Tony's screen work began on television in 1949, in 'One Man's Family', and his first movie appearance was in 1957, in *Oh, Men! Oh! Women!* He was soon a star, in popular movies such as *Will Success Spoil Rock Hunter?, Pillow Talk,* and *Let's Make Love* – in which he acted with Marilyn Monroe. Tony became a father for the first time at the advanced age of seventy-seven, when his second wife, Heather, gave birth to their daughter. He made his final film, *It's About Time,* the year he died, in New York, from pneumonia, following heart surgery.

Will Success Spoil Rock
Hunter? (1957)
No Down Payment (1957)
The Mating Game (1959)
Pillow Talk (1959)
The Adventures of
Huckleberry Finn (1960)
Let's Make Love (1960)
Lover Come Back (1961)
Boys Night Out (1962)
7 Faces of Dr. Lao (1964)
The Brass Bottle (1964)
Send Me No Flowers (1964)
Everything You Always Wanted
to Know About Sex (1972)
Down With Love (2003)

Basil **Rathbone**
6ft 1½in
(PHILIP ST. JOHN BASIL RATHBONE)

Born: **June 13, 1892**
Johannesburg, South Africa
Died: **July 21, 1967**

When he was three, Basil's family had to flee to England, because his father, Edgar, who was a mining engineer, was accused by the Boers of being a British spy. With his violinist wife, Anna, and their three children, they traveled by ship from Cape Town. Basil attended Repton School, in Derbyshire, where he developed his love for the theater. After working a year with an insurance company, Basil turned his attention to acting. His cousin Frank, gave him his start on the stage. While appearing in a series of Shakespeare's plays, Basil fell for Marion Foreman. They married in 1914 and had a son before Basil went to war – receiving the British Military Cross for his bravery. In 1921, he made his film debut, in *Innocent*. From 1923, he worked on the New York stage and by the late 1920s, was a Hollywood star. Basil was nominated for Supporting Oscars for *Romeo and Juliet* and *If I Were King*. His second wife, Ouida, was with him when he died of a heart attack, in New York.

Sin Takes a Holiday (1930)
David Copperfield (1935)
Anna Karenina (1935) The Last Days
of Pompeii (1935) Captain Blood (1935)
A Tale of Two Cities (1935)
Romeo and Juliet (1936)
Confession (1937) Tovarich (1937)
The Adventures of Robin Hood (1938)
If I Were King (1938)
The Dawn Patrol (1938)
Son of Frankenstein (1939)
The Hound of the Baskervilles (1939)
The Adventures of Sherlock
Holmes (1939) Tower of London (1939)
The Mark of Zorro (1940)
The Black Cat (1941) Crossroads (1942)
The Spider Woman (1944)
The Scarlet Claw (1944)
Frenchman's Creek (1944)
Pursuit to Algiers (1945) Terror By
Night (1946) Dressed to Kill (1946)
We're No Angels (1955)
The Court Jester (1955)
The Last Hurrah (1958)

Aldo **Ray**
6ft
(ALDO DARE)

Born: **September 25, 1926**
Pen Argyl, Pennsylvania, USA
Died: **March 27, 1991**

From an Italian American family, with four brothers and a sister, Aldo couldn't wait to enter the war. When he was eighteen, he joined the United States Navy and served win the Frogman unit until 1946. He briefly studied at the University of California at Berkeley, then settled in Crockett, with his first wife Shirley, with whom he had a daughter. He was elected Constable in the town, and while there, attended a movie casting session with his brother. They were more interested in him, and hired him for a small role in the 1951 sports drama, *Saturday's Hero*. He impressed Columbia and was offered a contract. He appeared in films using his birth name, Aldo DaRe, before co-starring in *The Marrying Kind*, as Aldo Ray. He was nominated for a Best Newcomer Golden Globe, for his work in the Kate Hepburn/Spencer Tracy movie, *Pat and Mike*. Aldo suffered a short-lived second marriage in 1954, but his career flourished in films like *Battle Cry*, *We're No Angels* and *The Naked and the Dead*. His third marriage ended in 1967. Aldo's film career continued and he worked with few breaks (unfortunately on mostly inferior material) up to the late 1980s. He died of throat cancer, in Martinez, California.

Saturday's Hero (1951)
The Marrying Kind (1952)
Pat and Mike (1952)
Battle Cry (1955)
We're No Angels (1955)
Nightfall (1957)
Men in War (1957)
The Naked and the Dead (1958)
God's Little Acre (1958)
The Siege of Pinchgut (1959)
The Day They Robbed the
Bank of England (1960)
Johnny Nobody (1961)
Sylvia (1965)
Nightmare in the Sun (1965)
What Did You Do in the War,
Daddy? (1966)
Welcome to Hard Times (1967)
Sweet Savage (1979)

Paula **Raymond**
5ft 6in
(PAULA RAMONA WRIGHT)

Born: **November 23, 1924**
San Francisco, California, USA
Died: **December 31, 2003**

The daughter of a leading attorney, when Paula was a child she looked like a movie star of the future. That it didn't happen as quickly as people expected was due to lack of natural acting talent. She studied dancing and music – including opera. When she and her mother were visiting Los Angeles in 1937, she was spotted by a 20th Century Fox talent scout. After taking up residence in the city and moving to Hollywood High School, she was given her film debut, in a 1938 comedy, *Keep Smiling*. Nothing more happened on the movie front for ten years, but she kept her hand in by appearing in local stage productions before completing legal studies at San Francisco Junior College. In 1944, she entered a two-year marriage which produced a daughter named Raeme. Leaving the baby with her mother, Paula returned to Hollywood, where she worked as a model. In 1947, she signed a contract with Paramount and was given an uncredited role in *Night Has a Thousand Eyes*. A busy period during the early 1950s saw her star with Dick Powell in the excellent, *The Tall Target*. Paula was also in the cult-movie, *The Beast from 20,000 Fathoms*. She was always nice to look at, but her luck ran out when, in 1962, she was a passenger in a car crash on Sunset Boulevard and was facially disfigured. After extensive surgery, she made a few more films up until 1994's *Mind Twister*. She then retired. Paula died at her West Hollywood home, of respiratory ailments.

Crisis (1950)
Duchess of Idaho (1950)
Devil's Doorway (1950)
Grounds for Marriage (1951)
Inside Straight (1951)
The Tall Target (1951)
The Sellout (1952)
The Bandits of Corsica (1953)
The Beast from
20,000 Fathoms (1953)
City That Never Sleeps (1953)
The Human Jungle (1954)

Ronald **Reagan**
6ft 1in
(RONALD WILSON REAGAN)

Born: **February 6, 1911**
Tampico, Illinois, USA
Died: **June 5, 2004**

Ronnie was born in an apartment above the town's bank. His parents were Nelle, who followed the 'Disciples of Christ' faith, and Jack Reagan, who gave him the nickname "Dutch". Ronnie attended Dixon High School, in the small town of that name, and was a part-time lifeguard at Rock River, where he saved seventy-seven people from drowning. At Eureka College, he majored in Economics and Sociology and he was a star performer in several sports. In 1932, he began his entertainment career on the radio. One of his first jobs was at the WHO station, in Des Moines, as commentator on Chicago Cubs' games. While on tour with them in California, he was given a screen test and then a contract with Warner Brothers. Appropriately, Ronnie made his film debut, in 1937, as a radio crime reporter, in *Love Is on the Air*. His own favorite film, and almost certainly his best, was *King's Row*, but he was employed in films and on TV until the mid-1960s, when he decided to concentrate on politics. Having been President of the Screen Actors Guild, he was Governor of California, until he became the 40th President of the United States of America. His two wives, Jane Wyman and Nancy Davis, were both actresses. After Suffering from Alzheimer's disease in later life, he died of pneumonia.

Brother Rat (1938)
Dark Victory (1939)
Knute Rockne All American (1940)
Santa Fe Trail (1940)
Nine Lives Are Not Enough (1941)
King's Row (1942)
Desperate Journey (1942)
That Hagen Girl (1947)
The Voice of the Turtle (1947)
John Loves Mary (1949)
The Hasty Heart (1949)
Louisa (1950)
Storm Warning (1951)
Cattle Queen of Montana (1954)
Tennessee's Partner (1955)
The Killers (1964)

Robert **Redford**
5ft 10in
(ROBERT CHARLES REDFORD JR.)

Born: **August 18, 1936**
Santa Monica, California, USA

Bob's mother, Martha, died in 1955. His father, Charles, eventually landed a top job at Standard Oil. After attending Van Nuys High School, Bob went to the University of Colorado in 1956, but lost his scholarship after getting drunk. With the money he'd saved from his vacation jobs, he went to Europe and painted. In 1958, he began studying Art at the Pratt Institute, but he switched to an acting career – enrolling at the American Academy of Dramatic Art. That year, he married for the only time, Lola Van Wagenen. They had four children, but divorced in 1985. In 1959, he got a small role on Broadway, in "Tall Story". He made his movie debut in 1962, in a low-budget independent called *War Hunt*. A leading role on Broadway in "Barefoot in the Park" in 1963, was his first big stage success. He had to wait somewhat longer for his breakthrough to true movie stardom, in *Butch Cassidy and the Sundance Kid*. In 1981, he won a Best Director Oscar, for *Ordinary People*. Bob has maintained his status as both director and star. Since 1996, he has had a steady relationship with the German-born painter, Sibylle Szaggers.

Inside Daisy Clover (1965)
The Chase (1966)
This Property Is Condemned (1966)
Barefoot in the Park (1967)
Butch Cassidy and
the Sundance Kid (1969)
Tell them Willie Boy Is Here (1969)
The Candidate (1972)
Jeremiah Johnson (1972)
The Way We Were (1973)
The Sting (1973)
All the President's Men (1976)
Brubaker (1980)
The Natural (1984)
Out of Africa (1985)
Sneakers (1992)
The Horse Whisperer (1998)
Spy Game (2001)
The Clearing (2004)
An Unfinished Life (2005)
Lions for Lambs (2007)

Lynn **Redgrave**
5ft 10in
(LYNN RACHEL REDGRAVE)

Born: **March 8, 1943**
London, England

The youngest of Sir Michael and Lady Rachel's talented trio of children, Lynn was educated at Queen's Gate School, in London. She later studied acting at the Central School of Speech and Drama. In 1962, she made her stage debut, at the Royal Court, in "A Midsummer Night's Dream". One year later, she made her film debut in the award winning *Tom Jones*. She joined the National Theater for three years, and worked with such top directors as Franco Zeffirelli and Laurence Olivier. She was nominated for a Best Actress Oscar, for her role in *Georgy Girl*. Lynn made her Broadway debut, in 1967, with Michael Crawford, in "Black Comedy". She married her manager, John Clark that year, and it lasted until 2000. They had three children. She has continued to appear on stage and screen, and like a good wine, she is better the older she gets. In 1999, she should have won an Oscar for her superb work opposite Ian McKellen in *Gods and Monsters*. In 2007, Lynn appeared on television in an episode of 'Desperate Housewives'.

Girl With Green Eyes (1964)
Georgy Girl (1966)
The Deadly Affair (1966)
The Virgin Soldiers (1969)
Everything You Always Wanted to
Know About Sex (1972)
The National Health (1973)
Getting It Right (1989)
Shine (1996)
Gods and Monsters (1998)
Strike! (1998)
The Annihilation of Fish (1999)
Deeply (2000)
How to Kill Your
Neighbor's Dog (2000)
Venus and Mars (2001)
My Kingdom (2001)
Spider (2002)
Unconditional Love (2002)
Charlie's War (2003)
Peter Pan (2003)
The White Countess (2005)
The Jane Austen Book Club (2007)

Sir Michael **Redgrave**
6ft 3in
(MICHAEL SCUDAMORE REDGRAVE)

Born: **March 20, 1908**
Bristol, Avon, England
Died: **March 21, 1985**

Michael's father, the silent film actor, Roy Redgrave, left his baby son and his wife – actress, Margaret Scudamore, when he was six months old. His mother married a wealthy tea planter whom the boy hated. At least it enabled him to be expensively educated, at the local Clifton College, and later graduate from Magdalene College, Cambridge. Before becoming an actor, in 1934, he had a brief career as a master at Cranleigh School in Surrey. In 1935, he married the actress, Rachel Kempson, despite being bisexual. They had three children. His first experience of film acting was in Hitchcock's *Secret Agent,* in 1936. It was a tiny role, but his next – for the same director – was in the classic *The Lady Vanishes.* Michael was nominated for a Best Actor Oscar, for his first American film – *Mourning Becomes Electra.* He secured stardom in excellent British films – *The Browning Version, The Importance of Being Earnest, The Dam Busters,* and *The Go-Between* – being my personal favorites. He died in Denham, Buckinghamshire, of Parkinson's disease.

The Lady Vanishes (1938)
The Stars Look Down (1940)
Kipps (1941) **Thunder Rock** (1942)
The Way to the Stars (1945)
Dead of Night (1945)
The Captive Heart (1946)
The Years Between (1946)
Mourning Becomes Electra (1947)
The Browning Version (1951)
**The Importance of
Being Earnest** (1952)
The Sea Shall Not Have Them (1954)
**The Night My Number
Came Up** (1955)
The Dam Busters (1955) **1984** (1956)
The Quiet American (1958)
The Wreck of the Mary Deare (1959)
The Innocents (1961)
**The Loneliness of
the Long Distance Runner** (1962)
Battle of Britain (1969)
The Go-Between (1970)

Vanessa **Redgrave**
5ft 11in
(VANESSA REDGRAVE)

Born: **January 20, 1937**
London, England

Vanessa was educated at The Alice Ottley School, in Worcester. She trained as an actress at the Central School of Speech and Drama – making her stage debut, at the Frinton Summer Theater, in Essex, in 1957 – and her West End debut, the following year. Her film debut was in 1958, when she appeared with her dad in *Behind the Mask.* Later, for the Royal Shakespeare Company she received great acclaim for her role of Rosalind, in "As You Like It" in 1961. She did some TV dramas and concentrated on stage work until 1966, when a flurry of activity on the movie front included her Oscar-nominated role in *Morgan,* and a contribution to the land-mark 'sixties film, *Blowup.* Five more nominations include a Best Supporting Actress Oscar, for *Julia.* She is the mother of Natasha and Joely Richardson, from her marriage to director, Tony. After almost thirty years together, she married the actor Franco Nero, in 2006. The couple have a son named Carlo. Vanessa has performed as a star and supporting actress in recent movies including *Atonement.*

**Morgan: A Suitable Case for
Treatment** (1966) **A Man for All
Seasons** (1966) **Blowup** (1966)
Camelot (1967) **The Charge of the
Light Brigade** (1968) **Isadora** (1968)
A Quiet Place in the Country (1969)
The Devils (1971)
The Trojan Women (1971)
Mary, Queen of Scots (1972)
The Seven-Per-Cent Solution (1976)
Julia (1977) **Yanks** (1979)
Prick Up Your Ears (1987)
Howard's End (1992)
Little Odessa (1994) **A Month by
the Lake** (1995) **Wilde** (1997)
Mrs. Dalloway (1997)
Cradle Will Rock (1999)
Girl, Interrupted (1999)
The Pledge (2001)
Crime and Punishment (2002)
Venus (2006) **Evening** (2007)
Atonement (2007)
Gud, lukt och henne (2008)

Ekaterina **Rednikova**
5ft 5in
(EKATERINA REDNIKOVA)

Born: **May 17, 1973**
Moscow, Soviet Union

Living under Communist rule wasn't all bad. Apart from the academic side of a state education, Ekaterina learned ice skating, dancing and piano during her formative years and proved to be a good swimmer. She was a graduate of the Russian Academy of Theater Arts, in Moscow, in 1994. While attending the Academy she appeared as Polina, in Dostoyevsky's "Gambler", and as Ariel in Shakespeare's "The Tempest". After graduating, she acted in Moscow theaters, in productions of "Beyond the Horizon", "Dark Lady of the Sonnets" as well as "A Streetcar Named Desire". She made her film debut at the age of sixteen, in *Babnik.* In 1995, she went to Rumania to appear with English and American actors, in a TV film – 'Roger Corman presents Hellfire'. A later theater release, *Border Blues,* was equally undistinguished. Ekaterina's film breakthrough was when she played the young mother, Katya, in *Vor* – which became famous internationally as *The Thief.* Her acting was superb and she was undoubtedly very beautiful. It won her a Russian Cinema Academy Award as Best Actress, and she was also honored with a Golden Eagle from Russian Movie Critics. Ekaterina had a four year hiatus from 2001, but came back strongly in 2005, when in the role of Zinaida Rapava, she co-starred with Daniel Craig in the superb television version of Robert Harris's novel, 'Archangel.' There have been some strong movie roles recently including *The Last Armored Train.* Her many overseas fans can only hope that she gets a chance to act in some good English-language films before it's too late.

Lady Peasant (1995)
The Thief (1997)
Falling Through (2000)
Balalayka (2000)
The Last Armored Train (2006)
The Man of No Return (2006)
Smersh (2007)
The Gift to Stalin (2008)
The Sovereign (2008)

Donna **Reed**
5ft 7in
(DONNA BELLE MULLENGER)

Born: **January 27, 1921**
Denison, Iowa, USA
Died: **January 14, 1986**

Donna was the oldest of five children. When she was sixteen, she left home and her local high school, to attend secretarial school at Los Angeles City College. When she was voted "Campus Queen" her photograph appeared in the local newspaper. It aroused interest among agents and studios and resulted in a successful screen test and a contract with MGM. In 1941, she made her film debut, in the studio's B-picture, *The Get-Away.* Later, Donna was fourth-billed below William Powell and Myrna Loy, in a *Thin Man* movie. In 1943, she married the make-up artist, William Tuttle. They divorced in 1945, and she married producer, Tony Owen, with whom she had four children. She was pretty, but didn't hit stardom until she co-starred with Jimmy Stewart in everyone's favorite movie, *It's a Wonderful Life.* A steady run of successful films kept her going until, in 1958, when she starred on television in her own successful vehicle, 'The Donna Reed Show' which ran until 1966. Before that, she had won a Best Supporting Actress Oscar, for *From Here to Eternity.* Her last movie was in 1974, when she co-starred with Walter Pidgeon, in *Yellow-Headed Summer.* In 1984, she took over the role of Miss Ellie, in 'Dallas', but fell ill after completing a season. She died in Beverly Hills, of pancreatic cancer.

Shadow of the Thin Man (1941)
Eyes in the Night (1942)
The Human Comedy (1943)
The Picture of Dorian Gray (1945)
They Were Expendable (1945)
It's a Wonderful Life (1946)
Green Dolphin Street (1947)
Saturday's Hero (1951)
Scandal Sheet (1952)
Hangman's Knot (1952)
Trouble Along the Way (1953)
From Here to Eternity (1953)
Three Hours to Kill (1954)
The Benny Goodman Story (1955)
Ransom! (1956)
Backlash (1956)

Oliver **Reed**
5ft 11in
(ROBERT OLIVER REED)

Born: **February 13, 1937**
Wimbledon, London, England
Died: **May 2, 1999**

Ollie was the son of Peter Reed, a racing correspondent, and his wife Marcia. His grandfather was the legendary actor, Sir Herbert Beerbohm Tree. Of even greater relevance was the fact that his uncle was the English film director, Sir Carol Reed – young Ollie was mad about movies! He wasn't so enamored with education – attending thirteen schools. He excelled at sports – coming third in the All England Cross Country race while at St. George's College. One of his jobs during school holidays, was as an exhibition fighter, on Mitcham Green. After two years National Service he became a film extra in 1958, in Norman Wisdom's *The Square Peg.* The earliest films he registered in began with *Paranoiac,* in 1963. He was a star by the time he wrestled nude with Alan Bates, in Ken Russell's adaptation of *Women in Love,* by D.H. Lawrence. He gave one of his best performances in Russell's controversial, *The Devils.* His admiration for Errol Flynn affected his career and his alcohol-fuelled escapades often led to tears. He died of a heart attack, drinking rum in a bar in Malta. Ollie's outrageous behavior was tolerated by two wives and countless female conquests. Many men envied him.

The Trap (1966)
The Jokers (1967)
I'll Never Forget What's'isname (1967)
Oliver! (1968) **The Assassination Bureau** (1969) **Women in Love** (1969) **The Devils** (1971)
Sitting Target (1972)
The Three Musketeers (1973)
Tommy (1975) **Royal Flash** (1975)
Burnt Offerings (1976)
Crossed Swords (1977)
The Brood (1979)
Lion of the Desert (1981)
Castaway (1986)
The Adventures of Baron Munchausen (1988)
The Return of the Musketeers (1989)
Funny Bones (1995)
Gladiator (2000)

Christopher **Reeve**
6ft 4in
(CHRISTOPHER D'OLIER REEVE)

Born: **September 25, 1952**
New York City, New York, USA
Died: **October 10, 2004**

Chris was the son of the poet, scholar, and novelist, Franklin D'Olier Reeve, who studied for a Master's degree in Russian at Columbia University. Chris's mother, Barbara, was a novelist, who had been a student at Vassar College. The pair were far too clever for the marriage to survive, and in 1956, Barbara took Chris and his brother Benjamin, to live in Princetown, where the boys attended Nassau Street School. Their mother married a stockbroker in 1959, and he gave the two boys a good education – starting with Princetown Country Day School. Chris was academically bright and a fine athlete. When he was nine, he began to develop his love of acting with a role in the school's production of "The Yeoman of the Guard". In the summer of 1962, he was taken on as an apprentice at the Williamstown Theater Festival. In 1963, Chris joined the Harvard Repertory Company. Later, at Cornell University, he got the chance to act in all sorts of plays. He toured Scotland and England and on his return, transferred for his senior year, to Juilliard. After TV roles, he made his film debut, in 1978, in *Gray Lady Down,* and was immediately cast as the ideal *Superman.* His career almost ended when he was paralyzed in a riding accident in 1995, and was confined to a wheelchair (which he used in his last roles) until his death from a heart attack, in Mount Kisco, New York. He and his wife Dana, co-founded the Paralysis Resource Center. They had a son named Will.

Superman (1978)
Somewhere in Time (1980)
Superman II (1980)
Deathtrap (1982)
Street Smart (1987)
Noises Off (1992)
The Remains of the Day (1993)
Speechless (1994)
Village of the Damned (1995)
Above Suspicion (1995)
A Step Toward Tomorrow (1996)

Keanu **Reeves**
6ft 1¼in
(KEANU CHARLES REEVES)

Born: September 2, 1964
Beirut, Lebanon

Keanu's English mother, Patricia, met his father, Sam, when she was working in Beirut. A sister Kim, was born in 1966. Sam turned out to be really bad news – abandoning his family and later serving a jail sentence in Hawaii, for selling heroin. Patricia married three more times, but none of them worked out. At the age of nine, Keanu had his first taste of acting, in a school production of "Damn Yankees" and two years later, he made his TV debut, in 'Night Heat'. It was an unsettling time for the youngster – by the early 1980s, he'd attended four different high schools including the Etobicoke School of the Arts, in Toronto – from which he was expelled. At De La Salle College, he excelled as an ice hockey goalie – and acquired a players' nickname, "The Wall". Appropriately, when he made his first movie, in 1986, it was with a role in the ice hockey film, *Youngblood,* which starred Rob Lowe. Keanu graduated from teen movies into adult films. For some of them, he won plaudits: for *Point Break* - he was voted "Most Desirable Male" in the MTV Movie Awards and for *The Matrix* – his Blockbuster Favorite Actor Award helped him towards his current A-list status.

River's Edge (1986)
The Night Before (1988)
Permanent Record (1988)
Dangerous Liaisons (1988)
Bill & Ted's Excellent Adventure (1989)
Parenthood (1989)
Point Break (1991)
My Own Private Idaho (1991)
Dracula (1992)
Much Ado About Nothing (1993)
Speed (1994)
A Walk in the Clouds (1995)
The Devil's Advocate (1997)
The Matrix (1999)
The Gift (2000)
Something's Gotta Give (2003)
Thumbsucker (2005)
A Scanner Darkly (2006)
The Lake House (2006)
Street Kings (2008)

Natacha **Régnier**
5ft 7in
(NATHALIE RÉGNIER)

Born: April 11, 1972
Ixelles, Brussels, Belgium

Natacha grew up in a suburb of the Belgian capital city of Brussels. She first revealed a talent when acting in school plays during her childhood and adolescent years. She then attended the Saint-Pierre d'Uccle College and spent a year at the Higher Institute of Performing Arts, in Brussels. After beginning her career touring in a number of stage productions, Natacha made her movie debut, in 1993, in a Belgian short called *The Motorcycle Girl.* She followed it with television work, and two years later, had a strong supporting role in the French romantic comedy, *Dis-moi oui.* She went to Paris, where she had a largely frustrating time with small roles in TV series and, until the comedy, *Encore* – for which she won Jean Vigo and Jean Carmet Awards, things moved slowly. Then, as in all good careers, she got her first important break. She was selected by the director, Erick Zonca, to star with another young actress, Édolie Bouchez, in his superb, *La Vie rêvée des anges.* The two shared the Best Actress Award at the 1998 Cannes Film Festival. She later married Yann Tiersen, who wrote the film's score and they had a daughter together. Natacha sang with Yann on an album of Georges Brassens songs, but they are no longer in harmony.

Dis-moi oui... (1995)
Encore (1996)
La Vie rêvée des anges (1998)
Il Tempo dell'amore (1999)
Les Amants Criminels (1999)
Everything's Fine,
We're Leaving (2000)
How I Killed My Father (2001)
Tomorrow We Move (2004)
Le Silence (2004)
Le Pont des Arts (2004)
Duplicity (2005)
Sunduk predkov (2006)
Poison Friends (2006)
La Raison du plus faible (2006)
Les Boîtes (2007)
That Day (2007)
Intrusions (2008)

Tara **Reid**
5ft 5in
(TARA REID)

Born: November 8, 1975
Wyckoff, New Jersey, USA

Tara was the daughter of teachers, Tom and Donna Reid, who also owned a day care center. She has two brothers and a sister. Tara had a precocious talent which was encouraged by her parents. Her very first experience of the world of show business was back in 1982, when she appeared on the children's television game show, 'Child's Play'. She was educated at Dwight D. Eisenhower Middle School, and as she grew older, she became a model – appearing in television commercials for McDonald's, Crayola and Jell-O. When she was twelve, she made her film debut, in a poor horror movie called *A Return to Salem's Lot.* She graduated from the Ramapo High School, in New Jersey, and then attended the Professional Children's School, in New York, where, among her contemporaries, were Christina Ricci, and Macauley Culkin. In the mid 1990s. Tara got a couple of roles in TV series before she portrayed Bunny Lebowski, in the Coen Brothers hit film, *The Big Lebowski.* A year later, she made her major film breakthrough, in *American Pie,* and starred in its sequel. The breakup of her engagement to the MTV DJ, Carson Daly, upset her greatly during the making of that film, but she recovered her composure and got her career back on track with light-hearted comedies such as *Knots* and the recent *7-10 Split.* Tara's brother, Patrick, runs a fashion store in Santa Monica, for which Tara acts as both a consultant and as an occasional guest model.

The Big Lebowski (1998)
Around the Fire (1999)
American Pie (1999)
Just Visiting (2001)
American Pie 2 (2001)
Van Wilder (2002)
Devil's Pond (2003)
Knots (2004)
If I Had Known
I Was a Genius (2007)
7-10 Split (2007)
Clean Break (2008)

John C. **Reilly**
6ft 1½in
(JOHN CHRISTOPHER REILLY)

Born: May 24, 1965
Chicago, Illinois, USA

The son of an Irish American father and a Lithuanian mother, John was the fifth of six children who were raised in the Catholic faith. John was a bit of a tearaway as a kid, but still managed to graduate from Chicago's Brother Rice High School for Boys. He soon found an outlet for his surplus energy, when he discovered acting. He enrolled at the Goodman School of Drama, at St. Paul University and eventually made his contribution to the Chicago drama scene after joining the famous Steppenwolf Theater. He made his film debut, with a strong supporting role in the dynamic, *Casualties of War*. During the 1990s, John established himself as a forceful character actor who also had a lovable side. In 1992, he married the film producer, Alison Dickey. They have two children. John was nominated for a Best Supporting Actor Oscar, for *Chicago* – in which he did all his own singing. He has continued to bring his special brand of acting to the screen and is especially good in the recent comedy, *Step Brothers*. His next film will be *Cirque du Freak*.

Casualties of War (1989)
State of Grace (1990) **Hoffa** (1992)
What's Eating Gilbert Grape? (1993)
The River Wild (1994)
Dolores Claiborne (1995)
Georgia (1995) **Sydney** (1995)
Boogie Nights (1997)
For Love of the Game (1999)
Magnolia (1999)
The Perfect Storm (2000)
The Anniversary Party (2001)
The Good Girl (2002)
Gangs of New York (2002)
Chicago (2002)
The Hours (2002) **Criminal** (2004)
The Aviator (2004)
A Prairie Home Companion (2004)
**Talladega Nights: The Ballad of
Ricky Bobby** (2004)
Year of the Dog (2007)
**Walk Hard: The Dewey
Cox Story** (2007)
Step Brothers (2008)

Kelly **Reilly**
5ft 6in
(KELLY REILLY)

Born: July 18, 1977
Kingston-Upon-Thames, Surrey, England

Kelly was from a working-class family background; her father was a policeman and her mother worked at the local hospital. Kelly decided to pursue an acting career in her teens after attending a stage performance of Bertold Brecht's play "The Resistible Rise of Arturo Ui". She was studying for her A-levels when, at the age of seventeen, she made her TV debut, in an episode of 'Prime Suspect' with Helen Mirren. Because of the lack of money in her family, Kelly wasn't able to go to drama school, but her winning personality enabled her to get regular work in television dramas . In 2000, she made her film debut, with a small role in the Ben Elton romantic comedy, *Maybe Baby*. A year later, after some pretty ordinary material, Kelly made a good impression with a featured role in the drama, *Last Orders*. A French/Spanish co-production, *L'Auberge espagnole,* gave her some international exposure and led to the Irish film, *Dead Bodies*. In 2004, Kelly became the youngest ever Best Actress nominee at the Olivier Awards, for her performance in the title role of "After Miss Julie" at Donmar Warehouse, in London. The year 2005, saw her breakthrough, and a sign of good things to come with her first starring role in, *Les Poupées russes,* and the key role of Caroline Bingley, in *Pride & Prejudice*. The Kelly Reilly movie line-up for 2009 suggests a very bright future for this charming actress. Her work in the British horror film, *Eden Lake,* is especially brilliant and her appearance as Mary Morstan in the new Guy Ritchie version of *Sherlock Holmes* is eagerly awaited.

Last Orders (2001)
L'Auberge espagnole (2002)
Dead Bodies (2003)
The Libertine (2004)
The Russian Dolls (2005)
Pride & Prejudice (2005)
Mrs. Henderson Presents (2005)
Puffball (2007)
Eden Lake (2008)
Me and Orson Welles (2008)

Lee **Remick**
5ft 6in
(LEE ANN REMICK)

Born: December 14, 1935
Quincy, Massachusetts, USA
Died: **July 2, 1991**

Like many Americans, Lee was a mixture of several nationalities, including English, Irish and a little German. Her father, Frank Remick owned a department store, and her mother, Margaret – a former New York actress, gave her daughter much early encouragement and moved with her to New York when Frank was posted to Washington. After Lee's early education at a private girl's school, Miss Hewitt's, she studied ballet at the Swaboda School of Dance, and joined the Powers modeling agency. In 1953, Lee was at Sardi's restaurant with her mother when quite by chance she was spotted by a playwright and given her Broadway debut in "Be Your Age" – which was a flop. She stuck it out with summer stock and television and eventually caught the eye of Elia Kazan, who gave her a small role in *A Face in the Crowd*. By 1958, she was married to the director, Bill Colleran (with whom she had two children) and her movie career had taken off. Five years later, Lee was nominated for a Best Actress Oscar for *Days of Wine and Roses,* which co-starred Jack Lemmon. She was a big star throughout the 1960s and 1970s. She made her last movie appearance in 1986, in the drama, *Emma's War*. From 1989, Lee fought a losing battle with cancer and died in Los Angeles, at the age of fifty-five.

The Long, Hot Summer (1958)
These Thousand Hills (1959)
Anatomy of a Murder (1959)
Wild River (1960)
Experiment in Terror (1962)
Days of Wine and Roses (1962)
The Wheeler Dealers (1963)
No Way to Treat a Lady (1968)
The Detective (1968)
Sometimes a Great Notion (1971)
A Delicate Balance (1973)
The Omen (1976)
Telefon (1977)
The Medusa Touch (1978)
The Europeans (1979)
The Competition (1980)

Michael **Rennie**
6ft 4in
(ERIC ALEXANDER RENNIE)

Born: **August 25, 1909**
Bradford, Yorkshire, England
Died: **June 10, 1971**

Michael grew up in the Bradford suburb of Idle. When he was eleven, he was sent to board at the Leys School, in Cambridge. For eight years after he left school, he floundered in a series of uninspiring jobs. The best of which were automobile salesman, and as manager of his uncle's rope factory. On his twenty-sixth birthday, he decided to become an actor, and in 1936, he had an uncredited role in the Alfred Hitchcock film, *Secret Agent*. He worked for various British repertory companies and had unbilled parts in ten movies before he was given his first leading role, in 1941, in *Tower of Terror*. During World War II, he joined the Royal Airforce Volunteer Reserve and worked as a flying instructor in Macon, Georgia. He reappeared on the British screen in such hits as *The Wicked Lady,* and by 1949, he had a Hollywood contract. Michael's landmark film was *The Day the Earth Stood Still*. He was already ill when, in 1970, he worked on his final film, *Assignment Terror*. His second wife was actress, Maggie McGrath. Michael died of emphysema, in Harrogate, Yorkshire – close to his birthplace.

Root of All Evil (1947)
Uneasy Terms (1948) Trio (1950)
The Black Rose (1950)
The 13th Letter (1951)
The Day the Earth Stood Still (1951)
The House in the Square (1951)
Phone Call from a Stranger (1952)
5 Fingers (1952)
Les Miserables (1952)
Single-Handed (1953)
Dangerous Crossing (1953)
The Robe (1953)
King of the Khyber Rifles (1953)
Princess of the Nile (1954)
Demetrius and the
Gladiators (1954)
Desirée (1954)
Soldier of Fortune (1955)
Island in the Sun (1957)
Third Man on the Mountain (1959)
Hotel (1967)

Jean **Reno**
6ft 2in
(JUAN MORENO Y HERRERA JIMÉNEZ)

Born: **July 30, 1948**
Casablanca, Morocco

His parents, who were from Andalusia, in Spain, had moved to Morocco to escape the dictatorship of General Franco. Jean's mother died when he was an adolescent, and when he was twelve, he and his younger sister were taken to live in France, and raised as Catholics. As he grew older, Jean made up his mind to become an actor. After he left school, he studied at the famous Cours Simon, in Paris. In 1979, he made his film debut in *L'Hypothèse du tableau volé*. He worked in French films and on television, but made his first impression on the international scene, in Luc Besson's *Le Grand bleu,* and he followed up in the same director's hit movies, *Nikita,* and *Léon*. Since then, Jean has featured in a number of high profile Hollywood films, such as *Mission Impossible* and *The Da Vinci Code*. He continues to make French movies – he's been nominated for three Césars – for *Le Grand bleu, The Visitors,* and *Léon*. His third wife is the actress Zofia Borucka, whom he married in 2006, with future French President, Nicolas Sarkozy, as his best man. In a rare error of judgement, Jean is in the cast of the ill-advised Steve Martin comedy, *The Pink Panther 2.*

Le Dernier combat (1983)
The Big Blue (1988)
Nikita (1990)
L'Homme au masque d'or (1991)
The Visitors (1993)
Léon (1994)
French Kiss (1995)
Beyond the Clouds (1995)
Mission Impossible (1996)
Roseanna's Grave (1997)
Ronin (1998)
The Crimson Rivers (2000)
Wasabi (2001)
Décalage horaire (2002)
Tais-toi (2003)
Empire of the Wolves (2005)
The Tiger and the Snow (2005)
The Da Vinci Code (2006)
Flyboys (2006)
Ca$h (2008)

Anne **Revere**
5ft 5in
(ANNE REVERE)

Born: **June 25, 1903**
New York City, New York, USA
Died: **December 18, 1990**

Anne was a direct descendant of Paul Revere – of American Revolution fame. After high school, she graduated from the famous Wellesley College for Women, in Massachusetts. She trained for the stage at New York's American Laboratory Theater and began acting in summer stock productions. By the late 1920s, she was very experienced. She made her Broadway stage debut, in 1931, in "The Great Barrington". After her success in the hit play, "Double Door", Anne went to Hollywood, and made her screen debut in the 1934 film version. There were no other movie offers for six years, so she returned to the stage. In 1940, as a famous stage actress, she was given a new start by RKO, in *One Crowded Night*. After that, her face was well known to audiences – even if her name wasn't. Anne won the Best Supporting Actress Oscar, for *National Velvet,* and was nominated for *The Song of Bernadette* and *Gentleman's Agreement*. Black-listed in 1951, for refusing to name Hollywood communists, she and husband Sam Rosen, who directed her on Broadway in "As You Like It", ran an acting school, until she returned for a couple of movies and some television work during the 1970s. Anne died of pneumonia, in Locust Valley, New York.

Remember the Day (1941)
Meet the Stewarts (1942)
The Meanest Man in the World (1943)
Old Acquaintance (1943)
The Song of Bernadette (1943)
Sunday Dinner for a Soldier (1944)
National Velvet (1944)
The Keys of the Kingdom (1944)
The Thin Man Goes Home (1944)
Fallen Angel (1945)
Dragonwyck (1946)
The Shocking Miss Pilgrim (1947)
Body and Soul (1947)
Gentleman's Agreement (1947)
The Great Missouri Raid (1951)
A Place in the Sun (1951)
Birch Interval (1976)

Fernando **Rey**
5ft 11in
(FERNANDO CASADO ARAMBILLET)

Born: **September 20, 1917**
A Coruña, Galicia, Spain
Died: **March 9, 1994**

The son of Colonel Casado Viega, a career soldier, young Fernando finished his schooling at eighteen and studied to be an architect in Madrid. He began to earn money as a film extra, starting with *Fazendo Fitas,* in 1935. The Spanish Civil War erupted the following year, and Fernando gave up his studies to commit himself to the film industry. Most of the fifty or so movies he made during the next twenty-five years, were either Franco government propaganda, or strictly censored. In 1957, Fernando had his first taste of freedom when he appeared in Vadim's *The Night Heaven Fell,* with Brigitte Bardot. His breakthrough was working with Luis Buñuel, in *Viridiana.* He won a Fotogramas de Plata, as Best Spanish Movie Performer, for Buñuel's *Tristana* and starred in the director's hugely successful, *The Discreet Charm of the Bourgeoisie.* Fernando was best known in America for *The French Connection* and its sequel. From 1960 until his death from cancer in Madrid, Fernando was married to the Argentine actress, Mabel Karr.

Viridiana (1961)
The Running Man (1963)
Backfire (1964)
El Greco (1966) **Tristana** (1970)
The French Connection (1971)
La Duda (1972) **The Discreet Charm
of the Bourgeoisie** (1972)
High Crime (1973)
Drama of the Rich (1974)
The Lady with Red Boots (1974)
Seven Beauties (1975)
French Connection II (1975)
The Eyes Behind the Wall (1977)
Elisa, My Love (1977)
The Obscure Object of Desire (1977)
Traffic Jam (1979)
The Hit (1984)
Our Father (1985)
Rustler's Rhapsody (1985)
Saving Grace (1985)
El Bosque animado (1987)
Pasodoble (1988)

Burt **Reynolds**
5ft 10in
(BURTON LEON REYNOLDS JR.)

Born: **February 11, 1936**
Waycross, Georgia, USA

Burt's father, Burton Reynolds Sr., was of half-Cherokee Indian descent. He was drafted into the US Army during World War II and Burt, his sister and his mother, lived for two years at Fort Leonard Wood, in the Missouri Ozarks. When his dad was sent to Europe, Burt and his family moved to Michigan. Burt attended school in Merritt until his dad returned from the war and they settled in Riviera Beach, Florida. He went to school at Lake Park and the Central Junior High, where he was a star footballer. This continued at Palm Beach High School and led to a college football scholarship to Florida State University. His career ended after a car crash. He went to acting classes and got his first stage role in "Outward Bound" which won him the 1956 State Drama Award. After about three seasons of summer stock, Joanne Woodward helped him find an agent. In 1959, Burt made his TV debut, in an episode of 'M Squad' and his film debut two years later, in *Angel Baby.* He was nominated for a Best Supporting Actor Oscar, for *Boogie Nights.* Burt's been married and divorced twice – both times to actresses – Judy Carne, and Loni Anderson. Over the past few years, he's appeared in a mixed bag of movies – the best of which is *Randy and the Mob.*

Deliverance (1972)
**Everything You Always Wanted to
Know About Sex** (1972)
The Longest Yard (1974)
Hustle (1975)
Smokey and the Bandit (1977)
The End (1978)
Hooper (1978)
Starting Over (1979)
Sharkey's Machine (1981)
Breaking In (1989)
Citizen Ruth (1996)
Boogie Nights (1997)
Pups (1999)
Mystery, Alaska (1999)
Snapshots (2002)
The Longest Yard (2005)
Randy and the Mob (2007)

Debbie **Reynolds**
5ft 2in
(MARY FRANCES REYNOLDS)

Born: **April 1, 1932**
El Paso, Texas, USA

The daughter of Raymond and Maxine Reynolds, Debbie had an older brother called Bill. The family went to live with Maxine's parents when Raymond lost his job as a carpenter during the Great Depression. Even so, they were surprisingly happy years, and eventually they moved to Burbank, when he got a job with the Southern Pacific Railroad. Debbie enjoyed her schooldays – excelling at sports and also enjoying music and the movies. In 1948, she entered a "Miss Burbank" contest, which she won. Warner Brothers offered her a contract, but her mother refused to let her be educated at the studio. She went to John Burroughs High School in Burbank, and in 1948, she made her screen debut with an uncredited role in *June Bride.* Warners let her go to MGM in 1950, and it was there that she established herself in musical comedies, including the classic *Singin' in the Rain.* In 1955, Debbie married the singer, Eddie Fisher. One of their two children is Carrie. Despite her divorce from him and two other failed marriages, Debbie remained upbeat and has kept on working. She has been seen mostly on television during the past few years – in series such as 'Kim Possible' and 'Will & Grace'.

The Daughter of Rosie O'Grady (1950)
Three Little Words (1950)
Two Weeks with Love (1950)
Singin' in the Rain (1952)
I Love Melvin (1953)
Susan Slept Here (1954)
Hit the Deck (1955)
The Tender Trap (1955)
The Catered Affair (1956)
Tammy and the Bachelor (1957)
The Mating Game (1959)
The Rat Race (1960)
The Second Time Around (1961)
How the West Was Won (1962)
The Unsinkable Molly Brown (1964)
Divorce American Style (1967)
**What's the Matter with
Helen?** (1971) **Mother** (1996)
In & Out (1997)

Marjorie **Reynolds**
5ft 4in
(MARJORIE GOODSPEED)

Born: **August 12, 1917**
Buhl, Idaho, USA
Died: **February 1, 1997**

Marjorie was a local doctor's daughter. Her parents took her to live in Los Angeles when she was young and she showed enough early talent to make her film debut at the age of six, in the uncredited role of a waif, in *Trilby.* She appeared in three more silent movies before 'retiring' until 1933, when she made *Wine, Women and Song.* In the meantime, Marjorie finished her education. Early work in Hollywood was as a girl in small uncredited roles. In 1937, after she married a Canadian, Jack Reynolds, she changed her luck and her name. She became a star of westerns, with cowboys, Tex Ritter, Roy Rogers, and unknowns like Bob Baker. In 1939, Marjorie was an extra in *Gone With the Wind.* Her big break was in the Astaire Crosby classic, *Holiday Inn,* and for two or three years, she enjoyed bigger films and was considered a star. Her movie career was over by the early 1950s, and from 1953, she became best known, as William Bendix's wife, in the TV series, 'The Life of Riley'. That year, she married her second husband, the actor John Whitney. Her last movie was *The Silent Witness,* in 1962. Marjorie died of heart failure, at Manhattan Beach, California.

Six-Shootin' Sheriff (1938)
Streets of New York (1939)
Enemy Agent (1940)
Up in the Air (1940)
Cyclone on Horseback (1941)
Dude Cowboy (1941)
Holiday Inn (1942)
Dixie (1943)
Up in Mabel's Room (1944)
Ministry of Fear (1944)
Bring on the Girls (1945)
Meet Me on Broadway (1946)
The Time of Their Lives (1946)
Monsieur Beaucaire (1946)
Heaven Only Knows (1947)
Bad Men of Tombstone (1949)
That Midnight Kiss (1949)
The Great Jewel Robber (1950)
His Kind of Woman (1951)

Ryan **Reynolds**
6ft 2in
(RYAN RODNEY REYNOLDS)

Born: **October 23, 1976**
Vancouver, British Columbia, Canada

Ryan's father, Jim Reynolds, was a food wholesaler in Vancouver. In his earlier life Jim had fought as a semi-professional boxer. Ryan's mother, Tammy, was a sales lady in a Vancouver retail store. Ryan was the youngest of four brothers. Beginning his career as a child actor, he made his first appearance on television, in an episode of the series, 'Hillside', in 1990. Three years later, he made his movie debut, when he starred in the Canadian film, *Ordinary Magic.* Ryan was educated locally in Vancouver, and at the age of eighteen, he graduated from Kitsilano Secondary School. For three years, he worked exclusively in TV shows, including an episode of 'The X Files'. He had supporting roles in a couple of decent comedies, *Life During Wartime* and *Dick,* and then really hit his stride in the thriller, *Finder's Fee.* His progress was rapid after that and he received recognition with a Young Hollywood Award in 2003, and the Teen Choice Award, for the "Most Scary Scene" – in *The Amityville Horror.* Having been previously involved with Canadian singer, Alanis Morissette, Ryan married Scarlett Johansson, in September, 2008.

Ordinary Magic (1993)
Life During Wartime (1997)
Dick (1999)
We All Fall Down (2000)
Finder's Fee (2001)
Van Wilder (2002)
Buying the Cow (2002)
The In-Laws (2002)
Foolproof (2003)
Harold & Kumar Go to
White Castle (2004)
Blade: Trinity (2004)
The Amityville Horror (2005)
Waiting (2005)
Just Friends (2005)
Smokin' Aces (2006)
The Nines (2007)
Chaos Theory (2007)
Definitely, Maybe (2008)
Fireflies in the Garden (2008)
Adventureland (2009)

Christina **Ricci**
5ft 1in
(CHRISTINA RICCI)

Born: **February 12, 1980**
Santa Monica, California, USA

Christina was the fourth child of Ralph Ricci – a psychiatrist who became a lawyer, and his wife Sarah – a real estate agent, who in her earlier days, had been a Ford Model. Although there is Italian in her name, she regards her ancestry as Scots-Irish. After the family moved to Montclair, New Jersey, she attended the Edgemont Elementary School. She had appeared in several commercials and had also made her film debut, in *Mermaids,* by the time she went to Montclair High School. When she was thirteen, her parents separated. She, and her two brothers and a sister stayed with their mother. The trauma effected Christina deeply – causing her serious emotional problems. She was sent to the Professional Children's School in New York, where she recovered her poise and developed the confidence needed to handle a career as an actress. She built up to star status in movies like *The Addams Family,* and its sequel – for both of which she was nominated for Saturn Awards. She won them, for *Casper* and *Sleepy Hollow,* and has since performed with distinction in powerful movies like *Monster.*

Mermaids (1990)
The Hard Way (1991)
The Addams Family (1991)
The Cemetery Club (1993)
Addams Family Values (1993)
Now and Then (1995)
Bastard Out of Carolina (1996)
The Last of the High Kings (1996)
The Ice Storm (1997)
Buffalo '66 (1998)
Fear and Loathing in
Las Vegas (1998)
The Opposite Sex (1998)
Pecker (1998) I Woke Up
Early the Day I Died (1998)
Sleepy Hollow (1999)
Prozac Nation (2001) Pumpkin (2002)
Anything Else (2003)
Monster (2003) Penelope (2006)
Black Snake Moan (2006)
Speed Racer (2008)
New York, I Love You (2008)

Joely **Richardson**
5ft 9in
(JOELY KIM RICHARDSON)

Born: **January 9, 1965**
London, England

Part of a great British theatrical family – Joely's dad was the film director, Tony Richardson, and her mother is Vanessa Redgrave. She first appeared on screen at three years of age – as a tiny extra in her father's movie, *The Charge of the Light Brigade*. At boarding school, in Santa Barbara, California, Joely showed great potential as a gymnast and was generally talented at sports. Despite her thespian pedigree, Joely's early ambition was to become a professional tennis player – she spent two years, during her time at high school in Pinellas Park, being coached at a Florida tennis academy. Unluckily for British female tennis, Joely returned to her family tradition and made her first adult film appearance, in the comedy/drama, *The Hotel New Hampshire*. She played her mother, when young, in *Wetherby,* and she did a television episode of 'Poirot' in 1989. By the early 1990s, Joely had established herself as a fine actress on the international scene. She was given good reviews for her work in *Sister My Sister*. In 1992, she married director, Tim Bevan, with whom she has a daughter named Daisy. They were divorced in 2001. In 2005, she was highly praised for her portrayal of Wallis Simpson, in the television drama, 'Wallis & Edward'. Since 2003, Joely has been seen in around ninety episodes of the TV drama, 'Nip/Tuck'.

The Hotel New Hampshire (1984)
Wetherby (1985) Drowning
by Numbers (1988)
Shining Through (1992)
Sister My Sister (1994)
Hollow Reed (1996)
101 Dalmatians (1996)
Event Horizon (1997)
Under Heaven (1998)
The Tribe (1998) Return to
Me (2000) The Patriot (2000)
The Affair of the Necklace (2001)
The Fever (2004)
The Last Mimzy (2007)
The Christmas Miracle of
Jonathan Toomey (2007)

Miranda **Richardson**
5ft 5in
(MIRANDA JANE RICHARDSON)

Born: **March 3, 1958**
Southport, Merseyside, England

Miranda's no relation to Joely and Natasha – she didn't even come from a theatrical background. Her father, William, worked as a marketing executive and her mother was a homemaker. At Southport High School for Girls, Miranda showed a remarkable talent for acting. By the time she left school, her original ambition to become a vet was shelved in preference for human drama. She attended Bristol Old Vic Theater School at the same time as Daniel Day-Lewis. After graduating, she made her London West End stage debut in 1981, at the Queen's Theater, in "Moving". For four years, Miranda learned everything she needed to know from the theater, and has never lost her fondness for it. She did eventually turn to the Cinema – and she made her film debut, as the last woman to be hanged in Britain – Ruth Ellis – in *Dance with a Stranger*. In 1986, Miranda began her long association with the classic TV comedy series, "Blackadder". She was cast by Steven Spielberg, in his *Empire of the Sun,* and became a film star. Miranda has twice been nominated for Oscars – as Best Supporting Actress for *Damage* – (which won her a BAFTA), and Best Actress for the T.S.Eliot biopic, *Tom & Viv*.

Dance with a Stranger (1985)
Empire of the Sun (1987)
The Bachelor (1991)
Enchanted April (1992)
The Crying Game (1992)
Damage (1992) Century (1993)
Tom & Viv (1994)
The Evening Star (1998)
The Apostle (1997) St. Ives (1998)
Sleepy Hollow (1999)
Blackadder Back & Forth (1999)
Spider (2002) The Hours (2002)
The Rage in Placid Lake (2003)
Falling Angels (2003)
The Phantom of the Opera (2004)
Wah-Wah (2005) Harry Potter and
the Goblet of Fire (2005)
Provoked (2006) Puffball (2007)
The Young Victoria (2009)

Natasha **Richardson**
5ft 9in
(NATASHA JANE RICHARDSON)

Born: **May 11, 1963**
London, England
Died: **March 18, 2009**

Natasha's parents, Tony Richardson and Vanessa Redgrave, named their first daughter after the heroine of "War and Peace" – the classic novel by Leo Tolstoy. Along with her younger sister, Joely, she made her screen debut, at four, in her father's production of *Charge of the Light Brigade*. She was educated at St. Paul's Girls' School, in Hammersmith, and after that, followed in the footsteps of her illustrious mother, by doing her training at the Central School of Speech and Drama, in London. She began her stage career at the West Yorkshire Playhouse, in Leeds and made her professional debut, in movies, in 1983, in a little seen drama called *Every Picture Tells a Story*. Her first film role of any note was in Ken Russell's weird and wonderful, *Gothic*. It was followed by the more conventional, *A Month in the Country*. In 1991, she was the Evening Standard's Best Actress, for *The Handmaid's Tale,* and *The Comfort of Strangers*. Fifteen years later, she picked up the same award, for *Asylum*. She has appeared on Broadway with great success. She won a Tony in 1998, as Best Actress in a revival of "Cabaret". Natasha was married to the actor, Liam Neeson, from 1994 until her tragic death following a skiing accident in Canada. The couple were devoted to each other and their two sons – Michael and Daniel.

Gothic (1985)
A Month in the Country (1987)
Patty Hearst (1988)
Fat Man and Little Boy (1989)
The Handmaid's Tale (1990)
The Comfort of Strangers (1990)
The Favour, the Watch and
the Very Big Fish (1991)
Widow's Peak (1994) Nell (1994)
The Parent Trap (1998)
Blow Dry (2001)
Waking Up in Reno (2002)
Asylum (2005)
The White Countess (2005)
Evening (2007) Wild Child (2008)

Sir Ralph **Richardson**
6ft
(RALPH DAVID RICHARDSON)

Born: **December 19, 1902**
Cheltenham, Gloucestershire, England
Died: **October 10, 1983**

Ralph's mother, Lydia, left his father when he was a baby and took him to live in Gloucester, where he was raised as a Roman Catholic. She hoped he would become a priest, but although he was educated at the Xaverian College, in Brighton, when he left in 1918, he preferred to work as a scene painter, prop man, and electrician, for the St. Nicholas Players, in that town. In 1921, he went to Lowestoft, where he made his professional acting debut in "Merchant of Venice". In 1924, he married Muriel Hewitt. Ralph continued as a stage actor – with the Birmingham Repertory and the Old Vic Company, until 1933, when he was persuaded to act in his first film *The Ghoul* – which starred Boris Karloff. Ralph was soon dividing his time between the stage and the movies. During the war he served as a Lieutenant Commander in the Royal Navy Reserve. After that he became a co-director of the Old Vic. Ralph was knighted in 1947. He appeared in several classic movies, including *Things to Come, The Four Feathers, The Fallen Idol, The Heiress, Richard III,* and *Doctor Zhivago.* Ralph's two Oscar nominations – as Best Supporting Actor – were for *The Heiress* and *Greystoke* – which was posthumous. He died of a stroke, in London.

Things to Come (1936) **The Man
Who Could Work Miracles (1936)
The Citadel** (1938) **Q Planes** (1939)
The Four Feathers (1939) **The Day Will
Dawn** (1942) **School for Secrets** (1946)
Anna Karenina (1948) **The Fallen
Idol** (1948) **The Heiress** (1949)
Outcast of the Islands (1952)
The Holly and the Ivy (1952)
Richard III (1955)
Our Man in Havana (1959)
Long Day's Journey Into Night (1962)
Doctor Zhivago (1965)
Khartoum (1966) **O Lucky Man!** (1973)
Time Bandits (1981)
**Greystoke: The
Legend of Tarzan** (1984)

Alan **Rickman**
6ft 1in
(ALAN SIDNEY PATRICK RICKMAN)

Born: **February 21, 1946**
Acton, London, England

The son of Bernard Rickman, an Irish Catholic, who worked in a factory, and his wife Margaret, who was a Methodist from Wales. Alan didn't have a very privileged upbringing. His dad died when he was eight – leaving his mother to raise the four children alone. Alan showed an early aptitude for art, and with examples of his calligraphy and water colors, he won a scholarship to Latymer Upper School, in London. He did some acting while he was there, but still opted to study at Chelsea College of Art, where he qualified as a graphic designer. In 1972, he attended RADA – supporting himself by working as a dresser for Nigel Hawthorne, and Sir Ralph Richardson. He graduated in 1974 and worked for repertory groups and appeared at the Edinburgh Festival. He then joined the Royal Shakespeare Company. His film career took off with *Die Hard* and *Robin Hood: Prince of Thieves.* Alan is a regular in the *Harry Potter* films, in which he portrays Severus Snape. He's looking forward to a long career in films. Alan's longtime partner is Rima Horton.

Die Hard (1988)
Quigley Down Under (1990)
Truly Madly Deeply (1990)
Closet Land (1991)
**Robin Hood: Prince of
Thieves** (1991)
Close My Eyes (1991)
Bob Roberts (1992)
Sense and Sensibility (1995)
Michael Collins (1996)
Judas Kiss (1998)
Dogma (1999)
Galaxy Quest (1999)
Blue Dry (2001)
The Sorcerer's Stone (2001)
The Search for John Gissing (2001)
The Prisoner of Azkaban (2004)
The Goblet of Fire (2005)
Snow Cake (2006)
Perfume (2006)
Nobel Son (2007)
Sweeney Todd (2007)
Bottle Shock (2008)

Molly **Ringwald**
5ft 8in
(MOLLY KATHLEEN RINGWALD)

Born: **February 18, 1968**
Roseville, California, USA

Molly is the daughter of Bob Ringwald, a blind jazz pianist, and his wife Adele, who was a chef from a Dutch background. Molly began her acting career at the age of five, when she played the 'dormouse' in a stage version of "Alice in Wonderland". A year later, she sang with her father's group, the Fulton Street Jazz Band, on an album titled, "I Wanna Be Loved By You". She began working in commercials for the local TV station – landing a guest spot on 'The New Mickey Mouse Club' and made her television acting debut, in an episode of 'Different Strokes', in 1980. It was also the year she performed as lead vocalist on the Disney album, "Yankee Doodle Mickey". Molly was educated at the Casa Roble High School, in Sacramento, and at fourteen, made her movie debut, in the comedy drama, *Tempest,* for which she had a Golden Globe nomination. Her big break came two years later, when she starred in John Hughes' coming of age movie, *Sixteen Candles* – qualifying her as an original member of the "Brat Pack". A second Hughes movie, *The Breakfast Club,* proved to be her biggest success. Having been one of America's top teenage actresses, her career faltered as she reached adulthood. She worked in France and married Valery Lameignère. They were divorced in 2002. Since her last two movies, in 2001, Molly's been mainly seen in television dramas. She married writer, Panio Gianopolis in 2007. The couple now have a daughter. In 2008, Molly became a regular in the TV drama, 'The Secret Life of the American Teenager'.

Tempest (1982)
Sixteen Candles (1984)
The Breakfast Club (1985)
Pretty in Pink (1986)
For Keeps (1988)
Betsy's Wedding (1990)
**Some Folks Call It a
Sling Blade** (1994)
Baja (1995)
In the Weeds (2000)
Cowboy Up (2001)

Thelma **Ritter**
5ft 3in
(THELMA RITTER)

Born: **February 14, 1905**
Brooklyn, New York City, New York, USA
Died: **February 5, 1969**

One of the very few actresses to be born on St. Valentine's Day, Thelma was a real sweetheart as a child – quite the opposite to her later screen persona. She began acting in plays at grade school and trained at the American Academy of Dramatic Arts. In 1927, she married Joseph Moran, with whom she had two children and was with him until her death. She worked with stock companies, and on radio shows. In 1946, director, George Seaton, was casting for his film, *Miracle on 34th Street,* and gave Thelma her film debut, with a small role. She was memorable in her next film, *A Letter to Three Wives,* even though she had very little screen time. Her rasping voice and cynical, but good-hearted personality, shone from every film she made. Thelma received the first of six Supporting Actress Oscar nominations, in 1950, for *All About Eve* – then for *The Mating Season, With a Song in My Heart, Pickup on South Street, Pillow Talk,* and *Birdman of Alcatraz* – she still has most nominations for that award without a win. She suffered a heart attack after her TV appearance on 'The Jerry Lewis Show.' Thelma died at her home in New York, nine days before her sixty-fourth birthday.

City Across the River (1949)
Father Was a Fullback (1949)
Perfect Strangers (1950)
All About Eve (1950)
The Mating Season (1951)
The Model and the Marriage
Broker (1951) With a Song in
My Heart (1952) Titanic (1953)
Pickup on South Street (1953)
Rear Window (1954)
Daddy Long Legs (1955)
Lucy Gallant (1955)
The Proud and Profane (1956)
Pillow Talk (1959) The Misfits (1961)
The Second Time Around (1961)
Birdman of Alcatraz (1962)
For Love or Money (1963)
A New Kind of Love (1963)
Move Over Darling (1963)

Emmanuelle **Riva**
5ft 3in
(EMMANUELLE PAULETTE RIVA)

Born: **February 24, 1927**
Chenimenil, Vosges, France

After leaving school, Emmanuelle worked as a seamstress. She went to Paris in 1953 to attend acting classes at Centre d'Art Dramatique de la rue Blanche. She passed with flying colors, and in 1954, she began working as an actress on the Paris stage. Having established herself during the mid-1950s in the theater, she was chosen by director, Alain Resnais, to star in his powerful film about the aftermath of the bombing of Japan – *Hiroshima mon amour.* It was also a love story, beautifully acted by Emmanuelle and Eiji Okada. She was nominated for a BAFTA and won the Étoile de Cristal from the Cinéma Français. Although not a conventional movie star, Emmanuelle landed challenging roles in films like *Léon Morin, Priest,* where she brought out the very best in Jean-Paul Belmondo. It was followed by the title role in Georges Franju's highly regarded film adaptation of Mauriac's novel, *Thérèse Desqueyroux.* Her portrayal won her the Volpi Cup – for Best Actress, at the Venice Film Festival. She has since graced a number of good films – the best of which are listed below. At the end of 2008, she marked the 50th Anniversary of *Hiroshima mon amour,* by visiting Japan.

Hiroshima mon amour (1958)
Kapò (1959) The Eighth Day (1960)
Léon Morin, Priest (1961)
Thérèse Desqueyroux (1962)
Thomas the Imposter (1964)
Risky Business (1967) J'irai comme un
cheval fou (1973) Along the Fango
River (1974) The Games of Countess
Dolingen (1980) Is there a Frenchman in
the House? (1981) Gli Occhi,
la bocca (1982) Liberté, la nuit (1983)
The Tribulations of Balthazar
Kober (1988) La Passion de
Bernadette (1989) Far from Brazil (1992)
Trois couleurs: Bleu (1993)
Shadow of a Doubt (1993)
Venus Beauty Institute (1999)
C'est la vie (2001) Eros Therapy (2004)
Mon fils à moi (2006)
Le Grand alibi (2008)

Jason **Robards**
5ft 10in
(JASON NELSON ROBARDS JR.)

Born: **July 26, 1922**
Chicago, Illinois, USA
Died: **December 26, 2000**

The son of Jason Robards Sr., a stage and early screen star, and Hope Glanville, he lived in New York as a child. A later move to Los Angeles, resulted in the break-up of his parents' marriage and caused him a great deal of trauma. It did not affect his athletic ability – at Hollywood High School, he was within a whisker of a 4-minute mile. After he graduated, in 1940, Jason joined the United States Navy, and he was on board the "USS Honolulu", when the Japanese attacked Pearl Harbor. He also saw action in the Pacific. After a short spell at the American Academy of Dramatic Arts, he made his stage debut, in 1947. Jason was a stage star when he made his TV debut in 1954, in 'The Man Behind the Badge'. His film debut, was in *The Journey.* Jason starred in a number of fine movies, including *The Ballad of Cable Hogue* and *Melvin and Howard.* He won Best Supporting Actor Oscars – for *All the President's Men* and *Julia.* His third wife was Lauren Bacall. He had completed thirty years of marriage, with his fourth wife, Lois, when he died of lung cancer, in Bridgeport, Connecticut.

The Journey (1959)
Long Day's Journey Into Night (1962)
A Thousand Clowns (1965)
A Big Hand for the Little Lady (1966)
Divorce American Style (1967)
The St. Valentine's Day
Massacre (1967)
Once Upon a Time in
the West (1968)
Isadora (1968)
The Ballad of Cable Hogue (1970)
Tora! Tora! Tora! (1970)
Pat Garrett & Billy the Kid (1973)
All the President's Men (1976)
Julia (1977)
Melvin and Howard (1980)
Something Wicked This
Way Comes (1983)
Reunion (1989) Parenthood (1989)
Philadelphia (1993) The Paper (1994)
Magnolia (1999)

Tim **Robbins**
6ft 4¹/₂in
(TIMOTHY FRANCIS ROBBINS)

Born: **October 16, 1958**
West Covina, California, USA

The son of the folk singer, Gil Robbins, and the actress, Mary Bledsoe, Tim grew up in Greenwich Village after his father moved there to perform with the folk group, "The Highwaymen". He and his two sisters and a brother were raised as Catholics. Tim's first interest in acting was at the age of twelve, when he joined the drama club at Stuyvesant High School. During his early teens, he got involved with theater with the New City and its Summer Street Theater. After graduating, he went to the State University of New York, a liberal arts college, in Plattsburgh. After two years, he studied at the UCLA Film School. In California, he began to get work - his first TV appearance was in 1979, as a slave, in an episode of 'Buck Rogers in the 25th Century'. Tim's movie debut was five years later, in *Toy Soldiers.* His reputation soared from the mid-1980s. He later directed *Bob Roberts,* and that same year, won a Golden Globe as an actor, for *The Player.* in 1996, he was Oscar-nominated as Best Director, for *Dead Man Walking.* He won an Oscar, as Best Supporting Actor, for *Mystic River.* In his private life, Tim has been in a relationship (they have two sons) for more than twenty years, with Susan Sarandon. The couple are not afraid to speak out on political issues.

The Sure Thing (1985)
Top Gun (1986) **Bull Durham** (1988)
Miss Firecracker (1989)
Jacob's Ladder (1990)
The Player (1992)
Bob Roberts (1992)
Short Cuts (1993)
The Hudsucker Proxy (1994)
The Shawshank Redemption (1994)
I.Q. (1994) **Nothing to Lose** (1997)
High Fidelity (2000)
Human Nature (2001)
Mystic River (2003) **Code 46** (2003)
The Secret Life of Words (2005)
Zathura: A Space Adventure (2005)
Catch a Fire (2006) **Noise** (2007)
The Lucky Ones (2008)
City of Ember (2008)

Julia **Roberts**
5ft 9in
(JULIA FIONA ROBERTS)

Born: **October 28, 1967**
Smyrna, Georgia, USA

Julia's father, Walter, worked as a vacuum cleaner salesman. Her mother, Betty, had spent some time as a real estate agent. They had both enjoyed acting in their early lives – performing in plays for the armed forces and co-founding the Atlanta Actors and Writers Workshop. Young Julia loved horses, and her ambition was to become a veterinarian, but after Campbell High School, in Smyrna, and Georgia State University, she decided to join her actress sister, Lisa, in New York. She registered with the Click Model Agency and took acting classes. In 1986, Julia made her film debut in *Blood Red,* which starred her brother, Eric, and wasn't released until 1989. By that time, she had acted on TV and established herself in movies. She was a big star by the time she was twice Oscar-nominated – for *Steel Magnolias,* and *Pretty Woman,* and she was already a mega-star when she was awarded both a BAFTA and Best Actress Oscar, for *Erin Brockovich.* Since July 2002, Julia's been married to her second husband – the movie cameraman, Danny Moder. They run a production company together and have three children – two of whom are twins. Her next film, *Duplicity,* looks like being something special.

Mystic Pizza (1988)
Steel Magnolias (1989)
Pretty Woman (1990)
Flatliners (1990)
The Pelican Brief (1993)
I Love Trouble (1994)
Michael Collins (1996)
Everyone Says
I Love You (1996)
My Best Friend's Wedding (1997)
Stepmom (1998)
Notting Hill (1999)
Erin Brokovich (2000)
America's Sweethearts (2001)
Ocean's Eleven (2001)
Mona Lisa Smile (2003)
Closer (2004)
Charlie Wilson's War (2007)
Fireflies in the Garden (2008)

Rachel **Roberts**
5ft 5in
(RACHEL ROBERTS)

Born: **September 20, 1927**
Llanelli, Carmarthenshire, Wales
Died: **November 26, 1980**

Rachel was brought up in a Baptist family. She later rebelled against this, but during her school years (in wartime Britain) she studied hard and earned a place at the University of Wales. While there, she decided on an acting career. She was accepted at the Royal Academy of Dramatic Art, in London, and surprisingly, (considering the rather serious nature of her future roles), she was awarded the Athene Seyler Award for Comedy. In 1951, Rachel made her stage debut – with Michael Redgrave – at the Old Vic – in "Twelfth Night". She continued to appear in Shakespearean roles – in "Othello", "Macbeth" and "Henry V" – to name just three. She made her film debut, in 1953, in *Valley of Song,* set in Wales. In 1955, Rachel married the actor, Alan Dobie, but by the time that finished, in 1961, she was a confirmed alcoholic. She worked on stage and didn't really register with film audiences until *Saturday Night and Sunday Morning* – for which she won the first of three BAFTAs. She was nominated for a Best Actress Oscar for *This Sporting Life.* After her divorce from Dobie, she married Rex Harrison. Their split in 1971, affected her very badly. Rachel died in Los Angeles, of a barbiturates overdose.

Valley of Song (1953)
Saturday Night and
Sunday Morning (1960)
Girl on Approval (1961)
This Sporting Life (1963)
A Flea in Her Ear (1968)
The Reckoning (1969)
Wild Rovers (1971)
Alpha Beta (1973)
The Belstone Fox (1973)
O Lucky Man! (1973)
Murder on the
Orient Express (1974)
Picnic at
Hanging Rock (1975)
Foul Play (1978)
Yanks (1979)
When a Stranger Calls (1979)

Cliff **Robertson**
5ft 11in
(CLIFFORD PARKER ROBERTSON III)

Born: **September 9, 1925**
La Jolla, California, USA

The son of Clifford Parker Robertson III, and his wife Audrey, Cliff was educated at the independent liberal arts school, Antioch College, in Yellow Springs, Ohio – where he appeared in school plays. Cliff's first movie appearances were uncredited roles in the 1943 war films, *We've Never Been Licked* and *Corvette K-225*. Cliff served in the Merchant Marine during World War II – seeing action in the South Pacific, the Mediterranean, France and the North Atlantic. After the war, he went to work as a reporter for the 'Springfield Daily News'. He joined a local playhouse and pretty soon, decided to give it a serious go, by studying drama at the Actors' Studio, in New York. He made his first impact on stage in Chicago, in "Mister Roberts". Theater and TV dominated the next few years, until he made his official film debut, in *Picnic*. He won a Best Actor Oscar for *Charly*, and is still active. Cliff was twice married and divorced – from actresses Cynthia Stone (Jack Lemmon's ex-wife) and Dina Merrill. He had a daughter with each of them.

Picnic (1955) **The Naked and the Dead** (1958) Gidget (1959) **Underworld U.S.A.** (1961) **The Interns** (1962) PT 109 (1963) **Sunday in New York** (1963) **The Best Man** (1964) 633 Squadron (1964) Masquerade (1965) **Up from the Beach** (1965) **The Honeypot** (1967) The Devil's Brigade (1968) Charly (1968) **Too Late the Hero** (1970) J.W.Coop (1972) **The Great Northfield Minnesota Raid** (1972) **Three Days of the Condor** (1975) Midway (1976) Obsession (1976) Brainstorm (1983) **Wild Hearts Can't Be Broken** (1991) Wind (1992) **Waiting for Sunset** (1995) **Family Tree** (1999) Spider-Man (2002) Spider-Man 2 (2004) **Spider-Man 3** (2007)

Edward G. **Robinson**
5ft 5in
(EMMANUEL GOLDENBERG)

Born: **December 12, 1893**
Bucharest, Rumania
Died: **January 26, 1973**

E.G's parents were Yiddish-speaking Jews, who emigrated to New York City when he was ten. He was educated at Townsend Harris High School and New York's City College. He made his first appearance on the amateur stage, in "Bells of Conscience", which he wrote himself. His acting won him a scholarship to the American Academy of Dramatic Arts, and after graduating, he changed his name to Edward G. Robinson. He made his Broadway debut, in 1915, followed by a bit part in a silent, *Arms and the Woman.* Apart from one featured silent role, he remained a stage actor. He married actress Gladys Lloyd, in 1927, and made his 'talkie' debut in 1929, with Claudette Colbert, in *The Hole in the Wall.* Despite over forty years of great screen work, from *Little Caesar* onwards, E.G. was never ever nominated for an Oscar, but he was voted Best Actor, for *House of Strangers,* at the 1949 Cannes Film Festival. Jane Robinson, his second wife, was with him when he died of cancer, in Hollywood.

Little Caesar (1931) **Smart Money** (1931) **Two Seconds** (1932) The Little Giant (1933) **The Whole Town's Talking** (1935) Barbary Coast (1935) **Bullets or Ballots** (1936) Kid Galahad (1937) **The Amazing Dr. Clitterhouse** (1938) Blackmail (1939) Brother Orchid (1940) **Larceny, Inc.** (1942) Flesh and Fantasy (1943) **Double Indemnity** (1944) **The Woman in the Window** (1944) Our Vines Have Tender Grapes (1945) Scarlet Street (1945) **The Stranger** (1946) **The Red House** (1947) All My Sons (1948) Key Largo (1948) **Night Has a Thousand Eyes** (1948) House of Strangers (1949) Black Tuesday (1954) Illegal (1955) **Seven Thieves** (1960) The Prize (1963) **The Cincinnati Kid** (1965) **Soylent Green** (1973)

Dame Flora **Robson**
5ft 10in
(FLORA MCKENZIE ROBSON)

Born: **March 28, 1902**
South Shields, Durham, England
Died: **July 7, 1984**

Flora was of Scottish descent. Her father was a ship's engineer. She was from a large family and had two brothers and four sisters – three of whom, including herself, would remain unmarried and childless. When she was only six-years old, Flora revealed an extraordinary talent for recitation, and would be taken by horse and carriage to perform in competitions – which she usually won. Educated at Palmer's Green High School, she later went to RADA to study acting, and in 1921, made her stage debut, in London. Flora's height gave her great stage presence, but more of a surprise was her success in the movies, which emphasized her very plain looks. When she made her film debut, in 1931, in *Dance Pretty Lady,* she wasn't in the title role. Flora created many great characters of history in her films – giving, in *Fire Over England,* what was for a long time, considered to be the definitive portrayal of Elizabeth I. Flora must have been disappointed that her only Oscar nomination, was as the Best Supporting Actress, in *Saratoga Trunk.* She continued working well into her seventies and died of cancer, at her home in Brighton, Sussex.

The Rise of Catherine the Great (1934) **Fire Over England** (1937) **Wuthering Heights** (1939) We Are Not Alone (1939) Invisible Stripes (1939) Poison Pen (1940) **The Sea Hawk** (1940) **Bahama Passage** (1941) Two Thousand Women (1944) **Saratoga Trunk** (1945) **Caesar and Cleopatra** (1945) The Years Between (1946) Black Narcissus (1947) Frieda (1947) **Good-Time Girl** (1948) Saraband for Dead Lovers (1948) **Romeo and Juliet** (1954) **Innocent Sinners** (1958) 55 Days at Peking (1963) **Guns at Batasi** (1964) Young Cassidy (1965) 7 Women (1966) **Clash of the Titans** (1981)

Patricia Roc
5ft 4in
(FELICIA MIRIAM URSULA HEROLD)

Born: **June 7, 1915**
St. Pancras, London, England
Died: **December 30, 2003**

Pat was the eldest of three sisters. One of them married the British tennis star, Fred Perry. Pat's parents were reasonably well off. Her father was from Holland, and her mother, who was half French, was born on the Isle of Jersey. Pat began her education at the Francis Holland School, in Regents Park, and at fourteen, she was sent to a boarding school in Broadstairs, Kent. She mostly enjoyed sporting activities and was especially fond of riding and swimming. When she was nineteen, Pat went to a finishing school in Paris. On her return to England, she was accepted at the Royal Academy of Dramatic Art, in London. She was seen in a stage play by a talent scout who worked for the film producer, Alexander Korda. This led to her film debut in 1938, with an uncredited bit part, in *The Divorce of Lady X,* starring Merle Oberon and Laurence Olivier. Pat then married a Canadian doctor, who was twenty years older than her and remained in London for most of World War II. In her twelfth movie, *Millions Like Us,* she made her first impact. By 1945, she had reached her peak in Britain, and went to Hollywood to act in the western, *Canyon Passage.* She returned home to feature in several Gainsborough films, and in 1949, moved to Paris, after marrying cinematographer, André Thomas. They had a son. After his death in 1954, she was a widow until 1962. She married a Viennese and retired. Pat died of kidney failure, in Switzerland.

Millions Like Us (1943)
Two Thousand Women (1944)
Love Story (1944)
Madonna of the Seven Moons (1945)
Johnny Frenchman (1945)
The Wicked Lady (1945)
Canyon Passage (1946)
The Brothers (1947)
So Well Remembered (1947)
Holiday Camp (1947) **Jassy** (1947)
One Night With You (1948)
Retour à la vie (1949)
Circle of Danger (1951)

Sam Rockwell
5ft 9in
(SAM ROCKWELL)

Born: **November 5, 1968**
Daly City, California, USA

Sam's parents – the actors Pete Rockwell and Penny Hess, divorced when he was five, and he was raised by his dad, in San Francisco. He used to visit his mother in New York during the summer and, when he was ten, he was loudly applauded for his cameo role, as Humphrey Bogart, in an East Village Improv comedy sketch, in which Penny starred. Sam attended the School of the Arts High School, in San Francisco, but dropped out before graduation. He got his high school diploma at an alternate high school, and rediscovered his love of acting – making his film debut, in the independent, *Clownhouse.* He went back to New York, where, for two years, he was trained at the William Esper Acting Studio. In 1994, Sam starred in a Miller Ice Beer commercial and made up his mind to concentrate on his film career. At the time of *The Green Mile* and *Galaxy Quest,* he'd 'made it'. He later won a Silver Bear in Berlin, for *Confessions of a Dangerous Mind.* In recent years, Sam has appeared in big films like *The Assassination of Jesse James* and *Frost/Nixon,* as well as some good Indies, such as *Snow Angels.*

Clownhouse (1989)
Last Exit to Brooklyn (1989)
In the Soup (1992)
Light Sleeper (1992)
Drunks (1995)
Box of Moon Light (1996)
Lawn Dogs (1997)
Jerry and Tom (1998)
Safe Men (1998)
A Midsummer Night's Dream (1999)
The Green Mile (1999)
Galaxy Quest (1999) **Heist** (2001)
Welcome to Collinwood (2002)
**Confessions of a
Dangerous Mind** (2002)
Matchstick Men (2003)
Joshua (2007)
Snow Angels (2007)
**The Assassination of
Jesse James by the Coward
Robert Ford** (2007) **Choke** (2008)
Frost/Nixon (2008) **Moon** (2009)

Ginger Rogers
5ft 4½in
(VIRGINIA KATHERINE MCMATH)

Born: **July 16, 1911**
Independence, Missouri, USA
Died: **April 25, 1995**

Of Scottish and Welsh ancestry, Ginger was brought up by her mother, Lela, in Kansas City. After remarrying John Rogers when Ginger was nine, Lela was theater critic for the Fort Worth Record, in Texas. Ginger considered teaching, but she won the Texas State Charleston Championship and a vaudeville tour. At seventeen, she married the first of five husbands, Jack Culpepper, a dancer – it was over in a few months. She made her Broadway debut, in 1929, in "Top Speed" and was signed to appear in "Girl Crazy". Ginger got a Paramount contract, but after some weak films, she left them. Her first good part was in *42nd Street,* but her great fame would come in her nine films, as Fred Astaire's partner, in the 1930s. She proved that she was more than a tap dancer, by winning a Best Actress Oscar, for *Kitty Foyle.* Other movies such as *Roxie Hart* and *The Major and the Minor* underlined that point. A reunion with Astaire, in *The Barkleys of Broadway,* although not nearly as good as some of their earlier efforts, proved that they were still magic together. She retired in 1987 and remained single until dying of congestive heart failure, in Rancho Mirage, California.

42nd Street (1933) **Gold Diggers of
1933** (1933) **Flying Down to Rio** (1933)
Twenty Million Sweethearts (1934)
The Gay Divorcee (1934) **Romance in
Manhattan** (1935) **Roberta** (1935)
Top Hat (1935) **Follow the Fleet** (1936)
Swing Time (1936)
Shall We Dance (1937) **Carefree** (1938)
**The Story of
Vernon and Irene Castle** (1939)
Bachelor Mother (1939)
Primrose Path (1940)
Kitty Foyle (1940) **Roxie Hart** (1942)
Tales of Manhattan (1942)
The Major and the Minor (1942)
I'll Be Seeing You (1944)
The Barkleys of Broadway (1949)
Monkey Business (1952)
Tight Spot (1955)

Mimi **Rogers**
5ft 8½in
(MIRIAM SOICKLER)

Born: **January 27, 1956**
Coral Gables, Florida, USA

The daughter of a Jewish father and an Episcopalian mother, Mimi graduated from high school at fourteen, and got involved with doing charity work. While underage, she accompanied her father to Tahoe, where she played blackjack and poker. In 1976, she married a Scientologist, James Rogers, who got the message through to her, and gave her his name. He must have realized that her statuesque beauty deserved a wider viewing, because eventually, she turned her attention to acting. In 1981, after divorcing Rogers, she got her first television work – in two episodes of 'Hill Street Blues'. Mimi did TV until 1983, when she made her film debut, in *Blue Skies Again.* It did little to further her film career, but three years later, she scored in a pair of hits, and the excellent thriller, *Someone to Watch Over Me.* In 1987, she began a three year marriage to Tom Cruise and introduced him to her religion. Since they parted, she has lived with, and later married, producer Chris Ciaffra. They have two children. Although she has a couple of interesting-sounding films in the pipeline, Mimi's most visible recent work has been on TV, as Meryl, in 'The Loop'.

Gung Ho (1986)
Street Smart (1987)
Someone to Watch Over Me (1987)
The Mighty Quinn (1989)
The Doors (1991)
Wedlock (1991)
The Rapture (1991)
Shooting Elizabeth (1992)
Killer (1994)
Far from Home: The Adventures of
Yellow Dog (1995)
Trees Lounge (1996)
The Mirror Has Two Faces (1996)
Austin Powers: International
Man of Mystery (1997)
Seven Girlfriends (1999)
Ginger Snaps (2000)
The Door in the Floor (2004)
Dancing in Twilight (2005)
Big Nothing (2006)
Frozen Kiss (2009)

Ruth **Roman**
5ft 5in
(NORMA ROMAN)

Born: **December 22, 1922**
Lynn, Massachusetts, USA
Died: **September 9, 1999**

Ruth grew up in the Boston suburb of Lynn. She began acting when she was nine years old, in local community theater productions. After high school, where she was an enthusiastic participant in school plays, she enrolled at the Bishop Lee Dramatic School, in Boston. She then went to Hollywood, where she made her first appearance – in an uncredited role in Frank Borzage's star-studded 1943 film, *Stage Door Canteen.* Ruth's first featured part was the following year, in a modest Ken Maynard B-western, called *Harmony Trail.* In 1945, she took the title role for Universal, in the serial, *Jungle Queen* – which wasn't very inspiring either. But Ruth stuck it out, even though bit parts were all she got, until her breakthrough film, the boxing classic, *Champion* – for which she was nominated for a Golden Globe. In 1956, after divorcing her first husband, Ruth was on her way home from the Cannes Film Festival with their son, Richard. They were both rescued when the "Andrea Doria" on which they were passengers, sank after a collision in the Atlantic. Ruth married twice more and worked for another thirty years – mainly on television. She died peacefully in her sleep at her home, in Laguna Beach, California.

Champion (1949)
The Window (1949)
Three Secrets (1950)
Dallas (1950)
Lightning Strikes Twice (1951)
Strangers on a Train (1951)
Tomorrow Is Another Day (1951)
Invitation (1952)
Young Man With Ideas (1952)
Blowing Wild (1953)
The Far Country (1954)
Down Three Dark Streets (1954)
Joe MacBeth (1955)
Great Day in
the Morning (1956)
Rebel in Town (1956)
Bitter Victory (1957)
The Killing Kind (1973)

Cesar **Romero**
6ft 2in
(CESAR JULIO ROMERO JR.)

Born: **February 15, 1907**
New York City, New York, USA
Died: **January 1, 1994**

For the early years of his existence, Cesar enjoyed a life of luxury provided by his wealthy Cuban parents, who owned a sugar import business. His education, at the Collegiate School, in Manhattan, and Riverdale Country School in the Bronx, went smoothly, and he added drama lessons to his studies. Cesar worked as a bank messenger until his skills as a dancer, got him work on Broadway, beginning with "Lady Do!", in 1927. Luckily he did, because when the Stock Market crashed in 1929, his parents lost most of their fortune. Cesar was able to support his family as both a speciality dancer and a straight actor – in plays like "Strictly Dishonorable" and "Dinner at Eight". His movie career got off to a poor start with *The Shadow Laughs,* in 1933. Luckily, it was quickly followed by parts in quality films. A unique character, he acted in musicals, comedies and westerns, for nearly sixty years. He was famous as 'The Joker' in film and TV versions of *Batman,* but his private life and his homosexuality remained a well-kept secret. Cesar quit acting in 1990, and died of bronchitis and pneumonia, in Santa Monica, California.

The Thin Man (1934)
Clive of India (1935)
Cardinal Richelieu (1935)
Diamond Jim (1935)
Happy Landing (1938)
The Little Princess (1939)
Dance Hall (1941)
Weekend in Havana (1941)
Tales of Manhattan (1942)
Orchestra Wives (1942)
Springtime in
the Rockies (1942)
Captain from Castile (1947)
Julia Misbehaves (1948)
FBI Girl (1951)
Vera Cruz (1954)
Ocean's Eleven (1960)
If a Man Answers (1962)
Donovan's Reef (1963)
Batman (1966)

Mickey **Rooney**
5ft 3in
(JOSEPH YULE JR.)

Born: **September 23, 1920**
Brooklyn, New York City, New York, USA

His father Joe, who was from Scotland, and his Kansas City-born mother, Nellie, were both in vaudeville. When Mickey was born, the pair were appearing in the long-running Brooklyn production of "A Gaiety Girl". By the time he was fifteen months old, he featured in their act, in a specially tailored tuxedo. His parents separated when he was four, and Nellie took her son to live in Hollywood. She helped him to get the role of Mickey Maguire, in a short film series based on a comic strip, "Toonerville Trolley". He claimed Walt Disney named Mickey Mouse after his character. In addition to the series, Mickey appeared in a number of juvenile roles. His first big film, was *A Midsummer Night's Dream,* when he played Puck, but an MGM contract and teaming up with Judy Garland, moved him forward. *Love Finds Andy Hardy* and *Boys Town,* made him a star. In 1942, he married Ava Gardner. After their divorce, he served in the military. When he returned as an adult actor, roles were more difficult to get, but he kept plugging away. Mickey was nominated for Oscars, for *Babes in Arms, The Human Comedy, The Bold and the Brave* and *The Black Stallion.* In 1983, he received a "Lifetime Achievement" Oscar. Mickey married his eighth wife, Jan Chamberlin, in 1978. She's been good for him – he is still making films in 2009!

A Midsummer Night's Dream (1935)
Ah, Wilderness! (1935)
Little Lord Fauntleroy (1936)
Captains Courageous (1937)
Slave Ship (1937)
Thoroughbreds Don't Cry (1937)
Love Finds Andy Hardy (1938) Boys
Town (1938) Babes in Arms (1939)
Girl Crazy (1943)
The Human Comedy (1943)
National Velvet (1944)
Words and Music (1948)
The Bridges at Toko-Ri (1954)
The Bold and the Brave (1956)
Baby Face Nelson (1957)
Requiem for a Heavyweight (1962)
The Black Stallion (1979)

Françoise **Rosay**
5ft 6in
(FRANÇOISE BANDY DE NALÈCHE)

Born: **April 19, 1891**
Paris, Ile-de France, France
Died: **March 28, 1974**

Françoise was the illegitimate daughter of actress, Marie-Thérèse Chauvin, whose stage-name was Sylviac. Françoise was blessed with an exquisite singing voice and when she left school she pursued an operatic career by studying at the Paris Conservatoire – making her debut, in the title-role of the opera, "Salammbô". She made her film debut, in 1911, in William Shakespeare's *Falstaff.* She married the French director, Jacques Feyder, and after a handful of silent films, went to Hollywood to appear in her first talkie, *The One Woman Idea.* She remained there to make French-language films with Charles Boyer, Maurice Chevalier and Buster Keaton. In 1931, Françoise returned to France and established herself as a popular actress – co-starring with Fernandel, and getting top billing, in 1933, in *Coralie et Cie.* She was directed by her husband in *Le Grand Jeu.* Her breakthrough came in *Carnival in Flanders* – after which she appeared with the cream of French Cinema, including Raimu, Louis Jouvet and Michel Simon. In 1938, Françoise was acknowledged by her natural father, Count François Bandy de Nalèche. During World War II, she lived in Switzerland, where she taught acting, in Geneva. In 1944, she made her first British film, *The Halfway House.* She retired in 1973, and died in Montgeron, a year later.

Carnival in Flanders (1935) The Robber
Symphony (1936) Jenny (1936) Dance
of Life (1937) Le Fauteuil 47 (1937)
Drôle de drame (1937)
People Who Travel (1938)
The Halfway House (1944)
Johnny Frenchman (1945)
Macadam (1946) Saraband for Dead
Lovers (1948) Quartet (1948)
September Affair (1950)
Women Without Names (1950)
The 13th Letter (1951)
The Red Inn (1951)
The Seven Deadly Sins (1952)
La Reine Margot (1954)
Me and the Colonel (1958)

Isabella **Rosellini**
5ft 8in
(ISABELLA FIORELLA ELETTRA GIOVANNA ROSSELLINI)

Born: **June 18, 1952**
Rome, Italy

Isabella and her twin sister, Isotta, are the daughters of the Italian film director, Roberto Rossellini – from his relationship with the great Swedish actress, Ingrid Bergman. She grew up in Paris and Rome – using her languages to get her first job, as a television reporter – for the Italian television corporation, RAI – in New York. Around that time, she made a few appearances in Italy, on Roberto Benigni's TV show 'The Other Sunday'. In 1976, Isabella made her film debut, in *A Matter of Time.* It starred Ingrid Bergman, Liza Minnelli and Charles Boyer, and was directed by Vincente Minnelli, who washed his hands of the finished product after studio interference. After *Il Prato,* for which she won a Silver Ribbon as Best New Actress from Italian Film Journalists, she married Martin Scorsese, and devoted herself to being his wife. After their divorce in 1982, she began to work as a model for Lancôme. A three year marriage to Jon Wiedemann, produced her only child, Elettra. *Blue Velvet* was the start of a long, productive international movie career.

Il Prato (1979) Il Pap'occhio (1980)
White Nights (1985)
Blue Velvet (1986) Zelly and Me (1988)
Cousins (1989) Wild at Heart (1990)
Caccia alla vedova (1991)
Death Becomes Her (1992)
The Innocent (1993)
Fearless (1993)
Wyatt Earp (1994)
Immortal Beloved (1994)
Big Night (1996)
The Funeral (1996)
Left Luggage (1998)
The Impostors (1998)
Roger Dodger (2002)
The Saddest Music in
the World (2003)
King of the Corner (2004)
Heights (2005)
La Festivo del chivo (2005)
Infamous (2006)
The Accidental Husband (2008)
Two Lovers (2008)

Katharine **Ross**
5ft 5¹/₂in
(KATHARINE JULIET ROSS)

Born: January 29, 1940
Hollywood, California, USA

The daughter of a naval officer, Katharine was raised in the town of Walnut Creek, California. She was educated at the local Las Lomas High School, followed by Santa Rosa College. She studied Drama at San Francisco's Actors' Workshop. She appeared in plays, including "The Devil's Disciple". In 1962, when she was acting in "The Balcony", Katharine was spotted by Edmond O'Brien, who hired her for her first television role, in his series, 'Sam Benedict'. It led to work in other television shows, among which were 'The Alfred Hitchcock Hour', 'Ben Casey' 'Wagon Train' and 'Gunsmoke'. The last named most probably clinched her film debut – a featured role in the wonderful James Stewart western, *Shenandoah*. For her work in another important film, *The Graduate,* Katharine received a Best Supporting Actress Oscar nomination. Despite the breakup of her first marriage, the 1960s and 1970s were good for her. Her ride on the handlebars of Paul Newman's bike in *Butch Cassidy and the Sundance Kid* is an iconic image of the American Cinema. For that movie she won a BAFTA Best Actress Award in tandem with *Tell Them Willie Boy Is Here.* She's married to actor Sam Elliott and has a daughter named Cleo.

Shenandoah (1965)
Mister Buddwing (1966)
Games (1967)
The Graduate (1967)
Hellfighters (1968)
Butch Cassidy and the
Sundance Kid (1969)
Tell Them
Willie Boy Is Here (1969)
The Stepford Wives (1975)
Voyage of the
Damned (1976)
The Final Countdown (1980)
Wrong Is Right (1982)
Redheaded Stranger (1986)
A Climate for Killing (1991)
Donnie Darko (2001)
Don't Let Go (2002)

Tim **Roth**
5ft 7in
(TIMOTHY SIMON SMITH)

Born: May 14, 1961
London, England

Tim's father, Ernie, was a journalist and a member of the British Communist Party. His mother, Anne, was a landscape painter and a teacher. After attending the Strand School, in Tulse Hill, where he began to perfect his skill of imitating accents, Tim studied at the Camberwell College of Art, in South London. During his time there, he turned his attention to acting. In 1982, he made his television debut in 'Made in Britain' – playing the role of a White-Power 'skinhead'. Two years later, Tim made his movie debut, in *The Hit* – which earned him a "London Evening Standard" 'Most Promising Newcomer' Award. By 1990, everybody knew him, and after he played Mr. Orange, in Quentin Tarantino's *Reservoir Dogs,* everbody feared him. There was further work for Tarantino, most notably in *Pulp Fiction.* Tim won a Best Supporting Actor BAFTA and was nominated for a Best Supporting Actor Oscar, for his very mean and nasty Archibald Cunningham, in *Rob Roy*. A man with a tattooed-arm, Tim's married to Nikki Butler, with whom he has two sons – Timothy and Cormac.

The Hit (1984)
The Cook the Thief his Wife
& Her Lover (1989)
Vincent & Theo (1990)
Rosencrantz & Guildenstern
Are Dead (1990)
Reservoir Dogs (1992)
The Perfect Husband (1993)
Pulp Fiction (1994)
Little Odessa (1994)
Captives (1994) Rob Roy (1995)
No Way Home (1996)
Everyone Says I Love You (1996)
Gridlock'd (1997)
Deceiver (1997)
Animals and the Tollkeeper (1998)
The Legend of the
Pianist on the Ocean (1998)
Vatel (2000) Invincible (2001)
The Beautiful Country (2004)
Youth Without Youth (2007)
The Incredible Hulk (2008)

Richard **Roundtree**
6ft 3in
(RICHARD ROUNDTREE)

Born: July 9, 1942
New Rochelle, New York, USA

Richard was born into an extremely poor but hardworking family. His father, John, was a garbage collector, and his mother, Kathryn, worked as a nurse. Following high school, he went to Southern Illinois University on a football scholarship. After that, he worked as a male model for the Ebony Magazine Fashion Fair. As an actor, Richard became a member of the New York Negro Ensemble Company and had early success, in "Man Better Man" and "Mau Mau Room". It was his stage portrayal of the black heavyweight boxing champion, Jack Johnson, in "The Great White Hope" that brought him to the attention of Hollywood. After his debut in the hilarious comedy, *What Do You Say to a Naked Lady?,* Richard made his first appearance, as John Shaft, in *Shaft,* and was nominated for a Golden Globe as Most Promising Newcomer. Although his 1970s movies were mostly of the so-called "blaxploitation" variety, he proved several times that he could play other roles. He was treated for breast cancer in the early 1990s, but in recent years, he's become something of a cult figure, and is working steadily. He has a son named John from his long marriage to his ex-wife Karen, and also has four daughters – three from an earlier marriage.

What Do You Say to a
Naked Lady? (1970)
Shaft (1971)
Shaft's Big Score! (1972)
Charlie One-Eye (1973)
Shaft in Africa (1973)
Earthquake (1974)
Man Friday (1975)
Q: The Winged Serpent (1982)
City Heat (1984) Maniac Cop (1988)
Once Upon a Time...When
We Were Colored (1995)
Se7en (1995)
George of the Jungle (1997)
Shaft (2000) Antitrust (2001)
Brick (2005)
All the Days Before Tomorrow (2007)
Speed Racer (2008)

Mickey **Rourke**
5ft 11in
(PHILLIP ANDRE ROURKE JR.)

Born: **September 16, 1956**
Liberty City, Florida, USA

The son of Philip and Anne Rourke, he moved with them to Florida when he was a young boy. Because of the tough nature of the 'Liberty City' area he was living in, Mickey took up boxing at Miami Boys Club. He won his first bout at the age of twelve, as a bantamweight and kept fighting as an amateur until being concussed during the Golden Gloves tournament. Mickey attended Miami Beach Senior High School. He studied at the Lee Strasberg Institute and began his film career in 1979, with a small role in Steven Spielberg's *1941*. Mickey established himself as a top actor around the time of *Body Heat* and *Diner*. He returned to boxing in 1991, as a professional – earning a million dollars from seven unbeaten fights – three KO's. After retiring, he needed serious work to repair his battered face. In later films he has taken on a whole new career as an interesting, world-weary character. Mickey's been married and divorced twice – both times to actresses. In his recent film, *The Wrestler*, he got himself in shape for an absolutely barn-storming performance. In the great tradition of come-back stories, Mickey won a BAFTA, and then narrowly missed a Best Actor Oscar.

Heaven's Gate (1980)
Body Heat (1981) Diner (1982)
Eureka (1983) Rumble Fish (1983)
The Pope of Greenwich Village (1984)
Year of the Dragon (1985)
Nine$^{1}/_{2}$ Weeks (1986)
Angel Heart (1987) Barfly (1987)
A Prayer for the Dying (1987)
Homeboy (1988) Francesco (1989)
White Sands (1992) Bullet (1996)
The Rainmaker (1997)
Buffalo '66 (1998) Thursday (1998)
Cousin Joey (1999) Shades (1999)
Animal Factory (2000) Spun (2002)
Once Upon a Time
in Mexico (2003)
Man on Fire (2004)
Sin City (2005) Domino (2005)
The Wrestler (2008) Killshot (2008)
The Informers (2009)

Jean-Paul **Rouve**
5ft 8in
(JEAN-PAUL ROUVE)

Born: **January 26, 1967**
Dunkerque, Nord, France

During his schooldays, Jean-Paul loved comedy. He took drama classes at the National Drama Center of Nord-Pas-De-Calaism. He was taught comedy by Isabelle Nanty, at Cours Florent, in Paris, which has produced some of the finest French actors and actresses, including Isabelle Adjani, Daniel Auteil, Sophie Marceau, and Audrey Tautou. Jean-Paul then joined the troupe, 'Robins des Bois' and they were given a spot on Cable TV's 'La Grosse Emission'. Jean-Paul made his first solo TV appearance in the series 'Julie Lescaut'. He eventually progressed to the French Cinema, where he had made his debut, in 1996, in the short comedy, *Le Souffleur*. His first feature was in 1998 – a small part in *Serial Lover*, and a year later, he was higher up the cast list in the drama, *Karnaval* – which was shot in his home town, Dunkerque. In 2003, he earned a César Award as Most Promising New Actor, for *Monsieur Batognole*. Since then he has worked in several top French films, including internationally acclaimed, titles such as *A Very Long Engagement* and *La Vie en Rose*.

Karnaval (1999)
Tanguy (2001)
Astérix & Obélix: Mission
Cléopâtre (2002)
Monsieur Batognole (2002)
Mon Idole (2002)
Moi César,
10 ans $^{1}/_{2}$, 1m39 (2003)
Mais qui a tué
Pamela Rose? (2003)
Podium (2004)
A Very Long Engagement (2004)
Un petit jeu
sans Conséquence (2004)
Je préfère qu'on reste ami (2005)
Bunker paradise (2005)
A Year in My Life (2006)
Nos jours heureux (2006)
La Vie en Rose (2007)
La Jeaune fille et les loups (2008)
Sans arme, ni haine,
ne violence (2008)

Gena **Rowlands**
5ft 6in
(VIRGINIA CATHRYN ROWLANDS)

Born: **June 19, 1930**
Madison, Wisconsin, USA

Gena grew up in Cambria, Wisconsin. Her father, Edwin, was a banker and state legislator, and her mother, Mary, a talented painter, who hailed from Arkansas. When Edwin was given a position in the U.S. Department of Agriculture, in 1939, the family spent nearly three years in Washington, D.C. Gena attended various schools before her father moved to Milwaukee. From 1947 until 1950, she attended the University of Wisconsin. Following her graduation, she went to New York, where she studied acting at the American Academy of Dramatic Arts. In 1952, Gena was an understudy in the original Broadway stage version of "The Seven Year Itch". In 1954, she married John Cassavetes, with whom she had four children and made ten films. For one of them, *Opening Night*, she won a Silver Berlin Bear. She made her TV debut in 1955, in 'Top Secret'. Since her film debut in 1958, Gena has produced many top-class performances and was Oscar nominated as Best Actress – for *A Woman Under the Influence*, and *Gloria*. Apart from her reputation in the industry, Gena is admired by the younger generation – she is Maggie Gyllenhaal's favorite actress.

The High Cost of Loving (1958)
Lonely Are the Brave (1962)
A Child Is Waiting (1963)
Tony Rome (1967) Faces (1968)
Gli Intoccabili (1968)
Minnie and Moskowitz (1971)
A Woman Under the Influence (1974)
Opening Night (1977)
The Brink's Job (1978)
Gloria (1980) Tempest (1982)
Love Streams (1984)
Once Around (1991)
Night on Earth (1991)
Silent Cries (1993)
Unhook the Stars (1996)
The Mighty (1998) Playing by
Heart (1998) The Weekend (1999)
The Notebook (2004)
The Skeleton Key (2005)
Broken English (2007)

Mark **Ruffalo**
5ft 9in
(MARK ALAN RUFFALO)

Born: **November 22, 1967**
Kenosha, Wisconsin, USA

Of French Canadian and Italian ancestry, Mark was one of four children born to Frank Ruffalo Jr., a construction painter, and his wife, Marie Rose, who worked as a hairdresser and stylist. His dad was a convert to the Bahá'í community and combined with the Italian traditions, the children enjoyed a warm and loving family home life. Mark was educated at First Colonial High School, in Virginia Beach, Virginia, and after his family moved to California, he studied at the Stella Adler Conservatory, in Los Angeles. After that, Mark co-founded the Orpheus Theater Company – supplementing his income by working as a bartender. Other work began to trickle in; in 1989, he appeared in an episode of 'CBS Summer Playhouse' and three years later, he co-starred in the movie, *Rough Trade*. His breakthrough came with his performance as Laura Linney's brother in *You Can Count on Me* – for which he won a 'New Generation Award' from the L.A. Film Critics and was named Best Actor at Montréal World Film Festival. Also in 2000, Mark married actress, Sunrise Coigney. They have three children. The eight years that followed have been filled with roles in quality films such as *My Life Without Me, Collateral, Zodiac,* and *The Brothers Bloom*.

A Gift from Heaven (1994)
The Last Big Thing (1996)
Safe Men (1998) A Fish in the
Bathtub (1999) Ride with the Devil (1999)
You Can Count on Me (2000)
The Last Castle (2001)
Windtalkers (2002)
My Life Without Me (2003)
We Don't Live Here Anymore (2004)
Eternal Sunshine of the Spotless
Mind (2004) 13 Going on 30 (2004)
Collateral (2004) Just Like Heaven (2005)
Rumor Has It... (2005)
All the King's Men (2006) Zodiac (2007)
Reservation Road (2007)
Blindness (2008)
The Brothers Bloom (2008)
What Doesn't Kill You (2008)

Charles **Ruggles**
5ft 6in
(CHARLES SHERMAN RUGGLES)

Born: **February 8, 1886**
Los Angeles, California, USA
Died: **December 23, 1970**

In 1904, Charlie began medical studies. Persuaded to act in summer stock, in "Nathan Hale", he caught the bug. His Broadway debut was in "Help Wanted" in 1914, and a year later, he made his film debut, in *Peer Gynt*. He was well established when his mother was shot dead by a bandit at her home. Until the talkies started, Charlie was mainly on stage, but with the coming of sound, his voice was heard for the first time in *Gentleman of the Press*. Charlie was in his early forties by that time and apart from his teaming with Mary Boland, starring roles were difficult to come by. His speciality were sympathetic, and often gently comical characters, in support of big stars like Maurice Chevalier, Cary Grant, Katherine Hepburn and Irene Dunne – one of whose films, *Invitation to Happiness,* was directed by his brother Wesley. Throughout the 1940s, he was in demand. He returned to the stage in 1949, and later, had his own TV show. Charlie made a few films in the 1960s, the best of which was *The Parent Trap*. He was twice married – firstly to the actress, Adele Rowland. He had divorced Marion, his second wife, only months before he died of cancer, at his home in Hollywood.

Charley's Aunt (1930)
The Smiling Lieutenant (1931)
One Hour with You (1932)
Love Me Tonight (1932)
Trouble in Paradise (1932)
If I Had a Million (1932)
Murders in the Zoo (1933)
Terror Aboard (1933)
The Pursuit of Happiness (1934)
Ruggles of Red Gap (1935)
Hearts Divided (1936)
Bringing Up Baby (1938)
Invitation to Happiness (1939)
Our Hearts Were Young
and Gay (1944)
Incendiary Blonde (1945)
A Stolen Life (1946)
The Parent Trap (1961)
Follow Me Boys! (1966)

Barbara **Rush**
5ft 6in
(BARBARA RUSH)

Born: **January 4, 1927**
Denver, Colorado, USA

Barbara was a gorgeous and talented kid. She made her stage debut aged ten, in "Golden Ball", at the Loberto Theater, in Santa Barbara. Throughout her school years, she was eager for the day when she would become a movie star. At the University of California, she won an award for her acting in "Little Foxes" and got a scholarship to study at the Pasadena Playhouse. Barbara was spotted in a production of "Anthony and Cleopatra" and signed by Paramount. Barbara's movie debut was in the rather feeble, *The Goldbergs,* in 1950, but her career began moving, in *The First Legion* – which was good. Her personal life was successful too. She married the handsome young movie actor, Jeffrey Hunter, and their son, Christopher, was born in 1952. She shone in lightweight vehicles and bigger budget films. *Bigger Than Life* and *The Young Lions,* were high profile. In the 1960s, she added her charming presence to a couple of Sinatra films – *Come Blow Your Horn* and *Robin and the 7 Hoods*. She married twice more – firstly to the publicist, Warren Cowan, with whom she had a daughter, Claudia. Since her divorce from Jim Gruzalski, in 1975, she's remained single. Barbara continued working and was seen on television as Ruth Camden, in several episodes of a recent series, '7th Heaven'.

The First Legion (1951)
When Worlds Collide (1951)
Flaming Feathers (1952)
It Came from Outer Space (1953)
Magnificent Obsession (1954)
The Black Shield of Falworth (1954)
Captain Lightfoot (1955)
Bigger Than Life (1956)
Oh, Men! Oh, Women! (1957)
No Down Payment (1957)
The Young Lions (1958)
Harry Black (1958)
The Young Philadelphians (1959)
Strangers When We Meet (1960)
Come Blow Your Horn (1963)
Robin and the 7 Hoods (1964)
Hombre (1967)

Geoffrey Rush
6ft
(GEOFFREY RUSH)

Born: **July 6, 1951**
Toowoomba, Queensland, Australia

Geoff's father, Roy, was an accountant in the Royal Australian Air Force. His mother, Merle, worked in a department store. They divorced when he was five, and he went with his mother to live with her parents. Geoff was educated at Everton Park State High School, where he did very little acting. Having decided on an acting career, he then joined the Queensland Theater Company, in Brisbane. In 1975, he studied mime at the famous Jacques Le Coq School, in Paris. After returning to Australia, he got an Art degree, from the University of Queensland, and then shared an apartment with Mel Gibson when he co-starred with him on the stage, in "Waiting for Godot". His movie debut was in *Hoodwink,* in 1981. Geoff did a lot of work in the theater and played supporting roles in Australian films until 1987 – after which he wasn't seen on the screen for eight years. It was his role in *Shine,* as David Helfgott, that fired his movie career and won him a Best Actor Oscar. He went international with *Les Misérables,* and was Oscar-nominated for *Shakespeare in Love* and *Quills.* Since 1988, Geoff has been married to the Australian actress, Jane Menelaus. They have two children.

Shine (1996)
Children of the Revolution (1996)
Les Misérables (1998)
Elizabeth (1998)
Shakespeare in Love (1998)
Quills (2000) Lantana (2001)
Frida (2002)
Swimming Upstream (2003)
Ned Kelly (2003)
Pirates of the Caribbean:
The Curse of the Black Pearl (2003)
Intolerable Cruelty (2003)
The Life and Death of
Peter Sellers (2004)
Munich (2005)
Candy (2006)
Pirates 2 (2006) Pirates 3 (2007)
Elizabeth:
The Golden Age (2007)
$9.99 (2008)

Jane Russell
5ft 7in
(ERNESTINE JANE GERALDINE RUSSELL)

Born: **June 21, 1921**
Bemidji, Minnesota, USA

Jane was the first of five children and the only daughter of Roy Russell, and his wife Geraldine. They both originated from North Dakota, and there were links to Canada and Germany through her grandparents. Her mother had been an actress and her father was a U.S. Army regular soldier during World War I. A temporary move to relatives in Canada was followed by a more permanent one to Burbank, California, where she went to school. Jane's mother sent her for piano lessons, but at Van Nuys High School, she began to take an interest in acting. After leaving school, she worked as a doctor's receptionist while getting occasional jobs as a photographer's model. Her mother recognized her potential as an actress, and persuaded Jane to study at Max Reinhardt's Theatrical Workshop and with the famous acting coach, Maria Ouspenskaya. Jane was nineteen when she was discovered by Howard Hughes, who promoted her generous bosom and showed it off in 1943, in a dull western, *The Outlaw.* Less dull was her marriage that year to high school sweetheart, Bob Waterfield. The Bob Hope comedy, *The Paleface,* and its sequel, brought Jane international attention. *Macao, Gentlemen Prefer Blondes,* and *The Revolt of Mamie Stover,* are the pick of her movies. Jane adopted three children with her first husband, and was married three times. Jane has long been fond of jazz and was a great fan and friend of the late Anita O'Day.

Young Widow (1946)
The Paleface (1948)
His Kind of Woman (1951)
The Las Vegas Story (1952)
Macao (1952)
Son of Paleface (1952)
Gentlemen Prefer
Blondes (1953) Foxfire (1955)
The Tall Men (1955)
Gentlemen Marry Brunettes (1955)
The Revolt of Mamie
Stover (1956) Waco (1966)
Darker Than Amber (1970)

Keri Russell
5ft 4in
(KERI LYNN RUSSELL)

Born: **March 23, 1976**
Fountain Valley, California, USA

Keri is the daughter of David Russell, a former executive with the Nissan Motors Company, and his wife Stephanie. Due to her father's work, Keri, her older brother, Todd, and her younger sister, Julie, moved home a lot when they were small – living and going to school in Texas, Arizona, and Colorado – where she attended the Highlands Ranch High School. Keri began her television career on 'The Mickey Mouse Club' – in 1991 – and with castmates, she recorded the album, "MMC". After she decided to pursue an acting career, she packed her bags and moved to Los Angeles – making her movie debut in the popular comedy, *Honey I Blew Up the Kid.* The next five years were spent acting on TV shows, before her next film appearance, in *Eight Days a Week.* In 1999, she won a Golden Globe for Best Performance by an Actress in a TV series, for 'Felicity', which ran until 2002, and led to more film work. In 2006, she was chosen by CoverGirl Cosmetics to be their new spokesman. She was also cast in one of her best roles, in *Waitress* – playing a pregnant woman. She married Shane Deary, on Valentine's Day, 2007, and she was soon actually pregnant. The couple have a little boy named River Russell Deary, and have recently moved into a brownstone house in Brooklyn. Keri is now back at work and is in three films scheduled for release in 2009 – one of which, *Wonder Woman,* is an animated movie, for which she provides the voice of the title character.

Honey I Blew Up the Kid (1992)
Eight Days a Week (1997)
Dead Man's Curve (1998)
Mad About Mambo (2000)
We Were Soldiers (2002)
The Upside of Anger (2005)
Mission Impossible III (2006)
Rohtenburg (2006)
Waitress (2007)
The Girl in the Park (2007)
August Rush (2007)
Bedtime Stories (2008)

Kurt **Russell**
5ft 10in
(KURT VOGEL RUSSELL)

Born: **March 17, 1951**
Springfield, Massachusetts, USA

Kurt's father, Bing Russell, was "Deputy Dan Foster", in the TV series, 'Bonanza'. His mother, Louise, was a dancer. Kurt first appeared on the big screen, with an uncredited part in the Elvis Presley film, *It Happened at the World's Fair*, in 1963. That same year, he had a small role in the television series, 'Sam Benedict'. He worked for Disney during his teens and for a while, until his career was cut short by injury, played minor league baseball. In 1979, he got good notices for playing Elvis Presley in the ABC TV-movie, 'Elvis'. That year, he married Season Hubley. They had a son, but were divorced in 1984. Kurt made his breakthrough into the world of adult movies, as anti-hero Snake Plissken, in *Escape from New York*. He followed up with prominent roles in big movies like *Silkwood*, *Big Trouble in Little China*, *Backdraft*, *Tombstone*, *Stargate*, *Vanilla Sky*, *Grindhouse* and *Death Proof*. Since 1983, he has been Goldie Hawn's partner. Their son Wyatt, is an actor. When Goldie's daughter, Kate Hudson, married rock star, Chris Robinson, Kurt assumed fatherly responsibilities and gave her away. In 2007, the year of her divorce, Kate cast Kurt in her short film, *Cutlass,* which she wrote and directed.

Follow Me, Boys! (1966)
Fools' Parade (1971) Now You See Him, Now You Don't (1972)
Used Cars (1980)
Escape from New York (1981)
The Thing (1982) Silkwood (1983)
The Mean Season (1985)
Big Trouble in Little China (1986)
Overboard (1987)
Tequila Sunrise (1988)
Winter People (1989)
Tango & Cash (1989) Backdraft (1991)
Unlawful Entry (1992)
Tombstone (1993) Stargate (1994)
Executive Decision (1996)
Breakdown (1997) Vanilla Sky (2001)
Dark Blue (2002) Miracle (2004)
Sky High (2005) Dreamer (2005)
Grindhouse (2007) Deathproof (2007)

Rosalind **Russell**
5ft 8in
(ROSALIND RUSSELL)

Born: **June 4, 1907**
Waterbury, Connecticut, USA
Died: **November 28, 1976**

Roz was the middle one of seven children, born to James and Clara Russell, who were Irish Catholics. Roz attended a Catholic school before deciding to pursue an acting career. She studied at the American Academy of Dramatic Arts, in New York. While working as a department store fashion model, she made her stage debut in 1926, in a revue, the "Garrick Gaieties". She did stock, before her Broadway debut, in 1932, in "Talent". She was on MGM's books for a while until her L.A. hit, "No More Ladies" resulted in her movie debut, in *Evelyn Prentice*. By the late 1930s, she was playing dramatic parts or screwball comedy with equal skill. She was Oscar-nominated for *My Sister Eileen*, *Sister Kenny*, *Auntie Mame,* and *Mourning Becomes Elektra*. Roz was married to Danish-born producer, Frederick Brisson – her only husband – from 1941 until she died from breast cancer, at their home in Beverly Hills.

Evelyn Prentice (1934)
Reckless (1935) China Seas (1935)
Trouble for Two (1936)
Craig's Wife (1936)
Night Must Fall (1937)
Four's a Crowd (1938)
The Citadel (1938)
The Women (1939)
His Girl Friday (1940)
Hired Wife (1940)
This Thing Called Love (1940)
They Met in Bombay (1941)
The Feminine Touch (1941)
Take a Letter, Darling (1942)
My Sister Eileen (1942)
Roughly Speaking (1945)
Sister Kenny (1946)
The Guilt of Janet Ames (1947)
Mourning Becomes Elektra (1947)
The Velvet Touch (1948)
Tell It to the Judge (1949)
A Woman of Distinction (1950)
Picnic (1955)
Auntie Mame (1958)
Gypsy (1962)

Theresa **Russell**
5ft 6½in
(THERESA PAUP)

Born: **March 20, 1957**
San Diego, California, USA

Theresa's sparkling beauty was first noticed by a photographer when she was twelve. She then worked as a model for childrens' wear, and when she attended Burbank High School, she showed natural talent for acting. When she was sixteen, she moved to New York, where she studied for two years at the Lee Strasberg Institute. In 1976, Theresa made her film debut, in Elia Kazan's *The Last Tycoon*. In her next film role, she co-starred with Dustin Hoffman in *Straight Time*. Theresa met her future husband, the British film director, Nicolas Roeg, when she worked with him and Art Garfunkel in *Bad Timing*. The pair married in 1982, had two sons, made some good movies together, but later divorced. In 1986, Theresa won the "Star of Tomorrow" Award given by the National Association of Theater Owners. In 1988, she was named Best Actress for *Track 29*. Considering that promise, her career has been uneven. She's kept busy and apart from a very disappointing period in the 1990s, her movie work has been rarely less than interesting. When she gets it right, it is challenging and memorable, like in *Impulse*, *Kafka*, and *The Believer*. In the past two years, her career seems to have got a second-wind with a featured role in *Spider-Man 3*, followed by two good films – including *Jolene*.

Straight Time (1978)
Bad Timing (1980)
Eureka (1984)
The Razor's Edge (1984)
Insignificance (1985)
Aria (1987)
Track 29 (1988)
Impulse (1990)
Kafka (1991)
Wild Things (1998)
The Believer (2001)
Passionada (2002)
Now and Forever (2002)
Save It for Later (2003)
Spider-Man 3 (2007)
Chinaman's Chance (2008)
Jolene (2008)

Rene **Russo**
5ft 8in
(RENE MARIE RUSSO)

Born: **February 17, 1954**
Burbank, California, USA

Rene had a tough early life. Her father, Nino, a motor mechanic and would-be sculptor, from a Sicilian background, deserted the family when she was two. From then on, Rene and her sister Toni, were raised by their mother, Shirley. When she was in junior high school, she was nicknamed "Jolly Green Giant" because of her height. She then attended Burroughs High School in Burbank, where one of her classmates was the future actor/director, Ron Howard. Rene dropped out of school in the tenth grade so she could help her family with an income. In 1972, when she was at a Rolling Stones concert, she was spotted by John Crosby, a scout, who helped her get on the books of the Ford Modeling Agency. Until the early 1980s, her smiling face regularly appeared on the covers of magazines like "Vogue". Rene then took acting lessons and began to get work in regional theaters in the L.A. area. In 1987 she made her TV debut, with a supporting role in 'Sable' and two years later, co-starred with Tom Berenger, in her first movie, *Major League*. Her big break was as detective, Lorna Cole, in the *Lethal Weapon* series. She's been married to Dan Gilroy since 1992. They have a daughter named Rose. One of Rene's last film roles was in the sporting drama, *Two for the Money,* co-starring Al Pacino and Matthew McConaughey. It was followed by the disappointing family comedy, *Yours, Mine and Ours.* Her many fans hope it won't be her last.

Major League (1989)
Mr. Destiny (1990)
Lethal Weapon 3 (1992)
In the Line of Fire (1993)
Outbreak (1995)
Get Shorty (1995)
Tin Cup (1996)
Ransom (1996)
Lethal Weapon 4 (1998)
The Thomas Crown Affair (1999)
Showtime (2002)
Big Trouble (2002)
Two for the Money (2005)

Ann **Rutherford**
5ft 6in
(THERESA ANN RUTHERFORD)

Born: **November 2, 1920**
Vancouver, British Columbia, Canada

Ann's father, the tenor, John Rutherford, was a former Metropolitan Opera singer. Her mother, Lillian Mansfield, had once aspired to be an actress. The family moved to California shortly after Ann was born and she made her stage debut there, at the age of five, in "Mrs. Wiggs of the Cabbage Patch". Ann appeared in radio shows and plays for nine years, before making her first film, *Carnival of Paris,* in 1934. When she was seventeen, she signed a contract with MGM, who made her famous as Polly Benedict, in the popular *Andy Hardy* series. She played other roles too – most memorably in the classics *A Christmas Carol,* and *Gone with the Wind.* Ann also starred in Glenn Miller's farewell film, *Orchestra Wives.* At the end of her movie career, she was featured in two major hits – *The Secret Life of Walter Mitty,* and *Adventures of Don Juan.* She then worked mainly on TV before retiring in 1975. Ann had two children with her first husband, David May. From 1953, she was married to producer, William Dozier. They were together until his death, in 1991.

You're Only Young Once (1937)
Of Human Hearts (1938)
Judge Hardy's Children (1938)
Love Finds Andy Hardy (1938)
Out West with
the Hardys (1938)
Dramatic School (1938)
A Christmas Carol (1938)
These Glamour Girls (1939)
Dancing Co-Ed (1939)
Gone with the Wind (1939)
Judge Hardy and Son (1939)
The Ghost Comes Home (1940)
Pride and Prejudice (1940)
Whistling in the Dark (1941)
Badlands of Dakota (1941)
Orchestra Wives (1942)
Whistling in Dixie (1942)
Bedside Manner (1945)
Murder in the
Music Hall (1946)
The Secret Life of Walter Mitty (1947)
Adventures of Don Juan (1948)

Dame Margaret **Rutherford**
5ft 3½in
(MARGARET RUTHERFORD)

Born: **May 11, 1892**
Balham, London, England
Died: **May 22, 1972**

Margaret was an only child. Her father, William Rutherford, suffered from serious mental illness. In 1883, he battered his father to death. Margaret wasn't pretty, and had resigned herself to being an 'old maid'. She loved the theater, but it was only after being talked into playing character roles in some amateur stage productions, that the idea grabbed her seriously. She became a student at the Old Vic before making her stage debut, at the age of thirty-three. Eight years later, she made her debut, in London's West End. Her film debut, was in 1936, in *Dusty Ermine.* For a few years, it was difficult to see how she could become such a beloved personality in British films. In 1941, she played Madame Arcati, on the London stage, in Noel Coward's "Blithe Spirit". When the screen version was made, hers was the first name to be penciled in on the cast list. Margaret won a Best Supporting Actress Oscar for *The V.I.P.s.* Around that time, she was perfect as Agatha Christie's Miss Marple, in three movies. She was married to the actor, Stringer Davis, from 1945, until her death from pneumonia, at their lovely country home, in Chalfont St. Peter, Buckinghamshire.

The Demi-Paradise (1943)
Blithe Spirit (1945)
Miranda (1948)
Passport to Pimlico (1949)
The Happiest Days of Your Life (1950)
The Magic Box (1951)
The Importance of
Being Earnest (1952)
Trouble in Store (1953)
The Runaway Bus (1954)
The Smallest Show on Earth (1957)
I'm All Right Jack (1959)
Murder She Said (1961)
On the Double (1961)
The Mouse on the Moon(1963)
Murder at the Gallop (1963)
The V.I.P.s (1963)
Murder Most Foul (1964)
Murder Ahoy (1964)

Meg **Ryan**
5ft 8in
(MARGARET MARY EMILY ANNE HYRA)

Born: **November 19, 1961**
Fairfield, Connecticut, USA

Meg was the daughter of Harry Hyra, a math teacher. Her mother, Susan Ryan, who had been an actress, was at one time a teacher of English, and later became a casting director for a brief period. Meg has two sisters and one brother, Andrew, who is a musician with the band, "Billy Pilgrim". She was raised as a Roman Catholic and attended the school her mother taught at – Saint Pius X, in Fairfield. Meg was later a graduate from the local Bethel High School. When she was eighteen, she acted in a commercial for a deodorant. Meg went to the University of Connecticut, to study Journalism, but while she was at New York University, she began getting plenty of work in TV commercials. She dropped out shortly before graduating and concentrated on an acting career, after making her movie debut, in *Rich and Famous.* She had a number of small roles before *Top Gun* accelerated her movie career. Two years later, she co-starred with Dennis Quaid, in the action film *Innerspace,* and in 1991, became his wife for ten years. They have a son named Jack. Meg was already a star because of *When Harry Met Sally,* and became even bigger, after *Sleepless in Seattle.* She has remained a big favorite and is still acting.

Top Gun (1986) **Promised Land** (1987)
Innerspace (1987) **D.O.A.** (1988)
The Presidio (1988)
When Harry Met Sally (1989)
The Doors (1991)
Prelude to a Kiss (1992)
Sleepless in Seattle (1993)
Flesh and Bone (1993)
When a Man Loves a Woman (1994)
I.Q. (1994) **French Kiss** (1995)
Restoration (1995)
Courage Under Fire (1996)
Addicted to Love (1997)
City of Angels (1998)
You've Got Mail (1998)
Proof of Life (2000)
Kate and Leopold (2001)
In the Land of Women (2007)
The Deal (2008)

Robert **Ryan**
6ft 4in
(ROBERT BUSHNELL RYAN)

Born: **November 11, 1909**
Chicago, Illinois, USA
Died: **July 11, 1973**

Bob was the only child born to Tim Ryan and his wife, Mabel. He graduated from Dartmouth College, in Hanover, New Hampshire, in 1932, having excelled as a sportsman – he was heavyweight boxing champion in all four years he attended. Following graduation Bob's first few jobs reflected the rather limited nature of his academic ability – he worked as a stoker on a ship, a ranch hand, and as a WPA worker. He then studied acting with Max Reinhardt, and in 1939, married a girl named Jessica, who would be his wife until her death, in 1972. He began his movie career with a bit part in the 1940 Bob Hope film, *The Ghost Breakers.* After serving in the United States Marines in World War II, as a drill instructor, Bob restarted his film career with his dynamic portrayal of an anti-Semitic soldier, in *Crossfire* – and was nominated for a Best Supporting Actor Oscar. Bob became a big star. His outstanding films include *The Set-Up, Bad Day at Black Rock, House of Bamboo, Odds Against Tomorrow, The Dirty Dozen, The Wild Bunch,* and his last – *The Iceman Cometh.* He worked until his death in New York, from lung cancer.

The Woman on the Beach (1947)
Crossfire (1947) **Berlin Express** (1948)
The Boy with Green Hair (1948) **Act of Violence** (1948) **Caught** (1949) **The Set-Up** (1949) **The Secret Fury** (1950)
Born to Be Bad (1950) **Flying Leathernecks** (1951) **The Racket** (1951)
On Dangerous Ground (1952)
Clash By Night (1952)
The Naked Spur (1953) **Inferno** (1953)
About Mrs. Leslie (1954)
Bad Day at Black Rock (1955)
House of Bamboo (1955) **The Proud Ones** (1956) **Men at War** (1957)
Odds Against Tomorrow (1959)
The Dirty Dozen (1967)
The Wild Bunch (1969)
Lawman (1971) **The Outfit** (1973)
Executive Action (1973)
The Iceman Cometh (1973)

Winona **Ryder**
5ft 4in
(WINONA LAURA HOROWITZ)

Born: **October 29, 1971**
Olmsted County, Minnesota, USA

Noni's father, Michael Horowitz, is an author and publisher. His parents were Jewish immigrants from Russia. Her mother, Cynthia, is also an author. Noni, who has a younger brother called Uri, was named after the nearby city of Winona. When she was seven, the family moved to a commune near Elk, in California – there was no electricity, so a lot of the daylight hours were spent reading. Three years later, they went to live in Petaluma, where she attended Kenilworth Middle School, and was the subject of bullying – because of her appearance – described as like a scrawny, effeminate boy. When she saw Sara Miles acting in *Ryan's Daughter,* she made up her mind to become an actress. After home schooling, she went to the American Conservatory, in San Francisco. Acting lessons restored her confidence and she changed her name to Ryder. Noni made her film debut, in 1986, in *Lucas.* Noni graduated from Petaluma High School in 1987, and within two years, was a star in the making. She was nominated for a Best Supporting Actress Oscar, for *The Age of Innocence* and a Best Actress Oscar, for *Little Women.* In 1996, her face had been used by Armani to promote his Manhattan stores. Somewhat bizarrely, Noni did community service in 2002, after she was convicted of shoplifting, at Saks Fifth Avenue store, in Beverly Hills. But this beautiful, talented actress has bounced back and is still capable of great things.

Lucas (1986) **Square Dance** (1987)
Beetlejuice (1988) **Heathers** (1989)
Great Balls of Fire (1989) **Edward Scissorhands** (1990) **Mermaids** (1990)
Night on Earth (1991) **Dracula** (1992)
The Age of Innocence (1993)
The House of the Spirits (1993)
Reality Bites (1994)
Little Women (1994)
The Crucible (1996)
Alien Resurrection (1997)
Girl, Interrupted (1999)
A Scanner Darkly (2006)
The Last Word (2008)

S

Ludivine **Sagnier**
5ft 3in
(LUDIVINE SAGNIER)

Born: July 3, 1979
La Celle-Saint-Cloud, Yvelines, France

Ludivine studied acting at Hieronimus Drama School, in Sèvres, in her teens. She had made her film debut at the early age of ten, in Alain Resnais' *Les Maris, les femmes, les amants.* The following year, she acted with Gérard Depardieu, in *Cyrano de Bergerac.* She continued to learn her profession at the Conservatoire d'Art Dramatique de Versailles. The promise she showed won her firsts in both the classic and modern theater. After some television roles of little consequence, Ludivine made her breakthrough as a grown-up actress with director François Ozon's *Water Drops on Burning Rocks,* and *8 femmes* – for which she shared a Silver Berlin Bear with six of France's top actresses. A year after that, Ozon's English-language film, *Swimming Pool,* thrust them both into the international spotlight. A Silver Hugo at the Chicago International Film Festival for *La Petite Lili,* confirmed her status as an actress. Her daughter, Bonnie, whose father is actor Nicolas Duvauchelle, was born in 2005. 2007 was a very strong year for Ludivine, with four excellent film offerings. Her latest movie, *Mesrine: Public Enemy No. 1* – is a powerful two-part crime biopic, about the notorious French gangster – Jacques Mesrine. Ludivine co-stars with Vincent Cassel and Mathieu Amalric.

Les Enfants du siècle (1999)
Water Drops on
Burning Rocks (2000)
My Wife is an Actress (2001)
8 femmes (2002)
Swimming Pool (2003)
La Petite Lili (2003)
Peter Pan (2003)
Paris, je t'aime (2006)
French California (2006)
Molière (2007)
Les Chansons d'amour (2007)
La Fille coupée en deux (2007)
Un secret (2007)
L'Instinct de mort (2008)
Mesrine: Public
Enemy No. 1 (2008)

Eva Marie **Saint**
5ft 4in
(EVA MARIE SAINT)

Born: July 4, 1924
Newark, New Jersey, USA

When Eva was at Bethlehem Central High School, in Delmar, New York, her ambition was to become a teacher, but when she studied at Bowling Green State University in Ohio, she had her first seductive taste of acting. It was enough to change her direction in life and during a summer vacation, she got a job at the NBC Studios in New York. After college, she worked in radio, and in 1946, made her television debut, in a production of 'A Christmas Carol' by Charles Dickens. In 1951, she married the television director, Jeffrey Hayden. Eva had two children with him and they are still together today. In 1953, after winning the Drama Critics Award for her acting in "The Trip to Bountiful", Eva was head-hunted by Hollywood. Her film debut was in one of the most admired movies of all time - *On the Waterfront* – for which she won an Oscar as Best Supporting Actress, in a role that was more than that. She was memorable in other films, including Alfred Hitchcock's *North by Northwest, The Russians Are Coming the Russians Are Coming* and *Grand Prix.* Eva continued to appear in movies, in supporting roles, up until three years ago, when she was last seen as Martha Kent, the adoptive mother of Clark, in *Superman Returns.*

On the Waterfront (1954)
That Certain Feeling (1956)
A Hatful of Rain (1957)
Raintree County (1957)
North by Northwest (1959)
Exodus (1960)
All Fall Down (1962)
36 Hours (1965)
The Sandpiper (1965)
The Russians Are Coming the
Russians Are Coming (1966)
Grand Prix (1967)
The Stalking Moon (1968)
Loving (1970)
Nothing in Common (1986)
Mariette in Ectstasy (1996)
Because of
Winn-Dixie (2005)
Superman Returns (2006)

George **Sanders**
6ft 1in
(GEORGE SANDERS)

Born: **July 3, 1906**
St. Petersburg, Russia
Died: **April 25, 1972**

George's English parents fled back to England with their two children at the start of the Russian Revolution. Like his older brother, Tom, (later the movie actor, Tom Conway) George was educated at the private Brighton College. After he left school, George went to work in a London advertising agency, where he met the young Greer Garson. She encouraged him to think about an acting career. He had the looks and the charm, so after a little coaching, he began to get small roles on the stage – starting with "Ballyhoo". While in Noel Coward's "Conversation Piece", in 1934, he made his first film appearance, in a Gracie Fields comedy, *Love, Life and Laughter.* In 1936, he was in Hollywood for *Lloyd's of London.* After that, George was the archetypal English cad in dozens of movies, including *Rebecca* and *Foreign Correspondent,* for Hitchcock. He won a Best Supporting Actor Oscar, for *All About Eve.* Despite success and four beautiful wives – of whom two were actresses, Zsa Zsa Gabor and Benita Hume – George was in Barcelona when he took his own life – because, as he said – he was bored!

Confessions of a Nazi Spy (1939)
Allegheny Uprising (1939)
The House of the Seven Gables (1940)
Rebecca (1940)
Foreign Correspondent (1940)
The Son of Monte Cristo (1940)
Man Hunt (1941) The Black
Swan (1942) This Land Is Mine (1943)
Appointment in Berlin (1943)
The Lodger (1944) Hangover
Square (1945) The Picture of
Dorian Gray (1945) The Strange Affair
of Uncle Harry (1945) The Private
Affairs of Bel Ami (1947) The Ghost and
Mrs. Muir (1947) Lured (1947)
Forever Amber (1947) The Fan (1949)
All About Eve (1950) Ivanhoe (1952)
Call Me Madam (1953)
Village of the Damned (1960)
The Quiller Memorandum (1966)
Warning Shot (1967)

Adam **Sandler**
5ft 10in
(ADAM RICHARD SANDLER)

Born: **September 9, 1966**
Brooklyn, New York City, New York, USA

Adam's father, Stanley Sandler, was an electrical engineer. His mother, Judy, was a teacher in a nursery school. They moved to Manchester, New Hampshire, when he was five and he began his schooling. At Manchester Central High School, Adam was a natural comic who had his class-mates in stitches. He was only seventeen when he went on stage at a Boston comedy club, and wowed the audience with his genius. When he was at New York University (from where he graduated in 1991 with a BA in Fine Arts) he would spend much of his free time performing in clubs. In his freshman year, Adam began appearing as Smitty, on 'The Cosby Show'. He made what looked like a disastrous start to his movie career in 1989, in *Going Overboard*. He did tons of TV work, but stuttered on the film front until, with *Airheads*, he got the recipe right. He was nominated for an American Comedy Award for *The Wedding Singer*, and for a Golden Globe for *Punch-Drunk Love*. Happy Madison Productions – named after two of his successes, is behind most of his films. In 2003, Adam married Jackie Titone. They now have a little daughter named Sadie - another is due. Two of his comedy discs have been certified "Gold".

Airheads (1994)
Billy Madison (1995)
Happy Gilmore (1996)
Bullet Proof (1996)
The Wedding Singer (1998)
The Waterboy (1998)
Big Daddy (1999)
Punch-Drunk Love (2002)
Mr. Deeds (2002)
Anger Management (2003)
50 First Dates (2004)
Spanglish (2004)
The Longest Yard (2005)
Click (2006)
Reign Over Me (2007)
I Now Pronounce You
Chuck & Larry (2007)
You Don't Mess with the Zohan (2008)
Bedtime Stories (2008)

Stefania **Sandrelli**
5ft 4in
(STEFANIA SANDRELLI)

Born: **June 5, 1946**
Viareggio, Tuscany, Italy

When she was fifteen, Stefania won a local beauty contest. She had a series of glamorous photographs taken on the beach at Viareggio, which were seen by the film director, Luciano Salce. He chose her to make her debut, in *The Fascist*, starring Ugo Tognazzi. She impressed enough to be cast in the classic comedy, *Divorce Italian Style*, which gave her a chance to work with Marcello Mastroianni. Stefania began a relationship with the musician, Gino Paoli, and in 1964, she gave birth to their daughter, Amanda. Stefania's career continued to flourish – allowing her to work with directors like Ettore Scola and Bernardo Bertolucci, and many great stars – including Vittorio Gassman, Catherine Deneuve, Gerard Depardieu and Simone Signoret. My own favorite Stefania Sandrelli films are: *I Knew Her Well, C'eravamo tanto amati, The Conformist,* and *The Family*. In 2005, She was presented with a Career Golden Lion at the Venice Film Festival. Her son, Vito and her actress daughter, Amanda, have given Stefania four grandchildren.

The Fascist (1961)
Divorce Italian Style (1961)
L'Aîné des Ferchaux (1963)
A Matter of Honor (1964)
I Knew Her Well (1965)
The Conformist (1970)
Delitto d'amore (1974)
C'eravamo tanto amati (1974)
Police Python 357 (1976)
Traffic Jam (1979)
La Chiave (1983)
Secret Secrets (1985)
The Family (1987)
The Little Devil (1988)
Stradivari (1989)
Lo zio indegno (1989)
Il male oscuro (1990)
Jamón, jamón (1992)
Stealing Beauty (1996)
La Cena (1998)
Waiting for the Messiah (2000)
One Last Kiss (2001)
The Perfect Day (2008)

Julian **Sands**
5ft 11in
(JULIAN SANDS)

Born: **January 4, 1958**
Otley, Yorkshire, England

He was one of five children born to Henry and Sarah Sands. At the age of seven Julian felt inspired to become an actor after seeing Laurence Olivier in the movie version of Richard III, on television. He later attended Lord Wandsworth College, a boarding school near Hook, Hampshire, where he first began acting. From then on, he concentrated on the tools of his trade at the Central School of Speech and Drama, in London. While he was there, he met his first wife, Sarah Jane Morris. In 1982, he made his film debut with a small role in *Privates on Parade*. Two years later, following some television work, Julian was fourth-billed in the powerful war drama, *The Killing Fields*. He had a romantic role in James Ivory's *A Room with a View,* but soon established himself as a sinister-looking guy in horror movies – probably scariest of all, in *Warlock*. In 1986, Julian abandoned his wife Sarah and their six-month-old son. Since 1990, he has been married to the Guinness heiress, Evgenia Citkowitz, who was first introduced to him by John Malkovich. Julian has done most of his recent work in the USA. It includes the role of Hector Matrick, in five episodes of the television-series, 'Lipstick Jungle'. He has several movies in production, one of which, *Cat City,* is to be released soon.

The Killing Fields (1984)
The Doctor and the Devils (1985)
A Room with a View (1985)
Wherever You Are (1988)
Warlock (1989)
Arachnophobia (1990)
Il sole anche do notte (1990)
Cattiva (1991)
Impromptu (1991)
Naked Lunch (1991)
The Browning Version (1994)
Leaving Las Vegas (1995)
Mercy (2000) Vatel (2000)
The Scoundrel's Wife (2002)
Her Name Is Carla (2005)
The Trial (2006)
Ocean's Thirteen (2007)
Blood and Bone (2009)

Chris **Sarandon**
6ft 1in
(CHRISTOPHER SARANDON)

Born: **July 24, 1942**
Beckley, West Virginia, USA

Chris was the son of Greek immigrant restaurateurs – Christopher and Mary Sarandon. He grew up with music as an important part of his life. While still at high school, he played drums in a band known as "The Teen Tones" – which toured with Gene Vincent and Bobby Darin. After he graduated from Woodrow Wilson High School, in Beckley, Chris attended West Virginia University. He studied Acting in Washington DC, at the Catholic University of America's Department of Drama. While there, he met his first wife, Susan Tomalin, later more famous than he was – as Susan Sarandon. It was Chris who helped get Susan her first break, when he took her to an audition. After working at Theater West Virginia, Chris headed for New York City, where he landed a role in the soap opera, 'The Guiding Light'. Following a couple of years acting on television, he made his film debut, in *Dog Day Afternoon.* He was nominated for a Best Supporting Actor Oscar and after that, he had twenty years of good employment – making several good movies – and becoming popular with teenage audiences – when he starred as a sexy vampire, in *Fright Night.* His TV work has been prolific. He has played Christ in a TV movie, and a couple of doctors, in 'Chicago Hope' and 'Felicity'. Following his divorce from Susan, Chris married twice more. He's been with his current wife, Joanna Gleason, since 1994.

Dog Day Afternoon (1975)
The Sentinel (1977)
The Osterman
Weekend (1983)
Fright Night (1985)
The Princess Bride (1987)
Child's Play (1988)
The Resurrected (1992)
Just Cause (1995)
The Vampyre Wars (1996)
Edie & Pen (1996)
Little Men (1997)
Loggerheads (2005)
My Sassy Girl (2008)
Multiple Sarcasms (2008)

Susan **Sarandon**
5ft 7in
(SUSAN ABIGAIL TOMALIN)

Born: **October 4, 1946**
New York City, New York, USA

Susan's father was Phillip Tomalin, an advertising executive and television producer, and his wife, Lenora. Her dad had been a nightclub singer during the Big Band era. Susan was the eldest of nine children born to the couple, and is of English, Welsh and Sicilian ancestry. She was raised as a Roman Catholic and after graduating from Edison High School in 1964, she worked with drama coach, Father Gilbert Hartke, at the Catholic University of America – she came away with a BA in Drama. In 1969, after accompanying husband Chris to a casting for the movie, *Joe,* she was given her film debut. Susan was kept busy until her breakthrough – in *The Rocky Horror Picture Show.* A Best Actress Oscar for *Dead Man Walking* after four previous nominations was scant reward for her consistent efforts. Susan's partner since 1988, has been actor Tim Robbins. They have two sons – Jack and Miles. Susan is currently a goodwill ambassador for UNICEF. She can be seen this year in a new movie, *The Greatest* – co-starring Pierce Brosnan.

Joe (1970) **The Front Page** (1974)
The Great Waldo Pepper (1975)
The Rocky Horror Picture Show (1975)
Pretty Baby (1978) **Atlantic City** (1980)
Tempest (1982) **The Hunger** (1983)
The Witches of Eastwick (1987)
Bull Durham (1988)
White Palace (1990)
Thelma & Louise (1991)
Light Sleeper (1992)
Lorenzo's Oil (1992)
The Client (1994) **Little Women** (1994)
Safe Passage (1994)
Dead Man Walking (1995)
Twilight (1998) **Stepmom** (1998)
Cradle Will Rock (1999)
Igby Goes Down (2002)
Noel (2002) **Shall We Dance** (2004)
Romance & Cigarettes (2005)
Enchanted (2007)
Speed Racer (2008)
Middle of Nowhere (2008)
The Greatest (2009)

Michael **Sarrazin**
6ft 2in
(JACQUES MICHEL ANDRE SARRAZIN)

Born: **May 22, 1940**
Québec City, Québec, Canada

The son of an attorney, Michael went to several schools before he became interested in acting at Loyola Junior College, in Montreal – appearing in a production of "The Winslow Boy" – and then deciding to make it his career. He attended the Canadian Drama Studio and became a professional actor at seventeen, in several historical documentaries for the NFBC. He worked at a Toronto Theater and was seen on Canadian television, and in two Canadian short films, *Selkirk of Red River* and *You're No Good.* In 1965, he was given a contract by Universal and played some roles in their TV productions while studying at the Actors Studio in New York. Two years later, he moved to Hollywood. He made his American film debut in the Bobby Darin western, *Gunfight at Abilene.* He worked with Jacqueline Bisset in *The Sweet Ride,* in 1968 – it wasn't just the start of a long and beautiful relationship, he was nominated for a Golden Globe as Most Promising Newcomer. Following a twenty year career, Michael's film roles are now fairly rare events and those he's been in during the past ten years have been of poor quality – like *FeardotCom.*

Gunfight in Abilene (1967)
The Flim Flam Man (1967)
Journey to Shiloh (1968)
Eye of the Cat (1969)
They Shoot Horses, Don't They? (1969)
Sometimes a Great Notion (1971)
The Pursuit of Happiness (1971)
Believe in Me (1971)
The Groundstar Conspiracy (1972)
The Life and Times of
Judge Roy Bean (1972)
Harry in Your Pocket (1973)
For Pete's Sake (1974)
The Reincarnation of
Peter Proud (1975)
The Gumball Rally (1976)
Caravans (1978)
Fighting Back (1982)
Viadukt (1983)
Joshua Then and Now (1985)
Captive Hearts (1987)

Peter **Sarsgaard**
6ft
(JOHN PETER SARSGAARD)

Born: **March 7, 1971**
Belleville, Illinois, USA

Pete first saw the light of day at Scott Airforce Base, in Illinois, where his father was an engineer. When he was ten, he lived in St. Louis, next door to a zoo and collected money for "Save the Elephant". He was raised as a Roman Catholic, and while attending Fairfield Prep – a Jesuit boys' school in Connecticut, he served as an altar boy. He took dancing lessons in his youth, then attended the liberal arts, Bard College. He gave up becoming a football player after suffering concussion more than once. By the age of twenty, he was a student at Washington University in St. Louis, Missouri, and it was there that he first discovered the joy of acting. Although he graduated with a degree in History, Pete had his mind set on something dramatic, so he went to study at the Tony Schreiber Studio in New York. In 1995, he had a role in an episode of TV's 'Law & Order'. Later that same year he made his movie debut when landing another small part, in the outstanding *Dead Man Walking*. Since then, Pete has appeared in over two dozen films – most of them are well above average. He and his partner, Maggie Gyllenhaal, are proud parents of a daughter named Ramona.

Dead Man Walking (1995)
The Man in the Iron Mask (1998)
Desert Blue (1998)
Boys Don't Cry (1999)
The Center of the World (2001)
Empire (2002)
The Salton Sea (2002)
K-19: The Widowmaker (2002)
Unconditional Love (2002)
Shattered Glass (2003)
Garden State (2004)
Kinsey (2004)
The Dying Gaul (2005)
The Skeleton Key (2005)
Flightplan (2005)
Jarhead (2005)
Year of the Dog (2007)
Rendition (2007)
Elegy (2008)
An Education (2009)

John **Savage**
5ft 9½in
(JOHN SMEALLIE YOUNGS)

Born: **August 25, 1949**
Long Island, New York, USA

As a youngster, John appeared in plays produced by the local Children's Theater Group, in Manhattan. After leaving school, he studied at the American Academy of Dramatic Arts, in New York City. He first made his name on the stage – being especially praised for his work in "One Flew Over The Cuckoo's Nest" – for which he won a Drama Circle Award. He had significant roles in other shows, including "Sensations" and "Fiddler on the Roof". In 1969, John made his film debut in *The Master Beater*. Three years later, he had his first big movie role, in the western, *Bad Company*. John's breakthrough movie was *The Deerhunter*, and the following year, he starred in a screen version of *Hair*. Success followed with regular frequency until the 1990s. When good parts were hard to get, he worked in supporting roles and Italian movies. In 1993, he married his present wife, the actress Sandi Schultz. Nowadays, John is still a very busy actor, but based on much of his recent output, quantity doesn't always mean quality.

Bad Company (1972)
The Killing Kind (1973)
Steelyard Blues (1973)
The Deerhunter (1978) **Hair** (1979)
The Onion Field (1979)
Inside Moves (1980)
Cattle Annie and Little Britches (1981)
The Amateur (1981)
Maria's lovers (1984)
Salvador (1986)
Do the Right Thing (1989)
The Godfather: Part III (1990)
Le Porte del Silenzio (1991)
Berlin '39 (1994)
The Crossing Guard (1995)
Little Boy Blue (1997)
A Corner of Paradise (1997)
The Thin Red Line (1998)
Summer of Sam (1999)
Dead Man's Run (2001)
Aimée Price (2005)
Iowa (2005)
Chatham (2008)
The Red Canvas (2008)

Telly **Savalas**
6ft
(ARISTOTELIS SAVALAS)

Born: **January 21, 1922**
Garden City, Long Island, New York, USA
Died: **January 22, 1994**

Telly was one of five children born to Greek Americans. His father, Nick, was the owner of a restaurant and his mother, Christina, was an artist. The family was so stubbornly traditional, when Telly first entered Sewahaka High School, in New York, he only spoke Greek. He graduated in 1940 and went to work as a lifeguard. His failure to rescue a man who was drowning haunted him for the rest of his life. From 1943 until 1946 he served in the U.S. Army, where he was a host on "Your Voice of America" radio program. On his return to civilian life he took courses in Broadcasting, English and Psychology at Columbia University School of General Studies. Telly then worked on a radio talk show, before joining ABC as an executive producer. It enabled him to start his acting career on TV, in the late 1950s and to make his film debut in 1961, in *Mad Dog Coll*. His humorous face and bald pate were popular long before he became 'Kojak' in 1973. His most famous film role was probably Archer Maggott, in *The Dirty Dozen*. Telly had five children from his three marriages – two with Julie, who survived him. He died of bladder cancer in Universal City, California, only a day after celebrating his seventy-second birthday.

The Young Savages (1961)
Cape Fear (1962)
Birdman of Alcatraz (1962)
The Interns (1962) **Love Is a Ball** (1963)
Battle of the Bulge (1965)
The Slender Thread (1965)
Beau Geste (1966)
The Dirty Dozen (1967)
The Scalphunters (1968)
Buona Sera, Mrs. Campbell (1968)
The Assassination Bureau (1969)
Mackenna's Gold (1969)
Crooks and Coronets (1969)
On Her Majesty's Secret Service (1969)
Kelly's Heroes (1970)
Violent City (1970)
Pretty Maids All in a Row (1971)
Lisa and the Devil (1973)

John **Saxon**
5ft 10½in
(CARMINE ORRICO)

Born: **August 5, 1935**
Brooklyn, New York City, New York, USA

John was the son of Italian Americans, Antonio and Anna Orrico. While attending New Utrecht High School, John appeared in several plays. He was walking along the street one day, when a fashion photographer advised him to take up modeling. His face was seen by Hollywood agent, Henry Wilson, who got him small roles in movies – starting in 1954, with *It Should Happen to You*. John was sent for acting lessons with Betty Cashman and after signing with Universal, he went to the famous coach Stella Adler. He made his film debut in one of the studio's program-fillers, *Girl in a Cage,* and was impressive when third-billed below Esther Williams and George Nader, in *The Unguarded Moment*. John had several good years just short of real stardom. He has kept busy through his willingness to work. John's made horror movies and comedies. and every so often, acted in Italian films. John never married, but has a son, Antonio, who was named after his dad. To see John in a good recent movie – made more than fifty years after his debut – take a look at *God's Ears*.

The Unguarded Moment (1956)
Rock, Pretty Baby (1956)
The Reluctant Debutante (1958)
The Restless Years (1958)
The Unforgiven (1960)
Agostino (1962) War Hunt (1962)
Mr. Hobbs Takes a Vacation (1962)
The Evil Eye (1963)
The Cardinal (1963)
The Cavern (1964)
Blood Beast from Outer Space (1965)
Death of a Gunfighter (1969)
Joe Kidd (1972)
Enter the Dragon (1973)
Black Christmas (1974)
Violent Naples (1976)
The Electric Horseman (1979)
Wrong Is Right (1982)
A Nightmare on Elm Street (1984)
From Dusk Till Dawn (1996)
Joseph's Gift (1998)
The Road Home (2003)
God's Ears (2007)

Greta **Scacchi**
5ft 9in
(GRETA GRACCO)

Born: **February 18, 1960**
Milan, Italy

Greta was the daughter of Luca Scacchi Gracco, an Italian painter, and his wife Pamela – a dancer who was born in England. She lived in Milan until her parents divorced when she was three and she was taken to England. When she was fifteen, her mother married a man called Giovanni Carsinga and the family moved to Australia. After three years, Greta went back to Europe – determined to become an actress. She joined the Bristol Old Vic Theater School at the same time as Miranda Richardson. Then the hard part began – looking for work. In between stage assignments, she acted in TV commercials. In 1982, she learned German for a leading role in Dominik Graf's *Das Zweite Gesicht – The Second Face.* Following *Heat and Dust,* she appeared on TV in Britain and Australia. She was involved with the singer, Tim Finn, until 1989. She has had a daughter with her ex-husband, Vincent D'Onofrio and a son fathered by her cousin, Carlo Mantegazza. Greta lives in Hurstpierpoint, Sussex, England.

The Second Face (1982)
Heat and Dust (1983)
Defence of the Realm (1985)
The Coca-Cola Kid (1985)
Burke & Wills (1985)
White Mischief (1987)
A Man in Love (1987)
Good Morning
Babylon (1987)
La Donna della luna (1988)
Presumed Innocent (1990)
Shattered (1991)
The Player (1992)
Salt on Our Skin (1992)
Country Life (1994)
Jefferson in Paris (1995)
Emma (1996)
Tom's Midnight Garden (1999)
Looking for Alibrandi (2000)
Festival in Cannes (2001)
Strange Crime (2004)
Beyond the Sea (2004)
Shoot on Sight (2007)
Brideshead Revisited (2008)

Roy **Scheider**
5ft 9in
(ROY RICHARD SCHEIDER)

Born: **November 10, 1932**
Orange, New Jersey, USA
Died: **February 10, 2008**

Roy was the son of Roy Bernhard Scheider, an auto mechanic, who was a German American Protestant, and Anna Crosson, who was Irish Catholic. He was educated at Columbia High School, in Maplewood, NJ. During his schooldays he was awarded two Theresa Helpburn Acting Awards. As a boy Roy suffered from rheumatic fever, and while recovering, took up boxing – which gave him his distinctive nose. He hung up his gloves to study acting at Rutgers University as well as at Franklin and Marshall College, in Lancaster, PA. After three years in the U.S. Air Force, he worked as a waiter before appearing in "Romeo and Juliet" at the New York Shakespeare Festival, in 1961. His film debut was in *The Curse of the Living Corpse,* in 1964. Roy burst onto the scene in the 1970s. He was in *Jaws* and was Oscar-nominated as Best Supporting Actor for *The French Connection* and Best Actor for *All That Jazz.* He was with his second wife, Brenda, when he died in Little Rock, Arkansas from multiple myeloma. Roy had three children. His final film, *Iron Cross,* will be released posthumously.

Klute (1971)
The French Connection (1971)
The Assassination (1972)
The Outside Man (1972)
The Seven-Ups (1973)
Sheila Levine is Dead and
Living in New York (1975)
Jaws (1975)
Marathon Man (1976)
Sorcerer (1977)
Last Embrace (1979)
All That Jazz (1979)
Still of the Night (1982)
Blue Thunder (1983)
2010 (1984) 52 Pick-Up (1986)
Cohen and Tate (1989)
The Russia House (1990)
Naked Lunch (1991)
Romeo Is Bleeding (1993)
The Rainmaker (1997)
Texas 46 (2002) The Poet (2007)

Maria Schell
5ft 3½in
(MARGARETE SCHELL)

Born: **January 15, 1926**
Vienna, Austria
Died: **April 26, 2005**

Maria was the eldest child of Hermann Schell, a Swiss playwright and poet, and the Austrian actress, Margarethe Noé von Nordberg. After studying at a religious institution in France, she started her acting career straight out of school – having received all the coaching she required from her mother. She was sixteen when she made her film debut in *Steinbruch* and later, she finished her education at a drama school, in Switzerland, during the war years. When peace returned, Maria studied in France before gaining valuable experience on stage in Vienna, Zurich, Berlin and Munich. In 1948, she appeared in an Austrian/German movie which, two years later, became her English language debut – *Angel with a Trumpet*. The title was very appropriate: she had a beautiful angelic face. Maria soon became popular in Europe, where she appeared in French, German, Italian and English films. It took a while until Hollywood recognized her qualities and cast her opposite Yul Brynner in *The Brothers Karamazov*. She was twice married and divorced – first to a German producer and secondly to an Austrian actor. She had two children. Maria died of pneumonia, in Preitenegg, Austria.

Angel with a Trumpet (1950)
The Magic Box (1951)
So Little Time (1952)
As Long as You're Near Me (1953)
The Heart of the Matter (1953)
Die Letzte Brücke (1954)
The Rats (1955)
Gervaise (1956)
Le notte bianche (1957)
The Brothers Karamazov (1958)
Une vie (1958)
The Hanging Tree (1959)
Cimarron (1960)
The Mark (1961)
The Devil by the Tail (1969)
The Odessa File (1974)
Superman (1978)
The First Polka (1979)
King Thrushbeard (1984)

Maximillian Schell
5ft 10in
(MAXIMILIAN SCHELL)

Born: **December 8, 1930**
Vienna, Austria

From the age of eight, Max grew up in Zurich, Switzerland. By the time he was eleven, he was writing and producing plays at his school. After the war, he completed his education at Munich University, where he studied Languages and Theatrical Science. He also became an accomplished pianist – of a high enough calibre to perform in concert with Leonard Bernstein. Max began acting on stage in 1952 – appearing in Basle, Essen and Berlin to name a few. In 1955, he made his film debut in *Kinder, Mutter und Ein General*. His international career kicked off with *The Young Lions*. After he had starred in the television version, in 1959, he won a Best Actor Oscar when *Judgement at Nuremberg* became a film. He was also nominated for *The Man in the Glass Booth* and *Julia* and, along with Arnie, is the most successful Austrian actor. Max has a daughter with the Russian actress, Natalya Andrejchenko. The couple acted in the movie, *Little Odessa*. He's currently filing for divorce. In recent years, Max has directed a number of films and operas.

Ein Mädchen aus Flandern (1956)
The Young Lions (1958)
Judgement at Nuremberg (1961)
Five Finger Exercise (1962)
The Condemned of Altona (1962)
The Reluctant Saint (1962)
Topkapi (1964)
Return from the Ashes (1965)
The Deadly Affair (1966)
The Castle (1968) Simón Bolivar (1969)
First Love (1970)
The Odessa File (1974)
The Man in the Glass Booth (1975)
St. Ives (1976) Cross of Iron (1977)
A Bridge Too Far (1977)
Julia (1977) The Chosen (1981)
Morgen in Alabama (1984)
The Rosegarden (1989)
The Freshman (1990)
A Far Off Place (1993) Justiz (1993)
Little Odessa (1994)
Festival in Cannes (2001)
The Brothers Bloom (2008)

Joseph Schildkraut
5ft 4in
(JOSEF SCHILDKRAUT)

Born: **March 22, 1896**
Vienna, Austro-Hungary
Died: **January 21, 1964**

Joseph's father, Rudolf, was one of the most famous actors in Vienna. The boy followed him onto the stage from the age of ten. His education was interrupted when the pair visited the USA in 1910, but after his return, he managed to fit in at high school and college in Berlin, before becoming an actor in Vienna with Max Reinhardt's company. In 1915, Joseph made his film debut in *Schlemihl* – a German film which featured his father. In 1921, the Schildkraut family emigrated to the USA. Joseph became a leading Broadway actor and made his first American movie in 1921 – D.W.Griffith's *Orphans of the Storm*. He worked for Cecil B. DeMille and as he was a fluent linguist - transferred to talking pictures without difficulty – starting with *The Mississippi Gambler,* in 1929. He was a strong character player and the highlight of his film career was a Best Supporting Actor Oscar for his role as Alfred Dreyfuss in *The Life of Emile Zola*. Apart from the reprise of his stage role, in "The Diary of Anne Frank", from 1949 onwards, Joseph worked mostly on television and in the theater. His autobiography, "My Father and I" was published in 1959. His first wife – until 1930, was the film actress, Elise Bartlett. There were two more before he died of a heart attack, in New York.

Viva Villa! (1934)
Cleopatra (1934)
The Crusades (1935)
The Garden of Allah (1936)
Slave Ship (1937)
Souls at Sea (1937)
The Life of Emil Zola (1937)
The Baroness and
the Butler (1938)
Marie Antoinette (1938)
Suez (1938)
The Man in the Iron Mask (1939)
The Rains Came (1939)
The Shop Around the Corner (1940)
Monsieur Beaucaire (1946)
The Diary of Anne Frank (1959)

Romy **Schneider**
5ft 3¹/₂in
(ROSEMARIE MAGDALENA ALBACH-RETTY)

Born: **September 23, 1938**
Vienna, Austria
Died: **May 29, 1982**

Romy's father Wolf, was an actor who was the son of the Viennese stage actress, Rosa Albach-Retty. Her mother, Magda Schneider, was also an actress, from Germany. When her parents divorced in 1945, Romy and her brother Wolfi were taken care of by their mother. Magda orchestrated her daughter's climb to fame and acted with her on stage. At the age of fifteen, Romy made her film debut in *Wenn der weisse Flieder wieder blüht*. She was soon a big favorite in movies about the history of German and Austrian royalty and in 1955, starred in the title role in *Sissi* – the first film in a romantic trilogy based on the life of Princess Elisabeth of Bavaria. In 1959, she fell in love with Alain Delon and went to live with him in France until 1963. She won a Best Actress César for *Une histoire simple*. Romy married twice, and had two children. After her son, David, died in a bizarre accident in 1981, when he was impaled on a fence, Romy sought solace in alcohol. Ten months later she was found dead in her Paris apartment. The coroner's verdict was cardiac arrest. Romy was hugely popular in France and was portrayed on a French postage stamp in 1998.

Mädchenjahre einer Königin (1954)
Sissi - Die junge Kaiserin (1956)
Scampolo (1958) Christine (1958)
Boccaccio '70 (1962)
Fire and Ice (1962) The Trial (1962)
Good Neighbor Sam (1964)
Triple Cross (1966)
The Swimming Pool (1969)
Les Choses de la vie (1970)
Max et les ferrailleurs (1971)
César et Rosalie (1972)
Ludwig (1972)
Le Mouton enragé (1974)
L'Important c'est d'aimer (1975)
Les Innocents aux
mains sales (1975)
Le Vieux fusil (1975)
Une histoire simple (1978)
Claire de femme (1979)

Arnold **Schwarzenegger**
6ft 2in
(ARNOLD ALOIS SCHWARZENEGGER)

Born: **July 30, 1947**
Thal bei Graz, Styria, Austria

The son of the local police chief, Gustav Schwarzenegger, and his wife, Aurelia, Arnie was raised as a Roman Catholic by strict parents – especially his father, who could be brutal at times. He had been a member of the Nazi party, but had no record of war crimes. It was a poor family and Arnie got most of his pleasure from playing sport. His soccer coach took him to a gym when he was fourteen years old and introduced him to his first barbell. After seeing movies starring Steve Reeves and Reg Park, Arnie took to body-building like a duck to water. Like all Austrian males at that time he did his National Service in the Austrian Army in 1965, and, without going AWOL, managed to win the "Junior Mr. Europe Contest|" in Stuttgart. He won the senior version two years later, and went to the USA – continuing weight training while looking for acting work. In 1970, the 'World's Strongest Man' made his film debut in *Hercules in New York*. He won a Golden Globe in 1977, for Best Acting Debut, in *Stay Hungry*. His accent was a problem to start with, but by the 1980s, audiences loved him, and he did comedy with an abundance of charm. After making *Terminator 3*, Arnie became Governor of California and hung up his acting boots. Since 1986, he's been married to Maria Shriver, a lady with Kennedy connections. They have four children.

Conan the Barbarian (1982)
The Terminator (1984)
Commando (1985)
Predator (1987)
The Running Man (1987)
Red Heat (1988) Twins (1988)
Total Recall (1990)
Kindergarten Cop (1990)
Terminator 2:
Judgement Day (1991)
Last Action Hero (1993)
True Lies (1994)
Eraser (1996)
The 6th Day (2000)
Terminator 3:
Rise of the Machines (2003)

Hanna **Schygulla**
5ft 7in
(HANNA SCHYGULLA)

Born: **December 25, 1943**
Kattowitz, Upper Silesia, Germany

Right in the middle of the horrors of World War II, the great joy for Hanna's mother, Antonie, was the birth of her daughter on Christmas Day. Shortly after that, her father, Josef, a German infantryman, was captured by American forces and held prisoner until 1948. After the war Hanna grew up in Munich and eventually, she studied German and Romance languages at its University. In her early twenties, she started taking acting lessons. Then, after establishing herself at the experimental Munich Action Theater, she met Rainer Werner Fassbinder, the charismatic, but volatile film director. He would be a huge influence on Hanna's career, which has included twenty-three of his movies. Hanna first appeared on the screen in a short – *Der Bräutigam, die Komödiantin und der Zuhälter*, in 1968. Her first Fassbinder film was *Liebe ist kälter als der Tod*. They acted together in Reinhard Hauff's *Mathias Kneissl*. Hanna lives in Paris, where she's is a popular chanteuse. Her recent movie, *The Edge of Heaven*, is a German/Turkish/Italian collaboration that has won several awards.

Liebe ist kälter als der Tod (1969)
Katzelmacher (1969) Götter der
Pest (1970) Mathias Kneissl (1970)
Warum läuft Herr R. Amok? (1970)
Händler der vier Jahreszeiten (1972)
Die Bitteren Tränen der Petra von
Kant (1972) The Clown (1976)
The Marriage of Maria Braun (1979)
The Third Generation (1979) Lili
Marleen (1981) False Witness (1981)
Antonietta (1982) Heller Wahn (1983)
A Love in Germany (1983)
Abraham's Gold (1990)
Warzawa. Année 5703 (1992)
Pakten (1995) Lea (1996)
The Girl of Your Dreams (1998)
Werkmeister Harmonies (2000)
Promised Land (2004)
Die Blaue Grenze (2005)
Friday or Another Day (2005)
Winter Journey (2006)
The Edge of Heaven (2007)

Annabella **Sciorra**
5ft 2in
(ANNABELLA GLORIA PHILOMENA SCIORRA)

Born: **March 29, 1960**
Wethersfield, Connecticut, USA

As her name and appearance suggests, Annabella has an Italian American father. Her mother, who was a fashion stylist, had French ancestry. Raised in New York City, after her father set up a business there as a veterinarian, Annabella was thirteen when she started training as an actress at the Hagen-Berghoff studios. After high school, Annabella attended the American Academy of Dramatic Arts. In 1988, she made her television debut in a mini series, 'The Fortunate Pilgrim'. A year later, she made her film debut in *True Love* and thought she'd found it when she married actor Joe Petruzzi. It lasted four years – by which time she'd established herself as an actress of note in such successful movies as *Jungle Fever, The Hand That Rocks the Cradle* and *Romeo is Bleeding*. After her divorce, there were more successes – a number of big budget productions and independent films – which she was happy to work in. For her TV acting, she received an Emmy nomination for playing Gloria Trillo, in 'The Sopranos'. Annabella has also acted on stage, at the Williamstown Theater Festival. Since 2006, she has concentrated on television.

Reversal of Fortune (1990)
The Hard Way (1991)
Jungle Fever (1991)
The Hand That Rocks the Cradle (1992)
Whispers in the Dark (1992)
The Night We Never Met (1993)
Romeo Is Bleeding (1993)
Mr. Wonderful (1993)
The Cure (1995)
The Addiction (1995)
The Funeral (1996)
Little City (1997)
Cop Land (1997)
Mr. Jealousy (1997)
What Dreams May Come (1998)
Above Suspicion (2000)
King of the Jungle (2000)
Domenica (2001)
Chasing Liberty (2004)
Twelve and Holding (2005)
Find Me Guilty (2006)

Paul **Scofield**
6ft 1in
(DAVID PAUL SCOFIELD)

Born: **January 21, 1922**
Hurstpierpoint, West Sussex, England
Died: **March 19, 2008**

Paul began appearing in plays during his five years at Varndean School for Boys, in the English seaside resort of Brighton. When he was seventeen, he started to train as an actor – firstly at the Croydon Repertory Theater School and in 1940, at the Mask Theater School, in London. During World War II, he toured with companies entertaining the British troops. In 1943, he married actress Joy Parker, with whom he had a couple of children. After Birmingham Repertory Company, Paul then moved to Stratford-upon-Avon, where he concentrated on the works of William Shakespeare. He was memorable in productions of "Henry V", "Love's Labour's Lost", "Measure for Measure", and "Hamlet" – becoming one of the greatest interpreters of the 'Bard' in the 20th Century and compared by the critics with Olivier. He was very cautious about moving into film work and his screen debut in 1955, as King Philip II of Spain, in *That Lady,* did not encourage him. Throughout the 1960s and 1970s, he chose his roles with extreme care. He won a Best Actor Oscar for *A Man for All Seasons,* but resisted any opportunity to become a conventional movie star. True to that stubborn character, he three times refused the offer of a knighthood. He was in around thirty films – his last in 1999, when he provided the voice of "Boxer" in an animated version of *Animal Farm.* Paul died of leukemia, at his home in Sussex.

Carve Her Name with Pride (1958)
The Train (1964)
A Man for All Seasons (1966)
Tell Me Lies (1968)
Bartleby (1970)
Nijinsky: Unfinished Project (1970)
King Lear (1971)
Scorpio (1973)
A Delicate Balance (1973)
When the Whales Came (1989)
Henry V (1989) Hamlet (1990)
Utz (1992) Quiz Show (1994)
The Crucible (1996)

Campbell **Scott**
6ft
(CAMPBELL SCOTT)

Born: **July 19, 1961**
New York City, New York, USA

George C. Scott's son – from his fourth marriage to Canadian actress, Colleen Dewhurst, Campbell appears to have inherited some talented genes. He first demonstrated that, when he acted in the play "Rosencrantz and Guildenstern are Dead" at John Jay High School. After graduating from Lawrence University, where he majored in Drama, Campbell set about fashioning a career of his own. He made his TV debut in 1987, in an episode of 'L.A. Law' and the same year, made his first movie appearance with a small role in *Five Corners.* One more movie got him listed as one of twelve "Promising New Actors of 1990". Campbell's work over the following eighteen years has amassed several award nominations, as well as a Best New Director Award, for *Big Night* – shared with its co-director, Stanley Tucci, but he has a way to go to emulate his dad by winning an Oscar – which he'd accept without much of an argument! Campbell's marriage to Anne, the mother of his son, Malcolm, ended in divorce in 2001.

Longtime Companion (1990)
The Sheltering Sky (1990)
Dying Young (1991)
Dead Again (1991) Singles (1992)
The Innocent (1993)
Mrs. Parker and the
Vicious Circle (1994)
Let It Be Me (1995)
The Daytrippers (1996)
Big Night (1996)
The Spanish Prisoner (1997)
The Impostors (1998) Hi-Life (1998)
Top of the Food Chain (1999)
Spring Forward (1999)
Other Voices (2000)
Roger Dodger (2002)
The Secret Lives of Dentists (2002)
Saint Ralph (2004)
The Dying Gaul (2005)
Loverboy (2005) Duma (2005)
The Exorcism of Emily Rose (2005)
Crashing (2007)
Music and Lyrics (2007)
Phoebe in Wonderland (2008)

George C. **Scott**
6ft 1in
(GEORGE CAMPBELL SCOTT)

Born: **October 18, 1927**
Wise, Virginia, USA
Died: **September 22, 1999**

George's father, George Dewey Scott, was an executive at the Buick Motor Company. His mother, Helena, died when George was eight, and he and his sister were raised by their father. During his high school years, he wrote short stories and his ambition was to be a novelist. When he was eighteen, he served for four years with the United States Marine Corps. He then enrolled at the University of Missouri, where he majored in Journalism. While he was at University, George appeared in several stage productions, including playing the lead in "The Winslow Boy". After about a year, he dropped out to work as a teacher – and acting in summer stock at every opportunity. He played "Richard III" at the 1957 New York Shakespeare Festival and his career took off. In 1958, he appeared on the live TV show 'Omnibus' and a year later, made his film debut in *The Hanging Tree*. George was nominated for Oscars, for *Anatomy of a Murder, The Hustler* and *The Hospital*. He refused to accept his Best Actor Oscar for *Patton*. George's final film was in Sidney Lumet's disappointing *Gloria,* in 1999. He married five times – lastly to the film actress Trish Van Devere – who was with him when he died in Westlake Village, California, following a burst abdominal aneurysm. He had six children.

The Hanging Tree (1959)
Anatomy of a Murder (1959)
The Hustler (1961)
The List of Adrian Messinger (1963)
Dr. Strangelove (1964)
Not with My Wife, You Don't (1966)
Petulia (1968) Patton (1970)
They Might Be Giants (1971)
The Last Run (1971)
The Hospital (1971) The New
Centurions (1972) Rage (1972)
Oklahoma Crude (1973)
Islands in the Stream (1977)
Movie Movie (1978)
The Changeling (1980) Taps (1981)
Malice (1993)

Lizbeth **Scott**
5ft 2in
(EMMA MATZO)

Born: **September 29, 1922**
Scranton, Pennsylvania, USA

The daughter of Slovakian immigrant parents, Lizabeth was educated at Central High School and Marywood College. She studied acting at Alvienne School of Drama in New York. Lizabeth worked in summer stock, did a bit of modeling, and even understudied Tallulah Bankhead on Broadway. In 1945, she was discovered by the producer, Hal Wallis, when she was dining out at the Stork Club. He got her a contract with Paramount, but before that, he gave her her film debut – when she starred in his independent production, *You Came Along*. Lizabeth had a uniquely husky voice and was considered by her studio as representing serious competition to the likes of Veronica Lake and Lauren Bacall. The fact that it never quite came off is no reflection on her many fine performances – demonstrated in a supporting role, where she out-acted the stars of *The Strange Love of Martha Ivers* – and when starring opposite Bogart, in the classic film noir, *Dead Reckoning*. Lizabeth featured in other notable films such as *Dark City* and *The Racket,* virtually retiring in 1957, after she starred with Elvis Presley, in *Loving You*. Lizabeth was seen on television during the 1960s, but made only one more movie appearance – in the Michael Caine crime drama, *Pulp*. She never married.

You Came Along (1945)
The Strange Love of
Martha Ivers (1946)
Dead Reckoning (1947)
Desert Fury (1947)
I Walk Alone (1948) Pitfall (1948)
Too Late for Tears (1949)
Easy Living (1949)
Paid in Full (1950)
Dark City (1950)
The Company She Keeps (1951)
Red Mountain (1951)
The Racket (1951)
Stolen Face (1952)
Scared Stiff (1953)
Silver Lode (1954)
The Weapon (1957)
Loving You (1957) Pulp (1972)

Randolph **Scott**
6ft 2in
(GEORGE RANDOLPH SCOTT)

Born: **January 23, 1898**
Orange County, Virginia, USA
Died: **March 2, 1987**

Randy was the only son (he had five sisters) of well-heeled parents, George and Lucille Scott. After attending the private Woodberry Forest School, he joined the Army in 1917, and served in France. After a brief military career, Randy went to Georgia Tech and finally, to the University of North Carolina. He then joined the textile firm which employed his father. Randy's dad knew Howard Hughes, and a letter from him resulted in his film debut in 1928, with a small role in *Sharp Shooters*. Randy gained stage experience at Pasadena Playhouse. A number of bit parts were followed by his appearance at the Vine Street Theater, in "Under a Virginia Moon". In the early 1930s, Randy starred in a series of Zane Grey westerns. He branched out into musicals, including *Roberta* and *Follow the Fleet* – with Astaire and Rogers – and screwball comedies like *My Favorite Wife* – with pal, Cary Grant. But he was always a cowboy at heart and that's how he finished his career, in *Ride the High Country*. Twice married, he died at his home in Beverly Hills, of heart and lung ailments.

Murder in the Zoo (1933)
The Last Round-Up (1934)
Roberta (1935) She (1935)
Follow the Fleet (1936)
The Last of the Mohicans (1936)
Go West Young Man (1936)
Jesse James (1939)
Frontier Marshal (1939)
Virginia City (1940)
My Favorite Wife (1940)
When the Daltons Rode (1940)
Western Union (1941) Belle Starr (1941)
The Spoilers (1942) Pittsburgh (1942)
The Desperadoes (1943)
Abilene Town (1946)
Home, Sweet Homicide (1946)
Albuquerque (1948) Santa Fe (1951)
Hangman's Knot (1952)
Ride Lonesome (1959)
Commanche Station (1960)
Ride the High Country (1962)

Zachary **Scott**
6ft 1in
(ZACHARY THOMSON SCOTT JR.)

Born: **February 21, 1914**
Austin, Texas, USA
Died: **October 3, 1965**

Zack was the son of a prominent local surgeon who was a distant relative of both George Washington and Marshal Bat Masterson. He intended to follow in his father's footsteps, but dropped out of medical studies at the University of Texas when he had his first taste of acting. He signed on as a cabin boy on a freighter and ended up in England. He remained there after he found work with a repertory theater. He returned to Texas and married his old sweetheart, Elaine Anderson – an aspiring actress, who encouraged him by joining him in stage productions in Austin. They were spotted by Alfred Lunt and given roles in Broadway plays. Warner Brothers were sufficiently impressed to give Zack the title role in his debut movie, *The Mask of Dimitrios.* By the time he appeared in *The Southerner* and *Mildred Pierce,* he was considered star material. It all went to plan until 1950, when a rafting accident, in which he was badly injured, coupled with divorce from Elaine, who married John Steinbeck, depressed him. Zack married actress Ruth Ford and acted on TV until shortly before dying of a brain tumor, in Austin, aged fifty-one.

The Mask of Dimitrios (1944)
The Southerner (1945) Mildred
Pierce (1945) Danger Signal (1945)
The Unfaithful (1947)
Cass Timberlane (1947)
Ruthless (1948)
Whiplash (1948)
Flaxy Martin (1949)
South of St. Louis (1949)
Flamingo Road (1949)
Guilty Bystander (1950)
Born to Be Bad (1950)
Pretty Baby (1950)
Lightning Strikes Twice (1951)
The Secret of Convict Lake (1951)
Stronghold (1951)
Let's Make It Legal (1951)
Bandido (1956)
The Young One (1960)
It'$ Only Money (1962)

Kristin **Scott Thomas**
5ft 6in
(KRISTIN SCOTT THOMAS)

Born: **May 24, 1960**
Redruth, Cornwall, England

Kristin's family is related to Captain Robert Falcon Scott, who explored the Antarctic regions at the beginning of the twentieth century . Her younger sister Serena is also an actress. Her father, a pilot in the Royal Navy, died in a flying accident in 1964. Her mother remarried another pilot, who died the same way – six years later. Kristin was educated at Cheltenham Ladies' College and later, St. Antony's Leweston School. She started drama school, but after she was told she'd never make it, she went to Paris as an au pair. Fluent in French, she attended ENSATT. In 1981, she married gynecologist Dr. François Olivennes. They separated seventeen years later. After graduating, she appeared on television, and made her film debut in 1986, with Prince, in *Under the Cherry Moon.* She acted in French movies, but made the big time in *Four Weddings and a Funeral.* She was nominated for a Best Actress Oscar for *The English Patient,* and has shone brightly ever since in a whole host of international films. The French movie, *Tell No One,* is first-class.

Agent Trouble (1987)
La Méridienne (1988)
A Handful of Dust (1988)
Force majeure (1989)
The Eyes of the World (1990)
The Bachelor (1991) Bitter Moon (1992)
Four Weddings and a Funeral (1994)
Un été inoubliable (1994)
Richard III (1995) Les Milles (1995)
Le Confessionnal (1995)
Angels and Insects (1995)
Mission Impossible (1996)
The English Patient (1996)
The Horse Whisperer (1998)
Life as a House (2001)
Gosford Park (2001)
Man to Man (2005)
Chromophobia (2005)
Keeping Mum (2005)
Tell No One (2006)
The Walker (2007)
I've Loved You So Long (2008)
Easy Virtue (2008)

Jean **Seberg**
5ft 6in
(JEAN SEBERG)

Born: **November 13, 1938**
Marshaltown, Iowa, USA
Died: **September 8, 1979**

Daughter of Lutheran parents – Edward Seberg and his wife Dorothy – Jean was twelve when she saw Marlon Brando in *The Men,* and made up her mind to become a film actress. She studied drama in her home town and appeared at the local theater in plays such as "Our Town" and "Picnic". Following a nationwide search, director, Otto Preminger, chose her as his *Saint Joan.* He was tough with her, and it was the worst possible start to her fledgling film career. After three films which were not very successful, she married a French lawyer, François Moreuil and went to live in Paris. It was lucky for her: she was cast by Jean-Luc Godard to play the American girlfriend of Jean-Paul Belmondo, in the film *À Bout de Souffle* – which was hailed as a masterpiece. It regenerated Jean's career and she was able to go back to Hollywood and act in some worthwhile American films, such as *Lilith* and *Paint Your Wagon.* In the late 1960s, she began to get very involved in political causes – most worryingly from J.Edgar Hoover's point of view – with the Black Panthers. After that, the pressure from the FBI caused her to split with her second husband, Romain Gary, and even more sadly, have a stillborn child. She married twice more, but turned to drugs and alcohol and finally, suicide in Paris.

Bonjour Tristesse (1958)
À Bout de Souffle (1960)
Let No Man Write
My Epitaph (1960)
L'Amant de cinq jours (1961)
In the French Style (1963)
Lilith (1964)
La Ligne de démarcation (1966)
A Fine Madness (1966)
Pendulum (1969)
Paint Your Wagon (1969)
Ondata di calore (1970)
Airport (1970)
L'Attentat (1972)
The Wild Duck (1976)
Le Bleu des origines (1979)

Kyra **Sedgwick**
5ft 5in
(KYRA MINTURN SEDGWICK)

Born: **August 19, 1965**
New York City, New York, USA

Descended from William Ellery – one of the fifty-six signatories to the Declaration of Independence – Kyra is the daughter of venture capitalist, Henry Sedgwick, and his Jewish wife, Patricia, who was a speech teacher. Kyra's younger brother, Robert, would also become an actor. Her parents divorced when she was six years old and her mother married an art dealer. She became half-sister to jazz guitarist, Mike Stern. Kyra was educated at private schools including Sarah Lawrence College and graduated from the Quaker school, Friends Seminary, in Manhattan. When she was sixteen she made her TV debut in the soap opera, 'Another World'. After that, she earned a Theater Degree from the University of California. Kyra made her movie debut in the romantic drama, *War and Love.* Bigger productions like *Born on the Fourth of July* soon came her way and in 1988, she had the good fortune to meet her soulmate, Kevin Bacon – when they acted together in the television movie, 'Lemon Sky'. The couple now have two children and live in Connecticut. In 2007, Kyra won a Golden Globe for the Best Performance by an Actress in a Television Series – in 'The Closer', for which she picked up several others. Kyra's next movie is the thriller, *Game.*

War and Love (1985)
Born on the Fourth of July (1989)
Mr. & Mrs. Bridge (1990)
Singles (1992)
Heart and Souls (1993)
Murder in the First (1995)
The Low Life (1995)
Phenomenon (1996)
Critical Care (1997)
Montana (1998)
What's Cooking (2000)
Personal Velocity: Three
Portraits (2002)
Behind the Red Door (2003)
Secondhand Lions (2003)
The Woodsman (2004)
Cavedweller (2004)
The Game Plan (2007)

George **Segal**
5ft 11in
(GEORGE SEGAL)

Born: **February 13, 1934**
Great Neck, Long Island, New York, USA

The son of George Segal Sr. and his wife Fanny, he was educated in Great Neck, during his junior years, before attending the appropriately named, George School - a private Quaker preparatory school near Newtown, Pennsylvania. While there he began performing a magic act, which made him very popular. George's next stop was Columbia University, where he helped form "Bruno Lynch and His Imperial Jazz Band" – in which he played banjo. George did two years army service, then married the first of three wives, Marion Sobel, in 1956, and had two daughters. In New York, he was janitor at an off-Broadway theater and appeared in a nightclub duo, "George Segal and Patricia Collins Singing Their Little Hearts Out". His stage debut was in "The Iceman Cometh". In 1961, he made his movie debut in *The Young Doctors.* He was nominated for a Supporting Oscar for *Who's Afraid of Virginia Woolf?* and won a Golden Globe for *A Touch of Class.* For twelve years, he's been married to Sonia Greenbaum. He's still busy acting.

King Rat (1965)
Who's afraid of Virginia Woolf? (1965)
The Quiller Memorandum (1966)
The St. Valentine's Day Massacre (1967)
Bye Bye Braverman (1968)
No Way to Treat a Lady (1968)
The Bridge at Remagen (1969)
Loving (1970) Where's Poppa? (1970)
The Owl and the Pussycat (1970)
Born to Win (1971)
The Hot Rock (1972)
Blume in Love (1973)
A Touch of Class (1973)
The Terminal Man (1974)
California Split (1974)
The Duchess and
the Dirtwater Fox (1976)
Fun with Dick and Jane (1977)
Who Is Killing the Great
Chefs of Europe? (1978)
Look Who's Talking (1989)
Flirting with Disaster (1996)
Heights (2005)

Emmanuelle **Seigner**
5ft 8in
(EMMANUELLE SEIGNER)

Born: **June 22, 1966**
Paris, France

Emmanuelle grew up in a creative family environment. She was the daughter of a photographer and a journalist. Her grandfather, Louis Seigner, was a distinguished character actor who served as chairman of the Comédie Française. Emmannuelle was educated at a convent school in Paris and during that time, earned extra pocket money due to being a tall fourteen-year-old beauty, by working as a model. After making it big time on the international catwalks and the covers of fashion magazines all over the world, Emmanuelle made her film debut in 1984, in *Year of the Jellyfish.* It was followed by a good role in Jean-Luc Godard's *Détective.* She was soon cast by Roman Polanski as Harrison Ford's missing wife, in his Paris-set thriller, *Frantic,* and she became the director's third wife, in 1989. They have two children – Morgane and Elvis. Four years later, she was one of the stars (with Hugh Grant and Kristin Scott Thomas) in Polanski's *Bitter Moon.* In 2006, after she became the lead singer in the band, "Ultra Orange", the group's name was changed to "Ultra Orange and Emmanuelle". Her next film to be released is *Giallo,* in which she stars wth Adrien Brody. She was recently in the comedy, *Le Code a changé.*

Détective (1985)
Frantic (1988)
Il Male oscuro (1990)
Bitter Moon (1992)
Le Sourire (1994)
Place Vendôme (1998)
The Ninth Gate (1999)
Buddy Boy (1999)
Laguna (2001)
Corps à corps (2003)
Os imortais (2003)
And They Lived
Happily Ever After (2004)
Backstage (2004)
Four Last Songs (2007)
La Vie en Rose (2007)
Le Scaphandre et
le papillon (2007)
Le Code a changé (2009)

Peter **Sellers**
5ft 8in
(RICHARD HENRY SELLERS)

Born: **September 8, 1925**
Southsea, Hampshire, England
Died: **July 24, 1980**

Peter's parents, Bill and Peg, worked in and ran an acting company. Peg spoiled him because her first child had died at birth. Through the Jewish branch of the family, he was a descendant of the boxer, Daniel Mendoza. Peter attended the Roman Catholic, St. Aloysius College, London. He joined the RAF when he was eighteen. In 1946, he set up a review in London, where he told off-color jokes, did impressions of celebrities, and played drums. In 1951, the year of his first marriage – to Anne Howe – he joined Harry Secombe and Spike Milligan in the 'Goon Show', a BBC radio comedy program. He and Milligan made a short, *Let's Go Crazy,* and a first feature, *Penny Points to Paradise.* Peter's movie ambitions started to bare fruit in *The Ladykillers,* and in *Tom Thumb.* He was nominated for Best Actor Oscars – for *Dr. Strangelove* and *Being There* – the latter providing a fine farewell to a film career which included *The Pink Panther* series and *Lolita* among its many highlights. Peter's third wife, actress Lynne Frederick, was with him when he died of a heart attack, in London.

The Smallest Show on Earth (1957)
The Naked Truth (1957) Tom
Thumb (1958) Carlton-Browne of the
F.O. (1959) The Mouse That
Roared (1959) I'm All Right Jack (1959)
The Battle of the Sexes (1959) Never Let
Go (1960) Two Way Stretch (1960)
Only Two Can Play (1962) Waltz of the
Toreadors (1962) Lolita (1962)
The Dock Brief (1962) The Wrong
Arm of the Law (1963) The Pink
Panther (1963) Heaven's Above (1963)
Dr. Strangelove (1964)
The World of Henry Orient (1964)
A Shot in the Dark (1964)
The Wrong Box (1966)
The Party (1968) Hoffman (1970)
The Return of the Pink Panther (1975)
Murder by Death (1976)
The Pink Panther Strikes Again (1976)
Being There (1979)

Michel **Serrault**
5ft 8½in
(MICHEL SERRAULT)

Born: **January 24, 1928**
Brunoy, Essone, France
Died: **July 29, 2007**

Michel's staunchly Catholic parents had him earmarked for the priesthood. As a young boy, his ambition was to become a clown in a circus, but he went along with their plan and endured several months in a seminary. He finally left when he decided that he couldn't face a lifetime of celibacy. Although he was turned down by the Paris Conservatoire, Michel made his stage debut in 1946, on a theater tour of the French-occupied sector of Germany. He did his National Service in the French Airforce, at Dijon, before in 1949, joining Robert Dhery's theater troupe. In 1953, he worked as a singer in cabaret – in a duo with his good friend, Jean Poiret. As a member of the Comédie Française, Michel acted in plays by Shakespeare and Molière. In 1954, he made his film debut in *Ah! les belles bacchantes.* His next was Henri-Georges Clouzot's masterly thriller, *Les Diaboliques.* He was exclusively in films made for the French market until *La Cage aux Folles* brought him world-wide fame and a César Award. Michel died of cancer at home, close to his birthplace, Honfleur. Michel was survived by his wife Jaunita, and his daughter, the actress and director, Nathalie Serrault.

Les Diaboliques (1956)
King of Hearts (1966)
L'Ibis rouge (1975)
Préparez vos mouchoirs (1978)
La Cage aux Folles (1978)
Garde à vue (1981)
Docteur Petiot (1990)
Ville à vendre (1992)
Bonsoir (1994)
Le Bonheur est
dans le Pré (1995)
Nelly et M. Arnaud (1995)
Beaumarchais l'Insolent (1996)
Artemisia (1997)
Rien Ne Va Plus (1997)
The Children of the
Marshland (1998)
Le Libertin (2000)
The Girl from Paris (2001)

Chloë **Sevigny**
5ft 8in
(CHLOË STEVENS SEVIGNY)

Born: **November 18, 1974**
Darien, Connecticut, USA

The daughter of David Sevigny, an interior painter of French ancestry, who had been an accountant, and his wife Janine, a Polish American. Chloë and her older brother Paul, were brought up strictly in the Catholic faith. While she was at Darien High School, she used to babysit the future actor, Topher Grace. When she was eighteen, Chloë moved into an apartment of her own in Brooklyn. She was spotted on the street in the East Village by a Sassy Magazine fashion editor and she went to work there as an intern. She later modeled for the magazine as well as for x-girl – the fashion label of Kim Gordon, of Sonic Youth. Chloë was described as the new "It-girl" in The New Yorker, and she was on the cover of Gigolo Aunts' 1994 album "Flippin' Out". It was only a question of time before filmmakers wanted her. She made her debut in the controversial film, *Kids.* Like several of her later films, it was independent – Art House style, which, given her pedigree, it's no surprise to see her support whenever she can. Along with her co-star, Hilary Swank, she received critical praise for her acting in *Boys Don't Cry* and she was nominated for a Best Supporting Actress Oscar. Her recent role in *Zodiac,* proved that she can shine in big-budget movies too. Since 2006, Chloë has featured in the television series, 'Big Love'. She lives in Manhattan.

Kids (1995)
Trees Lounge (1996)
Palmetto (1998)
Boys Don't Cry (1998)
A Map of the World (1999)
American Psycho (2000)
Ten Minutes Older: The Trumpet (2002)
Demonlover (2002)
Party Monster (2003)
Dogville (2003)
Shattered Glass (2003)
Melinda and Melinda (2004)
Manderlay (2005)
Broken Flowers (2005)
3 Needles (2005) Zodiac (2007)
The Killing Room (2009)

Jane **Seymour**
5ft 4in
(JOYCE PENELOPE WILHELMINA FRANKENBERG)

Born: **February 15, 1951**
Hayes, Middlesex, England

When she was seventeen, Jane adopted the name of Henry VIII's third wife. She was the eldest daughter of three girls born to John Frankenberg, an English Jewish obstetrician, and his wife Mieke van Trigt, a Dutch woman who had survived a Japanese prison camp during World War II. Jane was educated at the independent Arts Educational School, at Tring, in Hertfordshire. Apart from her beauty, she was unusual in having a brown right eye and a green left eye. Her first film appearance was in 1969, when she had an uncredited role in *Oh! What a Lovely War.* Jane's first starring role was as a Jewish girl in the war drama, *The Only Way.* She married Michael – son of director, Richard Attenborough – but it only lasted two years. She had consulted a psychic, who told her that she would be married three more times. She played the Bond girl, Solitaire, in *Live and Let Die.* For her TV work, Jane won an Emmy as Outstanding Supporting Actress, in 'Onassis: The Richest Man in the World', in 1988, and a Golden Globe for 'Dr.Quinn, Medicine Woman', in 1996. Since 1993, Jane has been married to Stacy Keach's brother, James. They have twin boys. Jane's love of children has led to involvement with UNICEF and Childhelp USA. Following a leading role in *After Sex,* Jane will be seen in the coming months in two American films – *The Assistants* and *Wake.*

The Only Way (1970)
Young Winston (1972)
Live and Let Die (1973)
Sinbad and the Eye of
the Tiger (1977)
Somewhere in Time (1980)
Oh Heavenly Dog (1980)
Lassiter (1984)
La Révolution Française (1989)
Touching
Wild Horses (2002)
Wedding Crashers (2005)
Blind Dating (2006)
After Sex (2007)
The Velveteen Rabbit (2007)

Delphine **Seyrig**
5ft 5in
(DELPHINE CLAIRE BELRIANE SEYRIG)

Born: **April 10, 1932**
Beirut, Lebanon
Died: **October 15, 1990**

Delphine was the daughter of two French expatriates – archeologist, Henri Seyrig, and his wife, Hermine de Saussure. Delphine spent her early childhood in Lebanon, Greece and the United States, before being sent to France, where she finished her education and studied drama at the Comédie de Saint-Étienne, and the Centre Dramatique de l'Est. In 1956, she went to the United States, where she attended Lee Strasberg's Actors Studio, in New York and made her film debut in *Pull My Daisy.* She performed on the stage in France until she was cast by director Alain Resnais in his landmark, *Last Year in Marienbad.* She won the Best Actress Award at the Venice Film Festival, for *Muriel,* and went on to work with Truffaut, Buñuel, and Marguerite Duras. She was fluent in three languages – which enabled her to work internationally. She married and divorced the American painter, Jack Youngerman. She died of lung cancer at her home in Paris.

Last Year in Marienbad (1961)
Muriel ou le temps d'un retour (1963
Accident (1967) La Musica (1967)
Stolen Kisses (1968)
The Milky Way (1969)
Donkey Skin (1970) Les Lèvres
rouges (1971) The Discreet Charm of
the Bourgeoisie (1972)
The Day of the Jackal (1973)
A Doll's House (1973)
Le Jardin qui
bascule (1974)
The Black Windmill (1974) Say it
with Flowers (1974) Aloïse (1975)
The Last Word (1975)
Jeanne Dielman, 23 Quai
du Commerce, 1080 Bruxelles (1975)
India Song (1975)
Son nom de Venise dans
Calcutta désert (1976)
Caro Michele (1976) On the
Move (1979) Chère inconnue (1980)
Freak Orlando (1981)
Letters Home (1986)

Tony **Shalhoub**
5ft 10in
(ANTHONY MARCUS SHALHOUB)

Born: **October 9, 1953**
Green Bay, Wisconsin, USA

Tony's father, Joe, came to America from Lebanon, when he was ten. He married a lady called Helen – who was a second-generation Lebanese-American. They were both Maronite Christians. Together, they opened a grocery store in the center of Green Bay and saw it succeed. One of Tony's older sisters first introduced him to acting when he was six, in her high school production of "The King and I". After graduating from Green Bay High School, Tony got a BA in Drama from USM, and a Master's from Yale School of Drama. After four seasons with the American Repertory Theater, he headed for New York, where he made his Broadway debut, in 1985, in "The Odd Couple". The following year, he worked on TV. His film debut was a small role in *Longtime Companion,* in 1990. He met his wife, Brooke Adams and they got married in 1992. Apart from his movie credits as an actor, Tony is also a director. He's also won an Emmy and a Golden Globe for his title-role in the TV-series, 'Monk' – in which he has completed more than a century of appearances.

Barton Fink (1991)
I.Q. (1994)
Big Night (1996)
Men in Black (1997)
Gattaca (1997)
A Life Less Ordinary (1997)
Primary Colors (1998)
Paulie (1998)
The Impostors (1998)
The Siege (1998)
A Civil Action (1998)
The Tic Code (1999)
Galaxy Quest (1999)
Spy Kids (2001)
The Man Who
Wasn't There (2001)
Impostor (2001)
Made-Up (2002)
Men in Black II (2002)
The Last Shot (2004)
The Great New Wonderful (2005)
Careless (2007)
1408 (2007)

Michael **Shannon**
6ft 3½in
(MICHAEL CORBETT SHANNON)

Born: **August 7, 1974**
Lexington, Kentucky, USA

Mike's father, Donald S. Shannon, was an accounting professor at DePaul University. His paternal grandfather was entomologist Raymond Corbett Shannon – from whom Mike got his middle name. His mother, Geraldine, was a lawyer. His parents divorced when he was very young but he was raised by both – in Kentucky and Chicago. After high school Michael started his stage career in Chicago, where he was one of the founders of the Red Orchid Theater and later worked with both The Next Lab and the Steppenwolf Theater Company. He made his television debut in 1992, in 'Angel Street'. The following year, he began his movie career with a small role in *Groundhog Day*. By the end of the 1990s, he'd established himself as a film actor as well as appearing on the London West End stage, in "Killer Joe", and "Woyzeck". Mike increased his credits with good Indie films such as *Jesus' Son* and began to get big budget work starting with *Pearl Harbor,* and following that with *Vanilla Sky*. After he co-starred with Ashley Judd, in *Bug,* his career took off. He was recently recognized for his efforts when he was nominated for a Best Supporting Actor Oscar, for *Revolutionary Road.* He's married to Kate Arrington and has a young daughter. Mike has a nose for good movies – so you'd better watch out!

Groundhog Day (1993)
Chicago Cab (1997) The Ride (1999)
Jesus' Son (1999)
The Photographer (2000)
Cecil B. Demented (2000)
Tigerland (2000) Vanilla Sky (2001)
High Crimes (2002)
8 Mile (2002) Bad Boys II (2003)
The Woodsman (2004)
Criminal (2004) Dead Birds (2004)
Bug (2006) World Trade Center (2006)
Let's Go to Prison (2006)
Shotgun Stories (2007) Blackbird (2007)
Before the Devil Knows
You're Dead (2007)
Revolutionary Road (2008)
The Missing Person (2009)

Omar **Sharif**
5ft 10in
(MICHEL SHALHOUB)

Born: **April 10, 1932**
Alexandria, Egypt

The son of a lumber merchant, Joseph Shalhoub (but no relation to Tony) and his wife, Claire, Omar was of Lebanese and Syrian extraction but was brought up as a Roman Catholic. He was educated at Victoria College in Alexandria and to finish off he gained a degree in Mathematics and Physics at Cairo University. After graduating, he joined his father's business. His good looks soon aroused the interest of local filmmakers and he became a big star of Egyptian cinema, after making his debut in 1954, in *Siraa Fil-Wadi*. His co-star in that film, Faten Hamamain, became his wife in 1955. He converted to Islam and adopted the name Omar al-Sharif. His first English-language movie was David Lean's *Lawrence of Arabia,* for which he was nominated for a Best Supporting Actor Oscar. Omar's been a popular star in a wealth of good movies for nearly half-a-century. He is the star of *J'ai oublié se te dire,* fifty-five years after he first appeared on the screen. Apart from his formidable movie achievements, Omar's also a world-class Bridge player.

Lawrence of Arabia (1962)
The Fall of the Roman Empire (1964)
Behold a Pale Horse (1964)
The Yellow Rolls Royce (1964)
Doctor Zhivago (1965)
The Night of the Generals (1967)
Funny Girl (1968) Mayerling (1968)
Mackenna's Gold (1969)
The Last Valley (1970)
The Horsemen (1971)
The Burglars (1971)
The Mysterious Island (1973)
The Tamarind Seed (1974)
Juggernaut (1974) Funny Lady (1975)
The Baltimore Bullet (1980)
Top Secret! (1984)
Grand Larceny (1987)
The Possessed (1988)
The Rainbow Thief (1990) Mayrig (1991)
588 rue paradis (1992)
The 13th Warrior (1999)
Monsieur Ibrahim (2003)
Hidalgo (2004)

William **Shatner**
5ft 9½n
(WILLIAM ALAN SHATNER)

Born: **March 22, 1931**
Montreal, Quebec, Canada

All four of Bill's grandparents were Jewish immigrants from Eastern Europe. His paternal grandfather, Wolf Schattner, had shortened the family name. Bill's father had a clothing manufacturing business in Montreal. His mother, Anna, looked after their home. Bill was educated at the Willingdon Elementary School, in Montreal and in 1952, graduated from McGill University with a degree in Commerce. In 1993, the student union building was renamed Schatner Building by students. Having made his first appearance on stage as Tom Sawyer, he made his film debut in 1951, in the Montreal-set, *The Butler's Night Off*. After University, Bill appeared in repertory productions until 1954, when he joined Stratford Ontario Shakespeare Company, and he became one of Canada's leading Shakespearean actors. He made his Broadway debut in "Tamberlaine the Great". After some TV work, Bill had his first major film role, in *The Brothers Karamazov*. In 1966, he was Captain Kirk in the first episode of the TV series, 'Star Trek'. It made him world famous and guaranteed him work for the next forty years. In 2004, Bill received a Golden Globe for his work in another long-running TV series, 'Boston Legal'. He now lives with his fourth wife, Elizabeth.

The Brothers Karamazov (1958)
The Explosive Generation (1961)
Judgement at Nuremberg (1961)
The Intruder (1962)
The Outrage (1964)
Incubus (1965)
Big Bad Mama (1974)
Kingdom of the Spiders (1977)
Star Trek: The Motion Picture (1979)
Star Trek: The Wrath of Khan (1982)
Star Trek: The Search for Spock (1984)
Star Trek IV: The Voyage Home (1986)
Bill and Ted's
Bogus Journey (1991)
Loaded Weapon 1 (1993)
Star Trek: Generations (1994)
Free Enterprise (1998)
Miss Congeniality (2000)

Helen **Shaver**
5ft 7in
(HELEN SHAVER)

Born: **February 24, 1951**
St.Thomas, Ontario, Canada

One of six sisters – Helen was also the unfortunate one. As a child she suffered from rheumatic fever and was confined to her bed for several of her early years. While she was ill, she focussed her mind on the dream of one day being famous. Happily, she recovered and after excelling as a young pianist, Helen became enough of an athlete to be pretty useful as a downhill skier. After high school, she attended acting classes and began her career on the Canadian stage. In 1971, she made her Canadian television debut in an episode of 'Dr. Simon Locke'. Four years later, she acted in her first movie – a Canadian/Mexican co-production – called *El Hombre desnudo*. Following a number of films in her own country, Helen made her American debut, in *The Amityville Horror*. In 1985, Helen won a Bronze Leopard Award at Locarno International Film Festival, in Switzerland, for *Desert Hearts*. It was memorable in other ways; she met her third husband, Steve Smith, who was key grip on the film, and she also got a call from Greta Garbo – praising her acting. In 1998, Helen started directing and won a Chicago Festival Children's Jury Award for a TV movie, 'Summer's End' – starring James Earl Jones. Other awards include Genies – for *In Praise of Older Women* and *We All Fall Down*.

Outrageous! (1977) **Who Has Seen the Wind** (1977) **In Praise of Older Women** (1978) **The Amityville Horror** (1979) **Harry Tracy, Desperado** (1982)
The Osterman Weekend (1983)
Desert Hearts (1985)
The Color of Money (1986)
The Believers (1987)
Tree of Hands (1989) **Bethune: The Making of a Hero** (1989)
Zebrahead (1992) **That Night** (1992)
Rowing Through (1996)
The Craft (1996)
The Wishing Tree (1999)
Bear with Me (2000)
We All Fall Down (2000) **Numb** (2007)

Robert **Shaw**
5ft 10in
(ROBERT ARCHIBALD SHAW)

Born: **August 9, 1927**
West Houghton, Lancashire, England
Died: **August 28, 1978**

One of five children born to Doctor Thomas Shaw and his wife, Doreen, Robert and his family went to live in Scotland when he was seven. Five years later, his dad committed suicide. The family moved to Truro in Cornwall, where he went to school. He became a teacher in Yorkshire before enrolling at RADA, in London. Robert's first movie appearance was a bit part in the 1951 Ealing comedy, *The Lavender Hill Mob*. He was fairly anonymous until the Bond film, *From Russia with Love*. He was nominated for a Best Supporting Actor Oscar for *A Man for All Seasons*. He was also a successful novelist and playwright. In 1963, he married his second wife, the actress Mary Ure. The couple had four children (he had nine in all) and he was depressed when she died, in 1976. He remarried and continued working, but his health was deteriorating. While driving with his third wife, Virginia and their baby son, Thomas, in County Mayo, Ireland, Robert suffered a heart attack and died.

A Hill in Korea (1956)
The Valiant (1962)
The Caretaker (1963)
From Russia with Love (1963)
Tomorrow at Ten (1964)
The Luck of Ginger Coffey (1964)
Battle of the Bulge (1965)
A Man for All Seasons (1966)
The Birthday Party (1968)
Battle of Britain (1969)
The Royal Hunt of the Sun (1969)
Figures in a Landscape (1970)
Young Winston (1972)
The Hireling (1973)
The Sting (1973)
The Taking of Pelham One Two Three (1974)
Jaws (1975)
Robin and Marian (1976)
Swashbuckler (1976)
Black Sunday (1977)
Force 10 from Navarone (1978)

Susan **Shaw**
5ft 4in
(PATSY SLOOTS)

Born: **August 29, 1929**
West Norwood, London, England
Died: **September 27, 1978**

Susan was from an ordinary working class background, but she was outstandingly pretty and ambitious. When she left school at fifteen, she began training as a clerk at the Ministry of Information, in London. Susan had a great personality and British films were crying out for new talent following World War II. She was spotted by a Rank Organization talent scout and enrolled at the Rank Charm School – which taught her how to act in front of the cameras. She was given her film debut in 1946, as a dancer, in *London Town,* and after a trio of small parts, she achieved star status when she was loaned out to Ealing Studios for a featured role in the impressive British classic, *It Always Rains on Sunday.* Not so lucky was her marriage to the German actor, Albert Lievens, who was twenty-three years older than her. Within two years, she was dating Bonar Colleano, with whom she had starred in *Pool of London.* Susan married him in 1954, and they had a son, Mark, who would become an actor. Four years later, Colleano died in a car crash on the way back from a theater appearance in Liverpool. It turned her into an alcoholic and after the 1963 film, *The Switch*, she retired from acting. Although regarded as one of the most beautiful actresses ever to emerge from England, Susan died lonely, broke and broken, from cirrhosis of the liver. Nobody from the film world attended her funeral, which was paid for by Rank.

It Always Rains on Sunday (1947)
My Brother's Keeper (1948)
London Belongs to Me (1948)
Quartet (1948)
Here Come the Huggetts (1948)
Train of Events (1949)
Waterfront Women (1950)
Five Angles on Murder (1950)
Wall of Death (1951)
Pool of London (1951)
The Intruder (1953)
The Good Die Young (1954)
Time Is My Enemy (1954)

Moira **Shearer**
5ft 6½in
(MOIRA SHEARER KING)

Born: **January 17, 1926**
Dunfermline, Fife, Scotland
Died: **January 31, 2006**

Moira was the daughter of a civil engineer and actor called Harold King. Because of her father's work, she moved around a lot – being educated in Scotland and England as well as in Africa (Ndola then Northern Rhodesia). She received her early training as a ballerina as a young girl, in Ndola, under the guidance of a former pupil of Italian maestro, Enrico Cecchetti. But it was in London in 1936, where she was coached by Flora Fairbairn and, most importantly, at the Nicholas Legat Studio that she developed into a dancer of international repute. After three years with Legat, she joined the Sadler's Wells Ballet School. Moira made her stage debut in 1941 with the newly-formed International Ballet. In 1942, she joined the Sadlers Wells Ballet Company and danced her first leading role, in "Les Sylphides" during her first season. She danced in more modern works over the war period, in several ballets created for her by Robert Helpmann, Ninette de Valois and Frederick Ashton. Moira's film debut, in *The Red Shoes,* made her an instant movie star – which she is said to have felt uncomfortable with – but it exposed the rather elitist art form of ballet to audiences all over the world. Moira then continued dancing – replacing the injured Margot Fonteyn in 1948, in Ashton's "Cinderella", at Covent Garden. She made a handful of films during the following twelve years, but retired after appearing in Michael Powell's controversial movie, *Peeping Tom.* She became a writer and reared a family – she had a son and three daughters with the journalist, author and broadcaster, Sir Ludovic Kennedy. Moira retired in 1987 and died in Oxford, of natural causes.

The Red Shoes (1948)
The Tales of Hoffmann (1951)
The Story of Three Loves (1953)
The Man Who Loved Redheads (1955)
Black Tights (1960)
Peeping Tom (1960)

Norma **Shearer**
5ft 1in
(EDITH NORMA SHEARER)

Born: **August 10, 1900**
Montréal, Québec, Canada
Died: **June 12, 1983**

Norma was the daughter of Andrew Shearer, a success in the construction industry, but an unhappy man in his marriage to her mother Edith. He was prone to manic depression. It was Edith who had high ambitions for Norma, firstly as a concert pianist. When her father's business collapsed, Edith moved into a boarding house with her two daughters, and Norma took a job – playing piano in a music store. Then, despite her physical shortcomings, Edith made up her mind to turn the girl into a film actress. She took her to auditions in New York until she got work as an extra. Norma had tenacity, she talked to D.W. Griffith when she was playing a small role in his 1920 film, *Way Down East.* He was totally unimpressed, but by 1925, she had an MGM contract and was given the star build up. In 1927, she married production head, Irving Thalberg, who used all his influence to make her a big star. In her first big talking picture, *The Divorcee,* she won the Best Actress Oscar. She was nominated five more times. Thalberg died in 1936, and a four-year adjustment to Norma's official age by the studio, began to look obvious – because of the youthful roles she continued to play. She retired in 1942 – after completing work on *Her Cardboard Lover* and married a young ski instructor. Her death in Woodland Hills, from pneumonia, followed a long illness.

The Trial of Mary Dugan (1929)
The Last of Mrs. Cheyney (1929)
Their Own Desire (1929)
The Divorcee (1930)
Let Us Be Gay (1930)
Strangers May Kiss (1931)
A Free Soul (1931)
Private Lives (1931)
Smilin' Through (1932) **Strange Interlude** (1932) **Riptide** (1934)
The Barretts of Wimpole Street (1934)
Romeo and Juliet (1936)
Marie Antoinette (1938)
Idiot's Delight (1939) **The Women** (1939)
Escape (1940)

Ally **Sheedy**
5ft 5in
(ALEXANDRA ELIZABETH SHEEDY)

Born: **June 13, 1962**
New York City, New York, USA

The daughter of John J. Sheedy Jr., a Manhattan advertising executive, who was from an Irish Catholic background, and his wife Charlotte – a Jewish writer and press agent, who was involved in the civil rights movement, Ally had a brother and a sister. She started ballet classes when she was six and danced with the American Ballet Theater until she was fourteen. When she was twelve, at Bank Street School, she wrote a best-selling children's book called "She Was Nice to Mice". After Columbia Grammar and Preparatory School, in New York, Ally studied Drama at the University of Southern California. In 1981, she made her TV debut, in an episode of 'CBS Afternoon Playhouse'. She was kept busy on the small screen until making her film debut, in *Bad Boys,* starring Sean Penn. She was an original 'Brat-Pack' member and matured into a fine actress in films like *High Art,* for which she won awards from Independent Spirit, Los Angeles Film Critics, and the National Society of Film Critics. In 1992, she married Angela Lansbury's actor nephew, David Lansbury. They have a daughter named Rebecca, but are currently filing for divorce.

Bad Boys (1983)
War Games (1983)
The Breakfast Club (1985)
Saint Elmo's Fire (1985)
Twice in a Lifetime (1985)
Short Circuit (1986)
Maid to Order (1987)
Betsy's Wedding (1990)
Fear (1990)
Only the Lonely (1991)
High Art (1998)
Sugar Town (1999)
The Autumn Heart (1999)
I'll Take You There (1999)
Just a Dream (2002)
Noise (2004)
Shooting Livien (2005)
Day Zero (2007)
Steam (2007)
Harold (2008)

Charlie **Sheen**
5ft 10in
(CARLOS IRWIN ESTÉVEZ)

Born: **September 3, 1965**
New York City, New York, USA

The son of the great movie actor, Martin Sheen, and the artist, Janet Templeton, Charlie has two brothers and a sister – all of whom are actors – using their original second name, Estévez. After his family went to live in Malibu, Charlie attended Santa Monica High School, where his prowess as pitcher and shortstop in the baseball team would prove useful in some of his films. With Martin as his dad, he could hardly ignore the movies. He started acting at the age of nine, and after being expelled from high school, he began his film career in 1984, in *Red Dawn*. Charlie appeared in big movies like *Platoon, Wall Street,* and *Young Guns,* but in the early 1990s, his career began to go into freefall. He was reported as being addicted to cocaine, and his first marriage, to Donna Peele, in 1995, was short-lived. The following year, Charlie became a born-again Christian, which brought a bit more stability into his life. In 2002, his marriage to actress Denise Richards produced two daughters. Four years later, that ended in divorce and a very acrimonious custody battle. He plays Charlie Harper, in the TV series, 'Two and a Half Men'.

Red Dawn (1984)
The Boys Next Door (1985)
Lucas (1986)
Ferris Bueller's Day Off (1986)
Platoon (1986) **No Man's
Land** (1987) **Wall Street** (1987)
Young Guns (1988) **Eight Men
Out** (1988) **Major League** (1989)
Cadence (1990) **Courage
Mountain** (1990) **The Rookie** (1990)
Hot Shots! (1991)
Beyond the Law (1992)
Loaded Weapon 1 (1993)
Hot Shots! Part Deux (1993)
The Chase (1994) **The Arrival** (1996)
Money Talks (1997)
Being John Malkovich (1999)
Good Advice (2001)
Deeper Than Deep (2003)
Scary Movie 3 (2003)
The Big Bounce (2004)

Martin **Sheen**
5ft 7in
(RAMON ANTONIO GERARD ESTÉVEZ)

Born: **August 3, 1940**
Dayton, Ohio, USA

The son of Francisco Estévez, a Spanish immigrant, and Mary Phelan, from County Tipperary, in Ireland – Martin, known as Ramón, (one of ten children – nine boys) was raised a Roman Catholic. His dad's job as sales representative for IBM, result- ed in the family living in Bermuda for a while. Martin, (the only one not born there) attended Mount Saint Agnes School. Back in the USA, he was educated at Chaminade High School in Dayton, before failing his entrance exam to the University of Ohio. His admiration for James Dean drew him to an acting career against his father's wishes. Martin acted on Broadway before his first TV role, in a 1961 episode of 'Route 66'. His film debut was in *The Incident,* in 1967. A forty-year career in movies has been highlighted by some fine portrayals in important productions such as *Badlands, Apocalypse Now, Gandhi, Wall Street, The American President* and *The Departed.* Martin and his wife Janet have been married since 1961. They are the parents of four actors – Charlie Sheen and the three Estévez siblings, Emilio, Renée and Ramon.

The Subject Was Roses (1968)
Catch-22 (1970) **Rage** (1972)
Badlands (1973)
The Cassandra Crossing (1976)
**The Little Girl Who Lives
Down the Lane** (1976)
Apocalypse Now (1979)
The Final Countdown (1980)
Ghandi (1982) **Enigma** (1983)
The Believers (1987)
Wall Street (1987) **Da** (1988)
When the Bough Breaks (1993)
Gettysburg (1993)
The American President (1995)
The War at Home (1996)
Entertaining Angels (1996)
A Texas Funeral (1999)
Catch Me If You Can (2002)
The Commission (2003)
Bobby (2006)
The Departed (2006)
Talk to Me (2007)

Michael **Sheen**
5ft 9in
(MICHAEL SHEEN)

Born: **February 5, 1969**
Newport, Gwent, Wales

Michael grew up in Port Talbot, in Wales. He was the only son of Meyrick and Irene Sheen, who worked in personnel manage- ment together. Meyrick earned extra money as a Jack Nicholson look-alike. Michael was educated at Glan Afan Comprehensive School, in Port Talbot. When he was sixteen he joined the National Youth Theater of Wales. After that he studied acting at the Royal Academy of Dramatic Art, in London. One of his first stage roles was as Mozart, in "Amadeus" at the Old Vic. In 1993, he joined the act- ing troupe, "Cheek By Jowl" and was nominated for the Ian Charleson Award for his acting in "Don't Fool With Love". His TV debut was that same year, when he starred in a mystery drama, 'Gallowglass'. Michael made his movie debut as Lodovico, in the Laurence Fishburne ver- sion of *Othello* and followed it with a good roles in *Mary Reilly* and *Wilde.* For five years after that, until *Heartlands,* Michael wasn't seen on the big screen. He con- centrated on the stage in plays such as "The Dresser" and "Look Back in Anger". In 2003 he portrayed Tony Blair, on TV, in 'The Deal' and played him again in the movie, *The Queen.* In the recent film, *Frost/Nixon,* Michael was a bit unlucky to be acting with Frank Langella, who was in top form as the disgraced president and was nominated for a Best Actor Oscar. Michael has a daughter from his relation- ship with Kate Beckinsale. In 2009, he was appointed OBE.

Othello (1995) **Mary Reilly** (1996)
Wilde (1997) **Heartlands** (2002)
The Four Feathers (2002)
Bright Young Things (2003)
Underworld (2003) **Dead Long
Enough** (2005) **Kingdom of
Heaven** (2005) **Underworld:
Evolution** (2006) **The Queen** (2006)
Blood Diamond (2006)
Music Within (2007) **Frost/Nixon** (2008)
**Underworld: Rise of
the Lycans** (2009)
The Damned United (2009)

Sam **Shepard**
6ft 1½in
(SAMUEL SHEPARD ROGERS III)

Born: **November 5, 1943**
Fort Sheridan, Illinois, USA

Sam's father, Samuel Shepard Rogers II, a teacher, had been a bomber pilot during the war. His mother, Elaine, was also a teacher. Reading and writing were instilled in Sam by his parents and although he dropped out of college, he was an educated man when he headed for New York City and began writing plays. He avoided the draft by pretending to be a heroin addict, and hung around in Greenwich Village. He had an early screen-writing credit with *Me and My Brother*, in 1968, and played drums in the band, 'The Holy Modal Rounders'. Their "Bird Song" was featured in *Easy Rider*. In 1970, Sam made his film debut in *Brand X,* but apart from stage acting, wasn't seen again until 1978, when *Days of Heaven* began a film career that has rarely failed to deliver the goods. Sam was nominated for a Best Supporting Actor Oscar, for *The Right Stuff* and since that year, 1983, Sam has been living with his occasional co-star, Jessica Lange. They have two children. For his work on TV, in 'Lily Dale' he won a Lone Star Film & Television Award and was nominated for an Emmy. Sam was seen on the big screen recently in the highly-rated crime drama, *Felon*.

Days of Heaven (1978)
Resurrection (1980) Raggedy Man (1981)
Frances (1982) The Right Stuff (1983)
Country (1984) Crimes of the
Heart (1986) Baby Boom (1987)
Steel Magnolias (1989)
Homo Faber (1991) Defenseless (1991)
Thunderheart (1992)
The Pelican Brief (1993)
Safe Passage (1994)
The Only Thrill (1997) Hamlet (2000)
The Pledge (2001) Swordfish (2001)
Black Hawk Down (2001) Leo (2002)
Blind Horizon (2003)
The Notebook (2004)
Don't Come Knocking (2005)
Bandidas (2006) The Assassination of
Jesse James (2007)
The Accidental Husband (2008)
Felon (2008)

Cybil **Shepherd**
5ft 8in
(CYBIL LYNNE SHEPHERD)

Born: **February 24, 1950**
Memphis, Tennessee, USA

The daughter of William Shepherd and his wife, Patty, Cybill had an ear for music and was five when she began singing along to Elvis Presley records. At nine, she was a member of the choir at Holy Communion Episcopal Church. At sixteen, she began vocal lessons with the coach from the Metropolitan Opera. That same year, she won the "Miss Teenage Memphis" contest - singing "Don't Think Twice It's All Right" and playing the ukulele. That exposure enabled her to become a successful model while she was still at East High School. In 1968, she was voted "Model of the Year". Her portrait on the cover of 'Glamour Magazine' caught the eye of film director, Peter Bogdanovich. Without any hesitation, he cast the inexperienced twenty-year-old – as Jacy Farrow – in his award-winning, *The Last Picture Show*. Cybill didn't give up her singing – she then featured jazz giant, Stan Getz, on her 1976 album "Cybill Getz Better" – and performed in New York. By the end of the 1970s, her career had slowed, but by 1985, she'd become a star all over again as Maddie Hayes, in the TV hit series 'Moonlighting'. It also did wonders for the newcomer, Bruce Willis. Her comedy series, 'Cybill' continued her success on the small screen. Twice married and divorced, Cybill has a daughter and twins. Much of Cybill's work during the past few years has been on television. Fans of her movies will be happy to know that she has four new ones lined up for release.

The Last Picture
Show (1971)
The Heartbreak Kid (1972)
Daisy Miller (1974)
Taxi Driver (1976)
Special Delivery (1976)
Silver Bears (1978)
The Lady Vanishes (1979)
Chances Are (1989)
Alice (1990)
Married to It (1991)
The Muse (1999)
Open Window (2006)

Ann **Sheridan**
5ft 5½in
(CLARA LOU SHERIDAN)

Born: **February 21, 1915**
Denton, Texas, USA
Died: **January 21, 1967**

A typical small town girl of the period, Ann was the daughter of a local automobile mechanic. She was the youngest of five children. When she grew up, she studied at North Texas Teachers' College, where she was a member of the girls' basketball team. One of her sisters sent a picture of her wearing a bathing suit, to Paramount Studios, who were running a "Search for Beauty" contest. She made her debut in the 1934 film of the same name, and signed a contract. After a dozen bit parts, the studio dropped her. She was unemployed until she was offered a contract by Warner Brothers, and was by then known as Ann. She appeared with Humphrey Bogart, in *The Black Legion* and went on to co-star with top stars – James Cagney, George Raft, Errol Flynn and Cary Grant. In 1939, she was named Max Factor's "Girl of the Year". By the mid-1950s, Ann's film career slowed, but she was seen on TV until 1967. She was married to three actors – the second of which was George Brent, but had no children. Ann died of cancer, in San Fernando Valley, California.

The Black Legion (1937) The Great
O'Malley (1937) San Quentin (1937)
Letter of Introduction (1938)
Angels with Dirty Faces (1938) They
Made Me a Criminal (1939)
Dodge City (1939)
Castle on the Hudson (1940)
It All Came True (1940)
Torrid Zone (1940)
They Drive By Night (1940)
City for Conquest (1940) Honeymoon
for Three (1941) The Man Who Came
to Dinner(1941) Kings Row (1942)
George Washington Slept Here (1942)
Edge of Darkness (1943) Shine On
Harvest Moon (1944)
One More Tomorrow (1946)
Nora Prentiss (1947)
The Unfaithful (1947) I Was a Male
War Bride (1949) Stella (1950)
Take Me to Town (1953)
Come Next Spring (1956)

Brooke **Shields**
6ft
(BROOKE CHRISTA CAMILLE SHIELDS)

Born: **May 31, 1965**
New York City, New York, USA

The daughter of Francis and Teri Shields, Brooke was a pretty baby, who appeared in an Ivory soap advertisement when she was an infant. She joined the Ford Model Agency, in New York, and in 1974, made her TV debut, in Arthur Miller's 'After the Fall'. Two years later, she made her film debut, in the horror film, *Communion.* Her break came in the French director, Louis Malle's essay on child prostitution in New Orleans – *Pretty Baby.* Brooke continued with her modeling career and when she was fourteen, she became the youngest-ever fashion model to grace the cover of Vogue magazine. She appeared in TV commercials for Calvin Klein Jeans – and even though her movies were a bit hit and miss, Brooke's was the most famous face around at the time. It was a huge error for her to star in a poor remake of *The Blue Lagoon,* in 1980, but she was wise to spend four years at Princetown University – from where she graduated in 1987, with a degree in French Literature. While she was studying, she took time off to appear in a Muppet movie. She had grown to her full adult height – which must have given casting directors a few problems at the time as well as frightening some of the shorter leading men. Her best break was on television, where in 1996, she began a successful four-year tenure in the title-role, of 'Suddenly Susan'. In 1997, she married the tennis champion, Andre Agassi, and it hit her hard when they were divorced two years later. She lives in New York with her second husband, TV writer, Chris Henchy, and their two daughters.

Communion (1976)
Pretty Baby (1978)
King of the Gypsies (1978)
Just You and Me, Kid (1979)
The Muppets Take Manhattan (1984)
Running Wild (1992)
Freaked (1993)
Freeway (1996)
The Misadventures of Margaret (1998)
The Weekend (1999)
Bob the Butler (2005)

Takashi **Shimura**
5ft 7in
(SHOJI SHIMAZAKI)

Born: **March 12, 1905**
Ikuno, Hyogo, Japan
Died: **February 11, 1982**

Takashi's background traces back to the samurai warriors. He grew up in the silver mining town of Ikuno, in southern Japan, Takashi's first experience of the theater world was when he visited the famous Takarazuka Grand Theater. He studied English at Kansai University before setting up an amateur drama group, called "Shichigatsu-za". In 1930, Takashi made his stage debut in Osaka, turned pro and toured with "Kindai-za". In 1934, he joined the Shinko Kinema Oizuni Studio, in Kyoto and began his film career, in *Chuji uridasu* in 1935. He married Masako, two years later and was a character actor until *Oshidori utagassen.* Too old for military service during World War II, he began to enjoy stardom and first acted for Akira Kurosawa in *Sugata Sanshiro.* He was the star of the director's propaganda film, *The Most Beautiful,* and became his second favorite actor – after Mifune – who Takashi first acted with in *Snow Trail.* He appeared in over two hundred films – the last one in 1980. He died of emphysema, in Tokyo.

Woman of Osaka (1936) **Chikemuri Takadanoba** (1937) **Oshidori utagassen** (1939) **Sugata Sanshiro** (1943) **They Who Step on the Tiger's Tail** (1945) **Those Who Make Tomorrow**(1946) **No Regrets for My Youth** (1946) **Snow Trail** (1947) **Drunken Angel** (1948) **A Silent Duel** (1949) **Stray Dog** (1949) **Scandal** (1950) **Rashômon** (1950) **Beyond Love and Hate** (1951) **The Idiot** (1951) **The Den of Beasts** (1951) **Vendetta of a Samurai** (1952) **Ikiru** (1952) **The Seven Samurai** (1954) **Godzilla** (1954) **I Live in Fear** (1955) **Bushido** (1956) **Macbeth** (1957) **The Hidden Fortress** (1958) **The Bad Sleep Well** (1960) **Sanjuro** (1962) **47 Samurai** (1962) **High and Low** (1963) **Japan's Longest Day** (1967)

Talia **Shire**
5ft 4in
(TALIA ROSE COPPOLA)

Born: **April 26, 1946**
Long Island, New York, USA

Talia was the youngest of three children born to an Italian American family. One of her brothers is the film director, Francis Ford Coppola. Talia's father, Carmine Coppola, had been first flautist under Arturo Toscanini, in the NBC Symphony Orchestra. He was also a composer. He'd met Talia's mother, Italia, when they were both studying at Juilliard. Because of her father's work, Talia moved many times – attending a number of Catholic schools. Because of her love for ballet, her first ambition was to become a choreographer. When she was nineteen, she accepted a scholarship to Yale School of Drama. Halfway through her second year, she dropped out and went to live in Los Angeles. Through her brother's contacts, she got small acting jobs, beginning with *The Wild Racers,* in 1968. In 1970, she married songwriter David Shire. With her new name, she acted in her brother's film, *The Godfather,* and was nominated as Best Supporting Actress for its sequel. Talia then co-starred with Sylvester Stallone in *Rocky,* for which she was Oscar-nominated as Best Actress. She had a son with Shire, and a son and a daughter from her second marriage, to producer, Jack Schwartzman.

The Godfather (1972)
Un homme est mort (1972)
The Godfather: Part II (1974)
Rocky (1976)
Rocky II (1979)
Rocky III (1982)
Rocky IV (1985) **Rad** (1986)
New York Stories (1989)
The Godfather: Part III (1990)
Bed & Breakfast (1991)
Caminho dos Sonhos (1998)
The Visit (2000)
The Whole Shebang (2001)
Family Tree (2003)
Dunsmore (2003)
Pomegranate (2005)
Looking for Palladin (2008)
Dim Sum Funeral (2008)

Elisabeth **Shue**
5ft 2in
(ELISABETH JUDSON SHUE)

Born: **October 6, 1963**
Wilmington, Delaware, USA

Lisa was born into money. Her father, James Shue, was a lawyer and real estate developer, who was also involved in Republican politics. Her mother, Anne was a vice president at the Chemical Banking Corporation. They divorced when Lisa was in fourth grade, but her educational progress was uninterrupted while she was growing up in New Jersey. After graduating from Columbia High School, in Maplewood, N.J., she attended the liberal arts Wellesley College, in Massachusetts and Harvard University. She withdrew from the latter to pursue an acting career – returning fifteen years later to complete her degree. During her time at High School, she acted in commercials for Burger King, DeBeers Diamonds, and Hellman's – so it was a natural step into movies. In 1982, she had a small role on TV in 'The Royal Romance of Charles and Diana'. Lisa's film debut came the following year, in *Somewhere, Tomorrow*, but it was her next movie – a featured role in *The Karate Kid* that put her on the road to stardom. Lisa is married to the movie and TV director and producer, Davis Guggenheim. They have two children.

The Karate Kid (1984)
Adventures in Babysitting (1987)
Cocktail (1988)
Back to the Future Part II (1989)
Back to the Future Part III (1990)
The Marrying Man (1991)
Soapdish (1991)
Twenty Bucks (1993)
Heart and Souls (1993)
Radio Inside (1994)
Underneath (1995)
Leaving Las Vegas (1995)
The Saint (1997)
Deconstructing Harry (1997)
Palmetto (1998)
Cousin Bette (1998)
Leo (2002) Mysterious Skin (2004)
Dreamer: Inspired by a
True Story (2005)
Gracie (2007)
Hamlet 2 (2008)

Sylvia **Sidney**
5ft 4in
(SOPHIA KOSOW)

Born: **August 8, 1910**
The Bronx, New York City, New York, USA
Died: **July 1, 1999**

Sweet Sylvia's father, Victor Kosow, was a Russian Jewish immigrant – her mother was Rumanian. After studying dancing as a child, Sylvia enrolled at the Theater Guild School, at the age of fifteen. She made her stage debut, in Washington, the following year, in "The Challenge of Youth". After a year or so on the stage, Sylvia made her film debut in 1927, in *Broadway Nights*. Her first talkie was *Thru Different Eyes,* in 1929. Despite her strong Bronx accent, she adjusted her speech quickly and was put under contract by Paramount. When the studio head, B.P. Schulberg fell in love with her and destroyed his marriage, she left and signed with Walter Wanger. Her first movie under his banner was the excellent *The Trail of the Lonesome Pine* – shot in early Technicolor. A series of good roles soon followed – including movies directed by Fritz Lang – *Fury,* and Alfred Hitchcock – *Sabotage.* Sylvia was nominated for a Best Supporting Actress Oscar for *Summer Wishes, Winter Dreams*, and worked on stage and television right up to the year she died of throat cancer, in New York. Sylvia was married three times – one of her husbands was actor, Luther Adler.

City Streets (1931)
An American Tragedy (1931)
Street Scene (1931)
Ladies of the Big House (1931)
The Miracle Man (1932)
Merrily We Go to Hell (1932)
Thirty Day Princess (1934)
The Trail of the
Lonesome Pine (1936) Fury (1936)
Sabotage (1936)
You Only Live Once (1937)
Dead End (1937)
You and Me (1938)
The Wagons Roll at Night (1941)
Blood on the Sun (1945)
The Searching Wind (1946)
Les Miserables (1952)
Summer Wishes,
Winter Dreams (1973)

Simone **Signoret**
5ft 6in
(SIMONE HENRIETTE CHARLOTTE KAMINKER)

Born: **March 25, 1921**
Wiesbaden, Germany
Died: **September 30, 1985**

Simone's father, André Kaminker, was a French Army officer who was stationed in Germany with the occupation forces after World War I. He and his wife, Georgette, took Simone and her two young brothers back to Paris in the mid-1920s. After she left school, Simone earned a teaching certificate in Latin and English, but acting had already become her passion. She studied acting with Solange Siccard, and after her father, (who was Jewish), fled to England in 1940, she adopted her mother's name. She made her film debut, in 1942, in *Le Prince Charmant.* She played small roles in films, without a permit during the Nazi occupation. In 1944, she married director, Yves Allégret, and first tasted fame in his film, *Woman of Antwerp.* Simone became one of the greatest French film stars of the post-war years – appearing in such classics as *La Ronde* and *Casque d'Or* – and won a Best Actress Oscar, for *Room at the Top.* In 1951, she married singer/actor, Yves Montand, with whom she frequently co-starred, until her death in Normandy, from pancreatic cancer.

Fantômas (1947) Woman of
Antwerp (1948) Gunman in the
Streets (1950) Manèges (1950)
La Ronde (1950) Casque d'Or (1952)
Thérèse Raquin (1953)
Les Diaboliques (1955)
La Mort en ce jardin (1956)
Les Sorcières de Salem (1957)
Room at the Top (1959)
Term of Trial (1962) Le Jour et
l'heure (1963) Ship of Fools (1965)
The Sleeping car Murders (1965)
The Deadly Affair (1966)
Games (1967)
The American (1969)
Army of Shadows (1969)
The Confession (1970) The Cat (1971)
La Veuve Couderc (1971)
Les Granges brulées (1973)
Police Python 357 (1976) Madame
Rosa (1977) L'Adolescente (1979)
Chère inconnue (1980)

Ron **Silver**
5ft 8½in
(RONALD SILVER)

Born: **July 2, 1946**
New York City, New York, USA

Ron's father, Irving, worked in the clothing business. His mother, May, was a teacher. Ron grew up in the Lower East Side of Manhattan and was educated at the Hebrew Institute. He later attended Stuyvesant High School and graduated from the University of Buffalo, with a Bachelor of Arts in Spanish and Chinese. He received a masters in Chinese History from St. John's University, and during that time, took acting lessons at the Herbert Berghof Studio, and also studied with Uta Hagen and Lee Strasberg. He could have become a diplomat or a politician (which he may do). As things transpired, following a spell of teaching Spanish for much of the 1960s, he became an actor. In 1973, Ron got good exposure in the cast of the stage satire, "El Grande De Coca-Cola". He moved to California and had a regular spot in the TV series, 'Rhoda'. In 1975, he began a twenty-two-year marriage to Lynne Miller, with whom he had two children. Ron made his film debut in 1976, in the comedy, *Tunnel Vision*, but his first important movie role was in the very serious drama, *Silkwood*. He has directed and produced for both films and television. On television in recent years, Ron was seen as Bruno Gianelli, in several episodes of 'The West Wing'. His latest movie role was in *Distance Runners,* which was shot in Shanghai, China.

The Entity (1981)
Best Friends (1982)
Silkwood (1983)
Garbo Talks (1984)
Enemies: A Love Story (1989)
Reversal of Fortune (1990)
Married to It (1991)
Mr. Saturday Night (1992)
Timecop (1994)
The Arrival (1996)
Danger Zone (1997)
Festival in Cannes (2001)
Ali (2001)
Find Me Guilty (2006)
The Ten (2007)
Distance Runners (2008)

Phil **Silvers**
6ft
(PHILIP SILVER)

Born: **May 11, 1911**
New York City, New York, USA
Died: **November 1, 1985**

Phil was the youngest of eight children born to a Jewish couple in Brooklyn. His father was one of the workers who built the original New York skyscrapers. When he was eleven, Phil was employed at a local movie theater to sing whenever the projector broke down. At fourteen, he left school to work in vaudeville as a stooge. In 1937, he began appearing in a series of musical shorts shot in New York, beginning with *Ups and Downs,* which starred June Allyson. Around that time, Phil appeared on Broadway, in a short-lived show called "Yokel". He must have been impressive because critics took a liking to him. He went to Hollywood on a wave of confidence and had a small part in the Rooney/Garland musical, *Strike Up the Band,* but his scenes were deleted. Later that year, he was featured in *Hit Parade of 1941.* For the next dozen or so years Phil was supporting comic in several musicals and worked with such stars as Betty Grable, Gene Kelly and Judy Garland. He also wrote the lyrics for the Sinatra hit, "Nancy (With the Laughing Face)". He had a big hit on Broadway in 1952, in "Top Banana", which won him a Tony. In 1955, he starred in 'The Phil Silvers Show' on TV. 'Sergeant Bilko' made him more famous than ever. Phil had five daughters with his second wife, Evelyn. He died of a heart attack, in Century City, California.

Roxy Hart (1942) Footlight
Serenade (1942) Coney Island (1943)
A Lady Takes a Chance (1943)
Four Jills in a Jeep (1944)
Cover Girl (1944)
Diamond Horseshoe (1945)
Don Juan Quilligan (1945)
A Thousand and One Nights (1945)
If I'm Lucky (1946)
Summer Stock (1950) Lucky Me (1954)
It's a Mad Mad Mad
Mad World (1963)
A Funny Thing Happened on the
Way to the Forum (1966)
Buona Sera, Mrs. Campbell (1968)

Alastair **Sim**
5ft 11in
(ALASTAIR SIM)

Born: **October 9, 1900**
Edinburgh, Scotland
Died: **August 19, 1976**

Alastair's father, Alexander Sim, was a Justice of the Peace as well as being a successful businessman in Edinburgh. His mother was the former Isabella McIntyre. Alexander owned and ran, among other things, an exclusive tailor's shop, which provided his son with his first job upon leaving George Heriot's School. He didn't last long as a suit maker – he trained as a teacher – supplementing his income by giving elocution lessons and finally being appointed as a drama coach and elocution lecturer at New College, Edinburgh University. His deep love for the theater took him to London in 1930, where, although he'd only ever acted in amateur productions, he was able to make his professional stage debut with a walk-on in "Othello", starring Paul Robeson. He did a season at the Old Vic then, in 1932, he married Naomi Plaskitt, with whom he had a daughter. Naomi was his wife until he died. In 1935, Alastair made his film debut in *The Riverside Murder.* After that he was kept too busy to do much in the theater. Prematurely bald, looking middle-aged at thirty, he became a big favorite with roles in *Green for Danger, Scrooge,* and the *St. Trinian's* films being most memorable. Alastair died of cancer, in London.

Cottage to Let (1941)
Waterloo Road (1945)
Green for Danger (1946)
Hue and Cry (1947)
Captain Boycott (1947)
London Belongs to Me (1948)
Stage Fright (1950)
The Happiest Days
of Your Life (1950)
Laughter in Paradise (1951)
Scrooge (1951)
Folly to Be Wise (1953)
An Inspector Calls (1954)
The Belles of St. Trinian's (1954)
Geordie (1955) Escapade (1955)
The Green Man (1956)
Blue Murder at St. Trinian's (1957)
School for Scoundrels (1960)

Jean **Simmons**
5ft 6in
(JEAN MERILYN SIMMONS)

Born: **January 31, 1929**
Crouch End, London, England

Jean went to Orange Hill School for Girls, in Edgware. She was evacuated to Somerset at the start of World War II, but returned to attend a dancing school. Producer Val Guest paid a visit to the school and Jean was selected to make her film debut in 1944, in *Give Us the Moon.* She became every British schoolboy's dream girl, as Estella, in *Great Expectations.* Following her first starring role, in *Uncle Silas,* Jean was nominated for a Best Supporting Actress Oscar, in Olivier's *Hamlet.* British filmgoers loved her and when they co-starred in *Adam and Evelyne,* Stewart Granger did too. He left his wife and married her in 1950. They went to Hollywood, where they co-starred in *Young Bess,* but by the time they got divorced in 1960, her career had totally outstripped his – with a list of credits which include *Guys and Dolls, The Big Country* and *Elmer Gantry.* She married Richard Brooks, who directed her Best Actress Oscar-nominated role, in *The Happy Ending.* They divorced in 1977. In the 1980s, she overcame alcoholism. Jean, who recently finished a starring role in the film, *Shadows in the Sun,* lives in Santa Monica, with her dog and two cats.

Great Expectations (1946)
Black Narcissus (1947)
Uncle Silas (1947) Hamlet (1948)
The Blue Lagoon (1949)
Adam and Evelyne (1949)
So Long at the Fair (1950)
The Clouded Yellow (1951)
Angel Face (1952) Young Bess (1953)
The Robe (1953) The Actress (1953)
The Egyptian (1954)
Footsteps in the Fog (1955)
Guys and Dolls (1955)
This Could Be the Night (1957)
Until They Sail (1957)
The Big Country (1958)
Home Before Dark (1959)
Elmer Gantry (1959)
All the Way Home (1963)
Life at the Top (1965)
The Happy Ending (1969)

Michel **Simon**
5ft 6in
(FRANÇOIS MICHEL SIMON)

Born: **April 9, 1895**
Geneva, Switzerland
Died: **May 30, 1975**

The son of a sausage-maker, Michel was born in the same year as the Cinema. When he was fifteen, he left home and went to Paris. In 1912, he began appearing as half of a comic duo, "Ribert & Simon" at the Casino in Montreuil-sous-Bois. In 1914, he was conscripted into the army, but released after contracting tuberculosis. He became an actor with Pitoëff's company and in 1924, Louis Jouvet cast him in "Jean de Lune". Michel made his first film appearance in 1924, in *La Galerie des monstres.* With the advent of sound, he imposed himself on the French Cinema in classics such as *L'Atlante, Drôle de drame* and *Le Quai des brumes.* It slowed a little during the 1950s, when he was partially paralyses after an accident involving make-up dye. He was soon active again – producing great performances right up to the year of his death from heart failure, at his home in Bry-sur-Marne, France.

La Chienne (1931) Boudu sauvé
des eaux (1932) L'Atlante (1934)
Le Bonheur (1934) Amants et
voleurs (1935) Le Mort en fuite (1936)
Drôle de drame (1937) Boys'
School (1938) Le Quai des
brumes (1938) La Fin du jour (1939)
Le Dernier tournant (1939)
Fric-Frac (1939) Circonstances
atténuantes (1939) Les Musiciens
de ciel (1940) Un ami viendra ce
soir (1946) Panique (1947)
Not Guilty (1947) Fabiola (1949)
La Beauté du diable (1950)
La Poison (1951)
The Virtuous Scoundrel (1953)
The Strange Desire of
Monsieur Bard (1954)
It Happened in Broad Daylight (1958)
Candide (1960) The Devil and
the Ten Commandments (1962)
The Train (1964)
Le Vieil homme et l'enfant (1967)
Blanche (1971) The Most Wonderful
Evening of My Life (1972)
L'Ibis rouge (1975)

Simone **Simon**
5ft 2in
(SIMONE THÉRÈSE FERNANDE SIMON)

Born: **April 23, 1910**
Marseille, Provence, Côte d'Azur, France
Died: **February 22, 2005**

The daughter of a French engineer, Henri Louis Fermin, and an Italian mother named Erma Giorcelli, Simone grew up in the city of Marseille. She went to Paris in 1931 and worked as an artist's model and briefly as a singer. Simone made her film debut that same year, in *Le Chanteur inconnu.* By 1935, she had appeared in fifteen movies and was very popular in France. Her ability to speak English got her a role in the Hollywood film, *Girls' Dormitory,* where she was billed above a young hopeful called Tyrone Power. She remained with 20th Century Fox until 1938, when she returned to France to star with Jean Gabin, in Jean Renoir's classic version of Zola's *La Bête humaine.* As World War II began, she went back to America and starred in *The Devil and Daniel Webster,* and *Cat People* and its sequel, but the fame they brought her did not translate into international stardom. Simone made her final film, *La Femme en bleu,* in 1973. Simone had many love affairs, but she never married. She died of natural causes, in Paris.

L'Étoile de Valencia (1933)
Les Beaux jours (1935)
Girls' Dormitory (1936)
Ladies in Love (1936)
Seventh Heaven (1937)
Josette (1938)
La Bête humaine (1938)
Cavalcade d'amour (1940)
The Devil and
Daniel Webster (1941)
Cat People (1942)
Mademoiselle Fifi (1944)
The Curse of the
Cat People (1944)
Johnny Doesn't
Live Here Any More (1944)
Pétrus (1946) La Ronde (1950)
Donne senza nome (1950)
Olivia (1951)
Le plaisir (1952)
I tre ladri (1954)
A Double Life (1954)

Frank **Sinatra**
5ft 7in
(FRANCIS ALBERT SINATRA)

Born: **December 12, 1915**
Hoboken, New Jersey, USA
Died: **May 14, 1998**

The only child of Sicilian fireman, Anthony Sinatra, and an Italian midwife/abortionist, Natalie Garaventi (known as Dolly), Frank left school early to set the bench mark for the art of crooning. He began his career with vocal group – the "Hoboken Four", in 1935. Four years later, he married Nancy Barbato and joined Harry James. In 1940, he stepped up a division with the Tommy Dorsey band and became the most famous popular singer in the world. He left in 1942, and after his film debut, in *Higher and Higher,* he was out on his own – with a Columbia records contract and movies – including the classic musical – *On the Town.* Vocal problems in 1950, and a hectic affair with Ava Gardner, whom he married in 1951 heralded a two-year slump, but he bounced back with an Oscar-winning portrayal in *From Here to Eternity. Young at Heart, Guys and Dolls, The Man with the Golden Arm, High Society* and *Pal Joey,* were a few screen gems he left us. There were also several great vocal albums. Despite increasingly poor health, Frank kept going until 1995. He died of heart and kidney disease and bladder cancer, in Los Angeles.

Higher and Higher (1943)
Step Lively (1944) **Anchors Aweigh** (1945)
It Happened in Brooklyn (1947)
Take Me Out to the Ball Game (1949)
On the Town (1949)
Meet Danny Wilson (1951)
From Here to Eternity (1953)
Suddenly (1954) **Young at Heart** (1954)
Not as a Stranger (1955)
Guys and Dolls (1955) **The Tender Trap** (1955) **The Man with the Golden Arm** (1955) **High Society** (1956)
The Joker Is Wild (1957) **Pal Joey** (1957)
Kings Go Forth (1958) **Some Came Running** (1958) **Can-Can** (1960)
Ocean's Eleven (1960) **The Manchurian Candidate** (1962) **Robin and the 7 Hoods** (1964) **Von Ryan's Express** (1965) **Tony Rome** (1967)
The Detective (1968)

Sir Donald **Sinden**
6ft
(DONALD ALFRED SINDEN)

Born: **October 9, 1923**
Plymouth, Devon, England

The son of a pharmacist, Alfred Sinden, and his wife Mabel, Donald's ambition when leaving school was to train as an architect. Two factors changed his plans: firstly, he acted in an amateur stage production, which he enjoyed. Then, when volunteering for military service, he was turned down because he was asthmatic, and was given the chance to entertain the troops with ENSA. He went to drama school, and made his professional debut, in 1942, at the Theater Royal Brighton, in "George and Margaret". In 1946, he joined the Shakespeare Memorial Theater. He was established as an actor by the time he was offered his film debut in *Portrait from Life,* in 1948. But it was five years after that, when he got regular movie roles, beginning with *The Cruel Sea,* and during a vintage year, appearing with Gable, Gardner and Kelly, in *Mogambo.* By the early 1960s, he'd starred in twenty films, but was then only seen on stage and TV for ten years. In 1963, he became a stalwart of the Royal Shakespeare Company – acting in a number of classics as well as modern comedies. He returned to films in *Villain,* and has been a supporting player in movies for another thirty years. In 1990, he acted in a solo presentation of "Oscar Wilde" and is still busy on television – most notably in the series, 'Judge John Deed'. Donald's wife for fifty-six years, Diana Mahony, died in 2004. They had two sons.

The Cruel Sea (1953)
Mogambo (1953)
A Day to Remember (1953)
Doctor in the House (1954)
The Beachcomber (1954)
Simba (1955)
Above Us the Waves (1955)
Eyewitness (1956)
Tiger in the Smoke (1956)
The Captain's Table (1959)
The Siege of Sidney Street (1960)
Villain (1971) **The Day of the Jackal** (1973) **The Island at the Top of the World** (1974)
The Accidental Detective (2003)

Jeremy **Sisto**
6ft 1¹/₂in
(JEREMY MERTON SISTO)

Born: **October 6, 1974**
Grass Valley, California, USA

Jeremy spent his first few years in Grass Valley, in Northern California. His father, Dick Sisto, was a farmer who became a jazz musician. Jeremy's mother, Reedy, was an actress. His parents divorced when he was six years old and after his mother married another actor, Jeremy and his older sister, Meadow, were raised in Chicago. There, he attended the Francis W. Parker School – founded by a champion of progressive education. When he was ten, he appeared in the video for the "Twisted Sister" track, "We're Not Gonna Take It". Through that mind-expanding and interesting exposure and enthusiastic encouragement from his sister, Jeremy got seriously interested in acting. When he was seventeen, he made his film debut in the crime drama, *Grand Canyon.* His big break was in Ridley Scott's *White Squall.* Since then, with his willingness to work in small-budget productions and to support independent filmmakers, Jeremy's had as much work as he wanted. Appearances in the TV-series 'Six Feet Under' did him no harm. He won a Special Jury Award at Cinequest San Jose Film Festival, for *The Movie Hero.* He was married for nine years to the actress, Marisa Ryan.

Grand Canyon (1991)
Clueless (1995)
White Squall (1996)
Oakland Underground (1997)
Suicide Kings (1997)
Without Limits (1998)
Trash (1999)
This Space Between Us (2000)
Takedown (2000)
Angel Eyes (2001)
May (2002)
Thirteen (2003)
The Movie Hero (2003)
Wrong Turn (2003)
One Point O (2004)
The Nickel Children (2005)
In Memory of My Father (2005)
Unknown (2006)
Waitress (2007)
Gardens of the Night (2008)

Red **Skelton**
6ft 1in
(RICHARD BERNARD SKELTON)

Born: **July 18, 1913**
Vincennes, Indiana, USA
Died: **September 17, 1997**

Red's father, a circus clown by the name of Joe Skelton, died only weeks before he was born. Raised by his mother, a cleaning woman, the youngster was a great help to her, taking a job selling newspapers when he was seven. One day, the actor, Ed Wynn, bought a paper from him and took him to meet the other members of his show. Within seven years, Red had begun his own career in vaudeville, minstrel shows, and even his dad's old circus. He was twenty-seven when he married his first wife, Edna Stillwell, who wrote a lot of his early material. When they divorced in 1943, Red was a big movie star. He'd made his debut in *Having Wonderful Time*. For twenty-five years, he retained his fan following – in popular films such as *Ziegfeld Follies, The Yellow Cab Man* and *Three Little Words*. When that ground to a halt, he had a good career on television. Red married twice more and in the 1970s, retired to paint pictures of clowns – which made him a second fortune. He died of pneumonia at his home in California.

Having Wonderful Time (1938)
Flight Command (1940)
The People vs. Dr. Kildare (1941)
Whistling in the Dark (1941)
Lady Be Good (1941)
Ship Ahoy (1942)
Maisie Gets Her Man (1942)
Panama Hattie (1942)
Whistling in Dixie (1942)
Du Barry Was a Lady (1943)
I Dood It (1943)
Whistling in Brooklyn (1943)
Bathing Beauty (1944)
Ziegfeld Follies (1946)
The Show-Off (1946)
Merton of the Movies (1947)
The Fuller Brush Man (1948)
A Southern Yankee (1948)
Neptune's Daughter (1949)
The Yellow Cab Man (1950)
Three Little Words (1950)
Excuse My Dust (1951)
Lovely to Look At (1952)

Tom **Skerritt**
6ft
(THOMAS ALDERTON SKERRITT)

Born: **August 25, 1933**
Detroit, Michigan, USA

Tom was the son of a businessman, Roy Skerritt and his wife, Helen. He graduated from Mackenzie High School, in Detroit, in 1953. After four years in the United States Airforce, Tom returned to Detroit, where he attended Wayne State University. It was there that he overcame a natural shyness by acting in plays. He joined the Dearborn Players, in Michigan, and for two years, appeared with them in summer stock. Tom then studied TV production at UCLA and was noticed by talent scouts when he appeared in the college production of "The Rainmaker". He married the first of his three wives in 1960, and two years later, he made his film debut, in *War Hunt*. For some time after that he was mainly seen on TV - in series such as 'Laramie', 'The Real McCoys', and 'My Three Sons'. His first big movie, was *MASH* – when he was third-billed below Donald Sutherland and Elliott Gould. Highlights of his career are his Captain Dallas, in *Alien* and as Viper in *Top Gun*. Since 1998, Tom's been happily married to Julie Tokashiki. In recent years, he's been seen on TV as William Walker, in the series, 'Brothers & Sisters'.

Those Calloways (1965)
MASH (1970)
Wild Rovers (1971)
Harold and Maude (1971)
Fuzz (1972)
Thieves Like Us (1974)
Big Bad Mama (1974)
The Turning Point (1977)
Ice Castles (1978) Alien (1979)
Silence of the North (1981)
Fighting Back (1982)
The Dead Zone (1983)
Top Gun (1986)
Maid to Order (1987)
Steel Magnolias (1989)
A River Runs Through It (1992)
Singles (1992) Contact (1997)
The Other Sister (1999)
Changing Hearts (2002)
Tears of the Sun (2003)
Swing (2003) Bonneville (2006)
The Velveteen Rabbit (2007)

Christian **Slater**
5ft 8½in
(CHRISTIAN MICHAEL LEONARD HAWKINS)

Born: **August 18, 1969**
New York City, New York, USA

Christian had the right background to become a movie star. His father, Mike, was an actor in soaps, and his mother, Mary Jo Slater – from whom he took his stage name – was a casting executive. In 1976, Christian made his first television appearance, in 'The Edge of Night'. He was educated at the private Dalton School, the Professional Children's School, and the LaGuardia High School of Music & Art and Performing Arts. In 1980, he made his Broadway debut in a revival of "The Music Man". In 1981, Christian appeared in a TV version of 'Sherlock Holmes', which starred Frank Langella. His film debut was in *The Legend of Billie Jean* – his co-star was Helen Slater – who is *not* his sister. His first important role was in *The Name of the Rose*. Christian has continued to impress on Broadway and in films. He shared an ensemble award at the Hollywood Film Festival, for *Bobby*. From 2000 he was married for six years to Ryan Haddon, from whom he is now divorced. They are both devoted to raising their son, Jaden, and daughter, Eliana.

The Legend of Billie Jean (1985)
The Name of the Rose (1986)
Tucker: The Man and
His Dream (1988) Heathers (1989)
The Wizard (1989)
Young Guns II (1990)
Pump Up the Volume (1990)
Robin Hood: Prince of
Thieves (1968)
Untamed Heart (1993)
True Romance (1993)
Interview with the Vampire (1994)
Murder in the First (1995)
Broken Arrow (1996)
Julian Po (1997) Hard Rain (1998)
Basil (1998)
Very Bad Things (1998)
The Contender (2000)
Who Is Cletis Tout? (2001)
Mindhunters (2004)
Bobby (2006)
He Was a Quiet Man (2007)
Lies & Illusions (2009)

Walter **Slezak**
6ft 3½in
(WALTER SLEZAK)

Born: **May 3, 1902**
Vienna, Austro-Hungary
Died: **April 21, 1983**

Walter was the son of the noted Viennese opera star, Leo Slezak, and the brother of Margarete, who was also a fine singer. After finishing his schooling, he studied Medicine for a while before dropping out to start work in a bank. His compatriot, Michael Curtiz, persuaded the amiable giant to appear in the 1922 film, *Sodom und Gomorrha*. After his twentieth German-language film – his first 'talkie' - in 1932 – Walter emigrated to the United States. His English was poor to begin with, but he managed to get small parts in several Broadway plays. In 1942, Walter married Johanna Van Ryn, who was his wife until his death. They had three children – one of them, Erika, became an actress. He made his American film debut in *Once Upon a Honeymoon* and for twenty years, was a well-loved actor in strong supporting roles including *Lifeboat, The Princess and the Pirate, The Inspector General* and *Call Me Madam*. In 1962, he published his autobiography entitled "What Time Is The Next Swan?" His last movie role was as Squire Trelawney, in the 1972 version of *Treasure Island*. Following a long spell of deteriorating health, Walter shot himself in the backyard of his home in Flower Hill, New York, two weeks before his eighty-first birthday.

Once Upon a Honeymoon (1942)
This Land Is Mine (1943) **The Fallen**
Sparrow (1943) Lifeboat (1944)
Till We Meet Again (1944)
The Princess and the Pirate (1944)
The Spanish Main (1945)
Cornered (1945) **Sinbad the**
Sailor (1947) **Born to Kill** (1947)
Riffraff (1947) **The Pirate** (1948)
The Inspector General (1949)
The Yellow Cab Man (1950)
People Will Talk (1951)
Call Me Madam (1953)
Come September (1961)
The Wonderful World
of the Brothers Grimm (1962)
Emil and the Detectives (1964)

Everett **Sloane**
5ft 7in
(EVERETT SLOANE)

Born: **October 1, 1909**
New York City, New York, USA
Died: **August 6, 1965**

Born into a wealthy Jewish family, Everett did well at school and went on to attend the University of Pennsylvania. Because of his passion for the stage, he dropped out when he was offered the chance to join a theater company. It didn't go too well at first and in the 1928, he became a runner on Wall Street. The 1929 stock market crash sent him scurrying back to the stage and by the early 1930s, he had established himself as an actor of promise. Fame would come Everett's way when he joined Orson Welles, at his fledgling Mercury Theater in 1937. Radio and stage plays followed, but it was Orson's *Citizen Kane* which brought varying degrees of stardom to its cast. Everett didn't have the looks for leading roles, but he was superb in character parts, especially as a jealous husband faced with the threat from a handsome younger man as in *The Lady from Shanghai*. His own marriage was an enduring one – Lillian Herman, with whom he had two children, was his wife from 1933 until his death. Everett's last movie was *The Disorderly Orderly*, and he went on working for one more year. Believing that he was going blind, he took his own life, at his home in Los Angeles.

Citizen Kane (1941)
Journey Into Fear (1943)
The Lady from Shanghai (1947)
Prince of Foxes (1949)
The Men (1950)
The Enforcer (1951)
Sirocco (1951)
The Desert Fox (1951)
The Blue Veil (1951)
The Sellout (1952)
Way of a Gaucho (1952)
The Big Knife (1955)
Patterns (1956)
Somebody Up There
Likes Me (1956)
Lust for Life (1956)
Marjorie Morningstar (1958)
Home from the Hill (1960)
The Disorderly Orderly (1964)

Alexis **Smith**
5ft 9in
(GLADYS SMITH)

Born: **June 8, 1921**
Penticton, British Columbia, Canada
Died: **June 9, 1993**

When she was a little girl, Alexis' family moved to Los Angeles and she was raised in the United States. At the age of ten, she appeared in the chorus of "Carmen" at the Hollywood Bowl. While at Hollywood High School, Alexis won a California State acting contest and she went to study drama at L.A. City College. After a screen test by Warner Bros., she got a contact. Her first screen appearance was in 1940, in one of the "Broadway Brevity" shorts – *Alice in Movieland*. Her height proved something of a barrier with so many small leading men in movies at that time. After nine uncredited roles, Alexis acted with three of the right stature – Flynn, MacMurray and Bellamy, in *Dive Bomber*. Errol was more than happy to repeat the pleasure, in *Gentleman Jim*. After that, even Bogart wasn't afraid of her – she appeared with him in *Conflict* and *The Two Mrs. Carrolls*. In 1944, she married Craig Stevens. They were still together when Alexis died of brain cancer in Los Angeles. The year she died, Alexis had a good role in Scorsese's *The Age of Innocence*.

Dive Bomber (1941)
The Smiling Ghost (1941)
Steel Against the Sky (1941)
Gentleman Jim (1942)
The Constant Nymph (1943)
The Adventures of Mark Twain (1944)
The Doughgirls (1944)
The Horn Blows at Midnight (1945)
Conflict (1945) **Rhapsody in Blue** (1945)
San Antonio (1945) **Of Human**
Bondage (1946) **The Two Mrs.**
Carrolls (1947) **The Woman in**
White (1948) **Whiplash** (1948)
South of St. Louis (1949)
Here Comes the Groom (1951)
The Turning Point (1952)
Split Second (1953) **The Sleeping**
Tiger (1954) **Beau James** (1957)
The Young Philadelphians (1959)
The Little Girl Who Lives Down the
Lane (1976) **The Trout** (1982)
The Age of Innocence (1993)

Kent **Smith**
6ft

(FRANK KENT SMITH)

Born: **March 19, 1907**
New York City, New York, USA
Died: **April 23, 1985**

The son of a hotelier, Kent was raised in a comfortable family environment. He had his first taste of show business as a child, when he assisted a magician. Kent was educated in New York and at a boarding school – Phillips Exeter Academy. Kent made his theatrical debut in 1929, in Baltimore. While completing his studies at Harvard University, he became one of the University Players, in West Falmouth. In 1932, he made his Broadway debut, in "Men Must Fight". He established himself on the New York stage, working with such big names as Ethel Barrymore and Lillian Gish. He went to Hollywood in 1936 to make his film debut, in MGM's *The Garden Murder Case*. It didn't result in a contract. Kent returned home, where three years later, he was cast in *Back Door to Heaven*, but suffered the humiliation of being replaced by Van Heflin, after shooting had begun. He married actress, Betty Gillette, and they had a daughter. Fame was his after he acted in the cult horror film, *Cat People* and he worked for thirty-five more years. He remarried in 1962, and died of heart disease in Woodland Hills, California.

Cat People (1942) **Hitler's
Children** (1943) **Forever and a Day** (1943)
This Land Is Mine (1943)
The Curse of the Cat People (1944)
The Spiral Staircase (1945)
Nora Prentiss (1947) **Magic Town** (1947)
The Voice of the Turtle (1947) **The
Fountainhead** (1949) **My Foolish
Heart** (1949) **The Damned Don't
Cry** (1950) **This Side of the Law** (1950)
Paula (1952) **Sayonara** (1957)
Imitation General (1958) **The
Badlanders** (1958) **Party Girl** (1958)
This Earth Is Mine (1959)
Strangers When We Meet (1960)
Susan Slade (1961) **The Balcony** (1963)
A Distant Trumpet (1964) **Youngblood
Hawke** (1964) **The Trouble with
Angels** (1966) **A Covenant with
Death** (1967) **Games** (1967)
Death of a Gunfighter (1969)

Dame Maggie **Smith**
5ft 5in

(MARGARET NATALIE SMITH)

Born: **December 28, 1934**
Ilford, Essex, England

Maggie's father, Nathaniel Smith, came from Newcastle-upon-Tyne, in north-east England. Her mother, Margaret, was a Scot from Glasgow. The family (including twin brothers) moved to Oxford in 1939, when her dad got a job as a public health pathologist at the University. Maggie left Oxford High School at sixteen, to join the Oxford Playhouse, where she was taught the basics of the acting profession. She appeared in many stage productions and acted at the Edinburgh Festival. She made her London debut in the aptly titled "Oxford Accents" and in 1955, began TV work. Maggie made a rather cautious entry into films, when, after her debut, in 1958's *Nowhere to Go* – there was a four year gap. Maggie's fine film portraits have so far yielded six Oscar nominations – she was voted Best Actress, for *The Prime of Miss Jean Brodie* and Best Supporting Actress, for *California Suite*. Maggie was married twice – first, to the distinguished actor, Robert Stephens, which resulted in two boys who have followed their parents into the acting profession.

The V.I.P.s (1963) **The Pumpkin
Eater** (1964) **Othello** (1965) **The Honey
Pot** (1967) **Hot Millions** (1968)
The Prime of Miss Jean Brodie (1969)
Travels with My Aunt (1972)
Murder by Death (1976)
Death on the Nile (1978)
California Suite (1978) **Quartet** (1981)
Clash of the Titans (1981)
Evil Under the Sun (1982)
The Missionary (1982) **A Private
Function** (1984) **A Room with a
View** (1985) **The Lonely Passion of
Judith Hearne** (1987) **Sister Act** (1992)
The Secret Garden (1993)
Washington Square (1997)
Tea with Mussolini (1999)
**Harry Potter and the Sorcerer's
Stone** (2001) **Gosford Park** (2001)
Ladies in Lavender (2004)
Keeping Mum (2005)
Becoming Jane (2007)
The Order of the Phoenix (2007)

Will **Smith**
6ft 2½in

(WILLARD CHRISTOPHER SMITH JR.)

Born: **September 25, 1968**
Philadelphia, Pennsylvania, USA

Will was the second of four children. He grew up in the city of Philadelphia and in Germantown, a neighborhood in the northwest of the city. His father, Willard, worked as a refrigeration engineer, and his mother, Caroline, was employed by the city's School Board. They raised their son as a Baptist, but divorced when he was thirteen. Will attended Overbrook High School, where he acquired the nickname, 'Fresh Prince' and used it when he helped form the hip-hop duo, "D.J. Jazzy & The Fresh Prince" during the 1980s. Ten years later, he was nearly bankrupt after the Internal Revenue Services went after him for unpaid income tax. It was lucky for him, when at just that time, NBC created a hit show around Will's personality - 'The Fresh Prince of Bel-Air'. It ran until 1996. In 1992, he made his film debut, in *Where the Day Takes You*. His breakthrough came with *Bad Boys*. That, and another film, *Men in Black*, have spawned successful sequels. Since then, his career has moved along nicely. He won Blockbuster awards for *Independence Day, Men in Black* and *Enemy of the State* and was twice nominated for Best Actor Oscars – for *Ali*, and *The Pursuit of Happyness*. Will had a son with his first wife, Sheree. He has a son, Jaden (who acted with him in *Happyness*), and a daughter, Willow, with his present wife – Jada Pinkett Smith.

**Where the Day
Takes You** (1992)
Six Degrees of Separation (1993)
Bad Boys (1995)
Independence Day (1996)
Men in Black (1997)
Enemy of the State (1998)
Men in Black Alien Attack (2000)
**The Legend of Bagger
Vance** (1964) **Ali** (2001)
Bad Boys II (2003)
I, Robot (2004) **Hitch** (2005)
The Pursuit of Happyness (2006)
I Am Legend (2007)
Hancock (2008)
Seven Pounds (2008)

Wesley **Snipes**
5ft 10in
(WESLEY TRENT SNIPES)

Born: **July 31, 1962**
Orlando, Florida, USA

Wesley's father was serving in the United States Airforce Reserve. He was taken to live in New York as a kid, and grew up on the streets of the South Bronx. Living in that tough neighborhood prompted him to take martial arts lessons from the age of twelve. Wesley eventually decided that the theater was his way out, but after he'd established himself at the High School for the Performing Arts, his mother took him back to Orlando. During his high school years, he renewed his interest in acting and got work in dinner theaters and also appeared in local stage productions. After graduating from high school, he attended the State University of New York, at Purchase. Wesley made his film debut, in *Wildcats*. In 1987, he was featured in Michael Jackson's video, "Bad". His appearance, in *Major League,* started a succession of hit movies, but brushes with the law – especially over tax matters, has hampered him. He is lucky to have a good home life with his second wife, the Korean painter, Nikki Park, and their four children. He's back in good form, with Richard Gere and Don Cheadle, in *Brooklyn's Finest.*

Wildcats (1986)
Streets of Gold (1986)
Major League (1989)
King of New York (1990)
Mo' Better Blues (1990)
New Jack City (1991)
Jungle Fever (1991)
The Waterdance (1992)
White Men Can't Jump (1992)
Rising Sun (1993)
Demolition Man (1993)
To Wong Foo
Thanks for Everything,
Julie Newmar (1995)
U.S. Marshals (1998)
Down in the Delta (1998)
Blade (1998)
The Art of War (2000)
ZigZag (2002)
Blade II (2002) Chaos (2005)
Brooklyn's Finest (2009)
Gallowwalker (2009)

Carrie **Snodgrass**
5ft 6in
(CAROLINE SNODGRESS)

Born: **October 27, 1946**
Park Ridge, Illinois, USA
Died: **April 1, 2004**

Carrie showed early promise as an actress during her high school years. She then blossomed even further at Northern Illinois University and it wasn't surprising when she switched to the Goodman Theater, in Chicago, to train for the stage. While she was there, she appeared in local theaters, in a variety of roles. In 1969, Carrie could be seen in no less than six different TV productions, starting with 'Judd for the Defense' and including 'The Virginian' and 'Marcus Welby, M.D'. She also managed an uncredited appearance in the cult film, *Easy Rider.* After more television work, she burst on to the movie screens, as Tina Balser, in *Diary of a Mad Housewife.* It earned her an Oscar nomination as Best Actress, and won her two Golden Globes – 'Best Actress' and 'Most Promising Newcomer'. She made one more film, the disappointing *Rabbit, Run,* before turning her back on Hollywood to devote her life to rock musician, Neil Young, and their son, who was born with cerebral palsy. Neil wrote a couple of songs in tribute to her – one of which was "A Man Needs a Maid" on the album, "Harvest". When he left her five years later, she tried to make a quick return to the top, but missed out on *Rocky* in 1977, because she demanded too much money. That, and a doomed affair with the film score composer, Jack Nitzsche didn't make life easier. Carrie died in Los Angeles, of heart failure, while awaiting a liver transplant.

Diary of a
Mad Housewife (1970)
The Fury (1978)
Pale Rider (1985)
Murphy's Law (1986)
L.A. Bad (1986)
Across the Tracks (1991)
The Ballad of Little Jo (1993)
8 Seconds (1994)
Blue Sky (1994)
Wild Things (1998)
In the Light of the Moon (2000)
Bartleby (2001)

Elke **Sommer**
5ft 7in
(ELKE SCHELTZ)

Born: **November 5, 1940**
Berlin, Germany

Elke was the daughter of a clergyman who died when she was in her teens. She showed talent as a painter as a young girl, and her gift for languages ear-marked her for a career with the United Nations. She worked as an au pair in England before, in the summer of 1958, while on holiday in Italy with her mother, she was crowned "Miss Viareggio" and invited to appear in a movie . It was a comedy starring Vittorio De Sica, called *Men and Noblemen.* She was given parts in a dozen Italian and German films before her first English-language appearance in *Don't Bother to Knock.* She was then featured in a war film, *The Victors,* and co-starred with Paul Newman in an entertaining thriller, set in Stockholm, titled *The Prize.* Elke made fifty more films, including the Peter Sellers classic – *A Shot in the Dark, The Wrecking Crew, Zeppelin* and *The Double McGuffin,* but the quality dropped off in the 1980s – especially some of the movies she made in Germany, including her last, *Flashback – Mörderische Ferien,* in 2000. Nowadays, she enjoys painting for much of the time and lives quietly in Los Angeles with her second husband, Wolf Walther.

Das Totenschiff (1959)
The Day it Rained (1959)
Don't Bother to Knock (1961)
The Victors (1963)
The Prize (1963)
A Shot in the Dark (1964)
Le Bambole (1965)
The Art of Love (1965)
The Corrupt Ones (1967)
Deadlier than the Male (1967)
The Invincible Six (1968)
The Wrecking Crew (1969)
Zeppelin (1971)
Lisa and the Devil (1973)
Einer von uns beiden (1974)
Ten Little Indians (1974)
Meet Him and Die (1976)
A Nightingale Sang in
Berkeley Square (1979)
The Double McGuffin (1979)
Der Mann im Pyjama (1981)

Gale **Sondergaard**
5ft 6in
(EDITH HOLM SONDERGAARD)

Born: **February 15, 1899**
Lichfield, Minnesota, USA
Died: **August 14, 1985**

The daughter of Danish parents, she grew up like most all-American girls, with a love for the movies. She studied acting at the Minneapolis School of Dramatic Arts, then joined the John Keller Shakespeare Company – with which she toured in "Hamlet", "The Merchant of Venice" and "Julius Caesar". By the age of thirty, she was a seasoned professional whose interesting personality would come to have great appeal to Hollywood filmmakers. She married her second husband, the writer/director, Herbert J. Biberman, and continued appearing in plays. In 1935, Gale was seen on stage by Mervyn LeRoy, and made her debut, in *Anthony Adverse* – her performance won her the very first Best Supporting Actress Oscar. She was nominated ten years later for *Anna and the King of Siam*. She was blacklisted in 1948 and only returned to acting in 1969, after which she appeared frequently on TV until making her last film, *Echoes*, in 1983. She died of cerebral vascular thrombosis, in Woodland Hills, California.

Anthony Adverse (1936)
Maid of Salem (1937)
Seventh Heaven (1937)
The Life of Emile Zola (1937)
Lord Jeff (1938)
Dramatic School (1938)
Never Say Die (1939) Juarez (1939)
The Cat and the Canary (1939)
The Bluebird (1940)
The Mark of Zorro (1940)
The Letter (1940)
The Black Cat (1941)
My Favorite Blonde (1942)
A Night to Remember (1943)
Appointment in Berlin (1943)
The Strange Death of
Adolf Hitler (1943)
The Spider Woman (1944)
Christmas Holiday (1944)
Anna and the King of Siam (1946)
The Time of their Lives (1946)
Road to Rio (1947)
East Side, West Side (1949)

Paul **Sorvino**
6ft 2in
(PAUL ANTHONY SORVINO)

Born: **April 13, 1939**
Brooklyn, New York City, New York, USA

Paul was the son of two Italian Americans, Ford Sorvino, a factory foreman, and his wife Marietta, As a youngster at school, he had a fine singing voice. He took singing lessons while working as a copywriter in a New York advertising agency and decided on a career in show business. He attended New York's American Musical and Dramatic Academy, where he became serious about acting. Paul made his Broadway debut in 1964, in the musical, "Bajour". He was thirty-one by the time he was offered his first movie role – in the comedy, *Where's Poppa?*, which starred George Segal. After another Segal film, *A Touch of Class,* and *The Gambler,* with James Caan, Paul's face became familiar to movie audiences, who didn't know his name. TV and film work made him famous, but his private life wasn't successful. In 1988, he and first wife, Lorraine Davis, divorced. Their three children are Mira and Michael, who are both actors and Amanda, who's a playwright. As he's suffered from severe asthma, Paul started the Paul Sorvino Asthma Foundation.

Where's Poppa? (1970)
The Panic in Needle Park (1971)
Made for Each Other (1971)
A Touch of Class (1973)
Shoot it Black, Shoot it Blue (1974)
The Gambler (1974)
Angel and Big Joe (1975)
Oh, God! (1977)
The Brink's Job (1978)
Cruising (1980)
Reds (1981) Melanie (1982)
The Championship Season (1982)
Dick Tracy (1990) Goodfellas (1990)
The Rocketeer (1991)
Nixon (1995) Romeo + Juliet (1996)
American Perfekt (1997)
Bulworth (1998) The Cooler (2003)
Mambo Italiano (2003)
Goodnight, Joseph Parker (2004)
Carnera: The
Walking Mountain (2008)
Repo! The
Genetic Opera (2008)

Mira **Sorvino**
5ft 10in
(MIRA KATHERINE SORVINO)

Born: **September 28, 1967**
Tenafly, New Jersey, USA

One of the three talented children born to actor Paul Sorvino and Lorraine Davis, a former actress who worked as a drama therapist with Alzheimer sufferers. During her years at Dwight-Englewood High School, she participated enthusiastically in theater productions. Against her father's wishes, Mira was intent on becoming an actress. At Harvard University, she continued with the development of those skills while majoring in East Asian Studies and graduated magna cum laude in 1989, with a prize winning thesis written during a year spent in Beijing. Mira also helped form the Harvard-Radcliffe Veritones, an 'a capella' group. She went to New York, where she spent three years struggling for work. She did well in a couple of TV dramas, and in 1994, a short documentary comedy about independent movies – *Everybody Just Stay Calm*. Mira's film career took off – winning a Best Supporting Actress Oscar for Woody Allen's *Mighty Aphrodite* – and appearing in such hits as *Beautiful Girls, The Grey Zone* and *Leningrad*. In 2004, she married the actor Christopher Backus. They have a daughter and a son. Mira will soon be seen in *Like Dandelion Dust.*

Barcelona (1994)
Quiz Show (1994)
Mighty Aphrodite (1995)
Blue in the Face (1995)
Beautiful Girls (1996)
Tarantella (1996)
Sweet Nothing (1996)
Romy and Michele's
High School Reunion (1997)
Mimic (1997)
The Replacement Killers (1998)
Lulu on the Bridge (1998)
At First Sight (1999)
Summer of Sam (1999)
The Triumph of Love (2001)
The Grey Zone (2001)
Between Strangers (2002)
Gods and Generals (2003)
The Final Cut (2004)
Reservation Road (2007)
Leningrad (2007)

Ann **Sothern**
5ft 1¹/₂in
(HARRIETTE ARLENE LAKE)

Born: **January 22, 1909**
Valley City, North Dakota, USA
Died: **March 15, 2001**

Ann's mother, who was a singing coach, was a big influence on her. After she graduated from Central High School, in St. Paul, Minnesota, Harriette Lake, as she was then known, went to live in New York. She made her film debut there in 1929, in *Broadway Nights.* In the meantime, her mother had relocated to Hollywood, where she was in demand at the birth of the talkies. The connection helped the newly named Ann Sothern, get bit parts in movies. She was on MGM's roster in 1930, but they used her only once and she returned to New York. It proved lucky. She soon starred on stage, in Rogers and Hart's "America's Sweetheart" and the studios beckoned. Ann made films for Columbia and RKO before signing an MGM contract in 1939. In 1949, she ended her second (and last) marriage to the actor Robert Sterling. During the 1950s, she concentrated on television work, but made a big screen comeback in the 1964 film, *The Best Man.* For her final film role, as Tisha Doughty, in *The Whales of August,* Ann was nominated for a Best Supporting Oscar. She died of heart failure at her home in Ketchum, Idaho.

Let's Fall in Love (1933)
Kid Millions (1934) Folies Bergère
de Paris (1935) Grand Exit (1935)
Walking on Air (1936)
Smartest Girl in Town (1936)
There Goes My Girl (1937)
Super-Sleuth (1937) Danger – Love
at Work (1937) Maisie (1939)
Fast and Furious (1939)
Brother Orchid (1940)
Maisie Was a Lady (1941)
Lady Be Good (1941)
Words and Music (1948)
A Letter to Three Wives (1949)
The Judge Steps Out (1949)
Shadow on the Wall (1950)
The Blue Gardenia (1953)
The Best Man (1964)
Lady in a Cage (1964) Sylvia (1965)
The Whales of August (1987)

Sissy **Spacek**
5ft 2in
(MARY ELIZABETH SPACEK)

Born: **December 25, 1949**
Quitman, Texas, USA

Sissy was a lovely Christmas Day gift for her parents, Edwin and Virginia Spacek. Her paternal grandfather, Arnold, served as Mayor of Granger, Texas. She enjoyed a country life while attending Quitman High School, but left home for New York City when she was in her teens. She was a singer in New York coffee houses before she even considered an acting career. She used the name 'Rainbo' and recorded a song, "Johnny You Went Too Far This Time", but decided to try for an acting career. Tuition at the Lee Strasberg Theatrical Institute was an important step which led to her film debut – two small roles in 1970's *Trash,* another small part in an episode of the television series, 'Love, American Style' and a bigger one on her movie debut, in *Prime Cut.* By 1973, she'd also appeared in 'The Waltons'. But just around the corner was a chance to shine with another young actor, Martin Sheen, in the impressive *Badlands.* Her six Oscar nominations – all as Best Actress, are: *Carrie, The Coal Miner's Daughter* (for which she won), *Missing, The River, Crimes of the Heart* and *In the Bedroom.* Sissy is married to a production designer, Jack Fisk. The couple have two children.

Prime Cut (1972)
Badlands (1973) Carrie (1976)
Welcome to L.A. (1976)
3 Women (1977) Coal Miner's
Daughter (1980) Heart Beat (1980)
Raggedy Man (1981) Missing (1982)
The River (1984) Marie (1985)
'night Mother (1986)
The Long Walk Home (1990)
Hard Promises (1991) JFK (1991)
The Grass Harp (1995)
Affliction (1997)
Blast from the Past (1999)
The Straight Story (1999)
In the Bedroom (2001)
Tuck Everlasting (2002)
A Home at the End of the
World (2004) Nine Lives (2005)
North Country (2005)
Hot Rod (2007) Lake City (2008)

Kevin **Spacey**
5ft 10¹/₂in
(KEVIN SPACEY FOWLER)

Born: **July 26, 1959**
South Orange, New Jersey, USA

Kevin. the youngest of three children, grew up in a tough situation for his family – especially his mother, Kathleen. His father, Tom had been accused of being a member of the American Nazi Party and found keeping a job difficult. They were subjected to frequent moves, but in 1963, they settled in California. Kevin attended Chatsworth High School, and because he had a good voice, starred in a senior production of "The Sound of Music". He took his mother's maiden name, Spacey, and attempted a career as a stand-up comic. From 1979 until 1981, he studied drama at Juilliard. His stage debut, that same year, was as a messenger, in "Henry VI" at the New York Shakespeare Festival. His first film role was five years later, in *Heartburn.* He won a best Supporting Oscar for *The Usual Suspects* and was voted Best Actor for *American Beauty.* He has been Artistic Director at London's Old Vic Theater, since 2003, and has taken up residency in England.

See No Evil, Hear No Evil (1989)
Dad (1989) Henry & June (1990)
Glengarry Glen Ross (1992)
Consenting Adults (1992)
Iron Will (1994) The Ref (1994)
Swimming with Sharks (1994)
The Usual Suspects (1995)
Outbreak (1995)
Se7en (1995)
A Time to Kill (1996)
L.A. Confidential (1997)
Midnight in the Garden of
Good and Evil (1997)
The Negotiator (1998)
American Beauty (1999)
The Big Kahuna (1999)
Ordinary Decent Criminal (2000)
The Shipping News (2001)
Austin Powers in
Goldmember (2002)
The United States of Leland (2003)
The Life of David Gale (2003)
Beyond the Sea (2004)
Superman Returns (2006)
21 (2008)

James **Spader**
5ft 10in
(JAMES TODD SPADER)

Born: **February 7, 1960**
Boston, Massachusetts, USA

The son of teachers, Todd and Jean Spader, Jimmy attended The Pike School – where his mother taught Art, and lived with his family on the Brooks School campus - where his father worked. Both schools were in Andover – just like his next – the private Phillips Academy. Jimmy left there when he decided to become an actor and moved to New York City, where he studied at the Michael Chekhov School. During those years, he took a variety of jobs in order to support himself – working as a yoga instructor and truck driver among others. In 1978, he made his film debut, in the comedy, *Team-Mates,* which was shot in Nassau County. There were a couple more low-grade movies and some TV work before Jimmy made a big impression as Steff, in *Pretty in Pink.* In 1989, he was voted Best Actor at the Cannes Film Festival, for *Sex, Lies, and Videotape.* He was married to Victoria Kheel, from 1987-2004. They had two sons. For the past four seasons, Jimmy's been seen regularly in the role of Alan Shore, in TV's 'Boston Legal'. His next movie appearance is in *Shorts.*

Pretty in Pink (1986)
Baby Boom (1987)
Less Than Zero (1987)
Wall Street (1987)
Jack's Back (1988)
Sex, Lies and Videotape (1989)
The Rachel Papers (1989)
Bad Influence (1990)
White Palace (1990)
True Colors (1991)
Storyville (1992)
Bob Roberts (1992)
The Music of Chance (1993)
Dream Lover (1994)
Wolf (1994)
Stargate (1994)
Crash (1996)
Critical Care (1997)
Curtain Call (1999)
Speaking of Sex (2001)
The Stickup (2001)
Secretary (2002)

Jill **St.John**
5ft 6in
(JILL ARLYN OPPENHEIM)

Born: **August 19, 1940**
Los Angeles, California, USA

Jill was the daughter of Betty Lou Oppenheim – an ambitious woman, who pushed her into performing from the age of five, when she began acting on stage and radio. In 1949, she made her first TV appearance – in a family show, 'Sandy Dreams'. Apart from show business, Jill enjoyed early fame because of her very high IQ of 162. She was even admitted to the University of California, in Los Angeles at the tender age of fourteen. Somehow she managed to juggle acting and academia and was regularly seen on television during the 1950s. She made her first movie appearance (uncredited) in 1952, in *Thunder in the East.* She was signed by Universal when she was sixteen, and her first featured role was in the teen musical comedy, *Summer Love.* From then on, Jill lent her special glamour to a whole series of movies – most notably as Tiffany Case, in the James Bond film, *Diamonds Are Forever.* Jill dated several famous men - among whom were Frank Sinatra and Henry Kissinger. In her spare time, Jill has written best-selling cookbooks. Her four husbands include the crooner Jack Jones and actor Robert Wagner, to whom she's been married since 1990. They both appear in her last film, *The Calling.* They live in Aspen, Colorado, where they enjoy skiing, and in Pacific Palisades, near Los Angeles, where Jill keeps several horses.

Summer Love (1958)
The Remarkable
Mr. Pennypacker (1959)
Holiday for Lovers (1959)
The Roman Spring of
Mrs. Stone (1961)
Tender Is the Night (1962)
Come Blow Your Horn (1963)
Who's Minding the Store? (1963)
Who's Been Sleeping in
My Bed? (1963) **Banning** (1967)
Tony Rome (1967)
Diamonds Are Forever (1971)
Sitting Target (1972)
Something to Believe In (1998)
The Trip (2002) **The Calling** (2002)

Robert **Stack**
6ft
(ROBERT LANGFORD MODINI STACK)

Born: **January 13, 1919**
Los Angeles, California, USA
Died: **May 14, 2003**

The son of James Langford Stack, who owned an advertising agency in Los Angeles, and Elizabeth Modini Wood, Bob went to live in Europe with his mother after his parents divorced when he was one year old. He went to school in Paris, and could speak fluent French and pretty good Italian before he spoke English. Bob was a quite outstanding sportsman. At the University of Southern California, he excelled at polo. He was successful when he took up Skeet Shooting and together with his brother, he won the Outboard Motor Championship – in Venice, Italy. Besides playing the saxophone and clarinet, he took acting lessons while at University and was the first actor to give Deanna Durbin a screen kiss in *First Love.* He became a star following *Mortal Storm.* From 1942, he was a gunnery instructor in the U.S. Navy. In 1952, he starred in the first 3-D film, *Bwana Devil.* For *Written on the Wind,* he was nominated for a Best Supporting Actor Oscar. In 1959, Bob started a TV career as Eliot Ness, in 'The Untouchables'. Bob was married to the actress Rosemarie Bowe, from 1956 until his death from a heart attack, in Beverly Hills, California. His two children included Elizabeth Stack, who was an actress.

First Love (1939)
The Mortal Storm (1940)
Badlands of Dakota (1941)
To Be or Not to Be (1942)
Eagle Squadron (1942)
A Date With Judy (1948)
Miss Tatlock's Millions (1948)
Bullfighter and the Lady (1951)
Sabre Jet (1953)
The High and the Mighty (1954)
House of Bamboo (1955)
Good Morning, Miss Dove (1955)
Great Day in the Morning (1956)
Written on the Wind (1956)
The Tarnished Angels (1958)
The Gift of Love (1958)
The Last Voyage (1960)
Airplane! (1980)

Sylvester **Stallone**
5ft 9in
(SYLVESTER GARDENZIO STALLONE)

Born: **July 6, 1946**
New York City, New York, USA

Sly was the son of an Italian immigrant – Frank Stallone, who was a professional hairdresser, and Jaci, an astrologer and promoter of women's wrestling. Sly grew up in Philadelphia, where he attended Lincoln High School. Sly's later education included Glenholme – a special needs boarding school, in Connecticut, the American College of Switzerland and the University of Miami – which he left before graduating, but received a BFA from in 1999. He went to New York to concentrate on an acting career and made his film debut in 1970, in the soft core porn movie, *The Party at Kitty and Stud's*. Four years later he made his orthodox film debut, in *The Lord's of Flatbush*. It took two more years for him to achieve true stardom, but when he did it was in *Rocky* – for which he was Oscar-nominated as Best Actor and Writer of Original Screenplay, only the third in film history (along with Charles Chaplin and Orson Welles) to be nominated for both awards. Its several sequels, and all-action movies like *Rambo,* have kept him at the top of the popularity charts for over thirty years. In 1997, he was voted Best Actor at the Stockholm Film Festival, for *Cop Land.* Sly has five children – three with his third wife, actress Jennifer Flavin.

The Lord's of Flatbush (1974)
Death Race 2000 (1975)
Rocky (1976) **F.I.S.T** (1978)
Paradise Alley (1978)
Rocky II (1979)
Nighthawks (1981)
Victory (1981) **Rocky III** (1982)
First Blood (1982)
Rambo: First Blood Part II (1985)
Rocky IV (1985)
Lock Up (1989)
Tango & Cash (1989)
Oscar (1991)
Cliffhanger (1993)
Demolition Man (1993)
Assassins (1995)
Cop Land (1997) **Shade** (2003)
Rocky Balboa (2006)
Rambo (2008)

Terence **Stamp**
6ft
(TERENCE STAMP)

Born: **July 22, 1939**
Stepney, London, England

The first of five children, Terry was the son of a Thames tugboat operator. His first screen idol was Gary Cooper, who he saw in *Beau Geste* when he was very young. He left school at sixteen and started his working life in advertising, where he met people who were interested in acting. He took a year's drama course at the Webber-Douglas School in London, and from there, worked in repertory companies. He made his film debut, in 1962, in *Term of Trial,* but more importantly, he was cast in the title role of *Billy Budd,* by Peter Ustinov, who'd seen him in a play called "Why the Chicken". The film brought stardom and a nomination for a Supporting Actor Oscar. *Far from the Madding Crowd* brought him romance with 'Swinging London's Darling', Julie Christie. After that, he was involved with Jean Shrimpton. Terry worked with Fellini and Pasolini, but when Jean left him, he dropped out and went to India. His next big film was *Superman.* Terry had enjoyed bachelorhood for nearly half a century when he finally got married in 2002 – to Elizabeth O'Rourke. Unfortunately, the habits of a lifetime proved to strong for Terry and they got divorced in April, 2008.

Term of Trial (1962)
Billy Budd (1962)
The Collector (1965)
Far from the Madding Crowd (1967)
Poor Cow (1967) **Blue** (1968)
Histoires extraordinaires (1968)
Teorema (1968)
Una Stagione all'inferno (1970)
The Mind of Mr. Soames (1970)
Superman (1978) **Superman II** (1980)
The Hit (1984) **Young Guns** (1988)
The Adventures of Priscilla,
Queen of the Desert (1994)
Tiré à part (1996) **The Limey** (1999)
Bowfinger (1999)
Ma femme est une actrice (2001)
These Foolish Things (2001)
Wanted (2008)
Get Smart (2008) **Yes Man** (2008)
Valkyrie (2008)

Lionel **Stander**
6ft
(LIONEL STANDER)

Born: **January 11, 1908**
The Bronx, New York City, New York, USA
Died: **November 30, 1994**

The first-born child of Russian Jewish immigrants, Lionel completed high school, and spent one year at the University of North Carolina, studying Accountancy with little enthusiasm. While he was there, he appeared in a student production of "The Muse and the Movies: A Comedy of Greenwich Village". Lionel started his working life with a New York newspaper. In 1926, he decided on an acting career and took drama lessons for two years. He made his professional stage debut in 1928, and his movie debut four years later, in *In the Dough.* He was married to his first wife, Lucy, and his bank-balance looked pretty healthy as a result of his demand as a character actor. Lionel appeared in film classics such as *Mr. Deeds Goes to Town* and *A Star Is Born,* and his gravelly voice was heard on the national radio shows of Eddie Cantor and Bing Crosby. A supporter of the studio unions during the 1930s, he was investigated by the HUAC. It did harm his career during the 1940s, but worse was to come. In 1951, he was black-listed and didn't make a movie for ten years. A delicious cameo in *Cul-de-sac,* his movie swan-song *The Last Good Time,* and his 'Max' in the popular TV-series, 'Hart to Hart', were some sweet memories he left us from his later career. He died of lung cancer, in Los Angeles. Lionel loved women and children – he had six wives and six kids!

We're in the Money (1935)
The Gay Deception (1935)
If You Could Only Cook (1935)
I Loved a Soldier (1936)
Mr. Deeds Goes to Town (1936)
A Star Is Born (1937) **The Last**
Gangster (1937) **The Crowd**
Roars (1938) **Hangmen Also Die** (1943)
Guadalcanal Diary (1943) **The Kid from**
Brooklyn (1946) **Unfaithfully Yours** (1948)
Cul-de-sac (1966) **The Cassandra**
Crossing (1976) **New York,**
New York (1977) **1941** (1979)
The Last Good Time (1994)

Harry Dean **Stanton**
5ft 8in
(HARRY DEAN STANTON)

Born: **July 14, 1926**
West Irvine, Kentucky, USA

Harry's father, Sheridan Stanton, was a tobacco farmer. His mother, Ersel, was a hairdresser. He had two younger brothers. After leaving Lafayette High School, in Lexington, Harry joined the United States Navy and saw action in Okinawa during World War II. From 1946 onwards, he studied Journalism and Radio Arts, at the University of Kentucky. During his time there, he appeared in a number of stage productions. He then enrolled at the Pasadena Playhouse and settled in Los Angeles. In 1954, Harry made his television debut, in an episode of 'Inner Sanctum'. His film debut, was three years later, in *Tomahawk Trail.* There was lots of TV and small roles in films until his career took off with the cult film, *Two-Lane Blacktop.* In the years that followed Harry's name graced a lot of good movies including *Paris Texas, Wild at Heart* and *The Green Mile* – and he's still making them. In his leisure time, he sings and plays his guitar in the Los Angeles area, with the "Harry Dean Stanton Band".

Two-Lane Blacktop (1971)
Cisco Pike (1972) Pat Garrett & Billy
the Kid (1973) Dillinger (1973)
Where the Lilies Bloom (1974)
Cockfighter (1974)
Rancho Deluxe (1984)
Farewell, My Lovely (1975)
The Missouri Breaks (1976)
Straight Time (1978) Alien (1979)
Wise Blood (1979) The Rose (1979)
Death Watch (1980)
Escape from New York (1981)
Repo Man (1984) Paris, Texas (1984)
UFOria (1985) One Magic
Christmas (1985) Pretty in Pink (1986)
Wild at Heart (1990)
She's So Lovely (1997)
The Mighty (1998)
The Straight Story (1999)
The Green Mile (1999)
Alpha Dog (2006)
Inland Empire (2006)
The Good Life (2007)
The Open Road (2008)

Barbara **Stanwyck**
5ft 5in
(RUBY CATHERINE STEVENS)

Born: **July 16, 1907**
Brooklyn, New York City, New York, USA
Died: **January 20, 1990**

Barbara had a miserable early life. She was the youngest child born to Byron Stevens and his wife, Catherine – who died when she was pushed from a moving trolley car by a drunk. By the time Barbara was four, her father had abandoned his family and Barbara was raised by a sister, and in foster homes. She worked in menial jobs when she was thirteen and then danced in speakeasies. At sixteen, she left Erasmus Hall High School to work as a fashion model. This led to her becoming a Ziegfeld Girl on Broadway. In 1926, her performance in a serious play, "The Noose", brought her to the attention of movie moguls. In 1927, she made her film debut in *Broadway Nights,* and married Frank Fay, who took her to Hollywood. Her first talkie was *Mexicali Rose,* in 1929. She never won an Oscar, but was nominated four times – for *Stella Dallas, Ball of Fire, Double Indemnity,* and *Sorry, Wrong Number.* She became a TV star in the 1960s – with her own show, followed by 'The Big Valley' and latterly, 'The Colbys'. Rumored to 'swing both ways' she never remarried after divorcing her second husband, Robert Taylor, in 1951. Barbara died in Santa Monica, California, of chronic lung disease and emphysema.

The Miracle Woman (1931)
Forbidden (1932) So Big! (1932)
The Bitter Tea of General Yen (1931)
Baby Face (1933) Annie Oakley (1935)
This Is My Affair (1937) Stella
Dallas (1937) Union Pacific (1939)
Golden Boy (1939) The Lady Eve (1941)
Meet John Doe (1941) Ball of
Fire (1941) Double Indemnity (1944)
My Reputation (1946) The Strange
Love of Martha Ivers (1946)
Sorry, Wrong Number (1948)
No Man of Her Own (1950)
Clash By Night (1952) Jeopardy (1953)
Titanic (1953) Executive Suite (1954)
The Violent Men (1955)
Trooper Hook (1957)
The Night Walker (1964)

Maureen **Stapleton**
5ft 3in
(LOIS MAUREEN STAPLETON)

Born: **June 21, 1925**
Troy, New York, USA
Died: **March 13, 2006**

Maureen was the daughter of a strict Irish American Catholic couple, John and Irene Stapleton, who separated during her early childhood. Maureen was educated at Troy High School, then at eighteen, she studied acting with Herbert Berghof, at the Actors' Studio. In 1946, she made her Broadway debut in Burgess Meredith's production of "Playboy of the Western World" – stepping in at the last minute because of a problem with the intended star, Anna Magnani's English. Maureen won a Tony when she starred in "The Rose Tattoo", but lost out to Magnani for the film role. She'd started acting on TV in 1948, but didn't make her film debut, until *Lonely Hearts,* ten years later. It brought her the first of four Best Supporting Actress Oscar nominations – the others being for *Airport, Interiors,* and *Reds* – for which she was successful. The second of Maureen's two husbands was the well-known screenwriter, Davis Rayfiel. She was terrified of flying and traveled by rail or ship whenever she needed to fulfill an engagement. She continued working until her last film appearance, in *Living and Dining.* After that, her health deteriorated rapidly. Apart from a long term drinking problem, Maureen was a heavy smoker and died of chronic pulmonary disease, at her home in Lenox, Massachusetts.

Lonely Hearts (1958)
The Fugitive Kind (1959)
A View from the Bridge (1961)
Bye Bye Birdie (1963)
Airport (1970)
Plaza Suite (1971)
Interiors (1978) Reds (1981)
Johnny Dangerously (1984)
Cocoon (1985)
The Money Pit (1986)
Heartburn (1986)
Sweet Lorraine (1987)
Made in Heaven (1987)
Nuts (1987)
The Last Good Time (1994)
Addicted to Love (1997)
Living and Dining (2003)

Alison **Steadman**
5ft 4in
(ALISON STEADMAN)

Born: **August 26, 1946**
Liverpool, England

Alison's parents were George and Marjorie Steadman. George worked as production controller for an electronics firm. She was educated at Childwall Valley High School, in Liverpool and then attended a business college where she trained as a secretary. She worked at the Liverpool Probation Service until she planned her escape via the East-15 Acting School, which she attended from 1966 until 1969. It was there that she met her future husband, the playwright, Mike Leigh. In 1971, she first appeared on television, in a dramatization of Guy de Maupassant's novel, 'Bel Ami'. She acted in Mike Leigh's stage plays, "The Jaws of Death" and "Wholesome Glory" – the latter marking her London debut, in 1973. She'd had a dozen years of TV and theater experience before making her film debut, in *Champions*. The big screen never quite became her regular medium, but she enhanced the movies she was seen in. Alison has been up for various awards and was named Best Actress for *Life Is Sweet,* by the United States National Society of Film Critics. She won an Olivier as Best Actress, the following year for 'The Rise and Fall of Little Voice'. She was awarded an OBE on New Year's Eve, 1999. For the past four years, most of Alison's acting roles have been in television dramas – most recently in the comedy series, 'Gavin & Stacey'. Her son, Toby, is an animator.

Champions (1984)
A Private Function (1984)
Coming Through (1985)
Clockwise (1986)
The Adventures of Baron
Munchausen (1988) Wilt (1989)
Shirley Valentine (1989)
Life Is Sweet (1990)
Secrets & Lies (1996)
Topsy-Turvy (1999)
Chunky Monkey (2001)
Happy Now (2001)
The Life and
Death of Peter Sellers (2004)
Confetti (2006)

Anthony **Steel**
6ft
(ANTHONY MAITLAND STEEL)

Born: **May 21, 1920**
Chelsea, London, England
Died: **March 21, 2001**

Tony spent his early years in India, where his father, Edward, was an officer in the Indian Army. He was sent to boarding school in Ireland and at eighteen, he attended Cambridge University. In the early part of World War II, he joined the Grenadier Guards. When he left, in 1945, he had achieved the rank of Major. Following that, Tony began his acting career with the Worthing Repertory and after a few stage roles, he made his screen debut, as an extra, in *Portrait from Life,* in 1948. There were several small movie roles before he became a star of the British Cinema after acting in a featured role, in *The Wooden Horse*. His matinee idol looks kept him in work throughout the 1950s, and most of his films from that time are a lot of fun. His hand was pierced by Errol Flynn's sword during the filming of *The Master of Ballantrae,* and he enjoyed showing the scar to people for nearly fifty years. He reached the peak of his career in *The Sea Shall Not Have Them*. There was a disastrous second marriage – to Anita Ekberg, which wore him down and marked his decline. He remarried in 1964, but sadly, he lived the last fifteen years of his life in London, alone and broke. Tony died of heart failure.

The Wooden Horse (1950)
The Mudlark (1950)
Laughter in Paradise (1951)
Another Man's Poison (1951)
Where No Vultures Fly (1951)
The Planter's Wife (1952)
Malta Story (1953)
The Master of Ballantrae (1953)
Albert R.N. (1953)
West of Zanzibar (1954)
The Sea Shall Not Have Them (1954)
Out of the Clouds (1955)
Storm Over the Nile (1955)
Valerie (1957)
A Question of Adultery (1958)
Harry Black (1958)
Honeymoon (1959)
A Matter of Choice (1963)

Barbara **Steele**
5ft 6in
(BARBARA STEELE)

Born: **December 29, 1937**
Birkenhead, Cheshire, England

Barbara showed exceptional artistic ability when she was quite young. She studied at Chelsea Art School, but instead of oil on canvas, Barbara would express an art form of a different and very exclusive kind – as a horror film actress. After gaining a year's stage experience with a repertory company, she began her film career in 1958, with a very small role in the British comedy, *Bachelor of Hearts*. Two years later, she starred in Mario Bava's classic Italian horror film, *Black Sunday*. In 1961, she went to America to star opposite Vincent Price, in Roger Corman's version of Edgar Allan Poe's, *Pit and the Pendulum*. She may have become typecast, but few actresses were able to play those roles like she could. Although she made several films in Italy – including an appearance in Fellini's *8½* – Barbara's voice wasn't heard, because of the Italian system of dubbing voices into their own language. From 1969 until 1978, she was married to the aptly-named writer – in view of her film career – James Poe. Today she lives in Los Angeles and after playing Dr. Julia Hoffman, in a 1991, TV-series, 'Dark Shadows', Barbara was absent from the screen until 1999. She can be seen again in the comedy thriller, *Her Morbid Desires*.

Black Sunday (1960)
Pit and the Pendulum (1961)
The Horrible Dr. Hitchcock (1962)
8½ (1962) The Ghost (1963)
The Long Hair of Death (1964)
The White Voices (1964)
Castle of Blood (1964)
The Monacle (1964)
Nightmare Castle (1965)
An Angel for Satan (1966)
Der Junge Törless (1966)
For Love and Gold (1966)
Shivers (1975)
I Never Promised You a
Rose Garden (1977)
Pretty Baby (1978)
Piranha (1978)
The Key Is in the Door (1978)
Her Morbid Desires (2008)

Mary **Steenburgen**
5ft 8in
(MARY NELL STEENBURGEN)

Born: **February 8, 1953**
Newport, Arkansas, USA

Mary's father, Maurice Steenburgen, was a freight train conductor and her mother, Nell, was a school-board secretary. From an early age, the only career Mary had in mind for herself was to become an actress. She appeared in several plays during her years at North Little Rock High School, and at the age of twenty, she moved to New York, to study drama. It was by sheer chance that, when looking for work, she was in Paramount's New York office and Jack Nicholson walked in. He liked her immediately and offered Mary her film debut, in his forthcoming, *Goin' South*. In 1980, she married the British film actor, Malcolm McDowell, whom she'd first met when they both appeared in *Time After Time*. Their daughter, Lilly, is an actress and son, Charlie, is a producer. Mary won a Supporting Oscar for *Melvin and Howard*, and for nearly thirty years, has continued to produce performances of a consistently high quality. Since 1995, she's been married to her second husband, the actor, Ted Danson.

Goin' South (1978)
Time After Time (1979)
Melvin and Howard (1980)
Ragtime (1981)
A Midsummer Night's
Sex Comedy (1982)
Cross Creek (1983)
Dead of Winter (1987)
The Whales of August (1987)
Miss Firecracker (1989)
Parenthood (1989)
Back to the Future Part III (1990)
What's Eating Gilbert Grape (1993)
Philadelphia (1993)
The Grass Harp (1995)
Powder (1995) Nixon (1995)
Nobody's Baby (2001)
Sunshine State (2002) Elf (2003)
Marilyn Hotchkiss Ballroom
Dancing & Charm School (2005)
Elvis and Annabelle (2007)
Nobel Son (2007)
The Brave One (2007)
Step Brothers (2008)

Rod **Steiger**
5ft 10in
(RODNEY STEPHEN STEIGER)

Born: **April 14, 1925**
Westhampton, New York, USA
Died: **July 9, 2002**

Rod was raised in the Lutheran religion by his alcoholic mother, who had been in a song and dance act with his father, Frederick, who'd left her before Rod was born. Rod left home at sixteen to serve in the U.S. Navy, where he saw combat on a destroyer in the Pacific. In 1946, he took advantage of the G.I. Bill of Rights to study Drama under Lee Strasberg and Elia Kazan at the Actors' Studio. He mastered 'The Method' and made his stage debut in "The Trial of Mary Dugan". His Broadway debut was in 1950, in "An Enemy of the People". Between 1948 and 1953, he is believed to have made around 250 TV appearances. Rod's film debut, was in 1951's *Teresa*. Oscar-nominated for *On the Waterfront* and *The Pawnbroker,* he won a Best Actor Oscar, for *In the Heat of the Night* and high praise for his work in at least a dozen more movies. Rod's five wives included actress, Claire Bloom. His final film *Poolhall Junkies,* was a good one. He died in Los Angeles, from pneumonia and kidney failure.

On the Waterfront (1954)
The Big Knife (1955) The Court-Martial
of Billy Mitchell (1955) Jubal (1956)
The Harder They Fall (1956)
Run of the Arrow (1957)
Across the Bridge (1957)
Cry Terror (1958) Al Capone (1959)
The Mark (1961)
The Pawnbroker (1964)
Doctor Zhivago (1965)
In the Heat of the Night (1967)
No Way to Treat a
Lady (1968) The Sergeant (1968)
The Illustrated Man (1969)
Three Into Two Won't Go (1969)
Waterloo (1970) Happy Birthday,
Wanda June (1971)
The Amityville Horror (1979)
Lion of the Desert (1981)
The Chosen (1981)
The Ballad of the Sad Cafe (1991)
Mars Attacks! (1996)
Poolhall Junkies (2002)

Sir Robert **Stephens**
6ft 2in
(ROBERT STEPHENS)

Born: **July 14, 1931**
Bristol, England
Died: **November 12, 1995**

Robert attended school in Bristol before studying Drama at the Bradford Civic Theater School. He began his career with The Caryl Jenner Mobile Theater, a touring company which had been formed in 1947, and traveled all over the United Kingdom – with the noble aim of bringing culture to the people. It gave young Robert a rich variety of roles to get his teeth into. He appeared on Broadway in 1959, and was nominated for a Tony Award for his leading role in "Epitaph for George Dillon". In 1960, he made his film debut, in *Circle of Deception*. On stage, his Shakespearean roles were critically acclaimed and in the 1960s, he was being touted as the natural heir to Sir Laurence Olivier. In 1967, he married another great British stage icon, Maggie Smith. They worked together in plays and in films, but after their break up, he quickly turned to drink. He is the father of actors Toby Stephens and Chris Larkin. Robert died from cancer, in London, the year he received a knighthood.

A Taste of Honey (1961)
The Queen's Guards (1961)
Lisa (1962) Cleopatra (1963)
The Small World of Sammy
Lee (1963) Morgan (1966)
Romeo and Juliet (1968)
The Prime of Miss
Jean Brodie (1969)
The Private Life of
Sherlock Holmes (1970)
Travels with My Aunt (1972)
Luther (1973)
The Asphyx (1973)
The Duellists (1977)
The Shout (1978)
Empire of the Sun (1987)
The Fruit Machine (1988)
Testimony (1988)
Henry V (1989)
Wings of Fame (1990)
Century (1993)
Searching for
Bobby Fischer (1993)
England, My England (1995)

Henry **Stephenson**
6ft 4in
(HENRY STEPHENSON GARROWAY)

Born: **April 16, 1871**
Grenada, British West Indies
Died: **April 24, 1956**

Henry was educated at the famous Rugby College, in England, before starting his stage career in London in the early 1890s. After establishing a reputation as a romantic leading man, his adventurous spirit took him to the United States, where he made his debut on Broadway, in 1901, in "A Message from Mars". Up until World War I, Henry divided his time between the London and New York stage. He made his film debut, in 1917 – in *The Spreading Dawn,* but was somewhat wasted in silents – making only five more before his first talkie, in 1932's Jean Harlow comedy, *Red-Headed Woman.* Unfortunately, he was already sixty-one years old and the roles offered to him were appropriate to his dignified and gentle personality. Over a seventeen year period, he appeared in no less than eighty-four movies – including such classics as *Little Women, Mutiny on the Bounty, Captain Blood, The Charge of the Light Brigade,* and towards the end of his career, a return to England for the definitive *Oliver Twist* – where the innate kindness Henry showed in the role of Mr. Brownlow, was the perfect counterpoint to the evil people Oliver was surrounded by. He had one child, a daughter, with Ann Shoemaker, a character actress, whom he was married to from 1918 until his death in San Francisco, after a short illness.

Little Women (1933)
The Richest Girl in the World (1934)
What Every Woman Knows (1934)
Mutiny on the Bounty (1935)
Captain Blood (1935) **The Charge of the Light Brigade** (1936)
Beloved Enemy (1936) **Marie Antoinette** (1938) **Suez** (1938)
The Adventures of Sherlock Holmes (1939) **This Above All** (1942)
Of Human Bondage (1946)
The Return of Monte Cristo (1946)
The Locket (1946) **Ivy** (1947)
Oliver Twist (1948) **Julia Misbehaves** (1948) **Enchantment** (1948)
Challenge to Lassie (1949)

Jan **Sterling**
5ft 6in
(JANE STERLING ADRIANCE)

Born: **April 3, 1921**
New York City, New York, USA
Died: **March 26, 2004**

The daughter of wealthy parents, Jan attended private schools before going to Europe when her mother remarried. She was taught by private tutors in Paris and London, where at fifteen, she took acting classes at Fay Compton's School. She returned to New York, and made her Broadway debut, in 1938, in "Bachelor Born". Jan continued working on stage in such shows as "Panama Hattie" and "Present Laughter". She married her first husband, actor John Merivale, in 1941. He remained with her until after she made her film debut in 1947, in *Tycoon* – billed as Jane Darian. The actress Ruth Gordon came up with Jan Sterling. Her first film under that name was *Johnny Belinda*. She made a name for herself playing tough women and won a National Board of Review Award for *Ace in the Hole.* She won a Golden Globe Award as Supporting Actress for *The High and the Mighty* and was nominated for an Oscar in that same category. She continued working after her movie fame evaporated and her second husband, Paul Douglas, passed away in 1959. Her last role was in 1988, in an episode of the TV-series, 'Baby Boom'. Jan died from a stroke at the Woodland Hills Home, in Los Angeles.

Johnny Belinda (1948)
Caged (1950) **Mystery Street** (1950)
The Mating Season (1951)
Appointment with Danger (1951)
Ace in the Hole (1951)
Rhubarb (1951)
Flesh and Fury (1952)
Sky Full of Moon (1952)
The High and the Mighty (1954)
Return from the Sea (1954)
Women's Prison (1955)
Female on the Beach (1955)
Man with the Gun (1955) **1984** (1956)
The Harder They Fall (1956)
Slaughter on Tenth Avenue (1957)
Kathy O' (1958)
The Incident (1967)
First Monday in October (1981)

Daniel **Stern**
6ft 4in
(DANIEL JACOB STERN)

Born: **August 28, 1957**
Bethesda, Maryland, USA

After graduating from Bethesda Chevy Chase High School, where he'd starred in "Fiddler on the Roof", Dan applied for an advertised job as a lighting engineer, at the Washington Shakespeare Festival. Instead, he was given a small role as a strolling lute player, in their production of "As You Like It". From there, he went to New York, where he took a few acting lessons before getting a series of roles in off-Broadway plays including, "Split", "Frankie and Annie", and "The Old Glory". In 1979, Daniel made his film debut, in British director Peter Yates' comedy drama, *Breaking Away*. Acting in Woody Allen's *Stardust Memories* further helped his cause and by the time he settled down to married life, with Laure Mattos, in 1981, things were moving along nicely. A good role in *Diner* secured his position. Dan has since tried his hand at directing, with a couple of TV-series, 'The Wonder Years' and 'Complete Savages', and the feature film, *Rookie of the Year*. Following a sticky patch during the past nine or ten years, Dan is back on form in the romantic comedy, *A Previous Engagement*. He and his wife Laure, have a son and two daughters.

Breaking Away (1979)
A Small Circle of Friends (1980)
Stardust Memories (1980)
Diner (1982)
Blue Thunder (1983)
Get Crazy (1983)
Hannah and Her Sisters (1986)
The Miralgo Beanfield War (1988)
Coupe de Ville (1990)
My Blue Heaven (1990)
Home Alone (1990)
City Slickers (1991)
Home Alone 2 (1992)
Rookie of the Year (1993)
City Slickers II:
The Legend of Curly's Gold (1994)
Bushwhacked (1995)
Very Bad Things (1998)
Viva Las Nowhere (2001)
The Last Time (2006)
A Previous Engagement (2008)

Mark **Stevens**
6ft
(RICHARD STEVENS)

Born: **December 13, 1916**
Cleveland, Ohio, USA
Died: **September 15, 1994**

While growing up in Cleveland, Mark showed great potential as an artist. When he left high school, he studied painting at an art college, which had a very active drama group. It had enough influence on him to push him towards a career in show business. His first job en route, was working as a radio announcer at a station in Akron, Ohio. Through that he developed his stage voice and got a number of roles in local plays. In 1942, Mark headed for Hollywood, where a year later, he became a contract player, named Stephen Richards, with Warner Brothers. He was given a series of bit parts, starting in 1943 with the Cary Grant – John Garfield war movie, *Destination Tokyo*. Until 1946, he was relatively unknown, but splitting from WB and changing his name to Mark Stevens, did the trick. 20th Century-Fox signed him and he became a star of a number of film-noir productions like *The Street With No Name,* and dramatic films such as *The Snake Pit*. The last fifteen years of his career, which ended in 1987, were spent in TV shows. Mark's wife from 1945-1962, was actress Annelle Hayes. He died of cancer in Majores, Spain.

Objective Burma! (1945)
God Is My Co-Pilot (1945)
Within These Walls (1945)
Pride of the Marines (1945)
From This Day Forward (1946)
The Dark Corner (1946)
I Wonder Who's
Kissing Her Now (1947)
The Street With No Name (1948)
The Snake Pit (1948)
Sand (1949)
Dancing in the Dark (1949)
Between Midnight
and Dawn (1950)
Target Unknown (1951)
The Lost Hours (1952)
Torpedo Alley (1953)
Jack Slade (1953)
Cry Vengeance (1954)
Timetable (1956)

Stella **Stevens**
5ft 5in
(ESTELLE CARO EGGLESTON)

Born: **October 1, 1936**
Yazoo City, Mississippi, USA

Stella married Herman Stevens when she was only fifteen. The couple soon had a son they named Andrew, but they were divorced after two years. Having made her big mistake early on, she focussed on her education – at Memphis State University – where she studied Medicine and first took an active interest in modeling and acting. In 1957, she starred as the female lead, Cherie, in the school production of "Bus Stop". After graduating, Stella's modeling work was the thing which brought her to the attention of Hollywood. She was discovered by a press-agent when she appeared in a fashion show, in the tea room of Goldsmith's Department Store, in Memphis. In 1959, she was given her film debut, with a bit part in *Say One For Me,* but she made her name in *Li'l Abner,* as Appassionata Von Climax. Stella posed for Playboy's January 1960 edition, and for the next decade or so, her face and figure were in demand – she co-starred with Elvis, Jerry Lewis and Dean Martin (separately), and worked in television series such as 'Surfside', 'Ben Casey' and 'General Hospital'. For several years now, Stella's been the partner of Bob Kulick, a guitarist and composer.

Li'l Abner (1959)
Man-Trap (1961)
Too Late Blues (1961)
Girls! Girls! Girls! (1962)
The Courtship of
Eddie's Father (1963)
The Nutty Professor (1963)
Advance to the Rear (1964)
The Silencers (1966)
Rage (1966)
How to Save a Marriage
and Ruin Your Life (1968)
Sol Madrid (1968)
Where Angels Go,
Trouble Follows (1968)
The Mad Room (1969)
The Ballad of Cable Hogue (1970)
Slaughter (1972)
The Poseidon Adventure (1972)
Nickelodeon (1976)

Alexandra **Stewart**
5ft 5in
(ALEXANDRA STEWART)

Born: **June 10, 1939**
Montréal, Québec, Canada

Although from Scottish stock, Alexandra grew up and went to school in Montréal. She was already fluent in French, when she left Canada in 1958, to study Art in Paris. She settled quickly in Europe and got caught up in the excitement of the French 'New Wave' of filmmaking. She took acting lessons and in 1959, was given her debut by the director/writer Jean Laviron, in his *Les Motards*. It was quickly followed by the first of six films for Pierre Kast – a comedy drama, *Le bel âge* – the cast of which included Jean-Claude Brialy. Alexandra had an uncredited appearance in Vadim's *Les Liaisons dangereuses* before starting her ride on the New Wave, in *L'Eau à la bouche.* She went to America for *Tarzan the Magnificent,* and *Exodus,* and then returned to France to work with Jean-Luc Godard, in *Ro.Go.Pa.G.,* Louis Malle, in *Le Feu follet,* as well as François Truffaut, in *The Bride Wore Black* and *Day for Night.* Alexandra had a daughter with Louis Malle. She lives in France nowadays and most of her film and television work is shot in Europe.

L'Eau à la bouche (1960)
Tarzan the Magnificent (1960)
Trapped by Fear (1960) Exodus (1960)
La Mort de Belle (1961) Les Mauvais
coups (1961) Ro.Go,Pa.G (1963)
The Endless Night (1963) Le Feu
follet (1963) Sweet and Sour (1963)
Thrilling (1965) The Wedding
March (1965) Mickey One (1965)
Law of Survival (1967)
Bye Bye, Barbara (1968)
The Bride Wore Black (1968)
Only When I Larf (1968)
Where Did Tom Go? (1971)
Zeppelin (1971)
Because of the Cats (1973)
Day for Night (1973)
Black Moon (1975)
Le Bon plaisir (1984) Frantic (1988)
Le Fils de Gascogne (1995)
Sous le Sable (2000)
Mon petit doigt m'a dit...(2005)
Fallen Heroes (2007)

James **Stewart**
6ft 3in
(JAMES MAITLAND STEWART)

Born: May 20, 1908
Indiana, Pennsylvania, USA
Died: **July 2, 1997**

Jimmy's parents, Alex and Elizabeth Stewart, owned a hardware store. He was the eldest of three children. After leaving Mercersburg Academy, Jimmy studied Architecture at Princeton University. While there, he met Joshua Logan, and joined his University Players.The company's stars included Margaret Sullavan and Henry Fonda – with whom he went to New York. He was given a screen test by MGM, who signed him, and he made his film debut, in 1934, with a bit part in *Art Trouble.* In *Born to Dance,* with Eleanor Powell, he attempted to sing. After being nominated for a Best Actor Oscar for *Mr. Smith Goes to Washington,* Jimmy was successful in 1941, for *The Philadelphia Story.* He also earned nominations for *It's a Wonderful Life, Harvey* and *Anatomy of a Murder.* His popularity remains undiminished thirty years after his final film, the Japanese-made, *A Tale of Africa.* He was happily married to Gloria Hatrick, from 1949 until, following some respiratory problems, he died in Los Angeles, of cardiac arrest .

Rose-Marie (1936) **Wife vs.**
Secretary (1936) **Born to Dance** (1936)
After the Thin Man (1936)
You Can't Take It with You (1938)
Mr. Smith Goes to Washington (1939)
Destry Rides Again (1939) **The Shop**
Around the Corner (1940)
The Mortal Storm (1940)
The Philadelphia Story (1940)
It's a Wonderful Life (1946)
Call Northside 777 (1948) **Rope** (1948)
The Stratton Story (1949)
Winchester '73 (1950)
Broken Arrow (1950) **Harvey** (1950)
Bend of the River (1952)
The Glenn Miller Story (1953)
Rear Window (1954)
The Man from Laramie (1955)
The Man Who Knew Too Much (1956)
Vertigo (1958) **Anatomy of a**
Murder (1959) **The Man Who**
Shot Liberty Valance (1962)
Shenandoah (1965)

Patrick **Stewart**
5ft 10in
(PATRICK STEWART)

Born: July 13, 1940
Mirfield, Yorkshire, England

Partrick was the son of Alfred Stewart, a Regimental Sergeant Major in the British Army. His mother worked as a weaver and textile worker in a Yorkshire mill. It was a tough time during World War II, with his dad being absent much of the time. When he did return home, he was abusive towards Patrick's mother. He was educated at Crowlees Church of England Junior and Infants' School and when he reached the age of eleven, Mirfield Secondary Modern. In 1955 he left school with the ambition to become an actor. He worked as a reporter on a local newspaper and whenever he could, he acted in plays performed at local theaters. When he was seventeen, Patrick took an acting course at the Bristol Old Vic Theater. He was already losing his hair, so he attended auditions wearing a rather unconvincing wig. He joined the Royal Shakespeare Company and appeared with them on Broadway. Patrick's film debut was in Trevor Nunn's adaptation of Henrik Ibsen's *Hedda.* His prowess as a great character actor saw him through the next two dozen years and he achieved fame as Captain Jean-Luc Picard, in the *Star Trek* films, and as Professor Xavier, in *X-Men.* Patrick was nominated for Golden Globes as Best Actor for two TV mini-series - 'Moby Dick' and 'The Lion in Winter'. Twice married – most recently to the producer, Wendy Neuss – he had two children. His son, Daniel, is an actor.

Hedda (1975) **Excalibur** (1981)
Dune (1984) **Life Force** (1985)
Code Name: Emerald (1985)
The Doctor and the Devils (1985)
Lady Jane (1986) **L.A. Story** (1991)
Robin Hood: Men in Tights (1993)
Star Trek: Generations (1994)
Let It Be Me (1995) **Star Trek: First**
Contact (1996) **Conspiracy Theory** (1997)
Dad Savage (1998) **Safe House** (1998)
Star Trek: Insurrection (1998)
X-Men (2000) **Star Trek:**
Nemesis (2002) **X2** (2003)
The Game of Their Lives (2005)

Julia **Stiles**
5ft 7½in
(JULIA O'HARA STILES)

Born: March 28, 1981
New York City, New York, USA

Julia's father, John O'Hara, was a teacher and businessman who ran a pottery in which her mother, Judith, worked at a wheel. They both were lapsed-Catholics. With her younger sister and brother, Julia was raised in the SoHo district of Manhattan. She was educated at Friends Seminary and took dancing classes. She became interested in acting when she was eleven. Julia appeared in La MaMa Theater Company productions and played the computer punk character, Erica Dansby, in the Public Broadcasting Services' 'Ghostwriter' in 1993 and 1994. Then, in 1996, she made her film debut, with a small role in *I Love You, I Love You Not.* Her first starring role was in the thriller, *Wicked.* For that film, she was named Best Actress at the Karlovy Vary Film Festival, in the Czech Republic. A year after that – closer to home, she shared the Most Promising Actress Award, for *10 Things I Hate About You.* That year, she graduated from New York Professional Children's School. She continued her career while studying, and in 2005, she left Columbia University, with a degree in English. Her importance in the three Bourne movies has increased with each outing. *The Bourne Ultimatum* allows her sufficient screen time to properly develop the character of Nicky Parsons.

The Devil's Own (1997)
Wicked (1998)
Wide Awake (1998)
10 Things I Hate
About You (1999)
Hamlet (2000)
State and Main (2000)
Save the Last Dance (2001)
The Business of Strangers (2001)
O (2001) **The Bourne Identity** (2002)
Mona Lisa Smile (2003)
The Prince & Me (2004)
The Bourne Supremacy (2004)
A Little Trip to Heaven (2005)
The Omen (2006)
The Bourne Ultimatum (2007)
Cry of the Owl (2009)

Ben Stiller

5ft 7in
(BENJAMIN EDWARD STILLER)

Born: **November 30, 1965**
New York City, New York, USA

Ben's father, Jerry Stiller, was Jewish, and his mother, Anne, was an Irish Catholic. Both of his parents were established actor/comedians. Young Ben was often taken onto the set with them and soon demonstrated that he had inherited their talent. When he was six, he made his first public appearance, on 'The Mike Douglas Show'. His older sister, Amy, had already done some acting and Ben was ten when he appeared as a guest in his mother's TV series, 'Kate McShane'. He appeared regularly with the First All Children's Theater, in New York, which provided valuable early experience. After he'd graduated from Calhoun School, Ben attended UCLA, then took acting lessons and landed a role on Broadway, in "The House of Blue Leaves". In 1987, he acted in a short, titled *Shoeshine,* and his first feature, *Hot Pursuit* – starring his dad. He has consistently delivered the goods for twenty years and his latest film, *Tropic Thunder,* shows off three aspects of his genius – director, writer and actor. Ben has two children with his wife, Christine.

Empire of the Sun (1987)
Next of Kin (1989) Highway to
Hell (1992) Reality Bites (1994)
Heavy Weights (1995)
Flirting with Disaster (1996)
The Cable Guy (1996)
There's Something About Mary (1998)
Your Friends & Neighbors (1998)
Permanent Midnight (1998)
Mystery Men (1999) The
Independent (2000) Meet the
Parents (2000) Zoolander (2001)
The Royal Tenenbaums (2001)
Along Came Polly (2004)
Starsky & Hutch (2004)
Dodgeball: A True
Underdog Story (2004)
Meet the Fockers (2004)
School for Scoundrels (2006)
Tenacious D in
The Pick of Destiny (2006)
Night at the Museum (2006)
Tropic Thunder (2008)

Dean Stockwell

5ft 6in
(ROBERT DEAN STOCKWELL)

Born: **March 5, 1936**
Hollywood, California, USA

Dean's parents were Harry Stockwell, who was an actor and singer, and Nina Olivette, who acted and danced. With such a pedigree, it was inevitable that Dean would make an early entrance into show business. When he was seven, this cute curly-haired kid started out on a sixty-year-long acting career. He signed a contract with MGM in 1944, and made his debut in 1945, with a small role in *Valley of Decision*. It was his role in his second film, *Anchors Aweigh* – as Kathryn Grayson's son – which showed off his acting talent. After that, he made progress as a juvenile – being the real star (although fourth-billed) in the title-role of *The Boy With Green Hair*. One of the few child actors to progress to an adult career, he was twice Best Actor at Cannes – for *Compulsion* and *Long Day's Journey Into Night*. Dean was Oscar-nominated for *Married to the Mob*. He was married and divorced twice and had a son and a daughter with his second wife, Joy.

Anchors Aweigh (1945)
The Green Years (1946)
The Romance of Rosy Ridge (1947)
Gentleman's Agreement (1947)
The Boy with Green Hair (1948)
Down to the Sea in Ships (1949)
The Secret Garden (1949)
Stars in My Crown (1950)
The Happy Years (1950) Kim (1950)
Cattle Drive (1951)
Gun for a Coward (1957)
Compulsion (1959)
Sons and Lovers (1960)
Long Day's Journey Into
Night (1962) Rapture (1965)
Psych-Out (1968) Tracks (1976)
Paris, Texas (1984) Dune (1984)
To Live and Die in L.A. (1985)
Blue Velvet (1986)
Married to the Mob (1988)
The Player (1992)
The Rainmaker (1997)
Air Force One (1997)
Buffalo Soldiers (2001)
The Manchurian Candidate (2004)

Eric Stoltz

6ft
(ERIC HAMILTON STOLTZ)

Born: **September 30, 1961**
Whittler, California, USA

The son of teachers, Jack and Evelyn Stoltz, Eric grew up in American Samoa, and Santa Barbara, California. He had an ear for music like his mother, who was a violinist. At the age of fourteen, he earned extra money by playing the piano for local stage shows. His sister, Catherine, is an opera singer. After San Marcos High School, he attended the University of Southern California, but dropped out in his junior year. He joined a repertory company with whom he went to Scotland and acted in plays at the Edinburgh Festival. In 1978, Eric made his first TV appearance, in 'The Grass Is Always Greener Over the Septic Tank'. In 1981, he began serious studies with Stella Adler and Peggy Feury, in New York. He made his movie debut, in *Fast Times at Ridgemont High,* the following year. He was nominated for a Golden Globe for *Mask*. After establishing himself as a movie actor, Eric has successfully turned to directing and producing - both for television and films – his short subject, *The Grand Design,* released in 2007, in which he also acts, is especially good.

Mask (1985)
Code Name: Emerald (1985)
Some Kind of Wonderful (1987)
Manifesto (1988)
Haunted Summer (1988)
Say Anything (1989)
Memphis Belle (1990)
The Waterdance (1992)
Pulp Fiction (1994)
Killing Zoe (1994)
Little Women (1994)
Rob Roy (1995) Fluke (1995)
The Prophecy (1995)
Kicking and Screaming (1995)
2 Days in the Valley (1999)
Jerry Maguire (1996)
Mr. Jealousy (1997) Hi-Life (1998)
It's a Shame About Ray (2000)
The House of Mirth (2000)
The Rules of Attraction (2002)
Happy Hour (2003)
The Butterfly Effect (2004)
The Lather Effect (2006)

Lewis **Stone**
5ft 10½in
(LEWIS SHEPARD STONE)

Born: **November 15, 1879**
Worcester, Massachusetts, USA
Died: **September 12, 1953**

Raised in a well-to-do American family in the second-biggest city in New England, Lew fought in the Spanish-American War in 1898. The effect of that experience turned him prematurely gray by the age of twenty. He began getting his first stage roles at the beginning of the 20th century and for a dozen or so years, he established himself in the American theater. He started his film career in 1914, in a William S. Hart western, *The Bargain*. Two years after that, he served in the cavalry during World War I. By the time he starred with Garbo and Gilbert in a *A Woman of Affairs,* he had acted in over fifty movies. He was nominated for an Oscar, for *The Patriot*. His prolific work continued through the 'talkies' era with another ninety films. Some – *Grand Hotel, Queen Christina* and *David Copperfield,* are classics. His third wife, Hazel, was with him when he died in Beverly Hills from a heart attack triggered by chasing some kids who were throwing stones at his garage.

The Big House (1930) Romance (1930) Inspiration (1931) The Phantom of Paris (1931) The Sin of Madelon Claudet (1931) Strictly Dishonorable (1931) Mata Hari (1931) Grand Hotel (1932) Night Court (1932) Letty Lynton (1932) Unashamed (1932) Men Must Fight (1933) The White Sister (1933) Bureau of Missing Persons (1933) Queen Christina (1933) The Mystery of Mr. X (1934) The Girl from Missouri (1934) Treasure Island (1934) David Copperfield (1935) China Seas (1935) Three Godfathers (1936) The Unguarded Hour (1936) Small Town Girl (1936) You're Only Young Once (1937) Andy Hardy's Dilemma (1938) Judge Hardy and Son (1939) Three Wise Fools (1946) State of the Union (1948) Scaramouche (1952) The Prisoner of Zenda (1953) All the Brothers Were Valiant (1953)

Sharon **Stone**
5ft 8½in
(SHARON VONNE STONE)

Born: **March 10, 1958**
Meadville, Pennsylvania, USA

The second of four children, Sharon was raised in a very strict family environment. With an IQ of 154, she was exceptionally bright and excelled during her teen years, at Saegertown High School and Edinboro University, in Pennsylvania, from where she graduated with a degree in Creative Writing and Fine Arts. When she was seventeen, Sharon entered, and won, the "Miss Pennsylvania" Beauty Contest. From that platform, she began a successful career as a Ford Model – appearing in magazines and television commercials for a variety of products. But after living in Europe, she decided to become an actress. In 1980, she made her film debut, with a bit part in Woody Allen's *Stardust Memories.* Sharon's film career took off with Arnold Schwarzenegger, in *Total Recall* and posed nude for Playboy. She became a fully-fledged star, in *Basic Instinct* – which produced an iconic image in the scene when she was being interrogated. She was later nominated for a Best Actress Oscar for *Casino* – which won her a Golden Globe, in 1996. The following year, Sharon won an Emmy Award, as Outstanding Guest Actress in the television drama series, 'The Practice'.

Irreconcilable Differences (1984) Beyond the Stars (1989) Total Recall (1990) He Said, She Said (1991) Basic Instinct (1992) Last Action Hero (1993) The Quick and the Dead (1995) Casino (1995) Last Dance (1996) Sphere (1998) The Mighty (1998) The Muse (1999) Beautiful Joe (2000) Broken Flowers (2005) Alpha Dog (2006) Bobby (2006) If I Had Known I Was a Genius (2007) When a Man Falls in the Forest (2007) The Year of Getting to Know Us (2008) $5 a Day (2008)

Madeleine **Stowe**
5ft 6½in
(MADELEINE MARIE STOWE MORA)

Born: **August 18, 1958**
Los Angeles, California, USA

Madeleine was the eldest of three girls born to Robert and Mireya Stowe. Her father, a civil engineer, was from Oregon, and her mother came from Costa Rica. She grew up in Eagle Rock, a working-class district of Los Angeles, but when she was ten, she showed enough natural musical talent to take piano lessons from the renowned music teacher, Sergei Tarnowsky. Following his death, she gave up any idea of a career in music. Instead, she studied Journalism and Cinema at the University of Southern California, and was soon performing in plays at the Solaris Theater in Beverly Hills. It was there that she was spotted by a movie agent. In 1978, he got Madeleine her first television role, in the crime series, 'Baretta'. After three years of TV she made her movie debut, in 1981, in the independent film *Gangster Wars*. Madeleine married the actor, Brian Benben, the following year. They run a ranch in Texas together. Her first major screen acting break came when she was cast opposite Richard Dreyfuss and Emilio Estevez, in the hit, *Stakeout*. International stardom looked hers for the asking after *The Last of the Mohicans, Short Cuts* and *Twelve Monkeys,* but her film career has faded during the past five years. In 2007, Madeleine was seen as Dr. Samantha Kohl, in several episodes of the television crime drama, 'Raines'. As of this moment there is nothing new lined up.

Stakeout (1987) Tropical Snow (1989) Worth Winning (1989) Revenge (1990) The Two Jakes (1990) Closet Land (1991) The Last of the Mohicans (1992) Short Cuts (1993) Blink (1994) China Moon (1994) Twelve Monkeys (1995) Playing by Heart (1998) The General's Daughter (1999) Impostor (2001) We Were Soldiers (2002)

Susan **Strasberg**
5ft 1in
(SUSAN ELIZABETH STRASBERG)

Born: **May 22, 1938**
New York City, New York, USA
Died: **January 21, 1999**

Susan was raised in a Jewish family. She was the daughter of the famed drama coach, Lee Strasberg and his actress wife, Paula Miller. She inherited their passion for acting, and was fifteen when she made her screen debut, on TV, in the 'Goodyear Television Playhouse'. In 1955, Susan made her stage debut, on Broadway, in the title role of "The Diary of Anne Frank". That same year, she had a good supporting role in her first movie, *Picnic,* and was nominated for a BAFTA as Most Promising Newcomer to Film. She returned to the stage - appearing with such luminaries as Richard Burton (with whom she had a passionate affair) and Helen Hayes. She alternated between the theater and films for the rest of her career – never quite achieving stardom on the screen, and won just one award – Best Actress at the Mar del Plata Film Festival, for *Kapò*. From 1965-68, she was married to the actor, Christopher Jones. They had a daughter named Jennifer. Susan was a close friend of Marilyn Monroe and appeared in three documentaries about her. Her last film was *Il Giardino dei ciliegi* – made in Italy in 1992. She died at her home in New York City after a long battle with breast cancer.

Picnic (1955)
The Cobweb (1955)
Stage Struck (1958)
Kapò (1959)
Taste of Fear (1961)
Hemingway's Adventures of
a Young Man (1962)
The High Bright Sun (1964)
The Trip (1967)
Psych-Out (1968)
The Name of the Game Is
Kill (1968) Chubasco (1968)
The Brotherhood (1968)
My Sister, My Love (1969)
Jailbird (1969)
The Legend of
Hillbilly John (1974)
In Praise of Older Women (1978)
The Delta Force (1986)

David **Strathairn**
6ft
(DAVID RUSSELL STRATHAIRN)

Born: **January 26, 1949**
San Francisco, California, USA

David's father, Tom Strathairn Jr., was a physician of Scottish ancestry and David, his brother, Tom, and sister, Anne, have Hawaiian blood from their mother, Mary. After Redwood High School in Larkspur, California, he graduated from Williams College in Williamstown, Massachusetts. It was there that he befriended the future screen writer, John Sales, with whom he'd work with frequently during his career. David appeared in stage productions while at the college, but first experienced professional show business, following study at Ringling Brothers Clown College in Venice, Florida, when he spent six months with a traveling circus. With actor friends, he founded a children's theater troupe and re-established contact with Sayles at the New Hampshire Playhouse. It led to his movie debut, when, in 1980, they collaborated in *Return of the Secaucus Seven*. Logan Goodman – whom he married, was a production assistant on the film. He started a family immediately, and built a reputation as a supporting actor. Surprisingly, his only nomination for an Oscar – was as Best Actor, in *Good Night, and Good Luck* – twenty-five years after his debut.

At Close Range (1986) Matewan (1987)
Eight Men Out (1988) Memphis
Belle (1990) City of Hope (1991)
A League of Their Own (1992)
Bob Roberts (1992) Sneakers (1992)
Passion Fish (1992) Lost in
Yonkers (1993) The Firm (1993)
The River Wild (1994)
Losing Isaiah (1995)
Home for the Holidays (1995)
L.A. Confidential (1997)
With Friends Like These... (1998)
A Midsummer Night's Dream (1999)
Limbo (1999) A Good Baby (2000)
Harrison's Flowers (2000) Blue
Car (2002) Missing in America (2005)
Good Night, And Good Luck (2005)
The Notorious Bettie Page (2005)
The Bourne Ultimatum (2007)
The Spiderwick Chronicles (2008)

Meryl **Streep**
5ft 6in
(MARY LOUISE STREEP)

Born: **June 22, 1949**
Summit, New Jersey, USA

Meryl is the daughter of a pharmaceutical company executive and a mother who worked as a graphic artist. At high school, Meryl was extremely popular and admired for her sporting prowess – including being the school's swimming champion. She won a scholarship to Yale University, where she studied for a Fine Arts degree and developed a reputation as a bright young actress. After acting lessons, she first established herself with a career on the New York stage and was twenty-eight when she made her film debut, in *Julia*. Meryl then won an Emmy for her portrayal of the German girl, Inga, in the acclaimed TV production, 'Holocaust'. Later that year, she married sculptor, Don Gummer, and gave birth to her son Henry, in 1979. She became a top movie actress with strong performances in films like *The Deerhunter, Manhattan,* and *Kramer vs. Kramer* – for which she won a Best Supporting Actress Oscar. She was nominated for *The French Lieutenant's Woman* and won for *Sophie's Choice*. She was also nominated for *Silkwood, Out of Africa, Ironweed, A Cry in the Dark, Postcards from the Edge, The Bridges of Madison County, One True Thing, Music of the Heart, Adaptation, The Devil Wears Prada* and *Doubt*. Meryl is a Superstar.

The Deer Hunter (1978) Manhattan (1979)
Kramer vs. Kramer (1979) Sophie's
Choice (1982) Silkwood (1983)
Out of Africa (1985) Ironweed (1988)
A Cry in the Dark (1988)
Postcards from the Edge (1990)
Defending Your Life (1991)
The House of the Spirits (1993)
The River Wild (1994) The Bridges of
Madison County (1995) Before and
After (1996) Marvin's Room (1996)
One True Thing (1998)
Music of the Heart (1999)
Adaptation (2002) The Hours (2002)
The Devil Wears Prada (2006)
Evening (2007) Rendition (2007)
Lion for Lambs (2008)
Mama Mia! (2008) Doubt (2008)

Barbra **Streisand**
5ft 5in
(BARBARA JOAN STREISAND)

Born: **April 24, 1942**
Brooklyn, New York City, New York, USA

Barbra's father, Emanuel was a Jewish immigrant from Vienna, who became a teacher. Her mother, Diana, worked as a secretary in a school. Barbra was educated at Bais Yakov School and Erasmus Hall High School, where she sang in the choir with Neil Diamond and was friendly with the future World Chess Champion, Bobby Fischer. She graduated fourth in her class in 1959. Barbra's mother urged her to train as a secretary because she didn't think her daughter was pretty enough for a show business career. But this girl had bags of talent and she soon proved her mother wrong. She started out as a nightclub singer and built up a big following when she performed at a gay bar – in Greenwich Village. In 1962, she made her Broadway debut with the small but visible role of Miss Marmelstein, in the musical, "I Can Get It for You Wholesale". That was also the year she signed a record contract with Columbia and appeared on the 'Ed Sullivan Show'. In 1963, she opened for Liberace, at Harrah's, in Lake Tahoe, and her first LP, "The Barbra Streisand Album" won two Grammys. The following year, she was on Broadway, as Fanny Brice, in "Funny Girl". It became her movie debut, and won her a Best Actress Oscar. She makes records and is also a producer and director. Her small number of films have usually been special. She was nominated for an Oscar for *The Way We Were*. Barbra's been married to James Brolin since 1998. Her first husband was Elliott Gould. They had a son named Jason.

Funny Girl (1968)
Hello, Dolly (1969)
What's Up, Doc? (1972)
The Way We Were (1973)
For Pete's Sake (1974)
Funny Lady (1975)
A Star Is Born (1976)
All Night Long (1981)
Yentl (1983) **Nuts** (1987)
The Prince of Tides (1991)
The Mirror Has Two Faces (1996)
Meet the Fockers (2004)

Woody **Strode**
6ft 4in
(WOODROW WILSON WOOLWINE STRODE)

Born: **July 25, 1914**
Los Angeles, California, USA
Died: **December 31, 1994**

He had Native American blood in his veins – partly Blackfoot and Cherokee. During his early years, Woody was an exceptional athlete. By the time he was studying at UCLA, he was not only one of the first African Americans to attend University, he was setting intercollegiate records for the decathlon – his shot-put and high jump marks were only slightly short of the world records at the time. In 1939, Woody starred for the UCLA Bruins football team - together with Kenny Washington, who became a professional footballer, and Jackie Robinson, who starred for the Brooklyn Dodgers and was inducted into the Baseball Hall of Fame. Woody then became a professional footballer with the Cleveland Rams (later the Los Angeles Rams) and for the Calgary Stampeders, in Canada. When his football days were over, he made a living from wrestling. In 1941, he married a girl from Hawaii called Luana and made an uncredited film debut, in the African-set war drama, *Sundown.* After two more bit parts, he wasn't seen on the screen again until 1951. Nothing much happened until *Pork Chop Hill,* but he made the most of supporting roles. He did star or was featured – most memorably in *Sergeant Rutledge* and *Spartacus* – for which he was nominated for a Golden Globe. His second wife, Tina, was with him when he died of lung cancer, at his home in Glendora, California.

Pork Chop Hill (1959) **The Last Voyage** (1960) **Sergeant Rutledge** (1960) **Spartacus** (1960) **The Sins of Rachel Cade** (1961) **The Man Who Shot Liberty Vallance** (1962) **Ghengis Khan** (1965) **7 Women** (1966) **The Professionals** (1966) **Black Jesus** (1968) **Once Upon a Time in the West** (1968) **The Unholy Four** (1970) **The Deserter** (1971) **Hit Men** (1972) **Keoma** (1976) **Kingdom of the Spiders** (1977) **Vigilante** (1983) **The Black Stallion Returns** (1983)

Mark **Strong**
6ft 2in
(MARCO GIUSEPPE SALUSSOLIA)

Born: **January 1, 1963**
Islington, London, England

The son of an Italian father and an Austrian mother, Mark's name was changed by deed poll when his mother decided that he shouldn't sound so foreign if he was going to grow up in the capital city of England. Even so, through her influence, he became fluent in German. When he was still a small boy, the family moved around a bit to different areas of London, and he changed schools several times. When he was eleven, Mark became a boarder at a school in the county of Norfolk, called Wymondham College. At that time he loved "The Clash" and was a singer in punk rock bands – "The Electric Hoax" and "Private Partner". His ambition was to be a lawyer, but after one year at Munich University, he took a joint English and Drama degree at Royal Holloway, University of London, and completed his training at Bristol Old Vic Theater School. Following stage experience he made his television debut, in an episode of 'After Henry', in 1989. Four more years of TV work elapsed before he made his movie debut, with a small role in *Century*. It was his portrayal of Mr. Knightley in the small screen adaptation of 'Emma', which first brought him fame, and the soccer-themed film, *Fever Pitch,* secured it. He acted with Penélope Cruz, then went international in films like *Sunshine*. In 2002, he acted on stage in "Twelfth Night" and was nominated for a Laurence Olivier Theater Award. Mark soon reached movie A-List fringes, in Polanski's *Oliver Twist, Syriana,* and now he's there – in Ridley Scott's *Body of Lies*. He's married and has two children.

Fever Pitch (1997)
The Man with Rain in His Shoes (1998)
Sunshine (1999) **To End All Wars** (2001) **Heartlands** (2002)
It's All About Love (2003)
Oliver Twist (2005)
Revolver (2005) **Syriana** (2005)
Tristan + Isolde (2006)
Scenes of a Sexual Nature (2006)
Stardust (2007) **RocknRolla** (2008)
Body of Lies (2008)

Margaret **Sullavan**
5ft 2½in
(MARGARET BROOKE SULLAVAN HANCOCK)

Born: **May 16, 1909**
Norfolk, Virginia, USA
Died: **January 1, 1960**

The daughter of a wealthy stockbroker, Margaret was educated at Chatham Episcopal Institute, a private boarding school where she became president of the student body. She moved to Boston to live with her half-sister and took dancing lessons. She started her acting career with the Harvard Dramatic Club – making her debut in 1929, in "Close Up". Margaret was then invited to join the University Players, in Falmouth. They gave her her professional stage debut, in their first offering, "The Devil in the Cheese". In 1931, she married the first of her four husbands, Henry Fonda – it lasted barely one year, during which, she first appeared on Broadway, in "A Modern Virgin". For a while, she was content to concentrate on stage work. Margaret was twenty-four when she went to Hollywood – making her film debut, in 1933, in *Only Yesterday*. She appeared in a number of excellent movies during the 1930s – one of which, *Three Comrades*, produced her only Best Actress Oscar Award nomination. She made her last screen appearance, in *No Sad Songs for Me*, but was on Broadway in the early 1950s, in "The Deep Blue Sea" and "Sabrina Fair". Margaret suffered from severe depression which was made worse as she grew older by increasing deafness. She was found dead in her hotel room in New Haven, after she had deliberately overdosed on barbiturates.

Only Yesterday (1933) Little Man,
What Now? (1934)
The Good Fairy (1935)
I Loved a Soldier (1936)
Next Time We Love (1936)
Three Comrades (1938)
The Shopworn Angel (1938)
The Shining Hour (1938)
The Shop Around the Corner (1940)
The Mortal Storm (1940)
Back Street (1941)
So Ends Our Night (1941)
Cry 'Havoc' (1943)
No Sad Songs for Me (1950)

Barry **Sullivan**
6ft 2½in
(PATRICK BARRY SULLIVAN)

Born: **August 29, 1912**
New York City, New York, USA
Died: **June 6, 1994**

Barry's father was the seventh son of his parents – and so was Barry! He took little interest in acting during his early years at school. It was when he attended Temple University, in Philadelphia – studying Law, he worked as an usher in a local theater and got his first close-up view of a stage. Because of his physique and good looks, he was tipped off about money-making opportunities in Broadway shows. He returned to New York, and after several walk-on parts, starting with "I Want a Policeman", he was given his first real opportunity to act, in the 1936 production of "Brother Rat". He gained experience by appearing in short comedies produced in Manhattan. His official film debut, was in a western, *The Woman of the Town*. His most important film role was in *The Bad and the Beautiful.* He was twice married. In 1987, after a Canadian film, *The Last Straw,* he retired. He died of a respiratory ailment in Sherman Oaks. His Daughter, Jenny is an actress and playwright.

The Woman of the Town (1943)
Lady in the Dark (1944)
Rainbow Island (1944)
And Now Tomorrow (1944)
Getting Gertie's Garter (1945)
Suspense (1946) Framed (1947)
The Gangster (1947)
Smart Woman (1948)
Bad Men of Tombstone (1949)
Any Number Can Play (1949)
The Great Gatsby (1949)
Tension (1949) The Outriders (1950)
Nancy Goes to Rio (1950)
Grounds for Marriage (1951)
Payment on Demand (1951)
Three Guys Named Mike (1951)
Inside Straight (1951) Cause for
Alarm! (1951) No Questions
Asked (1951) The Bad and the
Beautiful (1952) Jeopardy (1953)
Strategic Air Command (1955)
Queen Bee (1955) Another Time,
Another Place (1958) Light in
the Piazza (1962)

Francis L. **Sullivan**
5ft 8in
(FRANCIS LOFTUS SULLIVAN)

Born: **January 6, 1903**
Wandsworth, London, England
Died: **November 19, 1956**

From a wealthy Irish family, Francis was educated at private schools including the Jesuit boarding school, Stonyhurst, in Lancashire – whose alumni included Sir Arthur Conan Doyle and actor, Charles Laughton. Always a big fan of William Shakespeare during his schooldays, he made his stage debut in 1921, in Richard III, at the Old Vic in London. Francis then spent ten years learning his craft on the British stage. He befriended Agatha Christie – appearing in two of her 'Poirot' plays as well as the 'classics'. He made his film debut, in 1932, in a Sherlock Holmes mystery, *The Missing Rembrandt.* Two years later, after impressing in British films like *Chu-Chin-Chow*, Francis went to Hollywood to play Jaggers, in the first version of *Great Expectations*. Although not great, that and subsequent productions made him feel at home in America and he eventually became a U.S. citizen. He returned to England to act in David Lean classics *Great Expectations*, and *Oliver Twist*. His last performance was in 1955, as Captain Bligh, in an episode of 'General Electric Theater' on American TV. Francis died of a heart attack the following year.

F.P.I. (1933) Chu-Chin-Chow (1934)
The Return of Bulldog
Drummond (1934)
Mystery of Edwin Drood (1935)
Non-Stop New
York (1937) The Drum (1938)
The Citadel (1938)
21 Days Together (1940)
'Pimpernel' Smith (1941)
The Day Will Dawn (1942)
The Foreman Went to France (1942)
Caesar and Cleopatra (1945)
Great Expectations (1946)
The Man Within (1948)
Oliver Twist (1948)
The Winslow Boy (1948)
Joan of Arc (1948) The Red
Danube (1949) Night and
the City (1950) My Favorite
Spy (1951) Sangaree (1953)

Donald **Sutherland**
6ft 4in
(DONALD MCNICHOL SUTHERLAND)

Born: **July 17, 1935**
Saint John, New Brunswick, Canada

Donald's father, Frederick Sutherland, ran the St. John Gas and Electricity, and Bus Company. His mother was homemaker, Dorothy McNichol. When he was eleven, Donald was confined to bed for a whole year when he contracted rheumatic fever. Three years later, after a school trip to local radio station, CKBW, in Bridgewater, Donald became Canada's youngest-ever announcer and disc-jockey. He studied Engineering and Drama at the University of Toronto and graduated with a double major. Donald's involvement with the "UC Follies" and success in Shakespeare's "The Tempest", in Toronto, changed his mind about becoming an engineer. He went to London, where he studied acting at RADA, then spent nearly five years in the U.K. In 1962, he made his TV debut, in a BBC 'Studio Four' drama and made his film debut, with a bit part in *The World Ten Times Over,* in 1963. He progressed via *The Dirty Dozen* to star-billing in classics like *Klute* and *Don't Look Now*. All three wives were actresses – his present wife, Francine Racette, is the mother of his three young sons. Twins, Kiefer and Rachel, who are both in show business, are from his second wife, Shirley Douglas.

MASH (1970) **Kelly's Heroes** (1970)
Klute (1971) **Don't Look Now** (1973)
The Day of the Locust (1975)
1900 (1976) **The Eagle Has
Landed** (1976) **Invasion of the Body
Snatchers** (1978) **Murder By
Decree** (1979) **The First Great Train
Robbery** (1979) **Ordinary People** (1980)
Eye of the Needle (1981)
Threshold (1981) **Heaven Help Us** (1985)
A Dry White Season (1989)
Backdraft (1991) **JFK** (1991)
Six Degrees of Separation (1993)
Outbreak (1995) **A Time to
Kill** (1996) **The Assignment** (1997)
Fallen (1998) **Without Limits** (1998)
Panic (2000) **Aurora Borealis** (2005)
Pride & Prejudice (2005)
Land of the Blind (2006)
Reign Over Me (2007) **Fool's Gold** (2008)

Kiefer **Sutherland**
5ft 9in
(KIEFER WILLIAM FREDERICK.D.G.R.SUTHERLAND)

Born: **December 21, 1966**
London, England

Kiefer and his twin sister, Rachel, were born at St. Mary's Hospital, in Paddington, when both his actor parents – his father, Donald, and his mother, Shirley Douglas, were working in London. Kiefer was taken to live in Los Angeles when he was still a toddler – his parents divorced in 1970. Kiefer moved to Toronto with his mother in 1975 and was somehow totally unaware that his father was an actor until he was eighteen. He attended Crescent Town School and St. Clair Junior High School in East York, Ontario, before four different high schools – the last being Malvern Collegiate Institute, which has Glenn Gould, Norman Jewison, and Keanu Reeves among its alumni. Finally, he spent one semester at Regina Mundi Catholic College, in London, Ontario. He left Canada to work in commercials, in New York. In 1983, Kiefer made his film debut, in *Max Duggan Returns*. His first important screen role was in Canada, the following year, in *The Bay Boy*. In 1987, he married Camelia, the widow of Terry Kath, the legendary rock guitarist from "Chicago". They divorced in 1990. His films number more than seventy, but the list below covers the cream. Since 2001, Kiefer has been seen as Jack Bauer, in the TV-series, '24'.

The Bay Boy (1984) **At Close
Range** (1986) **Stand by Me** (1986)
Promised Land (1987)
The Lost Boys (1987)
Crazy Moon (1987)
Young Guns (1988) **1969** (1988)
Flashback (1990) **Young Guns II** (1990)
Flatliners (1990) **Article 99** (1992)
Twin Peaks: Fire Walk with Me (1992)
A Few Good Men (1992)
The Three Musketeers (1993)
Freeway (1996) **A Time to Kill** (1996)
Truth or Consequences, N.M. (1997)
Dark City (1998) **Ground
Control** (1998) **Desert Saints** (2000)
To End All Wars (2001) **Phone
Booth** (2002) **River Queen** (2005)
The Sentinel (2006)
Mirrors (2008)

John **Sutton**
6ft 2in
(JOHN SUTTON)

Born: **October 22, 1908**
Rawalpindi, British India
Died: **July 10, 1953**

John spent his early years in a part of British-ruled India which is now known as Punjab, Pakistan. When he was thirteen, he was sent to England to be educated at Wellington College, at Crowthorne, in Berkshire – a school which was founded by Queen Victoria in 1859, in memory of Britain's greatest military figure, the "Iron Duke". When he was eighteen, John set out to see the the world – traveling in China and the Far East, working as a big game hunter in various parts of Africa, and spending two years as a tea plantation manager in Kenya. When he returned to England in 1935, John made up his mind to go to Hollywood. He was immediately employed to give expert advice to the film industry on aspects of the British Empire. Being tall and handsome, he was given his first acting opportunity – in an uncredited part, in the 1936 film, *The Last of the Mohicans*. In the early 1940s, John was put under contract by 20th Century Fox, for whom he played strong supporting roles in such films as *Hudson's Bay* and *Jane Eyre*. Much of his later work was on TV. He died of a heart attack in France.

Four Men and a Prayer (1938)
Susannah of the Mounties (1939)
Bulldog Drummond's Bride (1939)
Tower of London (1939)
The Invisible Man Returns (1940)
Hudson's Bay (1941)
A Yank in the R.A.F. (1941)
My Gal Sal (1942) **Ten Gentlemen
from West Point** (1942)
Thunderbirds (1942) **Tonight We
Raid Calais** (1943) **Jane Eyre** (1944)
The Hour Before the Dawn (1944)
Claudia and David (1946)
Captain from Castile (1947)
The Counterfeiters (1948)
Mickey (1948)
The Three Musketeers (1948)
The Fan (1948) **Bagdad** (1949)
The Second Woman (1950)
Payment on Demand (1951)
My Cousin Rachel (1952)

Bo **Svenson**
6ft 5in
(BORIS LEE HOLDER SVENSON)

Born: **February 13, 1944**
Gothenburg, Västra Götalands län, Sweden

Bo's father, Birger Svenson, was a superb athlete who became the personal driver and bodyguard to King Gustaf of Sweden. In 1939-40, in the Finno-Russian Winter War, he fought on the side of the vastly outnumbered Finns. Bo's mother, Lola, who was from Russian stock, was an actress and singer, who at one time led her own dance band. When Bo left school, he made a big decision and emigrated to the United States without his family. He served for six years in the U.S. Marines, during which time he attended the University of Meiji, in Japan. A Black Belt, Bo became Far East Heavyweight Judo Champion in 1961. After being honorably discharged from the Marines, he studied for a Ph.D. in Metaphysics at UCLA. In his leisure time he played ice-hockey and drove racing cars. In 1967, he made his TV debut, in an episode of 'N.Y.P.D.' and after six years of exposure on the small screen, he made his film debut, in the biography of basketball star, Maurice Stokes, titled *Maurie*. His first high-profile movie was *The Great Waldo Pepper*. Being one of the tallest leading men, he inevitably got a large proportion of action roles, but he could show sensitivity and humor when given the chance. He was CEO of Motion Picture Group of America from 1984-95. After experiencing a hiatus during the 1990s, and some less than successful directing efforts, Bo bounced back with some good roles. He has three daughters with his wife, Lise.

The Great Waldo Pepper (1975)
Special Delivery (1976)
Counterfeit Commandos (1978)
North Dallas Forty (1979)
Day of Resurrection (1980)
Night Warning (1983)
The Delta Force (1986)
Heartbreak Ridge (1986)
Private Obsession (1995)
Kill Bill: Vol. 2 (2004)
Raising Jeffrey Dahmer (2006)
Chinaman's Chance (2008)
Jersey Justice (2008)

Hilary **Swank**
5ft 6in
(HILARY ANN SWANK)

Born: **July 30, 1974**
Bellingham, Washington, USA

Hilary's father, Stephen, was an officer in the Air Guard – a branch of the United States Airforce. Her mother, Judy, was a secretary who loved dancing. When she was six, she and her brother, Dan, grew up in a trailer park at Lake Samish, outside Bellingham, but Hilary already had her sights on something more glamorous. In 1984, after coaching by Suzy Sachs, she played 'Mowgli' in her school's production of "The Jungle Book". By the time she was attending Sehome High School, her talents were being used by Bellingham Theater Guild. She was a fine athlete – good enough to compete in Washington State's Swimming Championships, and ranking fifth in the State in gymnastics. Her parents were divorced when she was thirteen, and as soon as Hilary left high school, her mother took her to live in Los Angeles, to give her the best chance of an acting career. She spent a short time at South Pasadena High School, but left as soon as she began getting roles on TV. She made her film, debut in *Buffy the Vampire Slayer*, in 1992. Her athleticism came in useful in *The Next Karate Kid*, and it would prove even more so, later in her career. Hilary won her first Best Actress Oscar, for *Boy's Don't Cry*, and a second, for *Million Dollar Baby* – where she really had to get in top physical condition. She had married Rob Lowe's brother, Chad, in 1997, but it was all over in 2006. In her next film, *Amelia*, Hilary portrays the great American female pilot, Amelia Earhart.

The Next Karate Kid (1998)
Heartwood (1998)
Boys Don't Cry (1999)
The Gift (2000)
The Affair of the Necklace (2001)
Insomnia (2002)
The Core (2003) **11:14** (2003)
Red Dust (2004)
Million Dollar Baby (2004)
Freedom Writers (2007)
The Reaping (2007)
P.S. I Love You (2007)
Birds of America (2008)

Patrick **Swayze**
5ft 10in
(PATRICK WAYNE SWAYZE)

Born: **August 18, 1952**
Houston, Texas, USA

Patrick has two brothers and a sister. His father Jessie Swayze, worked in engineering and his mother, Patsy, is well known as a dancer and choreographer. Patrick was educated at St. Rose of Lima Catholic School, Oak Forest Elementary, Black Junior High, and Waltrip High – all in Houston. During that time, he was active as an ice skater and a classical ballet dancer. He studied Gymnastics at nearby San Jacinto College, before touring as Prince Charming in "Disney On Ice". At the age of twenty, he went to live in New York, were he attended the Harkness Ballet and Joffrey Ballet School. In 1975, he married his one-and-only wife, Lisa Niemi. He starred in the Broadway production of "Grease" before making his movie debut in 1979, in *Skatetown, U.S.A*. He studied at the Beverly Hills Playhouse and kept on appearing in films, but his first big success was on television, in the 1985 mini-series, 'North and South'. He reached star status when he played the instructor in the smash-hit, *Dirty Dancing*, and was nominated for a Golden Globe. After the deaths of his father and sister, Patrick had drink problems. In 1996, he was seriously injured while filming, and it interrupted his career. Since the new millennium, he has acted in some good movies. Diagnosed with pancreatic cancer, in January 2008, early response to treatment was hopeful, and he's working with genuine optimism, in a television series, 'The Beast'.

The Outsiders (1983)
Uncommon Valor (1983)
Red Dawn (1984) **Dirty Dancing** (1987)
Road House (1989) **Ghost** (1990)
Point Break (1991) **City of Joy** (1992)
Tall Tale (1995) **To Wong Foo Thanks for Everything, Julie Newmar** (1995)
Three Wishes (1995)
Letters from a Killer (1998)
Forever Lulu (2000) **Green Dragon** (2001) **Donny Darko** (2001)
Waking Up in Reno (2002)
11:14 (2003) **George and the Dragon** (2004) **Keeping Mum** (2005)

Tilda **Swinton**
5ft 10½in
(KATHERINE MATILDA SWINTON)

Born: **November 5, 1960**
London, England

Tilda is the daughter of a Scottish father, Major-General Sir John Swinton, and an Australian mother, Judith Balfour. She was in the same class as Diana, Princess of Wales, when she was a boarder at the exclusive West Heath Girls' School, in Seven Oaks, Kent. Her early education also included Fettes College, Edinburgh. In 1983, Tilda graduated from Cambridge University with a degree in English Literature. She began her theatrical career with the Traverse Theater, in Edinburgh, and later, she worked with the Royal Shakespeare Company. She made her film debut, in 1986, with a small part in Derek Jarman's *Caravaggio*. Three years later, he used her in a leading role in his *War Requiem*. Tilda's most memorable early film role was as the gender-bending *Orlando*. Since then, she's played some interesting and unorthodox characters. She was rewarded for her endeavors at the 2008 Academy Awards, when she won a Best Supporting Actress Oscar, for *Michael Clayton*. She lives in Nairn, with the Scottish painter, John Byrne, who is the father of her twins, but true to her non-conformist nature, she's in a relationship with Sandro Kopp, a New Zealand artist.

Friendship's Death (1987)
The Last of England (1988)
War Requiem (1989) The Garden (1990)
The Party: Nature Morte (1991)
Orlando (1992) Love Is the
Devil: Study for a Portrait of
Francis Bacon (1998) The War
Zone (1999) The Beach (2000)
The Deep End (2001) Vanilla Sky (2001)
Adaptation (2002) Young Adam (2003)
The Statement (2003)
Thumbsucker (2005) Constantine (2005)
Broken Flowers (2005)
The Chronicles of Narnia (2005)
Stephanie Daley (2006)
A Londoni férfi (2007) Michael
Clayton (2007) Julia (2008)
Burn After Reading (2008)
The Curious Case of
Benjamin Button (2008)

Gloria **Swanson**
4ft 11½in
(GLORIA MAY JOSEPHINE SVENSSON)

Born: **March 27, 1899**
Chicago, Illinois, USA
Died: **April 4, 1983**

Gloria's parents were Swedish and Polish Americans. Her father, Joseph Svensson, was a professional soldier. Her mother Adelaide's original name was Klanowski. Gloria was raised as a Lutheran and after attending Lake View High School, in Chicago, she started her working life as a sales clerk in a department store. On a visit to the local Essanay Studios, in 1914, she asked if she could be in a movie they were filming called *The Song of Soul*. She appeared as an extra. Gloria impressed the producer enough to get a steady flow of bit parts – one of which was in Chaplin's *His New Job*. Her debut was in the 1915 comedy *The Fable of Elvira and Farina and the Meal Ticket*. In a four year period she married two of her six husbands including Wallace Beery, and appeared in twenty-five films. Throughout the 1920s, Gloria was a major star and she was nominated for the first of three Best Actress Oscars for *Sadie Thompson*. The others were for *The Trespasser* and *Sunset Blvd.* That film marked the first time she'd been seen on the screen for nearly ten years, and her role as the faded former movie star, Norma Desmond, reflecting her own life, must have touched her heart. Although Gloria didn't win the Oscar it was an extraordinary performance and still much admired. During the 1960s she was seen quite regularly in television dramas. She made her last movie appearance in *Airport 1975*. In 1980 she published her memoirs – "Swanson on Swanson". Gloria died at her home in New York, of natural causes.

Queen Kelly (1929)
The Trespasser (1929)
Indiscreet (1931)
Tonight or Never (1931)
Perfect Understanding (1933)
Music in the Air (1934)
Father Takes a Wife (1941)
Sunset Blvd. (1950)
Three for Bedroom C (1952)
Mio figlio Nerone (1956)
Airport 1975 (1974)

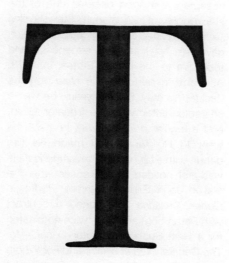

Russ **Tamblyn**
5ft 9in
(RUSSELL IRVING TAMBLYN)

Born: **December 30, 1934**
Los Angeles, California, USA

The son of the bit part actor, Eddie Tamblyn, Russ grew up in the very heart of Hollywood. At the age of ten, he was acting in a junior school play which happened to be seen by Lloyd Bridges, who cast him in his play "Stone Jungle". Russ took acting and dancing lessons and was soon appearing on local radio and in musical reviews. He made his film debut, in 1948, in *The Boy with Green Hair*. He had his first featured role the following year, in *The Kid from Cleveland,* and played young Saul, in the biblical epic, *Samson and Delilah*. At North Hollywood High School, Russ was their champion gymnast and a superb dancer. His first opportunity to demonstrate both of his talents was in *Seven Brides for Seven Brothers*. It impressed Venetia Stevenson, whom he married in 1956. Although Russ was best suited to musicals and actually helped Elvis Presley with his choreography for *Jailhouse Rock,* it was for a dramatic role, in *Peyton Place* that he received his only Oscar nomination – as Best Supporting Actor. Russ reached the peak of his fame as a movie star in the classic musical, *West Side Story*. For the next thirty years or so he worked in inferior films. In 1990, he resurfaced in sixteen episodes of David Lynch's TV-series, 'Twin Peaks'. In the movie version, he suffered the ignominy of having his scenes deleted from the final release print. Russ has been married three times. His daughter, Amber, is an actress.

Father of the Bride (1950)
As Young as You Feel (1951)
Take the High Ground (1953)
Seven Brides for Seven Brothers (1954)
Many Rivers to Cross (1955)
Hit the Deck (1955) **The Last Hunt** (1956)
The Fastest Gun Alive (1956)
Don't Go Near the Water (1957)
Peyton Place (1957)
High School Confidential (1958)
Cimarron (1960) **West Side Story** (1961)
**The Wonderful World of
the Brothers Grimm** (1962)
The Haunting (1963)

Akim **Tamiroff**
5ft 5in
(AKIM TAMIROFF)

Born: **October 29, 1899**
Tiflis, Georgia, Russian Empire
Died: **September 17, 1972**

Akim shared his birthplace with another Armenian, the great film director, Sergei Parajanov. As a youngster, Akim took little interest in acting, but because some friends saw the money-making potential in his distinctive features and deep voice, they urged him to apply for a place at the Moscow Art Theater School. He was accepted and soon became one of the star pupils of Constantin Stanislavsky. Akim then joined a touring company which gave him his first stage experience and took him to the United States, in 1923. After they'd performed in New York he decided to stay. For ten years, he was a character actor with the Theater Guild, and a regular on Broadway. In 1932, he went to Hollywood and made his film debut, with a bit part in *Okay, America!* He was first noticed by audiences when he played John Gilbert's servant, Pedro, in *Queen Christina*. He signed a contract with Paramount and was twice nominated for a Best Supporting Actor Oscar – for *The General Died at Dawn,* and *For Whom the Bell Tolls*. In *The Corsican Brothers* he was eventually slain after what is believed to be the longest duel on film. He became a close friend of Orson Welles when they worked on *Black Magic*. Akim acted in films and TV until 1992. His wife, Tamara, was with him when he died of cancer, at his home in Palm Springs, California.

Lives of a Bengal Lancer (1935)
China Seas (1935)
The Story of Louis Pasteur (1935)
Anthony Adverse (1936) **The General
Died at Dawn** (1936)
The Buccaneer (1938)
Union Pacific (1939) **The Corsican
Brothers** (1941) **Tortilla Flat** (1942)
Five Graves to Cairo (1943)
For Whom the Bell Tolls (1943)
The Miracle of Morgan's Creek (1944)
Black Magic (1949)
Touch of Evil (1958)
Romanoff and Juliet (1961)
The Trial (1962)

Jessica **Tandy**
5ft 3in
(JESSICA ALICE TANDY)

Born: **June 7, 1909**
London, England
Died: **September 11, 1994**

Born and raised in the Hackney district of London, Jessica was the youngest of three children. Her father, Harry Tandy, was a travelling salesman and her mother Jessie, taught in a school for mentally-handicapped children. Jessica received her secondary education at Dame Alice Owen's School in Islington – founded in 1613 and funded by the brewing industry – with which her father had connections. She appeared in plays at school and her parents enrolled her at the Ben Greet Academy of Acting. She made her stage debut at sixteen, in "The Manderson Girls". Over the next ten years, she established herself – performing with Olivier, in "Henry V" and with Gielgud, in "King Lear". In 1932, she married the young English actor Jack Hawkins, and made her film debut that year, playing the maid in *Indiscretions of Eve*. She didn't see another camera until 1938 – concentrating her efforts on the London stage. In 1942, she settled in the USA, marrying Hume Cronyn, whom she appeared with in *The Seventh Cross* as well as *The Green Years* and *Cocoon*. In 1947, Jessica won a Tony for her portrayal of Blanche Dubois, in the original Broadway production of "A Streetcar Named Desire". She became the oldest winner of an Oscar, when she was voted Best Actress, for *Driving Miss Daisy*. She was nominated for a Supporting Actress Oscar for *Fried Green Tomatoes*. She died of ovarian cancer in Easton, Connecticut.

The Seventh Cross (1946) **The Green
Years** (1946) **Dragonwyck** (1946)
Forever Amber (1947)
A Woman's Vengeance (1948)
The Desert Fox (1951)
The Light in the Forest (1958)
The Birds (1963) **Butley** (1974)
The World According to Garp (1982)
Cocoon (1985)
The House on Carroll Street (1988)
Driving Miss Daisy (1989)
Fried Green Tomatoes (1991)
Camilla (1994)

Jacques **Tati**
5ft 5in
(JACQUES TATISCHEFF)

Born: October 9, 1907
Le Pecq, Seine-et-Oise, France
Died: November 5, 1982

Jacques' father Georges-Emmanuel, was born when his own Russian-born father had been the ambassador to France. His mother was an elegant Dutch lady, named Marcelle Van Hoof. He had a privileged upbringing and was educated at private schools. When he and his older sister were children, their parents would take them to spend summer holidays on the Côte d'Azur in the south of France, and to the fashionable resorts of Normandy. He was good at sports – excelling at tennis, boxing and rugby. His love of mime found its first audience among his rugby fifteen, who he'd entertain in the changing room after the match. They were enthusiastic about his performances and persuaded him to try his luck in the Paris music halls. He was such a success, René Clément gave him his film debut, in 1932, in the short, *Oscar champion de tennis.* There were several two-reelers during the 1930s, but it was after the war that he began to think about becoming an actor. He had supporting roles in two movies before directing and acting in *L'Ecole des facteurs* – a homage to both Chaplin and Keaton. His first feature, *Jour de fête* won him the Best Director Award at Venice. The fact that he shot two versions – one in color – one in black and white, suggests his total lack of business acumen. He had more success with *Monsieur Hulot,* and his *Mon Oncle,* won him a Best Foreign Language Film Oscar. His next film, *Play Time,* took nine years to complete. It resulted in bankruptcy. His final film, *Traffic* was shot on a modest budget. He left a wife, Micheline and two grown children when he died in Paris, of pneumonia.

Sylvie et le fantôme (1946)
Le Diable au corps (1947)
Jour de fête (1949)
Les Vacances de
Monsieur Hulot (1953)
Mon Oncle (1958)
Playtime (1967)
Traffic (1971)

Audrey **Tautou**
5ft 3in
(AUDREY TAUTOU)

Born: August 9, 1976
Beaumont, Puy-de-Dôme, France

The eldest of four children, she has two sisters and a brother. Audrey grew up in Montluçon, in central France. Her father was a dental surgeon and her mother was a school teacher. With her cheeky humorous face, young Audrey showed a natural flair for comedy. She studied Literature at university, where her taste in music and the visual arts was eclectic. After that, she took acting classes at Cours Florent, in Paris. During 1996 and 1997, Audrey was seen in French TV dramas, and in 1998, she made her film debut, in a short, titled *La Vieille barrière.* She took part in a competition organized by Canal+ and won a Best Young Actress Award at the Bézier Festival. The film director, Tonie Marshall, gave her a role in the César winning film *Venus Beauty Institute,* and Audrey won the Prix Suzanne Bianchetti, as France's most promising film actress. She achieved international recognition when she starred in the title role of *Amélie.* Audrey then went to Indonesia to help with the preservation of a monkey sanctuary. In 2004, she joined the Academy of Motion Picture Arts and Sciences. After several successful French films, she acted opposite Tom Hanks, in *The Da Vinci Code.* Audrey is currently in the middle of filming *Coco avant Chanel* – a biography of the famous French fashion designer.

Venus Beauty Institute (1999)
Marry Me (2000)
Pretty Devils (2000)
Le Libertin (2000)
The Beating of a
Butterfly's Wings (2000)
Amélie (2001)
He Loves Me...He Loves
Me Not (2002)
The Spanish Apartment (2002)
Dirty Pretty Things (2002)
Not on the Lips (2003)
A Very Long Engagement (2004)
The Russian Dolls (2005)
The Da Vinci Code (2006)
Priceless (2006)
Hunting and Gathering (2007)

Elizabeth **Taylor**
5ft 2in
(ELIZABETH ROSEMOND TAYLOR)

Born: February 27, 1932
Hampstead, London, England

Liz's parents – Francis and Sara Taylor – were Americans who were resident in England. Her father was an art dealer and her mother had been an actress. Liz had an older brother named Howard. When she was three, she started taking ballet lessons and was settling down to life as an English girl. World War II changed all that – her parents took their young family to live in Los Angeles. In 1942, Liz was given a contract by Universal and made her film debut, in the comedy, *There's One Born Every Minute.* She moved to MGM to play Roddy McDowall's young friend, in *Lassie Come Home* and had her first big starring role, in *National Velvet.* Liz played her first grown-up part – opposite Robert Taylor, in *Conspirator,* in 1949. By the time she had her first dramatic success – in *A Place in the Sun,* she was halfway through her brief first marriage to Conrad Hilton Jr. There would be seven more over the next forty years – two of them with Richard Burton. From the mid-1950s, apart from her private life – which was exceptional – Liz was a massive star. She was nominated three times for Best Actress Oscars – *Raintree County, Cat on a Hot Tin Roof* and *Suddenly, Last Summer,* and she won it twice – for *BUtterfield 8* and *Who's Afraid of Virginia Woolf?* Upon the death of her great friend, Rock Hudson, Liz began her crusade on behalf of AIDS sufferers.

Lassie Come Home (1943)
National Velvet (1944) Life with
Father (1947) Julia Misbehaves (1948)
A Place in the Sun (1951)
Ivanhoe (1952) Giant (1956)
Raintree County (1957)
Cat on a Hot Tin Roof (1958)
Suddenly, Last Summer (1959)
BUtterfield 8 (1960) Cleopatra (1963)
The Sandpiper (1965) Who's Afraid
of Virginia Woolf? (1966)
The Taming of the Shrew (1967)
Reflections in a Golden Eye (1967)
The Only Game in Town (1970)
Under Milk Wood (1972)
Night Watch (1973)

Robert **Taylor**
5ft 11in
(SPANGLER ARLINGTON BRUGH)

Born: **August 5, 1911**
Filley, Nebraska, USA
Died: **June 8, 1969**

Bob's parents were Dr. Andrew Brugh and his wife Ruth. At Beatrice High School he was not only an outstanding athlete, he won several oratory awards and played cello in the school orchestra. The latter was his main passion, so after graduating he enrolled at Doane College in Crete, Nebraska, where he studied Music. He left there when he was twenty – going to Los Angeles where he followed in his father's footsteps by studying Medicine at Pomona College. He joined the campus theater group and was spotted by an MGM talent scout when he acted in the play, "Journey's End". He signed a 7-year contract with the studio, but it was a loan-out to Fox which provided his film debut in 1934 – the Will Rogers comedy, *Handy Andy*. His first big MGM role was opposite Greta Garbo, in *Camille*. His loyalty to his boss Louis B. Mayer, made him a major star on a modest salary. Films like *A Yank at Oxford, Johnny Eager* and *Bataan* made sure that he wasn't forgotten when he joined the US Naval Air Corps in 1943. During the war, he made a film called *Song of Russia*. In 1947, Bob testified before the HUAC – not only casting doubt on some actors but claiming that he did it against his will. The episode didn't affect his popularity and he continued as a star for another ten years. He was married twice – to Barbara Stanwyck, and Ursula Thiess, with whom he had two children. A heavy smoker, Bob died of lung cancer in Santa Monica, California.

Magnificent Obsession (1935)
Camille (1936) **A Yank at Oxford** (1938)
Three Comrades (1938) Waterloo
Bridge (1940) Johnny Eager (1942)
Bataan (1943) **High Wall** (1947)
The Bribe (1949) **Devil's Doorway** (1950)
Quo Vadis? (1951) Ivanhoe (1952)
Rogue Cop (1954) **Many Rivers to
Cross** (1955) **The Last Hunt** (1956)
The Law and Jake Wade (1958)
The Night Walker (1964)
Return of the Gunfighter (1967)

Rod **Taylor**
5ft 11in
(RODNEY STUART TAYLOR)

Born: **January 11, 1930**
Sydney, New South Wales, Australia

Born in the Sydney suburb of Lidcombe, Rod was the son of William Stuart Taylor, a steel construction contractor and his wife Mona, who was a writer of children's books. He studied engineering at Sydney Technical and Fine Arts College, but was drawn to an acting career when he saw Laurence Olivier and Vivien Leigh on stage during their Australian tour. While working as a designer, Rod began appearing in amateur plays and, in the early 1950s, was heard on the radio as Tarzan in a children's serial and in a popular soap 'Blue Hills'. In 1953, he made his film debut in a Chips Rafferty adventure, *King of the Coral Sea* and then played Israel Hands in *Long John Silver,* the sequel to Treasure Island. He went to the United States in 1954 and had a supporting role in the western, *Top Gun*. He supported in big pictures like *Giant* before his first starring role in George Pal's *The Time Machine* made him a star. Three years later, Alfred Hitchcock's *The Birds* consolidated that position. It lasted for ten years – Rod's final film of real quality was the Australian-made comedy drama, *The Picture Show Man*. Since then much of his work has been on television – most notably as Frank Agretti in 'Falcon Crest'. In 2007, he was featured in the horror film, *Kaw*. Rod has been married and divorced three times. His daughter is the CNBC anchor, Felicia Taylor. Rod will soon be seen as Winston Churchill, in the new Quentin Tarantino film – *Inglourious Basterds*.

World Without End (1956)
The Catered Affair (1956)
Giant (1956)
Raintree County (1957)
Ask Any Girl (1959)
The Time Machine (1960)
The Birds (1963) **The V.I.Ps** (1963)
Sunday in New York (1964)
Thirty-six Hours (1964)
Hotel (1967)
Zabriskie Point (1970)
Partizani (1974)
The Picture Show Man (1977)

Shirley **Temple**
5ft 2in
(SHIRLEY TEMPLE)

Born: **April 23, 1928**
Santa Monica, California, USA

Shirley was the daughter of banker, George Temple, and his wife Amelia, who would help shape her cute little girl's future. At the age of four, Shirley began appearing in a series of shorts called "Baby Burlesks". At the end of 1932, she made her first appearance in a feature film – *The Red-Haired Alibi*. She had twenty three titles to her credit before she was able to give a hint of her star quality – in *Little Miss Marker*. Although she had stiff competition from a slightly older, Jane Withers, Shirley sang "On the Good Ship Lollipop" in *Bright Eyes*. The innocence of that period was beautifully conveyed in a dozen or so films up to the beginning of World War II. Growing up was inevitable and apart from a couple of good teenage roles, the magic had disappeared. She was only seventeen when she met the soldier/actor, John Agar. They married in 1945, and appeared together in the John Ford western, *Fort Apache*. They had a daughter, but little else together and the year they divorced, Shirley met her second husband – a Californian businessman, Charles Alden Black. She made her final appearance in 1961 – on television, in the series – 'Shirley Temple's Storybook'. Her later roles included representative to the United Nations, and U.S. Ambassador to Ghana and later, Czechoslovakia.

Little Miss Marker (1934)
Bright Eyes (1934) **The Little
Colonel** (1935) **Curly Top** (1935)
The Littlest Rebel (1935)
Captain January (1936) **Poor Little
Rich Girl** (1936) **Dimples** (1936)
Stowaway (1936)
Wee Willie Winkie (1937)
Heidi (1937) **Rebecca
of Sunnybrook Farm** (1938)
The Little Princess (1939)
The Blue Bird (1940) **Since
You Went Away** (1944)
Kiss and Tell (1945)
**The Bachelor and
the Bobby-Soxer** (1947)
Fort Apache (1948)

Charlize **Theron**
5ft 9½in
(CHARLIZE THERON)

Born: **August 7, 1975**
Benoni, Gauteng, South Africa

Charlie was the only child of Charles Theron, who was successful with his own construction company, but a disastrous husband and father. Her mother, Gerda, who was of German descent, gave her daughter the love she needed. When she was thirteen, Charlie was sent away to a boarding school. Two years later, during a visit home, she witnessed her mother killing her abusive alcoholic husband with a shotgun, in self-defense. Charlie carried on with life – studying at the National School of the Arts in Johannesburg, and winning a year's work in Milan, Italy, as a model. She next went to New York, where she joined Pauline's Model Management. When the contract finished, she decided to stay – training as a dancer at the Joffrey Ballet School. Her dream ended when she suffered a knee injury. She was nineteen, but a bigger future lay ahead. Her mother gave her a one-way ticket to L.A. It was there, when she was having difficulty cashing a check in a bank, that she was spotted by a talent agent. Drama classes led to her movie debut – in direct-to-video *Children of the Corn III*. A twelve-year run of good films has made her a star. Charlie won a Best Acting Oscar, for *Monster* – one of the greatest displays of film acting I've ever seen. She was nominated again, for *North Country*. Since *Monster*, Charlie has been producer on four more films.

2 Days in the Valley (1996)
That Thing You Do! (1996) The Devil's Advocate (1997) The Cider House Rules (1999) The Yards (2000) Men of Honor (2000)
The Legend of Bagger Vance (2000) Sweet November (2001)
The Curse of the Jade Scorpion (2001) Trapped (2002) The Italian Job (2003) Monster (2003) The Life and Death of Peter Sellers (2004) North Country (2005) In the Valley of Elah (2007) Battle in Seattle (2007) Hancock (2008) The Burning Plain (2008)

David **Thewlis**
6ft 1in
(DAVID WHEELER)

Born: **March 20, 1963**
Blackpool, England

David was the son of Alec and Maureen Wheeler, who ran a small store. He was musically talented and in his teens, earned extra money by performing at Blackpool hotels, in a rock-band called "QED". He later played lead guitar in a punk-rock band known as "Door 66". David's music might quite easily have taken over his life if it wasn't for a friend who persuaded him to go to London and enroll at the Guildhall School of Music and Drama. He opted for Drama and graduated in 1985. When he went to register with the Actor's Union, there was already a "David Wheeler", so he adopted his mother's maiden name. In 1986, his guitar skills came in useful when he made his stage debut at the Greenwich Theater, in south east London, in "Buddy Holly at the Regal". His first film role was in *Road*, in 1987. Four years later he acted in Mike Leigh's terrific comedy/drama *Life Is Sweet,* and things looked promising. His marriage to the Welsh actress, Sara Sugarman didn't. In 1993, David received good notices for his performance in the Mike Leigh movie, *Naked* – and won the Best Actor Award at Cannes. Since then, David's shown his range as an actor and has also directed. In 2001, he found a true soul-mate in a Lancashire girl, Anna Friel, and they are the proud parents of Gracie.

Life Is Sweet (1991) Damage (1992)
The Trial (1993) Naked (1993) Black Beauty (1994) Total Eclipse (1995)
Restoration (1995) Dragonheart (1996) American Perfekt (1997)
Seven Years in Tibet (1997) The Big Lebowski (1998) Divorcing Jack (1998) Besieged (1998) Whatever Happened to Harold Smith? (1999)
Gangster No.1 (2000) Goodbye Charlie Bright (2001) Cheeky (2003) Timeline (2003) The Prisoner of Azkaban (2004) Kingdom of Heaven (2005) All the Invisible Children (2005) The New Word (2005) The Order of the Phoenix (2007)
The Boy in the Striped Pyjamas (2008) The Half-Blood Prince (2009)

Mélanie **Thierry**
5ft 4in
(MÉLANIE THIERRY)

Born: **July 17 1981**
St. Germaine en Laye, Paris, France

Mélanie was born with angelic looks and even at junior school in Paris, she seemed set for a career as a photo model. When she was twelve years old, she was taken on by the famous international agency, Karin Models. It resulted in her beautiful face gracing various magazine covers in France, Germany and Italy, and work for beauty and fashion accounts such as Alberta Ferretti, Hermès, and Max Factor. When she was seventeen she made her film debut, with a very visible role, in the blockbuster Italian production directed by Giuseppe Tornatore, called *The Legend of the Pianist on the Ocean*. She followed that with a modern French version of Victor Hugo's classic "The Hunchback of Notre Dame", entitled *Quasimodo d'El Paris*. It was directed by the comic/actor, Patrick Timsit, who, on his directorial debut, played the title-role and Melanie was cast as Esméralda. Her next film was another Italian production, shot in Prague, called *Canone inverso – making love*. She attempted light comedy without success, in *Jojo la frite,* but was back on track in the somewhat darker, *The Half Life of Timofey Berezin*. After the Sci-Fi thriller, *Chrysalis,* Mélanie made her Hollywood debut in the same genre – with Vin Diesel, in *Babylon A.D.* In March 2008, Mélanie had a starring role with her boyfriend, the French singer, Raphaël Haroche, in a dramatic video for his album, "Caravane". She will soon be seen in a new movie, *Le Dernier pour la route.*

The Legend of the Pianist on the Ocean (1998)
Quasimodo d'El Paris (1999)
Canone inverso – making Love (2000)
August 15 (2001)
Ne m'appelle plus BB (2002)
The Half Life of Timofey Berezin (2006)
Pardonnez-moi (2006)
Chrysalis (2007)
Babylon A.D. (2007)
Largo Winch (2008)

Terry-Thomas
5ft 11in
(THOMAS TERRY HOAR STEVENS)

Born: **July 14, 1911**
Finchley, London, England
Died: **January 8, 1990**

The son of wealthy parents, Terry went to private schools in London before Ardingley College, in West Sussex. He became a salesman for a meat company, where he had his first taste of show business. In his leisure time, he played the ukulele with a traditional jazz band. He also appeared in plays presented by the company's drama society. In 1935, Terry made his film debut with an uncredited part, in *One in a Million.* He married his first wife – actress Ida Patlanski, in 1938, but his career remained on a low level. Fourteen tiny film roles later a real drama – World War II, ensured that he wouldn't be unknown for much longer. He joined the Royal Signals, and became one of the "Stars in Battledress". In 1946, it propelled him into a West End review, "Piccadilly Hayride". Three years later, he appeared on TV, in 'How Do You View?'. What was wrong before was suddenly right. By the time he starred in his own series, 'Strictly T-T' his was one of the most famous faces in England. A new film career began with *Private's Progress,* and for the next few years moviegoers in Britain couldn't get enough. His last good role was the voice of 'Sir Hiss' in Disney's 1973 *The Jungle Book.* In the early 1980s, he retired to Ibiza with his second wife Belinda – living in poverty after the onset of his killer – Parkinson's disease. He went home to face death in Godalming, Surrey.

Private's Progress (1956)
The Green Man (1956)
Brothers in-Law (1957)
Lucky Jim (1957)
The Naked Truth (1957)
Blue Murder at St. Trinian's (1957)
Tom Thumb (1958)
Too Many Crooks (1959)
Carlton-Browne of the F.O. (1959)
I'm All Right Jack (1959)
School for Scoundrels (1960)
It's a Mad Mad
Mad Mad World (1964)
How to Murder Your Wife (1965)
La Grande vadrouille (1966)

Emma **Thompson**
5ft 8½in
(EMMA THOMPSON)

Born:**April 15, 1959**
Paddington, London, England

Emma was born into an acting family. Her father, Eric Thompson, was a television actor who was well-known for his fine speaking voice. His narration of the English version of the French Children's TV-series, 'The Magic Roundabout', was especially liked. Her mother Phyllida Law, who was Scottish, appeared in dozens of film and TV productions. Emma spent part of her early life in Scotland, but after the family moved back to London, she was educated at Camden School for Girls and Newnham College Cambridge, where she was a member of "Footlights" at the same time as Stephen Fry and Hugh Laurie. Emma signed with an agent before graduation and made her debut in the West End revival of "Me and My Girl". In 1984, she appeared with Fry and Laurie, as guest stars in the TV-sitcom 'The Young Ones'. Both she and Robbie Coltrane achieved national prominence in the cult series 'Tutti Frutti'. Emma made her film debut in *The Tall Guy,* in the same year she married Kenneth Branagh. They worked on several films, but her fame came with an Oscar winning performance, in *Howard's End.* She was nominated for *The Remains of the Day* and *In the Name of the Father.* In 2003, she married Greg Wise, her *Sense and Sensibility* co-star. The couple have a nine-year-old daughter, Gaia, and an adopted Rwandan son.

The Tall Guy (1989) Henry V (1989)
Impromptu (1991) Dead Again (1991)
Howard's End (1992) Peter's
Friends (1992) Much Ado About
Nothing (1993) The Remains of
the Day (1993) In the Name of
the Father (1993) Carrington (1995)
Sense and Sensibility (1995)
Primary Colors (1998)
Judas Kiss (1998) Love Actually (2003)
Imagining Argentina (2003)
Nanny McPhee (2005)
Stranger Than Fiction (2006)
The Order of the Phoenix (2007)
Brideshead Revisited (2008)
Last Chance Harvey (2008)

Billy Bob **Thornton**
6ft
(WILLIAM ROBERT THORNTON)

Born:**August 4, 1955**
Hot Springs, Arkansas, USA

Billy Bob was the eldest of four brothers born to a Methodist couple. His mother Virginia, who's psychic, predicted that he would work with Burt Reynolds. He did. His father Billy Ray, a history teacher and basketball coach, is of Irish stock. Billy Bob reckons he enjoyed some of his best quality time with his grandfather, Otis – a forest ranger. A few years later at high school, he was a good enough basketball player to merit a trial with the Kansas City Royals. He considered it seriously, but opted to study Psychology at Henderson University, in Arkadelphia. After only two semesters, he dropped out – heading for Los Angeles to pursue an acting career. It didn't come easily. After a series of fruitless auditions, he did get television work in the sitcom, 'Hearts Afire' and, in 1987, a small role in the film, *Hunter's Blood.* But advised by Billy Wilder, to become a screenwriter, he contributed film character dialogue and eventually wrote, directed and starred, in his own film, *Sling Blade.* It won him an Oscar – for Best Screenplay and a Best Actor nomination. He was nominated for a Best Supporting Actor Oscar for *A Simple Plan.* Most of his post-2000 films are excellent. In his personal life, his five ex-wives include actresses Toni Lawrence, Cynda Williams and Angelina Jolie. He's currently single.

One False Move (1992)
Dead Man (1995) The Stars Fell on
Henrietta (1995) Sling Blade (1996)
U Turn (1997) The Apostle (1997)
Primary Colors (1998) A Simple
Plan (1998) The Man Who Wasn't
There (2001) Daddy and
Them (2001) Bandits (2001)
Monster's Ball (2001)
The Badge (2002) Levity (2003)
Bad Santa (2003) Chrystal (2003)
The Alamo (2004)
Friday Night Lights (2004)
Bad News Bears (2005)
The Astronaut Farmer (2006)
Eagle Eye (2008)
The Informers (2009)

Ingrid **Thulin**
5ft 6¼in
(INGRID THULIN)

Born: **January 27, 1926**
Sollefteå, Västernorrlands län, Sweden
Died: **January 7, 2004**

Ingrid was the daughter of a fisherman in a small coastal village in northern Sweden. Although she attended ballet lessons when she was in junior school, there was little hint of her future career until after she went to live in Stockholm, at the age of seventeen. Even then, her early training at Påhlmans Commercial Institute resulted in a job as a clerk in an office. Towards the end of World War II, the very photogenic nineteen-year-old was persuaded to study acting with Gösta Tersurus and Koblanck. She revived her early interest in dancing with Lalla Cassel. In late 1947, Ingrid joined the Norrköping-Linköping Municipal Theater and had rave notices when she appeared in Kurt Weill's "One Touch of Venus". She made her film debut in 1948's *Känn dej som Hemma*. Around 1949, she attended the Royal Dramatic Theater's acting school in Stockholm. Two years later, she studied mime in Paris and while a resident there, appeared on stage in Jean Anouilh's play, "L'invitation au chateau". Returning home, she had a series of roles in minor Swedish movies before her first English language film – *Foreign Intrigue,* in 1956. Like many Swedish actors, her real fame came in Ingmar Bergman's films, beginning with *Wild Strawberries.* She later worked in France and Italy with some success – Visconti's *The Damned,* being a high point. She lived in Rome before returning to Stockholm – where she died of cancer.

Wild Strawberries (1957)
Brink of Life (1958)
The Face (1958)
Winter Light (1962)
The Silence (1963)
Return from the Ashes (1965)
La Guerre est finie (1966)
Hour of the Wolf (1968)
The Damned (1969)
Short Night of
the Glass Dolls (1971)
Cries and Whispers (1972)
The Cassandra Crossing (1976)

Uma **Thurman**
6ft
(UMA KARUNA THURMAN)

Born: **April 29, 1970**
Boston, Massachusetts, USA

Uma's father, Robert Thurman, was a scholar who eventually became professor of Indo-Tibetan Buddhist studies at Columbia University. Her mother Nena, was born in Mexico City to a German nobleman and his Swedish wife, who had posed for the nude statue which looks out over the harbor of Smygehuk. Nena worked as a fashion model. Uma's father gave her and her three brothers, a Buddhist upbringing. They spent some time in India where the Dalai Lama visited their home. Back in the USA, Uma was educated at Northfield Mount Hermon – a college prep boarding school where she had her first acting experience in school plays. After advice from talent scouts, she left to attend the Professional Children's School in New York. She left there before graduating and at fifteen, began a career with Click Models. In 1988, she made her movie debut, in the high school comedy *Johnny Be Good,* and had a good early role, as Cécile, in *Dangerous Liaisons.* She proved her acting ability in the flawed *Final Analysis* and she began to work with Tarantino, in *Pulp Fiction for which* she was nominated for a Best Supporting Actress Oscar. Her versatility – in comedy or drama is what keeps her at the very top of her profession as a movie star. She was briefly married to Gary Oldman. A second marriage to Ethan Hawke, ended in 2004, but resulted in a daughter and a son.

Dangerous Liaisons (1988)
Henry & June (1990)
Final Analysis (1992) Jennifer 8 (1992)
Mad Dog and Glory (1993)
Pulp Fiction (1994)
A Month by the Lake (1995)
Beautiful Girls (1996)
The Truth About Cats & Dogs (1996)
Gattaca (1997) Les Misérables (1998)
Sweet and Lowdown (1999)
Vatel (2000) The Golden Bowl (2000)
Tape (2001) Kill Bill: Vol.1 (2003)
Prime (2005) The Producers (2005)
The Life Before Her Eyes (2007)
Motherhood (2009)

Gene **Tierney**
5ft 7in
(GENE ELIZA TIERNEY)

Born: **November 20, 1920**
Brooklyn, New York City, New York, USA
Died: **November 6, 1991**

Gene was the daughter of an insurance broker, Howard Tierney, who was of Irish descent and his wife Belle, who had been a gym instructor. Gene had one older brother and a younger sister. She was educated at St. Margaret's School for Girls, in Westbury, Connecticut and the Unquowa School in Bridgeport, where her poem, "Night" was published in the school magazine. After that she was sent to the Brillantmont Finishing School in Lausanne, Switzerland where she became fluent in French. She was a debutante at seventeen, but she soon got bored with high society. Gene enrolled at the American Academy of Dramatic Arts and made her stage debut in "What a Life". Subsequent roles, which received favorable reviews led to her photo appearing in Harper's Bazaar. In 1939, Gene enjoyed a Broadway triumph in "The Male Animal". In 1940 she signed a contract with 20th Century Fox. They gave Gene her film debut in Fritz Lang's *The Return of Frank James.* In 1941, she married the fashion designer Oleg Cassini. After success in *Heaven Can Wait,* Gene went to the Hollywood Canteen when she was pregnant. She contracted German measles from a very thoughtless fan who visited her when she was infected. Gene's baby girl was born retarded. It led to mental problems and a suicide attempt. In the mid 1940s, she made three of her best pictures – *Laura, Leave Her to Heaven* and *The Ghost and Mrs. Muir.* After a brief come-back in the 1960s, she retired. Gene died at her home in Houston, Texas, of emphysema.

Tobacco Road (1941) The Shanghai
Gesture (1941) Heaven Can Wait (1943)
Laura (1944) Leave Her to Heaven (1945)
Dragonwyck (1946) The Razor's
Edge (1946) The Ghost and Mrs.
Muir (1947) Whirlpool (1949) Night and
the City (1950) The Mating Season (1951)
On the Riviera (1951) Never Let Me
Go (1953) Advise and Consent (1962)
Toys in the Attic (1963)

Maura **Tierney**
5ft 3in
(MAURA LYNN TIERNEY)

Born: **February 3, 1965**
Boston, Massachusetts, USA

Maura was raised in the Hyde Park district of Boston. Her father, Joe Tierney, was a long-serving Boston city councilman, who is now a lawyer. His wife Pat became a successful real estate agent. After high school, which is where she first became interested in acting, Maura went to New York where she studied at the Circle in the Square Theater School. Her first screen appearance was in 1987, in a television comedy, 'Student Exchange'. Maura's film debut, in *Dead Women in Lingerie,* was nothing to get excited about, but her next movie, *The Linguini Incident,* gave her hope for the future. Its director, Richard Shepard, had become a close friend of Maura's and went on to cast her in *Mercy.* In 1993, she married the actor Billy Morrissette – he directed her in his crime comedy movie, *Scotland, Pa.* In 1995, the TV-sitcom, 'NewsRadio' had her playing comedy and it landed her a role in Jim Carrey's *Liar Liar.* Other big movies which enhanced her reputation were – most notably, *Primal Fear, Primary Colors,* and *Instinct.* From 1999, Maura has starred on television, as Dr. Abby Lockhart, in 'ER'. In recent years, she's appeared in some very good short films such as *The Nazi,* and continued to add to her credit list – with *Baby Mama,* and *Finding Amanda,* being highly recommended viewing.

The Liguini Incident (1991)
White Sands (1992)
Mercy (1995)
Primal Fear (1996)
Liar Liar (1997)
Primary Colors (1998)
Oxygen (1999)
Instinct (1999)
Scotland, Pa. (2001)
Insomnia (2002)
Melvin Goes to Dinner (2003)
Welcome to Mooseport (2004)
Diggers (2006)
The Go-Getter (2007)
Semi-Pro (2008)
Baby Mama (2008)
Finding Amanda (2008)

Jennifer **Tilly**
5ft 5½in
(JENNIFER E.CHAN)

Born: **September 16, 1958**
Harbor City, California, USA

The second of four children, Jennifer's father was Chinese American, Harry Chan – a used-car salesman, and his wife, the former stage actress, Patricia Tilly. Following her parents' divorce, Jennifer was raised in British Columbia by her mother and stepfather. Marriage wasn't good news for Patricia and by the time Jennifer and sister Meg were teenagers, she was divorced again, so they moved to Victoria, Vancouver Island. There, Jennifer attended Belmont High School, before preparing for her acting career through a theater program at Stephens College, in Columbia, Missouri. She took her mother's second name and in 1983, she made her TV debut in an episode of 'Boone'. Jennifer's first movie was a 1984 romantic comedy, *No Small Affair.* Her first starring opportunity was in 1987, opposite Elliott Gould and Howard Hesseman, in the independent film, *Inside Out.* Jennifer later received high marks for her acting, in Woody Allen's *Bullets Over Broadway,* and was nominated for a Best Supporting Actress Oscar. She continues to give her support to independent filmmakers as well as shining in big movies. She is divorced from the writer, Sam Simon.

Inside Out (1987) **Far from
Home** (1989) **Let It Ride** (1989)
The Fabulous Baker Boys (1989)
Scorchers (1991)
Bullets Over Broadway (1994)
Man with a Gun (1995)
Edie & Pen (1996)
Bound (1996) **Liar Liar** (1996)
The Wrong Guy (1997)
Relax...It's Just Sex (1998)
Music from Another Room (1998)
Bruno (2000) **The Crew** (2000)
Dirt (2001) **The Cat's Meow** (2001)
Ball in the House (2001)
Second Best (2004) **Perfect
Opposites** (2004) **Saint Ralph** (2004)
**The Civilization of
Maxwell Bright** (2005)
Tideland (2005) **Intervention** (2007)
Return to Babylon (2008)

Meg **Tilly**
5ft 5½in
(MARGARET E. CHAN)

Born: **February 14, 1960**
Los Angeles County, California, USA

Jennifer's younger sister was raised by her mother Patricia, who was a schoolteacher, and her stepfather, John Ward. Although she was born on St. Valentine's Day, her early life was far from romantic. Her family lived in poor circumstances, and she has recalled physical, sexual and emotional abuse at the hands of her mother's partners, including Ward. Meg was a graduate from Esquimalt High School, in Victoria, British Columbia, and left for New York when she was eighteen. She was crazy about dancing as a teenager, and in the "Big Apple" she attended ballet school. It was her dancing ability which secured her first screen role, in Alan Parker's very popular 1980 film, *Fame.* After a serious back injury forced her to give up her dancing career, Meg turned her attention to acting. After a couple of TV roles, she starred with Matt Dillon in the drama *Tex.* She looked to be heading for serious stardom when she acted in the unusually effective sequel, *Psycho II* and the critical and commercial success, *The Big Chill.* Her first marriage – to Tim Zinneman, with whom she had two children, seemed to be going well. In 1986, Meg won a Golden Globe and was nominated for a Supporting Actress Oscar for *Agnes of God.* She divorced Zinneman and lived with the actor Colin Firth, with whom she had a son. In 1995, Meg acted in the TV film, 'Journey' and then retired. She married producer John Calley, who was thirty years her senior. Nowadays, she lives in British Columbia with her third husband Don – where she concentrates her life on raising her children. Meg has written and published, three books – "Porcupine", "Gemma" – and the semi-autobiographical, "Singing Songs".

Tex (1982) **One Dark Night** (1983)
Psycho II (1983) **The Big Chill** (1983)
Impulse (1984) **Agnes of God** (1985)
Masquerade (1988) **Valmont** (1989)
The Two Jakes (1990)
Leaving Normal (1992)
Body Snatchers (1993)
Sleep with Me (1994)

Ann Todd
5ft 5in
(ANN TODD)

Born: **January 24, 1909**
Hartford, Cheshire, England
Died: **May 6, 1993**

Ann's parents were from Aberdeen, in Scotland, but they were living 'south of the border' when she was born. They moved down to London shortly after that and because they were reasonably well off, they sent her to St. Winifred's, a boarding school for girls, in Eastbourne, East Sussex. While she was there Ann derived great pleasure from acting in school plays. She enrolled at the Central School in London, but lacking confidence, she initially trained to be a drama coach. She changed her mind in 1928, when she began to get walk-ons in West End productions. In 1931, Ann made her film debut, in *Keepers of Youth*. Apart from *Things to Come,* in which she had a small role and *South Riding,* in 1938, there was little to show for her first ten years as a film actress. Her first good part was opposite Robert Donat, in *Perfect Strangers,* and it was immediately followed by the popular psychological drama, *The Seventh Veil –* which owed much of its success to the presence of the new British screen idol, James Mason. After acting in a Hitchcock movie, *The Paradine Case,* Ann did her best work in a Victorian melodrama *So Evil My Love.* David Lean became husband number three and directed her in three films – the best of which was *Madeleine.* After 1960, her few appearances were in poorly made films, and stage productions. She also made travel documentaries. Ann acted for the last time, in an episode of 'Maigret' on television, in 1992. She died from a stroke the following year.

Perfect Strangers (1945)
The Seventh Veil (1945)
The Paradine Case (1947)
So Evil My Love (1948)
The Passionate Friends (1949)
Madeleine (1950)
The Sound Barrier (1952)
The Green Scarf (1954)
Time Without Pity (1957)
Taste of Fear (1961)
The Human Factor (1979)

Richard Todd
5ft 9in
(RICHARD ANDREW PALETHORPE TODD)

Born: **June 11, 1919**
Dublin, Ireland

Richard's father was an army doctor who before World War I, had played rugby for Ireland three times. The family moved to Devon in England when he was young and he was educated at Shrewsbury School. After that, Richard studied acting at the Italia Conti School, in London. In the late 1930s, he became a co-founder of the Dundee Repertory Company in Scotland. Richard's career was put on hold when he served in the King's Own Yorkshire Light Infantry and as a paratrooper during World War II. He returned to Dundee after the war, and then had his first major break when he starred on the London stage as Lachlan MacLachlan in "The Hasty Heart". He repeated his success on Broadway and returned to England to appear in the film version – for which he was nominated for a Best Actor Oscar. During that time, he had made an impressive film debut as the star of *For Them That Trespass.* He was given a leading role in Hitchcock's *Stage Fright,* and at that point in time, looked to have a big future. He went to Hollywood to make *Lightning Strikes Twice* and then became 'Robin Hood' for Walt Disney. His biggest films in America were *A Man Called Peter* and *The Virgin Queen.* Between those was his portrayal of Guy Gibson, in *The Dam Busters.* He was seen in supporting roles as the 1960s progressed, and was still acting in 2007.

The Hasty Heart (1949) Stage
Fright (1950) Flesh and Blood (1951)
Lightning Strikes Twice (1951)
The Story of Robin Hood and
His Merrie Men (1951)
The Sword and the Rose (1953)
Les secrets d'Alcove (1954)
A Man Called Peter (1955)
The Dambusters (1955)
The Virgin Queen (1955) D-Day the
Sixth of June (1956) Danger
Within (1959) Never Let Go (1960)
The Long and the
Short and the Tall (1961)
The Boys (1962) Asylum (1972)
House of the Long Shadows (1983)

Ugo Tognazzi
5ft 9in
(OTTAVIO TOGNAZZI)

Born: **March 23, 1922**
Cremona, Lombardy, Italy
Died: **October 27, 1990**

By the time he was ten, Ugo had lived for periods in towns and cities all over Italy. It was necessary because of his father's job as a traveling trouble-shooter for a big insurance company. Ugo left school in Cremona when he was fourteen, and up until World War II, he worked for a salami firm, at its production plant. His main leisure interest was the local theater, where he had opportunities to appear in amateur entertainments and stage plays. From 1940 he served in the Italian army – only returning home after the Armistice, in September, 1943. Ugo went to Milan in 1945, to join the Wanda Osiris Theatrical Company. He made his film debut in 1950 in *I cadetti di Guascogna,* but his biggest success was the comic duo he formed with Raimondo Vianello, which became popular on Italian television. Film stardom came ten years after his debut. *Il Federale* made him a star. He worked with all the best directors including Bertolucci, who helped him to a Best Actor Award at the Cannes Film Festival, for *La tragedia di un uomo ridicolo.* Three years earlier, Ugo had gained brief international fame, in *La Cage aux folles.* Ugo's final movie was made in the year he died in Rome, of a cerebral hemorrhage.

Il Federale (1961) La voglia
matta (1962) Ro.Go.Pa.G. (1963)
L'Ape regina (1963) I Mostri (1963)
Il magnifico cornuto (1965)
The Seventh Floor (1967)
Satyricon (1968)
The Conspirators (1969)
La supertestimone (1971)
In the Name
of the Italian People (1971)
La Grande bouffe (1973)
Romanzo popolare (1974)
Weak Spot (1975) Amici miei (1975)
Telefoni bianchi (1976) I nuovi
mostri (1977) First Love (1978)
The Cat (1978) La Cage aux folles (1978)
La tragedia di un uomo ridicolo (1978)
A Joke of Destiny (1983)

Marisa **Tomei**
5ft 6in
(MARISA TOMEI)

Born: **December 4, 1964**
Brooklyn, New York City, New York, USA

Marisa and her actor brother Adam, were the children of Italian Americans, Gary Tomei, a lawyer, and his wife Patricia, who was an English teacher. In their early years, she would give the two youngsters elocution lessons to help eliminate their strong Brooklyn accents. In 1982, Marisa graduated from Edward R. Murrow High School with a polished voice. She then attended Boston University, but dropped out after one year when she was offered a role in the CBS daytime drama, 'As the World Turns'. It led to her film debut, in 1984, with a small part in *The Flamingo Kid*. She was in a few modest movies before 1987, when a two-year run in another TV series 'A Different World', gave her the platform to move ahead with her film career. *Oscar,* where she supported Sly Stallone was the start, but *My Cousin Vinny* – in which she played Joe Pesci's foul-mouthed girfriend, was her break-through. Marisa won a Best Supporting Actress Oscar and moved onwards and upwards – via *Chaplin, The Perez Family, Unhook the Stars,* and a superb comedy *Slums of Beverly Hills.* Later film appearances and Broadway work confirm her position as a star. She was nominated for a Supporting Oscar, for *The Wrestler.*

My Cousin Vinny (1992)
Chaplin (1992) **Untamed Heart** (1993)
The Paper (1994) **Only You** (1994)
The Perez Family (1995) **Four
Rooms** (1995) **Unhook the
Stars** (1996) **Welcome to
Sarajevo** (1997) **Slums of Beverly
Hills** (1998) **Happy Accidents** (2000)
What Women Want (2000)
In the Bedroom (2001) **Someone
Like You** (2001) **The Guru** (2002)
Anger Management (2003) **Alfie** (2004)
**Marilyn Hotchkiss Ballroom
Dancing & Charm School** (2005)
Factotum (2005)
Danika (2006) **Wild Hogs** (2007)
**Before the Devil Knows You're
Dead** (2007) **War, Inc.** (2008)
The Wrestler (2008)

Lily **Tomlin**
5ft 8in
(MARY JEAN TOMLIN)

Born: **September 1, 1939**
Detroit, Michigan, USA

Lily was raised in a working-class neigh-borhood of Motown. Her parents, who were Southern Baptists from Kentucky, were Guy Tomlin, a factory worker, and his wife, Lillie Mae. Lily was educated at Cass Technical High School in her home town, from where she graduated in 1957. She was a pre-med student at Wayne State University, where she became interested in the theater and performing arts. After college Lily performed stand-up comedy in the city's clubs. Having perfected her act on a local basis, she was confident enough to go to New York City and do it again. In 1965 she made her first appear-ance on television, in 'The Merv Griffin Show'. In 1969, she was Ernestine, the gum-chewing switchboard operator, in 'Rowan & Martin's Laugh-In'. She was in her own show, 'Lily' in 1973 – with Alan Alda and Richard Prior and two years later, she made her film debut, as Linnea Reese in Robert Altman's *Nashville* – for which she received a Best Supporting Actress Oscar nomination. She was dynamic in several movies and was given top marks for the film of her 1991 one woman show, *The Search for Signs of Inteligent* (inten-tionally misspelt) *Life in the Universe*. It was written by her life partner – the writer, director, producer, Jane Wagner, and won Lily a Tony Award. In 2009, she appeared on TV in 'Desperate Housewives' and in the movie, *Pink Panther 2.*

Nashville (1975)
The Late Show (1977)
Nine to Five (1980)
All of Me (1984)
Big Business (1988)
Shadows and Fog (1992)
Short Cuts (1993)
Blue in the Face (1995)
Flirting with Disaster (1996)
Tea with Mussolini (1999)
The Kid (2000)
Orange County (2002)
I Love Huckabees (2004)
A Prairie Home Companion (2006)
The Walker (2007)

David **Tomlinson**
6ft 0¾in
(DAVID CECIL MACALISTER TOMLINSON)

Born: **May 7, 1917**
Henley-on-Thames, Oxfordshire, England
Died: **June 24, 2000**

The son of a lawyer, Clarence Tomlinson, David was educated at Tonbridge School in Kent. In 1935 he joined the Grenadier Guards, but within a year he got involved with amateur theatricals and had made up his mind to become an actor. For a time, he delayed any move towards profession-al status by working as a clerk in London. From the stage he was able to transfer to the cinema - making his film debut with an uncredited bit part in a comedy, *Garrison Follies*. During World War II, he served in the RAF as a Flight Lieutenant. He got so hooked on flying he carried on doing so in his private life after the war, and crashed his Tiger Moth near the back of his home. Uninjured, David continued with his film career. His cheerful demeanor was perfect for the British comedies which poured out of the studios in the 1940s. *Miranda* and *Here Come the Huggetts,* contain good examples of his style. David also showed his versatility in tense dramas like *So Long at the Fair* and *The Wooden Horse,* and remained a reliable second lead in some of Disney's best movies, before retiring in 1980. He was married to Audrey Freeman from 1943 until his death from a stroke, at his home in Mursley, Buckinghamshire.

Quiet Wedding (1941)
'Pimpernel' Smith (1941)
The Way to the Stars (1945)
Journey Together (1946)
I See a Dark Stranger (1946)
Miranda (1948)
My Brother's Keeper (1948)
Here Come the Huggetts (1948)
The Chiltern Hundreds (1949)
Landfall (1949)
So Long at the Fair (1950)
The Wooden Horse (1950)
Hotel Sahara (1951) **All for
Mary** (1955) **Three Men in a
Boat** (1956) **Tom Jones** (1963)
The Truth About Spring (1964)
Mary Poppins (1964)
The Love Bug (1968)
Bedknobs and Broomsticks (1971)

Franchot **Tone**
5ft 10in
(STANISLAS PASCAL FRANCHOT TONE)

Born: **February 27, 1905**
Niagara Falls, New York, USA
Died: **September 18, 1968**

The son of a pioneer in electrochemistry, Franchot was educated at the Hill School in Pottstown, Pennsylvania. At Cornell University, he studied romance languages and he was soon appearing in college plays. He was president of the drama club during his senior year. He had no interest in the family business so he joined a stock company – making his debut in Buffalo, in 1927, in "The Belt". He went to live in Greenwich Village, where he successfully auditioned for the New Playwrights' Theater, in 1929 – making his Broadway debut with Katharine Cornell, in "The Age of Innocence", that same year. With four years of successful stage work under his belt, Franchot was lured to Hollywood to make his film debut in 1932, in *The Wiser Sex,* which starred Claudette Colbert. Shortly after that, he was given a five-year contract by MGM. He was top-billed for the first time, in *Straight As the Way.* 1935 was the year he became a star – with good roles in *The Lives of a Bengal Lancer* and *Mutiny on the Bounty* – (for which he was Best Actor Oscar-nominated) and *Dangerous.* He married Joan Crawford, but the break-up in 1939 was the start of a serious drink problem. Three more wives didn't improve him. By 1951 he was relegated to TV. He looked ill in his 1960s films and died of lung cancer, in New York.

The Lives of a Bengal Lancer (1935)
Mutiny on the Bounty (1935)
Dangerous (1935)
The Unguarded Hour (1936)
Quality Street (1937)
Between Two Women (1937)
The Bride Wore Red (1937)
Three Comrades (1937)
Three Loves Has Nancy (1938)
Fast and Furious (1939)
Nice Girl? (1941)
Five Graves to Cairo (1943)
Dark Waters (1944)
I Love Trouble (1948)
Every Girl Should Be Married (1948)
Advise & Consent (1962)

Rip **Torn**
5ft 10in
(ELMORE RUEL TORN JR.)

Born: **February 6, 1931**
Temple, Texas, USA

"Rip" was a name taken by generations of Torn men and was passed on to him by his father – an agriculturalist, who was also called Elmore. Rip's mother's name was Mary. After high school, Rip graduated from Texas Agricultural and Mechanical University, in College Station – where he studied Acting. He moved to Hollywood where, in 1956, he made his film debut with an uncredited role in Elia Kazan's *Baby Doll.* Rip's first credited role was in *Time Limit,* starring Richard Widmark. In 1961, he divorced his first wife, and after working with Geraldine Page in *Sweet Bird of Youth,* he married her. They had three children and were together until her death in 1987. Rip has acted in many excellent movies and it is hard to understand why he was only once nominated for a Best Supporting Actor Oscar – in *Cross Creek.* He did win an American Comedy Award as 'Funniest Supporting Performer' – in the 'Larry Sanders Show', on TV, in 1992.

Time Limit (1957) **Pork
Chop Hill** (1959) **Sweet Bird of
Youth** (1962) **The Cincinnati
Kid** (1965) **Beach Red** (1967)
Coming Apart (1969) Tropic of
Cancer (1970) Payday (1973)
Birch Interval (1976)
The Man Who Fell to Earth (1976)
Nasty Habits (1977)
The Private Files of
J. Edgar Hoover (1977)
Coma (1978) The Seduction of
Joe Tynan (1979) Heartland (1979)
Cross Creek (1983)
Flash Point (1984) Songwriter (1984)
Extreme Prejudice (1987)
Beautiful Dreamers (1990)
Defending Your Life (1991)
Where the Rivers Flow North (1994)
Trial and Error (1997) **Men in
Black** (1997) **The Insider** (1999)
Wonder Boys (2000)
Rolling Kansas (2003) Eulogy (2004)
Dodgeball (2004)
Turn the River (2007)
Chatham (2008)

Totò
5ft 8in
(ANTONIO DE CURTIS)

Born: **February 15, 1898**
Naples, Campania, Italy
Died: **April 15, 1967**

Although he was the son of Guiseppe de Curtis (whose father was a Marquis) and his wife, Anna Clemente, Totò was raised in a poor area of Naples. He excelled at several sports during his early school years but neglected his education. A boxing injury paralyzed his nose and gave him his trade mark lop-sided look. He created a unique style of comedy which he took into the local music halls. In 1922, he went to live in Rome where he established himself in bigger theaters. In 1926, he began a passionate affair with a famous café-concert singer, called Liliana Castagnola. When he left her two years later, she committed suicide. After he met, and later married, Diana Rogliani, he named their daughter Liliana, in homage to her. He formed his own company with which he toured Italy. Totò's marriage vows were binding, but he lived an extremely free life outside it. Despite his weird appearance, women were crazy about him. In 1937, he made his movie debut, in *Fermo con le mani!* and was a star, who was described as an Italian Buster Keaton, until his death from a heart attack, in Rome.

Totò al giro d'Italia (1948)
Totò le Moko (1949)
Totò cerca casa (1949)
The Emperor of Capri (1949)
Napoli milionaria (1950)
Totò e le donne (1952)
The Gold of Naples (1954)
Totò, Peppino e i fuorilegge (1956)
The Big Deal (1958)
La Cambiale (1959)
You're on Your Own (1959)
Signori si nasce (1960)
Joyful Laughter (1960)
Letto a tre piazze (1960)
Chi si ferme è perduto (1960)
Totò, Fabrizi e i giovani
d'oggi (1960) Tototruffa (1961)
The Two Marshalls (1961)
Lo Smemorato di Collegno (1962)
The Two Colonels (1962)
La Mandragola (1965)

Audrey **Totter**
5ft 3in
(AUDREY TOTTER)

Born: **December 20, 1918**
Joliet, Illinois, USA

The daughter of an Austrian father, who had emigrated from Vienna, and a mother who was of Swedish heritage, Audrey began acting in plays when she was at junior school. Her early career was on the stage and also on radio in Chicago and New York. She went to Hollywood in 1944, where she was given a seven-year contract by MGM. For her film debut, she played a 'bad gal' role in a B-picture, *Main Street After Dark*. She played a supporting role in the John Garfield version of *The Postman Always Rings Twice* and got her big break from Robert Montgomery, when he cast her in his classic, *Lady in the Lake*. It was a good year for Audrey – she also starred with Claude Rains and Robert Taylor. Her career continued to progress when she played opposite Robert Ryan, in one of the best-ever boxing films, *The Set-Up*. In the early 1950s, television was beginning to lure audiences away from the movie theaters. And as with many other actors, the effect on Audrey was 'if you can't beat 'em, join 'em'. In 1954, she made her first small screen appearance in an episode of 'Four Star Playhouse'. Good film roles became scarce, but she did have an opportunity to act with movie legends George Raft, and Edward G. Robinson, in *A Bullet for Joey*. She retired in 1987 – living with her only husband, Doctor Leo Fred, until his death. Today, she resides in Woodland Hills, California.

The Cockeyed Miracle (1946)
Lady in the Lake (1947)
The Beginning or the End (1947)
The Unsuspected (1947)
High Wall (1947)
Alias Nick Beal (1949)
The Set-Up (1949)
Any Number Can Play (1949)
Tension (1949)
Under the Gun (1951)
The Blue Veil (1951)
FBI Girl (1951)
My Pal Gus (1952)
Women's Prison (1955)
A Bullet for Joey (1955)

Stuart **Townsend**
5ft 11in
(STUART TOWNSEND)

Born: **December 15, 1972**
Howth, County Dublin, Ireland

Stuart was the son of Peter Townsend, a professional golfer, (who was the winner of three European tour tournaments and was in the Ryder Cup teams of 1969 and 1971). Stuart's mother, Lorna, had been a model. Stuart was thirteen years older than his brother, Dylan, and fifteen years older than his sister, Chloe. He grew up in Dublin, where during his schooldays, he was developing into a useful boxer with no idea of ever becoming an actor. When he was eighteen, one of his many girlfriends suggested that he should go to the Gaiety School of Acting, in Dublin. While there, he appeared in a production of Brendan Behan's "Borstal Boy". The experience fired his enthusiasm to such an extent that after graduating, he and some friends founded their own theater company, and had a lot of fun. In 1993, Stuart made his screen debut, in a short film made in Ireland, called *Godsuit*. His first feature was *Trojan Eddie,* three years later, when his co-stars were Stephen Rea, and Richard Harris. In 1998, Stuart was judged Best Actor at the Fantafestival, in Rome, Italy, for his work in *Resurrection Man.* After making two movies together, Stuart and the actress, Charlize Theron, became engaged. Recently, he branched out – as producer and director on the well-received action drama, *Battle in Seattle,* which has his fiancé in a prominent role. Stuart also wrote the excellent screenplay.

Trojan Eddie (1996)
Shooting Fish (1997)
Under the Skin (1997)
Resurrection Man (1998)
Simon Magus (1999)
The Venice Project (1999)
Wonderland (1999)
Mauvaise Passe (1999)
About Adam (2000)
Trapped (2002) Shade (2003)
The League of Extraordinary
Gentlemen (2003)
Head in the Clouds (2004)
The Best Man (2005)
Chaos Theory (2007)

Lee **Tracy**
5ft 10in
(WILLIAM LEE TRACY)

Born: **April 14, 1898**
Atlanta, Georgia, USA
Died: **October 18, 1968**

Lee's father was a traveling railroad superintendent, and his mother had been a schoolteacher. He attended the Western Military Academy, in Alton, Illinois, but when his family relocated to New York he joined them. He studied Engineering at the liberal arts, Union College in Schenectady, where he also became seriously interested in acting. Lee joined a theater company following his graduation. His new career was interrupted by World War I, when he joined the Army. After he was discharged in 1918, Lee went to work as a U.S. Treasury Agent. It didn't last very long – two years later he was touring with stock companies and appearing in vaudeville shows. In 1926 he received the New York Drama Critics Award, for playing a song-and-dance-man in "Broadway". He had a reputation as a heavy-drinker, but it didn't prevent him from being offered a contract by Fox. He made his film debut in 1929, in *Big Time.* Lee then returned to Broadway, before beginning a run of good pictures, in 1932, including the famous film, *Dinner at Eight.* His reputation took over his life and MGM dropped him for bad behavior during the shooting of *Viva Villa!* in Mexico. Surprisingly, his 1938 marriage to Helen Thoms Wyse, survived until his death. Lee was nominated for a Best Supporting Actor Oscar for his portrayal of President Art Hockstader, in *The Best Man*. He died of cancer, in Santa Monica, California, three years later.

The Half Naked Truth (1932) Clear All
Wires! (1933) The Nuisance (1933)
Turn Back the Clock (1933)
Dinner at Eight (1933)
Bombshell (1933)
Advice to the Lovelorn (1933)
You Belong to Me (1934)
The Lemon Drop Kid (1934)
Carnival (1934) Two-Fisted (1935)
Behind the Headlines (1937)
Crashing Hollywood (1938)
Betrayal from the East (1945)
The Best Man (1964)

Spencer **Tracy**
5ft 10in
(SPENCER BONAVENTURE TRACY)

Born: **April 5, 1900**
Milwaukee, Wisconsin, USA
Died: **June 10, 1967**

The son of Irish Americans, John and Caroline Tracy, Spence attended seven different schools in Milwaukee and Kansas – where his father worked for a couple of years. He attended Marquette College where he got interested in acting through rooming with Pat O'Brien. They both left to enlist in the Navy in 1917, but Spence continued his education at Rippon College – where he starred in "The Truth". In 1923, he married Louise Treadwell, who would remain his wife, in name only, until his death. He went to New York with O'Brien and studied at the American Academy of Dramatic Art. John Ford saw him act in "The Last Mile" and Spence made his film debut in 1930 – with Humphrey Bogart, in Ford's *Up the River.* He was a star by 1933, but became a bigger one after MGM signed him in 1935 – winning back-to-back Oscars for *Captains Courageous* and *Boys Town.* First nominated for *San Francisco,* he was nominated on seven other occasions. In 1942, he began a love affair with Katherine Hepburn, after they starred in *Woman of the Year.* They co-starred several times and were devoted to each other until his death, from a heart attack, in Beverly Hills – after they'd acted in their last film together – *Guess Who's Coming to Dinner?*

Me and My Gal (1932)
20,000 Years in Sing Sing (1932)
Man's Castle (1933)
Dante's Inferno (1935)
Fury (1936) San Francisco (1936)
Captains Courageous (1937)
Boys Town (1938) Boom Town (1940)
Dr. Jekyll and Mr. Hyde (1941)
A Guy Named Joe (1943)
The Seventh Cross (1944) State of the
Union (1948) Edward, My Son (1949)
Adam's Rib (1949)
Father of the Bride (1950) Pat and
Mike (1952) Bad Day at Black
Rock (1955) The Last Hurrah (1958)
Inherit the Wind (1960) Guess Who's
Coming to Dinner? (1967)

Henry **Travers**
5ft 4in
(TRAVERS HEAGERTY)

Born: **March 5, 1874**
Berwick-Upon-Tweed, England
Died: **October 18, 1965**

Henry's father, Daniel, was a doctor who had settled in the north of England with his wife two years before their son was born. He left school at sixteen to train in an architect's office, but by his early twenties, he had moved down to London where he began getting small parts in stage plays and adopted the name Henry Travers. Before World War II, his was a famous name in the West End theater world, but in 1917 he made the decision to move to the USA. Henry repeated his success as a character actor on Broadway, and spent several years working with the Theater Guild. Henry's first film appearance came in 1933, when he was almost sixty years old – in *Reunion in Vienna.* Suddenly he was reaching a much bigger audience. His kindly features and bumbling personalty were very popular with moviegoers in the 1930s and 1940s. He received his only Oscar nomination – as Best Supporting Actor. in *Mrs. Miniver,* but his role as the angel Clarence, in *It's a Wonderful Life,* is the one people will always associate him with. Henry retired in 1949, and he died in Hollywood, of arteriosclerosis, sixteen years later, at the age of ninety-one.

The Invisible Man (1933)
Death Takes a Holiday (1934)
After Office Hours (1935)
The Sisters (1938)
Dodge City (1939)
Dark Victory (1939)
Stanley and Livingstone (1939)
Edison, the Man (1940)
High Sierra (1941)
Ball of Fire (1941)
Mrs. Miniver (1942)
Random Harvest (1942)
Shadow of a Doubt (1943)
The Moon Is Down (1943)
Madame Curie (1943)
None Shall Escape (1944)
The Bells of St. Mary's (1945)
The Yearling (1946)
It's a Wonderful Life (1946)
The Girl from Jones Beach (1949)

John **Travolta**
6ft 2in
(JOHN JOSEPH TRAVOLTA)

Born: **February 18, 1954**
Englewood, New Jersey, USA

John was the youngest of six children. His father Salvatore, had been a semi-pro football player who became a partner in a tire company. John's mother Helen, had been a singer in a radio vocal group – "The Sunshine Sisters". It was a Catholic family and Helen was forty-two when she gave birth to John. He was not an academic so after his junior year at Dwight Morrow High School, he dropped out to go to New York City and seek his fortune as a performer. In 1972, John appeared in an episode of the TV Series, 'Emergency'. One of his earliest stage roles was in the musical, "Grease". In 1975, he made his film debut in a poor horror film, titled *The Devil's Rain.* The following year, he played Billy Nolan in *Carrie.* John became an icon of American films when, as Tony Manero, he danced to the music of the Bee Gees, in *Saturday Night Fever,* and was nominated for a Best Actor Oscar. During the 1980s, his career took a downturn, but he bounced back with an Oscar-nominated role, in *Pulp Fiction.* John had remained a bachelor until 1991, when he married the actress, Kelly Preston, with whom he co-starred in *The Experts.* They had a son, Jett, (who died in January, 2009) and a daughter, Ella. John is a Scientologist.

Carrie (1976)
Saturday Night Fever (1977)
Grease (1978) Urban Cowboy (1980)
Blow Out (1981) Look Who's
Talking (1989) Pulp Fiction (1994)
Get Shorty (1995) Broken
Arrow (1996) Phenomenon (1996)
Face/Off (1997) Mad City (1997)
Primary Colors (1998)
The Thin Red Line (1998)
A Civil Action (1998)
The General's Daughter (1999)
Swordfish (2001) Austin Powers
in Goldmember (2002) Basic (2003)
The Punisher (2004) A Love Song for
Bobby Long (2004) Ladder 49 (2004)
Lonely Hearts (2006)
Wild Hogs (2007) Hairspray (2007)
The Taking of Pelham 123 (2009)

Claire **Trevor**
5ft 3in
(CLAIRE WEMLINGER)

Born: **March 8, 1910**
Bensonhurst, Long Island, New York, USA
Died: **April 8, 2000**

Claire was the only daughter of Noel Wemlinger, a Fifth Avenue merchant-tailor who was an immigrant from Paris, France. Her mother Betty, had been born in Belfast. Claire grew up in very comfortable circumstances. Well before the Great Depression began to affect her father's business, she'd attended Mamaroneck High School, and after starting classes at Columbia University, switched to Drama at the American Academy of Dramatic Arts. She began her acting career in summer stock at Ann Arbor, in 1932, and around that time she learned about filmmaking, in Vitaphone shorts, shot in Brooklyn. She moved to Hollywood and quickly made her mark. Her debut was in the western, *Life in the Raw,* in 1933. Two years later, after *Dante's Inferno* (co-starring Spencer Tracy) Claire's fanmail poured in. She was memorable in *Stagecoach,* and acquired the nickname "The Queen of Film Noir". She won a Best Supporting Actress Oscar for *Key Largo.* Claire, who was married three times, died of respiratory ailments at her home in Newport Beach, California.

Black Sheep (1935) **Dante's Inferno** (1935) **Dead End** (1937)
Second Honeymoon (1937)
The Amazing Dr. Clitterhouse (1938)
Stage Coach (1939)
Dark Command (1940)
Honky Tonk (1941) **Texas** (1941)
Crossroads (1942)
Street of Chance (1942)
Murder, My Sweet (1944)
Johnny Angel (1945)
Crack-Up (1946) **Born to Kill** (1947)
Raw Deal (1948) **The Velvet Touch** (1948) **Key Largo** (1948)
Best of the Badmen (1951)
Stop, You're Killing Me (1952)
The High and the Mighty (1954)
Man Without a Star (1955)
Lucy Gallant (1955)
The Mountain (1956)
Two Weeks in Another Town (1962)
How to Murder Your Wife (1965)

Jean-Louis **Trintignant**
5ft 8in
(JEAN-LOUIS TRINTIGNANT)

Born: **December 11, 1930**
Piolenc, Vaucluse, France

Son of a wealthy industrialist, Jean-Louis grew up in Piolenc and Aix-en-Provence. When he was twenty, he went to Paris to study drama. He made his stage debut in 1951, in "A Chacun selon sa faim", by Jean Mogin. By 1953, he was an established actor and toured in "Don Juan". The following year, in Paris, he acted in his first starring role, in Robert Hossein's play "Responsabilité Limitee". Jean-Louis' film debut was in 1955, in a short, titled *Pechineff* and his first feature film was *Si tous les gars du monde.* Before doing his army service in Algiers he made two more movies – one of them, *Et Dieu créa la femme,* launched Bardot to stardom, but didn't satisfy J-L artistically. Returning from duty he initially planned to quit acting, but offered the role of "Hamlet" in Paris, he changed his mind. That decision was a fruitful one – placing him with Belmondo and Delon, as young French actors of standing - but he outlasted both. Two best actor awards – a Silver Berlin Bear – for *L'Homme qui ment* and at Cannes, for *Z,* are scant reward for his fine acting. Stéphane Audran and the director Nadine Marquand, are his ex-wives.

The Game of Truth (1961) **The Easy Life** (1962) **The Seven Deadly Sins** (1962) **Il Successo** (1963)
Trans-Europ-Express (1966)
The Long March (1966)
A Man and a Woman (1966)
Paris brûle-t-il? (1966) **Les Biches** (1968)
L'Homme qui ment (1968)
Il grande silenzio (1968) **Z** (1969)
My Night at Maud's (1969)
Le Voyou (1970) **The Conformist** (1970)
Without Apparent Motive (1971)
The Assassination (1972) **The Last Train** (1973) **Love at the Top** (1974)
Cop Story (1975)
The Sunday Woman (1975)
Dirty Money (1978)
La Banquière (1980) **Under Fire** (1983)
Bunker Palace Hôtel (1989)
Three Colors Red (1994)
Fiesta (1995)

Marie **Trintignant**
5ft 6in
(MARIE JOSÉPHINE INNOCENTE TRINTIGNANT)

Born: **January 21, 1962**
Boulogne-Billancourt, Haute-de-Seine, France
Died: **August 1, 2003**

The daughter of Jean-Louis Trintignant and director/writer, Nadine Marquand – who was the daughter of the French film star, Christian Marquand – Marie was born to be an actress. She began at the age of four with a role in *Mon Amour, Mon Amour* which was directed by her mother. When she was eight-years old, the death of her baby-sister Pauline, sent her into her shell and for a time, she didn't speak. After she recovered from that trauma, her ambition was to be a veterinarian. But a year later, Marie could no longer ignore the family connections and appeared in *Ça n'arrive qu'aux autres* – with top stars, Marcello Mastroianni and Catherine Deneuve, and directed by Nadine. That experience and a subsequent Trintignant family movie with her father as the star, made up her mind. She was soon co-starring with the likes of Maximilian Schell and all her early shyness had vanished. She benefited from Claude Chabrol's experienced directing, in *Une affaire des femmes,* but her career almost ended when she was involved in a serious motor accident. Her private life was as fast as her film roles. Marie's four sons were by three different fathers, but at the end of 2003, her luck ran out. While working on a TV-movie 'Colette', at Neuilly-sur-Seine, a violent quarrel at her hotel with her rock-musician boy-friend, Bertrand Cantat, resulted in death through cerebral edema.

Série noire (1979)
La Terrazza (1980) **Les Îles** (1983)
L'Été prochain(1985)
Noyade interdite (1987)
La Maison de Jeanne (1988)
Une affaire des femmes (1988)
Wings of Fame (1990)
Alberto Express (1990) **Betty** (1992)
Hoffman's Hunger (1993)
Fugueuses (1995) **Les Apprentis** (1995)
Des nouvelles du bon Dieu (1996)
Le Cri de la soie (1996) **Ponette** (1996)
Le Cousin (1997) **Harrison's Flowers** (2000) **Janis et John** (2003)
Management (2003)

Stanley **Tucci**
5ft 8in
(STANLEY TUCCI)

Born: **November 11, 1960**
Peerskill, New York, USA

Stan was the son of Italian Americans – Stanley Sr., a high school art teacher, and Joan, whose career included secretarial work and writing. His sister, Christine, would become an actress. Stan was raised in Katonah, New York, where he attended John Jay High School and was an important member of the soccer and baseball teams. Stan excelled in the drama club and befriended Campbell Scott. After earning a B.A. at Purchase College, he made his Broadway debut in 1982, in "The Queen and the Rebels". His film debut, in 1985, was in John Huston's *Prizzi's Honor*. Following supporting roles in films and roles in television series such as 'Miami Vice', he shared the New York Film Critics Circle Award, as Best New Director, with his cohort, Campbell Scott, for their film, *Big Night*. Since then, Stan has won Best Actor Golden Globes, for 'Winchell' in 1998, and 'Conspiracy' in 2001. Stan made his first appearance in a Woody Allen film – *Deconstructing Harry*. He has managed to juggle careers as a film director and actor. Since 1995, Stan's managed a third successful career with his wife Kate. They have three children.

Fear, Anxiety and Depression (1989)
The Feud (1990) Billy Bathgate (1991)
Prelude to a Kiss (1992) Undercover
Blues (1993) The Pelican Brief (1993)
It Could Happen to You (1994)
A Modern Affair (1995)
The Daytrippers (1996) Big Night (1996)
Deconstructing Harry (1997)
A Life Less Ordinary (1997)
Montana (1998) The Impostors (1998)
A Midsummer Night's Dream (1999)
Joe Gould's Secret (2000)
Sidewalks of New York (2001)
Big Trouble (2002)
Road to Perdition (2002)
Spin (2003) The Terminal (2004)
Lucky Number Slevin (2006)
The Devil Wears Prada (2006)
The Hoax (2006) Four Last
Songs (2007) Blind Date (2008)
What Just Happened? (2008)

Forrest **Tucker**
6ft 4in
(FORREST MEREDITH TUCKER)

Born: **February 12, 1919**
Plainfield, Indiana, USA
Died: **October 25, 1986**

Tuck's parents were Forrest A. Tucker and his wife Doris. Being so tall, he never felt it was right to call himself "Junior". He got a job at the Chicago World's Fair in 1933 and after working all day, he performed as a singer during the evenings. After his family relocated to Arlington, Virginia, Tuck attended Washington-Lee High School and played semi-pro football. He won a Saturday night amateur contest at the Old Gayety Burlesque Theater in Washington, D.C. and although underage, he was hired by the owner as an M.C. In 1939, he went to Hollywood, where he was signed by Sam Goldwyn and made his film debut, in *The Westerner*. Tuck worked steadily in movies until 1942 when, after a good role in *Keeper of the Flame,* he joined the Army. After World War II, Tuck resumed his career in a B-musical *Talk About a Lady*. The high-point of his career was reached in *Sands of Iwo Jima*. During the 1950s, he remained a star – albeit in second features, but the rest of his working life was mainly on TV. He was married four times and died in Woodland Hills, California, of lung cancer and emphysema.

The Westerner (1940)
Keeper of the Flame (1942)
The Man Who Dared (1946)
Dangerous Business (1946)
Never Say Goodbye (1946)
The Yearling (1946)
Coroner Creek (1948)
Two Guys from Texas (1948)
The Last Bandit (1949)
Hellfire (1949) Brimstone (1949)
Sands of Iwo Jima (1949)
Rock Island Trail (1950)
California Passage (1950)
Crosswinds (1951) Rage at
Dawn (1955) Finger Man (1955)
The Vanishing American (1955)
Three Violent People (1956)
The Abominable Snowman (1957)
Fort Massacre (1958)
Auntie Mame (1958)
Chisum (1970)

Kathleen **Turner**
5ft 8in
(MARY KATHLEEN TURNER)

Born: **June 19, 1954**
Springfield, Missouri, USA

Kathleen's father Allen Turner, who grew up in China, was imprisoned by the Japanese during World War II. He later became a diplomat in the United States Foreign Service. He and his wife, Patsy, had three children. Due to her dad's work, Kathleen spent much of her early life in Canada, Venezuela, Cuba and England – where she became a keen gymnast, while attending the American School in London. She took lessons at the Central School of Speech and Drama – much to her father's disapproval. He died in 1972, and Patsy took the family back to the USA. Kathleen went to Missouri State University at the same time as John Goodman. Then, in 1977, she gained a Bachelor's Degree in Fine Arts from the University of Maryland, where she had appeared in a number of plays. She made her professional debut in 1978, in the NBC soap, 'The Doctors' and benefited from a star-making role on her film debut, in *Body Heat*. The 1980s and the early 1990s were prolific. She won Golden Globes for *Romancing the Stone* and *Prizzi's Honor* and she was nominated for a Best Actress Oscar, for *Peggy Sue Got Married*. In the mid-1990s, her career slowed when after a year of pain, she was diagnosed with rheumatoid arthritis. With modern treatment she has been able to continue – in 2006 she won a London Evening Standard Award for "Who's Afraid of Virginia Woolf". Kathleen's been married and divorced twice.

Body Heat (1981)
The Man with Two Brains (1983)
Romancing the Stone (1984)
Crimes of Passion (1984)
Prizzi's Honor (1985)
Peggy Sue Got Married (1986)
Switching Channels (1988)
The Accidental Tourist (1988)
The War of the Roses (1989)
Naked in New York (1993)
House of Cards (1993)
Serial Mom (1994)
The Real Blonde (1997)
The Virgin Suicides (1999)

Lana **Turner**
5ft 3in
(JULIA JEAN MILDRED FRANCES TURNER)

Born: **February 8, 1921**
Wallace, Idaho, USA
Died: **June 29, 1995**

Lana's father, John Virgil Turner, was a miner from Tennessee. Her Alabama-born mother, Mildred, was sixteen when Lana was born. They moved to San Francisco where the couple soon separated. In 1930, John was robbed of his winnings in a craps game and killed. The murder was never solved. The following year, Mildred took her daughter to Los Angeles and when she was a sixteen-year-old beauty at Hollywood High School, Lana was 'discovered'. During a break from classes she was seen sipping a Coke at the Top Hat Café, by a man from the Hollywood Reporter. Via actor Zeppo Marx, she was introduced to the film director, Mervyn LeRoy, and made her debut, in *They Won't Forget.* Lana was an MGM star by the beginning of the 1940s with credits including *The Postman Always Rings Twice.* Her lovers outnumbered her seven husbands – the first, to bandleader Artie Shaw, in 1940, lasted four months. After divorcing Lex Barker in 1957, she got involved with small-time gangster, Johnny Stompanato. Lana's fourteen-year-old daughter, Cheryl, stabbed him to death when he attacked her. Lana's courtroom performance helped prolong her flagging career and she was nominated for a Best Supporting Actress Oscar, for *Peyton Place.* Lana played her final film role in *Thwarted,* in 1991. She died at her home in Century City, California, of throat cancer.

They Won't Forget (1937)
Love Finds Andy Hardy (1938)
Rich Man, Poor Girl (1938)
Calling Dr. Kildare (1939)
Ziegfeld Girl (1941) Dr. Jekyll and
Mr. Hyde (1941) Honky Tonk (1941)
Johnny Eager (1942) The Postman
Always Rings Twice (1946)
Green Dolphin Street (1947)
The Three Musketeers (1948)
The Bad and the Beautiful (1952)
Betrayed (1954) Peyton Place (1957)
Imitation of Life (1959)
Madame X (1966)

John **Turturro**
6ft 1in
(JOHN MICHAEL TURTURRO)

Born: **February 28, 1957**
Brooklyn, New York City, New York, USA

John's father was Italian-born Nicholas Turturro, who worked as a carpenter and construction worker. His mother, a Sicilian named Katherine, had aspirations as a jazz singer. John was raised as a Roman Catholic. After high school John majored in Drama at the State University of New York and completed his Master of Fine Arts at Yale School of Drama. In 1983, he was in the title role of "Danny and the Deep Blue Sea" at the Eugene O'Neill Theater Center in Waterford, Connecticut. Repeating the role off-Broadway, he was seen by Spike Lee, who would later employ him in several films. John's first film appearance was as an extra in Martin Scorsese's *Raging Bull.* A number of small roles led to his breakthrough film, *To Live and Die in L.A.* It was the year he married the actress Katherine Borowitz. They have a son who was born during the shooting of *Barton Fink,* for which he won a Golden Palm at Cannes. During the 1990s, his success continued with a Golden Globe nomination for *Quiz Show.* He has written and directed, and continues to appear as an actor in top Hollywood productions.

To Live and Die in L.A. (1985)
Gung Ho (1986) The Color of
Money (1986) Five Corners (1987)
Do the Right Thing (1989)
Mo' Better Blues (1990)
Miller's Crossing (1990)
State of Grace (1990)
Barton Fink (1991) Brain Donors (1992)
Fearless (1993) Quiz Show (1994)
Unstrung Heroes (1995) Clockers (1995)
Box of Moon Light (1996) Grace of My
Heart (1996) The Truce (1997) The
Big Lebowski (1998) Rounders (1998)
Cradle Will Rock (1999) O Brother,
Where Art Thou? (2000) The Luzhin
Defence (2000) Fear X (2003)
Anger Management (2003) Secret
Passage (2004) Secret Window (2004)
The Good Shepherd (2006)
Transformers (2007)
What Just Happened (2008)
The Taking of Pelham 123 (2009)

U

Alanna **Ubach**
5ft 2in
(ALANNA NOEL UBACH)

Born: **October 3, 1975**
Downey, California, USA

Alanna was the daughter of Rodolo and Sidna Ubach, and is of Mexican and Puerto Rican descent. Her older sister, Athena, is also an actress. Alanna's career in show business started when she was four years of age, when she acted in an independent movie, *Los Alvarez.* While she was still a pupil at Lycée Français, in Los Angeles, in 1990, she made her first screen appearance, in the short film, *The Blue Men,* and two years later, acted in an episode of the TV-series, 'The Torkelsons'. Alanna was sixteen when she made her feature film debut, as Gloria, in *Airborne.* In 1993, she was nominated for a 'Young Artist Award' for her work in the television series, 'Beakman's World'. A year or so later, Alanna began to build her reputation with a role in the Danny DeVito comedy, *Renaissance Man,* and was more widely noticed when she played a lesbian, in *The Brady Bunch Movie.* Her comedic skills have been put to good use in films such as *Legally Blonde, Meet the Fockers,* and *Equal Opportunity.* She also wrote and directed a short film called *A Mi Amor Mi Dulce* – which was shown at a number of international film festivals. Alanna is unmarried but has two friendly canine companions – one of them is a bulldog named "Ready".

Airborne (1993)
Renaissance Man (1994)
The Brady Bunch Movie (1995)
Denise Calls Up (1995)
Freeway (1996) **Johns** (1996)
Clockwatchers (1997)
Enough Already (1998)
All of It (1998)
The Sterling Chase (1999)
Slice & Dice (2000)
Blue Moon (2000)
Legally Blonde (2001)
The Perfect You (2002)
Meet the Fockers (2004)
Waiting (2005)
Open window (2006)
Hard Scrambled (2006)
Equal Opportunity (2007)

Juri **Ueno**
5ft 5¾in
(JURI UENO)

Born: **May 25, 1986**
Kakogawa, Hyogo, Japan

When she was at school, Juri – from her nickname "Jurippe" – excelled at track and field, being especially good over the 100 metres sprints. Before she got her start as an actress, she had also mastered the tenor saxophone. When she left school at seventeen, she got work in TV commercials and small-screen dramas – starting with 'Seizon' and the 2003 family TV series, 'Teru teru kazoku'. That same year, she made her movie debut, in the romantic drama, *Josee, the Tiger and the Fish,* which along with *Swing Girls,* landed her the 'Best New Talent Prize' at the Yokohama Film Festival. For *Summer of Chirusoku,* and *Swing Girls,* she won the Sponichi 'Grand Prize New Talent Award' – at Mainich Film Concours. Whatever an actress needs for success Juri has it in abundance. With one exception, all her subsequent films have been both critical and box-office hits. On TV she has been equally successful – with a 'Best Lead Actress' prize at the 2007 Television Drama Academy Awards – for her title role in 'Nodame Cantabile'. It increased Juri's already high popularity rating and led to a role in another television triumph – as Ruka, a young motocross racer – in 'Last Friends'. The judges were on hand to give her the Best Supporting Actress Award. In 2008, Juri was named one of the "Women of the Year" by the Japanese version of Vogue magazine.

**Josee, the Tiger and
the Fish** (2003)
Summer of Chirusoku (2003)
Swing Girls (2004)
**Turtles Swim Faster than
Expected** (2005)
**Summer Time Machine
Blues** (2005)
Arch Angels (2006)
Sea Without Exit (2006)
Shiawase no suitchi (2006)
Rainbow Song (2006)
Kung Fu Kid (2007)
Naoko (2008)
Kodomo no kodomo (2008)

Tracey **Ullman**
5ft 5in
(TRACEY ULLMAN)

Born: **December 30, 1959**
Slough, Berkshire, England

Tracey was the daughter of Polish-born Antony Ullman, and his wife, Dorin – who had gypsy blood in her veins. Tracey's dad died at the early age of fifty, when she was six-years-old. She and her older sister, Patti, performed little shows to cheer their mother up and it wasn't too long before she'd remarried. Tracey's natural skills as a mimic were appreciated by the headmaster at her school. He recognized her potential and recommended her to a famous stage school, the Italia Conti Academy, in London. Tracey remained there until she was sixteen, which was when her career really began. She found work as a dancer in Berlin, in a German production of Lerner and Loewe's "Gigi". After that she joined the "Second Generation" – a group of dancers with whom she performed in variety shows. The exposure helped her get opportunities in West End musicals, including "Grease" and "The Rocky Horror Show". Through winning a competition at the Royal Court Theater, for 'Best Newcomer', Tracey was hot property, and in 1981, she had her own show on BBC television. Three years later Tracey made her movie debut, in Paul McCartney's rather self-indulgent, *Give My Regards to Broad Street.* In 1985, as a punk style singer, she performed in the "Live Aid" concert at Wembley Stadium. A second film role, in *Plenty,* resulted in a BAFTA nomination as Best Supporting Actress. In 1987, she settled in the United States. She's been a big hit on TV there but film roles have been limited. Tracey has two children with her husband, the producer, Allan McKeown.

Plenty (1985)
I Love You to Death (1990)
Robin Hood: Men in Tights (1993)
Household Saints (1993)
I'll Do Anything (1994)
Bullets Over Broadway (1994)
Panic (2000)
Small Time Crooks (2000)
A Dirty Shame (2004)
I Could Never Be Your Woman (2007)

Liv **Ullman**
5ft 8in
(LIV JOHANNE ULLMAN)

Born: **December 16, 1938**
Tokyo, Japan

Liv arrived in Tokyo, because her father was a Norwegian aircraft technician, who was working in Japan when she was born. When Japan entered World War II, her parents took her back to Trondheim, in Norway. Not long after that, Germany invaded and they packed their bags and sailed for Canada. She was educated in Toronto and New York. As a teenager, she began writing her own plays. Her first move towards a career was to go to England, where she trained for the stage at the Webber-Douglas Academy, in London. After graduating, Liv went to work in her mother-tongue, with the Stavanger Repertory Company. After playing the lead in "The Diary of Anne Frank", she went to Oslo, where she starred on the stage and appeared on Norwegian TV. In 1957, she made her film debut, with a small role in a locally-made comedy, *Fjols till fjells*. She married a psychiatrist in 1959 and had her first starring film role, in *The Wayward Girl*. In 1962, she went to Sweden to act in *Short Is the Summer*, with Bibi Andersson, and met Ingmar Bergman. After her divorce, Liv had an affair with him and starred with Bibi, in *Persona*. She was twice nominated for Best Actress Oscars – for *The Emigrants* and for Bergman's *Face To Face*. In 1974, Liv had starred in his TV-series, 'Scenes from a Marriage'. She began to work as a director, and in 2000, she was praised for *Faithless*. Liv was married and divorced twice. She had a daughter with Bergman.

Persona (1966)
Hour of the Wolf (1968)
Shame (1968)
A Passion (1969)
The Emigrants (1971)
The New Land (1972)
Cries and Whispers (1972)
Leonor (1975)
Face to Face (1976)
The Serpent's Egg (1978)
Autumn Sonata (1978)
Richard's Things (1980)
The Rosegarden (1989)

Skeet **Ulrich**
6ft
(BRIAN RAY TROUT)

Born: **January 20, 1970**
Lynchburg, Virginia, USA

Always small for his age, he was nick-named "Skeeter" in his early childhood, by his Little League baseball coach. Skeet was raised by his mother, in Concord, North Carolina, following his parents' divorce. He was given the name Ulrich, by his stepfather, the NASCAR driver and team owner, D. K. Ulrich. Skeet was a sickly child who not only endured bouts of pneumonia, when he was ten, he under-went an open heart surgery operation. He completely recovered, and at Northwest Cabarrus High School, he excelled as a soccer player. After he graduated, Skeet intended to study Marine Biology, at the University of North Carolina, but he went instead to New York University, where he studied acting at the Atlantic Theater Company, after being discovered by one of its founders, David Mamet. In 1989, Skeet appeared as an extra in a comedy *Weekend at Bernie's* – which was shot at Bald Head Island, near his home. It was another seven years before he was given his first real movie opportunities, as Bud Valentine, in *Boys,* and Chris Hooker, in *The Craft.* The latter was one of four good films he made in 1996. He was nominated for a Best Supporting Actor Saturn Award for *Scream,* by the Academy of Science Fiction, Fantasy and Horror Films. It was followed by a good role in *As Good as It Gets.* At the Academy Award party, Skeet met his future wife, the English-born actress, Georgina Cates. The couple had two children, but divorced in 2005. His next film appearances are in *Armored,* with Matt Dillon and Laurence Fishburn, followed by *For Sale by Owner.*

The Craft (1996)
The Last Dance (1996)
Albino Alligator (1996)
Scream (1996) **Touch** (1997)
As Good as It Gets (1997)
The Newton Boys (1998)
A Soldier's Sweetheart (1998)
Ride with the Devil (1999)
Takedown (2000)
Nobody's Baby (2001)

Deborah **Unger**
5ft 7in
(DEBORAH KARA UNGER)

Born: **May 12, 1966**
Vancouver, British Columbia, Canada

Deborah's father is a gynecologist and her mother is a nuclear scientist. She inherited the brains to match – studying Economics at the University of British Columbia before even thinking about a career. When she decided to become an actress, she was a little bit unusual in that she headed for Australia – where she became the first Canadian to be accepted into the Australian Institute of Dramatic Art, which is based in Sydney. She graduated in 1988. While living there, Deborah made her professional debut, in the 1989 TV mini-series, 'Bangkok Hilton' – co-starring Denholm Elliott and Nicole Kidman. She made her film debut, in 1990, in the Australian-shot drama *Till There Was You*. Her big break was that year, in *Blood Oath*. Deborah went back home and, after *Whispers in the Dark,* nothing happened for four years, until she became famous in director David Cronenberg's controversial film, *Crash*. She has since won special awards for her acting, in *Emile* and *One Point O*. Nowadays she regards herself as Canadian, and spends her time both in Los Angeles and Vancouver.

Blood Oath (1990)
Whispers in the Dark (1992)
Crash (1996)
No Way Home (1996)
The Game (1997) **Payback** (1999)
The Weekend (1999)
Sunshine (1999)
The Hurricane (1999)
Signs & Wonders (2000)
Ten Tiny Love Stories (2001)
The Salton Sea (2002)
Between Strangers (2002)
Leo (2002) **Thirteen** (2003)
Stander (2003) **Emile** (2003)
One Point O (2004)
A Love Song for
Bobby Long (2004)
White Noise (2005)
The Alibi (2006)
Silent Hill (2006)
88 Minutes (2007)
Shake Hands with the Devil (2007)

Mary **Ure**
5ft 5in
(MARY URE)

Born: **February 18, 1933**
Glasgow, Scotland
Died: **April 3, 1975**

Mary was the daughter of a civil engineer, Colin McGregor Ure, and his wife Edith. After her early education, Mary was sent to an independent establishment in York, called Mount School. When she finished Mary was already in love with the theater. She was accepted at the Central School of Speech and Drama in London, where she trained as an actress. In the 1950s she developed a reputation on the London stage and made her film debut, in *Storm Over the Nile.* Mary's theater work peaked with her appearance in John Osborne's 1956 play, "Look Back in Anger". Although he was married at the time, they began a relationship and after his divorce, in 1957, they married. Mary went to New York in 1958, to star in the Broadway production of the play and was nominated for a Best Actress Tony Award. She returned to England to co-star with Richard Burton and Claire Bloom in the film version, and there was every indication that she would become a big movie star – it was born out by her portrayal of Clara, in *Sons and Lovers* – for which she was nominated for a Best Supporting Actress Oscar. She began an affair with Robert Shaw, in 1959, when she was tired of Osborne's blatant philandering. The couple married in 1963 and had four children. Mary tried to combine motherhood with being an actress but Shaw was unable to cope with the idea of having a successful wife, and he certainly hampered her career. She sought solace in the bottle. After a disastrous first night in a London play, Mary met her untimely death through the lethal effects of alcohol and barbiturates.

Storm Over the Nile (1955)
Windom's Way (1957)
Sons and Lovers (1960)
The Mind Benders (1962)
**The Luck of
Ginger Coffey** (1964)
Custer of the West (1967)
Where Eagles Dare (1968)
A Reflection of Fear (1973)

Sir Peter **Ustinov**
5ft 11½in
(PETER ALEXANDER FREIHERR VON USTINOV)

Born: **April 16, 1921**
Swiss Cottage, London, England
Died: **March 28, 2004**

Peter's parents had connections to Russian nobility as well as to the Ethiopian Royal Family. His father Iona, had fought for Germany during World War I and met Nadia, his mother, in St. Petersburg. They went to England in 1921. Educated at Westminster School, Peter became fluent in five languages. He studied acting with Michael St. Denis at the London Theater Studio. His first stage appearance was in a 1939 revue, and he was with the Aylesbury Repertory Company before his film debut, in 1940, in a short titled *Hullo Fame.* In 1942, Peter played a German schoolboy, in *The Goose Steps Out.* He joined the Royal Sussex Regiment and in 1944, he wrote the screenplay and acted in *The Way Ahead.* Peter's first peacetime job was to write and direct the 1946 film, *School for Secrets,* which starred Ralph Richardson. Peter didn't act in another movie until 1949's flop, *Private Angelo.* Peter's first screen success was *Hotel Sahara.* He became famous for his portrayal of Nero, in *Quo Vadis,* and was a top character actor for the rest of his film career. He wrote successful plays – "The Love of Four Colonels" and "Romanoff and Juliet" – later a movie. Peter was writer/director on the film, *Billy Budd,* and won Best Supporting Actor Oscars – for *Spartacus* and *Topkapi.* Peter was three times married and had four children. He died of heart failure, in Switzerland.

Odette (1950) **Hotel Sahara** (1951)
Quo Vadis (1951)
Beau Brummell (1954)
We're No Angels (1955)
Lola Montès (1955) **Spartacus** (1960)
The Sundowners (1960)
Romanoff and Juliet (1961)
Billy Budd (1962) **Topkapi** (1964)
The Comedians (1967)
Blackbeard's Ghost (1968)
Hot Millions (1968)
Logan's Run (1976)
Death on the Nile (1978)
Lorenzo's Oil (1992) **Luther** (2003)

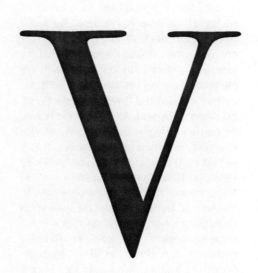

Brenda **Vaccaro**
5ft 5in
(BRENDA VACCARO)

Born: **November 18, 1939**
Brooklyn, New York City, New York, USA

Brenda grew up in Dallas, Texas, where her parents, Mario and Christine, co-founded the famous Mario's Restaurant. After graduating from Thomas Jefferson High School, she went to New York City, where she studied acting at the Neighborhood Playhouse. She made her Broadway debut in 1961, in the comedy, "Everyone Loves Opal". Her performance won her the Theater World Award. In 1963, Brenda made her first television appearance, in an episode of 'The Greatest Show on Earth'. It was followed by further TV work and other Broadway credits such as "Cactus Flower", "How Now, Dow Jones" and "The Goodbye People" – all three plays earned her Tony nominations. She made her film debut, in the underrated, *Where It's At,* and later that same year, appeared in the hit movie, *Midnight Cowboy.* She was nominated for Golden Globes for both. Her first starring role was in *Summertree,* with Michael Douglas and Jack Warden. Brenda's films were spread rather thinly compared with her work on TV. Surprisingly, for such a good actress, her only Oscar nomination was in 1975, for the less than satisfying, *Jacqueline Susann's Once Is Not Enough.* Three times married, she's been with her present husband, Guy Hector, since 1986.

Where It's At (1969)
Midnight Cowboy (1969)
Summertree (1971)
Death Weekend (1976)
Airport '77 (1977)
Capricorn One (1978)
Fast Charlie...the
Moonbeam Rider (1979)
The First Deadly Sin (1980)
Zorro, the Gay Blade (1981)
Water (1985)
Cookie (1989)
Love Affair (1994)
The Mirror Has
Two Faces (1996)
Sonny (2002)
The Boynton Beach
Bereavement Club (2005)

Rudy **Vallée**
5ft 8in
(HERBERT PRIOR VALLÉE)

Born: **July 28, 1901**
Island Pond, Vermont, USA
Died: **July 3, 1986**

Rudy was the son of parents from immigrant stock. His father, Charles Vallée was the son of French Canadians. His mother, Catherine, was the daughter of an Irish couple. "Rudy" (after a well-known 1920s saxophonist, Rudy Wiedoeft) was a nickname he acquired at high school when he took up the instrument. He began playing in local bands and added the clarinet to his repertoire. After high school, he had a brief spell in the U.S. Navy, but was discharged when it was discovered that he was only sixteen. He continued with his musical career and in the early 1920s, he performed with the Savoy Havana Band, in London, England. After returning home, he earned a degree in Philosophy at Yale University and then formed his own band, – featuring himself on vocals – "Rudy Vallée and his Connecticut Yankees". In 1928, he was married for three months to the first of his four wives. He was soon popular nationally as a crooner, due to his huge success on the radio. In 1929, he made his film debut, in *The Vagabond Lover.* His early film work was lightweight, but by the late 1930s, he had developed into a second lead, with a flair for comedy in films such as *Second Fiddle,* and most notably, the "screwball" classic, *The Palm Beach Story.* Rudy's third wife, Jane Greer, survived six months, but his film career went on for a further six years. There were a few more before he retired, in 1984. Rudy died of cancer, in North Hollywood.

Gold Diggers in Paris (1938)
Second Fiddle (1939) The Palm
Beach Story (1942) Happy Go
Lucky (1943) People Are
Funny (1946) The Bachelor and
the Bobby Soxer (1947)
I Remember Mama (1948)
So This Is New York (1948)
Unfaithfully Yours (1948)
My Dear Secretary (1949)
Mother Is a Freshman (1949)
The Beautiful Blonde from
Bashful Bend (1949)

Alida **Valli**
5ft 5in
(ALIDA MARIA LAURA VON ALTENBURGER)

Born: **May 31, 1921**
Pola, Istria, Italy
Died: **April 26, 2006**

Alida's parents were descended from two noble families from the old Austro-Hungarian Empire. On the more sinister side, Alida was a distant relative of the Italian fascist, Ettore Tolomei. It was at his home she went to stay, when at the age of fifteen she began studying in Rome, at the Centro Sperimentale di Cinematografia – a school for film-actors, which had been founded by Mussolini. She made her debut in *Il cappello a tre punte,* in 1934. She was veteran of a dozen films before making her breakthrough, in *Mille lire al mese,* in 1939, and two years later, she was voted Best Actress at Venice, for *Piccolo mondo antico.* Two roles opposite the young Rosanno Brazzi, gave her the title of Italy's number one actress. She went into hiding after refusing to appear in fascist propaganda. In 1944, she married Oscar Mejo – composer of "All I Want for Christmas is My Two Front Teeth"! Alida had a short Hollywood career. Her poor English proved a handicap when she starred in Hitchcock's *The Paradine Case* in 1947, but *The Third Man,* is considered a classic. In 1951, she returned to Italy – proving herself a formidable film actress for over half a century. She died in Rome.

Piccolo mondo antico (1941)
Addio Kira! (1942) We the Living (1942)
Apparizione (1943) Eugenia
Grandet (1947) The Third Man (1949)
The White Tower (1950) Walk Softly,
Stranger (1950) The Stranger's
Hand (1953) Senso (1954)
La grande strada azzurra (1957)
Il grido (1957) This Angry Age (1958)
Eyes Without a Face (1960)
The Long Absence (1961)
Ophélia (1963) The Paper Man (1963)
Oedipus Rex (1967)
Indian Summer (1972)
L'occhio nel labirinto (1972)
Cher Victor (1975)
The Cassandra Crossing (1976)
I Love You (1977) Suspiria (1977)
La luna (1979)

Raf **Vallone**
5ft 9in
(RAFFAELE VALLONE)

Born: **February 17, 1916**
Tropea, Calabria, Italy
Died: **October 31, 2002**

Raf's father, a lawyer, moved the family to Turin following the end of World War I, in November 1918. At school, he showed promise as a soccer player, but his father didn't approve of it as a career. To please his dad, Raf studied Law and Philosophy at Turin University, and to please himself, he took part in the Student World Soccer Championship – held in Vienna, in 1939. After graduating, he worked as a sports journalist then a music and film critic for "La Stampa". It was through the latter that he was given his film debut in 1942, with a small role in *We the Living*. Raf spent the next three years fighting with the Italian anti-fascist resistance. After the war, he continued as a journalist until, in 1949, he was offered a role he couldn't refuse, in the Art House favorite, *Bitter Rice* – made popular due to the physique of Silvana Mangano. Lux, gave him a contract and starred him in a series of Italian and French productions. The impact of *Two Women*, aroused interest in Hollywood. *A View from the Bridge* and *El Cid*, were a good start, but like many continental actors, true stardom was confined to his own country. Raf was married to Elena Varzi from 1952, until his death in Rome.

Bitter Rice (1949)
Under the Olive Tree (1950)
Path of Hope (1950)
The Forbidden Christ (1951)
Anna (1951) **Rome 11:00** (1952)
Thérèse Raquin (1953)
The Beach (1954)
The Sign of Venus (1955)
Love (1956) **Rose Bernd** (1957)
Two Women (1960) **A View from the Bridge** (1961) **El Cid** (1961)
Phaedra (1962) **The Cardinal** (1963)
The Secret Invasion (1964) **Nevada Smith** (1966) **The Italian Job** (1969)
The Kremlin Letter (1970)
A Gunfight (1971)
The Human Factor (1975)
Lion of the Desert (1981)
The Godfather: Part III (1990)

Courtney B. **Vance**
5ft 11in
(COURTNEY BERNARD VANCE)

Born: **March 12, 1960**
Detroit, Michigan, USA

Courtney's early education was at the private Detroit Country Day School, in Birmingham, Michigan. When he was growing up, he was a keen member of the Detroit Boys & Girls Club and he has continued to support the movement. When he attended Harvard University, he became involved in drama and appeared in several plays, before graduating with a Bachelor of Arts degree. By the time he graduated from Yale School of Drama, in 1986, with a Master of Fine Arts degree, he'd met the love of his life and future wife – Angela Bassett. Courtney had already started working as an actor at the Boston Shakespeare Company. He was nominated for Tony Awards – for an early stage appearance in "Fences" by August Wilson – and later, for his leading role in John Guare's "Six Degrees of Separation". He made his film debut, in the powerful Vietnam War movie, *Hamburger Hill*. He went on to impress in *Cookie's Fortune* and *Space Cowboys*. In 1990, he won an Obie award for the off-Broadway production of "My Children, My Africa". Since 2004, Courtney has been seen in three big TV-series – 'The American Experience', 'Law and Order: Criminal Intent' and most recently, the comedy/drama, 'State of Mind'. He is on the board of directors of The Actors Center, in New York City, and lives with Angela, whom he married in 1997 and their twins. The couple have co-authored a book – "Friends: A Love Story". Courtney has just completed work on a new movie, *Hurricane Season*.

Hamburger Hill (1987)
The Hunt for Red October (1990)
Beyond the Law (1992)
The Adventures of Huck Finn (1993)
Dangerous Minds (1995)
The Last Supper (1995)
Blind Faith (1998)
Ambushed (1998)
Cookie's Fortune (1999)
Space Cowboys (2000)
Nothing But the Truth (2008)

Lee **Van Cleef**
6ft 2in
(CLARENCE LEROY VAN CLEEF JR.)

Born: **January 9, 1925**
Somerville, New Jersey, USA
Died: **December 16, 1989**

Lee's father was Clarence Leroy van Cleef, Sr., an accountant. His mother was the former Marion Levinia van Fleet, who was something of a singer. Both were of Dutch origin. Lee was sixteen when World War II started, and in 1942, he dropped out of high school and enlisted in the United States Navy. Following the war, when he and his wife Patsy, had three children to raise, Lee took a job as an accountant. Amateur theatricals led to his professional debut in the original Broadway production of "Mister Roberts". He was seen on tour with the play in Los Angeles and cast as a villain in the classic western, *High Noon*. Lee had supporting roles (never sympathetic) in several more film and television westerns until, in 1962 he suffered serious injuries in a motor accident, and was out of action for three years. He re-emerged, bigger than ever, in the Spaghetti western, *For a Few Dollars More* – that film, and a dozen others, established him as a leading character actor, even though the quality of some of the films was not very high. One of the best films he acted in during his later career, was John Carpenter's *Escape from New York*. Lee died from a heart attack, in Oxnard, California. His widow, Barbara Havelone, was his third wife.

High Noon (1952)
The Lawless Breed (1953)
The Big Combo (1955)
Tribute to a Bad Man (1956)
China Gate (1957)
Gunfight at the O.K. Corral (1957)
The Tin Star (1957)
The Young Lions (1958)
The Bravados (1958)
Ride Lonesome (1959)
The Man Who Shot Liberty Vallance (1962)
For a Few Dollars More (1965)
The Good, the Bad and the Ugly (1966)
Death Rides a Horse (1967)
Days of Anger (1967)
Escape from New York (1981)

Jean-Claude **Van Damme**
5ft 9in
(JEAN-CLAUDE CAMILLE FRANÇOIS VAN VARENBURG)

Born: **October 18, 1960**
Berchem-Sainte-Agathe, Brussels, Belgium

Jean-Claude was the son of Eugène van Varenberg and his wife, Eliana. His father, who was an accountant and also owned a florist shop, enrolled him at a Shotokan Karate school when he was ten years old. At sixteen he studied ballet – which helped him later on when working on the choreography for his movies. He combined this with Karate and weight-lifting to build his physique. Jean-Claude had soon become known as "The Muscles from Brussels". In 1976 he won his first bout in Brussels and two years later, he won a big tournament in Antwerp. He retired in 1980, after beating the best in the world during a three-year career, when he won 15 out of 16 fights and was middleweight champion of Europe. He married the first of his four wives, Maria Rodrigues, and set about launching his film career. He began as an extra in 1983, in *Rue Barbare,* and by 1988 had earned a reputation as an action hero (if not as an actor) in the hit movie, *Bloodsport.* His ability to do his own stunts proved a great asset. Films such as *Double Impact, Nowhere to Run,* and *Hard Target,* secured his stardom. The movie *Time Cop* received the most critical acclaim of all his films. A period of cocaine addiction ended after he divorced his fourth wife. He is currently married (for the second time) to Gladys Portugues, a lady bodybuilder and fitness competitor, with whom he has two children.

Bloodsport (1988)
Universal Soldier (1992)
Hard Target (1993)
Timecop (1994)
Sudden Death (1995)
Maximum Risk (1996)
In Hell (2003)
Narco (2004)
Wake of Death (2004)
The Hard Corps (2006)
Sinav (2006)
Until Death (2007)
The Shepherd: Border
Control (2008)
JCVD (2008)

Trish **Van Devere**
5ft 4in
(PATRICIA DRESSEL)

Born: **March 9, 1943**
Tenafly, New Jersey, USA

After graduating from her local high school, Trish completed her education at Ohio Wesleyan University, a liberal arts college in Delaware. Following stage experience in the early 1960s, she made her television debut in 1965, in an episode of 'Search for Tomorrow'. Trish was next seen on the small screen in 1968, as Meredith Lord Wolek, in the original cast of 'One Life to Live'. Using the name Patricia Van Devere she made her film debut, in *The Landlord,* directed by Hal Ashby. It was an encouraging start to her movie career and five subsequent appearances confirmed that promise. She was nominated for a Golden Laurel Award as "Star of Tomorrow" for *Where's Poppa?* and a Golden Globe for Best Motion Picture Actress for *One Is a Lonely Number.* In the early 1970s she met the first man to refuse to accept an Academy Award, George C. Scott – when they appeared together in *The Last Run.* She married him in September, 1972, and helped to raise his eleven-year-old son, the future movie-actor, Campbell Scott. It was a sometimes difficult relationship with a larger than life character, and Trish may well have sacrificed her career because of her obvious love and devotion to the pair of them. She and George appeared together in four more movies – three of them – *The Day of the Dolphin, Movie Movie,* and *The Changeling* (for which Trish won a Canadian Genie Award as Best Foreign Actress) are very good. She was occasionally seen on television up until 1993 when she acted with George in 'Curacao'. Since his death in 1999, she appears to have retired from acting.

The Landlord (1970)
Where's Poppa? (1970)
The Last Run (1971)
One Is a Lonely Number (1972)
Harry in Your Pocket (1973)
The Day of the Dolphin (1973)
Movie Movie (1978)
The Changeling (1980)
Messenger of Death (1988)

Dick **Van Dyke**
6ft 1in
(RICHARD WAYNE VAN DYKE)

Born: **December 13, 1925**
West Plains, Missouri, USA

Dick's family was of Dutch origin. His father, Lauren Wayne van Dyke, was nicknamed "Cookie" because he worked for the Sunshine Biscuit Company. He had a great sense of humour which he passed on to his son. Dick started elementary school in Danville when he was five years old. Apart from a couple of years in Indiana, he received his education locally – attending Danville High School, where he acted in plays. He enlisted in the US Army Air Force, and during the war appeared in stage shows and worked as a DJ for the Armed Forces Radio. In 1948, Dick married Margie Willett, with whom he had four children. His career moved rather slowly until he started getting TV work in the mid-1950s. He made his stage debut in 1959 in the short-lived, "The Girls Against the Boys", but the following year's "Bye Bye Birdie" earned him a Tony Award as Best Featured Actor and resulted in his appearance in the screen version. 'The 'Dick Van Dyke Show' on TV, and the hit film *Mary Poppins* made him a star – even though his cockney accent was heavily criticized in Britain. Nevertheless, Dick's singing and dancing in the film were much appreciated and it remained his biggest success until *Chitty Chitty Bang Bang.* From the 1970s onwards his film work was limited and he made his living on television – ending with 'Diagnosis: Murder' – which ran from 1993 until 2001. Dick, who has seven grandchildren, lives with his longtime companion, Michelle Triola. He has remained a very busy actor.

Bye Bye Birdie (1963)
What a Way to Go! (1964)
Mary Poppins (1964)
The Art of Love (1965)
Divorce American Style (1967)
Fitzwilly (1967)
Chitty Chitty
Bang Bang (1968)
The Comic (1969)
Cold Turkey (1971)
Dick Tracy (1990)
Night at the Museum (2006)

Peter **Van Eyck**
6ft 2in
(GÖTZ VON EICK)

Born: **July 16, 1911**
Steinwehr, Pomerania, Germany
Died: **July 15, 1969**

After high school in Steinwehr, Peter went to Berlin to study Music. When he was twenty, he left Germany to live in Paris, London, North Africa and Cuba, before going to New York in the mid-1930s. He earned a living as a pianist in bars and nightclubs, and met the song-writer Irving Berlin, who hired him as stage manager. Before World War II started, Peter worked as an assistant director at Orson Welles' Mercury Theater. That experience gave him the idea to become an actor, and he headed for Hollywood where he drove trucks until he met Billy Wilder, who helped him get radio work, and later gave him roles in his movies. Peter made his film debut in 1943, in *Hitler's Children*, and had his first good role, in Wilder's *Five Graves to Cairo*. He became a US citizen and served in the army until the end of the war, when he returned to Germany. In 1949, he made his first German film, *Hallo Fräulein*. He was an ordinary guy in the French classic, *The Wages of Fear*, but was mostly cast as Nazis. Peter died of a blood infection, at his home in Zurich.

Hitler's Children (1943) **The Moon Is Down** (1943) **Five Graves to Cairo** (1943) **The Impostor** (1944) **Address Unknown** (1944) **Die Dritte von Rechts** (1950) **Königskinder** (1950) **Epilog** (1950) **The Desert Fox** (1950) **The Wages of Fear** (1953) **Single-Handed** (1953) **Le Grand jeu** (1954) **Mr. Arkadin** (1955) **Run for the Sun** (1956) **Attack** (1956) **Retour de manivelle** (1957) **The Girl Rosemarie** (1958) **The Snorkel** (1958) **Der Rest ist Schweigen** (1959) **Labyrinth** (1959) **The 1000 Eyes of Dr. Mabuse** (1960) **The World in My Pocket** (1961) **The Longest Day** (1962) **The Spy Who Came in from the Cold** (1965) **Assignment to Kill** (1968) **The Bridge at Remagen** (1969)

Jo **Van Fleet**
5ft 6½in
(JO VAN FLEET)

Born: **December 30, 1914**
Oakland, California, USA
Died: **June 10, 1996**

Jo was educated at the University of the Pacific in Stockton, California. Her interest in acting had started in high school plays during the 1930s, but it was only during World War II that she attended New York's Neighborhood Playhouse. Following top-flight instruction from Sanford Meisner and Uta Hagen, she made acting her career. She first appeared on the New York stage in 1944, but it was a featured role in "The Whole World Over" by the Russian playwright Konstantin Simonov, which brought her fame. During over 100 performances, she had the benefit of both Hagen and Meisner in the cast. In 1946, she married William Bales, with whom she had a son named Michael. In 1954, she won a Tony Award as Best Supporting Actress in "The Trip to Bountiful" – which starred Lilian Gish and Eva Marie Saint. Jo was forty years of age when she made her film debut, as James Dean's mother, in John Steinbeck's *East of Eden*. It won her an Oscar, as Best Supporting Actress, but it didn't lead to a flood of film offers. She needed the kind of roles she could get her teeth into, which explains her limited number of films. Apart from *East of Eden*, her best work is in *Rose Tattoo, Gunfight at the O.K. Corral* and *Wild River*. She made her last film, *Seize the Day,* in 1986, when deteriorating health forced her retirement. When she died at her apartment in Queens, New York, at the age of eighty-one, she was lying in bed chain-smoking.

East of Eden (1955) **The Rose Tattoo** (1955) **I'll Cry Tomorrow** (1955) **The King and Four Queens** (1956) **Gunfight at the O.K. Corral** (1957) **This Angry Age** (1958) **Wild River** (1960) **Cool Hand Luke** (1967) **I Love You, Alice B. Toklas!** (1968) **The Tenant** (1976) **Seize the Day** (1986)

Carice **Van Houten**
5ft 6in
(CARICE ANOUK VAN HOUTEN)

Born: **September 5, 1976**
Leiderdorp, Zuid-Holland, Netherlands

Carice is the daughter of Theodore van Houten, a writer and broadcaster, and his wife, Margje, who is on the board of Dutch Educational Television. Her younger sister, Jelka, is also an actress. She first became interested in movies when her father took her to see the 1927 Abel Gance silent classic, *Napoleon*. A little later, Carice developed a love of Charlie Chaplin's early work. During her high school years at St. Bonifatius College, in Utrecht, Carice frequently participated in the school drama presentations – most significantly, playing the leading role in "Tijl Uilenspieghel" by Hugo Claus. She next began a four year acting course at the Kleinkunstacademie, in Amsterdam. Its alumni include most of the top names in Dutch theater and films. Another skill she developed during that period was playing the clarinet to a high standard. In 1997, she starred in a short movie titled *3 ronden* and the following year, she acted in her first feature – *Ivoren wachters*. In 1999, Carice won a Golden Calf at the Nederlands Film Festival, as Best Actress in a TV-Drama, for 'Suzy Q'. In 2000, she sang and acted in the role of Polly, in the stage production of the "Threepenny Opera". Carice was first seen in the USA, when she starred in the psychological movie drama, *AmnesiA*. She won another Golden Calf for the same year's *Undercover Kitty,* and a third for her big international hit, *Black Book*. She is in a relationship with her co-star in that film, Sebastian Koch. In January 2008, Carice was named "Woman of the Year" by New York Magazine. She has some big movies currently in production.

Ivory Guardians (1998) **Storm in mijn hoofd** (2001) **AmnesiA** (2001) **Undercover Kitty** (2001) **Father's Affair** (2003) **Black Swans** (2005) **Lepel** (2005) **Knetter** (2005) **A Thousand Kisses** (2006) **Black Book** (2006) **Love Is All** (2007) **Dorothy Mills** (2008) **Valkyrie** (2008)

Peter **Vaughan**
6ft
(PETER OLM)

Born: **April 4, 1923**
Wem, Shrewsbury, Shropshire, England

The son of a bank clerk, Peter started his career with the Wolverhampton Repertory Company and then served in the British Army during World War II. In 1946, Peter joined Birmingham Repertory Company and later worked on the stage, mainly as a supporting actor. In 1952, he married the budding young actress, Billie Whitelaw, but while her career took off, he remained very much in the background. He continued to work on the stage until 1956, when he made his first screen appearance, on television, in an episode of 'Tales from Soho' – a series which featured his wife on a couple of occasions. Peter made his film debut in 1959, with an uncredited role – as a police constable, in the Kenneth More version of *The 39 Steps*. A year later, he played another policeman, a first credited film role, in *Village of the Damned*. He was ideal as Bill Sikes, in a TV serialization of 'Oliver Twist', but his movie career only really took off after his face hardened with age and he was third-billed, below Dustin Hoffman and Susan George, in *Straw Dogs*. After that, Peter was in demand and even made an impact in the Ronnie Barker TV comedy series, 'Porridge' and was also in the film version. He was seen most recently in Michael Caine's comedy drama, *Is Anybody There?* Peter lives in Mannings Heath, West Sussex, with his second wife, Lilias Walker.

Two Living, One Dead (1961)
Straw Dogs (1971) The Pied
Piper (1972) Savage Messiah (1972)
The MacKintosh Man (1973)
Zulu Dawn (1979) Time Bandits (1981)
Brazil (1985) The Remains of
the Day (1993) The Crucible (1996)
Les Miserables (1998)
The Legend of
the Pianist on the Ocean (1998)
An Ideal Husband (1999) Hotel
Splendide (2000) The Mother (2003)
The Life and Death of
Peter Sellers (2004)
Death at a Funeral (2007)
Is Anybody There? (2008)

Robert **Vaughn**
5ft 10in
(ROBERT FRANCIS VAUGHN)

Born: **November 22, 1932**
New York City, New York, USA

Both of Robert's parents were in show business. His father, Gerald, had a long career as a top radio actor. His mother, Marcella, was a stage actress. It was a Catholic family and his parents decided to separate when Robert was young. He was taken by his mother to live in Minneapolis. He was educated at North High School in the city and later majored in Journalism at the University of Minnesota, but after only a year there, he moved to Los Angeles. In L.A. he attended City College of Applied Arts and Sciences, where he earned a master's degree in Theater. Robert made his TV debut in 1955, in an episode of 'Medic' and his first film appearance was in an almost invisible uncredited role, in *The Ten Commandments* the following year. Robert was nominated for a Best Supporting Actor Oscar, for *The Young Philadelphians,* and was also one of *The Magnificent Seven*. From 1964 to 1968, he played his most famous role, Napoleon Solo, in TV's 'The Man from U.N.C.L.E'! In 1968, he was asked by the California Democratic Party to stand against Ronald Reagan. He refused. Robert has been married to Linda Staab since 1974. They have two adopted children and live in Connecticut. For Robert's many fans, a return to the small screen as Albert Stroller, in the series 'Hustle' has provided much pleasure.

Hell's Crossroads (1957)
No Time to Be Young (1957)
Good Day for a Hanging (1959)
The Young Philadelphians (1959)
The Magnificent Seven (1960)
Bullitt (1968) If It's Tuesday,
This Must Be Belgium (1969)
The Bridge at Remagen (1969)
Julius Caesar (1970)
The Man from
Independence (1974)
The Towering Inferno (1974)
Virus (1980) S.O.B. (1981)
BASEketball (1998)
Happy Hour (2003)
Scene Stealers (2004)

Vince **Vaughn**
6ft 5in
(VINCENT ANTHONY VAUGHN)

Born: **March 28, 1970**
Minneapolis, Minnesota, USA

Vince's dad, Vernon, was a salesman for a meat company. His mother, Sharon, who is Canadian, was a real estate agent and one-time stockbroker. They were of different faiths – Protestant and Catholic – and divorced in 1991. Vince graduated from Lake Forest High School, in Illinois, in 1988, where a promising athletic future had ended due to a motor accident, and he turned his attention to acting. In 1988, he appeared in a Chevrolet TV commercial and a year later, he did a season in the series 'China Beach'. After struggling in Hollywood for a while, Vince made his film debut, in *Rudy,* in 1993. His breakthrough came in the independent film, *Swingers*. Steven Spielberg's *The Lost World: Jurassic Park* elevated him to star level, but the quality of subsequent films varied dramatically until a series of hit comedies such as *Dodgeball*, *Wedding Crashers*, and *The Break-up,* made him an unofficial member of the Hollywood "Frat Pack" – meaning actors who frequently co-star in comedies. Vince broke the mould in Sean Penn's critically acclaimed adventure film, *Into the Wild*. Vince has visited soldiers in Afghanistan, Kuwait and Iraq, as part of the U.S.O. tour.

Rudy (1993) At Risk (1994)
Swingers (1996)
The Lost World:
Jurassic Park (1997)
A Cool, Dry Place (1998)
Return to Paradise (1998)
Clay Pigeons (1998)
The Cell (2000)
Made (2001)
Old School (2003)
I Love Your Work (2003)
Starsky & Hutch (2004)
Dodgeball: A True Underdog
Story (2004)
Thumbsucker (2005)
Mr. & Mrs. Smith (2005)
Wedding Crashers (2005)
The Gift: Life Unwrapped (2007)
Into the Wild (2007)
Four Christmases (2008)

Conrad **Veidt**
6ft 3in
(HANS WALTER CONRAD WEIDT)

Born: **January 22, 1893**
Potsdam, Germany
Died: **April 3, 1943**

Despite his noble bearing, Conrad grew up in a poor district of Berlin. Educated at the Hohenzollern Gymnasium, he had a passion for acting and hung around the theaters until he met Max Reinhardt, who gave him small stage roles. During World War I, Conrad toured the army camps to entertain the German soldiers. In 1917, he made his film debut, in *Spion*, and while continuing his stage career, he had his first leading role, in the film, *Das Rätsel von Bangalor*. From then on he appeared in dozens of silent dramas directed by such talents of the German cinema as Richard Oswald, Fritz Lang and Friedrich Murau – including *The Cabinet of Dr. Caligari*. He also made films in France. He was an unusual character who was described by his friends as "heterosexual when sober and homosexual when drunk". He signed for Universal in 1927, and began making films in Hollywood and Britain. Conrad married Illona Prager, a Jewess. They left Germany and settled in England, where his best films were Michael Powell's *The Spy in Black*, and *The Thief of Bagdad*. After impressive work in *A Woman's Face* and *Casablanca*, he made his final Hollywood film, *Above Suspicion*. Conrad died on a golf course in Los Angeles.

The Congress Dances (1931)
Rome Express (1932)
I Was a Spy (1933) Jew Süss (1934)
The Passing of the
Third Floor Back (1935)
Dark Journey (1937)
Under the Red Robe (1937)
The Spy in Black (1939)
Contraband (1940)
Escape (1940)
The Thief of Bagdad (1940)
A Woman's Face (1941)
Whistling in the Dark (1941)
The Men in Her Life (1941)
All Through the Night (1941)
Nazi Agent (1942)
Casablanca (1942)
Above Suspicion (1943)

Lupe **Velez**
5ft
(MARÍA GUADALUPE VÉLEZ DE VILLALOBOS)

Born: **July 18, 1908**
San Luis Potosi, Mexico
Died: **December 13, 1944**

The daughter of a Mexican army officer – killed in the Mexican Revolution, and a former opera singer, "Lupe" was a shortening of her second name, Guadalupe. After her father's death, Lupe, along with younger siblings – two sisters and a brother, fled Mexico and settled in San Antonio, Texas. Until she was sixteen she attended Our Lady of the Lake Convent school. She then worked in a department store as a sales assistant, but soon began to dream about seeing her cute face on the silver screen. She took dancing lessons and in 1924, made her stage debut in a musical entertainment, at a theater in Mexico. Two years later, she moved to Los Angeles and in 1927, had her first bit part - in a Charley Chase comedy – *What Women Did for Me*. Later that year she co-starred with Doug Fairbanks, in *The Gaucho*. A part-talkie, *Lady of the Pavements* made her a star, and for six years she had plenty of work in films with an exotic flavor. In 1933, Lupe married the screen Tarzan, Johnny Weissmuller, and before her career went downhill, she appeared in two funny films – *Palooka* and *Strictly Dynamite*. By the time of her divorce, in 1939, she was known as the "Mexican Spitfire" and she exploited that. She had also developed a liking for alcohol and drugs, and after she became pregnant, and was abandoned by the father, she committed suicide.

Lady of the Pavements (1929)
Where East Is East (1929)
Hell Harbor (1930) The Storm (1930)
East Is West (1930) The Squaw
Man (1931) Cuban Love
Song (1931) Kongo (1932)
The Half Naked Truth (1932)
Hot Pepper (1933) Palooka (1934)
Strictly Dynamite (1934) Stardust (1937)
High Flyers (1937) The Girl from
Mexico (1939) Mexican Spitfire (1940)
Mexican Spitfire's Baby (1941)
Honolulu Lu (1941)
Mexican Spitfire at Sea (1942)
Mexican Spitfire's Elephant (1942)

Lino **Ventura**
5ft 9¼in
(ANGIOLINO GIUSEPPE PASQUALE VENTURA)

Born: **July 14, 1919**
Parma, Italy
Died: **October 22, 1987**

Lino was a baby when his parents, Giovanni and Luisa, took him to Paris to seek a better life. He started school there and spoke Italian at home with a French accent. He had no interest in education and, to help his struggling parents, Lino quit school at the age of eight. He worked as an apprentice mechanic and earned extra cash from prize fighting – which gave him his beautiful nose. In 1942, he married Odette Lecomte. They had three children and the responsibility turned Lino into a Greco-Roman wrestler. He was European champion in 1950, but age and injury, bought it to an end. In 1953, he made his film debut in *Touchez pas au Grisbi* which starred Jeanne Moreau and Jean Gabin – who insisted on Lino for several movies. His best films are *Un témoin dans la ville*, *The Threepenny Opera*, *Armée des ombres* and *The Valachi Papers*. In 1982 he was nominated for a César for *Les Misérables*. He worked right up until his death from a heart attack, at his home in St-Cloud, Hauts-de-Seine, France.

Razzia (1955) Crime and
Punishment (1956) Maigret tend
un piège (1958) Ascenseur pour
l'échafaud (1958) Modigliani of
Montparnasse (1958)
Marie-Octobre (1959) 125 rue
Montmartre (1959) The Big Risk (1960)
Taxi to Tobrouk (1960)
The Last Judgement (1961)
Crooks in Clover (1963) Greed in
the Sun (1964) Second Breath (1966)
L'Armée des ombres (1969)
The Sicilian Clan (1969)
Last Known Address (1970)
The Valachi Papers (1972)
Le Silencieux (1973)
La Bonne année (1973)
L'Emmerdeur (1973) La Gifle (1974)
The French Detective (1975)
Illustrious Corpses (1976)
The Medusa Touch (1978)
Garde à vue (1981)
Les Misérables (1982)

Vera-Ellen

5ft 4in

(VERA ELLEN WESTMEIER ROHE)

Born: **February 16, 1921**
Norwood, Ohio, USA
Died: **August 30, 1981**

Vera-Ellen was the only child of Martin and Alma Rohe, who were both of German descent. Her father was a piano tuner, but there was little musical interest shown by his daughter until, at the age of nine, she became frail and unhealthy. The family doctor suggested that dancing might help and she was sent to the same Cincinatti studio as Doris Day. She loved it – became a lot stronger, and at sixteen, she won the Major Bowes Amateur Hour. She began working in the chorus at nightclubs and in 1939, she made her Broadway debut, in the Kern/Hammerstein musical, "Very Warm for May". In 1940, she met her first husband, the dancer Robert Hightower, when they both appeared in "Panama Hattie" – supporting Ethel Merman. Vera-Ellen got good notices in "A Connecticut Yankee" and was spotted by Sam Goldwyn. She made her film debut in the Danny Kaye vehicle, *Wonder Man*. After joining MGM, she danced with Gene Kelly in "Slaughter on Tenth Avenue" in *Words and Music*. They topped that in *On the Town*. Although she wasn't a major star, she had the pleasure of dancing with Fred Astaire in *Three Little Words* and *The Belle of New York,* and was delightful in *Call Me Madam*. She retired in 1957, after making her final movie appearance, in *Let's Be Happy,* but her later life was far from being a happy one. She suffered from anorexia and arthritis, and her daughter from her second marriage was a cot death victim. Vera-Ellen became a virtual recluse until her death in Los Angeles, from cancer.

Wonder Man (1945)
The Kid from Brooklyn (1946)
Three Little Girls in Blue (1946)
Carnival in Costa Rica (1947)
On the Town (1949)
Three Little Words (1950)
Happy Go Lovely (1951)
The Belle of New York (1952)
Call Me Madam (1953)
White Christmas (1954)
Let's Be Happy (1957)

Jan-Michael **Vincent**

5ft 10½in

(JAN-MICHAEL VINCENT)

Born: **July 15, 1944**
Denver, Colorado, USA

His parents, Lloyd and Doris, moved the family to Hanford, California, when Jan-Michael was in his teens. He attended Ventura College, in Southern California where he began to get seriously interested in acting. He made his film debut in 1964 in *Los Bandidos* – directed by its star, Robert Conrad. His career really got going in the late 1960s, when he was signed by Universal Studios and appeared in small roles on television, before a good feature part in the made-for-TV movie, 'Tribes' brought offers of bigger roles. He became popular in films such as *The Mechanic* – co-starring Charles Bronson and even more so after the cult classic, *White Line Fever*. After receiving praise for his work in the 1983 TV mini-series 'The Winds of War', Jan-Michael landed the role of Stringfellow Hawke in the exciting action-espionage series 'Airwolf'. He co-starred with Ernest Borgnine and had the distinction of being the highest paid actor in U.S. TV at that time. In 1996, he broke three vertebrae in his neck in a serious automobile accident – said to have been caused by drunken driving. His career and private life was on the slide from then on, but he did get a role in the critically acclaimed *Buffalo '66*. Jan-Michael's last movie was *White Boy*, in 2002. He has a daughter from his first marriage to Bonnie Portman. Since 2004, he has spent most of his time with his horses, on his ranch in Redwood, Mississippi.

Journey to Shiloh (1968)
The Undefeated (1969)
The Mechanic (1972)
Buster and Billie (1974)
Bite the Bullet (1975)
White Line Fever (1975)
Baby Blue Marine (1976)
Shadow of the Hawk (1976)
Big Wednesday (1978)
Hooper (1978) **Defiance** (1980)
Hard Country (1981)
Born in East L.A. (1987)
Buffalo '66 (1998)
Escape to Grizzly Mountain (2000)

Helen **Vinson**

5ft 5½in

(HELEN RULFS)

Born: **September 17, 1907**
Beaumont, Texas, USA
Died: **October 7, 1999**

Helen's father was a Texas oil man, and her early life was luxurious. She began a life-long love of horses in her early teens. Helen dabbled in acting when she was at high school, but it was after she went to the University of Texas at Austin, that her interest became serious. She was tall, with a charming personality and one evening in Austin, when she was watching a play, she was approached by March Culmore, a lady who worked as director of the Little Theater, in Houston. She took Helen under her wing and the enthusiastic pupil soon became a star of local productions. She went to New York, and had a big success on Broadway in a play called "Los Angeles". It was an apt title, because that's where she ended up, as a Warner Bros. player. She made her film debut, in *Jewel Robbery* and enjoyed twelve years of success – ending her career with a *Thin Man* movie. She retired in 1944. Her three husbands included the British Wimbledon tennis champion, Fred Perry, with whom she lived in England. She died of natural causes, in Chapel Hill, North Carolina.

Jewel Robbery (1932)
Two Against the World (1932)
They Call It Sin (1932) **I Am a Fugitive
from a Chain Gang** (1932)
Lawyer Man (1932) **Grand Slam** (1933)
The Little Giant (1933)
The Midnight Club (1933)
The Power and the Glory (1933)
The Kennel Murder Case (1933)
The Life of Vergie Winters (1934)
The Captain Hates the Sea (1934)
Broadway Bill (1934)
The Wedding Night (1935)
Private Worlds (1935)
Age of Indiscretion (1935)
Vogues of 1938 (1937)
Live, Love and Learn (1937)
In Name Only (1939)
Married and in Love (1940)
Nothing But the Truth (1941)
Chip off the Old Block (1944)
The Thin Man Goes Home (1944)

Monica **Vitti**
5ft 3½in
(MONICA VITTI)

Born: **November 3, 1931**
Rome, Italy

Monica grew up in Milan, where, as a teenager, she appeared in amateur stage productions. When she left school, she trained as a secretary, but following good reviews in "La Nemica", she went back to the city of her birth and enrolled at L'Accademia d'Arte Drammatica. After graduating, Monica joined an acting troupe which went on a tour of Germany. On her return, she made her Rome stage debut, in Machiavelli's "La Mandragola". In 1954, Monica made her first film, *Ridere Ridere Ridere*. A key moment for Monica was when she joined Antonioni's Teatro Nuovo di Milano, in 1957. She appeared in his production of "I Am a Camera" and she became famous in his landmark movie, *L'Avventura* – which was poorly received when it was first shown. A new wave was hitting European cinema and the French, who were at its forefront, reacted warmly to her next films, *La Notte*, and *L'Eclisse* and she made films there, with varying results. *Modesty Blaise,* with Terence Stamp, was her only attempt at an English language film. The *Phantom of Liberty,* directed by Luis Buñuel, was her only post-1960s movie to get distribution internationally. Monica was cautious in her love life. She lived with Roberto Russo for twenty-seven years before they married!

L'Avventura (1960)
La notte (1961) L'Eclisse (1962)
Château en Suède (1963)
Sweet and Sour (1963)
High Fidelity (1964)
The Red Desert (1964)
Il Disco volante (1964)
The Dolls (1965) Le fate (1966)
Girl with a Pistol (1968)
La Femme écarlate (1969)
Help Me My Love (1969)
Ninì Tirabusciò (1970)
The Couples (1970) Teresa la
ladra (1972) La Tosca (1973)
Polvere di stelle (1973)
The Phantom of Liberty (1974)
La Raison d'etat (1978)
Camera d'albergo (1981)

Marina **Vlady**
5ft 3in
(MARINA CATHERINE DE POLIAKOFF-BAIDAROV)

Born: **May 10, 1938**
Clichy, Haute-de-Seine, France

Marina was the youngest of four actress daughters of a Russian-born painter and his wife. She learned classical ballet as a child, but when her sister, Odile Versois, entered films, Marina followed. She and another sister, Olga, made their film debuts in 1944, in *Orage d'été*. At seventeen, Marina married actor/writer/director, Robert Hossein. He promoted her career by starring her in popular films like *Les Salauds vont en enfer* (The Wicked go to Hell), *Pardonnez nos offenses*, *La Nuit des espions* and *Toi, le venin,* which co-starred Odile. She had two sons – Igor and Pierre with Hossein, but they were divorced in 1959. Marina became a star of French and Italian movies. In 1963, she won the Best Actress Award at Cannes, for *L'ape regina*. One of the few English language films she acted in was *Chimes at Midnight* – directed by Orson Welles. Marina's third husband, the Russian poet/songwriter, Vladimir Vysotsky died of a drug overdose aggravated by alcoholism, in 1980. After that, she was mainly seen on French TV. Her fourth husband died in 2003.

Le infedeli (1953)
L'età dell'amore (1953)
Avant le déluge (1954)
Days of Love (1954)
Sins of Casanova (1955)
Le Crâneur (1955)
The Sorceress (1956)
Crime and Punishment (1956)
Toi, le venin (1958) La Sentence (1959)
La Nuit des espions (1959)
The Seven Deadly Sins (1962)
Les Bonnes causes (1963)
L'ape regina (1963) Sweet and
Sour (1963) Mona, l'étoile sans
nom (1965) An American Wife (1965)
Chimes at Midnight (1965)
Two or Three Things I Know
About Her (1967)
Winter Wind (1969) Time to Live (1969)
The Conspiracy (1973)
Que la fête commence... (1975)
Women (1977) Splendor (1989)
Anemos stin poli (1996)

Jon **Voight**
6ft 3in
(JONATHAN VINCENT VOIGHT)

Born: **December 29, 1938**
Yonkers, New York City, New York, USA

The son of professional golfer, Elmer Voytka, and his wife, Barbara, Jon was raised in the Roman Catholic faith. He attended Archbishop Stepiac High School for Boys, in White Plains. It was there that he became interested in acting – playing Puck, in "A Midsummer Night's Dream". In 1956, he went to the Catholic University of America in Washington D.C. where he majored in Art and designed the Cardinal on the floor of the basketball court. After graduating with a B.A. he moved to New York. In 1962, he married the actress Lauri Peters. Jon then acted in episodes of "Gunsmoke" and he didn't make his film debut until 1967, in *Fearless Frank*. *Midnight Cowboy* made him a star. In 1971, Jon married Marcheline Bertrand. One of their two children is Angelina Jolie. His next movie, *Deliverance,* was critically acclaimed – as was *The Odessa File* – and he won a Best Actor Oscar, for *Coming Home*. After a slow early 1980s, Jon got back on track in *Runaway Train,* for which he won a Golden Globe as Best Actor and was nominated for an Oscar. He shows no sign of slowing down. Nowadays he's an in-demand supporting player.

Midnight Cowboy (1969)
Out of It (1969) Catch-22 (1970)
Deliverance (1972) Conrack (1974)
The Odessa File (1974)
Der Richter und sein Henker (1975)
Coming Home (1978) Table for
Five (1983) Runaway Train (1985)
Desert Bloom (1986) Heat (1995)
Mission Impossible (1996)
Rosewood (1997) U Turn (1997)
The Rainmaker (1997)
The General (1998)
Enemy of the State (1998)
A Dog of Flanders (1999)
Pearl Harbor (2001)
Zoolander (2001) Ali (2001)
Holes (2003) National Treasure (2004)
Glory Road (2006)
Transformers (2007)
National Treasure 2 (2007)
Pride and Glory (2008)

Erich **Von Stroheim**
5ft 7in
(ERICH OSWALD STROHEIM)

Born: September 22, 1885
Vienna, Austro-Hungary
Died: **May 12, 1957**

The son of Jewish parents – Benko Stroheim, and his wife, Johanna, Erich would later claim to be of Austrian nobility – adding the 'Von' to his name and largely inventing his early life in an authorized biography. He did go to Hollywood at the beginning of World War I, and was a consultant on German fashions and culture. He made his film debut, in 1915, with an uncredited role in *The Country Boy*. For about three years, he learned everything he could about film-making from D.W. Griffith, and in 1919, he wrote, directed and acted in his own film *Blind Husbands*. His most famous work as a director was *Greed*, in 1924, but with the coming of sound, his inability to stick to budgets ended his career behind the camera and he concentrated on acting. He appeared in many American and European movies – the most famous being Jean Renoir's *La Grande Illusion*, filmed in France – and Billy Wilder's classic, *Sunset Boulevard*, for which he was nominated for a Best Supporting Actor Oscar. Erich was married several times – lastly to actress Denise Vernac, with whom he lived in Maurepas, France. Before he died, he was awarded the French Légion d'honneur.

The Great Gabbo (1929) The Lost Squadron (1932) Fugitive Road (1934) Crimson Romance (1934) La Grande Illusion (1937) Under Secret Orders (1937) Derrière la façade (1939) Pièges (1939) Threats (1940) Tempête (1940) I Was an Adventuress (1940) So Ends Our Night (1941) Gambling Hell (1942) Five Graves to Cairo (1943) The North Star (1943) The Great Flamarion (1945) The Devil and the Angel (1946) Portrait d'un assassin (1949) Sunset Boulevard (1950) Minuit...Quai de Bercy (1953) Alert au sud (1953)

Max **Von Sydow**
6ft 3¼in
(MAX CARL ADOLF VON SYDOW)

Born: April 10, 1929
Lund, Skåne län, Sweden

Max's father was an ethnologist and professor of folklore at the University of Lund. His mother was a teacher. He was raised as a Lutheran – he attended the Cathedral School of Lund, where from the age of nine, he was taught English and German. While at high school, Max and some of his friends formed their own theater company. In 1946, he did his two-year National Service before going to study at the Royal Dramatic Theater, in Stockholm. In 1951, he made his film debut, in *Miss Julie*. That same year he married the actress, Kerstin Olin, with whom he has two sons. He joined the Malmö Municipal Theater and met Ingmar Bergman, who was directing there. He made the first of twelve films for Bergman, *The Seventh Seal*. In 1965, Max launched his international career, when he played Jesus, in *The Greatest Story Ever Told*. He went on to appear in over eighty movies, in several languages. Since 1997, Max has been married to the French filmmaker, Catherine Brelet. They live in Paris. In 2009, he'll be seen in three new films.

The Seventh Seal (1957) Wild Strawberries (1957) Brink of Life (1958) The Face (1958) The Virgin Spring (1960) The Wedding Day (1960) Through a Glass Darkly (1961) The Mistress (1962) Winter Light (1962) The Greatest Story Ever Told (1965) Hawaii (1966) The Quiller Memorandum (1966) Hour of the Wolf (1968) Shame (1968) The Passion of Anna (1969) The Night Visitor (1971) The Emigrants (1971) The New Land (1972) The Exorcist (1973) Steppenwolf (1974) Three Days of the Condor (1975) Illustrious Corpses (1976) Death Watch (1980) Flash Gordon (1980) Conan the Barbarian (1982) Dune (1984) Pelle the Conqueror (1987) Father (1990) Oxen (1991) Hamsun (1996) Minority Report (2002) Le Scaphandre et le papillon (2007) Rush Hour 3 (2007)

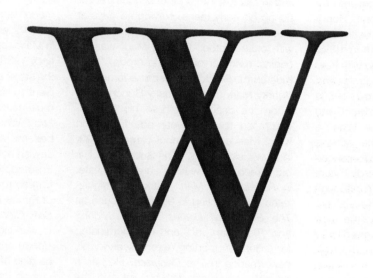

Robert **Wagner**
5ft 11in
(ROBERT JOHN WAGNER)

Born: February 10, 1930
Detroit, Michigan, USA

Bob's parents, a steel executive and his wife, relocated to Los Angeles when he was seven. Bob attended the Harvard Westlake Military School in the city and eventually graduated from Santa Monica High School – as Senior Class President. His first contact with the movie world was when he worked as a caddy for Clark Gable. He was dining with his family in Beverly Hills when he was discovered by a gay Hollywood talent scout, Henry Wilsson – who specialized in "beefcake". Bob was given his screen debut in 1950, in *The Happy Tears*. After signing with Fox, in 1953, he began to get starring roles and was firmly established by the mid-1950s after such films as *A Kiss Before Dying* and *Between Heaven and Hell*. When a four-year relationship with the actress Barbara Stanwyck ended, Bob romanced Joan Collins and Debbie Reynolds before marrying Natalie Wood, in 1957. Although divorced five years later, they re-married, had a daughter, and were together until her tragic early death. He transferred to TV with great success, in 'Hart to Hart', but is still active in movies such as the *Austin Powers* series. Bob has been married to the actress, Jill St. John, since 1990.

Halls of Montezuma (1950)
Prince Valiant (1954) Broken
Lance (1954) A Kiss Before Dying (1956)
Between Heaven and Hell (1956)
The Mountain (1956) The True Story of
Jesse James (1957) The
Hunters (1958) In Love and War (1958)
Sail a Crooked Ship (1961) The War
Lover (1962) The Condemned of
Altona (1962) The Pink Panther (1963)
Harper (1966) Madame Sin (1972)
The Towering Inferno (1974)
Midway (1976) Austin Powers:
International Man of Mystery (1997)
Wild Things (1998)
Something to Believe In (1998)
Austin Powers: The Spy
Who Shagged Me (1998)
Austin Powers: Goldmember (2002)
Man in the Chair (2007)

Mark **Wahlberg**
5ft 8½in
(MARK ROBERT MICHAEL WAHLBERG)

Born: June 5, 1971
Dorchester, Boston, Massachusetts, USA

Mark was youngest of the nine children of Donald Whalberg, a teamster, and his wife, Alma, who had various jobs including a spell in banking and working as a nurse's aide. It was a Catholic family environment, but his parents divorced when Mark was eleven. He attended, but didn't graduate, from Copley Square High School, in Boston. He wasn't academic and in fact got into a lot of serious trouble during his early teens, serving 45 days at Deer Island House of Correction. Along with older brother, Donnie, Mark was an original member of the pop group, "New Kids on the Block" and became famous in "Marky Mark and the Funky Bunch," with whom he used to strip to his briefs – which led to underwear ads for Calvin Klein. Mark's acting debut came in 1993, in a television movie, 'The Substitute'. His big screen debut was as an army private, in *Renaissance Man*. Mark was highly-rated for his acting in hit movies such as *The Basketball Diaries, Boogie Nights,* and *The Italian Job,* and was nominated for a Best Supporting Actor Oscar, for his performance in *The Departed*. He has a daughter and a son with his girlfriend, the Revlon model, Rhea Durham.

Renaissance Man (1994)
The Basketball Diaries (1995)
Fear (1996)
Traveller (1997)
Boogie Nights (1997)
The Big Hit (1998)
The Corruptor (1999)
Three Kings (1999)
The Yards (2000)
The Perfect Storm (2000)
Rock Star (2001)
The Italian Job (2003)
I Heart Huckabees (2004)
Four Brothers (2005)
Invincible (2006)
The Departed (2006)
Shooter (2007)
We Own the Night (2007)
The Happening (2008)
Max Payne (2008)

Anton **Walbrook**
6ft
(ADOLF ANTON WILHELM WOHLBRÜCK)

Born: November 19, 1896
Vienna, Austro-Hungary
Died: **August 9, 1967**

Although Anton was descended from ten generations of stage actors, his father earned a living as a clown in a circus. It was of little appeal to the handsome young Viennese, who after leaving school, took the opportunity to study with the actor and later, famous film and stage director, Max Reinhardt. Anton began his acting career on the Vienna stage, but he made his silent screen debut in Germany, in 1915, when he played a circus director, in *Marionetten*. Throughout the 1920s and early 1930s, Anton was hugely popular on the stage and in German films. In 1936, he went to Hollywood to work for RKO on a multi-national film, *The Soldier and the Lady*. When the Hitler threat in Germany became a reality, his position as a part Jewish homosexual, caused him to flee to England. There, he forged a big career in English movies, starting with his portrayal of Prince Albert, in *Victoria the Great* and *Sixty Glorious Years*. His linguistic gifts led to working in France – most notably in *La Ronde* and *Lola Montès*. The year before he died of a heart attack in Bavaria, Anton starred on German television in a warmly received drama, 'Robert und Elisabeth.'

The Pride of Third Company (1932)
Walzerkrieg (1933) Viktor und
Viktoria (1933) Maskerade (1934)
Die Englische Heirat (1934)
Der Student von Prag (1935)
The Soldier and the Lady (1937)
Victoria the Great (1937)
Sixty Glorious Years (1938)
The Murder in Thornton Square (1940)
Dangerous Moonlight (1941)
49th Parallel (1941)
The Life and Death
of Colonel Blimp (1943)
The Red Shoes (1948)
The Queen of Spades (1949)
La Ronde (1950) Le Plaisir (1952)
L'Affaire Maurizius (1954)
Oh...Rosalinda! (1955)
Lola Montès (1955) Saint Joan (1957)
I Accuse! (1958)

Christopher **Walken**
6ft
(RONALD WALKEN)

Born: **March 31, 1943**
Queens, New York City, New York, USA

Chris's father, Paul Walken, was a German immigrant. His mother, Rosalie, was from Scotland. They ran their own bakery and named Chris after their screen idol, Ronald Colman. Encouraged by their mother, Chris and his brothers, Kenneth and Glenn appeared as child actors on TV. Chris's debut (as Ronnie Walken), was in 1953, in 'The Wonderful John Acton'. He also appeared as an extra on 'The Colgate Comedy Hour' with Martin and Lewis. He was taught to act at the Professional Children's School in New York, and later attended Hofstra University, on Long Island. He made his film debut, in 1969, in *Me and My Brother.* A good dancer, Chris met his wife, Georgianne Thon, when he was touring in "West Side Story". They've been married for forty years. His career in movies is packed with great performances – few better than his dynamic role as Nick, in *The Deer Hunter,* for which he won a Best Supporting Actor Oscar. Twenty-four years later, Chris was nominated for the same award, for *Catch Me If You Can.*

Roseland (1977) **The Deer Hunter** (1978) **Last Embrace** (1979) **Heaven's Gate** (1980) **Brainstorm** (1983) **The Dead Zone** (1983) **A View to Kill** (1985) **At Close Range** (1986) **The Miralgo Beanfield War** (1988) **Biloxi Blues** (1988) **Homeboy** (1988) **King of New York** (1990) **Batman Returns** (1992) **True Romance** (1993) **Pulp Fiction** (1994) **Things to Do in Denver When You're Dead** (1995) **The Prophecy** (1995) **The Addiction** (1995) **Nick of Time** (1995) **Celluloide** (1996) **Basquiat** (1996) **The Funeral** (1996) **Last Man Standing** (1996) **Suicide Kings** (1997) **Blast from the Past** (1999) **Sleepy Hollow** (1999) **The Opportunists** (2000) **Scotland, Pa.** (2001) **Catch Me If You Can** (2002) **The Rundown** (2003) **Man on Fire** (2004) **Wedding Crashers** (2005) **Romance & Cigarettes** (2005) **Click** (2006) **Man of the Year** (2006) **Hairspray** (2007)

Robert **Walker**
6ft
(ROBERT HUDSON WALKER)

Born: **October 13, 1918**
Salt Lake City, Utah, USA
Died: **August 28, 1951**

Bob was the youngest of four sons. His father, Horace Walker, was news editor of a Salt Lake City newspaper. He was affected emotionally when his parents separated during his early childhood, and at junior school, he displayed uncontrolled aggression. As a form of therapy, Bob was introduced to acting, which helped him greatly. While attending the San Diego Army and Navy Academy, he appeared in a school play. His confidence was boosted by the good response and he entered an acting contest, at the Pasadena Playhouse, and won a prize. In 1938, a favorite aunt financed him for an acting course at the American Academy of Dramatic Art. While there, Bob met and fell in love with a young actress, Phyllis Isley (later better known as Jennifer Jones). They married in 1939, the year Bob made his film debut, with a small role in *Winter Carnival.* They had two sons – Robert Jr., and Michael, who became actors. Sadly for Bob, by the time he'd established himself as a movie actor, in *Since You Went Away,* his wife had fallen for the big-time movie producer, David O. Selznick. Bob soon pressed the self-destruct button and it was a surprise that he survived as long as he did. He began drinking heavily, had a nervous breakdown and a disastrous short second marriage. He also produced his greatest performance – in *Strangers on a Train.* Bob died in Los Angeles, from a reaction to prescription drugs.

Bataan (1943) **See Here, Private Hargrove** (1944) **Since You Went Away** (1944) **Thirty Seconds Over Tokyo** (1944) **The Clock** (1945) **Her Highness and the Bellboy** (1945) **What Next, Corporal Hargrove?** (1945) **The Sailor Takes a Wife** (1945) **Till the Clouds Roll By** (1946) **The Beginning or the End** (1947) **The Sea of Grass** (1947) **One Touch of Venus** (1948) **Vengeance Valley** (1951) **Strangers on a Train** (1951)

Dee **Wallace**
5ft 4¹⁄₂in
(DEANNA BOWERS)

Born: **December 14, 1948**
Kansas City, Kansas, USA

The daughter of Robert (an alcoholic who would commit suicide) and his wife, Maxine Bowers, Dee attended Wyandotte High School, in Kansas City. Dee was bright and creative. Apart from showing promise as a ballet dancer she graduated from the University of Kansas with a degree in Education. She had acted in various stage productions during her school years and was able to teach drama at Washington High School – before embarking on her own career as a professional actress. She was first seen in that guise in 1974, in an episode of the television sporting drama, 'Lucas Tanner'. Dee made her movie debut the following year, when she played a small role in *The Stepford Wives.* A bigger film exposure was in the Blake Edwards comedy, *10.* Her first important starring role was in 1982, as Mary, in the classic Steven Spielberg sci-fi fantasy *ET: The Extra-Terrestrial.* Strangely, considering her many excellent performances, that role yielded Dee her only Award nomination – a Saturn as Best Supporting Actress. For fifteen years until his death in 1995, she was married to the actor, Christopher Stone, and was known as Wallace-Stone. They had a daughter. Since 1998, Dee's been married to Skip Belyea. She now runs an acting studio.

All the King's Horses (1977) **The Hills Have Eyes** (1977) **10** (1979) **The Howling** (1981) **E.T: The Extra-Terrestrial** (1982) **Secret Admirer** (1985) **Critters** (1986) **My Family Treasure** (1993) **The Phoenix and the Magic Carpet** (1995) **The Frighteners** (1996) **A Month of Sundays** (2001) **Paradise** (2003) **The Lost** (2005) **American Blend** (2006) **Kalamazoo?** (2006) **Expiration Date** (2006) **Bone Dry** (2007) **Halloween** (2007) **The Blue Rose** (2007)

Eli **Wallach**
5ft 7in
(ELI WALLACH)

Born: **December 7, 1915**
Brooklyn, New York City, New York, USA

Eli was born in an Italian neighborhood. His parents, Abraham and Bertha Wallach were the only Jews in the area. Eli studied hard – graduating from the University of Texas at Austin before earning a Master of Arts from the City College of New York. He served in the United States Army as a staff sergeant in Hawaii, during World War II. Later, he was sent to Casablanca, and France, where his talent was used to entertain wounded servicemen in a show called "Is This the Army?". He made his Broadway debut in 1945, but it was the "method" acting technique, learned at the Neighborhood Playhouse, which won him fame and a career in movies. Through that ability, he appeared in a 1951 episode of TV's 'Lights Out', and it was the small screen and the stage, which kept him busy until his film debut, in Elia Kazan's *Baby Doll*. That performance won him a BAFTA as Most Promising Newcomer. His next win was an Emmy, for *Poppies Are Also Flowers,* ten years later. Eli's been married to the actress, Anne Jackson, for over fifty years. They have a son and two daughters – all three are in the business.

Baby Doll (1956) **The Lineup** (1958)
Seven Thieves (1960) **The Magnificent Seven** (1960) **The Misfits** (1961)
Hemingway's Adventures if a Young Man (1962) **How the West Was Won** (1962) **The Victors** (1963)
Act One (1963) **The Moon-Spinners** (1964) **Lord Jim** (1965)
The Poppy Is Also a Flower (1966)
How to Steal a Million (1966) **The Good, the Bad and the Ugly** (1966) **The Tiger Makes Out** (1967) **How to Save a Marriage and Ruin Your Life** (1968)
Mackenna's Gold (1969)
The People Next Door (1970)
Zigzag (1970) **Cinderella Liberty** (1973) **Nasty Habits** (1977)
Movie Movie (1978) **The Hunter** (1980)
Nuts (1987) **The Godfather: Part III** (1990)
Keeping the Faith (2000)
The Hoax (2006) **The Holiday** (2006)
New York, I Love You (2008)

J.T. **Walsh**
6ft 1in
(JAMES THOMAS PATRICK WALSH)

Born: **September 28, 1949**
New York City, New York, USA
Died: **February 27, 1998**

J.T. was one of four children born to Roman Catholic parents. His father, who was in the U.S. Military, was stationed in Germany – which explains how J.T. became fluent in German. When he was twelve, he was sent to the Jesuit boarding school, Clongowes Wood College, in County Clare, Ireland. On returning to the United States, he attended the University of Rhode Island, which is where he first developed his passion for acting and was the star of several stage productions. J.T. did a variety of jobs after graduating and one of them, as barman, in a Manhattan seafood restaurant, gave him the chance to practice his nice-guy personality – one that would be rarely seen in his movie roles. His professional career began in the 1970s, in off-Broadway shows. In 1982, he was first seen (briefly) on TV, in the drama, 'Little Gloria...Happy at Last'. The following year, J.T. made his film debut, with a small role in *Eddy Macon's Run.* For the next fifteen years he provided many unpleasant moments in several of more than fifty movie appearances. He was at the top of his game when dying from a heart attack, in La Mesa, California.

Hard Choices (1985)
The Beniker Gang (1985) **Power** (1986)
Hannah and Her Sisters (1986)
Tin Men (1987) **House of Games** (1987)
Good Morning, Vietnam (1987)
Tequila Sunrise (1988)
The Big Picture (1989) **Dad** (1989)
The Grifters (1990) **Narrow Margin** (1990)
The Russia House (1990)
Backdraft (1991) **Red Rock West** (1992)
A Few Good Men (1992)
Hoffa (1992) **Needful Things** (1993)
Blue Chips (1994)
The Last Seduction (1994)
The Client (1994)
Black Day Blue Night (1995)
The Low Life (1995)
Nixon (1995) **Sling Blade** (1996)
Breakdown (1997) **The Negotiator** (1998)
Pleasantville (1998)

Kay **Walsh**
5ft 4in
(KATHLEEN WALSH)

Born: **August 27, 1911**
London, England
Died: **April 16, 2005**

Kay and her sister, Peggy, grew up in the London district of Pimlico. Abandoned by their poor Irish parents, they were left with their grandmother, who raised them. Kay was crazy about dancing from the time she first saw the Astaires perform on the London stage. She left school at fifteen and was soon appearing in the chorus of popular revues, produced by Frenchman, André Charlot. In the late 1920s, Kay appeared on the New York stage and also danced in Berlin. In 1934, she made her film debut, with a bit part in the musical, *How's Chances,* and had a featured role in a comedy called *Get Your Man.* Neither were of great quality, nor were the dozen or so films she appeared in up to 1939, when she became the second of director David Lean's six wives. Her first film of any real value was when Lean co-directed – with its author, Noël Coward – the wartime flagwaver, *In Which We Serve.* The year before they divorced, Kay played Nancy in his classic version of *Oliver Twist.* Her only award was when she was voted Best Supporting Actress by the National Board of Review, for *The Horse's Mouth.* Kay's final film was *Night Crossing,* in 1981. She retired and lived in London until her death.

In Which We Serve (1942)
This Happy Breed (1944)
The October Man (1947)
Vice Versa (1948) **Oliver Twist** (1948)
Stage Fright (1950)
Last Holiday (1950)
The Magnet (1950)
The Magic Box (1951) **Encore** (1951)
The Stranger in Between (1952)
Meet Me Tonight (1952)
Young Bess (1953)
Lease of Life (1954)
Cast a Dark Shadow (1955)
Now and Forever (1956)
The Horse's Mouth (1958)
Tunes of Glory (1960)
Reach for Glory (1962)
He Who Rides a Tiger (1965)
The Ruling Class (1972)

M. Emmet **Walsh**
5ft 10in
(MICHAEL EMMET WALSH)

Born: **March 22, 1935**
Ogdensburg, New York, USA

Michael was the son of Harry Walsh Sr., and his wife, Agnes. His father worked as a customs agent. Michael attended Tilton School in New Hampshire, before earning a Business Degree at Clarkson University School of Business. He was an interesting character, even as a young man. The idea of a business career quickly evaporated after he made his television debut in 1969, with a small role in the series, 'N.Y.P.D'. It was followed by an equally small part on his film debut, in *Midnight Cowboy,* but the wagon was starting to roll. By the early 1970s, Michael was in demand – with TV roles – in 'Ironside', 'Bonanza', and 'The Sandy Duncan Show', supplementing his income from supporting film roles, in hits such as *What's Up, Doc?* With his natural talent and reliability, Michael's workload has never slowed down. He received an Independent Spirit award as Best Male Lead, for *Blood Simple,* and was recently judged one of the Best Ensemble Cast of *Man in the Chair,* at the Method Festival, in Calabasas, California.

Mikey and Nicky (1976)
Straight Time (1978)
The Jerk (1979) **Brubaker** (1980)
Ordinary People (1980)
Reds (1981) **Cannery Row** (1982)
The Escape Artist (1982)
Blade Runner (1982) **Fast-Walking** (1982)
Silkwood (1983) **Courage** (1984)
The Pope of Greenwich Village (1984)
Blood Simple (1984) **Fletch** (1985)
The Best of Times (1986) **Critters** (1986)
Harry and the Hendersons (1987)
The Mighty Quinn (1989)
Chattahoochee (1989) **Sundown: The
Vampire in Retreat** (1990) **Narrow
Margin** (1990) **White Sands** (1992)
Equinox (1992) **The Music of
Chance** (1992) **The Glass Shield** (1994)
Romeo + Juliet (1996) **Retroactive** (1997)
My Best Friend's Wedding (1997)
Twilight (1998) **Christmas in the
Clouds** (2001) **Man in the Chair** (2007)
Big Stan (2007) **Your Name Here** (2008)
Don McKay (2009)

Julie **Walters**
5ft 3in
(JULIA MARY WALTERS)

Born: **February 22, 1950**
Smethwick, West Midlands, England

Julie is the daughter of Thomas and Mary Walters. Her father was a builder and her mother, who was from an Irish Catholic background, worked as a postal clerk. Julie's secondary education, at Holly Lodge Grammar School for Girls, ended when she was expelled for inappropriate behavior. Her mother, who reasoned that Julie wasn't academically inclined, urged her to train as a nurse – which she did – at Birmingham's Queen Elizabeth Hospital. She eventually followed her boyfriend to Manchester, where she studied English and Drama at Manchester Polytechnic, at the same time as Pete Postlethwaite. She made her TV debut, in an episode of 'Second City Firsts', in 1975, but her first big success came with another contact from Manchester – comedienne, Victoria Wood. In 1978, they teamed up in a revue called "In at the Death", and four years later, co-starred in their own TV show, 'Wood and Walters'. Julie was nominated for a Best Actress Oscar, on her movie debut, in *Educating Rita* – which won her the first of her five BAFTAs. The second was for *Billy Elliot* – also nominated for a Best Supporting Actress Oscar. In 1988, Julie gave birth to a daughter, Maisie, after a twelve-year relationship with Grant Roffey. They married in 1997.

Educating Rita (1983)
Personal Services (1987)
Prick Up Your Ears (1987)
Buster (1988) **Stepping Out** (1991)
Just Like a Woman (1992)
Sister My Sister (1994)
Girls' Night (1998) **Billy Elliot** (2000)
**Harry Potter and the
Sorcerer's Stone** (2001)
**Harry Potter and
the Chamber of Secrets** (2002)
**Harry Potter and
the Prisoner of Azkaban** (2004)
Mickybo and Me (2004)
Driving Lessons (2006)
Becoming Jane (2007)
The Order of the Phoenix (2007)
Mamma Mia! (2008)

Sam **Wanamaker**
5ft 10½in
(SAM WANAMAKER)

Born: **June 14, 1919**
Chicago, Illinois, USA
Died: **December 18, 1993**

Sam was the son of Jewish immigrants, Morris and Molly Wanamaker. After he left high school, Sam began getting bit parts in summer stock productions, and was trained at the Goodman Theater, in Chicago. In 1937, he helped to build the stage of the famous Peninsula Theater, at Fish Creek, Door County, Wisconsin. Sam worked in travelling shows and eventually, appeared on Broadway. In 1940, he met and married Charlotte Holland, who was a star of radio soaps. He completed his education at Drake University, in Iowa, and in 1943, served for three years in the U.S. Army. On his return to civilian life, Sam resumed his stage career, before making his film debut, opposite the beautiful Lilli Palmer, in *My Girl Tisa.* Following work on the film, *Mr. Denning Drives North,* he was blacklisted by the House Un-American Activities Committee, and went to live and work in England. He established himself with the Shakespeare companies in both Liverpool and Stratford and restarted his film career in the 1960s. Despite many fine performances, there was only one award nomination – for the 1978 TV mini-series, 'Holocaust'. He died of cancer, in London. His daughter is actress Zoë Wanamaker.

My Girl Tisa (1948)
Give Us This Day (1949)
Mr. Denning Drives North (1952)
The Concrete Jungle (1960)
Taras Bulba (1962)
The Winston Affair (1963)
**The Spy Who Came in
from the Cold** (1965)
Warning Shot (1967)
The Billion Dollar Bubble (1976)
**Voyage of
the Damned** (1976)
Death on the Nile (1978)
Private Benjamin (1980)
The Competition (1980)
Irreconcilable Differences (1984)
Baby Boom (1987)
Judgement in Berlin (1988)
Secret Ingredient (1988)

Fred **Ward**
5ft 9¹/₂in
(FREDDIE JOE WARD)

Born: December 30, 1942
San Diego, California, USA

Fred, who is of part Cherokee ancestry, endured the sad death of his mother when he was thirteen years old. After leaving school, he spent three years in the United States Air Force. He was a boxer for a while when he returned to civilian life, but eventually became interested in acting. A drama course at the Herbert Berghof Studio, in New York, didn't lead to much work, and Fred went to Europe, where he used his rich voice to dub several Italian movies – specializing in "Spaghetti westerns" and first appearing on screen, in Roberto Rossellini's 1973 TV drama, 'L'età di Cosimo di Medici'. His movie debut came the following year, back in the USA, in *Ginger in the Morning*. Fred's first major film role was in Clint Eastwood's, *Escape from Alcatraz*. During the following thirty years, he's had no shortage of work. After being included in an ensemble prize, for *Short Cuts,* Fred was awarded a Special Jury Prize, at Chicago Film Festival, for *Train of Dreams.* He's been married twice and has a son called Django – named after the great Belgian jazz guitarist, Django Reinhardt.

Escape from Alcatraz (1979)
Southern Comfort (1981)
The Right Stuff (1983)
Silkwood (1983)
Uncommon Valor (1983)
Swing Shift (1984)
Secret Admirer (1985) Remo: The
First Adventure (1985) UFOria (1985)
Train of Dreams (1987)
Off Limits (1988) Big Business (1988)
Tremors (1990) Miami
Blues (1990) Henry & June (1990)
Thunderheart (1992)
The Player (1992)
Short Cuts (1993)
Naked Gun 33¹/₃: The Final Insult (1994)
Dangerous Beauty (1998)
Circus (2000) Road Trip (2000)
Sweet Home Alabama (2002)
Feast of Love (2007)
Exit Speed (2008)
Management (2008)

Rachel **Ward**
5ft 9in
(RACHEL CLAIRE WARD)

Born: September 12, 1957
Chipping Norton, Oxfordshire, England

Rachel's parents were Peter Ward and his wife, Claire Baring. Her grandfathers were William Ward, the 3rd Earl of Dudley, and Giles Baring, a member of the Baring banking family – who also played cricket for Cambridge University and first-class cricket for Hampshire. With a natural creative talent, Rachel attended the Byam Shaw School of Art, near where she was living, in North London. In 1973, she began working as a fashion model, and although having no training or acting experience, her beauty demanded to be seen by a much wider audience. During that period, Rachel briefly dated David, the son of Robert Kennedy. She made her television debut in the USA, in 1981, in an episode of 'Dynasty'. Her film debut, that same year, was in a terribly poor horror offering, called *Night School*. That title must have stayed in her head, because after being voted one of the ten most beautiful women in the United States, and marriage to the Australian actor, Bryan Brown, she attended acting classes at night. Rachel was out of circulation for three years, but on her return, acted in the award-winning Australian thriller, *Fortress.* Her decision to take acting seriously came too late. She appeared infrequently in movies after that, but established herself as a director and screenwriter. In 2001, Rachel won the Australian Film Institute Award, for Best Short Fiction Film – for *The Big House.* As an actress, Rachel has been seen most recently in six episodes of a popular Australian TV drama series, called 'Rain Shadow'. Rachel's daughter, Matilda Brown, has just started her career as an actress.

Sharky's Machine (1981)
Dead Men
Don't Wear Plaid (1982)
Against All Odds (1984)
Fortress (1986)
The Good Wife (1987)
After Dark, My Sweet (1990)
Wide Sargasso Sea (1993)
The Ascent (1994)

Jack **Warden**
5ft 9in
(JOHN H. LEBZELTER)

Born: **September 18, 1920**
Newark, New Jersey, USA
Died: **July 19, 2006**

Jack was the son of John Warden Lebzelter, and his wife, Lara. He wasn't happy at high school and was expelled for fighting. It seemed like a good career idea so he became a professional boxer. As Johnny Costello, he fought thirteen times. He followed that with spells as a nightclub bouncer, a deckhand, and a lifeguard. In 1938, he joined the United States Navy and spent three years in China. During World War II, he was a U.S. merchant marine, before becoming a paratrooper. Just before D-Day, he shattered his leg in a practice jump. Laid up in a hospital, he read a Clifford Odets play, and decided to become an actor. Using the G.I. Bill, he joined the Dallas Alley Theater, and performed in stage plays. He made his film debut, in 1950, with a bit part in *The Asphalt Jungle*. Working with Warren Beatty brought out the best in him – he was nominated for Best Supporting Actor Oscars, for both *Shampoo,* and *Heaven Can Wait.* Jack died in New York of heart and kidney failure. He was married to Vanda Dupre, from 1958 until his death.

The Bachelor Party (1957) 12 Angry
Men (1957) Run Silent Run Deep (1958)
The Sound and the Fury (1959)
That Kind of Woman (1959) The
Lawbreakers (1960) Wake Me When
It's Over (1960) Donovan's Reef (1963)
The Thin Red Line (1964) Blindfold (1965)
Bye Bye Braverman (1968)
Summertree (1971) The Apprenticeship
of Duddy Kravitz (1974) Shampoo (1975)
All the President's Men (1976)
Heaven Can Wait (1978) Death on
the Nile (1978) The Champ (1979)
Being There (1979) The Verdict (1982)
September (1987) The Presidio (1988)
Passed Away (1992) Bullets Over
Broadway (1994) While You
Were Sleeping (1995) Things to Do in
Denver When You're Dead (1995)
Mighty Aphrodite (1995)
The Island on Bird Street (1997)
Dirty Work (1998)

David **Warner**
6ft 2in
(DAVID WARNER)

Born: July 29, 1941
Manchester, England

David's father was a Russian Jew, Herbert Warner. His mother, Doreen, gave birth to him out of wedlock – which was considered a terrible sin in those dark days of wartime England. He eventually chose to live with his father, who ran a nursing home, and was raised by his stepmother. After eight different schools, due to frequent moves, he finished his education at the Feldon School, in Leamington Spa. David won a scholarship to London's Royal Academy of Dramatic Art. He made his professional acting debut in 1962, with a small role in "A Midsummer Night's Dream", at the Royal Court Theater. It was also the year of his film debut (uncredited) in *We Joined the Navy*. David became part of the Royal Shakespeare Company before his first notable screen role, in *Tom Jones*. He was nominated for a BAFTA, as Best British Actor, for *Morgan!* which was really the beginning of a forty-year story of success – in films, on stage and television. Married twice, he has a daughter, Melissa, with his second wife, Sheilah.

Tom Jones (1963)
Morgan! (1966) **The Bofors Gun** (1968)
A Midsummer Night's Dream (1968)
The Fixer (1968) **The Seagull** (1968)
The Ballad of Cable Hogue (1970)
From Beyond the Grave (1973)
A Doll's House (1973)
The Omen (1976) Providence (1977)
Cross of Iron (1977)
Age of Innocence (1977)
The Thirty Nine Steps (1978)
Silver Bears (1978)
Time After Time (1979)
The Man with Two Brains (1983)
The Company of Wolves (1984)
Waxwork (1988) Hanna's War (1988)
Hansel and Gretel (1988)
Tripwire (1990)
In the Mouth of Madness (1994)
Seven Servants (1996)
The Leading Man (1996)
Titanic (1997) Scream 2 (1997)
The Code Conspiracy (2001)
Ladies in Lavender (2004)

Lesley Ann **Warren**
5ft 8in
(LESLEY ANN WARREN)

Born: August 16, 1946
New York City, New York, USA

Lesley Ann was the daughter of a Jewish couple, whose original surname was Woronoff. Her father was a realtor and her mother, Margot, had sung in nightclubs prior to her marriage. She studied ballet from the age of six – right up to her high school days. During her senior year, she learned jazz technique, with Stella Adler, and then as a seventeen-year-old, studied at the Actors' Studio. She made her Broadway debut during that time, in the musical show, "110 in the Shade" and, although it flopped, she won the Theater World Award in 1965, for another musical, "Drat! The Cat!" It's lack of success didn't prove a problem, because she was then in the title-role in the TV remake of Rodgers and Hammerstein's "Cinderella" – which also featured Hollywood greats – Ginger Rogers, Walter Pidgeon, Celeste Holm and Jo Van Fleet. Two years later, Lesley Ann made her movie debut, in *The Happiest Millionaire,* but had to wait five more years for her next film role, in *Pickup on 101.* For the next ten years, most of her work was on television, but a return to movies saw her nominated for an Oscar – as Best Supporting Actress, in *Victor Victoria.* She has a son called Christopher from her first marriage. Lesley's husband since 2000, is Ronald Taft.

The Happiest Millionaire (1967)
Pickup on 101 (1972)
Race for the Yankee Zephyr (1981)
Victor Victoria (1982) Choose Me (1984)
Songwriter (1984)
Clue (1985) Cop (1988)
Worth Winning (1989)
Pure Country (1992)
Going All the Way (1997)
Marriage Material (1998)
The Limey (1999) Twin Falls
Idaho (1999) Delivering Milo (2001)
The Quickie (2001)
The Frenchman (2002)
Secretary (2002)
When Do We Eat? (2005)
The Shore (2005) Stiffs (2006)
10th & Wolf (2006)

Denzel **Washington**
6ft 0½in
(DENZEL HAYES WASHINGTON JR.)

Born: December 28, 1954
Mount Vernon, New York, USA

Denzel's father, Denzel Washington Sr., was a Pentecostal minister. His mother, Lennis, who was known as "Lynne", ran her own beauty parlor. His parents' began to have marital problems when Denzel was fourteen, and he and his sister were sent away to boarding school during the build-up to their divorce. Earlier, he was part of a boys club known as the "Red Raiders", and believed he would end up at Texas Tech – which was known by the same name. In the event, he earned his degree in Drama and Journalism, at Fordham University – where he excelled at basketball. After working in a summer camp YMCA, in Connecticut, Denzel was encouraged to consider an acting career. He studied at Lincoln Center campus, and starred in the title roles of "The Emperor Jones" and "Othello". A scholarship to the American Conservatory Theater, in San Francisco, made him ready. Denzel's TV debut was in 'Wilma' in 1977. His film debut was in *Carbon Copy,* in 1981. He was a mega-star by the 1990s – with two Oscars – Best Supporting Actor, for *Glory,* and Best Actor, for *Training Day.* Denzel was nominated for *Cry Freedom, Malcolm X* and *The Hurricane.* He married his wife, Pauletta, in 1983. They have four children.

Power (1986) **Cry Freedom** (1987)
Glory (1989) **Mo' Better Blues** (1990)
Mississippi Masala (1991)
Ricochet (1991) **Malcolm X** (1992) **Much Ado About Nothing** (1993) **The Pelican Brief** (1993) **Philadelphia** (1993) **Crimson Tide** (1995) **Devil in a Blue Dress** (1995)
Courage Under Fire (1996) **Fallen** (1998)
He Got Game (1998) **The Siege** (1998)
The Bone Collector (1999) **The Hurricane** (1999) **Remember the Titans** (2000) **Training Day** (2001)
John Q (2002) **Antwone Fisher** (2002)
Out of Time (2003) **Man on Fire** (2004)
The Manchurian Candidate (2004)
Inside Man (2006) **Deja Vu** (2006)
American Gangster (2007)
The Great Debaters (2007)
The Taking of Pelham 1 2 3 (2009)

Kerry **Washington**
5ft 4½in
(KERRY WASHINGTON)

Born: **January 31, 1977**
Bronx, New York City, New York, USA

Kerry's father was real estate broker. Her mother was a professor, who worked as an educational consultant. She is proud of her Native American ancestry. Kerry showed early promise as a performer and in her early teens, was part of the Tada! Youth Theater, at West 28th Street, in New York. Kerry was educated at the Spence School in Manhattan, and when she was twenty-one, graduated with a degree in Theater, from D.C.'s George Washington University. She had earlier polished up her acting skills at Michael Howard Studios, in the Chelsea arts district of the Big Apple – from where she graduated in 1994. She had celebrated that occasion by landing her first TV role, in an episode of 'ABC Afterschool Specials' – "Magical Make-Over". Kerry made her movie debut in the drama, *Our Song.* Her film career has built nicely over the past nine years and she's been recognized, with nominations and awards – the first being a 'Teen Choice Award' for *Save the Last Dance,* which was followed that same year with an Independent Spirit Award for Best Female Lead, in *Lift.* Since she hit the big-time, Kerry's won an Image Award for *Ray,* and was nominated – for *The Last King of Scotland.* She keeps slim and beautiful by working out, and the result is visible in most of her movies. She is single at the moment, but was engaged for three years to the actor, David Moscow.

Our Song (2000)
**Save the Last
Dance** (2001) **Lift** (2001)
Take the A Train (2002)
Bad Company (2002)
The United States of Leland (2003)
The Human Stain (2003)
She Hate Me (2004) **Ray** (2004)
Mr. & Mrs. Smith (2005)
Fantastic Four (2005)
The Last King of Scotland (2006)
The Dead Girl (2006)
I Think I Love My Wife (2007)
4: Rise of the Silver Surfer (2007)
Lakeview Terrace (2008)

Ken **Watanabe**
6ft 0¾in
(KENSAKU WATANABE)

Born: **October 21, 1959**
Uonuma, Japan

Ken's parents were of the intellectual kind; his father was an instructor in the art of Japanese calligraphy, and his mother taught various subjects in schools. Ken was academically capable of becoming a teacher himself, but after graduating from high school in 1978, he opted for a career as an actor. He moved to Tokyo, where he joined a theater troupe known as "En". His breakthrough role, which received plenty of critical and public praise, was as the hero of the play "Shimodani Mannencho Monogatari". It was directed by the highly talented, Yukio Ninagawa. After making his name on the Tokyo stage, Ken made his television debut in 1982, in 'Unknown Rebellion'. Two years later, he acted in his first movie, *MacArthur's Children.* He made both TV dramas and movies, where he was cast as a samurai, and things were fine until 1989, when he fell ill with a form of leukemia, during the making of *Heaven and Earth.* After several years undergoing chemotherapy, his health improved to the point that he was able to continue acting. He was later nominated for a Japanese Academy Award as Best Supporting Actor, in *Kizuna.* For his American debut movie, *The Last Samurai,* Ken was nominated for a Best Supporting Actor Oscar. In 2007, he won a Japanese Academy Award, as Best Actor, for *Memories of Tomorrow.* Married twice, he has an actor son named Dai.

MacArthur's Children (1984)
Tampopo (1985)
The Sea and Poison (1986)
Heaven and Earth (1990)
Kizuna (1998)
Hi wa mata noboru (2002)
T.R.Y. (2003)
The Last Samurai (2003)
Year One in the North (2005)
Ashes and Snow (2005)
Batman Begins (2005)
Memoirs of a Geisha (2005)
Memories of Tomorrow (2006)
Letters from Iwo Jima (2006)
Cirque de Freak (2009)

Sam **Waterston**
6ft 1in
(SAMUEL ATKINSON WATERSTON)

Born: **November 15, 1940**
Cambridge, Massachusetts, USA

Sam's father, George, who came from Leith, in Scotland, was a language teacher and semanticist. His mother, Alice, was a talented landscape painter, who was a proud descendant of one of the original "Mayflower" immigrants. Sam received his education at the private Brooks School, in Andover, Massachusetts, and the Groton School, in the same State. In 1958, he was awarded a scholarship to Yale, and also attended the Sorbonne, in Paris. After graduating from Yale with a BA, Sam took his first steps towards an acting career by working at the Clinton Playhouse, in Connecticut, and completed his training at the Actors Workshop, in New York. Sam's early work was in stage productions of the Shakespeare plays, "Much Ado About Nothing" and "Hamlet". In 1967, he made his film debut, with a small role in the Dick Van Dyke comedy, *Fitzwilly.* From 1970 onwards, his has been a familiar face in some important films – such as Woody Allen's *Crimes and Misdemeanors.* He was nominated for a Best Actor Oscar and a BAFTA, for his role in the powerful drama, *The Killing Fields,* and has a Golden Globe to his credit for a television-Series, 'I'll Fly Away'. He has appeared in more than 300 episodes of TV's 'Law & Order'. Sam has four children from two marriages – three with second wife, Lynn.

Generation (1969) **Three** (1969)
**Who Killed Mary What's 'Er
Name?** (1971) **The Great Gatsby** (1974)
Rancho Deluxe (1975)
Sweet Revenge (1976)
Capricorn One (1978)
Hopscotch (1980) **Heaven's Gate** (1980)
The Killing Fields (1984)
September (1987)
Welcome Home (1989)
Crimes and Misdemeanors (1989)
Mindwalk (1990)
The Man in the Moon (1991)
Serial Mom (1994)
The Journey of August King (1995)
The Proprietor (1996)
The Commission (2003)

Emily **Watson**
5ft 8in
(EMILY ANITA WATSON)

Born: **January 14, 1967**
Islington, London, England

Emily's father was an architect and her mother was a professor of English. After leaving school, she trained at the Drama Studio, in Ealing, not far from the famous old British film studio. She then followed her mother's path by earning a BA in English from Bristol University. Her next move was to pursue an acting career. In 1992, she joined the Royal Shakespeare Company - where, in 1995, she met her future husband, Jack Waters. Emily acted in several stage productions during that period, including "The Children's Hour", "Three Sisters," and "Much Ado About Nothing". Emily's film debut, in *Breaking the Waves,* was fortuitous in a number of ways. Helena Bonham-Carter suddenly pulled out of the project, and director, Lars von Trier, decided to take a chance with an "unknown". The result for Emily included Critics Circle Awards, from London, L.A. and New York, and an Oscar nomination as Best Actress. Her role as cellist, Jacqueline du Pre, in *Hilary and Jackie,* put her name on everyone's lips and earned a second Oscar nomination. Emily continues to impress in some big movies.

Breaking the Waves (1996)
Metroland (1997)
The Boxer (1997)
Hilary and Jackie (1998)
Cradle Will Rock (1999)
Angela's Ashes (1999)
The Luzhin Defence (2000)
Gosford Park (2001)
Punch-Drunk Love (2002)
Red Dragon (2002)
Equilibrium (2002)
The Life and Death of Peter Sellers (2004)
The Proposition (2005)
Wah-Wah (2005)
Separate Lies (2005)
Crusade in Jeans (2006)
Miss Potter (2006)
The Water Horse (2007)
Fireflies in the Garden (2008)
Synecdoche, New York (2008)
Cold Souls (2009)

Emma **Watson**
5ft 6in
(EMMA CHARLOTTE DUERRE WATSON)

Born: **April 15, 1990**
Paris, France

Emma is the daughter of two lawyers: an English father, Chris Watson, and a French mother, Jacqueline Luesby. She lived in Paris until she was five-years old. When her parents got divorced, Emma and her younger brother, Alex, moved with their mother, to Oxford, in England. From the autumn term of 1995, Emma attended Lynam's, which is the nursery school for the Dragon School, in Oxford. By the age of six, she was expressing a keen interest in poetry and won the Daisy Pratt poetry competition, a year later. From the age of eight she spent five happy years at the main school. She had already starred in plays, including "Arthur: the Young Years" and "The Happy Prince", when in 1999, she auditioned successfully for the role of Hermione Granger, in *Harry Potter and the Sorcerer's Stone.* Emma had no training as an actress, but was simply a 'natural'. The first film was a worldwide success and it was inevitable that she would star in subsequent productions of J.K. Rowling's best-selling novels. Meanwhile, Emma had to continue with her education – attending the private all-girls school, Headington, in Oxford and achieving top passes in her GCSE exams in 2006. Before that was out of the way, Emma had begun to look at ways of expanding her repertoire. She liked the sound of a BBC adaptation of 'Ballet Shoes', from a novel by Noel Streatfeild. In it, she played the eldest of three sisters. It was aired in the UK on Boxing Day 2007. Emma's performance was praised, but the film received the thumbs down from many critics.

Harry Potter and the Sorcerer's Stone (2001)
Harry Potter and the Chamber of Secrets (2002)
Harry Potter and the Prisoner of Azkaban (2003)
The Goblet of Fire (2005)
Harry Potter and the Order of the Phoenix (2007)
Harry Potter and the Half-Blood Prince (2009)

Naomi **Watts**
5ft 5in
(NAOMI ELLEN WATTS)

Born: **September 28, 1968**
Shoreham, Kent, England

Naomi's parents were certainly achievers. Her dad, Peter Watts, had borrowed fame from his association as road manager and sound engineer with the legendary pop group, "Pink Floyd". That fame rubbed off on young Amy. Her mother, 'Miv' was an antiques dealer. She also had the energy to work as a set and costume designer. Sadly, her parents split up when Naomi was four, and her dad died three years later. "Miv" was a typical hippie of the time and Naomi and her brother, Ben, lived a nomadic existence in Wales and various parts of England. Their grandmother was Australian, so in 1982, the family moved to Sydney. Naomi was entitled to citizenship, which was taken up, but she still considers herself British. When she attended North Sydney Girls High School, one of her classmates was Nicole Kidman. She had brief spells as a model, and in 1986, as a fashion editor – the year of her film debut in *For Love Alone.* She then acted on Australian television. Her breakthrough movie was *Under the Lighthouse Dancing* and she was soon taking Hollywood by storm. She was nominated for a Best Actress Oscar, for *21 Grams,* and won Saturn Awards for *The Ring,* and *King Kong.* She had her second child with actor, Liev Schreiber, in 2008, and has recently agreed to pose nude for the Australian artist, David Bromley.

Under the Lighthouse Dancing (1997)
Dangerous Beauty (1998) **Strange Planet** (1999) **Mulholland Drive** (2001)
Rabbits (2002) **The Ring** (2002)
Plots with a View (2002)
Ned Kelly (2003) **21 Grams** (2003)
We Don't Live Here Anymore (2004)
The Assassination of Richard Nixon (2004)
I Heart Huckabees (2004)
Ellie Parker (2005) **Stay** (2005)
King Kong (2005)
The Painted Veil (2006)
Eastern Promises (2007)
Funny Games U.S. (2007)
The International (2009)

David **Wayne**
5ft 7in
(WAYNE JAMES MCMEEKAN)

Born: **January 30, 1914**
Traverse City, Michigan, USA
Died: **February 9, 1995**

David, the son of an insurance executive, was raised in Bloomingdale, Michigan. After graduating from high school, he attended Western Michigan University, in Kalamazoo. In the mid-1930s, he worked in Cleveland, Ohio, as a statistician and began acting in local amateur theatrical productions. He then moved to New York where he took acting classes. In 1938, the year of his professional stage debut on Broadway, David was in two successive failures, "Escape the Night" and "Dance Night" but had a small role in a success – "The American Way". In 1941, he married the woman who would be his wife until his death, Jane Gordon. Before the U.S. entered World War II, he was rejected by his own army, but was able to serve in North Africa as an ambulance driver for the British. He was erroneously reported to have died at Tobruk, and eventually served with the U.S. forces. When peace returned, David resumed his acting career and was the first recipient of a Tony Award, in "Finian's Rainbow". David made his movie debut, in *Portrait of Jennie,* and his first impact, in *Adam's Rib.* He made 31 movies, several of which, like *How to Marry a Millionaire* are fondly remembered. He died of lung cancer, in Santa Monica.

Portrait of Jennie (1948)
Adam's Rib (1949) The Reformer and
the Redhead (1950) Stella (1950)
My Blue Heaven (1950) Up Front (1951)
M (1951) As Young as You Feel (1951)
With a Song in My Heart (1952)
Wait Till the Sun Shines, Nellie (1952)
We're Not Married (1952)
O. Henry's Full House (1952)
The I Don't Care Girl (1953)
How to Marry a Millionaire (1953)
Hell and High Water (1954)
The Tender Trap (1955)
The Three Faces of Eve (1957)
The Last Angry Man (1959)
The Andromeda Strain (1971)
The Front Page (1974)
Finders Keepers (1984)

John **Wayne**
6ft 4in
(MARION ROBERT MORRISON)

Born: **May 26, 1907**
Winterset, Iowa, USA
Died: **June 11, 1979**

Duke's father, Clyde Leonard Morrison, was the son of Marion Mitchell Morrison, who fought in the American Civil War. His wife, Mary, agreed to name their son after him. The Morrisons moved to California, and Duke went to school in Glendale, where his dad ran a pharmacy. It was a local fireman who first gave him the nickname, "Duke" and he was never again called Marion. After Wilson Middle School, Duke attended Glendale High School, where he was a member of the champion football team of 1924. He studied at the University of Southern California, but left when he got work as a prop man through the recommendation of Tom Mix. He was invited along with his USC teammates, to play football on-screen – beginning with *Brown of Harvard,* in 1926. Duke found fame as a cowboy, starting with *The Big Trail,* in 1930. He appeared in sixty films in that decade – mostly westerns, before his star-making role as the Ringo Kid, in John Ford's classic, *Stagecoach.* Duke won an Oscar for *True Grit.* He was a major film star until he died of lung and stomach cancer, in Los Angeles.

Stagecoach (1939) The Long Voyage
Home (1940) Reap the Wild Wind (1942)
The Spoilers (1942) Pittsburgh (1942) A
Lady Takes a Chance (1943) They Were
Expendable (1945) Fort Apache (1948)
Red River (1948) 3 Godfathers (1948)
Wake of the Red Witch (1948) She Wore
a Yellow Ribbon (1949) Sands of Iwo
Jima (1949) Rio Grande (1950)
The Quiet Man (1952) Hondo (1953)
The High and the Mighty (1954)
The Searchers (1956) Rio Bravo (1959)
The Horse Soldiers (1959)
The Alamo (1960) North to Alaska (1960)
The Comancheros (1961) The Man
Who Shot Liberty Valance (1962)
Hatari! (1962) Donovan's Reef (1963)
McLintock! (1963) In Harm's Way (1965)
The Sons of Katie Elder (1965)
El Dorado (1966) True Grit (1969) The
Cowboys (1972) The Shootist (1976)

Sigourney **Weaver**
5ft 11in
(SUSAN ALEXANDRA WEAVER)

Born: **October 8, 1949**
New York City, New York, USA

Sigourney was christened Susan by her parents – Sylvester Weaver, an NBC TV executive, and his wife, Elizabeth, an English-born former actress. When she was fourteen, she started using the name "Sigourney" after a character she had read about in F. Scott Fitzgerald's novel, "The Great Gatsby". Sigourney was educated at the Ethel Walker School, in Simsbury, Connecticut, before graduating with a BA in English from Stanford, in 1972. Two years later, she achieved an MFA at Yale School of Drama. While there, she acted in several plays and befriended the future playwright, Christopher Durang – who, in 1981, cast her in his comedy, "Beyond Therapy", off-Broadway. After a small role in *Annie Hall,* Sigourney became famous internationally for playing Ripley, in *Alien.* She was nominated for a Best Actress Oscar for its sequel, and in 1988, was up for both Best Actress – for *Gorillas in the Mist* and Best Supporting Actress – for *Working Girl.* Sigourney has remained in demand as a star name right up to today. Her private life has been successful too; she been married to Jim Simpson, since 1984 and has a daughter called Charlotte. Her next film is the sci-fi thriller, *Avatar.*

Alien (1979)
The Year of Living Dangerously (1982)
Ghostbusters (1984) Aliens (1986)
Gorillas in the Mist (1988)
Working Girl (1988)
Ghostbusters II (1989) Dave (1993)
Death and the Maiden (1994)
Copycat (1995)
The Ice Storm (1997)
Snow White: A Tale of Terror (1997)
Galaxy Quest (1999)
Heartbreakers (2001)
The Guys (2002) Holes (2003)
Imaginary Heroes (2004)
The Village (2004) Snowcake (2006)
The TV Set (2006) Infamous (2006)
The Girl in the Park (2007)
Be Kind Rewind (2008)
Vantage Point (2008)
Baby Mama (2008)

Clifton **Webb**
5ft 11in
(WEBB PARMALEE HOLLENBECK)

Born: **November 19, 1889**
Marion County, Indiana, USA
Died: **October 13, 1966**

Clifton was the son of Jacob Hollenbeck, and his wife, Mabelle. His parents were a disparate pair, Jacob hated the theater. Mabelle loved it, and used to take "Little Webb", as she called Clifton, to see plays on a regular basis. When he was seven, he appeared with the New York Children's Theater at Carnegie Hall. Mabelle encouraged him to learn to paint and he studied voice with the French baritone, Victor Maurel. He joined the Aborn Opera Company in Boston and appeared in their production of the operetta, "Mignon". By 1913, Clifton was a professional ballroom dancer and made his Broadway debut in "The Purple Road". He made his film debut in 1917 – as a dancer, in the fund raiser, *National Red Cross Pageant.* His first five movies were of little consequence but throughout the 1920s, he starred in several musicals and was a big star. Other than a short comedy, made in 1930, the first time his voice was heard on screen was in the classic film-noir, *Laura.* Clifton was fifty-five, but it didn't stop him from being nominated for three Oscars - for *Laura, The Razor's Edge* and *Sitting Pretty.* Clifton, who was privately gay, lived with his mother until she died at the age of ninety-one. His final movie – *Satan Never Sleeps,* in 1962, was below par. Clifton became a recluse until his death from a heart attack, at his home in Beverly Hills.

Laura (1944)
The Dark Corner (1946)
The Razor's Edge (1946)
Sitting Pretty (1948)
Mr. Belvedere Goes to College (1949)
Cheaper by the Dozen (1950)
Mr. Belvedere Rings the Bell (1951)
Dreamboat (1952) Titanic (1953)
Mister Scoutmaster (1953)
Three Coins in the Fountain (1954)
Woman's World (1954)
The Man Who Never Was (1956)
The Remarkable
Mr. Pennypacker (1959)
Holiday for Lovers (1959)

Jack **Webb**
5ft 10in
(JOHN RANDOLPH WEBB)

Born: **April 2, 1920**
Santa Monica, California, USA
Died: **December 23, 1982**

Jack was the son of a Jewish father, who left home before he was born. His Roman Catholic mother raised him as a Catholic in the poor Bunker Hill district of Los Angeles. From the age of six, he suffered from acute asthma. In his mother's rooming house, he was introduced to jazz via records owned by an ex-jazzman tenant. Jack was educated at Belmont High School and in 1932, made his film debut with an uncredited part in *Three On a Match.* Five years later, he played 'The Prisoner', in a television drama, 'Capital Punishment'. During World War II, he served on a B-26 Marauder in the United States Army Air Force. In 1945, he settled in San Francisco, where, a year later, he hosted 'The Jack Webb Show'. He married the singer/actress, Julie London, in 1947 and they were regularly seen together in Los Angeles jazz clubs. Jack's first significant film role was in *He Walked by Night.* In 1949, he began co-starring with Raymond Burr, in the radio drama series, 'Pat Novak for Hire'. Although he would contribute greatly to successful movies such as *The Men* and *Pete Kelly's Blues,* it was his television role, as Sergeant Joe Friday, in 'Dragnet', which made him a star. It ran for eight seasons from 1951, and during that time, he brought it to the big screen. In the late 1960s, he revived the series and was only seen on TV until he retired from acting in 1978. Jack died in West Hollywood, from a heart attack with his fourth wife, Opal, by his side.

He Walked by Night (1948)
The Men (1950)
Sunset Blvd. (1950)
Dark City (1950)
Halls of Montezuma (1950)
You're in the Navy Now (1951)
Appointment with Danger (1951)
Dragnet (1954)
Pete Kelly's Blues (1955)
The Drill Instructor (1957)
The Last Time
I Saw Archie (1961)

Johnny **Weissmuller**
6ft 3in
(JANOS WEISSMULLER)

Born: **June 2, 1904**
Freidorf, Banat, Austro-Hungary
Died: **January 20, 1984**

Johnny's parents were Peter and Elisabeth Weissmüller a poor couple who, in 1905, took their son to America to seek a better life. They settled in Windber, Pennsylvania, where Peter worked as a miner. In view of what happened later, it is surprising to learn that Johnny was struck down by polio when he was nine. He later took up swimming to combat the effects of the disease and the rest is history. His family moved to Chicago and Johnny was soon the star of the YMCA swimming team. His parents split up, but his life got better and better. After leaving school, he was seen by a coach at the Illinois Athletic Club and in 1921, he won the National Swimming Championships. Three gold medals at the 1924 Olympics in Paris, were followed by two more, in Amsterdam, four years later. After working as a swimwear model, he made his screen debut, in *Glorifying the American Girl,* in 1929. Two years later, a visit to Hollywood coincided with the actor who had been cast to play the title-role in *Tarzan the Ape Man,* falling ill. Johnny was hired after a screen test and became a sensation on his film debut. He never did much else, but he was certainly the best Tarzan in screen history. A charming guy, women loved him. His six wives included the "Mexican-Spitfire", Lupe Velez. Johnny retired from films in 1955, to run a small business in Fort Lauderdale. After suffering a series of strokes, Johnny died in Acapulco, Mexico, and is buried there.

Tarzan the Ape Man (1932)
Tarzan and His Mate (1934)
Tarzan Escapes (1936)
Tarzan Finds a Son! (1939)
Tarzan's Secret
Treasure (1941) Tarzan's
New York Adventure (1942)
Tarzan Triumphs (1943)
Tarzan's Desert Mystery (1943)
Tarzan and the Amazons (1945)
Swamp Fire (1946)
Jungle Jim (1948)
Devil Goddess (1955)

Rachel **Weisz**
5ft 7in
(RACHEL HANNAH WEISZ)

Born: **March 7, 1971**
London, England

Rachel first saw the light of day in London's City of Westminster – a stone's throw away from Big Ben. Her father, George Weisz, is a Hungarian-born Jew, who is an inventor. Her mother, Edith, was from Vienna. She started out as a teacher and later, became a psychotherapist. Her sister, Minny, grew up to be an artist. As the family were wealthy, they were able to send Rachel to private schools – firstly Benenden, in Kent, and finally to St.Paul's Girls' School, in London. She went on to graduate from Trinity Hall, Cambridge, with a 2:1 in English. At university, Rachel acted in several student stage productions and was also a founding member of the drama group known as "Cambridge Talking Tongues" – which won a Guardian Award at the Edinburgh Festival. She began her acting career in 1993, with a starring role in the television drama, 'Dirty Something'. It was followed by other small-screen work and, in 1995, her movie debut, in *Death Machine*. She progressed quickly to more demanding roles and, after several nominations, she was rewarded with a Best Supporting Actress Oscar and a Golden Globe, for the exceptional film, *The Constant Gardener*.

Stealing Beauty (1996)
Chain Reaction (1996)
Swept from the Sea (1997)
The Land Girls (1998)
I Want You (1998)
The Mummy (1999)
This Is Not an Exit: The Fictional World of Bret Easton Ellis (2000)
Beautiful Creatures (2000)
Enemy at the Gates (2001)
The Mummy Returns (2001)
About a Boy (2002)
The Shape of Things (2003)
Confidence (2003)
Runaway Judge (2003)
Constantine (2005)
The Constant Gardener (2005)
The Fountain (2006)
Definitely, Maybe (2008)
The Brothers Bloom (2008)

Raquel **Welch**
5ft 6in
(JO RAQUEL TEJADA)

Born: **September 5, 1940**
Chicago, Illinois, USA

Raquel was the eldest of three children born to a Bolivian immigrant, Armando Tejada, and his wife, Josephine – who was Irish-American. In 1940, the family settled in La Jolla, California, where little Raquel attended junior school and was first sent to dancing lessons. She was a beautiful teenager during her years at La Jolla High School – winning several beauty pageant titles including "Miss La Jolla" and "Miss San Diego". On a theater arts scholarship, she went to San Diego State College and in 1959, married her first husband, her high school sweetheart, Jim Welch. She spent the next few years raising their two children. Raquel worked as a weather girl on a local TV station and then split with her husband and moved to Dallas, where she did a bit of modeling and worked as a barmaid. In 1964, she went to Los Angeles and started getting work in TV shows and bit parts in movies – making her debut, as a call girl, in that year's *A House Is Not a Home*. Her big break came when she starred in *One Million Years B.C.* – which made her one of the iconic sex symbols of the 1960s. Aside from film work, in 1970, she starred with Tom Jones in her own musical spectacular, 'Raquel!' In 1984, she published her "Total Health and Fitness Program". She is separated from her fourth husband, Richard Palmer. Raquel's daughter, Tahnee, is an actress.

Le Fate (1966)
Fantastic Voyage (1966)
One Million Years B.C. (1966)
Fathom (1967)
Bedazzled (1967)
Bandolero! (1968)
Lady in Cement (1968)
100 Rifles (1969)
The Magic Christian (1969)
Hannie Caulder (1971)
The Last of Sheila (1973)
The Three Musketeers (1973)
Mother, Jugs & Speed (1976)
Crossed Swords (1977)
L'Animal (1977) **Tortilla Soup** (2001)
Legally Blonde (2001)

Tuesday **Weld**
5ft 4in
(SUSAN KER WELD)

Born: **August 27, 1943**
New York City, New York, USA

Tuesday was the daughter of Lathrop Motley Weld, and his fourth wife, Yosene – who was the daughter of Life magazine illustrator, William Balfour Ker. Tuesday had an older sister, Sarah, and a brother, David. When her husband died, when Tuesday was four, Yosene was under great financial pressure and put her little girl to work, as a child model. When she was twelve, she made her first appearance on television and had a bit role in Alfred Hitchcock's *The Wrong Man*. The pressure on the youngster to be the bread-winner for her family resulted in a nervous breakdown and alcohol abuse. Even so, her looks got her plenty of movie work, including the teen film, *Rock, Rock, Rock*. She left home when she was sixteen, and bought her own house. After attending the Hollywood Professional School, her career took off in the 1960s with a good role in one of Elvis' best films, *Wild in the Country*, and romance with "The King" off screen. She got even better as she matured. She was nominated for a Best Supporting Actress Oscar, for *Looking for Mr. Goodbar*, and for a BAFTA in the same category, for *Once Upon a Time in America*. Her three ex-husbands include Dudley Moore and the classical violinist, Pinchas Zukerman.

Rally 'Round the Flag, Boys! (1958)
The Five Pennies (1959)
Because They're Young (1960)
High Time (1960) **Return to Peyton Place** (1961) **Wild in the Country** (1961)
Bachelor Flat (1962) **Soldier in the Rain** (1963) **The Cincinnati Kid** (1965)
Lord Love a Duck (1966)
Pretty Poison (1968)
I Walk the Line (1970)
Play It As It Lays (1972)
Looking for Mr. Goodbar (1977)
Who'll Stop the Rain (1978)
Serial (1980) **Thief** (1981)
Author! Author! (1982)
Once Upon a Time in America (1984)
Heartbreak Hotel (1988)
Falling Down (1993)

Peter **Weller**
6ft
(PETER FREDERICK WELLER)

Born: **June 24, 1947**
Stevens Point, Wisconsin, USA

Pete's father, Frederick Weller, served in the United States Army as a helicopter pilot. Pete's mother, Dorothy, took care of their home. Due to his father's work, he spent several of his early years in Germany and other parts of the world. When the family finally settled in Texas, he attended Alamo Heights High School, in San Antonio and later, Texas State University, from where he graduated with a BA in Theater. He was gifted musically; a great fan of Miles Davis – while at university, he played trumpet in a campus band. He later performed in a jazz combo with Jeff Goldblum, in both a film, *The Adventures of Buckaroo Banzai,* and in Los Angeles clubs. Intent on an acting career, Pete went to New York City, where he studied at the American Academy of Dramatic Arts. Pete made his Broadway debut just two weeks after graduating, as David, in "Sticks and Bones". He made his film debut in *Butch and Sundance: The Early Days* and his first big impact, in *RoboCop,* for which he was nominated for a Saturn Award. In 1993, when he directed and acted in a short TV film, called 'Partners', he was nominated for an Oscar. Since 2006, Pete has been married to the actress, Shari Stowe.

Butch and Sundance:
The Early Days (1979)
Just Tell Me What
You Want (1980)
Shoot the Moon (1982)
Of Unknown Origin (1983)
The Adventures of
Buckaroo Banzai (1984)
Firstborn (1984)
A Killing Affair (1986)
RoboCop (1987)
Naked Lunch (1991)
Beyond the Clouds (1995)
Screamers (1995)
Mighty Aphrodite (1995)
Shadow Hours (2000)
Ivansxtc (2000)
The Hard Easy (2005)
Man of God (2005)

Orson **Welles**
6ft 1½in
(GEORGE ORSON WELLES)

Born: **May 6, 1915**
Kenosha, Wisconsin, USA
Died: **October 10, 1985**

The son of a successful inventor, Richard Head Welles, and his wife, Beatrice, who was a concert pianist and a suffragette, Orson was born into wealth and power. Much of that disappeared when his father abandoned his career to alcohol in 1919, and left home and in 1926, his mother died of jaundice. Orson was educated at the Todd School for Boys, in Woodstock, Illinois. The very year Orson graduated, his father died and with a small inheritance, the sixteen-year-old traveled to Europe. He claimed he was a Broadway star when he arrived at the Gate Theater, in Dublin. His story was accepted and he made his stage debut there, in "Jew Suss". He was soon acting on the New York stage. When he was nineteen, he married the socialite, Virginia Nicholson, and had a son. He set up his Mercury Theater Company and, in 1938, he achieved notoriety with a chilling broadcast of "The War of the Worlds". He then made the landmark movie, *Citizen Kane.* It brought him nominations as Best Actor and Director. He shared the screenplay Oscar with his co-writer, Herman Mankiewicz. Orson's three wives included Rita Hayworth. He was a living legend until dying of a heart attack, in Hollywood.

Citizen Kane (1941) **Journey Into**
Fear (1943) **Jane Eyre** (1944)
Tomorrow Is Forever (1946)
The Stranger (1946) **The Lady from**
Shanghai (1947) **Macbeth** (1948)
Black Magic (1949) **The Third**
Man (1949) **Prince of Foxes** (1949)
The Black Rose (1950) **The Tragedy of**
Othello: The Moor of Venice (1952)
Trent's Last Case (1952)
Three Cases of Murder (1955)
Mr. Arkadin (1955) **Moby Dick** (1956)
Man in the Shadow (1957) **The Long,**
Hot Summer (1958) **Touch of Evil** (1958)
Compulsion (1959) **The Trial** (1962)
A Man for All Seasons (1966)
I'll Never Forget What'sisname (1967)
The Immortal Story (1968)
Waterloo (1970)

Oscar **Werner**
5ft 9in
(OSKAR JOSEF BSCHLIESSMAYER)

Born: **November 13, 1922**
Vienna, Austria
Died: **October 23, 1984**

Oscar's parents got divorced when he was a young boy and he was raised by his mother. During his junior school years, he regularly performed in plays. He dropped out of high school to become the youngest ever actor to be taken on by the Burgtheater, in Vienna. By his late teens, he was able to gain experience in movie-acting through his uncle's contacts in the German film industry. His film debut, as Oskar Werner, in 1938, was in the German/Swedish co-production, titled *Geld fällt vom Himmel,* starring Signe Hasso. There were two more roles before Germany started World War II, and Oscar, who was a pacifist, was faced with a huge dilemma. He was eventually drafted into the German Army, where he feigned incompetence in order to avoid military action. He endangered himself further by marrying a half-Jewish actress, called Elisabeth Kallina. When their daughter was born, in 1944, Oscar and his family hid in a village in the Vienna Woods. After the war, he went back to the stage until making his first credited film appearance in 1948, in the German version of *Angel with the Trumpet.* Oscar's second wife, Anne, was the daughter of French actress, Annabella. He burst onto the film scene several years later, in *Jules et Jim* and was nominated for a Best Actor Oscar, for *Ship of Fools.* He died of a heart attack in Germany, but was buried in Liechtenstein.

Eroica (1949) **The Angel with the**
Trumpet (1950) **The Wonder Kid** (1951)
Decision Before Dawn (1951)
The Last Ten Days (1955)
Spionage (1955) **Mozart** (1955)
Lola Montès (1955)
Jules et Jim (1962)
Ship of Fools (1965)
The Spy Who Came in
from the Cold (1965)
Fahrenheit 451 (1966)
Interlude (1968)
The Shoes of the Fisherman (1968)
Voyage of the Damned (1976)

Mae West
5ft 1in
(MARY JANE WEST)

Born: **August 17, 1893**
Woodhaven, New York, USA
Died: **November 22, 1980**

Mae was the daughter of a prizefighter, "Battlin' Jack West", and his wife, Matilda – known as "Tillie" – who was from a German Jewish background. Mae was brought up as a Catholic. She had a younger brother and sister. She was five when she started singing at church socials. At fourteen, she began performing professionally, with the Hal Clarendon Stock Company. From 1911 until 1942, she was married to the only husband among her many lovers – Frank Wallace. From early in her career, Mae wore six-inch platform shoes which increased her height and gave her that unique walk. But it was her generous bosom that attracted male audiences. She acted in several plays she wrote herself – most of them had a risqué content – including her first success on Broadway, which she aptly titled "Sex". In 1927, she was prosecuted and sentenced to ten days for "corrupting the morals of youth". In 1932, she was given a contract by Paramount, and made her film debut with George Raft, in *Night After Night*. Mae's films were said to have saved the ailing studio from bankruptcy. Her next picture, *She Done Him Wrong,* with Cary Grant, made her a star. She was also on top form in the follow-up with Grant, *I'm No Angel,* and appeared with success opposite the great W.C. Fields, in *My Little Chickadee.* Mae's 1943 film, *The Heat's On,* was mediocre, and she didn't reappear on the screen until 1970, in *Myra Breckinridge.* Her final movie, *Sextette,* in 1978, was embarrassing. Mae died in Hollywood, from complications following a series of strokes.

Night After Night (1932)
She Done Him Wrong (1933)
I'm No Angel (1933)
Belle of the Nineties (1934)
Goin' to Town (1935)
Klondike Annie (1936)
Go West Young Man (1936)
Every Day's a Holiday (1937)
My Little Chickadee (1940)

Joanne Whalley
5ft 4in
(JOANNE WHALLEY)

Born: **August 25, 1964**
Salford, Manchester, England

Joanne grew up in the Lancashire town of Stockport. She began performing in school plays when she was a little girl and, with enthusiastic encouragement from her parents, she began getting work on television – beginning, in 1974, with a small role in the popular British series, 'Coronation Street'. When she was twelve, Joanne appeared in six episodes of 'Emmerdale Farm'. After leaving school, she continued on the small screen until making her film debut, with a cameo role as one of "Pink Floyd's" groupies, in Alan Parker's *The Wall.* Her first featured film role was in the biographical drama about Ruth Ellis – the last woman to be executed in Britain – *Dance with a Stranger.* In 1986, she was nominated for a BAFTA TV Award, as Best Actress, in 'Edge of Darkness'. Two years later, Joanna starred opposite Val Kilmer, in *Willow.* She married him and they had a son named Jack, and a daughter named Mercedes. In 1991, People magazine voted her one of the "50 Most Beautiful People in the World". For fourteen years, (the pair were divorced in 1996) she was known professionally as Joanne Whalley-Kilmer. Since *The Man Who Knew Too Little,* she uses her original name. She has stayed single since her marriage ended. On the career front, Joanne's recent movies have been disappointing.

Dance with a Stranger (1985)
No Surrender (1985)
The Good Father (1985)
Willow (1988)
To Kill a Priest (1988)
Scandal (1989)
Kill Me Again (1989)
The Big Man (1990)
Shattered (1991)
Storyville (1992)
The Secret Rapture (1993)
Trial by Jury (1994)
**The Man Who Knew
Too Little** (1997)
A Texas Funeral (1999)
The Guilty (2000)
Before You Go (2002)

Billie Whitelaw
5ft 2in
(BILLIE HONOR WHITELAW)

Born: **June 6, 1932**
Coventry, Warwickshire, England

Billie was the daughter of Gerry and Frances Whitelaw. She was raised in a poor family, in a disadvantaged area of Coventry. In 1942 she was evacuated to Liverpool following the heavy bombing of Coventry. She was bright enough to earn a place at Thornton Grammar School, in Bradford, Yorkshire. Around that time, she began performing as a child actor on the radio. After leaving school, she appeared in repertory in Leeds, and then went to London to study acting at the famous Royal Academy of Dramatic Art. In 1950 Billie made her London stage debut, and two years later, she appeared as Martha in the TV serial, 'The Secret Garden'. Her film debut was in 1953, when she played a small role as a waitress, in *The Fake.* was the start of several hardly-noticed parts in films, and up until 1960, Billie was best known for her stage and television work. After that, she was recognized as a film actress. BAFTA nominations started with *Hell Is a City.* She was named Best Supporting Actress for *Charlie Bubbles* and *Twisted Nerve.* Billie's two husbands were Peter Vaughan and Robert Muller.

The Flesh and the Fiends (1960)
Hell Is a City (1960) **Make Mine
Mink** (1960) **Mr. Topaze** (1961)
The Devil's Agent (1962)
The Comedy Man (1964)
Charlie Bubbles (1967)
Twisted Nerve (1968)
The Adding Machine (1969)
**Start the Revolution
Without Me** (1970)
Leo the Last (1970) **Gumshoe** (1971)
Eagle in a Cage (1972)
Frenzy (1972) **Night Watch** (1973)
The Omen (1976)
Leopard in the Snow (1978)
**An Unsuitable Job for a
Woman** (1982) **The Chain** (1984)
Maurice (1987) **The Dressmaker** (1988)
The Krays (1990) **Skallagrigg** (1994)
Deadly Advice (1994)
The Lost Son (1999) **Quills** (2002)
Hot Fuzz (2007)

Stuart **Whitman**
6ft
(STUART MAXWELL WHITMAN)

Born: **February 1, 1928**
San Francisco, California, USA

Stuart, who was the son of a realtor and his wife, once claimed to have attended twenty-six different schools – none of them famous. There wasn't too much to boast about on the academic side, but he did excel at football and boxing. In 1945, he began three years service in the U.S. Army Engineers. During that time, he fought, and won 32 bouts as a light-heavyweight. On his return to civilian life he spent two years at the Los Angeles City College, where he first became interested in acting. He then studied at the Los Angeles Academy of Dramatic Art, and fine-tuned his skills with Ben Bard and Michael Chekhov. Following a small role in *When World's Collide,* in 1951, he got uncredited work on TV and in movies. In 1952, Stuart began a fourteen-year marriage to Patricia LaLonde. They had four children. He built a career as a reliable supporting actor and eventually, a star. He reached his peak in the early 1960s, when he was nominated for a Best Actor Oscar, for *The Mark,* and featured in hit movies such as *Those Magnificent Men in Their Flying Machines* and *Sands of the Kalahari.* His last movie was in 1998.

Seven Men from Now (1956)
Johnny Trouble (1957) Hell Bound (1957)
Ten North Frederick (1958) The Decks
Ran Red (1958) The Sound and the
Fury (1959) These Thousand
Hills (1959) The Story of Ruth (1960)
Murder, Inc. (1960)
The Fiercest Heart (1961)
The Mark (1961)
The Comancheros (1961)
Convict 4 (1962) The Day and the
Hour (1963) Shock Treatment (1964)
Rio Conchos (1964)
Signpost to Murder (1964)
Those Magnificent Men in Their
Flying Machines (1965)
Sands of the Kalahari (1965)
An American Dream (1966)
Crazy Mama (1975) Eaten Alive (1977)
Delta Fox (1979)
Second Chances (1998)

James **Whitmore**
5ft 10in
(JAMES ALLEN WHITMORE JR.)

Born: **October 1, 1921**
White Plains, New York, USA
Died: **February 6, 2009**

Jim was the son of a park commission official, James Whitmore Sr., and his wife, Florence. Jim graduated from Amherst High School, in Amherst, New York, and later attended Yale University, where he was a member of the secret society, "Skull and Bones". During World War II, Jim served in the United States Marine Corps. Following acting classes, he appeared in a New Hampshire Players stage production of "The Milky Way" during the summer of 1947. It was the year he married Nancy Mygatt. He made his Broadway debut in the hit, "Command Decision". In the film-version, made by MGM that same year, 1948, his part was acted by Van Johnson. It did however, lead to Jim making his film debut, in the Columbia production of *The Undercover Man* – starring Glenn Ford. A distinguished movie career from then on – included a Best Supporting Actor Oscar nomination for *Battleground* – a role which Spencer Tracy turned down. A second nomination was for a Best Actor Oscar, in *Give 'em Hell, Harry!* Jim was still acting into his eighties. He died of lung cancer, at his home in Malibu, California

The Undercover Man (1949)
Battleground (1949)
The Asphalt Jungle (1950)
The Next Voice You Hear (1950)
Shadow in the Sky (1952)
Because You're Mine (1952)
Above and Beyond (1952)
Them! (1954) Battle Cry (1955)
Oklahoma! (1955) The Last
Frontier (1955) Crime in the
Streets (1956) The Eddy Duchin
Story (1956) The Restless Years (1958)
Who Was That Lady? (1960)
Nobody's Perfect (1968)
Planet of the Apes (1968)
The Split (1968) Tora! Tora! Tora! (1970)
Chato's Land (1972)
Where the Red Fern Grows (1974)
Give 'Em Hell, Harry! (1975) Nuts (1987)
The Shawshank Redemption (1994)
The Majestic (2001)

Forest **Whitaker**
6ft 2in
(FOREST STEVEN WHITAKER)

Born: **July 15, 1961**
Longview, Texas, USA

Forest's father, Forest Whitaker, Jr., was the son of a novelist. When their son was four, he and his wife, Laura, decided to move to Los Angeles, because of the racism they had to endure in Texas. They settled in Carson and in the new environment, he thrived as an insurance salesman and his wife was able to put herself through college – earning two Master degrees while raising Forest, his older sister and two younger brothers. Forest was educated at Palisades High School, where he was an all-league defensive tackle, in a team which included future NFL player, Jay Schroeder. After voice training he performed in musicals. In 1979, he went to Cal Poly, Pomona, on a football scholarship, but was sidelined due to an injury. Next was the music conservatory at USC, followed by drama studies at Berkeley. In 1982, he made his TV debut in an episode of 'Making the Grade'. His movie debut (as a footballer) was in that year's *Fast Times at Ridgemont High*. He has since built up a wealth of good work – winning the Best Actor Award at Cannes for his portrayal of jazz legend, Charlie Parker, in *Bird*. He topped that when he played Idi Amin, in *The Last King of Scotland* and won a Best Actor Oscar. His wife, Keisha, is a former model. They've two daughters.

Platoon (1986) Stakeout (1987)
Good Morning, Vietnam (1987)
Bloodsport (1988) Bird (1988) Johnny
Handsome (1989) Downtown (1990)
A Rage in Harlem (1991) The Crying
Game (1992) Consenting Adults (1992)
Body Snatchers (1993) Blown
Away (1994) Jason's Lyric (1994)
Smoke (1995) Species (1995)
Phenomenon (1996) Green
Dragon (2001) Phone Booth (2002)
Mary (2005) A Little Trip to
Heaven (2005) American Gun (2005)
The Last King of Scotland (2006)
The Air I Breathe (2007) The Great
Debaters (2007) Vantage Point (2008)
Street Kings (2008)
Winged Creatures (2008)

Richard **Widmark**
5ft 10in
(RICHARD WIDMARK)

Born: **December 26, 1914**
Sunrise, Minnesota, USA
Died: **March 24, 2008**

The son of a salesman, young Richard was a brilliant student. Following graduation from Princeton High School, in Illinois, he studied Speech & Political Science at Lake Forest College. He remained at the college after graduating – making a living by teaching Speech and Dramatics. He began his career as an actor in New York, in 1938, on the radio show 'Aunt Jenny's Real Life Stories'. In 1942, Richard married his first wife, Jean. He then acted in summer stock productions before making his Broadway debut, in 1943, in "Kiss and Tell". Due to a perforated eardrum, he was unable to join the military during World War II. He was acting on stage in Chicago when he was spotted by a 20th Century Fox talent scout and given a seven-year contract. His debut, in *Kiss of Death,* was a great way to begin – earning him a Best Supporting Actor Oscar nomination. That quality was maintained and he never gave anything other than his best in any of his sixty movies. Richard died in Roxbury, Connecticut, following a fall. His second wife, Susan, was by his side.

Kiss of Death (1947) **The Street with No Name** (1948) **Road House** (1948) **Yellow Sky** (1948) **Down to the Sea in Ships** (1949) **Night and the City** (1950) **Panic in the Streets** (1950) **No Way Out** (1950) **Halls of Montezuma** (1950) **Red Skies of Montana** (1952) **Don't Bother to Knock** (1952) **Pickup on South Street** (1953) **Take the High Ground** (1953) **Garden of Evil** (1954) **Broken Lance** (1954) **The Cobweb** (1955) **Backlash** (1956) **The Last Wagon** (1956) **The Trap** (1959) **Warlock** (1959) **The Alamo** (1960) **Judgement at Nuremburg** (1961) **How the West Was Won** (1962) **Cheyenne Autumn** (1964) **The Bedford Incident** (1965) **Madigan** (1968) **Death of a Gunfighter** (1969) **Murder on the Orient Express** (1974) **Twilight's Last Gleaming** (1977) **Rollercoaster** (1977) **Coma** (1978) **Against All Odds** (1984)

Diane **Wiest**
5ft 5in
(DIANE WIEST)

Born: **March 28, 1948**
Kansas City, Missouri, USA

Diane's father was dean of a college, who met her Scottish-born mother in Algiers. They also had two sons. Diane was keen on dancing during her childhood, but in her teens she took more interest in the theater – after appearing in high school plays. She studied the subject at the University of Maryland at Baltimore, but left in her third term in order to go on tour with a troupe which was specializing in Shakespeare plays. She returned to obtain a degree in Arts and Sciences. Diane acted in many stage productions before making her Broadway debut in 1971, in "Solitaire/Double Solitaire". She then worked with the Arena Stage, in Washington D.C. and later toured with them to the USSR. In 1975, Diane made her television debut, in 'Zalmen: or, The Madness of God' and five years later, made her film debut, with a small role in *It's My Turn.* She progressed to bigger parts and for *Hannah and Her Sisters,* won a Best Supporting Actress Oscar. There were two more nominations in the same category – for *Parenthood,* and *Bullets Over Broadway* – which won her another Oscar. Diane also won a Funniest Supporting Actress American Comedy Award, for *The Birdcage.* She's never married, but has two adopted children.

I'm Dancing as Fast as I Can (1982) **Independence Day** (1983) **Footloose** (1984) **Falling in Love** (1984) **Hannah and Her Sisters** (1986) **The Lost Boys** (1987) **September** (1987) **Parenthood** (1989) **Edward Scissorhands** (1990) **Little Man Tate** (1991) **Bullets over Broadway** (1994) **The Birdcage** (1996) **The Horse Whisperer** (1998) **Not Afraid, Not Afraid** (2001) **I Am Sam** (2001) **Merci Docteur Rey** (2002) **A Guide to recognizing Your Saints** (2006) **Dedication** (2007) **Dan in Real Life** (2007) **Synecdoche, New York** (2008) **Passengers** (2008)

Henry **Wilcoxon**
6ft 4in
(HARRY FREDERICK WILCOXON)

Born: **September 8, 1905**
Roseau, Dominica, British West Indies
Died: **March 6, 1984**

Henry's father, Robert Wilcoxon, was the manager of the Colonial Bank in Jamaica. His mother, Lurleene, had been a stage actress. She died when he was young and he had a dreadful childhood when he and his brother were sent to foster homes. Henry began his working life at the age of fourteen, as a pearl and salvage diver. He was educated in Jamaica, before being shipped off to boarding school at Ashford in Kent, England. After that Henry stayed in England, and took a job with a Bond Street tailor in London. He was far too good looking to spend his life cutting suits, so after some acting lessons, he made his London West End theater debut, in 1927, in "The Hundredth Chance". He joined the Birmingham Repertory and a few years of stage roles led to his film debut, in 1931, in *The Perfect Lady.* Paramount invited him for a screen test which impressed Cecil B. DeMille enough to star him in his epic film, *Cleopatra,* opposite Claudette Colbert. He was briefly married in 1936, but at the end of 1938, had a second wife, the actress Joan Woodbury. During World War II he served with the U.S. Coastguard. He was a supporting actor after the war and became a producer. He and Joan had three daughters and were together until his death from cancer, in Los Angeles.

Cleopatra (1934) **The Crusades** (1935) **The Last of the Mohicans** (1936) **The President's Mystery** (1936) **Souls at Sea** (1937) **If I Were King** (1938) **Mysterious Mr. Moto** (1938) **Chasing Danger** (1939) **Tarzan Finds a Son!** (1939) **That Hamilton Woman** (1941) **The Corsican Brothers** (1941) **The Man Who Wouldn't Die** (1942) **Mrs. Miniver** (1942) **Unconquered** (1947) **A Connecticut Yankee in King Arthur's Court** (1949) **Samson and Delilah** (1949) **The Greatest Show on Earth** (1952) **Scaramouche** (1952) **The War Lord** (1965) **Man in the Wilderness** (1971) **Caddyshack** (1980)

Cornel **Wilde**
6ft 1in
(CORNELIUS LOUIS WILDE)

Born: **October 13, 1915**
Budapest, Hungary
Died: **October 16, 1989**

The son of Hungarian Jewish immigrants, Béla Weisz and Renée Vojtech, Cornel spoke several languages and graduated from Townsend Harris High School, at fourteen. At City College of New York he completed the four-year course in three. Cornel qualified as a fencer for the United States team, ahead of the Berlin Olympics in 1936. He declined, in favor of accepting his first movie role, in a short film called *The Rhythm Party.* In 1937, he married his first wife, Patricia and they had a daughter. There were more uncredited roles before Cornel's skills at fencing were used to teach Laurence Olivier, for his Broadway production of "Romeo and Juliet" in 1940. Cornel's role in the play – as Tybalt, served as a launching pad for his Hollywood career, beginning with *High Sierra*. He was signed by 20th Century Fox and made his first appearance for them in 1941, in *The Perfect Snob*. It was a mutually beneficial partnership. He was nominated for a Best Actor Oscar, for *A Song to Remember* and did well for them in *Leave Her to Heaven, Forever Amber,* and *Roadhouse*. In 1951, he married Jean Wallace – acting with her in his films *Storm Fear* and *Beach Red*. Cornel died of leukemia, in Los Angeles.

High Sierra (1941) **Manila Calling** (1942)
Life Begins at Eight-Thirty (1942)
A Song to Remember (1945)
A Thousand and One Nights (1945)
Leave Her to Heaven (1945)
Centennial Summer (1946)
The Homestretch (1947)
Forever Amber (1947) **It Had to Be You** (1947) **The Walls of Jericho** (1948)
Roadhouse (1948) **Shockproof** (1949)
Two Flags West (1950) **The Greatest Show on Earth** (1952) **At Sword's Point** (1952) **Treasure of the Golden Condor** (1953) **Woman's World** (1954)
The Big Combo (1955) **The Scarlet Coat** (1955) **Storm Fear** (1955)
Beyond Mombasa (1956)
The Naked Prey (1966)
Beach Red (1967) **The Comic** (1969)

Gene **Wilder**
5ft 10½in
(JEROME SILBERMAN)

Born: **June 11, 1933**
Milwaukee, Wisconsin, USA

Gene was the son of a Russian-born Jewish immigrant, William Silberman, and his Chicago-born wife, Jeanne. When his mother fell ill with rheumatic fever, the eight-year-old was urged by the doctor to "make her laugh" which he did. Gene later endured racial and physical abuse at the Black-Foxe Military School, in Hollywood. After leaving there at fifteen, he performed at a local theater with a supporting role in a production of "Romeo and Juliet". He studied Communications and Theater Arts at the University of Iowa. In 1955, Gene went to England. to the Bristol Old Vic Theater School, and a year later, was a student at Herbert Berghof's Studio, in New York. He served with the U.S. Army Medical Corps until 1958, and lost his mother to ovarian cancer during that time. He continued with Berghof – acting and serving as a fencing choreographer in his British production of "Twelfth Night". Gene made his TV debut in 1962, in an episode of 'The Defenders' and his film debut five years later, in *Bonnie and Clyde*. It was his teaming with Mel Brooks in *The Producers* which launched his film career and earned an Oscar nomination, as Best Supporting Actor. He was nominated as writer for his screenplay, for *Young Frankenstein*. Married four times – his current wife, Karen, has been with him since 1991. In 2000, Gene made a full recovery from cancer.

Bonnie and Clyde (1967)
The Producers (1968)
Start the Revolution Without Me (1970) **Fun Loving** (1970)
Willy Wonka & the Chocolate Factory (1971)
Everything You Always Wanted to Know About Sex (1972)
Blazing Saddles (1974)
The Little Prince (1974)
Young Frankenstein (1974)
Sherlock Holmes' Smarter Brother (1975) **Silver Streak** (1976)
The Frisco Kid (1979) **Stir Crazy** (1980)
The Woman in Red (1984)
See No Evil, Hear No Evil (1989)

Michael **Wilding**
5ft 9in
(MICHAEL CHARLES GAUNTLETT WILDING)

Born: **July 23, 1912**
Westcliff-on-Sea, Essex, England
Died: **July 8, 1979**

Mike was raised in a creative family environment and after leaving school at fifteen he took art classes, before joining a London advertising agency. His interest in the theater led to several roles in amateur stage productions. His fascination with the cinema influenced his decision to join the art department of Gaumont British Pictures, located in Shepherd's Bush, in West London. Mike began getting bit parts in the studio's films – starting with the 1933 crime drama, *Channel Crossing*. He continued to work as a backroom boy until, six years later, he caught the eye of a producer and was given his first featured role, at Ealing Studios, in *There Ain't No Justice*. It was a slow road to stardom but along the way he married his first wife, Kay Young, and supported Tommy Trinder, in the comedy, *Sailors Three*. Due to health problems, Mike didn't serve his country and was able to work non-stop during World War II. In 1946 he struck up a friendship with Herbert Wilcox and his film star wife, Anna Neagle. They co-starred in six lightweight films (the best of them is *Spring in Park Lane)* which caught the imagination of the British public. Mike was most famous for marrying Elizabeth Taylor with whom he had two children. He was a pal of 'the Burtons', and was Margaret Leighton's husband until her sad lingering death in 1976. Mike fell to his death down a flight of stairs, at his home in Chichester, during an epileptic seizure.

The Remarkable Mr. Kipps (1941)
In Which We Serve (1942) **Piccadilly Incident** (1946) **The Courtneys of Curzon Street** (1947) **An Ideal Husband** (1947)
Spring in Park Lane (1948)
Stage Fright (1950) **The Lady with the Lamp** (1951) **Trent's Last Case** (1952)
The Egyptian (1954) **The Scarlet Coat** (1955) **Danger Within** (1959)
The World of Suzie Wong (1960)
The Best of Enemies (1962)
A Girl Named Tamiko (1962)
Waterloo (1970)

Tom **Wilkinson**
6ft 1in
(THOMAS JEFFREY WILKINSON)

Born: December 12, 1948
Leeds, West Yorkshire, England

Tom's father, Thomas Wilkinson Sr., was a farmer. In 1953 he emigrated to Canada with his family. Tom was in his teens when they all returned to England. His father ran a pub down in Cornwall and Tom went to the University of Kent at Canterbury, where he was an enthusiastic member of the Drama Society. After graduating from Kent with a degree in English and American Literature, Tom began to give serious thought to an acting career. He was soon a student at the Royal Academy of Dramatic Art, in London. In 1976, Tom made his film debut, in *Smuga cienia,* which was directed by the Polish genius, Andrzej Wajda. During the 1980s, he did mostly theater work – winning a London Critics Circle Best Supporting Actor Award in 1986, for "Ghosts", and was Best Actor in 1988, for "An Enemy of the People". Tom married his present wife, Diana, in 1988. They have two children. His status as a top actor in movies culminated with his nominations for a Best Actor Oscar, for *In the Bedroom,* and a Best Supporting Actor Oscar, for *Michael Clayton.*

Paper Mask (1990)
Prince of Jutland (1994) **Priest** (1994)
Sense and Sensibility (1995)
The Ghost and the Darkness (1996)
Smilla's Sense of Snow (1997)
The Full Monty (1997) **Wilde** (1997)
Oscar and Lucinda (1997)
The Governess (1998) **Rush Hour** (1998)
Shakespeare in Love (1998)
The Patriot (2000) **Chain of Fools** (2000)
In the Bedroom (2000) **Another**
Life (2001) **The Importance of Being**
Earnest (2002) **Girl with a Pearl**
Earring (2003) **Piccadilly Jim** (2004)
If Only (2004) **Eternal Sunshine of**
the Spotless Mind (2004) **Stage**
Beauty (2004) **A Good Woman** (2004)
Batman Begins (2005) **The Exorcism**
of Emily Rose (2005) **Separate**
Lies (2005) **Ripley Under Ground** (2005)
The Last Kiss (2006)
Michael Clayton (2007)
RocknRolla (2008)

Billy Dee **Williams**
6ft
(WILLIAM DECEMBER WILLIAMS)

Born: April 6, 1937
New York City, New York, USA

Billy's dad, William December Williams Sr., was a Texan who worked as a janitor. His wife, Loretta, was from Montserrat in the Leeward Islands. Billy and his twin sister, Loretta, were raised in Harlem, by their maternal grandmother. He was a good student at school and at the age of seven, began to realize his dream of becoming an actor, by appearing in a Broadway musical "Firebrand of Florence". Billy trained for the stage at the Harlem Actors' Workshop and won a scholarship to the National Academy of Fine Arts & Design, where he developed his life-long love of painting and went on to sell his work. He graduated from the School of Performing Arts in Manhattan – where his classmate was Diahann Carroll, who would play his wife in a 1980s TV soap, 'Dynasty'. Billy's movie debut, in *The Last Angry Man,* must have appeared to be a one-off. It was five more years before he was seen, in an episode of 'The Defenders' and various TV shows and eleven years, before his next film, *The Out of Towners.* After co-starring with Diana Ross, in *Lady Sings the Blues,* the momentum carried him forward. Billy was nominated for his work in TV's 'Brian's Song' and for the *Star Wars* movies. In 2009, he will celebrate his half-century as a movie actor. Billy has been married three times and had a son called Corey with his first wife, Audrey Sellers. His third wife, Teruko Nakagami, was previously married to the tenor sax jazz giant, Wayne Shorter.

The Last Angry Man (1959)
The Final Comedown (1972)
Lady Sings the Blues (1972)
Hit! (1973)
Scott Joplin (1977)
The Empire Strikes Back (1980)
Nighthawks (1981)
Marvin & Tige (1983)
Return of the Jedi (1983)
Batman (1989)
The Visit (2000)
Undercover Brother (2002)
Fanboys (2008)
iMurders (2008)

Esther **Williams**
5ft 8in
(ESTER JANE WILLIAMS)

Born: August 8, 1921
Los Angeles, California, USA

Esther was the daughter of Louis and Bula Williams. Even at her junior school she was fanatical about swimming, and by her teenage years, had become the National AAU Champion over 100 yards. From 1939-1941, Esther performed at the San Francisco World's Fair with Johnny Weismuller, in Billy Rose's "Aquacade". While working there, she fended off the advances of "Tarzan" by marrying Leonard Kovner, whom she met while studying at the University of Southern California. He lasted four years. Meanwhile, it was the perfect shop window, and Esther was noticed by MGM talent scouts. Although she didn't need a life-belt, her first film appearance was in a short called *Inflation.* Her first featured role was in *Andy Hardy's Double Life.* But it was as a swimmer, in movies starting with *Bathing Beauty,* that propelled Esther to Hollywood stardom. For around ten years, audiences all over the world couldn't get enough of her. She made her last film, *Magic Fountain,* in 1963, and concentrated on running her swimwear business. She had four children from her four marriages. Her husbands included her former co-star, Fernando Lamas, and she met her current spouse, Edward Bell, when she was attending the 1984 Olympic Games, in Los Angeles.

Andy Hardy's
Double Life (1942)
A Guy Named Joe (1943)
Bathing Beauty (1944)
Thrill of Romance (1945)
The Hoodlum Saint (1946)
Easy to Wed (1946)
This Time for Keeps (1947)
On an Island with You (1948)
Take Me Out to
the Ball Game (1949)
Neptune's Daughter (1949)
Pagan Love Song (1950)
Million Dollar Mermaid (1952)
Dangerous When Wet (1953)
Easy to Love (1953)
Jupiter's Darling (1955)
The Unguarded Moment (1956)

JoBeth **Williams**
5ft 7¼in
(MARGARET JOBETH WILLIAMS)

Born: **December 6, 1948**
Houston, Texas, USA

The daughter of an opera singer, Fredric Williams, JoBeth was attracted to the performing arts from an early age. As a bonus, she was kept in beautiful shape by her mother, Frances, who worked as a dietitian. After high school, JoBeth went to Brown University, where she studied to qualify as a child psychologist. Fortunately for her fans, the university, in Providence, was close to the Trinity Theater. JoBeth had soon become hooked on acting and she joined the Trinity Repertory Company. She took acting classes in tandem with voice lessons, which helped her to lose her strong Texas accent. In the 1970s she moved to New York to begin her career. It was actually in Boston where she landed her first TV role, in 1974 – in the childrens' program 'Jabberwocky'. JoBeth made an auspicious start to her film career when she played Phyllis, in *Kramer vs. Kramer*. It was quickly followed by more good roles including her Saturn Award-nominated performance in *Poltergeist,* and a Best Actress Award by Kansas City Film Critics for *American Dreamer.* In 1995, she was Oscar nominated (as director) for Best Short Film, *On Hope.* She was inducted into the Texas Film Hall of Fame in 2006. JoBeth has been married to her husband, director, John Pasquin, since 1982. They have two sons, Nick and Will.

Kramer vs. Kramer (1979)
Stir Crazy (1980)
The Dogs of War (1980)
Poltergeist (1982)
Endangered Species (1982)
The Big Chill (1983) Teachers (1984)
American Dreamer (1984)
Desert Bloom (1986)
Memories of Me (1988)
Welcome Home (1989)
Dutch (1991)
Me, Myself and I (1992)
Wyatt Earp (1994) Just Write (1997)
Little City (1997)
Fever Pitch (2005)
Crazylove (2005)
In the Land of Women (2007)

Michelle **Williams**
5ft 4in
(MICHELLE INGRID WILLIAMS)

Born: **September 9, 1980**
Kalispell, Montana, USA

Michelle was born into comfortable family circumstances; her father, Larry Williams, was a successful trader in stocks and commodities, and is a former Republican candidate for Montana. Her mother, Carla, kept house for three half siblings from her husband's previous marriage as well as raising Michelle and her younger sister, Paige. When she was nine, the family moved to San Diego, California. She attended Santa Fe Christian School, in Solana Beach. In 1993, Michelle made her first appearance on TV, in an episode of 'Baywatch' and a year later, made her film debut, in *Lassie.* When she was sixteen, she proved that she had inherited her father's genes – by winning the Robbins World Cup Trading Championship – she turned $10,000 into $110,000 during the course of one year. She had several good supporting roles during the late 1990s and after co-starring with Kirsten Dunst, in the comedy *Dick,* she was on the road to stardom. Michelle was nominated for a Best Supporting Actress Oscar, for *Brokeback Mountain* and went to live with its young star, Heath Ledger, with whom she had a daughter in 2005. The couple separated less than five months before his death.

Lassie (1994) Species (1995)
A Thousand Acres (1997)
Halloween: H20 (1998) Dick (1999)
But I'm a Cheerleader (1999)
Me Without You (2001)
Prozac Nation (2001)
The United States of
Leland (2003)
The Station Agent (2003)
Imaginary Heroes (2004)
Land of Plenty (2004)
The Baxter (2005)
Brokeback Mountain (2005)
The Hawk Is Dying (2006)
The Hottest State (2006)
I'm Not There (2007)
Incendiary (2008)
Deception (2008)
Wendy and Lucy (2008)
Synedoche, New York (2008)

Robin **Williams**
5ft 8in
(ROBIN MCLAURIM WILLIAMS)

Born: **July 21, 1951**
Chicago, Illinois, USA

Robin's father, Robert Williams, was a senior executive at Lincoln-Mercury. His mother, the former Laura Smith, had been a model prior to her marriage. Although she was a Christian Scientist, Robin was raised in the Episcopal Church. He grew up in Bloomfield Hills, Michigan, where he attended the Detroit Country Day School. After moving to Marin County, California, he overcame his shyness, in the drama department at Redwood High School. Along with Christopher Reeve, Robin was one of twenty students accepted into the 1973 freshman class at Juilliard, and they became close friends. Robin was first seen on TV in 1977, in two episodes of 'The 'Richard Prior Show'. Fame followed after he developed the character "Mork" which culminated in four years of 'Mork & Mindy'. In 1980, he made his film debut as *Popeye.* His numerous successes include Best Actor Oscar nominations, for *Good Morning, Vietnam, Dead Poets Society* and *The Fisher King.* He was named Best Supporting Actor for *Good Will Hunting.* Robin's two marriages have ended in divorce. He has two sons and a daughter.

The World According to Garp (1982)
The Survivors (1983) Moscow on the
Hudson (1984) The Best of Times (1986)
Seize the Day (1986)
Good Morning, Vietnam (1987)
Dead Poets Society (1989)
Awakenings (1990) Dead Again (1991)
The Fisher King (1991)
Mrs. Doubtfire (1993)
Jumanji (1995) The Birdcage (1996)
The Secret Agent (1996) Hamlet (1996)
Deconstructing Harry (1997)
Good Will Hunting (1997)
What Dreams May Come (1998)
Patch Adams (1998) Jakob the
Liar (1999) Bicentennial Man (1999)
One Hour Photo (2002) Insomnia (2002)
House of D (2004) The Big White (2005)
The Night Listener (2006)
Man of the Year (2006)
Night at the Museum (2006)
August Rush (2007)

Treat **Williams**
5ft 10in
(RICHARD TREAT WILLIAMS)

Born: **December 1, 1951**
Rowayton, Connecticut, USA

The son of Richard Norman Williams, a corporate executive, and his wife, Marion, who ran a successful antiques business, Treat attended the exclusive Kent School in Connecticut. After showing creative leanings, he went to Franklin & Marshall College, a private liberal arts school in Lancaster, Pennsylvania. During that period he worked during the summer break with the Fulton Repertory Theater, where he performed in classics, musicals, and contemporary works. After graduating, he went to live in Manhattan, where he was understudy for the Danny Zuko role, in "Grease". Following work in "Over There" – an Andrews Sisters-themed musical, Treat made his film debut, in 1976, in Richard Lester's comedy, *The Ritz*. A few supporting roles later he was the star of the film version of *Hair* – directed by Milos Forman. It got him a nomination for a New Star Golden Globe and two years after that he was nominated as Best Actor, for his work in *Prince of the City*. He has been in a number of excellent movies as well as the TV series, 'Everwood' and 'Heartland'. He has been happily married to Pam Van Sant since 1988. The couple have a son, Gill, and a daughter, Elinor.

The Eagle Has Landed (1976)
Hair (1979)
Prince of the City (1981)
Once Upon a Time in
America (1984)
Flash Point (1984)
Smooth Talk (1985)
Beyond the Ocean (1990)
Where the Rivers Flow North (1994)
Things to Do in Denver
When You're Dead (1995)
Mulholland Falls (1996)
The Devil's Own (1997)
Deep Rising (1998)
The Deep End of the Ocean (1999)
Skeletons in the Closet (2001)
Hollywood Ending (2002)
The Hideout (2007)
Il Nascondiglio (2007)
What Happens in Vegas (2008)

Nicol **Williamson**
6ft 3in
(NICOL WILLIAMSON)

Born: **September 14, 1938**
Hamilton, South Lanarkshire, Scotland

From a poor working-class family, Nicol still received great encouragement from his parents, Hugh and Mary Williamson. After leaving secondary school he went to study acting at the Birmingham School of Speech & Drama. In 1960 he started two years of invaluable experience with the Dundee Repertory Company, and a year later, he appeared at the Arts Theater, in Cambridge, and played his first role on the London stage. His first screen appearance was in 1963, in a short subject titled *The Six-Sided Triangle*. In 1964, Nicol enjoyed his first major success when he starred in John Osborne's "Inadmissable Evidence". Following its transfer to Broadway, he won a Tony as Best Actor and was later seen in the movie version, for which he was nominated for a Best Actor BAFTA. Osborne actually described him as "the greatest actor since Marlon Brando". His playing of Hamlet on stage and screen lent credence to that accolade. Nicol's first feature film role was as the star of the drama *The Borfors Gun,* for which he was also BAFTA nominated. From 1971-1977, his wife was Californian-born actress, Jill Townsend. Nicol's television appearances have been rare, but special, with his 1983 'Macbeth' (in the title role) and his portrayal of Lord Louis Mountbatten, in the 1986 bio-drama 'Lord Mountbatten: The Last Viceroy' being particularly memorable. He hasn't been seen since the 1997 film, *Spawn*.

The Bofors Gun (1968)
Inadmissable Evidence (1968)
The Reckoning (1969)
Laughter in the Dark (1969)
Hamlet (1969)
The Jerusalem File (1972)
The Wilby Conspiracy (1975)
The Seven-Per-Cent Solution (1976)
The Cheap Detective (1978)
The Human Factor (1979)
Excalibur (1981)
I'm Dancing as Fast as I Can (1982)
Return to Oz (1985)
Black Widow (1987)
The Hour of the Pig (1993)

Bruce **Willis**
5ft 11¾in
(WALTER BRUCE WILLIS)

Born: **March 19, 1955**
Idar-Oberstein, West Germany

Bruce was the son of David Willis, an American soldier who was stationed in Germany. When his father was discharged in 1957, he took his family back to the United States, where they settled in Penns Grove, New Jersey. He took a job as a welder in a factory and saw to it that Bruce received a good education which included Penns Grove High School. He suffered with a stutter during his early years and it was through getting involved with school plays, that he was able to overcome it. He eventually became president of the school council and graduated with supreme self-confidence. It didn't translate immediately into a worthwhile career – his first job was as a security guard. He entered the world of entertainment through playing harmonica with a band called "Loose Goose" and then studied Drama at Montclair State University, in New Jersey. In 1980, Bruce made his film debut, with an uncredited part in *The First Deadly Sin*. After playing David Addison Jr., in 'Moonlighting' his film career took off with *Blind Date*. He was a mega-star after *Die Hard* and its sequels and has never looked back. For thirteen years – from 1987, Bruce was married to Demi Moore. They had three children.

Blind Date (1987) Die Hard (1988)
In Country (1989) Die Hard 2 (1990)
Mortal Thoughts (1991) Billy
Bathgate (1991) The Last Boy
Scout (1991) Pulp Fiction (1994)
Nobody's Fool (1994) Die Hard: With a
Vengeance (1995) Twelve Monkeys
(1995) Last Man Standing (1996) The
Fifth Element (1997) The Jackal (1997)
Armageddon (1998) The Siege (1998)
The Sixth Sense (1999) The Story of
Us (1999) The Whole Nine Yards (2000)
Unbreakable (2000) Bandits (2001) Hart's
War (2002) Tears of the Sun (2003)
Hostage (2005) Sin City (2005) Alpha
Dog (2006) Lucky Number Slevin (2006)
16 Blocks (2006) Grindhouse (2007) Live
Free or Die Hard (2007) Planet
Terror (2007) Assassination of a High
School President (2008)

Chill **Wills**
6ft 2in
(CHILL THEODORE WILLS)

Born: **July 18, 1903**
Seagoville, Texas, USA
Died: **December 15, 1978**

His parents named him Chill, as an ironic comment on the fact that July 18th, was the hottest day of 1903. He was a brilliant singer as a child. He performed in vaudeville and tent shows from the age of twelve and was acting with stock companies by his early teens. From an early age, Chill was leader of the "Avalon Boys" group, with whom he performed in a number of film westerns – starting with *Bar 20 Rides Again* in 1935. He even did the bass voice for Stan Laurel, in *Way Out West*. He married ballet dancer, Hattie Chappelle, in 1928. The couple had three children and were together until her death in 1971. In 1938 he began to get acting roles in films like *Allergheny Uprising.* By the time he appeared in *Boom Town,* he was much in demand as a character actor in big films like *Meet Me in St. Louis, Leave Her to Heaven, Rio Grande* and *Giant.* Chill was nominated for a Best Supporting Actor Oscar for his role as 'Beekeeper' in *The Alamo.* In 1973, he married his second wife, Googie Novadeen, and continued working – making his last film *Poco... Little Dog Lost,* a year before he died of cancer, at his home in Encino, California.

Boom Town (1940)
The Westerner (1940)
Western Union (1941)
Honky Tonk (1941)
See Here, Private Hargrove (1944)
Meet Me in St. Louis (1944)
Sunday Dinner for a Soldier (1944)
Leave Her to Heaven (1945)
The Harvey Girls (1946)
The Yearling (1946)
Rio Grande (1950)
The City That
Never Sleeps (1953)
Giant (1956)
From Hell to Texas (1958)
The Alamo (1960)
The Deadly Companions (1961)
McLintock! (1963)
The Rounders (1965)
Pat Garrett & Billy the Kid (1973)

Luke **Wilson**
6ft
(LUKE CUNNINGHAM WILSON)

Born: **September 21, 1971**
Dallas, Texas, USA

Owen Wilson's younger brother, Luke, also attended St. Mark's School of Texas in Dallas. After that he branched out. He moved to Los Angeles to study at the private liberal arts school, Occidental College. It was there that he developed his passion for acting and was also a pretty useful track and field athlete – both at Occidental and after transferring to Texas Christian University in Fort Worth. In 1994, Luke made his film debut in the thirteen minute short, *Bottle Rocket,* and was with Owen in the feature-length version two years later. Luke progressed through half-a-dozen supporting parts in films and an episode of 'The X Files', before starring in a Canada/USA co-production, *Dog Park.* He struck gold in Wes Craven's comedy drama *Rushmore.* He has since had ten years of success – in small budget Indies like *Kill the Man,* family films such as *My Dog Skip,* and increasingly, big movies including *Charlie's Angels, Legally Blonde, The Royal Tenenbaums, 3:10 to Yuma* and most recently, *Henry Poole Is Here.* Luke was co-director with his brother, Andrew, and he wrote and starred in *The Wendell Baker Story.* It received the Best Film Award at the Vail Film Festival in Colorado.

Bottle Rocket (1996)
Telling Lies in America (1997)
Best Men (1997) Rushmore (1998)
Kill the Man (1999)
Blue Streak (1999) My Dog Skip (2000)
Preston Tylk (2000)
Charlie's Angels (2000)
Legally Blonde (2001)
The Royal Tenenbaums (2001)
The Third Wheel (2002)
Old School (2003)
Around the World in 80 Days (2004)
Anchorman (2004)
The Wendell Baker Story (2005)
The Family Stone (2005)
Mini's First Time (2006)
Idiocracy (2006)
You Kill Me (2007) Vacancy (2007)
3:10 to Yuma (2007)
Henry Poole Is Here (2008)

Owen **Wilson**
5ft 10½in
(OWEN CUNNINGHAM WILSON)

Born: **November 18, 1968**
Dallas, Texas, USA

Owen's father, Robert Wilson, worked as an advertising executive and ran a public service TV station. His mother is the well known photographer, Laura Cunningham. Owen's two brothers, Luke and Andrew also work in the film industry. The family is Roman Catholic from an Irish-American background. He was educated in Dallas at The Lamplighter School and at St. Mark's School of Texas. He was expelled from the latter while in the tenth grade and spent his junior and senior years at the New Mexico Military Institute, in Rosewell. He attended the University of Texas at Austin, where he befriended the future director and writer, Wes Anderson. Owen made his film debut in Wes' *Bottle Rocket,* which they co-wrote. It also starred his younger brother Luke. Owen appeared in nine movies with Ben Stiller, including *The Cable Guy, Meet the Parents, Zoolander* and *The Royal Tenenbaums.* Owen shared a Lone Star Award with Wes, for Best Screenplay, for *Rushmore,* and they were Oscar nominated for their writing on *The Royal Tenenbaums.* He and Luke are members of the "Frat Pack" an exclusive group of successful Hollywood comedy actors which includes Will Ferrell and Jack Black. Owen had a serious relationship with Kate Hudson, but is still unmarried.

Bottle Rocket (1996)
The Cable Guy (1996)
Armageddon (1998)
Permanent Midnight (1998)
The Minus Man (1999)
Shanghai Noon (2000)
Meet the Parents (2000)
Zoolander (2001)
The Royal Tenenbaums (2001)
Behind Enemy Lines (2001)
Shanghai Knights (2003)
Starsky & Hutch (2004)
The Life Aquatic with
Steve Zissou (2004)
You, Me and Dupree (2006)
The Darjeeling Limited (2007)
Drillbit Taylor (2008)
Marley & Me (2008)

Marie **Windsor**
5ft 9in
(EMILY MARIE BERTELSEN)

Born: **December 11, 1919**
Marysvale, Utah, USA
Died: **December 10, 2000**

Marie was the first of three children who were raised as Mormons by Lane and Etta Bertelsen. Her brother, Jerry, arrived eleven years later and sister, Louise, when she was seventeen, and in her first year at Brigham Young University in Provo, Utah. While studying there, Marie was crowned "Miss Utah" and decided to become an actress. She cultivated her voice when she worked as a telephone operator to pay for drama classes with the Russian-born acting legend, Maria Ouspenskaya. Marie began her career on the stage and also worked on the radio. She was signed by RKO and made her film debut with an uncredited part in a poor 1941 comedy, *Weekend for Three.* She acted in twenty-four such 'invisible' roles by the time she first had her name on the cast list for MGM in the 1947 comedy, *Song of the the Thin Man.* A year later she was third-billed below John Garfield and Thomas Gomez in the excellent *Force of Evil.* A kick-start to her career, it was the first of several film-noir roles in which Marie shone. She was married twice. Husband number two, Jack Hupp, was with her when she died in Beverly Hills, of congestive heart failure.

Force of Evil (1948) Hellfire (1949)
Dakota Lil (1950) The Showdown (1950)
The Little Big Horn (1951)
Two Dollar Bettor (1951)
Japanese War Bride (1952)
The Narrow Margin (1952)
The Sniper (1952) The Tall Texan (1953)
Trouble Along the Way (1953)
So this Is Love (1953)
The City That Never Sleeps (1953)
Hell's Half Acre (1954)
The Bounty Hunter (1954)
The Silver Star (1955)
No Man's Woman (1955)
The Killing (1956)
The Day of the Bad Man (1958)
Critic's Choice (1963)
Bedtime Story (1964)
Support Your Local Gunfighter (1971)
The Outfit (1973)

Paul **Winfield**
6ft 1½in
(PAUL EDWARD WINFIELD)

Born: **May 22, 1939**
Los Angeles, California, USA
Died: **March 7, 2004**

Paul's mother, Lois, was abandoned by his father. When he was eight, she married a construction worker called Clarence Winfield, and Paul was given his name. After high school, Paul continued with his education at the University of Portland, Stanford University, Los Angeles City College and UCLA. When Paul set out to start his acting career, parts for African Americans were as scarce as hen's teeth. Luckily for him, he was able to conceal the fact that he was gay, and following some work on the radio he made his television debut in 1965, in an episode of 'Perry Mason'. Typically for the time, Paul's movie debut was as an African servant, in an unfunny Pat Boone comedy, *The Perils of Pauline,* in 1967. His first featured role was in the Sidney Poitier film, *The Lost Man.* Society was changing and by the early 1970s Paul was working regularly. He was nominated for an Oscar as Best Actor, for his role as Nathan Lee Morgan in Martin Ritt's superb film, *Sounder.* Paul acted in the television series, 'Touched by an Angel' until the year before he died of a heart attack, in Los Angeles.

The Lost Man (1969)
Brother John (1971) Sounder (1972)
Trouble Man (1972)
Gordon's War (1973)
Conrack (1974) Hustle (1975)
Twilight's Last Gleaming (1977)
A Hero Ain't Nothin'
But a Sandwich (1978)
Carbon Copy (1981)
Star Trek: The Wrath of Khan (1982)
White Dog (1982)
The Terminator (1984)
Big Shots (1987)
The Serpent and
the Rainbow (1988)
Presumed Innocent (1990)
Cliffhanger (1993)
Mars Attacks! (1996)
Relax...It's Just Sex (1998)
Catfish in
Black Bean Sauce (1999)

Debra **Winger**
5ft 4in
(MARY DEBRA WINGER)

Born: **May 16, 1955**
Cleveland Heights, Ohio, USA

The daughter of a meat packer, Robert Winger, and his wife, Ruth, Debra was raised in the Orthodox Jewish religion. The family moved to California when she was five. She graduated from Oliver Wendell Holmes Junior High School, in 1970. She then spent a few months at a Kibbutz in Israel. Shortly after returning to the United States, Debra was involved in an automobile accident which caused her to be partially paralyzed and blind, for a worrying period of ten months. Although she was initially told that she would never see again, she resolved that if she did, she would go to Hollywood and become an actress. God was looking over her and after graduating from James Monroe High School in Sepulveda, California, she did just that. Despite an inauspicious start in the 1976 film, *Slumber Party '57,* Debra became well known for her appearances in television's 'Wonder Woman' and by the late 1970s, she began getting the parts she deserved. She co-starred with John Travolta in *Urban Cowboy,* and followed that with a pair of Best Actress Oscar-nominated roles – in *An Officer and a Gentleman,* and *Terms of Endearment.* Ten years after the second, she had her third Best Actress Oscar nomination – for *Shadowlands.* In 1986, she began a four year marriage to actor Timothy Hutton. Since 1996, she's been with her present husband, Arliss Howard. They have a son.

French Postcards (1979)
Urban Cowboy (1980)
An Officer and a Gentleman (1982)
Terms of Endearment (1983)
Legal Eagles (1986)
Black Widow (1987)
Betrayed (1988)
The Sheltering Sky (1990)
Leap of Faith (1992)
A Dangerous Woman (1993)
Shadowlands (1993)
Forget Paris (1995)
Big Bad Love (2001)
Radio (2003) Eulogy (2004)
Rachel Getting Married (2008)

Charles **Winninger**
5ft 6in
(KARL WINNINGER)

Born: **May 26, 1884**
Athens, Wisconsin, USA
Died: **January 27, 1969**

Charlie was the son of show business folk who toured in vaudeville. His parents had no time for education and Charlie left school when he was eight years old to join their act – "The Winninger Family Concert Company". He was working with his five brothers after his parents retired, but they soon went their separate ways – performing with a variety of stock and repertory companies. Charlie made his stage debut in 1910, in a musical comedy "The Yankee Girl". The girl was Blanche Ring, whom he married two years later. He toured with her and they appeared on Broadway together. In 1915, Charlie had his first experience of film making when he appeared in a two-reeler called *Mister Flirt in Wrong*. He acted in six more silent films but his heart was in the theater. Charlie was the original Cap'n Andy in the Jerome Kern and Oscar Hammerstein musical hit, "Showboat". It brought him to the attention of Hollywood and in 1930, he made his talkie debut in *Soup to Nuts*. It was the start of a prolific film career as a loveable character actor. He retired after playing Santa Claus in *The Miracle of the White Reindeer*, in 1960. His second wife Gertrude was with him when he passed away in Palm Springs, after a long illness.

The Bad Sister (1931) **The Sins of Madelon Claudet** (1931) **Show Boat** (1936) **Three Smart Girls** (1936) Café Metropole (1937) **The Go Getter** (1937) **You Can't Have Everything** (1937) Nothing Sacred (1937) **You're a Sweetheart** (1937) Hard to Get (1938) **Three Smart Girls Grow Up** (1939) Babes in Arms (1939) Destry Rides Again (1939) **Beyond Tomorrow** (1940) Little Nellie Kelly (1940) Ziegfeld Girl (1941) Coney Island (1943) A Lady Takes a Chance (1943) Flesh and Fantasy (1943) Sunday Dinner for a Soldier (1944) State Fair (1945) Father Is a Bachelor (1950) **The Sun Shines Bright** (1953)

Kate **Winslet**
5ft 6½in
(KATE ELIZABETH WINSLET)

Born: **October 5, 1975**
Reading, Berkshire, England

Kate is the daughter of Roger Winslet – a swimming-pool contractor, and his wife, Sally. Both of them had acted at one time or another. Her maternal grandparents, Archie and Linda Bridges, had founded and ran the Reading Repertory Company. Kate's uncle, Robert Bridges, appeared in the original West End stage production of "Oliver!" So it was on the cards that Kate and her two sisters, Beth and Anne, would become actresses. Kate began her journey at the Redroofs Theater School, in Maidenhead, Berkshire. She was bullied to start with but eventually became head girl. She acted in a Sugar Puffs television commercial before a small role in 'Shrinks' on TV, in 1991. Next came a co-starring role, in the BBC children's serial, 'Dark Season'. Her movie debut was in the excellent *Heavenly Bodies,* shot on location in New Zealand. By 1995, Kate was already a popular established name – with a Best Supporting Actress Oscar nomination for *Sense and Sensibility,* to her credit. She followed that with Best Actress nominations for *Titanic, Eternal Sunshine of the Spotless Mind* and *Little Children,* as well as a Supporting Actress nomination for *Iris.* She's had a child with each of her two husbands – the film directors Jim Threapleton and Sam Mendes. Kate's sensitive portrayal of a former concentration camp guard, in *The Reader,* won her a Best Actress Oscar.

Heavenly Creatures (1994) Sense and Sensibility (1994) Jude (1996) **Hamlet** (1996) Titanic (1997) **Hideous Kinky** (1998) Holy Smoke (1999) **Enigma** (2001) Iris (2001) **Plunge: The Movie** (2003) The Life of David Gale (2003) **Eternal Sunshine of the Spotless Mind** (2004) **Finding Neverland** (2004) Romance & Cigarettes (2005) Little Children (2006) All the King's Men (2006) The Holiday (2006) **The Reader** (2008) Revolutionary Road (2008)

Shelley **Winters**
5ft 4in
(SHIRLEY SCHRIFT)

Born: **August 18, 1920**
St. Louis, Missouri, USA
Died: **January 14, 2006**

Shelley's parents were Jewish. Jonas Schrift worked as a tailor's cutter. His wife, Rose Winter, sang in the chorus of The Municipal Opera Association of St. Louis. Shelley and her sister Blanche were taken to live in Brooklyn when she was three. She attended Thomas Jefferson High School, in New York. She had acted in high school plays, but first jobs included clerking at Woolworth's. She began acting lessons with Charles Laughton, and paid for them by working as a model in an art school and as a borscht belt vaudevillian. She made her Broadway debut in 1941, in "The Night Before Christmas" and her film debut two years later, in *There's Something About a Soldier.* Her big break came when she played Pat Kroll, in *A Double Life.* Shelley was nominated for a Best Actress Oscar for *A Place in the Sun* and won Supporting Oscars for *The Diary of Anne Frank* and *A Patch of Blue.* Her four husbands included actors – Vittorio Gassman and Anthony Franciosa. Shelley retired in 1999. She died in Beverly Hills.

A Double Life (1947) **Larceny** (1948) **Cry of the City** (1948) **The Great Gatsby** (1949) **Johnny Stool Pigeon** (1949) **Winchester '73** (1950) **South Sea Sinner** (1950) **He Ran All the Way** (1951) **A Place in the Sun** (1951) **Behave Yourself!** (1951) **The Raging Tide** (1951) **Meet Danny Wilson** (1951) **Phone Call from a Stranger** (1952) **Executive Suite** (1954) **I Am a Camera** (1955) **The Big Knife** (1955) **The Night of the Hunter** (1955) **I Died a Thousand Times** (1955) **The Diary of Anne Frank** (1959) **Odds Against Tomorrow** (1959) **Let No Man Write My Epitaph** (1960) **The Young Savages** (1961) **Lolita** (1962) **The Balcony** (1963) **A House Is Not a Home** (1964) **A Patch of Blue** (1965) **Harper** (1966) **Alfie** (1966) **The Scalphunters** (1968) **Buona Sera, Mrs. Campbell** (1968) **The Poseidon Adventure** (1972)

Googie **Withers**
5ft 3½in
(GEORGETTE LIZETTE WITHERS)

Born: **March 12, 1917**
Karachi, British India

She was the daughter of a career soldier in the British Army. Her mother was Dutch. Googie's unusual nickname is believed to have originated from her affectionate Hindi "amah" or nurse, in Karachi. Her family returned to England to live and she received her education (including acting training) at the Italia Conti Academy, in London. She was dancing in the chorus of a West End musical comedy, when she was spotted by a movie studio scout. In 1935, Googie was given her film debut, in *Windfall.* She was then offered work as an extra in *The Girl in the Crowd* – directed by Michael Powell, but when she arrived at the studio, a member of the cast had dropped out and Googie was third billed, as Sally. Googie was featured in Alfred Hitchcock's *The Lady Vanishes,* and also appeared in some of the famous Ealing Studios productions, including *Dead of Night,* and *Pink String and Sealing Wax.* When she was working on one of her best films, *It Always Rains on Sunday,* she fell in love with her handsome co-star, the Australian actor, John McCallum. They married in 1948 and in 1950, they had a daughter, Joanna, who also became an actress. Their son, Nicholas McCallum, is a production designer. For her work in her last film *Shine,* she was nominated for a share of a Screen Actors Guild Award for Outstanding Performance by a Cast. In 1998, Googie appeared in an Australian stage production of "An Ideal Husband".

Accused (1936) Her Last
Affaire (1936) Crown v. Stevens (1936)
Convict 99 (1938) The Lady
Vanishes (1938) One of Our Aircraft
Is Missing (1942) Dead of Night (1945)
Pink String and Sealing Wax (1946)
The Loves of Joanna
Godden (1947) It Always Rains
on Sunday (1947) Miranda (1948)
Night and the City (1950)
White Corridors (1951)
Time After Time (1986)
Country Life (1994)
Shine (1996)

Reese **Witherspoon**
5ft 1½in
(LAURA JEANNE REESE WITHERSPOON)

Born: **March 22, 1976**
New Orleans, Louisiana, USA

The former Betty Reese gave birth to her baby girl in the Southern Baptist Hospital in New Orleans. Reese's father, John Witherspoon, who was a specialist in ear, nose, throat, head and neck disorders, was known as an otolaryngologist. He worked for the U.S. Military in Wiesbaden, Germany, which is where Reese spent four of her early years. On the family's return to the United States, she went to school in Nashville, Tennessee, and was raised as an Episcopalian. When she was seven, she appeared in a TV commercial. Not long after that, she began acting lessons, and at eleven years of age, she was first in the 'Ten-State Talent Fair'. After the Harding Academy, she graduated from Harpeth Hall Girls' School. She then went to Stanford University, as an English Lit major, but left a year later to start her acting career. Reese made her film debut, in *The Man in the Moon,* for which she was nominated for the Young Artist Award – as 'Best Young Actress'. Other nominations were American Comedy Awards' Funniest Female Guest, in an episode of 'Friends', and Funniest Actress in a Motion Picture, for *Election.* Her greatest achievement is her Best Actress Oscar, for *Walk the Line.* For seven years, from 1999, Reese was married to Ryan Phillippe. They have two children, Ava and Deacon.

The Man in the Moon (1991)
A Far Off Place (1993)
Jack the Bear (1993) S.F.W. (1994)
Freeway (1996) Fear (1996)
Twilight (1998) Overnight Delivery (1998)
Pleasantville (1998)
Cruel Intentions (1999)
Election (1999) Best Laid Plans (1999)
American Psycho (2000)
Legally Blonde (2001)
The Importance of Being
Earnest (2002) Sweet Home
Alabama (2002) Vanity Fair (2004)
Walk the Line (2005)
Just Like Heaven (2005)
Penelope (2006) Rendition (2007)
Four Christmases (2008)

Anna May **Wong**
5ft 7in
(WONG LIU TSONG)

Born: **January 3, 1905**
Los Angeles, California, USA
Died: **February 2, 1961**

Anna May was one of seven children born to Chinese-American parents, Wong Liu Tsong and his wife Lee Gon Toy, who ran a laundry near Los Angeles' Chinatown. At Hollywood High School and in her daily life, she endured the racial prejudice of the time, but because of where she was living and the excitement generated by the infant film industry, she quickly became fascinated with Hollywood. She was only fourteen when she first took advantage of her good looks and the need for Chinese talent – playing a small role on her film debut, in 1919, in *The Red Lantern.* Her first major role was in 1922, as "Lotus Flower", in an Americanized version of "Madame Butterfly", known as *The Toll of the Sea.* By 1924, she played supporting roles in such huge international hits as Douglas Fairbanks', *The Thief of Bagdad.* Anna May moved to Europe in 1928, and acted in both German and British films – one of which was *Piccadilly.* She returned to America to appear in *Shanghai Express* with Marlene Dietrich, and played stereotypical parts until she was bitterly disappointed to lose out to Luise Rainer, for the role of O-Lan, in the film of Pearl Buck's novel, *The Good Earth.* There were some anti-Japanese propaganda films in the war years, TV work during the 1950s and 1960s, and a final film appearance – in *Portrait in Black.* Anna May died of a heart attack, in Santa Monica, California.

Piccadilly (1929)
Daughter of the Dragon (1931)
Shanghai Express (1932)
A Study in Scarlet (1933)
Java Head (1934) Tiger Bay (1934)
Limehouse Blues (1934) Daughter of
Shanghai (1937) Dangerous to
Know (1938) When Were You
Born (1938) King of Chinatown (1939)
Island of Lost Men (1939)
Lady from Chungking (1942)
Bombs Over Burma (1943)
Impact (1949)
Portrait in Black (1960)

Natalie **Wood**
5ft
(NATALIA NIKOLAEVNA ZAKHARENKO)

Born: **July 20, 1938**
San Francisco, California, USA
Died: **November 29, 1981**

Natalie's parents were Russian immigrants Nikolai and Maria Zakharenko. When Natalie was still a baby, the family settled in Santa Rosa, California, and changed their surname to Gurdin. During a 20th Century Fox film shoot in the town, little Natalie was taken by her mother to the location. She was cute enough to be used as an extra in two 1943 pictures – *Happy Land* and *The Moon Is Down*. Three years later, as Natalie Wood, she was featured in *Tomorrow Is Forever,* which starred Orson Welles. Her performance in the beautiful original version of *Miracle on 34th Street* turned her into a child star. Natalie gave many charming performances before she blossomed as a teenage actress, in *Rebel Without a Cause,* for which she was nominated for a Best Supporting Actress Oscar. Her two further nominations – for *Splendor in the Grass* and *Love with the Proper Stranger,* were as Best Actress. She retained her popularity throughout her two marriages to Robert Wagner, and it was on their yacht "Splendor" that she met her death when falling into the water.

Miracle on 34th Street (1947)
The Ghost and Mrs. Muir (1947)
Driftwood (1947) **Chicken Every Sunday** (1949) **Father was a Fullback** (1949) **No Sad Songs for Me** (1950) **Our Very Own** (1950)
The Jackpot (1950)
The Blue Veil (1951) **Just for You** (1952)
The Star (1952) **One Desire** (1955)
Rebel Without a Cause (1955)
The Searchers (1956) **A Cry in the Night** (1956) **The Burning Hills** (1956)
The Girl He Left Behind (1956) **Marjorie Morningstar** (1958) **Splendor in the Grass** (1961) **West Side Story** (1961)
Gypsy (1962) **Love with the Proper Stranger** (1963)
Sex and the Single Girl (1964)
The Great Race (1965)
Inside Daisy Clover (1965)
This Property Is Condemned (1966)
Bob & Carol & Ted & Alice (1969)

Alfre **Woodard**
5ft 3½in
(ALFRE ETTE WOODARD)

Born: **November 8, 1952**
Tulsa, Oklahoma, USA

Alfre was the youngest of three children born to African American parents. Her father, Marion Woodard, was an interior designer and described as something of an entrepreneur. Her mother, Constance, was a traditional homemaker. Alfre was raised in the Catholic faith and attended the private Bishop Kelley High School, in Tulsa. Having taken a keen interest in acting during her schooldays she studied Drama at Boston University. Following her graduation Alfre began looking for work as an actress, but things moved slowly. In 1978 she played her first role on television in the drama 'The Trial of the Moke', which had Samuel L. Jackson in the cast. She made her film debut in Robert Altman's comedy *HealtH,* in 1980. After a strong showing in *Cross Creek,* for which she was nominated for an Oscar – as Best Supporting Actress, she had to wait three years for her next film role – in *Extremities.* In 1983, she married Roderick Spencer, with whom she adopted two children. In 1987, Alfre won an ACE Award for her acting in 'Mandela'. Her television work has played a very big part in her acting career – 'Hill Street Blues', 'St. Elsewhere' and 'Desperate Housewives' being just three examples. In this medium she has won four Emmys. During 2008, Alfre, who is a Democratic Party activist, lent her support to Barack Obama.

Cross Creek (1983) **Extremities** (1986)
Scrooged (1988) **Miss Firecracker** (1989)
Grand Canyon (1991) **Passion Fish** (1992) **Rich in Love** (1993)
Heart and Souls (1993)
Bopha! (1993) **Blue Chips** (1994)
Crooklyn (1994) **How to Make an American Quilt** (1995) **Follow Me Home** (1996) **Primal Fear** (1996) **A Step Toward Tomorrow** (1996) **Star Trek: First Contact** (1996) **Down in the Delta** (1998) **Mumford** (1999)
Love & Basketball (2000)
K-PAX (2001) **Radio** (2003) **The Forgotten** (2004) **Something New** (2006)
Take the Lead (2006)

Donald **Woods**
5ft 9in
(RALPH L. ZINK)

Born: **December 2, 1906**
Brandon, Manitoba, Canada
Died: **March 5, 1998**

Don's parents moved south, to settle in California when he was in his early teens. Their decision proved important in terms of his future career. After high school he attended the University of California at Berkeley and following his graduation, he looked for work at the movie studios. Apart from physical labor – building sets, the only acting job he got was as an extra in the 1928 Mack Sennett silent comedy *Motorboat Mamas.* But the idea of becoming an actor was firmly implanted in his head. Don took acting lessons while doing any work he could get during the Great Depression. In 1933, he married Josephine Van de Horck. She would be his wife for sixty-five years. His good looks got him a part in a 1934 B-movie – *As the Earth Turns.* He then got featured roles in bigger pictures and appeared in three 1930s classics – *The Story of Louis Pasteur, A Tale of Two Cities* and *Anthony Adverse.* Don didn't quite have the stature or the personality for true stardom and much of his work remained in B-movies. During the 1940s he had supporting roles in two popular films – the award-winning *Watch on the Rhine,* and Danny Kaye's *Wonder Man.* Don was later a success in real estate. He died of natural causes, in Palm Springs, at the age of ninety-one.

Charlie Chan's Courage (1934)
The Case of the Curious Bride (1935)
The Story of Louis Pasteur (1935)
A Tale of Two Cities (1935)
Anthony Adverse (1936)
Romance on the Run (1938)
Danger on the Air (1938) **The Girl from Mexico** (1939) **Mexican Spitfire** (1940)
Sky Raiders (1941)
Watch on the Rhine (1943)
The Bridge of San Luis Rey (1944)
Wonder Man (1945)
Never Say Goodbye (1946)
Scene of the Crime (1949)
The Beast from 20,000 Fathoms (1953)
Moment to Moment (1965)
True Grit (1969)

James **Woods**
6ft
(JAMES HOWARD WOODS)

Born: **April 18, 1947**
Vernal, Utah, USA

Jimmy was thirteen when his father, Gail Peyton Woods – who was a U.S. Army intelligence officer, died following routine surgery. His mother, Martha then ran a pre-school establishment until she remarried. Jim was raised in Warwick, Rhode Island. He was educated at the local Pilgrim High School. An injury suffered in a collision with a plate glass window ruined his chances of joining the United States Air Force Academy and shattered his dream of becoming a fighter pilot. Following a score of 1580 in the SAT test, he majored in Political Science at the Massachusetts Institute of Technology. He was active as a member of the university's student theater group, "Dramashop" and both acted in and directed, several plays. Just before graduation in 1969, with his mother's rather cautious blessing, Jimmy dropped out in order to pursue an acting career. He made his television debut in 1971 in 'All the Way Home' a drama starring Joanne Woodward. Jimmy's film debut was in Elia Kazan's *The Visitors*. He first made an impact in *Night Moves* and was nominated for a Best Actor Oscar, for *Salvador* and as Best Supporting Actor, for *Ghosts of Mississippi*. Jimmy has been twice married and divorced.

The Visitors (1972) **Night Moves** (1975)
The Billion Dollar Bubble (1976)
The Onion Field (1979)
Eyewitness (1981) Split Image (1982)
Fast-Walking (1982) Videodrome (1983)
Once Upon a Time in America (1984)
Against All Odds (1984)
Joshua Then and Now (1985)
Salvador (1986) Best Seller (1987)
Cop (1988) True Believer (1989)
The Hard Way (1991) Diggstown (1992)
Casino (1995) Nixon (1995) Ghosts of
Mississippi (1996) Another Day in
Paradise (1997) True Crime (1999)
The Virgin Suicides (1999) Any Given
Sunday (1999) Riding in Cars with
Boys (2001) John Q (2002)
Northfork (2003) This Girl's Life (2003)
Pretty Persuasion (2005)

Joanne **Woodward**
5ft 4in
(JOANNE GIGNILLIAT TRIMMIER WOODWARD)

Born: **February 27, 1930**
Thomasville, Georgia, USA

Joanne was the daughter of Wade Woodward Jr., a vice president of Charles Scribner's Sons – the New York publisher. Her mother, the former Elinor Gignilliat, was descended from Huguenot stock. Elinor was movie crazy and she had a big influence on Joanne's future involvement in the medium. The family moved twice during her childhood – the first time to Marietta, Georgia, and secondly, after her parents divorced, to Greenville, South Carolina, where she graduated from the local high school. During her teenage years, Joanne entered and won several beauty contests. She starred in a number of plays at high school and also appeared in "The Glass Menagerie" at the Little Theater, in Greenville. Joanne majored in Drama at Louisiana State University, in Baton Rouge, before going to New York to begin her career. She acted on stage and made her television debut in 1952, in an episode of 'Tales of Tomorrow'. She made her film debut in the excellent western, *Count Three and Pray*. She won a Best Actress Oscar for *The Three Faces of Eve*. Joanne was nominated three more times – for *Rachel, Rachel, Summer Wishes, Winter Dreams* and *Mr. & Mrs. Bridge* – in which she co-starred with her husband, Paul Newman. They were happily married with three children until his death in 2008.

Count Three and Pray (1955) A Kiss
Before Dying (1956) The Three Faces of
Eve (1957) No Down Payment (1957)
The Long, Hot Summer (1958)
The Fugitive Kind (1959) The Sound and
the Fury (1959) From the Terrace (1960)
Paris Blues (1961) The Stripper (1963)
A New Kind of Love (1963)
A Big Hand for the Little Lady (1966)
Rachel, Rachel (1968) They Might Be
Giants (1971) The Effect of Gamma Rays
on Man-in-the-Moon Marigolds (1972)
Summer Wishes, Winter Dreams (1973)
The Drowning Pool (1975)
The End (1978)
The Glass Menagerie (1987)
Philadelphia (1993)

Monty **Wooley**
5ft 11in
(EDGAR MONTILLION WOOLEY)

Born: **August 17, 1888**
New York City, New York, USA
Died: **May 6, 1963**

Because Monty's father owned the Bristol Hotel in New York City, he enjoyed a life of luxury and privilege from the day he was born. He attended private schools and eventually Yale University, where he was a friend and classmate of Cole Porter. With Clifton Webb, they were members of New York's gay theatrical circle. Monty was an academic of such high standing, he became a professor/lecturer at Yale, in English and Dramatics. Aged forty-seven, he gave it all up to begin a career as an actor on Broadway. He made his debut in the Rogers and Hart musical "On Your Toes", which starred Ray Bolger, and had an uncredited role in that same year's film, *Ladies in Love.* He made his official movie debut in *Live, Love and Learn,* and was a popular larger-than-life character actor until the early 1940s. Monty repeated his stage success as the eccentric wheel-chair-bound, Sheridan Whiteside, in *The Man Who Came to Dinner* and was nominated for an Oscar as Best Actor, in *The Pied Piper.* He rounded off a vintage Wooley year, in *Life Begins at Eight-Thirty.* A Best Supporting Actor Oscar nomination for *Since You Went Away,* spelt the end of Monty's brief stardom. He made his final film appearance in 1955, in *Kismet,* and died of a heart and kidney ailment, in Albany, New York, eight years later.

Live, Love and Learn (1937)
Arsène Lupin Returns (1938)
The Girl of the Golden West (1938)
Three Comrades (1938)
Lord Jeff (1938) Young Dr. Kildare (1938)
Midnight (1939) Never Say Die (1939)
Man About Town (1939)
Dancing Co-Ed (1939)
The Man Who Came to Dinner (1942)
The Pied Piper (1942)
Life Begins at Eight-Thirty (1942)
Holy Matrimony (1943)
Since You Went Away (1944)
The Bishop's Wife (1947)
Miss Tatlock's Millions (1948)
As Young as You Feel (1951)

Fay **Wray**
5ft 3in
(VINA FAY WRAY)

Born: **September 15, 1907**
Cardston, Alberta, Canada
Died: **August 8, 2004**

During her childhood, Fay moved with her family to the United States and lived for a time in Arizona and Colorado. She was in her early teens when she moved to Los Angeles. While she was at Hollywood High School she began working as an extra at the studios, and made her film debut, in 1923, in the two-reeler, *Gasoline Love*. Fay appeared in more than thirty silent films before co-starring with Eric von Stroheim, in his 1928 part-sound melodrama *The Wedding March*. The following year she co-starred with George Bancroft and Richard Arlen in her first true sound movie, *Thunderbolt*. She co-starred with Lionel Atwill, in a classic horror-film *Doctor X*, but her real claim to movie immortality was as Ann Darrow, in the original *King Kong*. Fay would always be associated with that role. She married three times and had three children. Fay was a month away from her 97th birthday when she died in her sleep, at her Manhattan apartment.

Thunderbolt (1929) Pointed Heels (1929)
Dirigible (1931) The Finger Points (1931)
Doctor X (1932) The Most Dangerous
Game (1932) The Vampire Bat (1933)
Mystery of the Wax Museum (1933)
King Kong (1933) Below the Sea (1933)
Ann Carver's Profession (1933)
The Woman I Stole (1933) Shanghai
Madness (1933) One Sunday
Afternoon (1933) The Bowery (1933)
The Clairvoyant (1934) Once to Every
Woman (1934) Viva Villa! (1934)
Black Moon (1934) The Affairs of
Cellini (1934) The Richest Girl in the
World (1934) Woman in the Dark (1934)
Mills of the Gods (1934) They Met in
a Taxi (1936) It Happened in
Hollywood (1937) Murder in Greenwich
Village (1937) Melody for Three (1941)
Adam Had Four Sons (1941)
Treasure of the Golden Condor (1953)
Melody for Three (1953)
Small Town Girl (1953)
Queen Bee (1955) Hell on Frisco
Bay (1955) Crime of Passion (1957)

Robin **Wright Penn**
5ft 6in
(ROBIN VIRGINIA GAYLE WRIGHT)

Born: **April 8, 1966**
Dallas, Texas, USA

Robin is the daughter of Fred Wright, who was an executive with a pharmaceutical company, and his wife Gayle, who worked for Mary Kay cosmetics. When she was a young girl her parents relocated to San Diego, California. When she was fourteen Robin began working as a model in San Diego and at fifteen, she was dating actor Charlie Sheen. She also modeled in both Paris and Tokyo before landing her first acting role on television, in 1983, in an episode of 'The Yellow Rose'. She made her film debut three years later in *Hollywood Vice Squad*, while maintaining her TV presence as Kelly, in the long-running series 'Santa Barbara'. Robin moved up a couple of notches in the movie league when she played 'Buttercup' in the charming fantasy, *The Princess Bride*. A two-year marriage to her 'Santa Barbara' co-star, Dane Witherspoon, ended in divorce, in 1988. Her relationship with Sean Penn began when they acted together in *State of Grace*. Robin's many nominations include one for a Golden Globe as Best Supporting Actress, in *Forrest Gump*. Prior to getting married, in April, 1996, she and Sean Penn had a daughter, Dylan and a son named Hopper.

The Princess Bride (1987)
State of Grace (1991)
The Playboys (1992)
Forrest Gump (1994)
Moll Flanders (1996)
Hurlyburly (1998)
Message in a Bottle (1999)
How To Kill Your
Neighbor's Dog (2000)
The Pledge (2001)
White Oleander (2002)
The Singing Detective (2003)
A Home at the End
of the World (2004)
Nine Lives (2005) Sorry, Haters (2005)
Breaking and Entering (2006)
Hounddog (2007) Beowulf (2007)
What Just happened (2008)
New York, I Love You (2008)
State of Play (2009)

Jeffrey **Wright**
5ft 11in
(JEFFREY WRIGHT)

Born: **December 7, 1965**
Washington, D.C., USA

Jeff's father died when he was a year old and he was raised by his aunt and his mother, who worked in the legal department of United States Customs. After graduating from St. Alban's School for Boys, in Washington, Jeff earned a Bachelor's Degree in Political Science, at Amherst College, in Massachusetts. Although he won an acting scholarship to New York University, he only attended for a brief period – deciding instead to begin his career as a professional actor. After stage work off and on-Broadway, Jeff made his film debut in 1990, in *Presumed Innocent*, starring Harrison Ford. For the next five years, Jeff worked in the theater and acted in 'The Young Indiana Jones Chronicles" on TV. In 1996, he shot to stardom in the movie biography about the New York graffiti artist – Neo-Expressionist painter, Jean-Michel *Basquiat*. Jeff has since been seen in high profile movies such as *Ali*, *The Manchurian Candidate*, *Syriana*, and two Bonds – *Casino Royale* and *Quantum of Solace*. In 2004, Jeff won a Golden Globe as Best Supporting Actor, in the TV mini-series, 'Angels in America'. He has a son named Elijah with his wife, actress Carmen Ejogo.

Faithful (1996)
Basquiat (1996)
Critical Care (1997)
The Giraffe (1998)
Crime and Punishment
in Suburbia (2000)
Shaft (2000)
Ali (2001)
The Manchurian Candidate (2004)
Broken Flowers (2005)
Syriana (2005)
Casino Royale (2006)
The Invasion (2007)
Blackout (2007)
The Adventures of Young
Indiana Jones: Scandal of
1920 (2008)
W. (2008)
Quantum of Solace (2008)
Cadillac Records (2008)

Teresa **Wright**
5ft 3in
(MURIEL TERESA WRIGHT)

Born: **October 27, 1918**
Manhattan, New York City, New York USA
Died: **March 6, 2005**

Sweet Teresa was the daughter of Arthur Wright, an insurance agent, and his wife, Martha. She was raised in Maplewood, New Jersey, where she attended the local Columbia High School and developed her passion for acting. During the summer months, Teresa would spend as much time as possible, near Cape Cod, where she appeared in Provincetown Theater presentations. After graduating from Columbia in 1938, she headed for New York, where she was employed as an understudy to Dorothy McGuire and Martha Scott, in the Broadway version of Thornton Wilder's "Our Town". In 1939, Teresa was a regular in the play "Life with Father". During that stint she was discovered by a Goldwyn scout, and cast as Bette Davis' daughter, for her film debut in *The Little Foxes.* She was nominated for a Best Supporting Actress Oscar and given a five-year contract. A year later she was nominated as Best Actress, for *The Pride of the Yankees* and *was* Best Supporting Actress, for *Mrs. Miniver.* She rarely took any roles that were ordinary. Before Teresa rejected the studio system she had added *Shadow of a Doubt, The Best Years of Our Lives* and *The Men,* to her list of credits. Teresa's two husbands were both screen writers. She had two children. She died of a heart attack in New Haven, Connecticut.

The Little Foxes (1941)
Mrs. Miniver (1942) The Pride of the
Yankees (1942) Shadow of a
Doubt (1943) Casanova Brown (1944)
The Best Years of Our Lives (1946)
Pursued (1947) The Imperfect
Lady (1947) The Trouble with
Women (1947) Enchantment (1948)
The Capture (1950) The Men (1950)
Something to Live For (1952) The Steel
Trap (1952) Count the Hours (1953)
The Actress (1953) Track of the
Cat (1954) The Search for Bridey
Murphy (1956) The Restless Years (1958)
The Happy Ending (1969)
Roseland (1977) The Rainmaker (1997)

Jane **Wyman**
5ft 2½in
(SARAH JANE MAYFIELD)

Born: **January 5, 1917**
St. Joseph, Missouri, USA
Died: **September 10, 2007**

Jane was the daughter of a laborer, Manning Mayfield, who died at twenty-seven, and his wife Hope, who had filed for divorce a year earlier. Five-year-old Jane was surplus to requirements, and was left with foster parents when her mother moved to Cleveland. It was a miserable childhood and when, at eleven, she was taken to southern California, it didn't get better. As a teenager she settled in Saint Joseph, Missouri, where she attended Lafayette High School. Jane started a career as a radio singer and added three years to her age in order to get work. She was fifteen when she moved to Hollywood – appearing as an extra in Eddie Cantor's 1932 comedy, *The Kid from Spain.* She was finally credited for the first time in a 1936 short – entitled *The Sunday Round-Up.* Jane went almost unnoticed until 1937, and it would be several years before she would be a star. *The Lost Weekend, The Yearling, Johnny Belinda* – for which she won a Best Actress Oscar, *The Blue Veil* and *Magnificent Obsession,* are her best works. Jane's four husbands included Ronald Reagan. She died from arthritis and diabetes, in Palm Springs, California.

The King and the Chorus Girl (1937)
Slim (1937) Wide Open Faces (1938)
The Crowd Roars (1938) Brother
Rat (1938) Gambling on the High
Seas (1940) My Love Came Back (1940)
Larceny Inc. (1942) My Favorite
Spy (1942) Princess O'Rourke (1943)
Crime by Night (1944)
The Lost Weekend (1945)
One More Tomorrow (1946)
Night and Day (1946) The Yearling (1946)
Cheyenne (1947) Magic Town (1947)
Johnny Belinda (1948) A Kiss in
the Dark (1949) Stage Fright (1950)
The Glass Menagerie (1950)
The Blue Veil (1951) Just for You (1952)
So Big (1953) Magnificent
Obsession (1954) Lucy Gallant (1955)
All That Heaven Allows (1955) Miracle in
the Rain (1956) Pollyanna (1960)

Keenan **Wynn**
5ft 10in
(FRANCES XAVIER ALOYSIUS JAMES J. KEENAN WYNN)

Born: **July 27, 1916**
New York City, New York, USA
Died: **October 14, 1986**

Keenan was born into a show business family - the most prominent of whom was his father – Jewish burlesque comedian Ed Wynn. His mother, Hilda, was an Irish Catholic actress whose father, Frank Keenan, had specialized in the tragic Shakespearean roles. It was from him that her son took his stage name. There was money enough to send young Keenan to private schools including the famous St John's Military Academy, in Lake Geneva, Wisconsin. After deciding on a serious acting career as opposed to his father's comedy, he made his stage debut in "Accent of Youth" with the Lakewood Players, in Maine. At twenty-one he made his Broadway debut – in "Hitch Your Wagon" and met his first wife, Eve Abbott, who became his manager. After his movie debut, in 1942's *Somewhere I'll Find You,* Keenan had a busy screen career (more than 130 films) until the year of his death in Los Angeles, from pancreatic cancer.

The Clock (1945) Week-End at the
Waldorf (1945) Easy to Wed (1946) The
Cock-Eyed Miracle (1946) The
Hucksters (1947) The Three
Musketeers (1948) That Midnight
Kiss (1949) Annie Get Your Gun (1950)
Three Little Words (1950) Royal
Wedding (1951) Kind Lady (1951) Angels
in the Outfield (1951) Phone Call from a
Stranger (1952) The Belle of New
York (1952) Holiday for Sinners (1952)
All the Brothers Were Valiant (1953)
Kiss Me Kate (1953) The Long, Long
Trailer (1953) The Marauders (1955)
The Man in the Gray Flannel Suit (1956)
Joe Butterfly (1957) A Time to
Love and a Time to Die (1958)
The Perfect Furlough (1958)
That Kind of Woman (1959)
A Hole in the Head (1959) Dr.
Strangelove (1964) The Great
Race (1965) Warning Shot (1967)
Point Blank (1967)
Mackenna's Gold (1969)
The Mechanic (1972)

Y

Michael **York**
5ft 11in
(MICHAEL HUGH JOHNSON)

Born: March 27, 1942
Fulmer, Buckinghamshire, England

Michael's father, Joseph, was an army man, who in civilian life, became executive of Marks and Spencer department stores. His mother Florence was a keen pianist. Michael was educated in Kent, at Bromley Grammar School and at fourteen, he had his first stage role – in a production of "The Yellow Jacket". Following a few acting lessons, he made his London West End stage appearance in 1959, with one of the smaller parts in "Hamlet". Michael read English at University College, Oxford and performed with both the Dramatic Society and the University College Players. After graduating with a degree in English, he worked with Dundee Repertory Company and then joined the National Theater. With the latter, he appeared in Franco Zeffirelli's 1965 production of "Much Ado About Nothing". In 1967, he made his film debut in a Dutch movie, *Confessions of Love*. Michael's first British film was the Liz Taylor/Richard Burton movie, *The Taming of the Shrew* – directed by Zeffirelli. He soon served the Italian master once again, in *Romeo and Juliet.* That was the year of his marriage to Patricia McCallum – with whom he lives in California. Michael really made his name internationally, in *Cabaret* and *The Three Musketeers,* and his movie career has been ticking over, without too many fireworks, ever since then.

The Taming of the Shrew (1967)
Accident (1967)
The Strange Affair (1968)
Romeo and Juliet (1968)
Justine (1968)
Something for Everyone (1970)
Cabaret (1972)
England Made Me (1973)
The Three Musketeers (1973)
The Four Musketeers (1974)
Murder on the Orient Express (1974)
Logan's Run (1976)
The Riddle of the Sands (1979)
Austin Powers: International
Man of Mystery (1997)
Borstal Boy (2000) Austin Powers in
Goldmember (2002)

Susannah **York**
5ft 6¹⁄₂in
(SUSANNAH YOLANDE FLETCHER)

Born: January 9, 1941
London, England

Because of the dangers presented by the London Blitz, Susannah was evacuated to Scotland soon after her birth. She began to act in junior school and when she was nine, she enjoyed the audiences' laughter when she played an ugly sister in a production of "Cinderella". She studied acting at the Royal Academy of Dramatic Art in London, where she was a winner of The Arthene Seyler and Ronson Awards. She was especially proud of her portrayal of Norah, in Ibsen's "A Doll's House", during her final term. She landed a role in an episode of the ITV 'Television Playhouse' in 1959, and within a few months, had made her film debut, in a Norman Wisdom comedy called *There Was a Crooked Man.* In the spring of 1960, she married her only husband, the young actor, Michael Wells and that same year, was seen with Alec Guinness, in *Tunes of Glory.* After working with her, Alec remarked that Susannah was "the best thing in films since Audrey Hepburn". She knew the value of good photographs to promote herself – using masters like Cornel Lucas. She was one of John D. Green's era-defining, "Birds of Britain". Her career rocketed, but her husband's didn't, and they divorced in 1980. She was a star by the time she was seen as Sophie Western, in *Tom Jones,* and was nominated for an Oscar – for They Shoot Horses, Don't They? After that, the good film roles were few and far between.

There Was a Crooked Man (1960)
Tunes of Glory (1960)
The Greengage Summer (1961)
Freud (1962) Tom Jones (1963)
Sands of the Kalahari (1965)
Kaleidoscope (1966)
A Man for All Seasons (1966)
Sebastian (1968)
The Killing of Sister George (1968)
Battle of Britain (1969) They Shoot
Horses, Don't They? (1969)
Images (1972) The Shout (1978)
Superman (1978) A Summer
Story (1988) The Gigolos (2006)
Franklyn (2008)

Burt **Young**
5ft 8in
(JERRY DE LOUISE)

Born: April 30, 1940
New York City, New York, USA

The son of Michael and Josephine De Louise, Burt grew up in the Queen's district of New York City. The environment and the characters who inhabited it, gave him plenty of material for his future career. In high school plays, Burt had already shown signs of having acting talent. After he left, he served for two years in the United States Marines – from 1957-1959. Burt then worked in a series of dead-end jobs, including as a salesman and carpet cleaner, before attempting a career as a boxer. He then got married and soon had a daughter to support, so he decided to become an actor. With the help of the G.I. Bill, Burt received the best possible start by training with the famous drama coach Lee Strasberg at the Actor's Studio. In 1970, he made a less than auspicious movie debut, in the horror film *Carnival of Blood,* but from then on, he was in demand whenever there was a need for an Italian-American tough guy – which was every few months. His first taste of fame was as Sylvester Stallone's brother-in-law, Paulie, in the massive hit, *Rocky.* It earned him a Best Supporting Actor Oscar nomination and work in every one of the sequels. Burt appeared in Italian movies and rounded off his boxing experience in the biography of Primo Carnera.

Chinatown (1974)
The Gambler (1974) Rocky (1976)
Rocky II (1979) Once Upon a
Time in America (1984)
Back to School (1986)
Las Exit to Brooklyn (1989)
Americano rosso (1991)
Berlin '39 (1994)
She's So Lovely (1997) One
Deadly Road (1998) Mickey Blue
Eyes (1999) Blue Moon (2000)
Very Mean Men (2000)
The Boys of Sunset Ridge (2001)
Land of Plenty (2004)
Transamerica (2005)
Rocky Balboa (2006)
The Hideout (2007) Carnera:
The Walking Mountain (2008)

Gig **Young**
6ft 1in
(BYRON ELSWORTH BARR)

Born: **November 4, 1913**
St. Cloud, Minnesota, USA
Died: **October 19, 1978**

Gig's parents, John and Emma Barr took the family to live in Washington D.C. His acting talent developed at high school. After graduation, he appeared in a number of amateur plays and then got a scholarship to Pasadena Community Playhouse. Performing in "Pancho", he and the future Superman George Reeves, were spotted by a talent scout from Warner Bros. They both signed Supporting Player contracts and Gig made his film debut, in 1940, using the name Byron Barr, in the comedy *Misbehaving Husbands*. That year, he married the first of his five wives. After thirteen more supporting roles, he played a character called "Gig Young" in *The Gay Sisters*. The name was adopted. During World War II, he served with the U.S. Coast Guard. He became a freelance and had a series of good roles. He was nominated for a Best Supporting Actor Oscar, for *Come Fill the Cup*. His likeness to the alcoholic character he played in the film, didn't harm his career and he was again nominated – for *Teacher's Pet*. He won an Oscar for *They Shoot Horses, Don't They?* In 1978 he wed his fifth wife, Kim Schmidt. Three weeks later they were found dead in their apartment. Gig apparently had shot Kim before turning the gun on himself.

The Gay Sisters (1942) Air Force (1943)
Old Acquaintance (1943) Escape Me
Never (1947) The Woman in White (1948)
The Three Musketeers (1948)
Wake of the Red Witch (1948)
Lust for Gold (1949)
Tell It to the Judge (1949)
Target Unknown (1951) Only the
Valiant (1951) Come Fill the Cup (1951)
City That Never Sleeps (1953)
Young at Heart (1954) The Desperate
Hours (1955) Desk Set (1957)
Teacher's Pet (1958) Ask Any Girl (1959)
The Story on Page One (1959)
That Touch of Mink (1962)
They Shoot Horses, Don't They? (1969)
Bring Me the
Head of Alfredo Garcia (1974)

Karen **Young**
5ft 10in
(KAREN YOUNG)

Born: **September 29, 1958**
Pequannock Township, New Jersey, USA

Karen was the eldest of six children born to a New Jersey stonemason and his wife. She was bright and fairly academic during her early high school years, and the signs of acting talent had yet to surface. After graduating, Karen studied at Douglass College for Women, part of the long-established Rutgers University – The State University of New Brunswick, where she majored in Writing and English Literature. After graduating with a BA, she made the decision to move to New York City and become an actress. To this end she joined the Image Theater, where she majored in Drama. In 1983, she was given the starring role of Kathleen, in a good, low-budget movie thriller called *Handgun*. Shortly after that she was fifth-billed in the excellent war drama *Birdy*. The only let-down during that early period, was the 1987 movie *Jaws: The Revenge*. Luckily for Karen, she already had decent titles to her name and she proceeded onwards and upwards. In 1992, she made her directorial debut with a short, titled *A Blink of Paradise*. That year was also when she married actor, Tom Noonan. They had a son and a daughter and acted together in *The Wife*, which he wrote and directed. Karen was seen regularly in recent years in the TV series 'The Sopranos'. The pick of Karen's later film work is in *Restless*.

Handgun (1983)
Maria's Lovers (1984)
Birdy (1984)
Nine 1/2 Weeks (1986)
Heat (1986)
Criminal Law (1988)
Torch Song Trilogy (1988)
The Boy Who Cried Bitch (1991)
Hoffa (1992)
The Wife (1995)
Daylight (1996)
Pants on Fire (1998)
Joe the King (1999)
Mercy (2000)
Factotum (2005)
Heading South (2005)
Restless (2008)

Loretta **Young**
5ft 6in
(GRETCHEN YOUNG)

Born: **January 6, 1913**
Salt Lake City, Utah, USA
Died: **August 12, 2000**

Loretta was raised as a Roman Catholic. She made her film debut at the age of three, in *The Primrose Ring*. Her parents separated when she was four years old so she and her three sisters were taken by their mother to live in Los Angeles. Loretta was nearly fourteen when she entered the Ramona Convent Secondary School to complete her education. A year later, she took over a role intended for her sister, Polly, in *Naughty But Nice,* and from that point on, she was the family's star. Her first all-talkie was *The Squall*, in 1929. In 1930, she married the actor, Grant Withers, but one year later, they divorced. The upheaval didn't effect Loretta's career – she played in dozens of emotional dramas – opposite the top male stars of the day. *Taxi*, with James Cagney, and *Man's Castle*, opposite Spencer Tracy, are two examples. She then joined 20th Century Pictures and co-starred with Ronald Colman and Tyrone Power. She won a Best Actress Oscar, for *The Farmer's Daughter* and retained her popularity until 1953, when she became a regular on TV with 'The Loretta Young Show'. It won several Emmys and ran until 1961. Loretta retired in 1989, and died of ovarian cancer at her sister's home, in Los Angeles.

Taxi (1932) Zoo in Budapest (1933)
The Life of Jimmy Dolan (1933)
Man's Castle (1933)
Bulldog Drummond Strikes Back (1934)
Clive of India (1935) The Crusades (1935)
Love Is News (1937) Suez (1938)
The Story of Alexander Graham
Bell (1939) The Doctor Takes a
Wife (1941) Bedtime Story (1941)
China (1943) Along Came Jones (1945)
The Stranger (1946)
The Farmer's Daughter (1947)
The Bishop's Wife (1947)
Rachel and the Stranger (1948)
The Accused (1949)
Mother Is a Freshman (1949)
Come to the Stable (1949)
Cause for Alarm! (1951)

Robert Young
6ft
(ROBERT GEORGE YOUNG)

Born: **February 22, 1907**
Chicago, Illinois, USA
Died: **July 21, 1998**

Robert's father was an immigrant from Ireland. He married an American girl and they settled in Los Angeles. Robert was educated at Abraham Lincoln High School and when he was seventeen, he met his future wife, Betty Henderson. He graduated in 1925 and started his working life as a bank clerk. He began to get involved with amateur theatricals and when he lost his job, he did the rounds of the Hollywood studios – working as an extra, in *The Campus Vamp,* in 1928. In 1930, he signed a contract with MGM. Robert was considered a "B" actor for a couple of years, but his winning personality resulted in promotion and roles opposite female stars such as Crawford, Shearer, Rainer, and Hayes. One of his most memorable roles occurred towards the end of his MGM contract, as *H.M.Pelham Esq.* He appeared in several hit films, of which *Claudia, The Enchanted Cottage,* and *Crossfire,* were outstanding. In 1949, his film career slackened off, but he found new fame on radio's 'Father Knows Best' – which transferred to TV in 1956, and ran until 1960. He was forgotten until re-emerging as 'Marcus Welby M.D.' nine years later. Contrary to his cheerful screen personality, he was a depressive character and dependent on alcohol. In 1991, he tried to commit suicide. He eventually died of respiratory failure, in Westlake Village.

Men Must Fight (1933)
The House of Rothschild (1934)
Remember Last Night? (1935)
Secret Agent (1936)
The Bride Wore Red (1937)
Three Comrades (1938) **Maisie** (1939)
Northwest Passage (1940)
The Mortal Storm (1940)
Western Union (1941) **Journey for Margaret** (1942) **Claudia** (1943)
The Canterville Ghost (1944)
The Enchanted Cottage (1945)
Crossfire (1947) **Sitting Pretty** (1948)
That Forsyte Woman (1949)
The Second Woman (1950)

Roland Young
5ft 6in
(ROLAND YOUNG)

Born: **November 11, 1887**
London, England
Died: **June 5, 1953**

Roland's parents were what was referred to in Victorian and Edwardian times, as Upper Class. He was educated at one of England's oldest and most highly-respected private schools – Sherborne, in Dorset. Even in his schooldays, Roland's interest in theater was paramount. Whenever he could, he attended plays in London's West End. When he was eighteen, he started at the Royal Academy of Dramatic Art. His debut on the London stage, was in 1908, in "Find the Woman". His reputation soon spread to the United States where, four years later, he made his Broadway debut, in "Hindle Wakes". He starred in two plays specially written for him by Clare Kummer and then served two years in the U.S. Army. At the end of World War I, Roland returned and married Marjorie Kummer – Clare's daughter. He made his film debut, in 1922, as Dr. Watson in *Sherlock Holmes* and his talkie debut, in *The Unholy Night,* in 1929. He signed a contract with MGM and was much in demand as a supporting player – *Ruggles of Red Gap* and *David Copperfield* are fine examples. As a star, he is most fondly remembered for *Topper* and its sequels. From 1950 onwards, he was mainly seen on TV. When Roland died at home in New York City, his second wife, Patience DuCroz, was at his bedside.

The Squaw Man (1931) **Lovers Courageous** (1932) **Pleasure Cruise** (1933) **David Copperfield** (1935)
Ruggles of Red Gap (1935)
Give Me Your Heart (1936)
The Man Who Could Work Miracles (1936) **King Solomon's Mines** (1937) **Topper** (1937)
Ali Baba Goes to Town (1937)
The Young in Heart (1938)
Topper Takes a Trip (1938)
Star Dust (1940) **Irene** (1940)
The Philadelphia Story (1937)
Topper Returns (1941)
Tales of Manhattan (1942)
And Then There Were None (1945)
The Great Lover (1949)

Sean Young
5ft 10in
(MARY SEAN YOUNG)

Born: **November 20, 1959**
Louisville, Kentucky, USA

Sean's parents were Donald Young – a TV newsman and journalist, and Lee Guthrie, who had successful careers as a screen-writer and as a PR Executive. Sean was educated at Cleveland Heights High School, in Ohio, and the Interlochen Arts Academy, in Michigan. Following Sean's graduation from the latter, she attended the American Ballet school, in New York City, and for a time, worked as a model and professional dancer. In 1980, she made her film debut, in *Jane Austen of Manhattan.* Two years later, Sean's first leading role was opposite Harrison Ford, in Ridley Scott's *Blade Runner,* which divided the critics, but pleased audiences. It was good for Sean, who had a fine run during the 1980s – (apart from losing the role of Vicki Vale in *Batman,* after breaking her arm in a riding accident) - with starring roles in *Dune, No Way Out* and *Wall Street* keeping her name on the hit-list. The 1990s began promisingly, in *Ace Ventura: Pet Detective,* but by the end of the decade, personality clashes contributed to a barren spell – apart from her marriage to Robert Lujan, with whom she had two children. Since their divorce in 2002, Sean has attempted a come-back, but much of the material has been uninspiring. In January 2008, she attended a rehab program for alcohol abuse, but four months later, she not only competed, she placed fourth against professional drivers, in a "Demolition Derby" in Tennessee!

Stripes (1981)
Blade Runner (1982)
Dune (1984) **No Way Out** (1987)
Wall Street (1987)
The Boost (1988)
Cousins (1989)
Once Upon a Crime... (1992)
Blue Ice (1992)
Fatal Instinct (1993)
Ace Ventura: Pet Detective (1994)
Mirage (1995) **Men** (1997)
Out of Control (1998)
Mockingbird Don't Sing (2001)
Parasomnia (2008)

Z

Grace **Zabriskie**
5ft 2¹/₂in
(GRACE ZABRISKIE)

Born: **May 17, 1941**
New Orleans, Louisiana, USA

Grace's father was the founder of 'Lafitte's in Exile' – a cafe and bar on Bourbon Street. When she was little, it would be a watering hole for giants of the literary world, Gore Vidal, Tennessee Williams and Truman Capote. Grace's grandparents were teachers. They supplemented her education, and (without formal training) she was able to teach at an academy for black teenage dropouts. In the early 1960s, she went to live in Atlanta, Georgia – singing folk songs at artists' hangouts and learning silk-screen printmaking. Her confidence was high after her public performances and she was able to head for Hollywood and get roles in Walt Disney TV productions – starting in 1978, with 'The Million Dollar Dixie Deliverance' and one episode of 'Disneyland'. That same year, she made an inauspicious start to her film career, in an absurdly titled comedy, *They Went That-Away & That Away*. Luckily, her role was so small she was hardly noticed! It wasn't the case with her next film, *Norma Rae* – still a small part, but that, together with *The Big Easy,* got her good notices. David Lynch cast her in *Wild at Heart*. He gave her another role two years later and yet again, in his recent, *Inland Empire*. A highly creative woman, Grace and her daughter Marion produce visual arts for 'Arthaus' in Los Angeles.

The Private Eyes (1981)
An Officer and a Gentleman (1982)
Nickel Mountain (1984)
The Big Easy (1987) Rampage (1988)
Drugstore Cowboy (1989)
Wild at Heart (1990)
My Own Private Idaho (1991)
Fried Green Tomatoes (1991)
Twin Peaks: Fire Walk
with Me (1992) Drop Zone (1994)
The Passion of Darkly Noon (1995)
A Family Thing (1996)
Bastard Out of Carolina (1996)
George B. (1997)
Trash (1999) A Texas Funeral (1999)
Inland Empire (2006)
Careless (2007)

Billy **Zane**
6ft
(WILLIAM GEORGE ZANE JR.)

Born: **February 24, 1966**
Chicago, Illinois, USA

Of Greek ancestry, Billy's parents, William and Thalia Zane anglicized their surname, Zanikopolous. Apart from founding a school for medical technicians, they were both enthusiastic amateur actors with their local theatrical group. In his early teens, he attended the Harand Camp of the Theater Arts, at Elkhart Lake, in Wisconsin. Billy and his older sister Lisa, who is also an actress, were raised in the Greek Orthodox religion. Billy's education included the prestigious American School, at Montagnola, Lugano, in Switzerland. After graduating from the Francis W. Parker School, in Chicago, he set off for California to start his acting career. A few weeks later, he was making his film debut in *Back to the Future*. He reprised the role in 1989 – the same year that he made a dynamic appearance, in *Dead Calm*. In 1991, Billy played John Justice Wheeler, in five episodes of the TV-series 'Twin Peaks'. His role in the blockbuster, *Titanic* brought him international recognition. *I Woke Up Early the Day I Died,* which he produced, won him the Best Actor Award at the B-Movie Festival in Syracuse, New York. His singing voice has been heard in Broadway musicals like "Chicago". From 1988 to 1995, Billy was married to the Australian actress, Lisa Collins.

Back to the Future (1985)
Critters (1986) Dead Calm (1989)
Back to the Future Part II (1989)
Memphis Belle (1990)
Blood and Concrete (1991)
Orlando (1992)
Sniper (1993) Only You (1994)
Tales from the Crypt: Demon
Knight (1995) Head Above
Water (1996) Titanic (1997)
I Woke Up Early the
Day I Died (1998) Susan's
Plan (1998) The Believer (2001)
CQ (2001) Big Kiss (2004)
The Valley of the Wolves (2006)
Fishtales (2007)
Love N' Dancing (2008)
The Hessen Affair (2009)

Renée **Zellweger**
5ft 4in
(RENÉE KATHLEEN ZELLWEGER)

Born: **April 25, 1969**
Katy, Texas, USA

Renée's father was Emil Zellweger – a Swiss-born engineer, who worked in the Texas oil-refining business. Her mother, the former Kjeefrid Andreassen, had been a nurse and midwife in Norway. Renée has a brother named Drew, who became a marketing executive. At junior high school, she was active in a number of sports – including soccer, basketball and baseball. At Katy High School she was a gymnast and a cheerleader and eventually, she got interested in acting through becoming a member of the drama club – appearing in several school plays and being voted the "Best Looking" in her class. Renée then majored in English language at the University of Texas at Austin. She took acting classes and began getting work in TV commercials. She made her small screen debut, in 1992, in 'A Taste for Killing' – which was shot in Galveston. Renée made her film debut, two years later, in *Reality Bites* – which marked Ben Stiller's directorial debut. Her first starring role was in *Love and a .45*. By the mid-1990s, she was appearing in top movies such as *Jerry Maguire,* and well on her way to the summit which was reached in *Nurse Betty*. She proved her ability to do an English accent, in *Bridget Jones's Diary* – earning a Best Actress Oscar nomination – as she did for *Chicago*. She won a Best Supporting Oscar for *Cold Mountain*. In 2005, her seven-month marriage to the country singer, Kenny Chesney, ended.

Reality Bites (1994) Love and
a .45 (1995) Empire Records (1995)
The Whole Wide World (1996)
Jerry Maguire (1996) Deceiver (1997)
A Price Above Rubies (1998) One True
Thing (1998) Nurse Betty (2000)
Me, Myself & Irene (2000)
Bridget Jones's Diary (2001)
Chicago (2002) Cold Mountain (2003)
Cinderella Man (2005)
Miss Potter (2006) Leatherheads (2008)
Appaloosa (2008)
New in Town (2009)
My One and Only (2009)

Anthony **Zerbe**
5ft 10in
(ANTHONY JARED ZERBE)

Born: May 20, 1936
Long Beach,California, USA

The son of Arthur Lee Van Zerbe and his wife, Catherine, Anthony grew up in the Long Beach area. He was educated at Ponoma College in Claremont, California, and was a graduate of the Erhard Seminars Training Scheme, based in San Francisco. In 1953, Anthony went to live in New York City, where he was inspired to become an actor on seeing Paul Newman and Joanne Woodward, in the Broadway production of "Picnic". He then studied acting at the Stella Adler Theater Studio. After serving in the United States Airforce from 1959 to 1960, he resumed his career with determination. In 1962, he married his present wife, Arnette Jens. He began getting television roles – starting in 1963, with 'Naked City' and 'Route 66'. After a bit of a struggle, he made his film debut with a small part in the western *Cool Hand Luke* – which starred his first inspiration – Paul Newman. He quickly secured his position as a character actor, in another top western – *Will Penny*. By 1971, Anthony was co-starring with its star Charlton Heston - in *The Omega Man*. For forty years, he has kept busy with TV work, and good roles in some excellent movies – a 'Bond' among them.

Cool Hand Luke (1967)
Will Penny (1968)
The Molly Maguires (1970)
The Liberation of L.B. Jones (1970)
The Omega Man (1972)
The Life and Times of Judge
Roy Bean (1972)
Papillon (1973)
The Laughing Policeman (1973)
Farewell My Lovely (1975)
Rooster Cogburn (1975)
The Turning Point (1977)
Who'll Stop the Rain (1978)
The Dead Zone (1983)
See No Evil, Hear No Evil (1989)
Licence to Kill (1989)
Star Trek: Insurrection (1998)
The Matrix Reloaded (2003)
The Matrix Revolutions (2003)
Veritas, Prince of Truth (2006)

Catherine **Zeta-Jones**
5ft 8in
(CATHERINE JONES)

Born: September 25, 1969
Swansea, West Glamorgan, Wales

Catherine's father, David Jones, owned a candy factory in Swansea. Her mother, Patricia, was Irish. Catherine was raised as a Roman Catholic. She began performing at family get-togethers as a child, and when she was ten, she appeared in entertainments provided by the members of the congregation at her local church. She made her stage debut, at the Grand Theater, Swansea, in the title role of "Annie". When her parents won £100,000 at Bingo, the family moved to a better part of town. Catherine attended Dumbarton House School. She left there early to start a three-year-course at the Arts Education School in Chiswick, near London. While there, Catherine completed a program in musical theater. When Mickey Dolenz of the "Monkees" was visiting Wales, he was so impressed he invited her to join him on tour. In 1987, she starred in the London West End production of "42nd Street". Three years later, Catherine added her Greek grandmother's name – Zeta, and made her film debut, in *1001 Nights.* From 1991, Catherine attracted national attention when acting in the TV-series, 'The Darling Buds of May'. In 1992, her duet with David Essex, on the single "True Love Ways" reached 38 in the U.K. charts. Her movie career took off after *The Mask of Zorro,* and reached its peak with her Oscar-winning performance in *Chicago.* She's been married to Michael Douglas since 2000. They have two children.

Splitting Heirs (1993)
The Mask of Zorro (1998)
Entrapment (1999)
High Fidelity (2000)
Traffic (2000)
America's Sweethearts (2001)
Chicago (2002)
Intolerable Cruelty (2003)
The Terminal (2004)
Ocean's Twelve (2004)
The Legend of Zorro (2005)
No Reservations (2007)
Death Defying Acts (2007)
The Rebound (2009)

Mai **Zetterling**
5ft 3in
(MAI ELISABETH ZETTERLING)

Born: May 24, 1925
Västerås, Västmansland län, Sweden
Died: **March 17, 1994**

Like a lot of Swedes in the 1920s, Mai's parents were the victims of economic problems. When she was four, they emigrated to Australia, where she went to school and learned English with an Aussie accent. The family returned to Sweden in 1933 and she continued at school. After acting classes, she made her film debut, in 1941, with a small role in the comedy, *Lasse-Maja.* The pretty teenager was encouraged to improve her technique, so in 1942, she began a three-year course at the Royal Dramatic Theater in Stockholm. Towards the end of her studies, Mai gained wider attention when she was cast by Alf Sjöberg, in *Torment* – which was written by Ingmar Bergman. In 1944, she married the Norwegian ballet dancer/actor Tutte Lemkow, with whom she had two children. Four years later, Mai starred in Bergman's third film as a director - *Night Is My Future.* Before that, she made her English language film debut – in Basil Dearden's *Frieda.* She acted in films in Sweden and England, but made a permanent move to London after divorcing Lemkow. Three best films of the time, are two comedies – Danny Kaye's *Knock on Wood* and *Only Two Can Play,* with Peter Sellers, and a drama, *Seven Waves Away* – with Tyrone Power. She married writer David Hughes, with whom she collaborated on two directing ventures – *Loving Couples,* and *Night Games* (from her own novel) which was banned from the Venice Film Festival. She returned to acting in the 1990s. Mai died of cancer, in London.

Torment (1944)
Frieda (1947)
Portrait from Life (1948)
Night Is My Future (1948)
Quartet (1948)
The Ringer (1952)
Desperate Moment (1953)
Knock on Wood (1957)
Seven Waves Away (1957)
Only Two Can Play (1962)
Morfars resa (1993)

Ziyi **Zhang**
5ft 5in
(ZHANG ZI-YI)

Born: **February 9, 1979**
Beijing, China

Zi means "child" – Yi means "joy" – which her parents believed she was. Ziyi began training at the Beijing Dance Academy from eleven years of age. It was a strict boarding school, and she was far from happy there. Much better was her next school, the top Chinese acting college, the Central Academy of Drama. It was there that she established herself as a fine young actress and grew into a beautiful, photogenic young woman. When she was nineteen, Ziyi made her movie debut, in Yimou's *The Road Home,* which won the Silver Bear Award at the 2000 Berlin Film Festival. She'd become internationally known after her supporting role, in the hugely successful film, *Crouching Tiger, Hidden Dragon.* For that performance, she won the 'Independent Spirit' Award, as well as the Toronto Film Critics Prize, as Best Supporting Actress. Her next film, *Hero,* was also highly praised and it led to an opportunity to work with Jackie Chan, in her first American movie – *Rush Hour 2.* As she didn't speak any English, Jackie acted as translator. Ziyi was nominated for a Best Actress BAFTA for *House of Flying Daggers.* Her sweet voice can be heard on the soundtrack. She demonstrated her dancing skills when she acted in *Princess Raccoon,* and more nominations came her way for *Memoirs of a Geisha.* The face of Garnier and Maybelline, Ziyi's love-life is the subject of much rumor. Recently she has been linked with an Israeli, Vivi Nero – who is a shareholder in Time-Warner. See her with Dennis Quaid, in *The Horsemen.*

The Road Home (1999)
**Crouching Tiger Hidden
Dragon** (2000) **Rush Hour 2** (2001)
Musa the Warrior (2001)
Hero (2002) **Purple Butterfly** (2003)
House of Flying Daggers (2004)
2046 (2004) **Yasmin Flower** (2004)
Princess Raccoon (2005)
Memoirs of a Geisha (2005)
Legend of the Black Scorpion (2006)
Forever Enthralled (2008)
The Horsemen (2009)

Vicki **Zhao**
5ft 5½in
(ZHAO WEI)

Born: **March 12, 1976**
Wuhu, Anhui province, China

Vicki was the daughter of Zhao Jiahai, an appliance designer, and his wife, Wei Qiying, who worked as a teacher. Vicki has an older brother called Zhao Jian. After finishing her secondary schooling, Vicki decided to become a schoolteacher. With this goal in mind she attended and graduated from Shi Fan Fu Xiao and the Teachers' College High School. Before she even had a chance to look for a job something happened which would set her on an entirely different career path. In 1993, a film crew arrived in Wuhu to shoot a film called *Hua Hun,* starring Gong Li. They offered Vicki work as an extra and the experience caused her to make up her mind to become an actress. She enrolled at a film arts school in Shanghai, and in 1995, she appeared in the television series 'Yu Tian You Gu Shi' and made her official movie debut, in *Penitentiary Angel* – she still considers her performance less than satisfactory, but she kept on improving. Two years later, Vicki was accepted at the Beijing Film Academy after she passed her entrance exams with flying colors. While there, she starred in the TV series 'My Fair Princess' and 'Old House Has Joy'. She graduated from Beijing in 2000 and set off on the road to movie stardom. She kept her face in front of audiences with more TV appearances – which won her Golden Eagle Awards as Best Actress. In 2005 Vicki won a Best Actress Golden Goblet at the Shanghai International Film Festival – for *A Time to Love.*

Penitentiary Angel (1995)
Behind the Forbidden City (1996)
The Duel (2000)
Shaolin Soccer (2001)
Chinese Odyssey (2002)
So Close (2002)
Green Tea (2003)
Godess of Mercy (2003)
A Time to Love (2005)
The Postmodern Life of My Aunt (2006)
The Longest Night (2007)
Red Cliff (2008)
Red Cliff: Part II (2009)

Sonja **Ziemann**
5ft 5in
(ALICE TONI SELMA ZIEMANN)

Born: **February 8, 1926**
Eichwalde bei Berlin, Germany

Sonja was the daughter of a Berlin tax consultant. At the age of ten she began to study dancing under the famous Russian-born dancer and choreographer, Tatjana Gsovsky. In 1940, Sonja finished normal schooling to concentrate on ballet, and after completing the course one year later, she had her first professional engagement at the renowned Berliner Plaza. She had a good singing voice and soon made an impact in operettas and musical shows. During World War II, she remained in Berlin, to study at the UFA Studio Acting School and in 1942, made her film debut in a German film called *Windstoss,* which was shot in Florence, Italy. She later established herself with German cinema audiences in the sentimental 'Heimatfilms' *Shwarzwaldmädel* and *Grün ist die Heide.* Sonja attempted to escape this type-casting when she appeared in the British film, *Made in Heaven,* but until 1958, it was usually more of the same. She then made four good films – *Battle Inferno, A Matter of WHO, The Secret Ways,* and *The Bridge at Remagen.* There was plenty of drama in her private life; her second husband, Marek Hlasko, committed suicide, her son died of cancer seven months later, and her companion, Martinius Adolff, was killed in a plane crash in 1974. In 1989, Sonja married the Swiss actor, Charles Régnier, who died in 2001. She survived it all and lives in Tegernsee, in Bavaria.

Paths in Twilight (1948)
Die Freunde meiner Frau (1949)
Made in Heaven (1952)
**Ich war ein hässliches
Mädchen** (1955) **Opera Ball** (1956)
Frühling in Berlin (1957)
The Eighth Day of the Week (1958)
Darkness Fell on Gotenhafen (1959)
Battle Inferno (1959)
Strafbataillon 999 (1960)
A Matter of WHO (1961)
The Secret Ways (1961)
Der Traum von Lieschen Müller (1961)
Her Most Beautiful Day (1962)
The Bridge at Remagen (1969)

Efrem **Zimbalist Jr.**
6ft
(EFREM ZIMBALIST JR.)

Born: **November 30, 1918**
New York City, New York, USA

The reason young Efrem decided against a career in music must have been that he would have had a lot to live up to. His father was Russian-born, Efrem Zimbalist Sr., who was one of the foremost classical violinists of his time. And Efrem's mother was the Rumanian-born Alma Gluck – a talented soprano who was very famous in operatic circles at the beginning of the 20th century, when she was a member of the Metropolitan Opera, in New York City. Young Efrem chose the right path. He did well at high school before attending the Yale School of Drama, from where he graduated in 1940. He went on to study at the Neighborhood Playhouse and worked as a page at NBC radio. But his dramatic entrance was interrupted by World War II and when his service was over, a friend of the family – Garson Kanin, gave him his professional stage debut, in "The Rugged Path" which starred Spencer Tracy. Efrem worked hard with the American Repertory Theater – appearing in classic plays like "Henry VIII', "Androcles and the Lion" and "Hedda Gabler". He made his film debut in *House of Strangers,* but it was his stage presentations which won him the plaudits – including the New York Drama Critic's Award and Pulitzer Prize for Menotti's "The Consul" in 1950. Sadly, it was the year his wife Emily (mother of his two children) died of cancer. He quit film acting until 1957, but TV shows like '77 Sunset Strip' and 'The F.B.I.' made him famous. Efrem was working – mainly on television until 2004. He lives in Santa Barbara, California, with his second wife, Stephanie.

House of Strangers (1949)
Band of Angels (1957)
The Deep Six (1958)
Too Much,Too Soon (1958)
Girl on the Run (1958)
Home Before Dark (1958)
The Crowded Sky (1960)
A Fever in the Blood (1961)
Wait Until Dark (1967)
Airport 1975 (1974)
Hot Shots! (1991)

Preity **Zinta**
5ft 4in
(PREITY ZINTA)

Born: **January 31, 1975**
Shimla, Himachal Pradesh, India

The aptly-named, Preity, was the daughter of a Hindu Rajput couple – Durganand Zinta, an officer in the Indian Army, and his wife, Nilprabhia. When she was thirteen, her parents were involved in a serious automobile accident. Her father was killed and her mother suffered injuries which resulted in her being bedridden for two years. The tragedy had a deep impact on Preity and her two brothers, and all three matured rapidly. She was educated at The Convent of Jesus and Mary – a boarding school, where she excelled at basketball and developed a love of literature. After graduating, Preity attended St. Bede's College, from where she emerged with an honors degree in English. She later earned a postgraduate degree in Criminal Psychology, before becoming a model. After appearing in TV commercials, she made her film debut, in *From the Heart* and was nominated for a Best Supporting Actress Filmfare Award. Preity decorated a few more films before playing a teenage single mother, in *Kya Kehna,* and was again nominated – this time as Best Actress. For *Armaan,* she was nominated as "Best Villain". Her first Filmfare Award as Best Actress came for her role in the tear-jerker, *Kal Ho Naa Ho.* It was the top-grossing Indian film overseas. Apart from films, Preity has performed in concerts in Canada and England. In 2003, she stood firm against the Indian Mafia in the Bharat Shah case. She is a modern woman.

From the Heart (1998) **Premante
Idera** (1998) **Raja Kumarudu** (1999)
Kya Kehna (2000)
Mission Kashmir (2000)
Chori Chori Chupke Chupke (2001)
Do Your Thing (2001) **My Heart Is
Yours** (2002) **Armaan** (2003) **Koi...Mil
Gaya** (2003) **Kal Ho Naa Ho** (2003)
Lakshya (2004) **Veer-Zara** (2004)
Salaam Namaste (2005)
Heartthrob (2006)
The Last Lear (2007)
Heaven on Earth (2008)
Heroes (2008)

George **Zucco**
5ft 10in
(GEORGE ZUCCO)

Born: **January 11, 1886**
Manchester, Lancashire, England
Died: **May 28, 1960**

George's Greek father ran an export-import business in Manchester. His dear mother had been a lady-in-waiting to Queen Victoria. As a boy, George enjoyed entertaining his family, and whenever an opportunity arose, appeared in amateur stage productions. In 1907, he married Frances Hawke, and took her to Canada, where they performed at provincial theaters - and were well-known for a routine, "The Suffragette". When war began in Europe, he returned to serve in the Yorkshire Regiment and suffered injuries to his arm, which was to remain partially paralyzed. He became a leading actor on the London stage and in 1931, made his film debut, in *The Dreyfus Case.* George remarried and in 1935, went to the USA, where he played Disraeli, in "Victoria Regina". George made the first of many Hollywood films, *Sinner Takes All,* but his most famous role was as Moriarty, in *The Adventures of Sherlock Holmes.* In the late 1940s, he was mostly in B-films. In 1951, George fell ill when filming began on *David and Bathsheba.* He retired and died of pneumonia, in Hollywood, nine years later.

**The Man Who Could Work
Miracles** (1936) **Sinner Takes All** (1936)
After the Thin Man (1936) **Souls at
Sea** (1937) **Madame X** (1937) **Arsène
Lupin Returns** (1938) **Lord Jeff** (1938)
Suez (1938) **Charlie Chan in
Honolulu** (1938) **The Adventures of
Sherlock Holmes** (1939) **The Cat and
the Canary** (1939) **The Hunchback of
Notre Dame** (1939) **New Moon** (1940)
Arise, My Love (1940)
The Monster and the Girl (1941)
Topper Returns (1941)
A Woman's Face (1941) **My Favorite
Blonde** (1942) **The Black Swan** (1942)
Sherlock Holmes in Washington (1943)
The Seventh Cross (1944)
**Week-End at the
Waldorf** (1945) **Captain from
Castile** (1947) **The Pirate** (1948)
The Secret Garden (1949)

Bibliography

Since the expansion and wide use of the Internet, research has become less and less reliant on printed books as a source of information on whatever subject one is writing about. In my case, the Wikipedia and IMDb sites proved an invaluable and rapid means of gathering facts and figures as well as background detail. Add to this a whole host of fansites – both official and unofficial and I soon had a wealth of material to work from. Even so, perhaps because of the era I'm from, I couldn't help using my library of movie books and magazines, to double check information and sometimes rediscover little details that may not be well known to modern writers on the subject. The following are books which have provided me with a lot of the inspiration and extremely useful references.

BORDWELL David –
Planet Hong Kong: Popular Cinema And The Art Of Entertainment
Harvard University Press 2000
COWIE Peter – *Swedish Cinema*
A.Zwemmer Ltd 1966
GILLESPIE David – *Russian Cinema*
Harlow: Longman 2003
HALLIWELL Leslie – *Film Guides*
Paladin Grafton Books 1977-2005
HAYWARD Susan –
French National Cinema
Routledge 1993
MALTIN Leonard – *Movie Guide*
Plume/Penguin 1992-2008
Picture Show Annuals –
The Amalgamated Press 1929-1960
QUINLAN David – *Quinlan's Illustrated Directory of Film Stars*
B.T. Batsford 1981-2000
Radio Times Guide to Films –
BBC Worldwide 2000

RAHEJA Dinesh/KOTHARI Jitendra –
Indian Cinema: The Bollywood Saga
Lustre Press 2003
RICHIE Donald/ANDERSON Joseph –
The Japanese Film: Art and Industry
Princeton University Press 1982
SHIPMAN David – *The Great Movie Stars The Golden Years*
Angus & Robertson 1970
SHIPMAN David – *The Great Movie Stars The International Years*
Angus & Robertson 1980
SPEED F. Maurice – *Film Review Annuals*
MacDonald & Co 1945-1963
WINCHESTER Clarence –
The World Film Encyclopedia
The Amalgamated Press 1933
WINCHESTER Clarence –
Winchester's Screen Encyclopedia
Winchester Publications 1948
WOOD Mary P – *Italian Cinema*
Berg 2005

Lightning Source UK Ltd.
Milton Keynes UK
10 November 2009

146062UK00001B/8/P